THE HANDBOOK OF
MULTISENSORY PROCESSES

THE HANDBOOK OF MULTISENSORY PROCESSES

Edited by: Gemma A. Calvert

Charles Spence

Barry E. Stein

A BRADFORD BOOK
THE MIT PRESS
CAMBRIDGE, MASSACHUSETTS
LONDON, ENGLAND

This book was set in Baskerville by ICC and was printed
and bound in the United States of America.

Library of Congress Cataloging-in-Publication Data

The handbook of multisensory processes / edited by Gemma A. Calvert, Charles Spence,
    Barry E. Stein.
        p.   cm.
    "A Bradford Book."
    Includes bibliographical references and index.
    ISBN 0-262-03321-6
    1. Senses and sensation—Handbooks, manuals, etc.   2. Intersensory effects—Handbooks,
manuals, etc.   I. Calvert, Gemma A.   II. Spence, Charles.   III. Stein, Barry E.

QP431.H286   2004
152.1—dc22

                                                                            2004042612

10 9 8 7 6 5 4 3 2 1

CONTENTS

VIII PERSECTIVES DERIVED FROM CLINICAL STUDIES

INTRODUCTION

One of the enduring interests of both neuroscientists and philosophers of science concerns how we perceive the external world, and speculation about the underlying processes involved has been ongoing since long before the advent of formal scientific disciplines (e.g., see Aristotle's *De Anima*). The rapid pace of technological developments in recent years has markedly advanced research in all the disciplines in which perception is a topic of interest, and which are loosely captured by the term *neuroscience*. However, much of the history of perceptual research can be characterized as a "sense-by-sense" approach, in which researchers have focused on the functional properties of one sensory modality at a time. These efforts have produced an enormous amount of information about sensory perception at every level of analysis, from the single-cell level to the level of phenomenology. We know far more about each of the senses than could possibly have been imagined by the early philosophers, who nevertheless posed some of the most fundamental questions about the mechanisms underlying our ability to perceive.

However, it is interesting to note that with the specialization of modern research and the tendency to focus on the functional properties of individual senses, an early perspective was set aside, namely, that perception is fundamentally a multisensory phenomenon. There can be no doubt that our senses are designed to function in concert and that our brains are organized to use the information they derive from their various sensory channels cooperatively in order to enhance the probability that objects and events will be detected rapidly, identified correctly, and responded to appropriately. Thus, even those experiences that at first may appear to be modality-specific are most likely to have been influenced by activity in other sensory modalities, despite our lack of awareness of such interactions. Indeed, mounting evidence now suggests that we are rarely aware of the full extent of these multisensory contributions to our perception.

Researchers now recognize that the everyday environment, outside the highly controlled laboratory of the scientific researcher, engenders a constant influx of sensory information in most of the sensory pathways. The brain's task is to sort through the massive and multiple streams of information it receives and to couple those signals that, regardless of their modality, should be related to one another because they are derived from a common event. At the same time, the brain also needs to keep separate the signals derived from different perceptual events. The final decision concerning what a particular event or object is, and what should be done with (or about) it, is frequently an operation requiring the synthesis of information derived from multiple sensory channels. Thus, to fully appreciate the processes underlying much of sensory perception, we must understand not only how information from each sensory modality is transduced and decoded along the pathways primarily devoted to that sense, but also how this information is modulated by what is going on in the other sensory pathways.

The recognition that a multisensory perspective is necessary to enhance our understanding of sensory perception has led many scientists to adopt a different research strategy in recent years. The result has been the emergence of a distinct field of scientific endeavor that has been loosely designated multisensory integration or multisensory processing. At the same time, an international organization, the International Multisensory Research Forum (IMRF), has been formed that is dedicated to promoting these efforts and has helped to spur progress in this emerging field. Indeed, there has been a dramatic upsurge over the last decade in the number of research programs directed toward understanding how the brain synthesizes information from the different senses, and this expansion of interest shows no sign of abating. This situation in turn has led to a growing awareness that multisensory processes are quite common and profoundly affect our appreciation of environmental events. The rapid growth of this field has not been restricted to an individual technique, discipline, species, or perspective; advances in multiple species have been made at the level of the single neuron, networks of neurons, neural modeling, development, and also psychophysics. These efforts have yielded data suggesting the presence of remarkable constancies in some of the underlying principles by which the brain synthesizes the different sensory inputs that are available to it, indicating their broad applicability in very different ecological circumstances. These principles appear to be operative regardless of the specific combination of senses being assessed. Thus, some of the same principles governing the synthesis of visual and auditory information apply equally well to other combinations of the spatial senses, and may even apply to the chemical senses (such as gustation and olfaction) as well. To take but one example close to the hearts of the editors of this volume, the multisensory response enhancement first reported at the single-cell level in the cat (see Stein & Meredith, 1993, for a review) has subsequently been documented in domains as diverse as the combination of olfactory and gustatory cues in flavor perception (e.g., Dalton, Doolittle, Nagata, & Breslin, 2000) and the hemodynamic responses of the human brain to congruent versus incongruent audiovisual speech stimuli (Calvert, Campbell, & Brammer, 2000). It will be particularly interesting in future research to determine how these principles affect the perception of multisensory signals that are critical for social interaction in the animal kingdom (see, e.g., Hughes, 1998; Partan & Marler, 2000).

Closely related, and of general concern at the perceptual level, is how the brain weighs the inputs it receives from the different senses in producing a final perceptual output or experience. This is an issue with a rich history in experimental psychology. It has been known for some time that when conflicting signals are presented via the different sensory modalities, the emergent percept is typically dominated by the most persuasive sensory cue in that particular context (e.g., Rock & Victor, 1964; Welch & Warren, 1980). These sorts of dominance effects have been reported in a number of species (see, e.g., Wilcoxin, Dragoin, & Kral, 1971), and recent computational modeling has revealed how they may actually reflect an optimal integration of what are inherently noisy perceptual inputs (e.g., Ernst & Banks, 2002).

Because the relevant literature on multisensory processing is spread across multiple disciplines, it has become increasingly fragmented in recent years. Providing a single source for descriptions of the most notable advances in these diverse areas has been a central motivation in preparing this book. We hope that by bringing together in one place as much of this disparate information as we can, we will provide researchers with a convenient source of knowledge with which to examine how data from very different experimental paradigms relate to one another. This organization allows readers to examine what is known of the principles of multisensory integration that operate at the level of the individual neuron, as well as those that operate at the level of neural networks and thereby encompass many neurons in multiple brain structures. These principles can then be related to the final perceptual and behavioral products that are initiated by multisensory stimuli. It also provides a means of understanding much of the thinking that has guided the construction of computational models of multisensory processes in the past few years.

By juxtaposing discussions of how different brain areas come to be capable of processing their respective sensory information as a consequence of development and sensory experience, and how the brain is able to coordinate the different reference schemes used by the different senses so that stimuli can be localized regardless of their modality of input, we hope to provide some insight into the monumental biological problems inherent to building a system of sensors that can be used synergistically. In addition, discussions about the fascinating cases of synesthesia and the susceptibility of multisensory information processing to various kinds of brain damage provide us with an appreciation of the magnitude of individual variability in these multisensory processes, even among members of the same species.

Organization of the book

This handbook is organized around eight key themes, with each chapter presented as a state-of-the-art review by leading researchers in the field. Although the chapters are grouped into sections that might appear to be independent of one another, the grouping is merely one of convenience. Many of the themes and models discussed actually exceed the organizational framework of particular sections, and many of the problems and solutions are referenced in multiple sections.

PART I: PERCEPTUAL CONSEQUENCES OF MULTIPLE SENSORY SYSTEMS
The chapters in Part I focus primarily on multisensory contributions to perception in humans. Included are chapters on the multisensory recognition of objects (Newell), multisensory contributions to the perception of movement (Soto-Faraco and Kingstone), multisensory flavor perception (Stevenson and Boakes), and multisensory texture perception (Lederman and Klatzky). Many of the chapters highlight studies documenting the perceptual consequences of conflicting cues in different senses, such as the ventriloquism effect (Woods and Recanzone) and the cross-modal dynamic capture effect (Soto-Faraco and Kingstone). The various newly discovered multisensory illusions, such as the "freezing" illusion (Vroomen & de Gelder, 2000), the "double flash" illusion (Shams, Kitamani, & Shimojo, 2000), and the "bouncing balls" illusion (Sekuler, Sekuler, & Lau, 1997), are also discussed at some length in several of the chapters (e.g., Shams, Kamitani, and Shimojo; Vroomen and de Gelder). Studying such illusions has helped scientists to understand some of the rules by which the senses interact even if their particular perceptual products do not enhance perceptual performance. Such laboratory conditions of sensory "conflict" also raise important questions about which responses on the part of the participants reflect the genuine products of multisensory integration and which reflect decisions or response-related strategies instead (e.g., see the chapters by Soto-Faraco and Kingstone and by Marks).

Finally, while the impact of prior experience on multisensory integration is addressed most thoroughly in animal studies (see the section on cross-modal plasticity), Stevenson and Boakes provide some fascinating evidence suggesting that our previous experience with particular combinations of tastes and smells in particular foodstuffs may affect the nature of the multisensory interactions that emerge in the perception of flavor. Thus, future studies of multisensory flavor perception may provide a particularly fascinating window into the way in which the multisensory interactions that govern our perception and behavior are molded by the particular sensory environments in which we develop.

Part II: Is Speech a Special Case of Multisensory Integration?
The multisensory perception of speech has already garnered more than its fair share of analysis and commentary in the literature in recent years (e.g., Campbell, Dodd, & Burnham, 1998; Dodd & Campbell, 1987; Massaro, 1998). When current views of speech research are brought under one roof, it is possible to see how some of the rules of audiovisual integration derived for speech perception fit the broader context of multisensory integration. A question that then emerges is whether the processes of multisensory integration taking place in the case of speech are somehow special. We are fortunate to have contributions from researchers on both sides of this debate. In particular, the chapters incorporated here address the issue of whether the type of multisensory integration that influences speech perception is fundamentally different from other forms of multisensory integration. Taking a computational approach to audiovisual speech perception, Massaro argues that data on the McGurk effect can be easily described by a general pattern recognition algorithm—in this case, the fuzzy logical model of perception—which indicates that speech is simply another case of audiovisual integration. A contrary stance is taken by Fowler, who expounds the gestural theory of speech perception. Fowler argues that the results from modality-specific auditory speech experiments are in direct contrast to the conclusions drawn from Massaro's studies based on auditory-visual speech perception experiments. Meanwhile, Munhall and Vatikiotis-Bateson review studies assessing whether the spatial and temporal constraints affecting multisensory speech perception are the same as for other types of audiovisual integration. In their chapter, Bernstein, Auer, and Moore investigate the neural sites specialized for the processing of speech stimuli. Finally, Sarah Partan broadens the discussion by reviewing what is currently known about multisensory contributions to animal communication.

Part III: The Neural Mechanisms Underlying the Integration of Cross-Modal Cues
Part III directly approaches the neural mechanisms underlying multisensory integration. A number of model species (e.g., rat, cat, monkey) are used to explore what is known about multisensory processing in the midbrain and cortex. The section begins with two chapters dealing with what is perhaps the best-known model of multisensory integration, the cat superior colliculus (SC) neuron. The first chapter, by Stein, Jiang, and Stanford, discusses the principles guiding the integration of visual, auditory, and somatosensory information in SC neurons and the consequences of multisensory integration on overt orientation. It also introduces the inherent problem in maintaining alignment among sensory representations when the peripheral sensory organs move with respect to one another (a longstanding problem in neuroscience research; e.g., see Pöppel, 1973). This issue is dealt with in regard to the alignment of cortical maps in Part VI. The neural data that have been obtained in SC neurons are then evaluated and modeled in the chapter by Anastasio and Patton, who apply a quantitative Bayesian perspective to the underlying processes. This analysis is followed by a series of chapters dealing with the many cortical regions in which convergent sensory information is processed. Kaas and Collins initiate this discussion

with an overview of the monkey cortex and the possible anatomical substrates for multisensory convergence. Schroeder and Foxe, who also use the nonhuman primate model, show that multisensory influences can be exerted very early in the stream of cortical information processing, an issue that has proved to be particularly contentious in the last few years (e.g., Rockland & Ojima, 2003; Falchier, Clavagnier, Barone, & Kennedy, 2002). The rich variety of multisensory interactions should become apparent as one reads the chapter by Rolls, in which the chemical as well as special senses in this model are dealt with. Parker and Easton discuss the integral role of learning and memory in dealing with multisensory events in monkeys, and Meredith provides a broad overview of the neural mechanisms of integration in cat cortex that impact a variety of physiological measures of sensory processing. Finally, Barth and Brett-Green show that the multisensory convergence of sensory information is present in several areas of the rat cortex previously thought to be modality-specific. These several chapters use various models to illustrate how different regions of the brain integrate multisensory information in performing their various roles.

PART IV: MULTISENSORY MECHANISMS IN ORIENTATION
Some of the early themes in Part III are revisited in Part IV in order to deal specifically with the behavioral consequences of multisensory integration. The research in this section is heavily dependent on the nonhuman primate model, as reflected in each of the chapters included here. In the first two chapters, Van Opstal and Munoz discuss how the integration of auditory and visual information at the level of the individual neuron speeds shifts of gaze and thereby facilitates the localization of external events, and Diederich and Colonius discuss both manual and eye movement control within this context. Lackner and DiZio then address the utility of multisensory integration in the broader circumstances in which body orientation and movement must be controlled. Fogassi and Gallese discuss similar issues, but from the perspective of how an organism's action influences the integration of multisensory cues, and Graziano, Gross, Taylor, and Moore evaluate the role of multisensory neurons in initiating protective movements in response to approaching targets. Then Ishibashi, Obayashi, and Iriki show the existence of multisensory neurons specifically involved in tool use and demonstrate that the experience of using a tool can change the properties of these multisensory neurons. Finally, Cohen and Andersen deal with an inherent problem in coordinating cues from different senses to locate an external event: because each sensory modality uses a different coordinate system to represent space, the brain has had to find an efficient way of interrelating these schemes in order to use cross-modal cues cooperatively.

PART V: HUMAN BRAIN STUDIES OF MULTISENSORY PROCESSES
The introduction of modern neuroimaging techniques has enabled researchers to examine the neural consequences of multisensory integration in the human brain (e.g., Calvert et al., 1997; Macaluso, Frith, & Driver, 2000). The chapters in Part V span a range of human imaging techniques, including electroencephalography (EEG), magnetoencephalography (MEG), positron emission tomography (PET), and functional magnetic resonance imaging (fMRI). The excellent spatial resolution of methods such as PET and fMRI has been exploited to localize the neuronal networks involved in multisensory integration, while the superior temporal resolution of electromagnetic techniques such as EEG and MEG has yielded vital insights into the time course of multisensory interactions during distinct cross-modal operations. Using these studies, researchers are now beginning to construct a picture of multisensory integration in humans that includes parallel stages of convergence at both early (see the chapter by Fort and Giard) and late (see the chapters by Calvert and Lewis and by Raij and Jousmäki) stages of information processing in what have

traditionally been considered primary sensory areas, as well as in the better-known multisensory cortical regions. It is interesting that despite the considerable variability among the different techniques, paradigms, and analytic strategies used, similar principles of multisensory integration reported at the cellular level in nonhuman species appear to be operative in large populations of neurons in humans. These processes also appear to be sensitive to attentional state (see the chapters by Fort and Giard, Eimer, and Macaluso and Driver), and the emotional context of an experience may reflect the synthesis of cross-modal cues as readily as the detection and localization of events (see Chapter 35, by O'Doherty, Rolls, and Kringelbach, and Chapter 36, by de Gelder, Vroomen, and Pourtois).

PART VI: THE MATURATION AND PLASTICITY OF MULTISENSORY PROCESSES
Many of the multisensory processes discussed in previous parts require postnatal sensory experience to emerge, and this part deals with these factors. A number of animal models have been used in these studies with the objective of manipulating experience in one sensory modality and determining its consequence on perception in other modalities. Part VI begins with a chapter by King, Doubell, and Skaliora on the impact of experience on aligning the visual and auditory maps in the ferret midbrain. These issues, and the presumptive neural circuits involved in effecting this spatial register between the visual and auditory maps in the midbrain, are then dealt with in the owl in Chapter 38, by Gutfreund and Knudsen. In Chapter 39, by Wallace, these issues are extended beyond the spatial register of visual and auditory midbrain maps to the impact of experience on the ability of neurons to synthesize cross-modal cues. Together, these chapters help clarify the ontogeny of the fundamental multisensory processes in the midbrain and their impact on overt orientation. The discussion then moves from orientation to perception. Chapter 40, by Lickliter and Bahrick, and Chapter 41, by Lewkowicz and Kraebel, discuss the maturation of multisensory processing in human infants, providing a timely update on Lewkowicz and Lickliter's (1994) seminal edited volume on this topic. These authors deal with some longstanding controversies regarding whether perception develops from a state in which the senses are differentiated at birth and then become integrated later, or vice versa. Examples from multiple species are brought to bear on these arguments, thereby demonstrating that many of the principles underlying multisensory processes are highly conserved across species.

PART VII: CROSS-MODAL PLASTICITY
The chapters in Part VII address some of the basic issues about the possible equivalence of brain regions thought to be genetically crafted to deal with input from a given sensory modality. In Chapter 42 Sur describes experiments in which early surgical intervention forces signals from one sense to be directed to the cortex normally used to deal with information from another. The ability of these cortices to deal with these redirected inputs is striking and raises questions about the driving force behind brain specialization. Using the results from animal experiments, Rauschecker examines the consequences of depriving the brain of information from one sense on the functional properties of other senses. This is an issue that is of particular concern for those who have lost the use of one sensory system (such as the blind or deaf), and the consequences for human perception and performance are examined in detail in the chapters by Röder and Rösler and by Bergeson and Pisoni.

PART VIII: PERSPECTIVES DERIVED FROM CLINICAL STUDIES
What happens to the multisensory processes underlying human perception when the normal processes of multisensory integration break down? That is the topic addressed by the chapters assembled in this final part of the handbook. Làdavas and

Farnè in Chapter 50 and Maravita and Driver in Chapter 51 discuss what happens when brain damage results in attentional deficits such as extinction and neglect. Persons with these deficits can fail to respond to a variety of sensory stimuli situated in the side of space contralateral to their brain lesion. Synesthesia, a condition in which a particular sensory event in one modality produces an additional sensory experience in a different modality, provides some fascinating insights into the multisensory brain. Research in this area has progressed very rapidly in the last few years with the advent of increasingly sophisticated psychophysical paradigms, which, combined with neuroimaging technologies, are now providing some provocative insights into the differences in the connections and patterns of brain activation in synesthetic, as compared to nonsynesthetic, individuals. These results have led to the development of a variety of neurocognitive theories of synesthesia, which are discussed in Chapter 53, by Mattingley and Rich, and in Chapter 54, by Ramachandran, Hubbard, and Butcher.

REFERENCES

Aristotle (1977). *De anima (On the soul),* translated by H. Lawson-Tancred. London: Penguin Books.

Calvert, G. A., Campbell, R., & Brammer, M. J. (2000). Evidence from functional magnetic resonance imaging of crossmodal binding in the human heteromodal cortex. *Current Biology, 10,* 649–657.

Calvert, G. A., Bullmore, E. T., Brammer, M. J., Campbell, R., Williams, S. C., McGuire, P. K., et al. (1997). Activation of auditory cortex during silent lipreading. *Science, 276,* 593–596.

Campbell, R., Dodd, B., & Burnham, D. (Eds.) (1998). *Hearing by eye: Part 2. The psychology of speechreading and audiovisual speech.* London: Taylor & Francis.

Dalton, P., Doolittle, N., Nagata, H., & Breslin, P. A. S. (2000). The merging of the senses: Integration of subthreshold taste and smell. *Nature Neuroscience, 3,* 431–432.

Dodd, B., & Campbell, R. (Eds.) (1987). *Hearing by eye: The psychology of lip-reading.* Hillsdale, NJ: Erlbaum.

Ernst, M. O., & Banks, M. S. (2002). Humans integrate visual and haptic information in a statistically optimal fashion. *Nature, 115,* 429–433.

Falchier, A., Clavagnier, S., Barone, H., & Kennedy, H. (2002). Anatomical evidence of multimodal integration in primate striate cortex. *The Journal of Neuroscience, 22,* 5749–5759.

Hughes, H. C. (1998). *Sensory exotica: A world beyond human experience.* Cambridge, MA: MIT Press.

Lewkowicz, D. J., & Lickliter, R. (Eds.) (1994). *The development of intersensory perception: Comparative perspectives.* Hillsdale, NJ: Erlbaum.

Macaluso, E., Frith, C., & Driver, J. (2000). Modulation of human visual cortex by crossmodal spatial attention. *Science, 289,* 1206–1208.

Massaro, D. W. (1998). *Perceiving talking faces.* Cambridge, MA: MIT Press.

Partan, S., & Marler, P. (2000). Communication goes multimodal. *Science, 283,* 1272–1273.

Pöppel, E. (1973). Comments on "Visual system's view of acoustic space." *Nature, 243,* 231.

Rock, I., & Victor, J. (1964). Vision and touch: An experimentally created conflict between the two senses. *Science, 143,* 594–596.

Rockland, K. S., & Ojima, K. (2003). Multisensory convergence in calcarine visual areas in macaque monkey. *International Journal of Psychophysiology* (special issue on multisensory processing), *50,* 19–28.

Sekuler, R., Sekuler, A. B., & Lau, R. (1997). Sound alters visual motion perception. *Nature, 385,* 308.

Shams, L., Kamitani, Y., & Shimojo, S. (2000). What you see is what you hear: Sound-induced visual flashing. *Nature, 408,* 788.

Stein, B. E., & Meredith, M. A. (1993). *The merging of the senses.* Cambridge, MA: MIT Press.

Vroomen, J., & de Gelder, B. (2000). Sound enhances visual perception: Cross-modal effects of auditory organization on vision. *Journal of Experimental Psychology: Human Perception and Performance, 26,* 1583–1590.

Welch, R. B., & Warren, D. H. (1980). Immediate perceptual response to intersensory discrepancy. *Psychological Bulletin, 3,* 638–667.

Wilcoxin, H. C., Dragoin, W. B., & Kral, P. A. (1971). Illness-induced aversions in rat and quail: Relative salience of visual and gustatory cues. *Science, 171,* 826–828.

I PERCEPTUAL CONSEQUENCES OF MULTIPLE SENSORY SYSTEMS

1 The Cross-Modal Consequences of the Exogenous Spatial Orienting of Attention

CHARLES SPENCE AND JOHN McDONALD

Introduction

Our attention is often captured by the sudden and unpredictable sensory events that frequent the environments in which we live. For instance, we will normally turn our heads if someone suddenly calls our name at a crowded cocktail party. Similarly, if a mosquito lands on our arm, our eyes will be drawn immediately to the source of the unexpected tactile event. In these and many other such situations, objects that are initially processed in one sensory modality "grab" our attention in such a way as to enhance the sensory processing of stimuli presented in other modalities at the same spatial location. The cross-modal consequences of the involuntary orienting of our spatial attention is an area that has been extensively researched in recent years and is the subject of this review.

Research has demonstrated that the reflexive overt orienting of our attention conveys immediate cross-modal benefits: Not only do we *see* visual events more accurately at the fovea than in the periphery of our visual fields, but perhaps more surprisingly, we also *hear* and *feel* more acutely if we look—or even if we simply prepare to look—in the direction of nonvisual sensory stimulation (e.g., Driver & Grossenbacher, 1996; Gopher, 1973; Honoré, 1982; Honoré, Bourdeaud'hui, & Sparrow, 1989; Kato & Kashino, 2001; Rorden & Driver, 1999). While many researchers have focused their attention on the nature and consequences of these cross-modal shifts in specifically overt attention (i.e., involving shifts of the eyes, head, or body to better inspect an event of interest; e.g., Amlôt, Walker, Driver, & Spence, 2003; Jay & Sparks, 1990; Perrott, Saberi, Brown, & Strybel, 1990; Whittington, Hepp-Reymond, & Flood, 1981; Zambarbieri, Beltrami, & Versino, 1995; Zambarbieri, Schmid, Prablanc, & Magenes, 1981; Zambarbieri, Schmid, Magenes, & Prablanc, 1982), others have investigated the consequences of the covert shifts of attention that may occur prior to, or in the absence of, any overt orienting.

Covert shifts of attention take place very rapidly following the presentation of a peripheral sensory event, occurring prior to any shift of the sensory receptors themselves. Under normal circumstances, there is a close coupling between overt and covert orienting (e.g., Jonides, 1981a; Posner, 1978), with covert shifts of attention typically preceding any overt orienting response (e.g., Klein, Kingstone, & Pontefract, 1992; Rafal, Henik, & Smith, 1991; Rizzolatti, Riggio, Dascola, & Umiltà, 1987; Shepherd, Findlay, & Hockey, 1986), and both being controlled, at least in part, by the same neural structures (such as the superior colliculus; see Desimone, Wessinger, Thomas, & Schneider, 1992; Groh & Sparks, 1996a, 1996b; Robinson & Kertzman, 1995; Stein & Meredith, 1993; Stein, Wallace, & Meredith, 1995; Thompson & Masterton, 1978).

Psychologists have known for many years that the presentation of a spatially nonpredictive visual stimulus, or cue, can lead to a rapid but short-lasting facilitation of responses to visual targets subsequently presented at the cued location (or elsewhere on the cued side), even in the absence of any overt orienting toward the cue itself (e.g., Jonides, 1981b; Posner & Cohen, 1984). Similar intramodal cuing effects following the presentation of a nonpredictive cue have also been reported in subsequent years between auditory cue and target stimuli (e.g., McDonald & Ward, 1999; Spence & Driver, 1994), and more recently, between tactile cue and target stimuli as well (Spence & McGlone, 2001).

In most situations, these cuing effects appear to reflect the consequences of a transient shift of attention to the cued location rather than a passive sensory effect per se (see Posner & Cohen, 1984; but see also Tassinari, Aglioti, Chelazzi, Peru, & Berlucchi, 1994, for a sensory explanation of some facilitatory cuing effects reported in earlier visual cuing studies). Because the cues were spatially nonpredictive with regard to the likely target location in these early studies, researchers concluded that spatial attention can be oriented involuntarily, and at least somewhat automatically, to the location of a cuing event. In line with the majority of previous research on this topic, we will refer to this as exogenous attentional orienting (as compared to the endogenous orienting that occurs following the presentation of a spatially predictive peripheral, or central symbolic, cue; e.g., see Driver & Spence, 2004; Klein & Shore, 2000; Spence & Driver, 1994; Wright & Ward, 1994).

Having provided evidence that exogenous shifts of attention to visual, auditory, and tactile cues can facilitate responses to targets presented subsequently in the same modality, the obvious question arises as to whether such shifts of *covert* attention can also facilitate responses to targets presented in sensory modalities other than that of the cue. Would, for example, an exogenous shift of attention to a sound on the left facilitate responses to subsequent visual targets appearing on that side? Any such cross-modal cuing effect might reflect the existence of a supramodal attentional mechanism, a finding that would have important implications at both the theoretical and applied levels (see, e.g., Spence, 2001). The evidence suggesting that the presentation of auditory or tactile cues can trigger an *overt* shift of visual attention in the cued direction provides at least prima facia evidence that this might be the case. However, as is often the case in the field of experimental psychology, proving (to the satisfaction of all) what is intuitively obvious to the majority of people has taken rather longer than one might have expected! Part of the problem with research in this area has often been the adoption of inappropriate experimental designs that have either used response measures that are relatively insensitive to the manipulation of attention or else do not satisfactorily rule out nonattentional explanations (such as simple detection latencies; see below). Meanwhile, other studies have incorporated experimental setups that failed to maximize the possibility of detecting any cuing effect present because the cue and target stimuli on ipsilaterally cued trials were presented from different spatial locations.[1]

A further problem has been an overreliance on particular experimental paradigms with relatively few attempts to understand why different groups of researchers have found different patterns of cross-modal cuing effects in their different experimental paradigms

(see Ward, Prime, & McDonald, 2002, on this point). Over the past decade, contradictory and often seemingly incompatible findings have emerged from the laboratories of Lawrence Ward, John McDonald, and their colleagues, on the one hand, and Charles Spence, Jon Driver, and their colleagues, on the other (see, e.g., Spence & Driver, 1997a; Ward, 1994; Ward, McDonald, & Golestani, 1998; Ward, McDonald, & Lin, 2000). Although these differences were originally attributed to methodological problems with the particular studies involved, recent work has confirmed the validity and robustness of each pattern of results, at least within the particular experimental paradigms in which they were tested. Fortunately, as the various different research groups have argued over the "true" nature of the cross-modal links in covert spatial attention that exist between the different sensory modalities, a number of important methodological and theoretical advances have emerged from the debate in this area. What is more, and as we hope to show in this chapter, there is now convincing empirical evidence that the covert orienting of exogenous attention that is triggered by the presentation of auditory, visual, or tactile cue stimuli can facilitate the perception of target stimuli presented subsequently at the cued location, no matter what their sensory modality. In fact, cross-modal cuing effects have now been demonstrated behaviorally between all possible combinations of auditory, visual, and tactile cue and target stimuli under a subset of experimental testing conditions.

The way is now open, therefore, for researchers to start investigating a number of theoretically more interesting issues in this area, among them the following: (1) the precise nature of the relationship between mechanisms underlying exogenous shifts of attention to auditory, visual, and tactile stimuli (McDonald & Ward, 2003a); (2) the possible modulation of cross-modal cuing effects by top-down, or endogenous, attentional factors (e.g., McDonald & Ward, 1999; Spence, 2001); (3) the effects of posture change on cross-modal covert attentional orienting (e.g., Driver & Spence, 1998; Kennett, Spence, & Driver, 2002); and (4) the underlying reasons behind the different patterns of cross-modal cuing effects reported in different experimental paradigms (i.e., over and above any simple methodological limitations inherent in particular studies; Prime, McDonald, & Ward, 2003; Ward et al., 2002). Cognitive neuroscientists have also begun to investigate some of the neural underpinnings (and consequences) of the cross-modal orienting of covert exogenous spatial attention (e.g., Kennett, Eimer, Spence, & Driver, 2001; Macaluso, Frith, & Driver, 2000; McDonald, Teder-Sälejärvi, Heraldez, &

---

[1]In this chapter, the terms *ipsilaterally cued* and *contralaterally cued* are used to refer to trials on which the target was presented on the same versus opposite side as the cue, respectively.

Hillyard, 2001; McDonald, Teder-Sälejärvi, Di Russo, & Hillyard, 2003; McDonald & Ward, 2000), an area that has led to the posing of some challenging questions concerning what exactly the difference is between cross-modal exogenous attentional orienting and multisensory integration (see Macaluso, Frith, & Driver, 2001; McDonald, Teder-Sälejärvi, & Ward, 2001; Spence, McDonald, & Driver, 2004). In this chapter we highlight the current state of understanding regarding the nature and consequences of the exogenous cross-modal covert orienting of spatial attention at both the behavioral and neural levels (see Driver & Spence, 2004, for a related discussion of this cross-modal question specifically for the case of endogenous spatial orienting).

Early cross-modal cuing studies of exogenous spatial attention

The first studies to have investigated the cross-modal covert orienting of exogenous spatial attention typically assessed the consequences of the presentation of a peripheral sensory event in one modality on speeded detection latencies for targets presented subsequently in another modality from either the same or opposite side of fixation (e.g., Buchtel & Butter, 1988; Butter, Buchtel, & Santucci, 1989; Farah, Wong, Monheit, & Morrow, 1989; Klein, Brennan, D'Aloisio, D'Entremont, & Gilani, 1987). These cross-modal cuing studies were based on the seminal experiments reported by Mike Posner and colleagues in Oregon (Posner & Cohen, 1984) that had shown an apparently reliable speeding up of behavioral responses to visual targets when they were presented from the same location as a spatially nonpredictive visual cue shortly beforehand (at stimulus onset asynchronies [SOAs] in the range of 0–100 ms).[2]

Early studies of the cross-modal consequences of covert spatial attentional orienting revealed that the presentation of spatially nonpredictive auditory cues also led to the facilitation of detection latencies for visual targets presented on the side of the cue (e.g., Buchtel & Butter, 1988; Farah et al., 1989; Klein et al., 1987). However, by contrast, the peripheral presentation of visual cues was found to have no spatially specific effect on auditory target detection latencies (e.g., Buchtel & Butter, 1988; Klein et al., 1987). These results provided some of the first empirical evidence for the existence of asymmetric audiovisual attentional cuing effects. In fact, the same asymmetric pattern of cuing effects has now been replicated in a number of more recent cross-modal cuing studies using both the simple detection task (e.g., Reuter-Lorenz & Rosenquist, 1996; Schmitt, Postma, & de Haan, 2000, 2001), as well as other kinds of discrimination tasks (e.g., Schmitt et al., 2000, 2001; Spence & Driver, 1997a; see below).

Subsequent research has, however, revealed a number of potential problems with the use of the simple speeded detection response measure in cross-modal attention research. First, simple auditory detection latencies often appear insensitive to the distribution of spatial attention, even when the shift of attention has been elicited by the presentation of an auditory cue (e.g., Buchtel, Butter, & Ayvasik, 1996; Spence & Driver, 1994). This may be because people can base their detection responses on very "early" tonotopic representations of the auditory targets, in which information about the spatial location of the stimulus is simply not made explicit (cf. McDonald & Ward, 1999; Rhodes, 1987; Spence & Driver, 1994). This contrasts with the earliest sensory representations of visual and somatosensory stimuli that are inherently spatiotopically organized, one retinotopically and the other somatotopically (though Spence & McGlone, 2001, recently suggested that tactile simple detection latencies may also be insensitive to the spatial distribution of attention).

Perhaps more important, many researchers have questioned whether, even when facilitatory effects are reported in such cross-modal cuing experiments, they actually reflect the beneficial effects of a shift of covert spatial attention on perceptual processing at the cued location. Instead, it has been argued, they may simply reflect the consequences of criterion shifts taking place at the cued (and/or the uncued) location, and/or speed-accuracy trade-offs. Participants might therefore respond more rapidly on ipsilaterally cued trials simply because less target-related information is required to respond (i.e., their criterion for responding to targets at the cued location might be lower than for targets at the uncued location; e.g., see Spence & Driver,

---

[2]Somewhat ironically, given the impact of these findings on the field, a number of researchers have subsequently failed to demonstrate any facilitatory effect from spatially nonpredictive visual cues on visual target detection latencies (e.g., Tassinari et al., 1994), leading to the claim that any facilitatory effects that may be elicited by a visual cue are often masked by an inhibitory aftereffect that is also triggered by the cue (particularly if the cue is extinguished prior to target onset; see Maruff, Yucel, Danckert, Stuart, & Currie, 1999). In fact, visual inspection of Posner and Cohen's (1984) results (see their Fig. 32.2, p. 536) reveals that the facilitatory effect in their original study disappeared as soon as the cue was extinguished, to be rapidly replaced by an inhibitory aftereffect commonly known as inhibition of return (IOR; see Klein, 2000; Spence, Lloyd, McGlone, Nicholls, & Driver, 2000).

1997b).[3] Given such limitations regarding the appropriate interpretation of studies that have used a simple detection response measure, the majority of researchers in more recent years have started to examine the cross-modal consequences of involuntary, or exogenous, spatial attentional orienting by means of changes in a participant's performance on speeded discrimination tasks instead, where both the speed and accuracy of a participant's responding can be assessed (see Spence, 2001, for a review).

One of the most popular speeded discrimination tasks to have been used by researchers over the past 15 years has been the spatial discrimination task (e.g., Schmitt et al., 2000, 2001; Ward, 1994). For example, in a frequently cited series of experiments reported by Lawrence Ward, participants were required to make speeded left-right discrimination responses to auditory targets (auditory task) or visual targets (visual task) following the peripheral presentation of a spatially nonpredictive auditory cue, a spatially nonpredictive visual cue, both cues, or no cue (at SOAs of 100, 200, 550, or 1050 ms). Ward found that visual cues facilitated responses to ipsilaterally presented auditory targets at the shorter SOAs, but that auditory cues failed to influence response latencies to ipsilaterally presented visual targets at any SOA,[4] despite the fact that the auditory cues did facilitate response latencies to ipsilaterally cued

auditory targets at the shortest SOAs. This audiovisual asymmetry in cross-modal cuing effects was the opposite of that observed in the simple detection studies reported earlier, and also the opposite of that observed in subsequent studies using Spence and Driver's (1997a, 1999) orthogonal cuing paradigm (see below).

Ward's (1994) findings were initially met with some skepticism (e.g., Spence & Driver, 1997a), partly because of their apparent inconsistency with other results, and partly because of a potential methodological problem that affects this kind of spatial discrimination task. While the decision to use a spatial discrimination task is not, in and of itself intrinsically problematic, the majority of studies that have utilized such tasks (including Ward's study) have resulted in experimental paradigms in which the dimension on which the cue was varied and the dimension on which participants were required to respond overlapped. Consequently, the cuing effects reported in such studies are open to an alternative nonattentional interpretation in terms of response priming, or stimulus-response compatibility effects. Specifically, the presentation of the lateralized cue may simply have primed the response associated with the side of the cue (i.e., a left response may have been primed by the presentation of a cue on the left, and a right response by the presentation of the cue on the right; see Simon, 1990, on this issue).[5] Consequently, participants may have responded to ipsilaterally cued targets more rapidly than contralaterally cued targets in such experiments simply because the appropriate response had been primed in the former case and the inappropriate manual response had been primed in the latter case.

---

[3]A lowering of a participant's criterion for responding to targets on the cued side would be expected to lead to a speeding up of response latencies, with a corresponding increase in errors (see, e.g., Klein et al., 1987, Experiment 5, for one such example of a speed-accuracy trade-off). This pattern of behavioral results can be contrasted with the more commonly held view of a perceptual facilitation due to attentional orienting that would lead to a speeding up of response times, with a concomitant reduction in the number of errors that are made (or, at the very minimum, no increase in errors). The problem for studies incorporating a simple detection response is that no measure of error rates is provided, and hence the criterion-shifting explanation cannot be ruled out (see Duncan, 1980; Müller & Findlay, 1987; Shaw, 1980; Sperling & Dosher, 1980).
[4]However, the peripheral presentation of a cue typically leads to at least two distinct effects on a participant's performance. First, there is the spatial cuing effect, which is the focus of the present chapter. Second, there is an equally important and often behaviorally more dramatic alerting effect that is also triggered by the presentation of the cue (e.g., Niemi & Näätänen, 1981; Posner, 1978). Typically, alerting effects facilitate responses to all stimuli, regardless of their location, although this increased facilitation often comes at the cost of an increase in errors. Although Posner (1978) suggested that there may be a cross-modal asymmetry in alerting effects to stimuli of different sensory modalities, Ward (1994) demonstrated a clear cross-modal alerting effect from auditory (and visual) cues on visual (and auditory) targets (e.g., see Ward,

1994, Figs. 2 and 3, pp. 250 and 251). Similar cross-modal alerting effects have also been reported in the majority of subsequent cross-modal cuing studies. They will not be discussed further in the present chapter, in light of the inherently nonspatial nature of such effects.
[5]This problem of interpretation for spatial cuing studies that used overlapping cue and response dimensions is emphasized by the fact that a very similar experimental paradigm was used by researchers in the early 1970s to investigate a different research question related to stimulus-response compatibility effects. For example, Simon and Craft (1970) reported that participants made speeded left-right discrimination responses to visual targets presented on a screen more rapidly when the presentation of target was accompanied by a spatially nonpredictive auditory cue presented to the same side rather than to the opposite side over headphones. While the auditory and visual stimuli were presented simultaneously in Simon and Craft's study, similar stimulus-response compatibility effects were also reported by Bernstein and Edelstein (1971) when the auxiliary auditory stimuli were presented up to 45 ms after the onset of the lateralized visual target.

Ward (1994) considered response priming as a possible explanation for his cross-modal cuing results but argued that any such response priming effect would have led to an auditory cuing effect on visual discriminations as well as the visual cuing effect on audition that he found. By contrast, Spence and Driver (1997a) raised the possibility that even Ward's null result might be attributable to response priming, because the visual cues were presented much closer to fixation than the auditory targets. In particular, they suggested that even on ipsilaterally cued trials, the auditory cues and targets may have primed (or been associated with) opposite response tendencies. For example, an auditory cue on the left may have primed a left response, whereas a visual target on the left may have been coded in terms of a right response (at least initially) because the target was located on the right with respect to the cue (cf. Nicoletti & Umiltà, 1989; Umiltà & Nicoletti, 1985). Spence and Driver argued that the response tendencies generated on these ipsilaterally cued trials might therefore have been the same as on the contralaterally cued trials, thereby potentially canceling each other out and leaving no net cross-modal cuing effect.

Ward and his collaborators, however, have subsequently demonstrated that the cross-modal asymmetry reported in Ward's (1994) original study still occurs when these potential problems are avoided. For example, Ward et al. (1998) found the same pattern of asymmetric cuing effects in subsequent experiments when the cue and target were presented from exactly the same lateral eccentricity. Moreover, in a different study, Ward et al. (2000) also replicated the asymmetry using an experimental procedure (implicit spatial discrimination; McDonald & Ward, 1999) that ruled out any response priming explanation more directly (see below).

Two important points therefore emerge from this early debate over Ward's (1994) asymmetric cross-modal cuing results. First, response priming by the cue may be problematic on certain spatial discrimination tasks, and steps should be taken to avoid such problems, for example, by using techniques such as the orthogonal spatial cuing task or the implicit spatial discrimination task discussed below. Second, although a study may be methodologically confounded, this does not necessarily mean that the conclusions based on that study might not still turn out to be correct. Having demonstrated the robustness of the cross-modal cuing asymmetry first reported by Ward (1994) in subsequent studies, it therefore now becomes increasingly important to try to determine precisely why auditory cues have no effect on visual discrimination performance under at least certain experimental conditions.

Ward and his collaborators (Ward et al., 1998, 2000) have argued that auditory-on-visual cuing effects can be modulated by top-down control processes. In Ward's (1994) original study, the cue modality was unpredictable and the cuing environment complex (five different possible cue types could be presented on any trial). Ward et al. (2000) therefore suggested that participants might not have fully processed the locations of the auditory cues under such circumstances. According to the account of Ward et al., auditory-on-visual cuing effects would be expected to emerge when tested under more simple experimental conditions, such as when the cue and target modalities are fixed and predictable (see also McDonald & Ward, 2003a; Mondor & Amirault, 1998; and Spence, 2001, for a discussion of the role of the complexity of the stimulus environment, both that of the cue and that of the target, on the pattern of cross-modal cuing effects observed). Indeed, Schmitt et al. (2000) demonstrated a cross-modal cuing effect from auditory cues on visual left-right spatial discrimination responses (as well as the effect of visual cues on auditory discrimination responses already documented by Ward, 1994) under conditions where the cue (and target) modalities were fixed throughout each block of experimental trials. Symmetric audiovisual cuing effects have also been reported in the more recently developed implicit spatial discrimination task (McDonald & Ward, 1997; 2003a, 2003b; see below).

Cross-modal cuing studies using the orthogonal spatial cuing paradigm

Ambiguities concerning the appropriate interpretation of these early cross-modal cuing studies led Spence and Driver (1994, 1997a) to develop a modified version of the spatial discrimination task. They eliminated any possibility that the cue could prime the appropriate response in their task by making participants respond on a dimension (or direction) that was orthogonal to that on which they were cued. In the majority of their studies, Spence and Driver presented spatially nonpredictive auditory and visual cues from either the left or the right of a central fixation point on each trial. However, the auditory and/or visual targets were presented from one of four locations situated directly above or below the cue location on either side (Fig. 1.1A provides a schematic outline of the experimental setup used in many of Spence and Driver's studies). Participants in these experiments were required to make a speeded spatial discrimination response regarding the elevation (upper vs. lower) of the targets, regardless of the side and sensory modality of their presentation. Consequently, the left or right cues could not differentially affect responses on

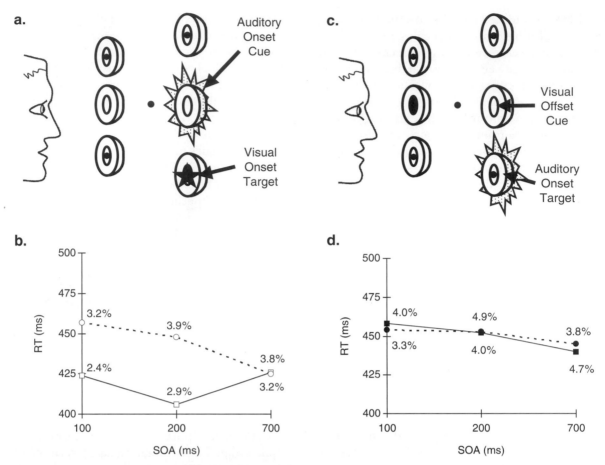

FIGURE 1.1   (*A*) Schematic illustration of the orthogonal spatial-cuing paradigm popularized by Spence and Driver (1994, 1997). Participants sit in front of an array of four target loudspeaker cones, one positioned above and one below fixation on either side of central fixation. Target lights (LEDs) are situated at the center of each of these loudspeaker cones. In the study shown, an auditory pure-tone cue was presented from either the left or the right at eye level shortly before presentation of a visual target requiring a speeded manual elevation discrimination response. (*B*) Typical pattern of cross-modal spatial-cuing effects from one such experiment (Spence & Driver, 1997; Experiment 1). The graph highlights the more rapid, and somewhat more accurate (error rates are shown numerically next to the associated RT value), responses on the visual target elevation discrimination task on ipsilaterally cued trials (represented by open squares connected by solid lines) as opposed to contralaterally cued trials (open circles connected by dotted lines). (*C*) Diagram highlighting the stimuli presented in another study (Spence & Driver, 1997; Experiment 4), in which the offset of a visual cue from either the left or right of fixation was used as the visual cue, followed shortly afterward by the presentation of an auditory white noise target, again requiring a speeded manual elevation discrimination response. (*D*) Diagram highlighting the null effect of visual cues on auditory elevation discrimination responses in this orthogonal spatial-cuing task. Ipsilaterally cued trials are represented by solid squares connected by the solid line, while contralaterally cued trials are represented by solid circles connected by dotted lines. Error rates are shown numerically next to the corresponding RT values.

ipsilaterally versus contralaterally cued trials, since any response bias elicited by a cue should affect responses on both types of trial equally.

In their first cross-modal cuing experiment, Spence and Driver (1997a; Experiment 1) found that the peripheral presentation of a spatially nonpredictive auditory cue led to a short-lasting facilitation of elevation discrimination responses latencies to auditory targets as well as to visual targets (Fig. 1.1*B*). This cross-modal cuing effect was observed despite the fact that participants were explicitly and repeatedly instructed to ignore the auditory cues as much as possible. What is

more, they were given more than 1000 trials on which to try to overcome any tendency they might have had to orient covertly toward the cue. Performance was also somewhat more accurate on ipsilaterally cued trials than on contralaterally cued trials, thus allowing Spence and Driver to rule out a speed-accuracy trade-off account of their findings.[6]

---

[6]Spence and Driver (1997a, Experiment 1) did not monitor the eye position of the participants in their original study. Therefore, one cannot rule out the possibility that their spatial cuing effect might reflect overt rather than covert

In their more recent research, Driver and Spence (1998) further investigated the spatial specificity of this specific cross-modal cuing effect by presenting auditory cues and visual targets from one of two locations on either side of fixation (one placed 13 degrees from central fixation, the other 39 degrees from fixation) (Fig. 1.2). Spence and Driver found that participants responded more rapidly and accurately to visual targets presented from LEDs directly above (or below) the auditorily cued loudspeaker (at SOAs of 100–150 ms), with performance falling off as the cue-target separation increased, even if the cue and target both fell within the same hemifield. Thus, the presentation of an auditory cue led to a spatially specific cross-modal facilitation of visual elevation discrimination responses, akin to the spatially specific cuing effects reported previously in intramodal studies of covert orienting within both vision and audition (e.g., Rorden & Driver, 2001; Tassinari et al., 1987) and subsequently replicated in a number of other cross-modal cuing studies (Frassinetti, Bolognini, & Làdavas, 2002; Schmitt et al., 2001). Driver and Spence (1998) have also shown that visual targets by the auditorily cued loudspeaker are discriminated more rapidly and accurately than lights by the other (noncued) loudspeakers when participants deviate their gaze 26 degrees to either side of central fixation throughout a whole block of trials (while keeping their head fixed in a straight-ahead position), thus showing that these cross-modal cuing effects update so that when posture changes, covert exogenous attention is still directed to the correct environmental location.

Having demonstrated a cross-modal cuing effect from auditory cues on visual elevation discrimination responses, Spence and Driver (1997a) went on to investigate whether the peripheral presentation of a spatially nonpredictive visual cue would also lead to a facilitation of responses to ipsilaterally presented auditory targets (see Fig. 1.1C). In fact—and in direct contrast with the results reported by Ward (1994)—Spence and Driver found no such spatially specific effect of visual cues on auditory elevation discrimination responses (see Fig. 1.1D). Importantly, this null effect of visual cues on auditory target discrimination responses was replicated in a number of different experiments using the orthogonal spatial cuing design, hence demonstrating the

---

orienting to the cued location, or else some unknown combination of the two effects. However, subsequent studies have revealed that the facilitatory effect of auditory cues on visual elevation discrimination responses is robust to the monitoring of eye movements (and to the removal of all trials in which an eye movement was detected), thus supporting a covert orienting account of their results (e.g., see Driver & Spence, 1998).

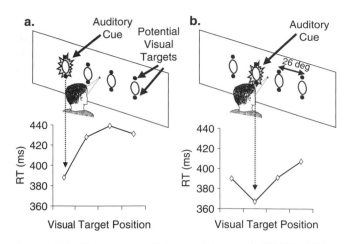

FIGURE 1.2 The setup in Driver and Spence's (1998) within-hemifield study of cross-modal spatial attention. On each trial, a spatially nonpredictive auditory cue was presented from one of four loudspeaker cones placed at eye level. Two loudspeakers were situated on either side of central fixation, separated horizontally by 26 degrees. Visual targets consisted of the brief offset of one of eight LEDs (otherwise continuously illuminated), one placed directly above and another directly below each of the four loudspeaker cones. (A) In the situation shown, the auditory cue was presented from the outer left loudspeaker cone. The results (lower panel) indicate that the presentation of an auditory cue from an outer loudspeaker cone led to a spatially specific shift of attention that facilitated visual elevation discrimination response latencies maximally for visual targets presented from directly above and below the auditorily cued location. Of note, there was little advantage for a visual target presented ipsilateral to the cue but from a less eccentric stimulus location when compared with performance on visual targets presented contralateral to the cue. (Similar results were found following the presentation of a target from the outer right loudspeaker.) (B) A similarly spatially specific cross-modal spatial-cuing effect was also demonstrated following the presentation of an inner (left) auditory cue. Once again, visual discrimination performance was facilitated maximally for targets presented at the auditorily cued location, with no benefit for visual targets presented from a more eccentric location on the ipsilaterally cued side when compared with performance on visual targets presented at the same distance from the cue on the side contralateral to the cue. (Similar results were found following the presentation of a target from the inner right loudspeaker.)

robustness of this null effect (at least in the orthogonal cuing paradigm). For example, Spence and Driver (1997a, Experiment 6) assessed auditory elevation discrimination performance at a much wider range of SOAs following the onset of the visual cue in order to try and rule out the possibility that the time course of visual cuing effects on auditory target discrimination responses might simply be different from those reported following an auditory cue. However, no effect of visual cues on auditory elevation discrimination responses was found at any of the SOAs tested (in the range of 100–550 ms) when the possible confounding effect of overt orienting had been ruled out (i.e., by ensuring continuous central fixation by means of an eye position monitor, and throwing out all trials on which participants either moved their eyes or else blinked).

Spence and Driver (1997a) also varied the nature of the visual cuing events that they used in order to try and demonstrate a cross-modal influence of visual cues on auditory discrimination responses. For example, they assessed the consequences of the presentation of visual cues consisting of visual offsets (Experiments 4–6), rather than the onset cues more commonly used in cross-modal cuing studies, and they also assessed the consequences of the presentation of cues consisting of the onset of a highly salient 3 × 3 array of high-luminance yellow LEDs on one side of fixation or the other (Experiments 3, 5, and 6). However, none of these manipulations elicited a significant cross-modal cuing effect. That is, no consistent evidence of a significant cross-modal spatial cuing effect from visual cues on auditory elevation discrimination responses was found in any of the four experiments that were conducted. Spence and Driver and others (e.g., Schmitt et al., 2000; Spence & Driver, 1999, 2000; Vroomen, Bertelson, & de Gelder, 2001) have also replicated the null effect of visual cues on auditory elevation discrimination responses in several further studies, including those that have incorporated more complex cuing environments (Fig. 1.3; cf. Ward et al., 2000). The asymmetric cross-modal cuing effects reported in Spence and Driver's studies also mirrored the findings reported earlier by researchers using simple detection response measures (e.g., Buchtel & Butter, 1988; Klein et al., 1987; Schmitt et al., 2000, 2001).

Spence and Driver (1997a, 1999) interpreted the null effect of visual cues on auditory target elevation discrimination performance as supporting the existence of asymmetric cross-modal links in exogenous spatial attention between essentially distinct (i.e., separate) auditory and visual exogenous attentional systems (see Schmitt et al., 2000, for a similar theoretical standpoint). Spence and Driver argued that whereas the presentation of a spatially nonpredictive peripheral auditory cue would lead to a shift of both the auditory and visual attentional systems, the presentation of visual cues appeared only to trigger a shift of the visual spatial attention system, not of the auditory attention system.

Cross-modal cuing between audition, touch, and vision

In the years following their original cross-modal cuing study, Spence, Driver, and their colleagues went on to investigate the nature of any cross-modal links in exogenous spatial attention between other combinations of

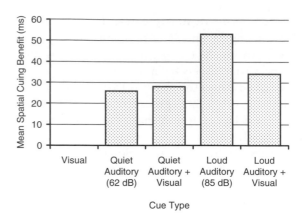

FIGURE 1.3 The results of another of Spence and Driver's (1999) orthogonal spatial-cuing studies that used a setup very similar to the one shown in Figure 1.1. Participants were required to make speeded elevation discrimination responses to a series of auditory targets presented shortly after one of five different types of cue (at stimulus onset asynchronies of either 50 ms or 250 ms). The mean spatial-cuing benefit is defined as performance on contralaterally cued trials minus performance on ipsilaterally cued trials for each cue type. Once again, a null effect of visual cues on auditory elevation discrimination responses was found (a 0 ms effect in this case). Meanwhile, unimodal auditory cues resulted in a significant cross-modal spatial-cuing effect, with the magnitude of the cuing effect modulated by the intensity of the cue. Interestingly, the simultaneous presentation of the visual cue had no effect on the cuing effect elicited by the quieter cue (62 dB, A), but resulted in a reduction in the cuing effect associated with the louder auditory cue (85 dB, A).

sensory modalities, using variations on their orthogonal spatial cuing design (e.g., Kennett et al., 2001, 2002; Spence, Nicholls, Gillespie, & Driver, 1998). For example, Spence et al. reported a series of experiments demonstrating that the peripheral presentation of a tactile cue to the index finger of either the left or right hand would elicit a cross-modal shift of both visual and auditory attention toward the position of the cued hand in space (Figs. 1.4A and B). Similarly, Spence et al. also reported that the peripheral presentation of either a spatially nonpredictive auditory or visual cue could facilitate a participant's ability to discriminate continuous from pulsed vibrotactile stimuli presented to the ipsilateral hand (Figs. 1.4C and D). A similar pattern of symmetric cross-modal cuing effects between vision and touch has now been reported in a number of other studies (Chong & Mattingley, 2000; Kennett, 2000; Kennett & Driver, 1999; Kennett et al., 2001, 2002; see also Tan, Gray, Young, & Irawan, 2001), supporting the robustness of the cross-modal cuing effects found between touch and audition or vision.

Kennett et al. (2002) have also demonstrated subsequently that if participants hold their hands in a crossed hands posture (Fig. 1.5), then a vibrotactile cue

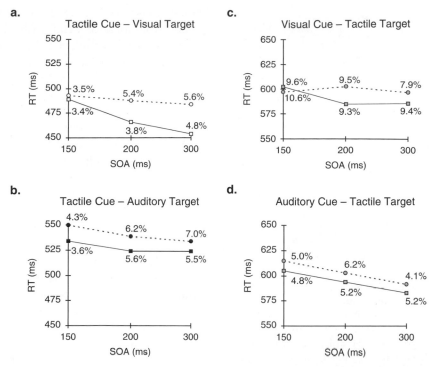

FIGURE 1.4 The results of a study by Spence et al. (1998) of cross-modal links in exogenous spatial attention between touch, vision, and audition. (A) Diagram showing the cross-modal facilitation of visual elevation responses following the presentation of a spatially nonpredictive tactile cue to either the left or the right hand (Spence et al., 1998; Experiment 3). Ipsilaterally cued trials are indicated by open squares connected by solid lines and contralaterally cued trials by open circles connected by dotted lines. Error rates are shown next to the associated RT value. (B) Tactile cues also facilitated elevation discrimination responses for auditory targets presented ipsilateral (solid squares connected by solid lines) as opposed to contralateral (solid circles connected by dotted lines) to the cue (Spence et al., 1998; Experiment 3). (C) In another experiment, Spence et al. (1998; Experiment 2) demonstrated that continuous versus pulsed discrimination latencies for tactile stimuli presented to one or the other hand were also facilitated by the presentation of a visual cue by the stimulated hand (ipsilateral trials, gray squares connected by solid lines) versus the unstimulated hand (gray circles connected by dotted lines). (D) Finally, Spence et al. (1998; Experiment 1) also demonstrated that continuous versus pulsed tactile discrimination latencies could be facilitated by the presentation of an auditory cue on the ipsilaterally cued side (gray squares connected by solid lines) as opposed to the contralaterally cued side (gray circles connected by dotted lines).

presented to the left hand will facilitate visual discrimination responses for targets on the participant's right (i.e., on the opposite side to the facilitation reported in the uncrossed posture, though in the correct external location). Cross-modal cuing effects therefore seem to result in the facilitation of information processing for all stimuli at the correct externally cued location, regardless of their modality and regardless of the person's posture. These results suggest that covert shifts of attention operate on a multisensory representation of space that is updated as posture changes (see Spence et al., in press, for a fuller discussion of this issue).

Cross-modal cuing studies using the implicit spatial discrimination paradigm

While Spence and Driver were extending their orthogonal cuing paradigm beyond the audiovisual pairing that they had originally studied, John McDonald,

Lawrence Ward, and their colleagues were highlighting a possible methodological problem with the paradigm. They noted that the vertical distance between targets in the orthogonal spatial cuing paradigm must be large enough for participants to be able to discriminate the elevation of the targets reliably. Consequently, the cue and target stimuli have often had to be presented from different positions not only on contralaterally cued trials, but on ipsilaterally cued trials as well. This is particularly noticeable for the combination of visual cues and auditory targets, given the difficulty that most humans have in discriminating the elevation from which auditory stimuli are presented. For example, in Spence and Driver's (1997) experiments, auditory and visual targets were presented from approximately 24 degrees above or below the cued location. Ward et al. (2000, p. 1264; see also Prime et al., 2003; Spence, 2001) speculated that the spatial focusing of attention in response to a highly localizable visual cue might be too narrowly

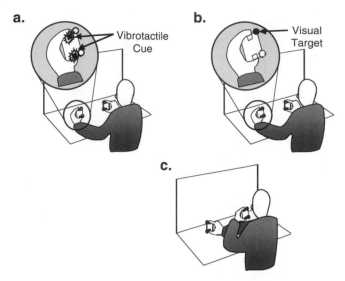

a. Vibrotactile Cue

b. Visual Target

c.

FIGURE 1.5   The setup used in studies by Kennett et al. (2002) of cross-modal links in spatial attention between vision and touch. Participants held two foam cubes, one in each hand. Two vibrotactile stimulators (solid rectangles) and two LEDs (open circles) were embedded in each cube, near the thumb and index finger. (A) On each trial, participants were presented with a vibrotactile cue from the pair of vibrotactile stimulators placed in one of the foams cube. (B) A short time later one of the four target LEDs was illuminated. Participants were required to make speeded elevation discrimination responses (by raising the toe or heel of their right foot) in response to the visual targets presented either from the "top," near the index finger of either hand, or from the "bottom," near either thumb. (C) Schematic view of the posture adopted by participants in the crossed-hands condition.

distributed to influence the processing of auditory targets in such tasks, whereas the spatial focusing of attention in response to a less localizable auditory cue might be broad enough to influence the processing of visual targets under comparable conditions (Fig. 1.6).[7]

In light of this possible limitation with the orthogonal spatial cuing paradigm, McDonald and Ward (1999) developed an alternative paradigm, called the implicit spatial discrimination task, in which the spatial component of the task was maintained while ensuring that the cue and target stimuli could be presented from exactly the same locations (hence maximizing the possibility of finding any cuing effects). In the implicit spatial discrimination task, participants are required to respond to targets presented from certain spatial locations

(known as Go trials), but not to stimuli at one or more other spatial locations (known as No-Go trials). In the original version of the task, depicted in Figure 1.7, participants were instructed to respond to the onset of targets presented to the left and right of fixation, and to refrain from responding to the onset of targets presented at fixation itself (McDonald & Ward, 1999, 2003a; Ward et al., 2000).

In subsequent versions of the implicit spatial discrimination task, participants have been required to discriminate between peripheral targets on the basis of a modality-specific feature instead (such as the frequency of auditory targets or the color of visual targets) while still refraining from making any response to target stimuli presented at fixation (McDonald et al., 2001; McDonald & Ward, 2003a, 2003b). Nevertheless, the crucial feature of each version of the implicit spatial discrimination task was that the location of target stimuli was still relevant to the participant's task, even though the participant's responses themselves were explicitly based on some other nonspatial criterion (such as onset detection, frequency, or color). Thus, just as in the orthogonal spatial cuing paradigm, the implicit spatial discrimination task maintains a spatial component to the participant's task while avoiding any problems associated with possible response priming by the cue. Later versions of the implicit spatial discrimination task also satisfy the definition of orthogonal cuing because the response dimension is independent of, and orthogonal to, the cuing dimension.

The implicit spatial discrimination task was originally used to investigate the intramodal consequences of the exogenous orienting of covert attention to auditory cues (McDonald & Ward, 1999), but it has since been used to gather both behavioral and electrophysiogical data on the cross-modal consequences of exogenous shifts of attention. As mentioned earlier, Ward et al. (2000) used this task in an attempt to replicate Ward's (1994) original audiovisual asymmetry. Separate groups of participants responded to auditory targets and to visual targets. As in Ward's original study, the targets in each task were preceded on a trial-by-trial basis by either a visual cue, an auditory cue, both types of cues, or no cue (i.e., both cue modality and cue type were unpredictable). The results of this study replicated Ward's original results in the crucial cross-modal conditions; namely, the presentation of peripheral visual cues led to a short-lasting facilitation of response latencies to auditory targets, but the presentation of peripheral auditory cues failed to have a significant influence on response latencies to the visual targets (Fig. 1.8). Importantly, eye position was carefully monitored for each participant and stimulus-response compatibility effects were eliminated.

---

[7]In fact, Spence and Driver (1994, 1997a) chose to use 2000 Hz pure tones as the auditory cues in their experiments precisely because they were unlocalizable in terms of their elevation (see Roffler & Butler, 1968; Spence & Driver, 1997a, Experiment 2), thus perhaps exacerbating this difference between the localizability of stimuli in different sensory modalities (e.g., Fisher, 1962; Warren, 1970).

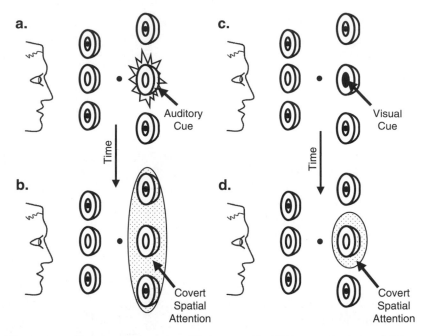

FIGURE 1.6   Schematic illustration of how spatially nonpredictive cues in different sensory modalities—here, audition (*A*) and vision (*C*)—might elicit attentional capture effects of different spatial specificity, thus providing one explanation for why auditory cues may facilitate elevation discrimination responses for visual targets (*B*), while visual cues may fail to elicit any significant effect on auditory elevation discrimination latencies (*D*).

McDonald and Ward (2003a) conducted a further series of reaction-time experiments in which the cue and target modalities were both fixed (unlike their earlier work, which involved unpredictable cue modalities). In their first experiment, a cue appeared from a single modality that was known in advance and a subsequent target appeared from a different sensory modality that was also known in advance. Thus, the conditions were similar to those in most unimodal spatial cuing studies except that the cue occurred in a sensory modality that was completely irrelevant to the participant's task (see Schmitt et al., 2000, for similar left-right discrimination

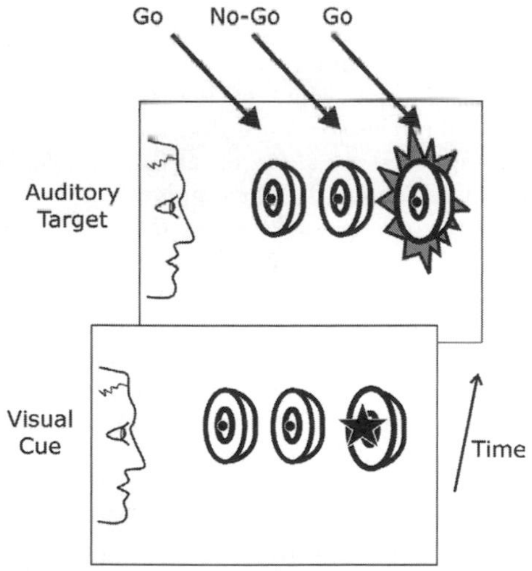

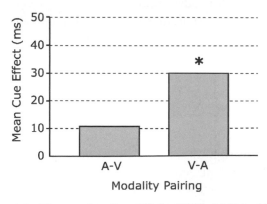

FIGURE 1.7   Schematic illustration of the implicit spatial discrimination task introduced by McDonald and Ward (1999). Participants sit in front of an array of three loudspeaker cones on which LEDs are fixed. Participants are asked to respond to targets appearing to the left or right side of fixation (Go trials) but to refrain from responding to targets appearing at fixation (No-Go trials). In this illustration, a visual cue precedes an auditory target from the same location (i.e., an ipsilaterally-cued trial).

FIGURE 1.8   The results of a study by Ward, McDonald, and Lin (2000) that replicated Ward's (1994) audiovisual cuing study using the implicit spatial discrimination task. The data shown are from the 100-ms SOA of each condition. An asterisk denotes a significant effect by the Bonferroni *t*-test. The cross-modal cuing effect was significant in the visual cue–auditory target (V-A) condition but not in the auditory cue–visual target (A-V) condition, highlighting the robustness of Ward's (1994) original pattern of asymmetrical results.

experiments under conditions of predictable cue and target modality presentation). Participants were instructed to respond to peripheral targets while trying to refrain from responding to central targets. McDonald and Ward again found that visual cues facilitated response latencies on the implicit spatial discrimination task for auditory targets presented ipsilateral to the cue, thereby providing additional evidence for the cross-modal cuing effect that has not as yet been found in orthogonal spatial cuing studies (e.g., Schmitt et al., 2000; Spence & Driver, 1997a, 1999; Vroomen et al., 2001). Moreover, McDonald and Ward now found that auditory cues facilitated implicit spatial discrimination latencies to ipsilateral visual targets as well (Fig. 1.9A). Once again, eye position was monitored; thus, the effects appeared to reflect exclusively the covert orienting of spatial attention.

One possible nonattentional explanation for the results obtained by McDonald and Ward is that the cues affected the participant's criterion for responding to targets differentially on ipsilaterally cued as opposed to contralaterally cued trials. To rule out this possibility, McDonald and Ward (2003a, 2003b) conducted a further experiment in which participants discriminated between red and green visual targets that appeared to the left or right of fixation while withholding responses to visual targets appearing at fixation. A spatially nonpredictive auditory cue was presented prior to the appearance of every target. By requiring the participants to discriminate between different peripheral targets, McDonald and Ward were able to rule out a criterion-shifting explanation of their results by testing explicitly for a speed-accuracy trade-off in their data. Critically, response latencies were faster on ipsilaterally cued trials than on contralaterally cued trials, and there was no evidence of a speed-accuracy trade-off (Fig. 1.9B).

McDonald et al. (2001) used a similar experimental design to investigate the crucial missing link in exogenous cross-modal attention further. In their experiment, participants discriminated between low-frequency and high-frequency auditory targets that were presented to the left or right of fixation while ignoring auditory targets that were presented at fixation. Prior to the appearance of each target, a visual cue was presented randomly to the left or right of fixation (at cue-target SOAs of 100–300 ms). The behavioral results showed a clear cross-modal cuing effect: Responses latencies were significantly shorter on ipsilaterally cued trials than on contralaterally cued trials, and once again, there was no evidence of a speed-accuracy trade-off (Fig. 1.9C). This study therefore provided the first unequivocal behavioral evidence that exogenously orienting attention to a

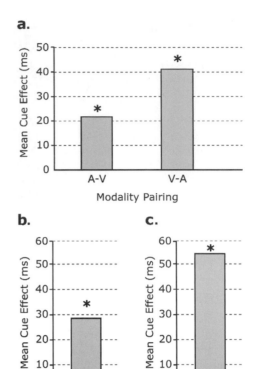

FIGURE 1.9 The results of recent implicit spatial discrimination experiments in which both the cue and target modalities were fixed. Cues were spatially nonpredictive with regard to the likely target location. Asterisks denote a significant effect according to the Bonferroni t-test. The data shown are from 100-ms SOA trials. (A) RT data from a Go/No-Go version of the task (McDonald & Ward, 2003b, Experiment 1). The mean cueing effects were significant for both the visual cue–auditory target (V-A) condition and the auditory cue–visual target (A-V) condition. (B) RT data from a modified version of the A-V task in which participants discriminated between green and red visual targets that appeared at peripheral locations and ignored visual targets at fixation (McDonald & Ward, 2003b, Experiment 3). The cuing effect was significant, with no evidence of a speed–accuracy trade off. (C) RT data from a modified version of the V-A task in which participants discriminated between high-frequency and low-frequency auditory targets that appeared at peripheral locations and ignored auditory targets at fixation (McDonald et al., 2001). The cuing effect was again significant, with no evidence of a speed–accuracy trade-off (95% correct on both ipsilaterally cued and contralaterally cued trials).

visual cue can modulate the processing of subsequent auditory targets.[8]

The fact that cross-modal cuing effects have now been demonstrated between all possible combinations

---

[8]Further support for the notion of Ward et al. (2000) that spatial relevance may enhance the magnitude of any cross-modal cuing effects reported comes from a comparison of the study of McDonald et al. with those reported by Mondor and

of auditory, visual, and tactile cue and target stimuli does not, however, mean that cross-modal cuing effects will occur in every task or under all testing conditions (McDonald & Ward, 2003a; Spence, 2001; Ward et al., 1998, 2000). For, as we have already seen, certain performance measures, such as simple auditory detection latencies, may be insensitive to the orientation of spatial attention. In addition, Ward and McDonald have argued that certain cross-modal cuing effects (specifically, from auditory cues to visual targets) may be harder to demonstrate in more complex cue-target environments. A number of results now also support the suggestion that cross-modal cuing effects appear to be both larger and more robust under conditions where "space" is somehow relevant to the participant's task (than in nonspatial tasks; see McDonald & Ward, 1999; Spence, 2001). Space can be made relevant either by requiring participants to make a spatial discrimination response regarding the target (as in the orthogonal spatial cuing task) or by instructing participants only to respond to targets coming from certain spatial locations (as in the implicit spatial discrimination task).

The two spatial discrimination paradigms reviewed thus far both manage to make space relevant to the participant's task while avoiding stimulus-response compatibility issues such as response priming. Each of these tasks appears to have its own advantages. The implicit spatial discrimination task has the important methodological advantage that the cue and target stimuli can be presented from exactly the same location on ipsilaterally cued trials, hence maximizing any cross-modal cuing effects that might be present. However, as yet this task has only been used to investigate cross-modal links between audition and vision. Meanwhile, the orthogonal spatial cuing paradigm has been used to demonstrate cross-modal cuing effects between all possible combinations of auditory, visual, and tactile cue and target stimuli with the exception of visual cues and auditory targets. Therefore, the orthogonal spatial cuing paradigm may be a more appropriate paradigm for investigating the effects of peripheral cues on visual and tactile target performance (where the elevation separation between upper and lower targets need not be

large), but one can run into problems when using this paradigm to investigate the effects of cross-modal attention on auditory discrimination performance, for which elevation separation between targets has to be much greater, owing to the poor elevation discrimination ability in audition in humans (Roffler & Butler, 1968).

Prime, McDonald, and Ward (2003; Ward et al., 2002) have begun to examine the visual-on-auditory cuing effect in closely matched implicit spatial discrimination and orthogonal spatial cuing experiments. In one such study, a visual cue was presented to the left or right of fixation along the horizontal meridian shortly before an auditory target was presented from one of five loudspeaker cones (at an SOA of either 100 ms or 500 ms). A pair of loudspeaker cones was positioned 15 degrees above and below the visual cue display on each side of fixation, and a single loudspeaker cone was positioned directly in front of the observer. In the implicit spatial discrimination condition, participants ignored targets appearing at fixation and pressed the same response button for lateralized targets appearing above and below fixation. In the orthogonal spatial cuing condition, participants ignored targets appearing at fixation and pressed different response buttons for the lateralized targets appearing above and below fixation (i.e., they were making speeded elevation discrimination responses). Response latencies were shown to be shorter for ipsilaterally cued trials than for contralaterally cued trials at the 100 ms SOA, but only for the implicit spatial discrimination condition (although a criterion-shifting explanation of these facilitatory effects cannot be ruled out). Interestingly, response latencies were actually significantly longer for ipsilaterally cued trials than for contralaterally cued trials in the orthogonal spatial cuing condition. The reason for this inhibitory cuing effect is unclear, although a similar effect was reported in another previous study by Ward et al. (1998).[9] Nevertheless, this difference in cuing results depending on the participant's task highlights the potential importance of processing requirements in the generation of cross-modal cuing effects.

Psychophysical studies of cross-modal exogenous cuing effects

The reaction time studies described so far have demonstrated that the exogenous orienting of attention to a stimulus in one sensory modality can facilitate

---

Amirault (1998, Experiment 1). Mondor and Amirault used an experimental design that was very similar to that of Ward et al., but without the spatial relevance component (i.e., participants had to respond to all targets). Whereas Ward et al. found cross-modal cuing effects in their experiment when space was relevant to the task, Mondor and Amirault did not (except under conditions where the cue was predictive with regard to the likely location of the upcoming target, and so endogenous attentional orienting mechanisms were presumably involved).

---

[9]Spence (2001) suggested that this unusual result may be related to the use of a highly localizable white noise cue (as opposed to the hard-to-localize pure-tone cue used in the majority of other previous orthogonal spatial cuing studies; see also Fig. 1.6 on this point).

responses to stimuli in other sensory modalities that happen to be presented at the same location a short time afterward. However, it is very difficult to know from such results where exactly in the stream of information processing the facilitatory effect is occurring. In particular, the studies discussed so far do not answer the question of whether cross-modal cuing effects represent a facilitation of the preparation and/or execution of a participant's responses (i.e., without requiring any enhancement of the participant's perceptual experience), or whether they also demonstrate a genuine enhancement in perceptual processing (e.g., Hawkins et al., 1990; Luce, 1986; Watt, 1991).[10]

In order to learn more about the processes underlying the facilitatory effects demonstrated in cross-modal cuing studies, researchers have now started to use signal detection theory (see Green & Swets, 1996; Macmillan & Creelman, 1991, for an introduction) to separate the effects of cross-modal cuing on perceptual sensitivity (i.e., d') from their effects on response-related processing (specifically criterion shifts). McDonald, Teder-Sälejärvi, Di Russo, and Hillyard (2000) reported one such study in which participants sat in front of two arrays of LEDs, one on either side of fixation (Fig. 1.10A). On each trial, a bright flash of red light was presented from four red LEDs on either the left or right of fixation. In half of the trials, this was preceded by a brief flash of green light from a single LED in the center of the LED array (the green light flash was absent in the remainder of trials). Participants had to judge whether or not the green target had been presented at the location of the red stimulus.[11] A spatially nonpredictive auditory cue was presented from one side or the other

a.

Fixation

Speaker

LEDs

b.

FIGURE 1.10   (A) Schematic illustration of the audiovisual apparatus used by McDonald et al. (2000). Small light displays were fixed to the bottom of two loudspeaker cones, one situated to the left and one to the right of a central fixation point. (The illustration is not drawn to scale.) (B) Mean data for all participants on one of the signal detection experiments reported by McDonald et al. (Experiment 2). In all graphs, black bars represent ipsilaterally cued trials and gray bars represent contralaterally cued trials.

---

[10]This viewpoint is nicely illustrated by the following quote from Roger Watt's (1991) book, *Understanding Vision*: "My own opinion is that studies based on reaction times should be treated much as one would regard a region on a map which was marked with the legend 'Centaurs abide here.' The point is that present information is not to be relied on too heavily, but rather as an indication of something of interest and perhaps, adventure" (p. 213).

[11]In this study, the red flash of light served both as a mask and as a postcue indicating the potential location of the target stimulus. The target could only occur at the postcued location; thus, there was no uncertainty about where the target may have occurred. By contrast, postcues were presented at multiple locations in some of the earlier signal detection studies of intramodal visual attention (e.g., Downing, 1988; Müller & Humphreys, 1991), thereby raising the possibility that the measures of perceptual sensitivity were confounded with difficulties in localizing the target itself (cf. Hawkins et al., 1990; Luck et al., 1994). The single-postcue technique avoids such confounds. Note also that by postcuing a single location, the technique also implicitly establishes some degree of spatial

100–300 ms before the interval when the target might be presented. McDonald et al. found that the parameter β was lower for targets on ipsilaterally cued trials than on contralaterally cued trials, thus providing evidence for a spatially specific criterion shift elicited by the auditory cue. More important, however, McDonald et al. also found that both accuracy and perceptual sensitivity, as measured by d', was higher for visual stimuli

---

relevance to the task. Essentially, participants are asked whether a target appeared at a specific location rather than at any location. As we have seen already, the establishment of spatial relevance appears to be one important factor in producing reliable auditory and audiovisual cuing effects (cf. McDonald & Ward, 1999; Spence, 2001).

that appeared at the cued location than for visual stimuli that appeared contralateral to the cue (Fig. 1.10*B*). This result demonstrates that cross-modal cuing modulates stimulus processing at a perceptual level (see also Frassinetti et al., 2002, for similar results).

Kato and Kashino (2001) have also used signal detection theory to investigate the effects of spatially nonpredictive visual cues on auditory perceptual judgments (i.e., the reverse situation to that examined by McDonald, Teder-Sälejärvi, Di Russo, et al., 2000). Participants in their study were presented with a series of visual cues unpredictably from 30 degrees to either side of central fixation. The participants were instructed to make an eye movement in the direction of the visual cue and to respond to the direction of motion (left-to-right vs. right-to-left) of auditory broadband noise targets presented binaurally over headphones. Perceptual sensitivity (*d'*) was higher for auditory targets presented on the cued side at SOAs that were too short for participants to have executed an eye movement toward the visual cue by the time that the auditory target was presented (i.e., at 0 ms and possibly also 100 ms SOA; see Rorden & Driver, 1999). As in the study by McDonald, Teder-Sälejärvi, Di Russo, et al. (2000) study, Kato and Kashino also reported a significantly higher criterion on ipsilaterally cued trials, which suggested that the cue also elicited a spatially specific shift in the participant's criterion for responding on ipsilaterally cued versus contralaterally cued trials.

Therefore, taken together, these two studies (Kato & Kashino, 2001; McDonald, Teder-Sälejärvi, Di Russo, et al., 2000) demonstrate that the peripheral presentation of either an auditory or a visual cue leads both to a lowering of the criterion for responding at the cued location and to a genuine improvement in perceptual sensitivity at the ipsilaterally cued relative to the contralaterally cued location. Given the benefits of the signal detection theory approach in determining the source of any facilitatory effects, it seems likely that we will see an increasing dependence on such measures of perceptual sensitivity in the coming years. In this regard, it would be interesting to extend the approach to investigate the perceptual consequences of the cross-modal cuing between audition and touch and between vision and touch (cf. Chong & Mattingley, 2000; Kennett et al., 2001, 2002; Spence et al., 1998).

Electrophysiological evidence for exogenous cross-modal spatial attention

A number of research groups have also started to collect information about the consequences of cross-modal attention from measures of electrical brain signals called event-related potentials (ERPs). Not only can this approach help to elucidate some of the brain structures where target-related information processing is being modulated cross-modally by the presentation of the cue, it can also help to demonstrate the genuinely perceptual nature of such cross-modal cuing effects (see Luck et al., 1994). The rationale for this approach and the neural underpinnings of ERPs are described in more detail in Chapter 34, by Martin Eimer, and so will not be reiterated here. Instead, we will simply focus on the results of a number of recent ERP studies that have provided dramatic evidence that the exogenous orienting of attention to a stimulus in one modality can modulate the neural sensory responses to stimuli in another modality. Such cross-modal ERP effects have been observed in reaction time studies with auditory cues and visual targets (McDonald & Ward, 2000), tactile cues and visual targets (Kennett et al., 2001), and visual cues and auditory targets (McDonald, Teder-Sälejärvi, Heraldez, et al., 2001). In each case, orienting attention in one sensory modality appeared to modulate neural activity in brain areas that are considered to be modality-specific for the target modality.

McDonald and Ward (2000) investigated the effect of the involuntary covert orienting of attention to auditory cues on the neural processing of subsequent visual target using the basic implicit spatial discrimination task. Manual responses to visual targets were faster on ipsilaterally cued trials than on contralaterally cued trials at shorter SOAs (100–300 ms) but not at longer SOAs (900–1100 ms). The cuing effects on the ERPs elicited by the visual targets followed a similar time course. Figure 1.11*A* shows the visually evoked ERPs for both ipsilaterally cued and contralaterally cued trials. At the short SOA, the ERPs were more negative on valid trials than on invalid trials between 200 and 400 ms after the appearance of the visual target. This negative difference extended to the contralateral occipital scalp (Fig. 1.11*B*), suggesting that the exogenous covert orienting of attention to the auditory cue modulated neural activity in modality-specific visual cortex. The absence of any ERP differences in the time range of the earlier P1 and N1 components indicated that the effect of cross-modal attentional cuing on activity in the visual cortex occurred after the initial sensory processing of the target had been completed. McDonald and Ward speculated that the enhanced occipital negativity might depend on feedback from higher, multisensory areas.

A more recent ERP study investigated the neural basis of cross-modal spatial attention in a task where attentional orienting to a nonpredictive auditory cue was found to improve visual target detectability

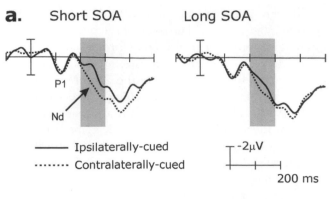

a.

Short SOA   Long SOA

P1

Nd

—— Ipsilaterally-cued   ┬ -2μV
········ Contralaterally-cued   ┼
                                    200 ms

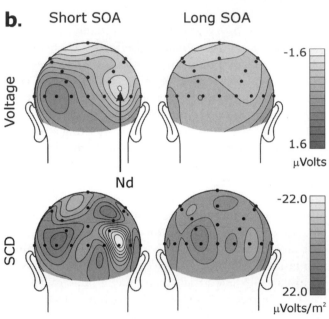

b.

Short SOA   Long SOA

Voltage

-1.6

1.6

μVolts

Nd

SCD

-22.0

22.0

μVolts/m²

FIGURE 1.11   ERP results from McDonald and Ward's (2000) auditory cue–visual target experiment. (*A*) Grand-averaged ERPs to visual target stimuli over the occipital scalp (electrodes PO7 and PO8), averaged across left and right targets. Negative voltages are plotted upward. Each tick on the *x*-axis represents 100 ms and on the *y*-axis represents a 2-μV voltage change. Mean ERP amplitudes were computed separately for ipsilaterally and contralaterally cued target ERPs in the time range indicated by the gray bars (200–300 ms poststimulus). (*B*) Contour maps of voltage and source current density (SCD) distributions of the enhanced negativity (or negative difference, Nd). The mean ERP amplitude in the ipsilaterally cued condition was subtracted from the mean ERP amplitude in the contralaterally cued condition to compute the Nd in the 200–300 ms interval. The voltage maps show a spatially "blurry" picture of the currents coming from the brain, because much of the current is diffused by the skull. The SCD maps show the estimated radial current flows into and out of the head, thereby providing a less spatially smeared picture of the currents coming from the brain. Both maps are collapsed across ERPs for left and right targets and averaged so that the right side of the map represents scalp sites contralateral to the target location and the left side represents scalp sites ipsilateral to the target location.

(McDonald, Teder-Sälejärvi, Di Russo, & Hillyard, 2003). Figure 1.12*A* shows the ERPs to the left of visual field stimuli on both ipsilaterally cued and contralaterally cued trials. As in McDonald and Ward's (2000) speeded discrimination task, the visually evoked ERPs were more negative on ipsilaterally cued trials than on contralaterally cued trials. This effect began 80–100 ms earlier than the effect reported by McDonald and Ward and consisted of at least two phases. The first phase was initially focused over the parietal scalp between 120 and 140 ms after stimulus onset, shifting to the occipital scalp between 150 and 170 ms after stimulus onset (Fig. 1.12*B*). The second phase was focused over the frontocentral scalp and extended to the contralateral occipital scalp between 240 and 260 ms after stimulus onset. Inverse dipole modeling suggested that the cerebral sources of the first phase were located in the superior temporal cortex and the fusiform gyrus of the occipital lobe (Fig. 1.12*C*). The superior temporal cortex has been identified as a site of multisensory convergence and multisensory integration (e.g., Calvert, Campbell, & Brammer, 2000). Interestingly, the superior temporal dipoles appeared to be active before the occipital dipoles were. This spatiotemporal sequence of dipole activity was in accord with McDonald and Ward's (2000) speculation that cross-modal attention effects on visual cortical activity depend on feedback from higher, multisensory areas (cf. Driver & Spence, 2000). More specifically, an involuntary shift of attention to sound appears to modulate visual-evoked brain activity first in multimodal cortex and subsequently in modality-specific visual cortex.

Cross-modal effects have also been found in an experiment in which attention was cued to the left or right hand by a spatially nonpredictive tactile stimulus prior to the appearance of a visual target presented from near to the left or right hand (Kennett et al., 2001). ERPs were recorded from eight electrodes over the frontal, central, parietal, and lateral occipital scalp. There were no cue effects on the P1 component, but, as in the other studies that we have already discussed, the ERPs to visual targets were more negative on ipsilaterally cued trials than on contralaterally cued trials following the P1. A biphasic negativity was found at central electrodes, with the first phase occurring between 110 and 180 ms after stimulus onset and the second phase occurring between 220 and 300 ms after stimulus onset. An enhanced negativity was also observed at lateral occipital electrodes in the latency range of the N1 component. Thus, the results of Kennett et al. also support the view that exogenously orienting attention to a nonvisual cue modulates visually evoked activity in modality-specific visual cortex.

The most contentious issue in the literature on the cross-modal cuing of attention has been settled by recent

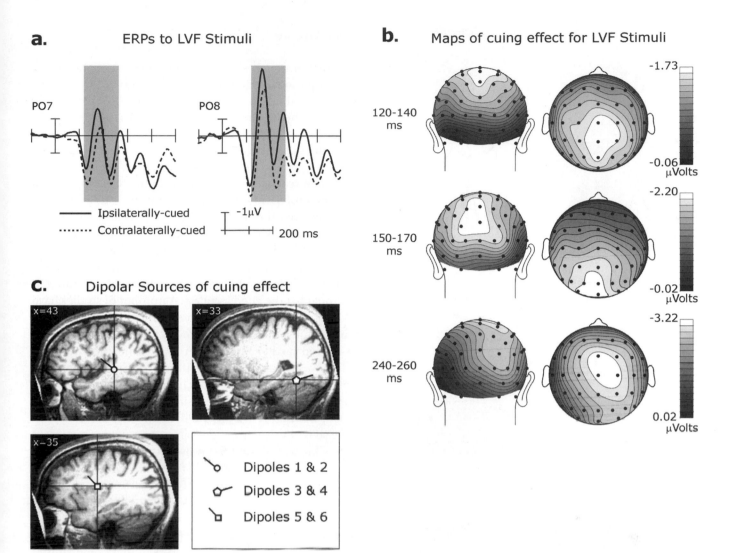

a. ERPs to LVF Stimuli

PO7

PO8

—— Ipsilaterally-cued

········ Contralaterally-cued

$-1\mu V$

200 ms

b. Maps of cuing effect for LVF Stimuli

120-140
ms

-1.73

-0.06
µVolts

150-170
ms

-2.20

-0.02
µVolts

240-260
ms

-3.22

0.02
µVolts

c. Dipolar Sources of cuing effect

x=43

x=33

x−35

○— Dipoles 1 & 2

⬠— Dipoles 3 & 4

▫— Dipoles 5 & 6

FIGURE 1.12 ERP results from the signal detection experiment of McDonald et al. (2003). Data are shown for left visual field stimuli only, but the data for right auditory targets were similar. (A) Grand-averaged ERPs to left visual field stimuli at electrodes over the occipital scalp (electrodes PO7 and PO8). Negative voltages are plotted upward. Each tick on the x-axis represents 100 ms and on the y-axis represents a 2-µV voltage change. Mean ERP amplitudes were computed separately for ipsilaterally and contralaterally cued target ERPs in three time ranges (120–140 ms, 150–170 ms, and 240–260 ms post-stimulus) that are spanned by the gray bars. (B) Scalp voltage topographies of the enhanced negativity in three time ranges. The maps were created by subtracting the ERPs to contralaterally cued targets from the ERPs to ipsilaterally cued targets and plotting the difference. The first two time ranges correspond to the early and late portions of the first phase of the enhanced negativity. The third time range corresponds to the second phase of the enhanced negativity. (C) Projections of calculated dipolar sources onto corresponding brain sections of an individual participant. The dipoles were based on grand-averaged ERP data. Dipoles 1 and 2 (shown as circles) were located in the superior temporal lobe (Talairach coordinates of $x = \pm43$, $y = -32$, $z = 9$). Dipoles 3 and 4 (shown as pentagons) were located in the fusiform gyrus of the occipital lobe ($x = \pm33$, $y = -58$, $z = -5$). Dipoles 5 and 6 (shown as squares) were located in perisylvian parietal cortex near the post-central gyrus ($x = \pm35$, $y = -25$, $z = 35$). The dipole model accounted for 97.6% of the variance in voltage topography over the 120–260 ms interval following stimulus onset.

ERP evidence. Namely, McDonald, Teder-Sälejärvi, Heraldez, et al. (2001) have provided ERP evidence of the effect of auditory cues on visual target processing. As in the auditory-visual ERP study by McDonald and Ward (2000), ERPs were more negative on ipsilaterally cued trials than on contralaterally cued trials (Fig. 1.13A). The earliest portion of the enhanced negativity (120–140 ms after target onset) was focused over the ipsilateral pari-

etal scalp, whereas a later portion of the enhanced negativity (220–260 ms after target onset) was focused over the midline frontocentral scalp (Fig. 1.13B). No dipole source modeling was performed, but it is conceivable that the neural source of the early enhanced negativity was generated outside of auditory cortex (perhaps in the parietal lobe), whereas the later enhanced negativity was generated in auditory cortex itself.

a.   ERPs to Left Auditory Targets

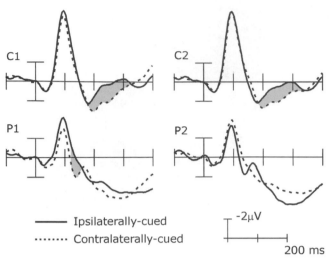

——— Ipsilaterally-cued
········ Contralaterally-cued

$-2\mu V$

200 ms

b.   Maps of Cuing Effect for Left Auditory Targets

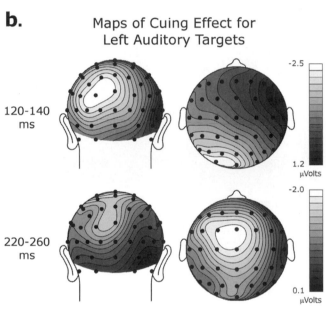

120–140 ms

220–260 ms

-2.5
1.2
μVolts

-2.0
0.1
μVolts

FIGURE 1.13 ERP results from the visual cue–auditory target experiment of McDonald et al. (2001). Data are shown for left auditory targets only. The data for right auditory targets were similar (A) Grand-averaged ERPs to left auditory targets following ipsilateral and contralateral cues. Negative voltages are plotted upward. Each tick along the x-axis represents 100 ms and on the y-axis represents a 2-μV voltage change. Electrodes C1 and C2 were placed over the central scalp, and electrodes P1 and P2 were placed over the parietal scalp. The waveforms were averaged over low-frequency and high-frequency tones. Mean ERP amplitudes were computed separately for ipsilaterally and contralaterally cued target ERPs in the time ranges indicated by the gray shading between ERP waveforms (120–140 ms post-stimulus at parietal electrodes, P1 and P2, and 220–260 ms post-stimulus for central electrodes, C1 and C2). (B) Scalp voltage topographies of the enhanced negativities in two time intervals. The maps were created by subtracting the ERPs to contralaterally cued targets from ERPs to ipsilaterally cued targets, averaging over low-frequency and high-frequency tones, and plotting the difference.

Conclusions

Interest in the cross-modal consequences of the covert orienting of exogenous spatial attention has grown rapidly in the past few years. An impressive array of behavioral and electrophysiological studies have now been published on the topic, and a number of important findings documented. Despite a number of early disagreements in this area, it now appears that a consensus view has been reached by researchers in the field. In particular, the empirical evidence currently available supports the view that the presentation of a spatially nonpredictive auditory, visual, and/or tactile cue can lead to a covert shift of exogenous spatial attention in the cued direction that will facilitate the processing of auditory, visual, and/or tactile targets subsequently presented at (or near to) the cued location. A number of studies have shown that this performance benefit is primarily focused at just the cued location and falls off as the target is moved farther and farther away from the cue, even when the cue and target stimuli are presented within the same hemifield (e.g., see Chong & Mattingley, 2000; Driver & Spence, 1998; Frassinetti et al., 2002; Kennett, 2000; Kennett & Driver, 1999; Schmitt et al., 2001). In everyday life, such exogenous covert orienting would probably be followed by an overt eye movement toward the cued location in order to fixate the event of interest. However, in the majority of studies reviewed in this chapter, the participants were instructed to keep their eyes on central fixation, thus resulting in a dissociation between covert and overt attentional orienting.

Several recently published cross-modal cuing studies have demonstrated that the cross-modal orienting of spatial attention can result in an enhancement of perceptual processing for targets presented at the cued location (Kato & Kashino, 2001; Frassinetti et al., 2002; McDonald, Teder-Sälejärvi, Di Russo, et al., 2000). Moreover, a number of researchers have now shown that cross-modal cuing effects also result in the modulation of neural activity in modality-specific regions of cortex associated with the target modality (Kennett et al., 2001; Macaluso et al., 2000; McDonald, Teder-Sälejärvi, Heraldez et al., 2001; McDonald et al., 2003; McDonald & Ward, 2000).

The suggestion that the existence of cross-modal cuing effects may reflect the consequences of a covert shift of a supramodal attentional system in the direction of the cue was first put forward 15 years ago by Martha Farah and her colleagues (Farah et al., 1989, pp. 469–470). However, this claim was based on a single experiment in which auditory cues were shown to facilitate simple detection latencies for visual targets presented on the cued side in patients suffering from parietal brain damage. Farah et al. did not provide any evidence that visual or tactile cues could elicit an exogenous shift of spatial attention, and so failed to provide sufficient evidence to support their claim. Moreover, the majority of the subsequently published data (typically showing asymmetric cross-modal cuing effects) appeared to be inconsistent with the supramodal attention view, and so it soon fell out of favor.

In the years since the original study by Farah et al., researchers have argued for the existence of various different kinds of attentional control systems. For example, Mondor and Amirault (1998) proposed the existence of entirely modality-specific attentional systems (with any cross-modal cuing effects simply reflecting the engagement of endogenous attentional mechanisms). Meanwhile, Spence and Driver (1997a) argued for the existence of separate-but-linked attentional systems instead (see also Schmitt et al., 2000, for a similar view), and others have suggested some combination of modality-specific and supramodal attentional systems (e.g., Posner, 1990, pp. 202–203; Ward, 1994; see also Buchtel & Butter, 1988).

Given that cross-modal cuing effects have now been demonstrated between all (nine) possible combinations of auditory, visual, and tactile cue and target stimuli (at least under certain experimental conditions), the available evidence would appear to provide a reasonable degree of support for the original suggestion by Farah et al. (1989) that cross-modal covert attentional orienting effects may actually reflect the operation of a supramodal attentional system. It is important to realize, however, that the putative existence of a supramodal attentional spotlight does not, in and of itself, necessitate that cross-modal cuing effects should always be found between all possible pairs of sensory modalities, no matter what the paradigm used. For, as we have already seen, a variety of top-down factors, from the complexity of the cuing situation to the relevance of space to the participant's task, can influence the magnitude of any cross-modal cuing effects observed (e.g., McDonald & Ward, 2000; Mondor & Amirault, 1998; Spence, 2001). Although the idea that top-down factors might modulate exogenous cuing effects reported is a relatively new one, it would be very surprising if they did not exert any influence, given the extensive literature on the *contingent* nature of attentional capture effects within purely visual attentional cuing paradigms (see Yantis, 1996, 2000, for reviews).

It is also important to note that differences between the senses in terms of the relative ease with which auditory, visual, and tactile stimuli can be localized will likely mean that the distribution of attentional facilitation will be somewhat different, depending on the modality (and

hence the localizability) of the cuing event used (Spence, 2001; see also Fig. 1.6). Additionally, any differences in transduction latencies between the senses (see Spence & Driver, 1997a; Spence & Squire, 2003) will presumably also result in modality-specific differences in the time course of cross-modal cuing effects, depending on the particular cue-target modality combination being investigated. Therefore, our view is that while attention may well be controlled by a supramodal attentional mechanism, it will nevertheless exhibit some modality-specific features, given the differences in the spatiotemporal processing of stimuli in each of our senses.

Several of the seminal investigations into the nature of any cross-modal links in spatial attention presented peripheral spatial cues that were also informative (i.e., predictive) with regard to the likely target location (e.g., Buchtel & Butter, 1988; Butter et al., 1989). A number of researchers have subsequently argued that these early studies may have confounded the effects of exogenous and endogenous attentional orienting (e.g., Spence & Driver, 1996; see also Pashler, 1998). Spence and Driver went so far as to suggest that the findings of these particular studies had no necessary implications for the possible existence of any cross-modal links in spatial attention. More recently, however, researchers have been able to study each type of spatial attention in relative isolation, by using specifically designed experimental paradigms. For example, spatially nonpredictive peripheral cues have been used to investigate the cross-modal consequences of purely exogenous covert orienting (as highlighted in the majority of experiments reviewed in this chapter), while spatially predictive symbolic cues have been used to investigate the cross-modal consequences of purely endogenous covert spatial attention (e.g., Lloyd, Merat, McGlone, & Spence, 2003; Spence & Driver, 1996; Spence, Pavani, & Driver, 2000; see Driver & Spence, 2004, for a recent review). Now that a better understanding of each of these types of attention in isolation has been developed, it will be important for researchers to begin to investigate how the two forms of attention interact to control behavior, as they inevitably do in the majority of the more ecologically relevant situations outside of the experimenter's laboratory. One need only think of the cocktail party example with which we started this chapter: the endogenous direction of our attention to a particular speaker can be overridden by the exogenous attentional capture that takes place when someone else suddenly calls our name. Studying the interaction between these top-down and bottom-up factors constantly competing to control the spatial distribution of attention will represent a particularly fruitful as well as challenging area for future cross-modal research.

REFERENCES

Amlôt, R., Walker, R., Driver, J., & Spence, C. (2003). Multimodal visual-somatosensory integration in saccade generation. *Neuropsychologia, 41*, 1–15.

Bernstein, I. H., & Edelstein, B. A. (1971). Effects of some variations in auditory input upon visual choice reaction time. *Journal of Experimental Psychology, 87*, 241–247.

Buchtel, H. A., & Butter, C. M. (1988). Spatial attention shifts: Implications for the role of polysensory mechanisms. *Neuropsychologia, 26*, 499–509.

Buchtel, H. A., Butter, C. M., & Ayvasik, B. (1996). Effects of stimulus source and intensity on covert orientation to auditory stimuli. *Neuropsychologia, 34*, 979–985.

Butter, C. M., Buchtel, H. A., & Santucci, R. (1989). Spatial attentional shifts: Further evidence for the role of polysensory mechanisms using visual and tactile stimuli. *Neuropsychologia, 27*, 1231–1240.

Calvert, G. A., Campbell, R., & Brammer, M. J. (2000). Evidence from functional magnetic resonance imaging of crossmodal binding in the human heteromodal cortex. *Current Biology, 10*, 649–657.

Chong, T., & Mattingley, J. B. (2000). Preserved cross-modal attentional links in the absence of conscious vision: Evidence from patients with primary visual cortex lesions. *Journal of Cognitive Neuroscience, 12*(Suppl.), 38.

Desimone, R., Wessinger, M., Thomas, J., & Schneider, W. (1992). Attentional control of visual perception: Cortical and subcortical mechanisms. *Cold Spring Harbor Symposia on Quantitative Biology, 55*, 963–971.

Downing, C. (1988). Expectancy and visual-spatial attention: Effects on perceptual quality. *Journal of Experimental Psychology: Human Perception and Performance, 14*, 188–202.

Driver, J., & Grossenbacher, P. G. (1996). Multimodal spatial constraints on tactile selective attention. In T. Inui & J. L. McClelland (Eds.), *Attention and performance XVI: Information integration in perception and communication* (pp. 209–235). Cambridge, MA: MIT Press.

Driver, J., & Spence, C. J. (1994). Spatial synergies between auditory and visual attention. In C. Umiltà & M. Moscovitch (Eds.), *Attention and performance: Conscious and nonconscious information processing* (Vol. 15, pp. 311–331). Cambridge, MA: MIT Press.

Driver, J., & Spence, C. (1998). Crossmodal links in spatial attention. *Philosophical Transactions of the Royal Society, Section B, 353*, 1319–1331.

Driver, J., & Spence, C. (2000). Multisensory perception: Beyond modularity and convergence. *Current Biology, 10*, R731–R735.

Driver, J., & Spence, C. (2004). Crossmodal links in endogenous spatial attention. In C. Spence & J. Driver (Eds.), *Crossmodal space and crossmodal attention*. Oxford, England: Oxford University Press.

Duncan, J. (1980). The demonstration of capacity limitation. *Cognitive Psychology, 12*, 75–96.

Farah, M. J., Wong, A. B., Monheit, M. A., & Morrow, L. A. (1989). Parietal lobe mechanisms of spatial attention: Modality-specific or supramodal? *Neuropsychologia, 27*, 461–470.

Fisher, G. H. (1962). Resolution of spatial conflict. *Bulletin of the British Psychological Society, 46*, 3A.

Frassinetti, F., Bolognini, N., & Làdavas, E. (2002). Enhancement of visual perception by crossmodal visuo-auditory interaction. *Experimental Brain Research, 147*, 332–343.

Gopher, D. (1973). Eye-movement patterns in selective listening tasks of focused attention. *Perception & Psychophysics, 14*, 259–264.

Green, D. M., & Swets, J. A. (1966). *Signal detection theory and psychophysics*. New York: Wiley.

Groh, J. M., & Sparks, D. L. (1996a). Saccades to somatosensory targets: 2. Motor convergence in primate superior colliculus. *Journal of Neurophysiology, 75*, 428–438.

Groh, J. M., & Sparks, D. L. (1996b). Saccades to somatosensory targets: 3. Eye-position dependent somatosensory activity in primate superior colliculus. *Journal of Neurophysiology, 75*, 439–453.

Hawkins, H. L., Hillyard, S. A., Luck, S. J., Mouloua, M., Downing, C. J., & Woodward, D. P. (1990). Visual attention modulates signal detectability. *Journal of Experimental Psychology: Human Perception and Performance, 16*, 802–811.

Honoré, J. (1982). Posture oculaire et attention selective a des stimuli cutanes [Eye position and selective attention to cutaneous stimuli]. *Neuropsychologia, 20*, 727–730.

Honoré, J., Bourdeaud'hui, M., & Sparrow, L. (1989). Reduction of cutaneous reaction time by directing eyes towards the source of stimulation. *Neuropsychologia, 27*, 367–371.

Jay, M. F., & Sparks, D. L. (1990). Localization of auditory and visual targets for the initiation of saccadic eye movements. In M. A. Berkley & W. C. Stebbins (Eds.), *Comparative perception: Vol. I. Basic mechanisms* (pp. 351–374). New York: Wiley.

Jonides, J. (1981a). Towards a model of the mind's eye's movement. *Canadian Journal of Psychology, 34*, 103–112.

Jonides, J. (1981b). Voluntary versus automatic control over the mind's eye's movement. In J. Long & A. Baddeley (Eds.), *Attention and performance* (Vol. 9, pp. 187–203). Hillsdale, NJ: Erlbaum.

Kato, M., & Kashino, M. (2001). Audio-visual link in auditory spatial discrimination. *Acoustical Science & Technology, 22*, 380–382.

Kennett, S. A. (2000). *Links in spatial attention between touch and vision*. Unpublished doctoral dissertation, Birkbeck College, University of London.

Kennett, S. & Driver, J. (1999). *Exogenous tactile-visual attention within hemifields: Increased spatial specificity when arms are visible*. Poster presented at the Experimental Psychology Society Workshop on Crossmodal Attention and Multisensory Integration, Oxford, England, October 1–2.

Kennett, S., Eimer, M., Spence, C., & Driver, J. (2001). Tactile-visual links in exogenous spatial attention under different postures: Convergent evidence from psychophysics and ERPs. *Journal of Cognitive Neuroscience, 13*, 462–468.

Kennett, S., Spence, C., & Driver, J. (2002). Visuo-tactile links in covert exogenous spatial attention remap across changes in unseen hand posture. *Perception & Psychophysics, 64*, 1083–1094.

Klein, R. (2000). Inhibition of return: Who, what, when, where, how and why. *Trends in Cognitive Sciences, 4*, 138–147.

Klein, R., Brennan, M., D'Aloisio, A., D'Entremont, B., & Gilani, A. (1987). *Covert cross-modality orienting of attention*. Unpublished manuscript.

Klein, R. M., Kingstone, A., & Pontefract, A. (1992). Orienting of visual attention. In K. Rayner (Ed.), *Eye movements and visual cognition: Scene perception and reading* (pp. 46–65). New York: Springer-Verlag.

Klein, R. M., & Shore, D. I. (2000). Relationships among modes of visual orienting. In S. Monsell & J. Driver (Eds.), *Control of cognitive processes: Attention and performance XVIII* (pp. 195–208). Cambridge, MA: MIT Press.

Lloyd, D. M., Merat, N., McGlone, F., & Spence, C. (2003). Crossmodal links in covert endogenous spatial attention between audition and touch. *Perception & Psychophysics, 65,* 901–924.

Luce, R. D. (1986). *Response times.* New York: Oxford University Press.

Luck, S. J., Hillyard, S. A., Mouloua, M., Woldorff, M. G., Clark, V. P., & Hawkins, H. L. (1994). Effects of spatial cuing on luminance detectability: Psychophysical and electrophysiological evidence for early selection. *Journal of Experimental Psychology: Human Perception and Performance, 20,* 887–904.

Macaluso, E., Frith, C., & Driver, J. (2000). Modulation of human visual cortex by crossmodal spatial attention. *Science, 289,* 1206–1208.

Macaluso, E., Frith, C. D., & Driver, J. (2001). A reply to McDonald, J. J., Teder-Sälejärvi, W. A., & Ward, L. M. "Multisensory integration and crossmodal attention effects in the human brain." *Science, 292,* 1791.

Macmillan, N. A., & Creelman, C. D. (1990). *Detection theory: A user's guide.* Cambridge, England: Cambridge University Press.

Maruff, P., Yucel, M., Danckert, J., Stuart, G., & Currie, J. (1999). Facilitation and inhibition arising from the exogenous orienting of covert attention depends on the temporal properties of spatial cues and targets. *Neuropsychologia, 37,* 731–744.

McDonald, J. J., Teder-Sälejärvi, W. A., Di Russo, F., & Hillyard, S. A. (2000, October). *Looking at sound: Involuntary auditory attention modulates neural processing in extrastriate visual cortex.* Poster presented at the Annual Meeting of the Society for Psychophysiological Research. San Diego, CA.

McDonald, J. J., Teder-Sälejärvi, W. A., Di Russo, F., & Hillyard, S. A. (2003). Neural substrates of perceptual enhancement by cross-modal spatial attention. *Journal of Cognitive Neuroscience, 15,* 1–10.

McDonald, J. J., Teder-Sälejärvi, W. A., Heraldez, D., & Hillyard, S. A. (2001). Electrophysiological evidence for the "missing link" in crossmodal attention. *Canadian Journal of Experimental Psychology, 55,* 143–151.

McDonald, J. J., Teder-Sälejärvi, W. A., & Hillyard, S. A. (2000). Involuntary orienting to sound improves visual perception. *Nature, 407,* 906–908.

McDonald, J. J., Teder-Sälejärvi, W. A., & Ward, L. M. (2001). Multisensory integration and crossmodal attention effects in the human brain. *Science, 292,* 1791.

McDonald, J. J., & Ward, L. M. (1997, March). *Covert orienting between modalities.* Poster presented at the annual meeting of the Cognitive Neuroscience Society, Boston.

McDonald, J. J., & Ward, L. M. (1999). Spatial relevance determines facilitatory and inhibitory effects of auditory covert spatial orienting. *Journal of Experimental Psychology: Human Perception and Performance, 25,* 1234–1252.

McDonald, J. J., & Ward, L. M. (2000). Involuntary listening aids seeing: Evidence from human electrophysiology. *Psychological Science, 11,* 167–171.

McDonald, J. J., & Ward, L. M. (2003a). *Crossmodal consequences of involuntary spatial attention and inhibition of return.* Manuscript submitted for publication.

McDonald, J. J., & Ward, L. M. (2003b, April). *Crossmodal consequences of involuntary spatial attention and inhibition of return.* Poster presented at the annual meeting of the Cognitive Neuroscience Society, New York.

Mondor, T. A., & Amirault, K. J. (1998). Effect of same- and different-modality spatial cues on auditory and visual target identification. *Journal of Experimental Psychology: Human Perception and Performance, 24,* 745–755.

Müller, H. J., & Findlay, J. M. (1987). Sensitivity and criterion effects in the spatial cuing of visual attention. *Perception & Psychophysics, 42,* 383–399.

Müller, H. J., & Humphreys, G. W. (1991). Luminance-increment detection: Capacity-limited or not? *Journal of Experimental Psychology: Human Perception and Performance, 17,* 107–124.

Nicoletti, R., & Umiltà, C. (1989). Splitting visual space with attention. *Journal of Experimental Psychology: Human Perception and Performance, 15,* 164–169.

Niemi, P., & Näätänen, R. (1981). Foreperiod and simple reaction time. *Psychological Bulletin, 89,* 133–162.

Pashler, H. E. (1998). *The psychology of attention.* Cambridge, MA: MIT Press.

Perrott, D. R., Saberi, K., Brown, K., & Strybel, T. Z. (1990). Auditory psychomotor coordination and visual search performance. *Perception & Psychophysics, 48,* 214–226.

Posner, M. I. (1978). *Chronometric explorations of mind.* Hillsdale, NJ: Erlbaum.

Posner, M. I. (1990). Hierarchical distributed networks in the neuropsychology of selective attention. In A. Caramazza (Ed.), *Cognitive neuropsychology and neurolinguistics: Advances in models of cognitive function and impairment* (pp. 187–210). Hillsdale, NJ: Erlbaum.

Posner, M. I., & Cohen, Y. (1984). Components of visual orienting. In H. Bouma & D. G. Bouwhuis (Eds.), *Attention and performance: Control of language processes* (Vol. 10, pp. 531–556). Hillsdale, NJ: Erlbaum.

Prime, D. J., McDonald, J. J., & Ward, L. M. (2003). *When crossmodal attention fails.* Manuscript submitted for publication.

Rafal, R., Henik, A., & Smith, J. (1991). Extrageniculate contributions to reflex visual orienting in normal humans: A temporal hemifield advantage. *Journal of Cognitive Neuroscience, 3,* 322–328.

Reuter-Lorenz, P. A., & Rosenquist, J. N. (1996). Auditory cues and inhibition of return: The importance of oculomotor activation. *Experimental Brain Research, 112,* 119–126.

Rhodes, G. (1987). Auditory attention and the representation of spatial information. *Perception & Psychophysics, 42,* 1–14.

Rizzolatti, G., Riggio, L., Dascola, I., & Umiltà, C. (1987). Reorienting attention across the horizontal and vertical meridians: Evidence in favor of a premotor theory of attention. *Neuropsychologia, 25,* 31–40.

Robinson, D. L., & Kertzman, C. (1995). Covert orienting of attention in macaques: III. Contributions of the superior colliculus. *Journal of Neurophysiology, 74,* 713–721.

Roffler, S. K., & Butler, R. A. (1968). Factors that influence the localization of sound in the vertical plane. *Journal of the Acoustical Society of America, 43,* 1255–1259.

Rorden, C., & Driver, J. (1999). Does auditory attention shift in the direction of an upcoming saccade? *Neuropsychologia, 37,* 357–377.

Rorden, C., & Driver, J. (2001). Spatial deployment of attention within and across hemifields in an auditory task. *Experimental Brain Research, 137,* 487–496.

Schmitt, M., Postma, A., & de Haan, E. (2000). Interactions between exogenous auditory and visual spatial attention. *Quarterly Journal of Experimental Psychology, 53A,* 105–130.

Schmitt, M., Postma, A., & de Haan, E. (2001). Cross-modal exogenous attention and distance effects in vision and hearing. *European Journal of Cognitive Psychology, 13,* 343–368.

Shaw, M. L. (1980). Identifying attentional and decision-making components in information processing. In R. S. Nickerson (Ed.), *Attention & Performance* (Vol. 8, pp. 277–296). Hillsdale, NJ: Erlbaum.

Shepherd, M., Findlay, J. M., & Hockey, R. J. (1986). The relationship between eye movements and spatial attention. *Quarterly Journal of Experimental Psychology, 38A,* 475–491.

Simon, J. R. (1990). The effects of an irrelevant directional cue on human information processing. In R. W. Proctor & T. G. Reeve (Eds.), *Stimulus-response compatibility* (pp. 31–86). Amsterdam: Elsevier Science.

Simon, J. R., & Craft, J. L. (1970). Effects of an irrelevant auditory stimulus on visual choice reaction time. *Journal of Experimental Psychology, 86,* 272–274.

Spence, C. (2001). Crossmodal attentional capture: A controversy resolved? In C. Folk & B. Gibson (Eds.), *Attention, distraction and action: Multiple perspectives on attentional capture* (pp. 231–262). Amsterdam: Elsevier.

Spence, C. J., & Driver, J. (1994). Covert spatial orienting in audition: Exogenous and endogenous mechanisms facilitate sound localization. *Journal of Experimental Psychology: Human Perception and Performance, 20,* 555–574.

Spence, C., & Driver, J. (1996). Audiovisual links in endogenous covert spatial attention. *Journal of Experimental Psychology: Human Perception and Performance, 22,* 1005–1030.

Spence, C., & Driver, J. (1997a). Audiovisual links in exogenous covert spatial orienting. *Perception & Psychophysics, 59,* 1–22.

Spence, C., & Driver, J. (1997b). On measuring selective attention to a specific sensory modality. *Perception & Psychophysics, 59,* 389–403.

Spence, C., & Driver, J. (1999). A new approach to the design of multimodal warning signals. In D. Harris (Ed.), *Engineering psychology and cognitive ergonomics: Vol. 4. Job design, product design and human-computer interaction* (pp. 455–461). Hampshire, England: Ashgate.

Spence, C., & Driver, J. (2000). Attracting attention to the illusory location of a sound: Reflexive crossmodal orienting and ventriloquism. *NeuroReport, 11,* 2057–2061.

Spence, C., Lloyd, D., McGlone, F., Nicholls, M. E. R., & Driver, J. (2000). Inhibition of return is supramodal: A demonstration between all possible pairings of vision, touch and audition. *Experimental Brain Research, 134,* 42–48.

Spence, C., McDonald, J., & Driver, J. (2004). Crossmodal exogenous spatial attention and multisensory integration. In C. Spence & J. Driver (Eds.), *Crossmodal space and crossmodal attention.* Oxford, England: Oxford University Press.

Spence, C., & McGlone, F. P. (2001). Reflexive spatial orienting of tactile attention. *Experimental Brain Research, 141,* 324–330.

Spence, C., Nicholls, M. E. R., Gillespie, N., & Driver, J. (1998). Cross-modal links in exogenous covert spatial orienting between touch, audition, and vision. *Perception & Psychophysics, 60,* 544–557.

Spence, C., Pavani, F., & Driver, J. (2000). Crossmodal links between vision and touch in covert endogenous spatial attention. *Journal of Experimental Psychology: Human Perception and Performance, 26,* 1298–1319.

Spence, C., & Squire, S. B. (2003). Multisensory integration: Maintaining the perception of synchrony. *Current Biology, 13,* R519–R521.

Sperling, G., & Dosher, B. A. (1986). Strategy and optimization in human information processing. In K. Boff, L. Kaufman, & J. Thomas (Eds.), *Handbook of Perception and Performance* (Vol. 1, pp. 2-1–2-65). New York: Wiley.

Stein, B. E., & Meredith, M. A. (1993). *The merging of the senses.* Cambridge, MA: MIT Press.

Stein, B. E., Wallace, M. T., & Meredith, M. A. (1995). Neural mechanisms mediating attention and orientation to multisensory cues. In M. S. Gazzaniga (Ed.), *The cognitive neurosciences* (pp. 683–702). Cambridge, MA: MIT Press.

Tan, H. Z., Gray, R., Young, J. J., & Irawan, P. (2001). Haptic cuing of a visual change-detection task: Implications for multimodal interfaces. In M. J. Smith, G. Salvendy, D. Harris, & R. J. Koubek (Eds.), *Usability evaluation and interface design: Cognitive engineering, intelligent agents and virtual reality,* Vol. 1 of *Proceedings of the 9th International Conference on Human-Computer Interaction* (pp. 678–682). Mahwah, NJ: Erlbaum.

Tassinari, G., Aglioti, S., Chelazzi, L., Marzi, C. A., & Berlucchi, G. (1987). Distribution in the visual field of the costs of voluntarily allocated attention and of the inhibitory after-effects of covert orienting. *Neuropsychologia, 25,* 55–71.

Tassinari, G., Aglioti, S., Chelazzi, L., Peru, A., & Berlucchi, G. (1994). Do peripheral non-informative cues induce early facilitation of target detection? *Vision Research, 34,* 179–189.

Thompson, G. C., & Masterton, R. B. (1978). Brain stem auditory pathways involved in reflexive head orientation to sound. *Journal of Neurophysiology, 41,* 1183–1202.

Umiltà, C., & Nicoletti, R. (1985). Attention and coding effects in S-R compatability due to irrelevant spatial cues. In M. I. Posner & O. S. M. Marin (Eds.), *Attention and performance* (Vol. 11, pp. 457–471). Hillsdale, NJ: Erlbaum.

Vroomen, J., Bertelson, P., & de Gelder, B. (2001). Directing spatial attention towards the illusory location of a ventriloquized sound. *Acta Psychologica, 108,* 21–33.

Ward, L. M. (1994). Supramodal and modality-specific mechanisms for stimulus-driven shifts of auditory and visual attention. *Canadian Journal of Experimental Psychology, 48,* 242–259.

Ward, L. M., McDonald, J. A., & Golestani, N. (1998). Crossmodal control of attention shifts. In R. Wright (Ed.), *Visual attention* (pp. 232–268). New York: Oxford University Press.

Ward, L. M., McDonald, J. J., & Lin, D. (2000). On asymmetries in cross-modal spatial attention orienting. *Perception & Psychophysics, 62,* 1258–1264.

Ward, L. M., Prime, D. J., & McDonald, J. J. (2002). Converging operations revisited: The case of attention. *Abstracts of the Psychonomic Society, 7,* 56.

Warren, D. H. (1970). Intermodality interactions in spatial localization. *Cognitive Psychology, 1,* 114–133.

Watt, R. J. (1991). *Understanding vision.* London: Academic Press.

Welch, R. B., & Warren, D. H. (1986). Intersensory interactions. In K. R. Boff, L. Kaufman, & J. P. Thomas (Eds.),

Handbook of perception and performance: Vol. 1. Sensory processes and perception (pp. 25-1–25-36). New York: Wiley.

Whittington, D. A., Hepp-Reymond, M. C., & Flood, W. (1981). Eye and head movements to auditory targets. *Experimental Brain Research, 41,* 358–363.

Wright, R. D., & Ward, L. M. (1994). Shifts of visual attention: An historical and methodological overview. *Canadian Journal of Experimental Psychology, 48,* 151–166.

Yantis, S. (1996). Attentional capture in vision. In A. F. Kramer, M. G. Coles, & G. D. Logan (Eds.), *Converging operations in the study of visual selective attention* (pp. 45–76). Washington, DC: American Psychological Association.

Yantis, S. (2000). Goal-directed and stimulus-driven determinants of attentional control. In S. Monsell & J. Driver (Eds.), *Control of cognitive processes: Attention and performance XVIII* (pp. 73–103). Cambridge, MA: MIT Press.

Zambarbieri, D., Beltrami, G., & Versino, M. (1995). Saccade latency toward auditory targets depends on the relative position of the sound source with respect to the eyes. *Vision Research, 35,* 3305–3312.

Zambarbieri, D., Schmid, R., Prablanc, C., & Magenes, G. (1981). Characteristics of eye movements evoked by presentation of acoustic targets. In A. Fuchs & W. Becker (Eds.), *Progress in oculomotor research* (pp. 559–566). Amsterdam: Elsevier/North-Holland.

Zambarbieri, D., Schmid, R., Magenes, G., & Prablanc, C. (1982). Saccadic responses evoked by presentation of visual and auditory targets. *Experimental Brain Research, 47,* 417–427.

2 Modulations of Visual Perception by Sound

LADAN SHAMS, YUKIYASU KAMITANI, AND SHINSUKE SHIMOJO

Introduction

Perception has traditionally been viewed as a modular function, with the different sensory modalities operating largely as separate and independent modules. To the degree that this thesis holds, it has contributed to progress in both empirical and theoretical research on the perceptual brain, yet to the degree that it has been overemphasized, it has masked the need for intensive research on cross-modal interactions. Perhaps for this reason multisensory integration has been one of the least studied areas of research in perception. As a result, prior to the very recent surge of interest in this topic, knowledge about multisensory integration and cross-modal interactions remained largely at the level of phenomenology. Even at this level, however, many important questions remain unanswered. Because vision has traditionally been viewed as the dominant modality (Howard & Templeton, 1966; Welch & Warren, 1986), most studies have focused on the effects of visual stimulation on perception in other modalities, and consequently the effects of other modalities on vision are not as well understood.

Vision alters other modalities

In normal people, the effects of cross-modal integration are made apparent under cleverly designed artificial conditions. The McGurk effect (McGurk & MacDonald, 1976) exemplifies such a condition. The McGurk effect is a perceptual phenomenon in which vision alters speech perception (for example, a sound of /ba/ tends to be perceived as /da/ when it is coupled with a visual lip movement associated with /ga/). The perceived spatial location of a sound source is also known to be drastically influenced by visual stimulation. This effect is known as the *ventriloquist effect* (Howard & Templeton, 1966) and is a common experience in daily life, such as when one is watching movies on television or at the cinema and voices are perceived to originate from the actors on the screen despite a potentially large spatial discrepancy between the image and the sound source.

It has been shown that tactile location can also be "captured" by visual location (Pavani, Spence, & Driver, 2000; Rock & Victor, 1964). All these effects emphasizing the strong influence of visual signals on other modalities (and a weak or absent reverse cross-modal effect) have been consistent with the commonsense notion that humans are primarily vision-dominant animals.

Sound alters temporal aspects of vision

Some later findings, however, revealed that visual perception could also be altered by other modalities, particularly in the temporal domain. Perceived duration (Walker & Scott, 1981) or rate (Gebhard & Mowbray, 1959; Shipley, 1964; Welch, Duttonhurt, & Warren, 1986) of a visual stimulus was shown to be influenced by accompanying sound signals. A recent study found that visual temporal resolution can be either improved or degraded by sounds, depending on the temporal relationship between the visual and auditory stimuli (Scheier, Nijwahan, & Shimojo, 1999). When two lights were turned on at different locations with a small temporal delay (in the range of −60 to 60 ms), the accuracy of temporal order judgments between the two lights was better with a sound preceding and another sound following the visual stimuli (A-V-V-A time order) than with a no-sound condition. Conversely, the subjects' performance became worse (as compared with the no-sound condition) when two sounds were inserted between the two visual stimuli (V-A-A-V time order). These results are consistent with the findings of another study which found that a flash is perceived earlier when it is preceded by a sound and later when it is followed by a sound, compared with a condition in which they occur simultaneously (Fendrich & Corballis, 2001).

A great body of behavioral findings on the cross-modal interactions summarized above can be accounted for by the modality appropriateness hypothesis (Choe, Welch, Guilford, & Juola, 1975; Fisher, 1968; Howard & Templeton, 1966; Kaufman, 1974; Welch & Warren,

1986). This hypothesis postulates that the modality that is most appropriate or reliable with respect to a given task is the modality that dominates the perception in the context of that task. Vision has a higher spatial resolution, hence its dominance in spatial tasks, whereas audition has a higher temporal resolution, hence its dominance in temporal tasks. The dominance of vision in the ventriloquist effect and the visual capture of tactile stimulation, and the dominance of audition in temporal tasks, are consistent with this hypothesis.

Sound alters other aspects of vision

Alteration of vision by sound, however, turned out to be not limited to temporal aspects of the visual stimuli. Auditory perceptual organization can affect perceptual organization in the visual domain (O'Leary & Rhodes, 1984). A sudden sound can improve the detection of a subsequent flash at the same location (McDonald, Teder-Sälejärvi, & Hillyard, 2000). The perceived intensity of a visual stimulus has recently been shown to be enhanced by the presence of sound (Stein, London, Wilkinson, & Price, 1996). An abrupt sound can improve the identification of a synchronously presented visual target embedded in a series of distractors (Vroomen & de Gelder, 2000).

A recent study has illustrated that the presence of a sound can alter the interpretation of an ambiguous visual motion event (Sekuler, Sekuler, & Lau, 1997). Two identical visual targets moving across each other can be perceived either to bounce off or to stream through each other, since their trajectory would be nearly identical. Nonetheless, the majority of observers report a perception of streaming, not bouncing motion. However, if a brief sound is added at the moment the targets visually coincide, visual perception is strongly biased in favor of a bouncing motion (Sekuler et al., 1997). The sound has to have a sharp onset to induce this effect (K. Watanabe & S. Shimojo, personal communication). The ecological origin of this phenomenon may be the following: The multisensory experience of collision events in the natural environment could lead to cross-modal associative learning via synchronized stimulation of sensory modalities. Recent studies on this phenomenon have revealed some unexpected properties. For example, a transient sensory stimulus biases visual perception toward bouncing, irrespective of its modality: a brief visual flash and a brief touch were found to induce bouncing perception as well (Watanabe, 2001; Watanabe & Shimojo, 1998).

Auditory "capture" of visual structure

We recently reported a cross-modal effect demonstrating that the alteration of vision by sound is not limited to minor modulation of perceived intensity or situations of ambiguity in the visual stimulus. In the "sound-induced illusory flash," or for short, "illusory flash effect" (Shams, Kamitani, & Shimojo, 2000, 2002), sound radically changes the phenomenological quality of the percept of a nonambiguous visual stimulus. When a single brief visual flash is accompanied by multiple auditory beeps, the single flash is perceived as multiple flashes, as shown in Figure 2.1. Control conditions,

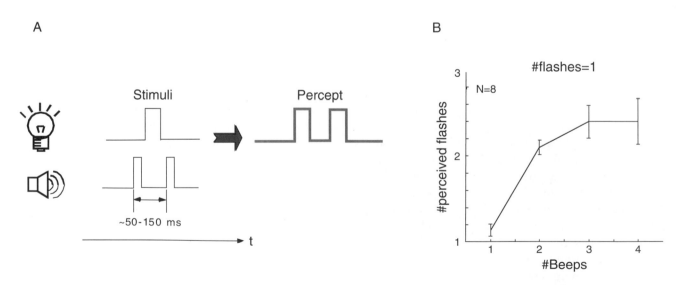

FIGURE 2.1 Sound-induced illusory flash effect. (A) Schematics of the sound-induced illusory flash. When a single flash is accompanied by two (or more) beeps, it is erroneously perceived as two (or more) flashes. (B) The average number of perceived flashes across eight observers is plotted against the number of beeps, for trials in which the visual stimulus consisted of one single flash. Observers reported seeing two or more flashes when the single flash was accompanied by two or more beeps.

catch trials, and many other observations indicate that the illusory flashing phenomenon is indeed a perceptual illusion and is not due to the difficulty of the task or to some cognitive bias caused by sound (Shams et al., 2000, 2002). The illusory double flash is perceptually very similar to a physical double flash. Furthermore, the illusion is not affected by the observer's knowledge about the physical stimulus, and is robust to variations in stimuli parameters. The temporal tuning of this effect was also measured by varying the relative timing of the visual and auditory stimuli. The illusory flash effect declined from 70 ms separation onward; however, it occurred strongly so long as the beeps and flash were within approximately 100 ms (Shams et al., 2002). Also interesting is the fact that the alteration of vision by sound in this study was found to be asymmetrical with respect to the number of events. Alteration of vision by sound occurred strongly only when a single flash was coupled with multiple beeps, but not when multiple flashes were paired with a single beep: multiple flashes were not perceived as one in the presence of a single beep. A similar dependency on the temporal structure of stimuli seems to have been at work in another study, which investigated the effect of vision on hearing (Saldaña & Rosenblum, 1993). A continuous sound (bowing a cello) was modulated by a discontinuous visual stimulus (plucking a cello), whereas a discontinuous sound (plucking) was not affected by the continuous visual stimulus (bowing). These findings, taken together, seem to suggest that cross-modal interactions depend at least partly on the structure of the stimuli.

A later study tackled another question related to the effect of sound on vision in the illusory flash effect: Is the illusory flash effect due to a mere fluctuation in brightness or to the creation of independent visual tokens? The study found that the sound-induced flashes can be perceived at different spatial locations from the real ones, and thus as independent visual tokens, when combined with a visual apparent-motion display (Kamitani & Shimojo, 2001). Two visual objects were flashed at different locations and separated by a temporal interval such that apparent motion was perceived between them. Each visual flash was accompanied by a beep, and another beep was presented between the flashes/beeps. Subjects reported that an illusory flash associated with the second beep was perceived at a location between the real flashes. This is analogous to the cutaneous "rabbit" illusion, in which trains of successive cutaneous pulses delivered to widely separated locations produce sensations at many in-between points (Geldard & Sherrick, 1972). Thus, the illusion can be referred to as sound-induced visual "rabbit."

Because no "rabbit" effect was observed when only visual stimuli were presented in a similar manner, the sound-induced visual rabbit seems to be a uniquely cross-modal effect.

Sound alters vision in motion perception

Perhaps a more direct test of the validity of the modality appropriateness hypothesis is to test the dominance (or nonmalleability) of vision in a spatial task. Motion perception involves an important spatial element and would provide an interesting framework for testing the effects of sound on vision in a spatial task. Whereas many studies have previously investigated cross-modal effects in motion perception, most of them have concentrated on the effects of visual motion on auditory motion perception (Aspell, Bramwell, & Hurlbert, 2000; Mateeff, Hohnsbein, & Noack, 1985; Soto-Faraco, Lyons, Gazzaniga, Spence, & Kingstone, 2002) (see also Soto-Faraco & Kingstone, Chap. 4, this volume) and reported the improvement in the auditory motion detection in the presence of a visual motion in the same direction.

One very recent study reported an influence of auditory motion on visual motion perception (Meyer & Wuerger, 2001). The visual stimulus was a dynamic random dot display in which the degree of motion coherence of the dots was varied, and the auditory stimulus consisted of a binaural tone presented from two speakers that simulated horizontal motion from left to right or vice versa. The investigators found that auditory motion biased the subjects' perceived direction of visual motion of the no-coherent-motion display in a direction consistent with the auditory motion.

Another recent study (Shams, Allman, & Shimojo, 2001) investigated this issue using a different method. Instead of using an ambiguous or subthreshold visual motion display, they used a brief (unambiguous) stationary visual stimulus. Eye movements were monitored during the session so that any artifact related to or created by them could be detected. In a subsequent experiment, other artifacts such as response and cognitive biases were addressed. Taken together, the data indicate that a moving sound does significantly affect visual perception by inducing motion in a stationary visual stimulus. It was also found that the moving flash did not have a significant effect on the percept of the stationary sound. These findings are important, because the observed direction of the cross-modal interactions cannot be uniquely predicted by the modality appropriateness hypothesis. Another theory must be proposed to account for the observations.

Modularity reexamined: Neural evidence

The mechanisms underlying the effects of sound on visual perception are not extensively studied or understood. It is not clear at what level of perceptual processing these cross-modal effects take place. These interactions may occur at subcortical regions, visual cortical areas, or polysensory associative cortical areas.

Event-related potential (ERP) recording provides an appropriate methodology for tackling this question because of its high temporal resolution. Schröger and Widdman (1998) used ERP recording to explore the site of audiovisual interactions. They used an odd-ball paradigm, and found no early interactions between the auditory and visual processes. They interpreted their results as suggesting that audiovisual integration occurs somewhere beyond the modality-specific areas but before the decision-making stage. They pointed out, however, that the lack of evidence for early modulation in their study could have been due to the fact that their task relied on memory mechanisms and thus might not have been appropriate for uncovering early sensory interactions. Giard and Perronet (1999) used ERP recording to tackle the same question using a pattern recognition task. They reported very early cross-modal effects in the occipital area and interpreted these results as a modulation of activity in the "sensory-specific" visual cortical areas by sound. In their study, however, they used two visual deformation patterns (a circle deforming into a horizontal or vertical ellipse) that unfolded over a course of 230 ms, and the subjects were trained in advance to associate each of the two deformation patterns with a specific tone. Therefore, it is not clear whether their results generalize to situations in which subjects are not trained to associate specific visual stimuli with specific auditory stimuli, or where the visual stimulus is a static image as opposed to a deforming pattern.

We recorded ERPs in a framework based on the illusory flash effect in order to examine the locus in the brain associated with alterations of visual perception by sound (Shams, Kamitani, Thompson, & Shimojo, 2001). Unlike the two studies just mentioned, the task used in our study was a simple perceptual task not involving memory. More important, the subjects were not instructed a priori to associate a certain visual stimulus with a certain auditory stimulus. The stimuli were extremely simple—brief tones and flashes. We employed a flash visual-evoked potential (VEP) paradigm and introduced a sound stimulus to examine whether sound would modulate the VEPs. Our prior psychophysical observation had shown that the illusory flash effect is significantly stronger in the periphery than in the fovea.

In order to search for any physiological correlation with this perceptual effect, we recorded VEPs for flashes presented in the fovea and the periphery separately. As can be seen in Figure 2.2, the data indicated extensive and early modulation of VEPs by sound in the illusion trials (the majority of the peripheral trials), in contrast to the lack of modulation of VEPs by sound in the nonillusion trials (the majority of the foveal trials). In a more recent analysis, we compared the time-frequency amplitudes of the illusion trials in the periphery with the no-illusion trials in the periphery and found significant auditory-visual interactions only in the illusion trials (Bhattacharya, Shams, & Shimojo, 2002). These results suggest a clear neurophysiological correlate for the perception of the illusory flash. Modulations of VEPs by sound occurred as early as ~140 ms after the onset of the second beep (or 170 ms after the onset of the flash) (Shams, Kamitani, et al., 2001). Considering that ERPs prior to 200 ms post-stimulus are believed to be due to the activity in the modality-specific pathways (Giard & Peronnet, 1999), these modulations appear to occur in the visual pathway. Most interesting is the finding that similar modulations were induced by sound and by an additional physical flash (Shams, Kamitani, et al., 2001). Comparison of the difference waves revealed a striking similarity between the activity associated with an illusory second flash and that of a physical second flash (Fig. 2.2). This similarity suggests that similar brain mechanisms underlie these two percepts. Because the evoked response to a physical flash involves activity in the visual cortex, this implies that the representation of the illusory flash also involves activity in the visual cortex.

The results of this study suggest that sound affects processing at the level of the "visual" cortex. These findings contradict a longstanding modular view of perceptual processing. For a long time—arguably for more than a century—the general belief was that the different modalities operated largely independently of each other, and only at some higher level such as the association cortex did the information from various modalities converge and get combined.

Some recent studies utilizing functional imaging, transcranial magnetic stimulation (TMS), or magnetoencephalography (MEG) also have provided evidence that the areas that have traditionally been viewed as modality-specific are modulated by signals from other modalities. For example, Sathian and colleagues (Sathian, Zangaladze, Hoffman, & Grafton, 1997; Zangaladze, Epstein, Grafton, & Sathian, 1999) have shown that an area of the extrastriate visual cortex is active during tactile discrimination of grating orientation. Macaluso, Frith, and Driver (2000) have reported

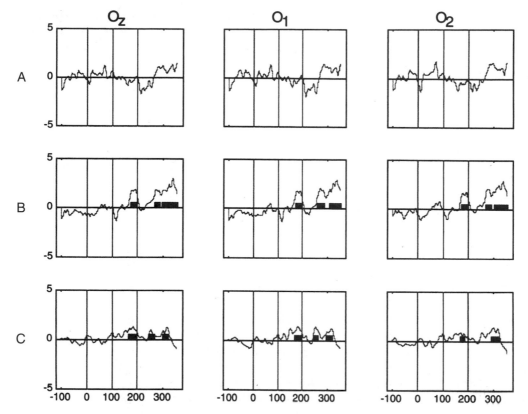

FIGURE 2.2   Auditory-visual interactions reflected in the ERP difference waves. Each row in this figure corresponds to a type of difference waves, and each column corresponds to one electrode. The horizontal and vertical axes denote time in milliseconds with respect to the onset of the (first) flash, and brain potential in μV, respectively. The gray lines represent the mean amplitudes across participants, and the black blocks denote the time intervals in which the amplitudes are significantly different from zero ($P < 0.05$). (A) The difference waves corresponding to subtraction of unimodal conditions from the bimodal condition (AV − [A + V]) in the fovea. (B) The difference waves AV − [A + V] in the periphery. (C) The difference waves corresponding to the subtraction of the double flash condition from the single flash condition, both in the periphery.

that activation of the human visual area V5 is enhanced in the presence of accompanying tactile stimulation. Sams et al. (1991) have reported that lipreading syllables that are inconsistent with the auditory syllables (as in McGurk's effect) modifies activity in human auditory cortex. Calvert et al. (1997) have shown that silent lipreading (purely visual) leads to activity in auditory cortical areas BA 41/42. Also, after comparing auditory-visual (bimodal) speech perception with auditory or visual (unimodal) speech perception, they reported enhancement of visual area V5 in the bimodal condition (Calvert et al., 1999). Amedi, Malach, Hendler, Peled, and Zohary (2001) have reported activity in a visual object–related region, the lateral occipital complex, during haptic object recognition.

Interestingly, recent anatomical studies suggest a cortical pathway that may underlie the early cross-modal modulations in visual cortical areas indicated in the ERP studies mentioned above. Very similar findings were reported by two independent laboratories that conducted anatomical studies of projections to

area V1 in monkey (Falchier, Clavagnier, Barone, & Kennedy, 2002; Rockland & Ojima, 2001). One group used anterograde tracers and reported direct projections from auditory parabelt regions to peripheral V1 and V2 (Rockland & Ojima, 2001). In the other study (Falchier et al., 2002), the investigators used retrograde tracers injected separately in foveal and peripheral regions of V1 and found extensive projections from the primary auditory cortex and the caudal parabelt to peripheral V1, in contrast to very sparse projections to foveal V1. They also reported projections from multi-modal area STP to peripheral V1. The projections from the auditory cortex and STP to peripheral V1 appeared to constitute a significant proportion of the total projections to V1 (respectively 8% and 41% of that from the visual movement complex to V1). Intriguingly, the difference between the projections to the peripheral and foveal regions reported in these studies are highly consistent with the differential effects between the fovea and periphery that we have observed in our psychophysical and ERP studies. If there are extensive projections from auditory areas (and to a lesser extent from multisensory areas) to V1 and V2 in the periphery but not in the fovea, then it is not surprising that both the illusory flash effect and the illusory motion effect are strong only in the periphery,[1] and that ERP results suggest a modulation of the activity in visual areas by sound only in the periphery and not in the fovea.

Summary

Vision may be the most important modality in the perceptual world of humans. Nonetheless, visual perception is not exempt from cross-modal influences. Although the effects of sound on vision in temporal tasks[2] have been documented for a long time, the discovery of cross-modal influences on vision during nontemporal tasks is rather new. A recent study has revealed that vision can be radically altered by sound in a nontemporal task, even when there is no ambiguity in the visual stimulus.

Studies investigating the brain areas involved in multisensory integration have indicated that the activity in areas traditionally considered to be modality-specific can be modulated by cross-modal signals. Again, the visual cortex has not proved an exception to this rule, having been shown to be affected by tactile and auditory stimulation. The majority of the strong cross-modal effects on visual perception occur only or much more strongly when the visual stimulus is in the peripheral visual field. The recent primate neuroanatomical studies reporting direct projections from auditory and multisensory areas to the peripheral representations of early visual areas are consistent with these findings.

REFERENCES

Amedi, A., Malach, R., Hendler, T., Peled, S., & Zohary, E. (2001). Visuo-haptic object-related activation in the ventral visual pathway. *Nature Neuroscience, 4*(3), 324–330.

---

[1]The results of various controls and observations reject the possible role of alternative factors such as eye movement or pupillary constriction that may affect perception more strongly in the periphery than in the fovea. For example, the illusory flash effect is stronger with shorter flash durations, persists with very large disk size, and degrades with a decrease in disk contrast (Shams et al., 2002). In the illusory motion effect, no eye movement was detected by EOG, the illusory and nonillusory trials had indistinct EOGs, and the effect persisted even with large disk size.

[2]Such as judging the duration of a signal, or the temporal order of two signals.

Aspell, J. E., Bramwell, D. I., & Hurlbert, A. C. (2000). Interactions between visual and auditory movement perception in a direction discrimination task. *Perception, 29*(Suppl.), 74.

Bhattacharya, J., Shams, L., & Shimojo, S. (2002). Sound-induced illusory flash perception: Role of gamma band responses. *NeuroReport, 13,* 1727–1730.

Calvert, G. A., Brammer, M. J., Bullmore, E. T., Campbell, R., Iversen, S. D., & David, A. S. (1999). Response amplification in sensory-specific cortices during crossmodal binding. *NeuroReport, 10*(12), 2619–2623.

Calvert, G. A., Bullmore, E. T., Brammer, M. J., Campbell, R., Williams, S. C., McGuire, P. K., et al. (1997). Activation of auditory cortex during silent lipreading. *Science, 276,* 593–596.

Choe, C., Welch, R., Guilford, R., & Juola, J. (1975). The "ventriloquist effect": Visual dominance or response bias? *Perception & Psychophysics, 18,* 55–60.

Falchier, A., Clavagnier, S., Barone, P., & Kennedy, H. (2002). Anatomical evidence of multimodal integration in primate striate cortex. *Journal of Neuroscience, 22*(13), 5749–5759.

Fendrich, R., & Corballis, P. M. (2001). The temporal cross-capture of audition and vision. *Perception & Psychophysics, 63*(4), 719–725.

Fisher, G. (1968). Agreement between the spatial senses. *Perceptual and Motor Skills, 126,* 849–850.

Gebhard, J. W., & Mowbray, G. H. (1959). On discriminating the rate of visual flicker and auditory flutter. *American Journal of Psychology, 72,* 521–528.

Geldard, F. A., & Sherrick, C. E. (1972). The cutaneous rabbit: A perceptual illusion. *Science, 178,* 178–179.

Giard, M. H., & Peronnet, F. (1999). Auditory-visual integration during multimodal object recognition in humans: A behavioral and electrophysiological study. *Journal of Cognitive Neuroscience, 11*(5), 473–490.

Howard, I. P., & Templeton, W. B. (1966). *Human spatial orientation.* London: Wiley.

Kamitani, Y., & Shimojo, S. (2001). Sound-induced visual "rabbit." *Journal of Vision, 1*(3), 478a.

Kaufman, L. (1974). *Sight and mind.* New York: Oxford University Press.

Macaluso, E., Frith, C. D., & Driver, J. (2000). Modulation of human visual cortex by crossmodal spatial attention. *Science, 289,* 1206–1208.

Mateeff, S., Hohnsbein, J., & Noack, T. (1985). Dynamic visual capture: Apparent auditory motion induced by a moving visual target. *Perception, 14,* 721–727.

McDonald, J. J., Teder-Sälejärvi, W. A., & Hillyard, S. A. (2000). Involuntary orienting to sound improves visual perception. *Nature, 407,* 906–908.

McGurk, H., & MacDonald, J. W. (1976). Hearing lips and seeing voices. *Nature, 264,* 746–748.

Meyer, G. F., & Wuerger, S. M. (2001). Cross-modal integration of auditory and visual motion signals. *NeuroReport, 12,* 2557–2560.

O'Leary, A., & Rhodes, G. (1984). Cross-modal effects on visual and auditory object perception. *Perception & Psychophysics, 35*(6), 565–569.

Pavani, F., Spence, C., & Driver, J. (2000). Visual capture of touch: Out-of-the-body experiences with rubber gloves. *Psychological Science, 11*(5), 353–359.

Rock, I., & Victor, J. (1964). Vision and touch: An experimentally created conflict between the two senses. *Science, 143,* 594–596.

Rockland, K. S., & Ojima, H. (2001). *Calcarine area V1 as a multimodal convergence area.* Paper presented at the Society for Neuroscience meeting, San Diego, CA.

Saldaña, H. M., & Rosenblum, L. D. (1993). Visual influences on auditory pluck and bow judgments. *Perception & Psychophysics, 54*(3), 406–416.

Sams, M., Aulanko, R., Hämäläinen, M., Hari, R., Lounasmaa, O., Lu, S.-T., & Simola, J. (1991). Seeing speech: Visual information from lip movements modifies activity in the human auditory cortex. *Neuroscience Letters, 127,* 141–145.

Sathian, K., Zangaladze, A., Hoffman, J. M., & Grafton, S. T. (1997). Feeling with the mind's eye. *NeuroReport, 8,* 3877–3881.

Scheier, C. R., Nijwahan, R., & Shimojo, S. (1999). *Sound alters visual temporal resolution.* Paper presented at the Investigative Ophthalmology and Visual Science meeting, Fort Lauderdale, FL.

Schröger, E., & Widmann, A. (1998). Speeded responses to audiovisual signal changes result from bimodal integration. *Psychophysiology, 35,* 755–759.

Sekuler, R., Sekuler, A. B., & Lau, R. (1997). Sound alters visual motion perception. *Nature, 385,* 308.

Shams, L., Allman, J., & Shimojo, S. (2001). *Illusory visual motion induced by sound.* Paper presented at the Society for Neuroscience meeting, San Diego, CA.

Shams, L., Kamitani, Y., & Shimojo, S. (2000). What you see is what you hear. *Nature, 408,* 788.

Shams, L., Kamitani, Y., & Shimojo, S. (2002). Visual illusion induced by sound. *Cognitive Brain Research, 14,* 147–152.

Shams, L., Kamitani, Y., Thompson, S., & Shimojo, S. (2001). Sound alters visual evoked potentials in humans. *NeuroReport, 12*(17), 3849–3852.

Shipley, T. (1964). Auditory flutter-driving of visual flicker. *Science, 145,* 1328–1330.

Soto-Faraco, S., Lyons, J., Gazzaniga, M., Spence, C., & Kingstone, A. (2002). The ventriloquist in motion: Illusory capture of dynamic information across sensory modalities. *Cognitive Brain Research, 14,* 139–146.

Stein, B. E., London, N., Wilkinson, L. K., & Price, D. D. (1996). Enhancement of perceived visual intensity by auditory stimuli: A psychophysical analysis. *Journal of Cognitive Neuroscience, 8,* 497–506.

Vroomen, J., & de Gelder, B. (2000). Sound enhances visual perception: Cross-modal effects of auditory organization on vision. *Journal of Experimental Psychology: Human Perception and Performance, 26*(5), 1583–1590.

Walker, J. T., & Scott, K. J. (1981). Auditory-visual conflicts in the perceived duration of lights, tones, and gaps. *Journal of Experimental Psychology: Human Perception and Performance, 7*(6), 1327–1339.

Watanabe, K. (2001). *Crossmodal interaction in humans.* Unpublished doctoral dissertation, California Institute of Technology, Los Angeles.

Watanabe, K., & Shimojo, S. (1998). Attentional modulation in perception of visual motion events. *Perception, 27*(9), 1041–1054.

Welch, R., & Warren, D. (1986). Intersensory interactions. In K. Boff, L. Kaufman, & J. Thomas (Eds.), *Handbook of perception and human performance: Vol. I. Sensory processes and human performance.* New York: Wiley.

Welch, R. B., Duttonhurt, L. D., & Warren, D. H. (1986). Contributions of audition and vision to temporal rate perception. *Perception & Psychophysics, 39*(4), 294–300.

Zangaladze, A., Epstein, C. M., Grafton, S. T., & Sathian, K. (1999). Involvement of visual cortex in tactile discrimination of orientation. *Nature, 401*(6753), 587–590.

3 Cross-Modal Interactions Evidenced by the Ventriloquism Effect in Humans and Monkeys

TIMOTHY M. WOODS AND GREGG H. RECANZONE

Introduction

The external world is filled with objects of interest and importance, many of which can be defined by several different sensory modalities. For example, an object generally has a specific shape and color, makes a distinctive noise under certain conditions, has a particular texture and weight, and in some cases has a characteristic smell and taste. Normally, all of these sensory attributes can be readily discerned and combined by an observer to form a unified percept of a single object. Even when the input from one sensory modality is discordant with that from other modalities, it may nevertheless be judged as consistent, and juxtaposed to form a congruent item. However, when multiple sensory attributes convey contradictory information, or when the input from one sensory modality is significantly different from the input from the others, the consequent perception is of two or more distinct objects. The manner in which information from different sensory modalities is combined to form single or multiple objects is intriguing, but there is no clear understanding of the "rules" that govern multisensory integration at the level of perception or at the level of the nervous system.

One way in which this issue is investigated is to manipulate the sensory stimuli significantly enough so that the information taken in is inconsistent with a single object. This results in the percept of a "normal" single object, an "unusual" single object, or two (or more) separate objects. Multiple studies have been performed in which discordant auditory, visual, and/or somatosensory information is presented to an observer and the resulting perception is measured (Hay, Pick, & Ikeda, 1965; Pick, Warren, & Hay, 1969; Thomas, 1940; see also Welch & Warren, 1980). In experiments such as these, the influence of one stimulus modality on another can be elucidated, and the level of congruency of inputs necessary for the perception of one versus multiple

objects can be inferred. These studies have led to a better understanding of how different sensory modalities are integrated, but they have not provided data regarding the underlying neuronal mechanisms of this integration.

In separate experiments, the activity of central nervous system (CNS) structures has been measured during the presentation of multisensory stimuli, and several brain regions have been identified that respond to two or more sensory modalities. However, these experiments do not directly address how the global neuronal activity relates to the perception of multisensory stimuli. This lacuna is largely due to the lack of an effective animal model that can be used to identify not only the areas of the brain that are responsive to multisensory stimuli, but also the fundamental characteristics of the neurons themselves. Such a model would allow the neuronal activity at the level of the single neuron to be correlated directly with the various stimuli. Ideally, this information could be incorporated into a model wherein the animal signifies its perception of a single object or multiple objects (or other perceptual details) while multisensory stimulus parameters are actively manipulated during neuronal recording. Such data would be eminently useful in determining how the human brain creates cogent perceptions from the innumerable stimuli that it is presented with daily.

This chapter focuses on studies of auditory and visual cross-modal interactions at the perceptual level in humans and monkeys in order to conceptualize simple neuronal models of sensory integration necessary for the perception of multisensory objects. Issues central to the interactions and integration of auditory and visual stimuli in human subjects are presented and reviewed, and evidence that an appropriate animal model can be developed which can then be used to perform direct analyses on the relationship between neural activity and perception is presented.

35

The ventriloquism effect

One of the best-studied sensory interactions between auditory and visual stimuli in human subjects is how they relate to the perception of extrapersonal space. When a visual stimulus is presented simultaneously with an auditory stimulus but at a slightly disparate spatial location, the resulting percept is that both stimuli originate at the location of the visual stimulus. This phenomenon was termed the ventriloquism effect by Howard and Templeton (1966) because it recalls the illusion created by ventriloquists when the words they produce in the absence of lip movements are perceived to originate from the mouth of a puppet that is in motion simultaneous with the speech (see Vroomen & de Gelder, Chap. 9, this volume). A similar illusion is experienced when viewing modern television and movies, where the visual input is in front of the observer but the auditory input is from the surround. Even with sophisticated multiple-speaker sound systems, there are very few locations where a person can sit and have the auditory cues appropriate for the sources of the visual images. For example, observers usually assign the locations of different actors' voices to different locations on a television screen (i.e., each actor's mouth), even though all acoustic stimuli may originate from a single speaker located off the screen. This illusion is very compelling despite the cognitive knowledge that it is fundamentally untrue. How powerful this illusion is can be demonstrated by a simple test—closing one's eyes and trying to localize different voices or other sounds emanating from the television set to any particular part of the screen. It is virtually impossible. The absence of visual input prevents the perception of auditory spatial location that is provided by the audiovisual interaction under normal circumstances, and the illusion is nullified.

Several previous studies have investigated the key features of the stimulus parameters necessary to generate the perception of the ventriloquism illusion (see Bertelson, 1999; Welch, 1999; Vroomen & de Gelder, Chap. 9, this volume). Some of these parameters are intuitive, based on the experience of the ventriloquist's act. The percept that the ventriloquist's dummy is speaking results from the fact that (1) the ventriloquist's lips are not moving, (2) the dummy's "lips" are moving, (3) the dummy's "voice" is different from the ventriloquist's and appropriate for the dummy's persona, and (4) the dummy and the ventriloquist are in close spatial register relative to the spatial acuity of the auditory system. The compellingness of the auditory and visual stimuli specific to the ventriloquism effect has been examined using human voices and videos of humans speaking (Driver, 1996; Thurlow & Jack, 1973; Warren, Welch, & McCarthy, 1981), as well as puppets of varying degrees of detail (Thurlow & Jack, 1973). These studies have shown that the more "appropriate" the visual stimulus, such as the detail of the puppet and the synchrony between the auditory and visual stimuli, the more compelling is the illusion. However, the illusion does not rely solely on this feature, and may also be seen with arbitrarily paired stimuli (discussed later). Others have examined the spatial relationship of the two stimuli (e.g., Jack & Thurlow, 1973) and found that, in general, small spatial disparities between the visual and auditory stimuli generated the effect more reliably than larger spatial disparities. Similarly, the temporal domain of the stimuli was also found to be important. Thurlow and Jack (1973) found that temporal disparities of merely a few hundred milliseconds completely eliminated the illusory effect.

Model of the neural substrate of polysensory integration

The auditory and visual interactions in the ventriloquism effect are consistent with findings in similar experiments investigating the percept of limb placement under conditions in which the visual percept is shifted in space (Hay et al., 1965; see Welch & Warren, 1980). Subjects with displaced visual input (commonly accomplished by wearing prism spectacles) mislocalized their limb position, even when informed to use proprioceptive input in making the judgments. The phenomenon in which visual input overwhelms other sensory input to construct perception has been termed *visual capture* (Hay et al., 1965).

In order to account for the visual sensory dominance of both auditory and proprioceptive input, it has been hypothesized that the sensory modality that has the highest acuity for the stimulus parameter being investigated dominates the percept. This has been termed the *modality appropriateness* hypothesis (Welch, 1999; Welch & Warren, 1980) and simply states that, when a stimulus of two or more discordant sensory modalities are presented, the modality with the greater resolution will have a stronger influence on the percept than the modality with lesser resolution. In regard to spatial location, the visual modality has much greater resolution than audition or proprioception, and therefore vision often (though not always) dominates the assessment of location so that the two stimuli are perceived to originate from the position of the visual stimulus.

Spatial acuity in the visual system has been described in a variety of ways. For example, vernier acuity describes the ability of normal human subjects, under the appropriate conditions, to detect that two lines are not continuous even when the lines are displaced by less than 1 minute of arc. However, when a person is required to determine the absolute location of a visual stimulus, the spatial acuity is measured as a greater value (i.e., not as refined). For example, asking subjects to turn their head in order to "point their nose" toward a 200 ms duration visual stimulus resulted in estimates that ranged over a space of 1 or 2 degrees (Recanzone, Makhamra, & Guard, 1998). This is also true of auditory localization. Judging whether two noise bursts are from the same or different locations results in a spatial resolution threshold of only a few degrees (e.g., Recanzone et al., 1998; Stevens & Newman, 1936). However, when human subjects are asked to turn their head to the sound source location, the behavioral estimates display greater variability (Carlile, Leong, & Hyams, 1997; Makous & Middlebrooks, 1990; Recanzone et al., 1998). The ability to localize sounds is also dependent on the stimulus parameters, with stimuli well above detection threshold more easily localized than stimuli near detection threshold (Su & Recanzone, 2001) and stimuli with a greater spectral bandwidth (e.g., noise bursts) easier to localize than stimuli with narrow spectral bandwidth (e.g., pure tones). For example, the range of estimates when localizing 4 kHz tones can be as much at 20–30 degrees (Recanzone et al., 1998).

An intriguing issue is how the modality appropriateness hypothesis can be translated into neural terms. A sensory stimulus can be represented along any particular stimulus attribute as a normal distribution of neural activity. In the case of visual space, this could be shown by the activity of visual neurons, for example, in the primary visual cortex (V1), that have receptive fields that overlap with the stimulus location. The population response, therefore, would be centered in the region of the brain corresponding to the representation of the location of the stimulus, with some response from nearby neurons that have receptive fields that only partially overlap with the actual stimulus. Ignoring the influence of neurons inhibited by such a stimulus, the population response in V1 would result in the representation distribution shown in Figure 3.1A (dashed line). A similar type of representation can be envisioned for the auditory system (Fig. 3.1A, solid line), although it would be much coarser because of the reduced spatial acuity of the system. Exactly how auditory space is represented is unclear, but in the primate superior colliculus (SC), auditory receptive fields are generally aligned with visual receptive fields, although they are much

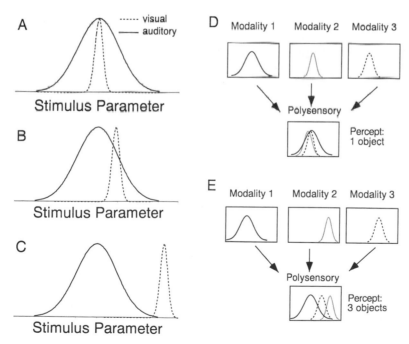

FIGURE 3.1   Distribution of multisensory representations. (A) Schematized representation of auditory (solid line) and visual (dashed line) stimuli that are perfectly in register as a function of some stimulus parameter to form the percept of a single object. (B) As in A, but with a slight offset of visual and auditory stimuli. In this example, the two stimuli are in adequate congruency for fusion, and a single object is perceived. (C) As in A and B, but with a significant disparity between visual and auditory stimuli. In this example, the lack of congruency between the two stimuli results in the perception of two separate objects. (D) Three sensory stimuli from distinct modalities may be combined to form the perception of one object (D) or multiple objects (E), depending on the consonance of the individual inputs over the stimulus parameter.

larger (e.g., Jay & Sparks, 1984; Wallace, Wilkinson, & Stein, 1996). In any case, when the auditory object is at the same location in space as the visual object, these two representations would overlap and the percept would presumably be one of a single object. If the visual stimulus was presented at progressively disparate spatial locations, initially there would be reasonable agreement in the location estimates between the two modalities, and the percept would be based on the better estimate by the visual system (Fig. 3.1B). If, however, the two representations were in clear disagreement (Fig. 3.1C), the two stimuli would be perceived as different objects.

The representations schematized in Figure 3.1A–C need not be restricted to spatial representations alone but could also be considered a function of time. Even stimuli presented from the same place but at different times would be perceived as two distinct objects (or events) rather than only one. Other sensory attributes—for example, the intensity or temporal rate of the stimuli—could be represented as well. The auditory modality is believed to have greater temporal acuity than the visual modality. Consequently, consistent with the modality appropriateness hypothesis, the auditory stimulus drives the percept of discordant auditory and visual stimuli in the temporal domain. Examples of such illusions are the findings that the flicker-fusion threshold of visual stimuli can be increased when the visual stimuli are presented simultaneously with auditory stimuli (Ogilvie, 1956; Shipley, 1964), and at low temporal rates auditory stimuli will dominate the percept of visual stimuli (Shams, Kamitani, & Shimojo, 2000; Welch, DuttonHurt, & Warren, 1986) and visual motion (Sekuler, Sekuler, & Lau, 1997; Watanabe & Shimojo, 2001). Furthermore, increasing the intensity of an auditory stimulus gives rise to the percept that a visual stimulus has greater brightness (Stein, London, Wilkinson, & Price, 1996).

How these sensory attributes may be combined in polysensory brain areas is schematized in Figures 3.1D and E. The representation along any particular stimulus parameter is aligned for a single object (Fig. 3.1D, top panels). The nature of this neural representation is currently unclear; for example, it may be based on the firing rate or timing of individual or populations of neurons. Regardless, when the peak energy of all sensory inputs occurs at the same location along a particular sensory parameter (but with different degrees of variance), the resulting percept is that of a single object (Fig. 3.1D, bottom panel). When different objects are presented to the senses, their peak activities are not aligned in space (Fig. 3.1E, top panels), and the percept that results is of two or more different objects (Fig. 3.1E,

bottom panel). It is reasonable to speculate that the polysensory areas themselves might therefore be responsible for combining inputs from different sensory modalities and parsing this information into different object categories based on a variety of stimulus parameters.

Although such a neural model is attractive for its simplicity, little is known about how these representations of multisensory stimuli may relate to perception. Lacking the tools to visualize the CNS at the neuronal level in the intact human, it would be extremely prudent to use an animal model to elucidate these issues. To date, however, there is no capable animal model that can assuredly link multisensory stimuli directly to perception, particularly to the sensory interactions that lead to illusions such as the ventriloquism effect, or visual capture. Over the past two decades great strides have been made in identifying CNS structures in the primate that respond to two or more sensory modalities. Multisensory neurons have been found in the parietal (e.g., Andersen, Snyder, Batista, Buneo, & Cohen, 1998; Andersen, Snyder, Bradley, & Xing, 1997; Hyvarinen, 1982), frontal (e.g., Bruce, Desimone, & Gross, 1981; Graziano, Reiss, & Gross, 1999; Russo & Bruce, 1994), and temporal lobes (e.g., Cusick, 1997; Cusick, Seltzer, Cola, & Griggs, 1995; Hikosaka, Iwai, Saito, & Tanaka, 1988; Watanabe & Iwai, 1991; Watson, Valenstein, Day, & Heilman, 1994) of the cerebral cortex, as well as in the insula (Bushara, Grafman, & Hallett, 2001) and the SC (Jay & Sparks, 1984; Wallace et al., 1996).

Given these insights into where multisensory processing occurs in the brain, the need for a suitable animal model to bridge the gap in knowledge between neuron and perception remains, but is slightly closer to resolution. One problem associated with animal models of multisensory perception is the generation of the appropriate task that will directly and clearly answer the given question. A further complication is determining the animal model in which to perform the experiments, though both issues are intimately related. Insofar as many of the stimuli used in previous studies included human speech, which is likely not compelling to many other species, it is probably more appropriate to ascertain how these illusions occur using less complex stimuli, such as tones and noise bursts in the auditory realm and small spots of light in the visual realm. Simple stimuli such as these are easily transferred to the percepts of animals. They can also be standardized to activate both primary sensory areas as well as multisensory areas in the brain, and can be effective in generating cross-modal interactions (e.g., Bertelson, 1999; Radeau & Bertelson, 1978).

The temporal and spatial dependency of the ventriloquism effect

To this end, more recent experiments on humans have defined the spatial and temporal parameters of simple stimuli that influence the ventriloquism effect (Slutsky & Recanzone, 2001). In these experiments, human subjects were first asked to determine whether a visual and auditory stimulus occurred at the same time or whether some temporal disparity existed between the two stimuli. A light-emitting diode (LED) light source and either a noise burst or 1 kHz tone was presented directly in front of the subjects. The visual and auditory stimuli were of the same duration (200 ms), but the onsets of the two stimuli could vary, from the visual stimulus leading the auditory stimulus by 250 ms to the auditory stimulus leading the visual stimulus by 200 ms (Fig. 3.2A). The task was a two-alternative, forced-choice task, and subjects were asked to respond using a switch to indicate whether they perceived the two stimuli to be presented at exactly the same time ("same") or one stimulus to be presented before the other ("different"), but the subjects were not required to report the order. The results revealed several important findings. First, there was no difference between sessions in which noise stimuli were presented and sessions in which tone stimuli were presented. Thus, the neuronal mechanisms of the auditory input necessarily span a very broad frequency range. Second, when the auditory stimulus was presented before the visual stimulus, subjects were more likely to detect these as different than when the same temporal disparity was presented, except that the visual stimulus preceded the auditory stimulus (Fig. 3.2B). The difference in performance between stimulus modalities was on the order of 50 ms. For example, auditory stimuli leading visual stimuli by 100 ms generated the same magnitude of difference in the perception of the timing of the two stimuli as visual stimuli leading auditory stimuli by 150 ms. Third, the ability to perceive the two stimuli as different was nearly 100% by the time the temporal disparity reached 250 ms (for 200 ms duration auditory and visual stimuli).

The second experiment showed that there was a clear interaction between the spatial and temporal parameters. It was hypothesized that, if an auditory stimulus is clearly perceived as originating from a different location than a visual stimulus (e.g., Fig. 3.1C), then there should be less of an interaction versus when the auditory stimulus is not well discriminated spatially from the location of the visual stimulus (e.g., Fig. 3.1A or B). This was indeed found to be the case (Fig. 3.2C). In this experiment, subjects were presented with one auditory stimulus directly in front of them along the azimuthal

A. Paradigm

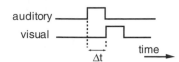

B. Temporal Discrimination

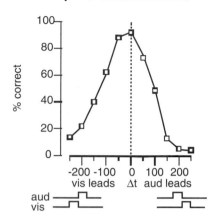

C. Temporal - Spatial Interactions

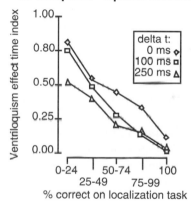

FIGURE 3.2 The ventriloquism effect in humans. (A) The paradigm employed to produce the ventriloquism effect in humans. Auditory stimuli consisted of either a 1 kHz tone or broadband noise of 200 ms in duration. The visual stimulus was a flash from an LED of the same duration. The visual stimulus could occur within a range of 250 ms prior to to 250 ms after the auditory stimulus (Δt). Subjects responded "same" or "different," depending on their perception of the congruence of the stimuli. (B) Temporal interactions between auditory and visual stimuli. Subjects were better able to determine differences in stimulus onsets when the auditory stimulus preceded the visual stimulus. The performance shown to the right of the vertical dashed line was better than that to the left. (C) Temporal and spatial interactions in the ventriloquism effect. Stimuli that were difficult to localize spatially (abscissa) were more likely to produce the ventriloquism illusion (ordinate). Note also that the closest temporal correspondence between stimuli showed the greatest ventriloquism effect across spatial locations. (Figures adapted from Slutsky & Recanzone, 2001.)

axis and a second auditory stimulus to the left or right at different eccentricities. Subjects were asked to determine if the two stimuli were presented from the same or different locations. On interleaved trials, visual stimuli were also presented at different temporal disparities, but always from directly in front of the subject. The ventriloquism effect was then measured by how well the visual stimulus influenced the perception of the auditory location at each temporal disparity. Auditory stimuli that were clearly discerned as spatially separate from the visual stimulus (for example, at 12 degrees of eccentricity) showed very little, if any, illusion effect, even at temporal disparities of 0 ms. Similarly, when the spatial disparity was very small and the human subjects could not reliably separate the auditory stimuli from the location of the visual stimulus located straight ahead (less than 24% correct when only auditory stimuli were presented), even large temporal disparities (up to 250 ms) generated the illusory effect on approximately 50% of the trials. Thus, there is a clear interaction between the spatial and temporal disparity of the two stimuli in generating the percept of a single object.

These results are consistent with the schematized model shown in Figure 3.1. When the two stimulus representations are sufficiently far apart, either in time or in space, there is a difference in the location (or time) signal for each stimulus by the two sensory processors (Figs. 3.1C and E). As a matter of course, this leads to the perception of two distinct events. The fact that time and space both influence perception is completely compatible with such a neuronal model, because the influence of unimodal inputs to polysensory brain areas will clearly have both temporal and spatial integration constraints at the neurophysiological level.

The ventriloquism aftereffect

Under particular circumstances, the ventriloquism effect produces longlasting changes in the perception of acoustic space, a phenomenon called the *ventriloquism aftereffect* (Canon, 1970; Radeau & Bertelson, 1974). In the classic paradigm, human subjects are asked to localize sounds in complete darkness, and then are presented with a period of training. During this period, acoustic and visual stimuli are presented simultaneously, but at disparate locations. One method by which this is accomplished is to have the subjects wear displacing prisms over their eyes so that the visual world is shifted to the left or right, thus displacing the perception of the visual stimulus relative to the auditory stimulus. A second method is to use a pseudophone, which is a dummy speaker that is not at the same location as the auditory stimulus. In both cases, after a period of as

little as 5 minutes of such training, the subjects are asked to localize auditory stimuli, again in the absence of visual stimuli. In the posttraining session the subject commonly mislocalizes the auditory stimulus in the same direction that the visual stimulus was perceived to be. For example, if the subject wore prisms that displaced the visual stimulus 10 degrees to the left, after training the subject would consistently report that the auditory stimulus was shifted to the left as well. In these examples, the visual stimulus is the distracter, and the spatial perception of auditory stimuli is altered in the direction of the spatially disparate visual stimulus.

In a more recent study, the stimulus parameters necessary to generate the aftereffect were measured using simple auditory and visual stimuli (Recanzone, 1998). Subjects were asked to localize either auditory stimuli alone or visual stimuli alone in an otherwise completely dark room by turning their head toward the location of the stimulus. Head movements were always performed after stimulus offset, so the stimulus itself could not guide the response during the head movement. Following this pretraining measurement of their auditory localization ability, subjects were asked to perform a different task during a training session wherein both auditory and visual stimuli were repeatedly presented, and subjects were to release a button when they detected that the auditory stimulus had increased or decreased in intensity. A visual stimulus was also presented simultaneously with the auditory stimulus, but the subjects were told that the visual stimulus had nothing to do with the task. Unknown to the subjects, the visual stimulus was displaced spatially by 8 degrees from the auditory stimulus on every trial. Thus, while the two stimuli were presented from various locations throughout frontal space during a session, the visual stimulus maintained a consistent spatial disparity with the auditory stimulus. The subjects were then asked to localize auditory stimuli, again in the dark with no accompanying visual stimuli, and the results from the pre- and posttraining periods were compared.

Typical results from these experiments are shown in Figure 3.3. In the pretraining phase, subjects displayed relatively accurate localization ability, as shown by the distribution of estimates near the target, but not very precise localization ability, as evidenced by the range of responses (Fig. 3.3A). This performance was consistent throughout frontal space (Fig. 3.3B) and was reliable across subjects. After training, there was a clear shift in the percept of the location of the auditory stimulus in the direction of the light during the training session, that is, toward the distracter stimulus. In the case of visual stimuli presented 8 degrees to the right of the auditory stimulus during training, the estimates during

A. Estimates at Two Locations

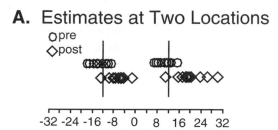

○ pre
◇ post

-32 -24 -16 -8 0 8 16 24 32
Degrees from Midline

B. Single Session Results

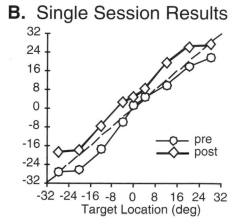

pre ○
post ◇

Target Location (deg)

C. No Effect with Large Spatial Disparity

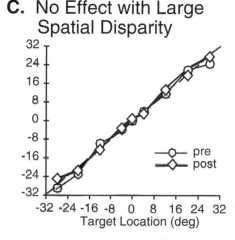

pre ○
post ◇

Target Location (deg)

FIGURE 3.3   Spatial dependence of the ventriloquism effect in humans. (*A*) Estimates of stimulus location before (circles) and after (diamonds) training with a consistent audiovisual disparity. Vertical lines indicate target location. Note the shift in localization estimates after training. (*B*) Single session estimates before (○) and after (◇) disparity training. Dashed line depicts correspondence between the given estimate (ordinate) and target location (abscissa). Note consistent shift in responses after training. (*C*) Spatial disparity dependence of ventriloquism effect. Identical conventions as *B*. Note the lack of a shift in the perception of acoustic space after training with greater than 8 degrees of disparity between stimuli. (Figures adapted from Recanzone, 1998.)

the posttraining period to auditory-alone stimuli were also shifted to the right, by approximately the same magnitude as the trained disparity. Similarly, when trained with visual stimuli to the left of auditory stimuli,

the posttraining estimates of auditory spatial location were shifted to the left. Of note, if there was no spatial disparity between the visual and auditory stimulus during the training period, there was also no shift in the auditory-alone localization between the pre- and posttraining periods.

Several other interesting aspects of this aftereffect were also discovered. If the visual and auditory stimuli were not presented simultaneously but were instead presented in a nonoverlapping manner, no effect was observed, displaying the temporal dependency of the illusion. Furthermore, the effect was not reliant on the head movement task itself and was prominent in multiple other paradigms. For example, subjects asked to indicate spatial location by moving a lever instead of moving their heads were just as likely to be influenced by the distracter stimulus, resulting in the same altered perception of acoustic space. Finally, there was a robust frequency dependence of the effect. Experiments employing acoustic stimuli that differed by two or more octaves in frequency between training and sound localization sessions generated the illusion for stimuli at the trained frequency, but not at the untrained frequency two octaves apart (Recanzone, 1998). This result indicates that the neuronal mechanisms underlying these effects are restricted in frequency.

Another factor influencing the demonstration of the ventriloquism aftereffect in humans was whether the subjects perceived the two stimuli as independent or fused during the training period. For example, when the auditory and visual stimuli were not perceived as originating from the same location during training, no aftereffect was observed. This was tested by using broadband noise as the acoustic stimulus, for which human subjects have fine spatial acuity, instead of tonal stimuli, which are much more difficult to localize spatially. During these sessions, in which the noise stimulus was discerned as incongruent with the visual stimulus, there was no perceptual fusion of the two stimuli during the training session, and no aftereffect was observed.

The ventriloquism aftereffect was also limited by the spatial disparity of the sensory stimuli. As shown in Figure 3.3*B*, repeated presentation of the paired auditory and visual stimuli at a spatial disparity of 8 degrees resulted in the persistence of that spatial fusion in the following sound localization paradigm. However, doubling this spatial disparity failed to influence the subsequent perception. Figure 3.3*C* shows the lack of any effect under these conditions. In fact, in every experiment in which subjects reported that they knew the visual stimulus was shifted to the left (or the right) of the auditory stimulus during the training session, no aftereffect was observed. Thus, akin to the ventriloquism effect, there is a clear spatial and temporal dependency on the generation of the ventriloquism aftereffect. It appears that the two illusions are intimately linked: if the experimental parameters during the training session are sufficient to produce the ventriloquism effect, then the persistence of this illusion over time, the ventriloquism aftereffect, is also generated. However, if the spatial and/or temporal parameters of the two stimuli do not adequately overlap (Figs. 3.1C and E), the subject perceives two distinct stimuli, the perception of the location of one stimulus is not influenced by the distracter, and the aftereffect is not generated.

The foundation has now been laid for the manifestation of the persistence in time of the ventriloquist effect—the ventriloquist aftereffect. Not only is the aftereffect illusion demonstrable in humans, it is repeatable, and restricted by certain variables such as space, time, and frequency. However, the neural substrates for this illusion cannot be elucidated directly in humans. The following section describes results obtained in an animal model designed to investigate the ventriloquism aftereffect, compares these results with results of studies in humans, and presents preliminary results suggesting likely cortical loci underlying the illusion.

Ventriloquism aftereffect experiments in nonhuman primates

The ventriloquism aftereffect is demonstrable in species other than man (Woods & Recanzone, 2000). The macaque monkey (*M. mulatta*) is a useful animal model of human neurobiology and behavior because of the many similarities between the two species in basic sensory perception, including the detection and discrimination of a variety of auditory and visual stimulus parameters. The incorporation of biological and behavioral metrics in studies undertaken on monkeys necessarily mimics to some degree the human condition. The impetus for the present set of experiments was to determine whether the same auditory-visual interactions in the spatial domain observed in humans also occur in monkeys. If so, it should be possible to use this animal model to investigate the putative neural locus for such visually mediated auditory plasticity.

One problem inherent in using animal models in studying perceptual illusions is in how to appropriately reward the animal. Human subjects are willing to perform experiments in the absence of feedback, and thus are given no information about their performance during the session. Animal subjects, including monkeys, that perform operant conditioning paradigms, however, must be rewarded for correct trials and unrewarded for

incorrect trials. The problem is how to reward an animal under stimulus conditions in which it may or may not be experiencing an illusion. Animals may learn to respond in a manner that elicits a reward regardless of their perception, and therefore they may give misleading information to the experimenter. We reasoned that one way to overcome this problem with the ventriloquism effect in monkeys was to measure whether the animal experienced the aftereffect. Because the temporal and spatial dependencies of the auditory and visual stimuli appear to be the same for the two effects, if we could demonstrate the aftereffect in monkeys, it could be inferred that the monkey experienced the ventriloquism effect during the training session.

To overcome obstacles inherent in awake monkey experiments, the ventriloquism aftereffect paradigm was slightly altered from that described earlier. Briefly, monkeys were trained to make saccades to one of two visual targets spanning the midline, or move a horizontal lever to the left or right to indicate the perceived side from which an acoustic stimulus originated. This served as the sound localization session. Acoustic stimuli emitted from speakers closer to the midline were naturally more difficult to lateralize; thus a psychometric function could be generated as a baseline for sound localization ability for each experimental day (Fig. 3.4). Following this, auditory and visual stimuli were presented simultaneously and repeatedly from the identical locations, or at a consistent disparity of 4 degrees to either the left or right. Monkeys indicated when the intensity of the acoustic stimulus increased by releasing a lever, thus theoretically they were not behaviorally attending to the specific location of the stimuli during the training session. These sessions consisted of 60–350 presentations of paired audiovisual stimuli at several different spatial locations spanning a range of ±30 degrees and lasting 20–60 minutes. Immediately after the training session, sound localization acuity was measured again in the same manner as initially, and the corresponding psychometric function was calculated (Fig. 3.4B). The only difference between this session and the baseline session was that no penalty (time out) was incurred for an incorrect response when the sound came from the two speakers closest to the midline. Hence, the monkey received positive feedback (rewards) whether it correctly perceived the location of the stimulus or was under the influence of the aftereffect illusion. The psychometric functions obtained after the training session were compared with the baseline psychometric functions to determine the shift in the perception of acoustic space (Fig. 3.4C), as will be described.

Conceptually, following the baseline sound localization performance session, the monkey was presented

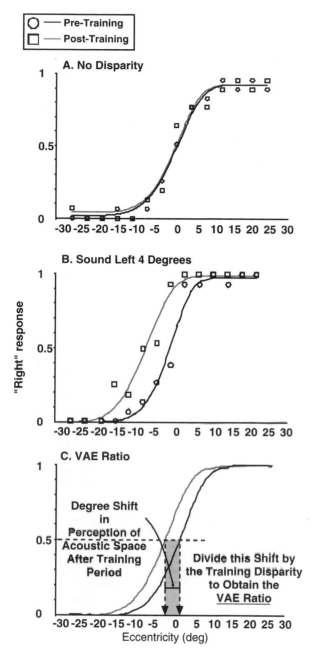

○ — Pre-Training
□ — Post-Training

A. No Disparity

B. Sound Left 4 Degrees

"Right" response

C. VAE Ratio

Degree Shift
in
Perception of
Acoustic Space
After Training
Period

Divide this Shift by
the Training Disparity
to Obtain the
VAE Ratio

Eccentricity (deg)

with more than 20 minutes of a consistent disparity between the sound and the light, which should fuse the perception of stimulus location for both stimuli. In the sound left condition, the acoustic stimulus was presented to the left of the visual stimulus (−4 degrees) during the training session. Similarly, the acoustic stimulus was presented to the right of the LED (+4 degrees) in the sound right condition, and from the same location in space in the no-disparity or control conditions. Following sound left training, the perception of acoustic space should be shifted toward the light direction, or right, and following sound right training, the perception of acoustic space should be shifted to the left. As a matter of course, training sessions within which audiovisual stimuli originated from the identical location in space should incur no perceptual plasticity.

The monkey's perception of acoustic space was indeed altered in the course of the present experiments. Figure 3.4 shows representative examples of fitted psychometric functions obtained under the described design. Psychometric functions are depicted as a normalized measure of responses of "right" (indicated by rightward saccade or lever push); consequently a data point left of the midline that carries a value of zero represents perfect performance, as does a 1 at a point to the right of the midline. Sound left training should shift this function to the left (Fig. 3.4*B*) because the monkey would consistently report the perceived location of a stimulus to the right (in the direction of the visual stimulus during the training period). It follows that sound right training should shift the second psychometric function to the left. In control or no-disparity sessions, there should be no difference in the functions before and after training (Fig. 3.4*A*).

To evaluate these results in greater detail, a specific metric was used that incorporated the observed shift in the perception of acoustic space compared to the actual disparity of audiovisual stimuli during the training session. This produces a ventriloquism aftereffect ratio, or VAE ratio (Fig. 3.4*C*). The VAE ratio was determined

FIGURE 3.4 Fitted psychometric functions from sound localization tasks in monkeys. In each panel, the abscissa depicts the location of speakers to the left (negative numbers) and right (positive numbers) of the midline (0). The ordinate depicts performance measured as the normalized responses of stimulus location to the right of the midline. Circles represent data points in the baseline sound localization session (pretraining) and squares represent individual data points following disparity training (posttraining). (*A*) No disparity. Representative psychometric functions from a no disparity experiment in which the sounds and lights were presented from the same location during the training period. Note the psychophysical congruity, showing consistent acoustic space perception. (*B*) Sound left condition. Representative psychometric functions obtained before and after a training period in which the sound stimulus was consistently presented 4 degrees to the left of the visual stimulus. Note the shift in the

posttraining psychometric function to the left, indicative of a shift in perception toward the right, consistent with visual capture to the right of the midline. (*C*) VAE ratio calculation. Idealized psychometric functions pre- and posttraining exhibiting the manner in which VAE ratios were obtained. The difference between the performance level of 0.5 (horizontal dashed line) in the posttraining condition was divided by the visual-auditory disparity presented during training, or by 4 degrees in the control condition. A VAE ratio of 1 or −1 thus indicates a shift in the perception of acoustic space of the same magnitude as the disparity during training. Shaded area represents a perfectly matched shift in the psychometric function of 4 degrees.

by dividing the difference in the location corresponding to 0.50 performance between the pre- and post-training psychometric functions and dividing this difference by the disparity presented during the training period (or by 4 degrees in the no-disparity condition). Since the audiovisual disparity was 4 degrees, a complete and perfectly matching shift in acoustic space perception would be the equivalent. Accordingly, a VAE ratio of 1 represents a perfectly matched shift in the psychometric function to the right (i.e., [4/4], sound right condition) and a VAE ratio of −1 a matched shift to the left (i.e., [−4/4], sound left condition). A VAE ratio of zero corresponds to no change in the perception of acoustic space. These experiments should indicate whether monkeys, like humans, are susceptible to the visual spatial capture of the auditory stimulus (the ventriloquism effect), and whether this illusion persists after training (the ventriloquism aftereffect).

The vast majority of experiments resulted in shifts of acoustic space perception in the expected direction. The magnitude of the shift varied considerably, however. As shown in Figure 3.5A, the median VAE ratios were ±0.6 in the sound left and the sound right conditions and 0.1 in the no-disparity conditions (including controls). These results demonstrate consistent behavioral performance between pre- and post-training sessions in the no-disparity condition, and the tendency for disparity between the acoustic and the visual stimuli to result in the expected shift in acoustic space perception. Thus, the visual stimulus captured the acoustic stimulus in a similar manner to that shown in humans, in that the observed realignment of auditory space approximated the actual disparity between stimuli.

The amount of time of disparate audiovisual stimulus exposure during training sessions did not significantly affect the results. The shortest training sessions, approximately 20 minutes, were just as likely to result in a perceptual shift in the expected direction as the longest, 60 minutes. Sessions shorter than 20 minutes were not performed because of the amount of time required to present adequate stimulus repetitions from each speaker location. Sessions greater than 60 minutes were troublesome for behavioral reasons, and not further investigated.

Interestingly, the spatial acuity associated with the acoustic stimulus greatly affected the ability to alter perception (Fig. 3.5B), similar to human studies described above. For example, a broadband noise stimulus that could be localized very accurately by the monkey during the initial sound localization session did not produce a shift in acoustic space perception, similar to the finding in humans. During disparity training, the

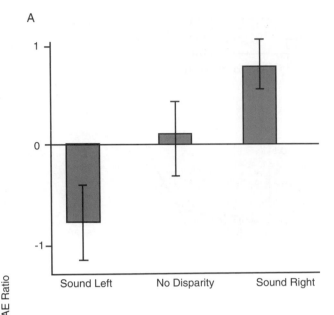

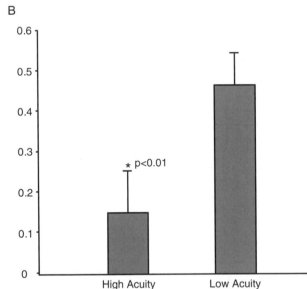

FIGURE 3.5 (A) VAE ratios summary. The median ± standard deviation of VAE ratios by training condition. Note that the median VAE ratios signify shifts in the perception of acoustic space in the expected direction for sound left (-0.6 ± 0.7; $n = 27$) and sound right (0.6 ± 0.5, $n = 21$) conditions, and no shift in the no-disparity (0.1 ± 0.5; $n = 34$) conditions. A Wilcoxon signed-rank test was applied to VAE ratios acquired after sound left, sound right, and no-disparity training. The rank sums were found to be significantly different (sound left vs. no-disparity training $p = 0.0042$; sound right vs. no-disparity training, $p = 0.0079$; sound left vs. sound right, $p \leq 0.0001$). (B) Dependence of VAE ratio magnitude on spatial acuity of the acoustic stimulus. Data across sessions using different acoustic stimuli were grouped according to the pretraining acuity thresholds. Sessions using stimuli the monkey could easily localize (threshold < 3 degrees) showed a smaller ventriloquism aftereffect, indicated by the VAE ratios, than sessions using tone stimuli that could not be localized as well (threshold > 3 degrees). These differences were statistically significant (t-test; $p = 0.0105$). Error bars show the standard error of the mean.

light would have obviously come from a different point in space than the sound, rendering visual capture impossible. However, auditory stimuli that were more difficult to localize were much more likely to result in a perceptual shift, putatively because it was difficult or impossible to discern the audiovisual disparity, leading to the ventriloquism effect during the training period. Consequently, stimuli that yielded spatial discrimination thresholds of more than 3 degrees resulted in significantly greater visual capture (Fig. 3.5B).

Therefore, just as in humans, the ventriloquism aftereffect in monkeys was dependent on the spatial salience of stimuli in terms of fusion. This brings up two further interesting similarities between results in humans and in monkeys. First, increasing the spatial disparity between auditory and visual stimuli to 8 degrees instead of 4 degrees failed to produce the aftereffect. This was true even for stimuli that consistently created the aftereffect in the experiments using 4 degrees of disparity. This disparity (8 degrees) did, however, result in the aftereffect in humans. The difference between subjects may be due to greater spatial acuity in the behaviorally trained monkeys or slight differences in the paradigms used. Regardless, the results demonstrate a strong spatial dependence of the aftereffect in both models. Second, varying the acoustic stimuli by two octaves between sessions canceled out the aftereffect in monkeys. Again, as in the human studies, the ventriloquism effect likely occurred for the trained frequency (although this was not specifically tested), yet did not lead to the aftereffect illusion because of the significant difference in the stimuli.

These experiments represent an effective animal model for the demonstration of a polysensory illusion based on the similarity in results between human and monkey subjects. In neither case was the length of time that the ventriloquism aftereffect persists investigated. However, in the absence of matching audiovisual inputs, it may be assumed that the aftereffect would persist indefinitely. When human subjects emerged from the experimental chamber and received the normal correlated sensory inputs from the environment for 20 minutes, the aftereffect illusion was extinguished (unpublished observations). This was specifically tested experimentally in monkeys by performing a second training session with no disparity between auditory and visual stimuli following the initial demonstration of the aftereffect. As expected, this training resulted in the realignment of acoustic space perception (see Fig. 3.4A). The temporal dependence of the aftereffect, that is, whether the audiovisual stimuli occurred simultaneously or were offset during training, was not analyzed in monkeys. However, the similarities shown

between the results in monkeys and the results in humans to this point strongly suggest the aftereffect would be temporally sensitive in both species.

The next logical step from these experiments is to investigate the neuronal activity at different brain regions before, during, and after the experience of the ventriloquism aftereffect illusion. Theoretically, this will help to explain the neuronal areas and mechanisms underlying the illusion in humans. The final section of this chapter discusses issues central to these conceptions.

Functional implications of the ventriloquism illusion

The prevalence of the aftereffect illusion evidenced in both humans and macaque monkeys suggests that there are long-term changes in the representation of acoustic space after a relatively brief period of exposure to spatially disparate auditory and visual stimuli in both primate species. The foundation of this altered perception is certainly neuronal plasticity. The representation of the two spatially disparate stimuli in polysensory brain areas is overlapped but not perfectly matched prior to the training session (Fig. 3.6A). The representation is adapted to the new input as the training session progresses, giving rise to the new, fused, spatial representation (Fig. 3.6B). As stated previously, in the ventriloquism effect, the location of the auditory stimulus is influenced by the disparate location of the visual stimulus (Fig. 3.6B). Finally, and most poignantly for the present discussion, the spatial representation acquired during the training session persists over time to display the ventriloquism aftereffect (Fig. 3.6C). This can be envisioned as a change in the spatial representation of auditory inputs in polysensory brain areas to coregister with the visual input, and thus is an example of rapidly induced neuronal plasticity. Similar types of plasticity have been observed in development, for example, in the SC of ferrets (King, Parsons, & Moore, 2000) and in the auditory midbrain of barn owls (Knudsen & Brainard, 1995; see also Cohen & Knudsen, 1999).

Spatial representational plasticity occurring over such a short time course has not been documented in adults, although it is well known that neuronal responses can be altered in the short term by a variety of manipulations. For example, the position of the eyes in the orbits directly influences the spatial response properties of neurons in the primate parietal lobe (e.g., Andersen et al., 1997) and in auditory neurons in the inferior colliculus (Groh, Trause, Underhill, Clark, & Inati, 2001). Thus, while short-term plasticity has not directly been shown to occur in the representations of extrapersonal space in the brain, some basic neuronal

A. Pre-Training

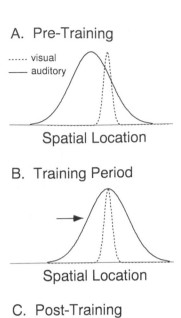

····· visual
—— auditory

Spatial Location

B. Training Period

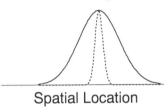

Spatial Location

C. Post-Training

Spatial Location

FIGURE 3.6   Progression of spatial representations during the ventriloquism effect and aftereffect. (*A*) Before training, the representations of the auditory (solid line) and visual (dashed line) stimuli are slightly displaced concomitant with the actual disparity of the stimuli. (*B*) During the training period, the representation of the auditory stimulus is shifted toward the visual stimulus (arrow) until it is completely fused, resulting in the ventriloquism effect. (*C*) After training, even in the absence of disparate visual input, the perception of the auditory stimulus location remains shifted in the trained direction, resulting in the ventriloquism aftereffect.

mechanisms are known to exist that can produce rapid changes in receptive field properties of neurons sensitive to auditory-visual interactions. Perceptional illusions such as the ventriloquism aftereffect indicate that rapid plastic changes are taking place in spatial representations in the brain. A significant dilemma related to this issue is that the brain structures that underlie the plasticity associated with the illusion are unclear. Some evidence suggests that acoustic space is represented in both unimodal auditory areas, where certain cortical fields display greater spatial sensitivity than others (Recanzone, Guard, Phan, & Su, 2000; Tian, Reser, Durham, Kustov, & Rauschecker, 2001; Woods, Su, & Recanzone, 2001), and in multisensory parietal areas.

A promising candidate area for direct involvement in the neural changes associated with the ventriloquism aftereffect is the parietal lobe, where individual neurons respond to multiple sensory stimuli. The parietal lobe has been implicated in aligning spatial frames of reference, for example, eye-centered, head-centered, body-centered, and environment-centered (see Andersen et al., 1998; Karnath, 1997; Phan, Schendel, Recanzone, & Robertson, 2000; Robertson, Treisman, Friedman-Hill, & Grabowecky, 1997; Ruff, Hersch, & Pribram, 1981). Lesions of the parietal lobe result in neglect symptoms, and these symptoms can be auditory, visual, or both (see De Renzi, Gentilini, & Barbieri, 1989; Phan et al., 2000; Posner, Walker, Friedrich, & Rafal, 1984; Soroker, Calamaro, & Myslobodsky, 1995). Auditory and visual interactions have been studied in a patient with bilateral parietal lobe lesions, and the results in this patient are consistent with the modality-specificity hypothesis (Phan et al., 2000). In this subject, auditory spatial acuity was greater than visual spatial acuity, which is in direct opposition to normal. Interestingly, when auditory and visual stimuli were presented to this individual in a manner that produced the ventriloquism effect in nonlesioned subjects, the reverse of the ventriloquism effect resulted. Whereas the perception of spatial location of a visual stimulus is not usually affected by auditory stimuli in normal humans, the lesioned subject was better able to tell that a visual stimulus changed location if an auditory stimulus also changed location simultaneously. The reverse pattern was also observed: normal subjects were less able to sense that an auditory stimulus changed location if the visual stimulus remained stationary, and the lesioned subject was less influenced by the visual stimulus. These experiments provide support for the modality appropriateness hypothesis, but they also indicate that the regions of the parietal lobe lesioned in this patient are probably not the polysensory areas where this integration occurs.

A final issue is what the underlying neural mechanisms are that lead to the aftereffect in the unimodal condition. If one assumes that the polysensory brain regions have a shifted spatial representation of one stimulus modality relative to the others in the presence of the illusion, how does this influence the percept of a single sensory modality presented in isolation? One possibility is that the polysensory areas are the regions that define the spatial location of both unimodal and multisensory stimuli. In this case, even though the unimodal information has not been altered, the perception based on the function of the polysensory area is altered. Alternatively, it could be that the polysensory areas are providing feedback to the unimodal areas and affecting the change at those locations. In this scenario, one would expect neurons in the unimodal areas to be altered after the training period and to better represent the percept rather than the actual stimulus location. It is currently unclear which of these two alternatives is correct, or indeed whether there is a single polysensory area for all stimulus attributes or multiple polysensory areas processing different stimulus attributes independently. Experiments in our laboratory are pursuing this interesting issue.

REFERENCES

Andersen, R. A., Snyder, L. H., Batista, A. P., Buneo, C. A., & Cohen, Y. E. (1998). Posterior parietal areas specialized for eye movements (LIP) and reach (PRR) using a common coordinate frame. *Novartis Foundation Symposium, 218,* 109–122.

Andersen, R. A., Snyder, L. H., Bradley, D. C., & Xing, J. (1997). Multimodal representation of space in the posterior parietal cortex and its use in planning movements. *Annual Review of Neuroscience, 20,* 303–330.

Bertelson, P. (1999). Ventriloquism: A case of cross modal perceptual grouping. In G. Aschersleben, T. Bachmann, & J. Musseler (Eds.), *Cognitive contributions to perception of spatial and temporal events* (pp. 357–362). New York: Elsevier.

Bruce, C., Desimone, R., & Gross, C. G. (1981). Visual properties of neurons in a polysensory area in superior temporal sulcus of the macaque. *Journal of Neurophysiology, 46,* 369–384.

Bushara, K. O., Grafman, J., & Hallett, J. M. (2001). Neural correlates of auditory-visual stimulus onset asynchrony detection. *Journal of Neuroscience, 21,* 300–304.

Canon, L. K. (1970). Intermodality inconsistency of input and directed attention as determinants of the nature of adaptation. *Journal of Experimental Psychology, 84,* 141–147.

Carlile, S., Leong, P., & Hyams, S. (1997). The nature and distribution of errors in sound localization by human listeners. *Hearing Research, 114,* 179–196.

Cohen, Y. E., & Knudsen, E. I. (1999). Maps versus clusters: Different representations of auditory space in the midbrain and forebrain. *Trends in Neuroscience, 22,* 128–135.

Cusick, C. G. (1997). The superior temporal polysensory region in monkeys. *Cerebral Cortex, 12,* 435–468.

Cusick, C. G., Seltzer, B., Cola, M., & Griggs, E. (1995). Chemoarchitectonics and corticocortical terminations within the superior temporal sulcus of the rhesus monkey: Evidence for subdivisions of superior temporal polysensory cortex. *Journal of Comparative Neurology, 360,* 513–535.

De Renzi, E., Gentilini, M., & Barbieri, C. (1989). Auditory neglect. *Journal of Neurology, Neurosurgery and Psychiatry, 52,* 613–617.

Driver, J. (1996). Enhancement of selective listening by illusory mislocation of speech sounds due to lip reading. *Nature, 381,* 66–68.

Graziano, M. S. A., Reiss, L. A. J., & Gross, C. G. (1999). A neuronal representation of the location of nearby sounds. *Nature, 397,* 428–430.

Groh, J. M., Trause, A. S., Underhill, A. M., Clark, K. R., & Inati, S. (2001). Eye position influences auditory responses in primate inferior colliculus. *Neuron, 29,* 509–518.

Hay, J. C., Pick, H. L., Jr., & Ikeda, K. (1965). Visual capture produced by prism spectacles. *Psychonomic Science, 2,* 215–216.

Hikosaka, K., Iwai, E., Saito, H., & Tanaka, K. (1988). Polysensory properties of neurons in the anterior bank of the caudal superior temporal sulcus of the macaque monkey. *Journal of Neurophysiology, 60,* 1615–1637.

Howard, I. P., & Templeton, W. B. (1966). *Human spatial orientation.* New York: Wiley.

Hyvarinen, J. (1982). Posterior parietal lobe of the primate brain. *Physiological Review, 62,* 1060–1129.

Jack, C. E., & Thurlow, W. R. (1973). Effects of degree of visual association and angle of displacement on the "ventriloquism" effect. *Perceptual and Motor Skills, 37,* 967–979.

Jay, M. F., & Sparks, D. L. (1984). Auditory receptive fields in primate superior colliculus shift with changes in eye position. *Nature, 309,* 345–347.

Karnath, H.-O. (1997). Spatial orientation and the representation of space with parietal lobe lesions. *Philosophical Transactions of the Royal Society of London, 353,* 1411–1419.

King, A. J., Parsons, C. H., & Moore, D. R. (2000). Plasticity in the neural coding of auditory space in the mammalian brain. *Proceedings of the National Academy of Sciences, USA, 97,* 11821–11828.

Knudsen, E. I., & Brainard, M. S. (1995). Creating a unified representation of visual and auditory space in the brain. *Annual Review of Neuroscience, 18,* 19–43.

Makous, J. C., & Middlebrooks, J. C. (1990). Two-dimensional sound localization by human listeners. *Journal of the Acoustical Society of America, 87,* 2188–2200.

Ogilvie, J. C. (1956). Effect of auditory flutter on the visual critical flicker frequency. *Canadian Journal of Psychology, 10,* 61–69.

Phan, M. L., Schendel, K. L., Recanzone, G. H., & Robertson, L. C. (2000). Auditory and visual spatial localization deficits following bilateral parietal lobe lesions in a patient with Balint's syndrome. *Journal of Cognitive Neuroscience, 12,* 583–600.

Pick, H. L., Jr., Warren, D. H., & Hay, J. C. (1969). Sensory conflict in judgments of spatial direction. *Perception & Psychophysics, 6,* 203–205.

Posner, M. I., Walker, J. A., Friedrich, F. A., & Rafal, R. D. (1984). Effects of parietal lobe injury on covert orienting of visual attention. *Journal of Neuroscience, 4,* 1863–1874.

Radeau, M., & Bertelson, P. (1974). The after-effects of ventriloquism. *Quarterly Journal of Experimental Psychology, 26,* 63–71.

Radeau, M., & Bertelson, P. (1978). Cognitive factors and adaptation to auditory-visual discordance. *Perception & Psychophysics, 23,* 341–343.

Recanzone, G. H. (1998). Rapidly induced auditory plasticity: The ventriloquism aftereffect. *Proceedings of the National Academy of Sciences, USA, 95,* 869–875.

Recanzone, G. H., Guard, D. C., Phan, M. L., & Su, T. K. (2000). Correlation between the activity of single auditory cortical neurons and sound localization behavior in the macaque monkey. *Journal of Neurophysiology, 83,* 2723–2739.

Recanzone, G. H., Makhamra, S. D. D. R., & Guard, D. C. (1998). Comparison of relative and absolute sound localization ability in humans. *Journal of the Acoustical Society of America, 103,* 1085–1097.

Robertson, L. C., Treisman, A., Friedman-Hill, S. R., & Grabowecky, M. (1997). The interaction of spatial and object pathways: Evidence from Balint's syndrome. *Journal of Cognitive Neuroscience, 9,* 254–276.

Ruff, R. M., Hersch, N. A., & Pribram, K. H. (1981). Auditory spatial deficits in the personal and extrapersonal frames of reference due to cortical lesions. *Neuropsychologia, 19,* 435–443.

Russo, G. S., & Bruce, C. J. (1994). Frontal eye field activity preceding aurally guided saccades. *Journal of Neurophysiology, 71,* 1250–1253.

Sekuler, R., Sekuler, A. B., & Lau, R. (1997). Sound alters visual motion perception. *Nature, 385,* 308.

Shams, L., Kamitani, Y., & Shimojo, S. (2000). What you see is what you hear. *Nature, 408,* 788.

Shipley, T. (1964). Auditory flutter-driving of visual flicker. *Science, 145,* 1328–1330.

Slutsky, D. A., & Recanzone, G. H. (2001). Temporal and spatial dependency of the ventriloquism effect. *NeuroReport, 12,* 7–10.

Soroker, N., Calamaro, N., & Myslobodsky, M. S. (1995). Ventriloquist effect reinstates responsiveness to auditory stimuli in the "ignored" space in patients with hemispatial neglect. *Journal of Clinical and Experimental Neuropsychology, 17,* 243–255.

Stein, B. E., London, N., Wilkinson, L. K., & Price, D. D. (1996). Enhancement of perceived visual intensity by auditory stimuli: A psychophysical analysis. *Journal of Cognitive Neuroscience, 8,* 497–506.

Stevens, S. S., & Newman, E. B. (1936). The localization of actual sources of sound. *American Journal of Psychology, 48,* 297–306.

Su, T. K., & Recanzone, G. H. (2001). Differential effect of near-threshold stimulus intensities on sound localization performance in azimuth and elevation in normal human subjects. *Journal of the Association for Research in Otolaryngology, 3,* 246–256.

Thomas, G. J. (1940). Experimental study of the influence of vision on sound localization. *Journal of Experimental Psychology, 28,* 163–177.

Thurlow, W. R., & Jack, C. E. (1973). Certain determinants of the "ventriloquism effect." *Perceptual and Motor Skills, 36,* 1171–1184.

Tian, B., Reser, D., Durham, A., Kustov, A., & Rauschecker, J. P. (2001). Functional specialization in rhesus monkey auditory cortex. *Science, 292,* 290–293.

Wallace, M. T., Wilkinson, L. K., & Stein, B. E. (1996). Representation and integration of multiple sensory inputs in primate superior colliculus. *Journal of Neurophysiology, 76,* 1246–1266.

Warren, D. H., Welch, R. B., & McCarthy, T. J. (1981). The role of visual-auditory "compellingness" in the ventriloquism effect: Implications for transitivity among the spatial senses. *Perception & Psychophysics, 30,* 557–564.

Watanabe, J., & Iwai, E. (1991). Neuronal activity in visual, auditory and polysensory areas in the monkey temporal cortex during visual fixation task. *Brain Research Bulletin, 26,* 583–592.

Watanabe, K., & Shimojo, S. (2001). When sound affects vision: Effects of auditory grouping on visual motion perception. *Psychological Science, 12,* 109–116.

Watson, R. T., Valenstein, E., Day, A., & Heilman, K. M. (1994). Posterior neocortical systems subserving awareness and neglect: Neglect associated with superior temporal sulcus but not area 7 lesions. *Archives of Neurology, 51,* 1014–1021.

Welch, R. B. (1999). Meaning, attention, and the "unity assumption" in the intersensory bias of spatial and temporal perceptions. In G. Aschersleben, T. Bachmann, & J. Musseler (Eds.), *Cognitive contributions to perception of spatial and temporal events* (pp. 371–387). New York: Elsevier.

Welch, R. B., DuttonHurt, L. D., & Warren, D. H. (1986). Contributions of audition and vision to temporal rate perception. *Perception & Psychophysics, 39,* 294–300.

Welch, R. B., & Warren, D. H. (1980). Immediate perceptual response to intersensory discrepancy. *Psychological Bulletin, 88,* 638–667.

Woods, T. M., & Recanzone, G. H. (2000). Visually mediated plasticity of acoustic space perception in behaving macaque monkeys. *Society of Neuroscience, Abstracts, 26.*

Woods, T. M., Su, T. K., & Recanzone, G. H. (2001). Spatial tuning as a function of stimulus intensity of single neurons in awake macaque monkey auditory cortex. *Society of Neuroscience, Abstracts, 27.*

4 Multisensory Integration of Dynamic Information

SALVADOR SOTO-FARACO AND ALAN KINGSTONE

Introduction

Movement, like orientation or shape, is a fundamental property in perception. For that reason, being able to detect and determine the direction in which objects are moving confers a great deal of adaptive power on organisms. Indeed, almost all everyday situations contain dynamic information, and, accordingly, the failure to perceive motion (the clinical syndrome of cerebral akinetopsia) renders everyday life tasks difficult and even dangerous (e.g., Zihl, von Cramon, & Mai, 1983). The issue addressed in this chapter concerns the integration of motion information across sensory modalities. The advantage provided by multisensory integration of motion signals becomes obvious in naturalistic environments, where the combination of auditory and visual motion cues can provide more accurate information than either modality alone. For example, an animal rushing across a cluttered forest floor will provide a potential observer with neither a clear visual signal nor an unambiguous auditory one about the direction of motion, but together the two sensory modalities can help the observer determine directional information more accurately.

Because dynamic information pervades everyday life environments, it may be surprising to learn that past research on multisensory integration rarely included moving events for investigation. For instance, the classic example to illustrate the behavioral consequences of multisensory integration is the *ventriloquist illusion,* which consists of mislocalizing a sound toward a concurrent visual event presented at a different location (e.g., Howard & Templeton, 1966). In the laboratory this illusion is often studied with a single stationary sound and a single stationary light, although real-world experiences of ventriloquism typically involve movement, such as movement of the mouth of a puppet or of items on a cinema screen.

In this chapter, we review research that has addressed multisensory interactions in the domain of motion perception. We consider both the influence of static events in one sensory modality on the perception of motion by another sensory modality, and the interactions between two moving events in different modalities. We also present data from our laboratory to support the argument that, as with other perceptual dimensions, the representation of dynamic properties of external objects is achieved by integration that occurs, at least in part, at an early level of processing. We also discuss potential dominance relationships between sensory modalities in the motion integration process.

Multisensory integration between static and dynamic events

THE INFLUENCE OF STATIC EVENTS ON THE PERCEPTION OF APPARENT MOTION   Early investigations of motion events were directed at studying how static stimulation in one sensory modality could influence the experience of apparent motion in another sensory modality (e.g., Gilbert, 1939; Hall & Earle, 1954; Hall, Earle, & Crookes, 1952; Maass, 1938; Zietz & Werner, 1927). In one of the first experiments in this area, Zietz and Werner asked participants to judge whether the presentation of two objects flashed at alternating locations produced the impression of motion (apparent motion, or phi phenomenon). The different shape of the two objects, an arrow and a ball, and the long interstimulus interval (ISI) of 780 ms were, in principle, unfavorable for the perception of apparent motion. However, when sound bursts were presented at the same time as the onset of the visual events, the perception of apparent motion was facilitated, whereas when sound bursts were presented at irregular rhythms—that is, out of synchrony with the visual events—the appearance of visual motion was greatly weakened or eliminated altogether. Other studies in the same tradition have reinforced the conclusion that auditory and even tactile events can influence the threshold ISI at which visual apparent motion is experienced (e.g., Gilbert, 1939; Hall & Earle, 1954; Hall et al., 1952; Maass, 1938).

Later studies by Allen and Kolers (1981) and Ohmura (1987) reexamined the influence that stimulation in one modality has on the perception of apparent motion in another modality. Contrary to earlier results, visual apparent-motion thresholds were found to be unaffected by spatially static sounds. However, both Allen and Kolers as well as Ohmura reported that light flashes modulated the temporal range at which auditory apparent motion occurred (although in different ways). Allen and Kolers (Experiment 2, Study 1) found that a flash presented simultaneously with the onset of the first sound in the apparent-motion stream inhibited the perception of auditory apparent motion, whereas a flash presented simultaneously with the onset of the second sound in the apparent-motion stream had no effect. Ohmura found that a flash presented at any moment (coincident with either of the two sounds or between them) enlarged the range of ISIs at which auditory apparent motion was experienced, relative to a no-flash baseline.

The Influence of Static Events on the Perceived Trajectory of Motion   The studies just described addressed the influence of stimulation in one modality on the range of interstimulus intervals at which apparent motion was experienced in another modality. Additional studies have found cross-modal influences on other dimensions of motion, including its trajectory (Berrio, Lupiánez, Spence, & Martos, 1999; Hall & Earle, 1954, Hall et al., 1952; Sekuler & Sekuler, 1999; Sekuler, Sekuler, & Lau, 1997; Shimojo et al., 2001; Watanabe & Shimojo, 2001) and velocity (Manabe & Riquimaroux, 2000). For example, Sekuler et al. presented visual displays consisting of two disks moving toward each other, coinciding, and then moving apart. These displays were ambiguous and could be seen as two disks that either crossed through or bounced off each other. A brief sound presented at the same time or shortly before the point of coincidence enhanced the perception of bouncing as compared to a no-sound condition or when a sound was presented well before or after the moment of coincidence.

Other findings also suggest, if indirectly, that the direction in which auditory stimuli appear to move can be influenced by input from the visual modality (Lakatos, 1995; Mateef, Hohnsbein, & Noack, 1985). Mateef et al. investigated the Filehne illusion, in which a static visual background appears to move in the direction opposite to a moving visual target, and included a static sound as part of the background. They observed that, contrary to the typical Filehne illusion, a central static sound often appeared to move in the same direction as the visual target. This observation suggests that the direction of visual motion can induce the perception of directional motion in audition.

Multisensory integration between moving events

The studies discussed so far have investigated multisensory interactions between static information in one sensory modality and moving events in another modality. Very different questions arise when one considers the real-world situation in which information about object motion comes from two or more sensory modalities simultaneously (e.g., the sight and sound of a passing car, or the sight of a fleeing animal and the sound of its footsteps). Only a small number of studies have addressed this issue (Allen & Kolers, 1981; Kitagawa & Ichihara, 2002; Meyer & Wuerger, 2001; Soto-Faraco, Lyons, Gazzaniga, Spence, & Kingstone, 2002; Soto-Faraco, Spence, & Kingstone, 2002, in press; Staal & Donderi, 1983; Wuerger, Hofbauer, & Meyer, 2002; Zapparoli & Reatto, 1969).

Early Studies   Zapparoli and Reatto (1969) tested the ability of observers to perceive stroboscopic movement under several cross-modal conditions, including apparent motion of sounds and lights presented synchronously but in conflicting directions. The results from this study were limited to a selection of descriptive reports about what the participants' subjective experiences were when presented with the displays. Some of these reports clearly indicated that apparent-motion streams in different modalities (even in different directions) were experienced as a unitary event with a common direction.[1] However, an obviously important concern with the observations of Zapparoli and Reatto (1969; see also Anstis, 1973) is that they are based solely on introspective verbal reports, and therefore the generality of the data is questionable and difficult to reproduce (see discussion in Allen & Kolers, 1981).

---

[1] On this point, Zapparoli and Reatto (1969, p. 262) wrote, "This impression [of unification of trajectories] is also obtained by presenting the two stroboscopic movements which in the individual sensorial fields take place in opposite directions. . . ." These observations are paralleled by the reports of Anstis (1973), in a study addressing adaptation to spatial rearrangement of auditory input. For six days, the author wore microphones on each hand that were connected directly to stereo headphones on his own ears. Among the various observations reported by Anstis we find the following (p. 338): "Crossing my hands over appears to reverse sounds left-to-right, especially with closed eyes. A car driving past from left to right sounded as if it were moving from right to left. Just as it passed me, I opened my eyes. Vision immediately dominated over the contradictory auditory message: the car appeared to jump round and rush back in the opposite direction!"

Allen and Kolers (1981, Experiment 2, Studies 2 and 4) used a more objective approach to the question of multisensory interactions between auditory and visual dynamic stimuli. They assessed the range of stimulus onset asynchronies (SOAs) over which apparent motion was experienced in one modality (audition or vision) as a function of the directional congruency of an apparent-motion stream in a different modality (vision or audition, respectively). One clear finding from Allen and Kolers's study was that the directional congruency of apparent motion in an irrelevant modality did not modulate motion perception in the target modality over and above the effects found when using static distractors (see discussion in the previous section). In another study, Staal and Donderi (1983) reported an experiment very similar to one of the conditions tested by Allen and Kolers (1981, Experiment 2, Study 4). Staal and Donderi measured the threshold of visual apparent-motion both in isolation and when an irrelevant auditory apparent motion stream moved in the same or opposite direction as the lights. They found that the threshold for visual apparent motion was greater in the silent condition than in either sound condition, again regardless of the relative directions in which the events in the two modalities moved. From these two studies, and contrary to the observations of Zapparoli and Reatto (1969) and Anstis (1973), it seems that directional congruency across modalities has little influence on the perception of moving events. Indeed, according to Allen and Kolers's interpretations, the influence of moving stimuli is not different from that of static events.

However, the interpretation of these early results is difficult, given the important methodological differences between them. More important, spatial confounds may limit considerably the generality of their conclusions (especially conclusions regarding the null influence of directional information of one modality on the perception of motion in the other modality). In particular, in both Allen and Kolers's (1981) and Staal and Donderi's (1983) experiments, visual stimuli were presented in front of the observer and the auditory stimuli were presented through headphones, thus creating a situation of spatial mismatch that may be less than optimal for multisensory integration (Stein & Meredith, 1993; Welch, 1999; Welch & Warren, 1980). As Staal and Donderi point out in their discussion (p. 102), the spatial relationship between visual and the auditory stimuli was not clear. Therefore, the evidence regarding cross-modal influences between dynamic events provided by these studies must remain equivocal. One particular question that arises from these studies is whether multisensory integration can occur for dynamic properties

(such as direction of motion) in addition to the interactions already explained by the influence of static events.

RECENT STUDIES Recently there has been renewed interest in multisensory interactions in the domain of motion (Kitagawa & Ichihara, 2002; Meyer & Wuerger, 2001; Soto-Faraco, Lyons, et al., 2002; Soto-Faraco, Spence, & Kingstone, 2002, in press; Wuerger et al., 2002). Meyer and Wuerger (2001) examined the potential influence of auditory motion on the discriminability of visual motion direction in the absence of spatial confounds. In their study, participants had to discriminate the global direction of motion (left or right) of a random dot kinematogram (RDK) at different coherence levels. RDK coherence ranged from 0% (every dot moved in a random direction) to 32% (32 out of every 100 dots moved in the same predetermined direction). In the critical trials, an irrelevant white noise source could move to the left or right (in potential congruency or conflict with the global visual movement). Meyer and Wuerger's results revealed a general response bias (of up to 30%) toward the direction of the irrelevant auditory movement when the RDK was ambiguous (coherence of 0%). At high coherence levels (when visual motion direction was unambiguous), no further effects of auditory congruency were found over and above the mentioned decision bias. These data suggest that the major contribution to the cross-modal directional effects observed were due to decisional processes and that there was little influence of auditory directional information on early processing stages of visual motion[2] (Aspell, Bramwell, & Hurlbert, 2000, and Wuerger et al., 2002, reached a similar conclusion).

Kitagawa and Ichihara (2002) have recently reported a study that addressed multisensory interactions between auditory and visual motion in the depth plane using cross-modal adaptation aftereffects. They used a looming/receding square as the visual motion stimulus and a tone increasing/decreasing in amplitude as the auditory motion stimulus. After adaptation to a looming visual event, a steady tone was perceived as slightly decreasing in intensity (and adaptation to a receding visual event produced the contrary result). Adaptation to the auditory stimulus did not produce any significant

---

[2]In Meyer and Wuerger's (2001) experiment, intermediate levels of visual motion coherence (i.e., when discrimination was difficult) showed a detrimental effect of *congruent* auditory motion. This result is intriguing, as it seems to point to the conclusion that auditory motion inhibits the perception of congruent visual motion. The final interpretation of this result remains unclear.

visual aftereffects. These results suggest that multi-sensory interactions in motion direction occur, and that there is an asymmetry between auditory and visual modalities. However, it is not clear whether this interaction occurred at an early level of processing (the interpretation favored by the authors) or whether it is the product of later processes related to decision or response stages (as in the study by Meyer & Wuerger, 2001; see also the discussion under Levels of Processing in Cross-Modal Dynamic Capture, later in this chapter).

In conclusion, recent studies reveal the existence of cross-modal effects involving the direction of motion. However, while some scientists have found that these interactions stem from late stages of processing, the evidence for early perceptual interactions has not been clearly established.

TABLE 4.1

Summary of studies on cross-modal integration in motion perception

	TM	DM	Attribute Tested	Study	Outcome
Cross-modal influences from static distracter events on the perception of target motion	V	A	Threshold/optimal impression of apparent motion	Allen & Kolers, 1981*; Gilbert, 1939; Hall & Earle, 1954; Hall et al., 1952; Maass, 1938; Ohmura, 1987*; Zietz & Werner, 1927	*A can influence the threshold/velocity/trajectory in which V apparent motion is perceived, but not always (*).*
			Perceived velocity	Manabe & Riquimaroux, 2000	
			Perceived trajectory/bouncing	Hall & Earle, 1954; Hall et al., 1952; Sekuler & Sekuler, 1999; Sekuler et al., 1997; Shimojo et al., 2001; Watanabe & Shimojo, 2001	
		T	Threshold/optimal impression of apparent motion	Gilbert, 1939	*T can influence the threshold of visual apparent motion and the perceived bouncing of two moving disks.*
			Perceived trajectory/bouncing	Berrio et al., 1999; Shimojo et al., 2001	
	A	V	Threshold/optimal impression of apparent motion	Allen & Kolers, 1981*; Ohmura, 1987[†]	*V events influence A motion by decreasing (*) or shifting up (†) the threshold of A apparent motion.*
Cross-modal influences between moving target and distracter events	A	V	Threshold/optimal impression of apparent motion	Allen & Kolers, 1981	*No influence.*
	V	A	Direction of motion	Anstis, 1976	*Capture.*
	V	A	Threshold/optimal impression of apparent motion	Allen & Kolers, 1981*; Staal & Donderi, 1983[†]	*No influence (*) or inhibition in case of conflict (†).*
			Direction of motion discrimination	Meyer & Wuerger, 2001; Wuerger et al., 2002	*A motion biases decisions on V motion.*
	A/V	V/A	n/a	Zapparoli & Reatto, 1969	*Opposite motion seems in same direction.*
			Direction of motion in depth	Kitagawa & Ichiara, 2002	*V adapters influence A motion perception, but not vice versa.*
	P/V	V/P	Direction of motion discrimination	Klein, 1977	*30% decrement in P motion when V motion in conflict. 8% decrement in the reverse situation.*

Note: Table summarizes the studies reviewed in the introduction to this chapter.
Abbreviations: TM, target modality; DM, distracter modality; A, audition; P, proprioception; T, touch; V, vision.

Cross-modal dynamic capture

In the following sections we discuss data from our own laboratory that target several questions about multisensory integration between moving stimuli. First, we summarize some experiments examining whether these multisensory interactions reflect the integration of motion information or if they can be explained by known integration processes involving static events alone. Then we describe a study addressing whether multisensory integration of motion can occur at a perceptual level. Finally, we present some recent data regarding cross-modal dynamic capture beyond the audiovisual case, and discuss the results within the broader issue of modality dominance.

Potential interactions between dynamic events in different modalities were studied by assessing how the perceived direction of an apparent-motion stream in one modality is affected by the presentation of an apparent-motion stream in a different modality (Soto-Faraco, Lyons, et al., 2002). The basic setup was composed of two loudspeakers placed 30 cm from each other and two light-emitting diodes (LEDs) attached to the loudspeaker boxes (Fig. 4.1A). Each trial consisted of the presentation of two tones (50-ms duration each, 150-ms SOA) that made up an auditory apparent-motion stream going from left to right or from right to left. The two LEDs were illuminated in sequence (for 50-ms duration each, 150-ms SOA) to produce visual apparent motion in either the same or opposite direction as the sounds. Participants performed an unspeeded decision on the direction of the sound (left/right) after each display and were instructed to ignore the visual stimulus (but maintain central fixation). There were four possible types of trials (mixed in random order): congruent-synchronous, conflicting-synchronous, congruent-asynchronous, and conflicting-asynchronous (Fig. 4.1B).

The results in this task (Fig. 4.1C), now replicated over many different studies (Soto-Faraco, Lyons, et al., 2002; Soto-Faraco, Spence, & Kingstone, 2002, in press), was that accuracy reached nearly perfect levels on the synchronous-congruent trials, but participants reported the sound direction incorrectly on as many as half of the synchronous-conflicting trials. On the asynchronous trials, however, there was no congruency effect, and sound direction was reported accurately on virtually all of the trials, regardless of whether visual apparent motion was congruent or conflicting. This dramatic decrement in the auditory motion task when concurrent visual motion was directionally conflicting with the target sound could reflect that the visual stimuli interfered with auditory motion processing. As a consequence, participants resorted to guessing and therefore performed at chance levels. Another potential explanation is that visual stimuli "captured" sound motion, thereby producing an illusory reversal of direction on half of the synchronous-conflicting trials (just as described in earlier studies using subjective reports; Zapparoli & Reatto, 1969). The latter interpretation is suggested by the phenomenological experience when performing the task. It is also favored by the results of another experiment using the same method but in which participants had to rate the confidence of their directional judgments. Contrary to the interference account, which would predict low confidence in the condition where performance was reduced (at chance), the confidence ratings remained high. Moreover, when low-confidence responses were excluded from the analysis, cross-modal dynamic capture did not decrease (it actually increased slightly).[3]

These data from Soto-Faraco, Spence, and Kingstone (in press) support the Zapparoli and Reatto's (1969; see also Anstis, 1973) phenomenological report that sound motion often appears to move in the same direction as visual motion, even when the two streams are presented in opposite directions. The data of Soto-Faraco et al. extend this observation in several ways. First, they provide an objective measure rather than a subjective verbal report, and therefore the effects can be quantified and compared. Second, the asynchronous condition provided a baseline measure of sound motion discrimination in the presence of visual motion. This is an important control condition, as it shows that the direction of auditory motion was not ambiguous at all and that participants were not confused about which modality they were supposed to respond to. Finally, the finding that congruency effects disappeared in the asynchronous condition is in keeping with the temporal window of audiovisual integration found in other studies, whereby multisensory integration breaks down for asynchronies larger than 200 ms or 300 ms (e.g., Bertelson, 1998).

In summary, the results described suggest the existence of strong cross-modal interactions between dynamic events, and in principle, they are in agreement

---

[3]This result has been replicated twice. On both occasions, less than 22% of the responses were excluded from the analysis, and the data included corresponded to responses that had obtained a confidence rating of at least 4 on a 5-point confidence scale (1 being *guessing* and 5 being *positive*). Confidence ratings were equivalent across conditions.

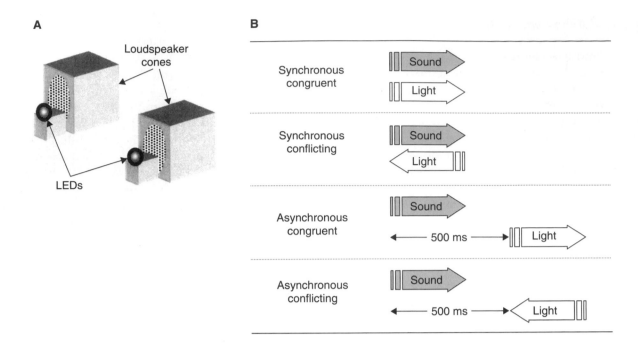

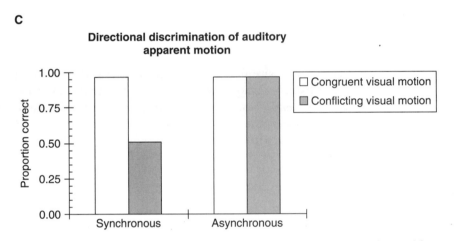

FIGURE 4.1 (*A*) Schematic view of the setup used in the cross-modal dynamic capture experiment (the response pedals are not shown). (*B*) Summary chart of the four types of trials included. The arrowheads indicate the direction in which light and sound apparent-motion streams were presented in each trial type (the example shows only the trials in which sounds moved to the right). (*C*) Average accuracy in discriminating the direction of auditory apparent motion (left vs. right) as a function of directional congruency and synchrony of irrelevant visual apparent motion.

with previous reports of cross-modal congruency effects between motion signals (e.g., Anstis, 1973; Kitagawa & Ichihara, 2002; Meyer & Wuerger, 2001; Zapparoli & Reatto, 1969). However, at least two important questions still need to be addressed. First, can these results be explained as the consequence of cross-modal interactions in the perceived *location* of static sounds without the need to invoke the quality of motion (e.g., Allen & Kolers, 1981)? In other words, it is important to address whether motion actually plays a role over and above interactions between static events. Second, what is the level or levels of processing at which these motion

congruency effects occur—perceptual or postperceptual? As seen in the previous section, the answer to this question is still unclear. We will deal with each of these two questions in turn.

The critical role of motion in cross-modal dynamic capture

Most of the studies investigating the influence between moving stimuli in different modalities have used apparent motion as their dynamic stimuli (Allen & Kolers, 1981; Soto-Faraco, Lyons et al., 2002; Soto-Faraco,

Spence, & Kingstone, 2002, in press; Zapparoli & Reatto, 1969). Apparent-motion streams typically consist of two events presented to different spatial locations with a timing that generates a reliable impression of movement.[4] However, the ventriloquist illusion offers an alternative explanation to cross-modal dynamic capture when obtained using apparent-motion streams. In the ventriloquist illusion a spatially static sound is often mislocalized toward a concurrent static visual event presented at a different position (e.g., Bertelson, 1998; Howard & Templeton, 1966). Based on this static venriloquism effect, one could argue that in cross-modal dynamic capture it is the perceived location of each individual sound in the auditory apparent-motion stream, rather than the direction of motion itself, that is biased toward the location of the individual light flashes. If this were the case, the cross-modal effects between motion signals would merely represent another instance of intersensory bias between static, rather than dynamic, features (e.g., Allen & Kolers, 1981).

In order to determine whether the cross-modal dynamic capture effect reflects classic static ventriloquism or whether it reveals the integration of motion information across modalities, we evaluated the role of motion in this phenomenon. Our working hypothesis was that if experiencing motion plays a critical role in cross-modal dynamic capture, then we can conclude that integration processes exist for dynamic events as well as integration processes for static events. We tested this hypothesis in various ways.

A first strategy to address the role of motion in cross-modal dynamic capture consisted of assessing directly the amount of ventriloquism obtained for each single component of the auditory apparent-motion stream and comparing it with the capture obtained using dynamic displays (Soto-Faraco, Spence, & Kingstone, in press). In the static condition participants discriminated the location—left versus right—of a single sound while ignoring a single light flash presented either to the same or the opposite location (synchronously or asynchronously). The dynamic condition was just like the one described above (two apparent-motion streams, one visual and one auditory, combining the directional congruency and synchrony factors). The results revealed an average of 53% capture in the dynamic condition (percent correct on congruent trials minus percent correct on conflicting trials) versus a 16% capture in the static condition (Fig. 4.2A). This result showed that the

amount of ventriloquism observed for a single sound was nowhere near the magnitude obtained when using the dynamic stimuli. In a follow-up experiment to control for potential differences in perceptual load between dynamic and static displays (one sound and one flash versus two sounds and two flashes, respectively), the auditory apparent-motion directional discrimination task was combined with double distracter flashes presented at the same location (to the left or to the right, so the visual stimuli did not induce motion). Again, the capture was minimal (18%),[5] confirming that only when visual distracters contained dynamic information was cross-modal dynamic capture observed in full.

A second test used the conditions of the initial experiment but adopted a range of different SOAs between the two events of the apparent-motion streams (from 100 ms to 950 ms). The rationale was that, as the ISI between the two events of the auditory and the visual apparent-motion streams increased, the experience of motion should decrease.[6] Accordingly, if motion is a key component of cross-modal dynamic capture, the magnitude of the effect should decrease as SOA increases. If motion plays no role, however, then this manipulation should not affect performance. The results indicated that the magnitude of cross-modal capture decreased as SOA increased, thus clearly supporting the critical role of motion (Fig. 4.2B). Together, these results suggest that the presence of motion is critical to observing full cross-modal dynamic capture and that simple static ventriloquism can, at best, account for only a small portion of the total effect.

The final piece of evidence supporting the view that motion is crucial to the cross-modal dynamic capture effect comes from the study of a split-brain patient, J.W. (Soto-Faraco, Lyons, et al., 2002). As a consequence of interhemispheric disconnection, visual information is no longer shared between J.W.'s two hemispheres. When presented with visual apparent motion across the midline, J.W. is still aware of the individual light

---

[4]Apparent motion has been studied extensively in vision and to some extent in audition and touch as well (e.g., Burtt, 1917a, 1917b; Kirman, 1974; Kolers, 1964; Wertheimer, 1912).

[5]There is a potential concern that ceiling effects in the asynchronous condition may weaken the interpretation of the significant interaction between the dynamic and the static condition in this experiment. It is important to note, however, that these results converge with the data from the other tests addressing the role of motion.
[6]The relationship between SOA and perception of apparent motion has been demonstrated extensively and described initially within Korte's laws (Korte, 1915). However, we confirmed this for our own paradigm in a separate experiment. The best quality of visual and auditory apparent motion was obtained with an SOA of 100 ms. It was slightly less with an SOA of 150 ms, and it declined thereafter.

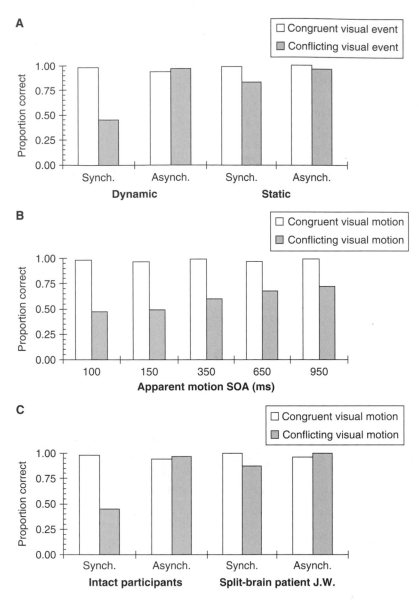

FIGURE 4.2   (A) Accuracy in discriminating the direction of auditory apparent motion as a function of visual apparent motion in dynamic trials and in discriminating the spatial location of single sound as a function of a light flash in static trials. In either case, visual distractors could be congruent or conflicting (in direction or location, respectively) and synchronous or asynchronous with respect to the target auditory event. (B) Accuracy in discriminating the direction of auditory apparent motion (left-to-right or right-to-left) as a function of the congruency in the direction of irrelevant visual apparent motion presented simultaneously. Results are plotted as a function of the temporal separation between the first and the second sound plus light pairings (apparent motion SOA). (C) Accuracy in discriminating the direction of auditory apparent motion as a function of the congruency (congruent vs. conflicting) and synchrony (synchronous vs. asynchronous by 500 ms) of visual apparent motion in intact participants and in patient J.W.

flashes within either hemispace, but he does not experience visual apparent motion (e.g., Gazzaniga, 1987). Yet auditory processing is unaffected in commissurotomized patients.[7] This peculiar combination of

Importantly, however, he was unable to perceive the direction of visual apparent motion across the midline when the two flashes were presented in a rapid succession (100 ms ISI), confirming previous observations (Gazzaniga, 1987). Finally, we made sure that J.W. could perceive the direction of visual apparent motion if it did not cross the midline, showing that he performed nearly perfect on a vertical (up vs. down) direction discrimination task presented to one hemifield alone.

[7]We ran a series of tests on J.W. to ensure that he was aware of 50 ms light flashes at either side of the midline and that he was able to make a left-right localization correctly.

conditions afforded us the opportunity to test whether or not the experience of motion is critical for the occurrence of cross-modal dynamic capture. According to the hypothesis that cross-modal dynamic capture is the consequence of integration of *dynamic* information, J.W.'s perception of auditory motion should not be affected by the visual stimulation when it crosses the midline, because in that situation J.W. will not experience visual motion. In other words, J.W. should perform more accurately than healthy observers in the cross-modal dynamic capture paradigm. In accord with this prediction, the results revealed that J.W. was largely spared from cross-modal dynamic capture (Fig. 4.2*C*), with only a marginal trend of a congruency effect in the synchronous condition being observed (12%). The magnitude of cross-modal dynamic capture in J.W. was nowhere near the strength that is observed when testing intact individuals (around 50%). This supports the view that the dramatic reduction in the magnitude of cross-modal dynamic capture in J.W. reflects an inability to experience the flashing lights as a moving event, and therefore their failure to influence the perception of auditory direction of motion.

Considered together, the data point to the conclusion that the experience of motion is critical for cross-modal dynamic capture to occur, and therefore this illusion reflects the integration of dynamic information. This suggests a dissociation between multisensory integration of static versus dynamic events. On the one hand, the classic ventriloquist illusion reflects multisensory integration of perceived location between spatially static events. On the other hand, cross-modal dynamic capture reflects multisensory integration of the perceived direction of motion between dynamic events. The difference in magnitude between simple ventriloquism and cross-modal dynamic capture may help to explain why everyday situations, which typically involve motion, usually produce capture across larger spatial distances than when tested in the laboratory with static stimuli (e.g., Bertelson & Aschersleben, 1998).

Levels of processing in cross-modal dynamic capture

Many of the studies considered so far, including the ones just described, appear to indicate the existence of strong congruency effects between motion signals in different modalities. One further question that arises from the literature regards the processing mechanisms involved in the occurrence of these cross-modal effects. Some investigators have stressed a decisional component as the underlying mechanism for cross-modal dynamic congruency effects (i.e., Meyer & Wuerger,

2001), whereas others have argued that the effects can occur during earlier (i.e., perceptual) stages (Kitagawa & Ichihara, 2002; Soto-Faraco, Lyons, et al., 2002; Soto-Faraco, Spence, & Kingstone, 2002, in press). This is an important distinction as it addresses directly a classic question about the processing level at which interactions between sensory modalities occur (e.g., Bertelson, 1998; Caclin, Soto-Faraco, Kingstone, & Spence, 2002; Choe, Welch, Gilford & Juola, 1975; Soto-Faraco, Spence, & Kingstone, in press; Welch, 1999; Welch & Warren, 1980, 1986). Multisensory integration at a perceptual level would imply that inputs from the two modalities are combined at early stages of processing, and only the product of the integration process is available to conscious awareness. On the other hand, a postperceptual level of explanation would imply that inputs from the two modalities are available independently, with congruency effects arising from later output processes, such as response interference (from the ignored modality), decisional biases, and, more generally, cognitive biases (or strategies).

Indeed, response bias induced by the irrelevant modality can account for the effects observed in experiments where information in the irrelevant modality possesses some form of congruency relationship with the responses available in the task. The idea here is that while participants are preparing a response to the target modality, the input from the irrelevant modality might activate the incorrect response to a certain degree (in case of conflicting input), in some cases so strongly that an incorrect response would be produced. Cognitive biases can represent another potential, albeit more subtle, postperceptual source of congruency effects. In intersensory conflict situations observers are, regardless of the instructions to ignore the irrelevant visual stimulation, usually aware that discrepancies may occur between auditory and visual motion streams (this situation has been called *transparent* by some authors, e.g., Bertelson & Aschersleben, 1998). This is important, because even if irrelevant information is neutral with respect to the responses available, there is no guarantee that the irrelevant, "to-be-ignored" visual stimulation is actually ignored. Rather, it could promote strategies and adjustments in the form of criterion shifts for certain response categories.

The influence of these late output processes on the integration of visual and auditory motion signals was highlighted in the study by Meyer and Wuerger (2001), the results of which showed that upon presentation of highly ambiguous visual motion, auditory motion can drive responses. On the other hand, the evidence for the existence of multisensory integration processes between motion signals at the perceptual level is still weak.

Some evidence is based on purely phenomenological methods (Anstis, 1973; Zapparoli & Reatto, 1969). Other reports base the evidence for perceptual interactions on the absence of effects when the two inputs are desynchronized (Soto-Faraco, Spence, Fairbank, et al., 2002) or on the modulation of congruency effects by factors that are unlikely to be sensitive to response interference (for example, the fact that motion is experienced or not; Soto-Faraco, Lyons, et al., 2002). The recent study of Kitagawa and Ichihara (2002) argued for the perceptual nature of the cross-modal interactions between motion signals in the depth plane based on the presence of adaptation aftereffects. As several authors have noted, however, even when using adaptation aftereffects, the role of postperceptual factors is not necessarily ruled out (see, e.g., Bertelson & Aschersleben, 1998; Choe et al., 1975; Welch, 1999). Indeed, in the task used by Kitagawa and Ichihara, the criterion to decide the direction of the target sound motion (increasing/decreasing) may have shifted as a function of the direction of the adapting stimulus (looming/receding). It appears, then, that the evidence for perceptual integration is not altogether compelling. Postperceptual accounts are viable because conditions for response interference were present or because the conditions of intersensory conflict were transparent, or both (e.g., Bertelson & Aschersleben, 1998; Bertelson, 1998; Choe et al., 1975; Welch, 1999; Welch & Warren, 1980).

In the case of static ventriloquism, the controversy over perceptual versus postperceptual components has existed for many decades, for the same reasons as noted earlier (see Choe et al., 1975; Radeau & Bertelson, 1976; Welch, 1999). However, in a recent study to address this controversy, Bertelson and Aschersleben (1998; see also Caclin et al., 2002) demonstrated that the perceptual basis of ventriloquism can be addressed using a psychophysical staircase methodology (e.g., Cornsweet, 1962). The key aspects in that study were that the staircase procedure was combined with a task in which the irrelevant stimulus dimensions were neutral with respect to the available responses, and the intersensory conflict situation was not transparent (in the critical trials, participants were not aware of the discrepancy between the two sources of stimulation).

To test whether the congruency effects observed between auditory and visual motion signals (cross-modal dynamic capture) have a perceptual component, Soto-Faraco, Spence, and Kingstone (2002) applied the method of psychophysical staircases while controlling for response bias. The task was to decide if two apparent-motion streams presented simultaneously, one visual and the other auditory, had the same or different directions. Because the response dimension was orthogonal to the direction of the stimuli presented, the role of response competition was neutralized. The SOA between the two components of the visual and the auditory apparent-motion streams was modified according to the staircase procedure. (That is, the two apparent-motion streams were always synchronous, but the temporal lag between the first sound/light and the second sound/light was manipulated.) This method was used to estimate the point of perceptual uncertainty regarding same/different direction judgments, that is, the SOA at which it was no longer possible to distinguish between displays containing visual and auditory streams moving in the same direction and displays containing visual and auditory streams moving in opposite directions. In this region of uncertainty, the information about whether visual and auditory inputs were in conflict was, by definition, not available to the participants for conscious deliberation (i.e., the condition of nontransparency was met).

The staircases consisted of a continuum of auditory apparent-motion streams where the SOA between the two sounds that formed the stream ranged from −1000 ms (left-to-right direction) to +1000 ms (right-to-left direction). For any auditory motion stream in the continuum, a visual motion stream was also presented simultaneously. The direction of the visual apparent-motion streams was fixed along the continuum (always left to right or always right to left), although the SOA varied accordingly to match the duration of the auditory streams. In this way, half of the trials in the continuum contained same-direction displays and the other half contained different-direction displays (Fig. 4.3A).

Four staircases were used combining the starting point and the relative directions of visual and auditory streams. One staircase started with left-to-right sounds and the visual motion always had a right-to-left direction (Fig. 4.3A, top). A second staircase began with right-to-left sounds and the visual motion always had a right-to-left direction (Fig. 4.3A, bottom). Similarly, there was a staircase beginning with left-to-right sounds with left-to-right visual streams, and a staircase beginning with right-to-left sounds with left-to-right visual streams. That is, two of the staircases started at the same-direction extreme of the continuum and the other two started at the different-direction extreme.

The staircases starting from a same-direction extreme moved one step down after each *same* response and one step up after each *different* response. The converse modification rule was applied to the staircases starting from the different-direction extreme. All staircases were run intermixed randomly in a single block. The staircases were stopped after 60 trials each, and the average SOA for the last ten trials of each staircase was assessed as an

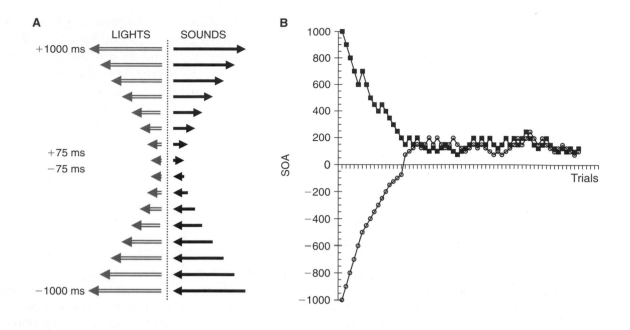

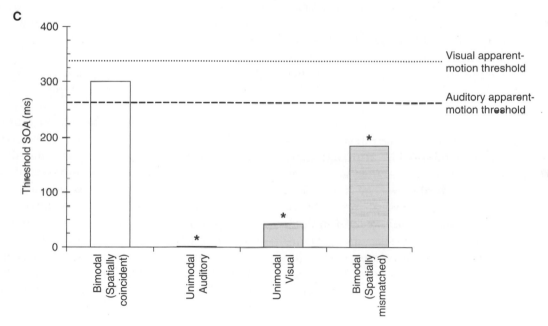

FIGURE 4.3 (*A*) Summary chart representing two of the staircases used (the other continuum was equivalent, except that visual stimuli were presented in a left-to-right direction). The arrowheads represent the direction of motion and the size of the arrows represents the SOA between the first and the second event of an apparent-motion stream. Visual and auditory streams were always presented synchronously and the trajectories were spatially matching (they are represented separately for the sake of clarity; see text for details). One staircase started from the top of the continuum (different-direction extreme) and the other staircase began from the bottom of the continuum (same-direction extreme). (*B*) Representative results of one participant for the two staircases in *A*. Empty symbols represent the SOA at each successive trial in the staircase starting at the same-direction extreme (bottom) of the staircase. Filled symbols represent the SOA at each successive trial in the staircase starting at the opposite-direction extreme (top) of the staircase. (*C*) The bars represent the average threshold SOA for different types of staircases: *left bar*, same/different discrimination in bimodal staircases with spatially coincident auditory and visual motion; *middle bars*, left/right discrimination in unimodal (auditory and visual) staircases; *right bar*, same/different discrimination in bimodal staircases when visual stimulation originated away from the loudspeakers (just left and right of central fixation). The dotted lines represent the average threshold SOA for the perception of apparent motion in audition (thick line) and vision (thin line). The stars indicate significant differences with respect to the bimodal spatially coincident threshold.

estimation of the uncertainty threshold (Cornsweet, 1962).[8]

An example of the results for two of the staircases of one participant are shown in Figure 4.3B. Typically, the staircases starting at the different-direction extreme began to level off before the staircase midpoint was reached. That is, participants started to classify about half of the displays as same-direction, despite all the displays in those staircases contained different-direction streams. In the staircases starting at the same-direction extreme, however, participants responded *same* all the way until the staircase crossed the midpoint (after which the direction of the two apparent-motion streams became *different*) and continued past the midpoint until an SOA, where *different* responses began to occur and the staircase stabilized. Note that for this second type of staircase, the SOAs that range beyond the midpoint up to where responses stabilized indicate the region of SOAs within which the illusion of cross-modal dynamic capture occurred. This region encompassed the SOA of 150 ms used in the experiments reported in the previous section.

There were no statistical differences between the thresholds obtained with the different staircases. The average point of perceptual uncertainty across participants and staircases converged at 300 ms (Fig. 4.3C, first bar on the left). This threshold for cross-modal dynamic capture was significantly higher than the average SOA at which observers could discriminate the direction of motion for auditory (1.1 ms) and visual (41.6 ms) apparent-motion streams when they were presented in isolation (Fig. 4.3C, the second and third bars, respectively). In a related experiment, the psychophysical threshold for apparent motion was assessed for the visual and auditory streams that had been used in the staircases. As Figure 4.3C shows (top and bottom lines, respectively), the threshold for cross-modal dynamic capture (300 ms) fell within the range of visual and auditory apparent motion. This provides independent support for the idea, discussed in the previous section, that motion plays a critical role in the cross-modal dynamic capture illusion.

Is it possible that performance was worse in the bimodal same/different staircases than in the unimodal left/right staircases because of the larger number of stimuli contained in the bimodal displays, or because participants had to attend to two stimuli modalities rather than one? To answer these questions we tested another group of participants in the bimodal staircases (same/different task), with the single exception that the LEDs used to generate the visual apparent-motion stream were placed next to each other in the center of the setup, 15 cm away from the loudspeaker cones. Under these conditions, the attentional load and task difficulty were equal to those of the original staircases (if not higher, because of the spatial mismatch between audio and visual information). But here, and consistent with a perceptual interpretation of the results, the threshold of cross-modal dynamic capture was dramatically reduced (Fig. 4.3C, bar on the right).

In summary, the staircase experiments demonstrate that cross-modal dynamic capture occurs in an experimental context that excludes response competition and potential top-down influences induced by an awareness of cross-modal conflict. These data provide strong support for the existence of early perceptual integration between auditory and visual motion signals.

Cross-modal dynamic capture across audition, touch, and vision

Traditionally, behavioral research on multisensory interactions in the domain of motion has concentrated on audiovisual combinations, studying the effects of one modality on the other (vision on audition or audition on vision). Few studies have addressed the interactions in both directions (audition on vision *and* vision on audition). Additionally, when it comes to motion, the literature has largely ignored the role of other modalities, such as touch and proprioception.[9] The study of each possible intersensory pairing is clearly important, because it is simply not valid to extrapolate how other combinations of modalities will interact from the study of a single modality combination (see, for

---

[8]Averaging over the last steps of the staircase, after the staircase has reached a plateau, is the usual procedure to establish the threshold performance (point of uncertainty in the present case). Occasionally investigators have used the average location of reversals to estimate this point of uncertainty (e.g., Bertelson & Aschersleben, 1998). These calculations were also performed in this study, with equivalent results (see Soto-Faraco, Spence, & Kingstone, 2002, for complete analyses and discussion).

[9]Indeed, this imbalance is present in most areas of multisensory research. An illustrative example is found in the study of spatial biases, which emphasizes audiovisual interactions (the ventriloquist illusion) despite evidence that ventriloquist-like effects can also occur between audition and touch (Caclin et al., 2002), audition and proprioception (Fisher, cited in Howard & Templeton, 1966; Pick, Warren, & Hay, 1969), and vision and proprioception (Botvinick & Cohen, 1998; Hay, Pick, & Ikeda, 1965; Nielsen, 1963; Pavani, Spence, & Driver, 2000; Pick et al., 1969). Moreover, direct comparisons across several pairs of modalities simultaneously have been extremely rare in the literature (see Pick et al., 1969, and Warren & Pick, 1970, for two exceptions).

TABLE 4.2

Average capture effect (congruent-conflicting accuracy) in every pairing of auditory, tactile, and visual motion

Target Modality	Distracter Modality			
	Audition	Touch	Vision	**Avg.**
Audition	—	36.2%*	46.4%*	**41.3%**
Touch	14.4%*	—	44.0%*	**29.4%**
Vision	2.9%	1.3%	—	**2.1%**
Avg.	**8.6%**	**18.7%**	**45.2%**	—

Note: Results of the Soto-Faraco et al. (2000) study. The percentages shown in the center cells are the result of subtracting the conflicting from the congruent trials in the synchronous condition, for the combination of modalities given by the row and column. Those percentages marked with an asterisk are significantly different from zero ($p \leq 0.05$). The averages in the column on the far right represent an estimation of how much a modality is susceptible to capture by others. The averages in the bottom row represent an estimation of how much a particular modality is able to capture others.

example, Pick, Warren, & Hay, 1969; Soto-Faraco, Spence, Fairbank, et al., 2002, on this point).

One of the first studies to address the effects of a static event in one modality on the perception of motion in another modality, outside the audiovisual case, was Gilbert's (1939) experiment on the effects of an electric shock on the threshold for visual apparent motion. More recently, various researchers have addressed the effects of brief vibrotactile stimuli on the perceived trajectory of a moving visual stimulus (Berrio et al., 1999; Shimojo et al., 2001), replicating the "bouncing disks" phenomenon (Sekuler et al., 1997) using a vibrotactile stimulus instead of a sound. Regarding the cross-modal studies addressing multisensory integration between two dynamic sources, several authors have investigated cross-modal interactions in the perception of motion between auditory and visual stimuli in both ways: audition on vision and vision on audition (Allen & Kolers, 1981; Kitagawa & Ichihara, 2002; Ohmura, 1987). Studies addressing modality combinations other than audiovisual simply have not, to the best of our knowledge, been published.

CROSS-MODAL DYNAMIC CAPTURE COMBINING SOUNDS, TOUCHES, AND LIGHTS In this section we present data from several recent experiments from our laboratory in which the investigation of cross-modal dynamic capture was extended beyond the audiovisual case to explore the potential interactions between dynamically presented sound, touch, and visual stimulation (Soto-Faraco, Kingstone, & Spence, 2000).[10]

Six experiments were carried out, one for each of the six potential combinations of target and distracter modalities, using cross-modal pairings of audition, touch, and vision. The original setup described earlier in this chapter was slightly modified to incorporate tactile stimulation: participants rested their index fingers on vibrotactile stimulators placed on a foam cube near the loudspeakers and LEDs and responded using two foot pedals that were placed beneath their right and left feet. In each experiment, participants had to discriminate the direction of motion of the target modality while ignoring distracter apparent motion in another modality.

The results were clear: auditory apparent motion was strongly influenced by visual apparent motion (46%, replicating previous results) and by tactile apparent motion (36%); tactile apparent motion was modulated by visual apparent motion (44%) and, to a smaller degree, by auditory apparent motion (15%); and, finally, visual apparent motion was uninfluenced by auditory or tactile apparent motion (Table 4.2). The capture effects always occurred in the synchronous condition but not in the control asynchronous condition, indicating that participants were not confused about which target modality demanded a response.

This array of data raises several interesting issues about multisensory integration of dynamic events. First, it indicates that cross-modal dynamic capture is a widespread phenomenon that can be observed using visuo-tactile and audiotactile combinations, and therefore it is not particular to audiovisual interactions. Moreover,

---

[10]Reports of tactile apparent motion are almost as old as Werthemer's (1912) famous paper on the visual appearance of motion (the phi phenomenon). Benussi (1913, 1914), Burtt (1917b), and many other authors since then (see Hulin, 1927, for a review of the early studies; Kirman, 1974; Lakatos

& Shepard, 1997; Sherrick & Rogers, 1966, for more recent examples) have studied tactile apparent motion experimentally. Furthermore, tactile, auditory, and visual apparent motion seem to follow the same constraints (e.g., Lakatos & Shepard, 1997).

the existence of audiotactile interactions indicates that a direct involvement of visual motion is not even necessary for cross-modal dynamic capture to occur (this is in agreement with other multisensory integration effects; see Caclin et al., 2002; Welch, 1999). Second, multisensory interactions between dynamic events appear to be asymmetric phenomena. That is, the fact that cross-modal dynamic capture occurs for a pair of modalities in one direction (e.g., vision captures audition) does not necessarily mean that the capture will occur in the other direction (e.g., audition does not capture vision). This result argues against an interpretation of cross-modal dynamic capture based on the existence of a processing bottleneck that would preclude the simultaneous perception of two independent motion streams in different sensory modalities.

MODALITY DOMINANCE AND CROSS-MODAL DYNAMIC CAPTURE Asymmetries like the one just described for vision and audition are common in the multisensory integration literature regarding static stimuli (e.g., Pick et al., 1969; Radeau & Bertelson, 1976, 1987; Rock & Harris, 1967). Of particular interest is the study of Pick et al. (1969; see also Warren & Pick, 1970), in which six potential combinations of target and distractor modalities (from vision, audition, and proprioception) were tested within a single paradigm. The results of the study showed that vision significantly influenced the localization performance in proprioception and audition; proprioception influenced audition and audition influenced proprioception (but to a lesser extent); and finally, proprioception and audition did not significantly influence visual performance. This pattern of results closely mirrors the results just described using apparent motion (Soto-Faraco et al., 2000), with the exception that Soto-Faraco et al. used tactile rather than proprioceptive stimulation (although the proprioceptive stimuli used by Pick et al. did actually include a tactile component; see Caclin et al., 2002, on this point).

In the domain of multisensory integration of moving events, asymmetries were also reported in the past. Allen and Kolers (1981, Experiment 2) and Ohmura (1987) observed that the threshold of visual apparent motion was unaffected by simultaneous sounds, whereas the threshold of auditory apparent motion was modulated by visual stimulation (although, as discussed in the introduction to this chapter, the results of the two studies were discrepant about the exact nature of the interaction). Additionally, some researchers have presented phenomenological reports of cross-modal dynamic capture which noted that, when sound and visual motion were directionally conflicting, sounds appeared to move in the direction of the visual motion rather than the other

way around, therefore suggesting an asymmetry in favor of visual information (Anstis, 1973; Zapparoli & Reatto, 1969). This dominance of vision in the domain of motion is in agreement with the data presented here. It also accords with the recent results of Kitagawa and Ichihara (2002), who found that visual motion (looming/receding) adaptors produced auditory intensity (raising/falling) aftereffects, whereas the auditory intensity adapters did not produce visual motion aftereffects. It is noteworthy that, despite the important methodological differences among all these studies, the direction of the asymmetries found is fairly consistent.[11]

Other studies, however, point to the possibility that this pattern of asymmetries may be malleable by showing that visual motion can be influenced by auditory information (e.g., Meyer & Wuerger, 2001; Zietz & Werner, 1927). Although their methodologies varied widely, these studies coincided in one important aspect; they measured multisensory dynamic interactions under conditions in which the visual motion signal was at or below threshold levels. In particular, Meyer and Wuerger (2001) observed a small influence of auditory motion on visual motion discrimination only when the visual motion was highly ambiguous (coherence of the random dot kinematogram was between 5% and 15%). The experiment of Zietz and Werner (1927) was also based on the fact that the visual displays could barely generate any sensation of movement. It is clear, then, that visual motion perception can be influenced by input in another modality when it is ambiguous (note that the finding of Sekuler et al. [1997] would also fall in this category).

---

[11]Further evidence of asymmetries outside the audiovisual case in previous cross-modal studies of dynamic events is nonexistent and can only be inferred from experiments addressing other issues. In a study by Klein (1977), the congruency effect in accuracy for proprioceptive motion judgments with motion visual distractors was noticeably larger than the congruency effect in the reverse condition (visual target motion with proprioceptive distractor motion), suggesting a potential asymmetry. In another study, Sherrick (1976) reported the results of a temporal order judgment (TOJ) experiment in which two sounds were delivered to alternate ears or two touches were delivered to alternate hands. Although he did not study apparent motion directly, the conditions tested were very close to the ones used in the audiotactile experiments of Soto-Faraco et al. (2000) described in this section. In Sherrick's experiment, TOJs in one modality (auditory or tactile) were measured as a function of the congruency of simultaneous input presented in the other modality. From the graphs presented by Sherrick (1976, pp. 153–154) it can be inferred that the influence of irrelevant touch on auditory TOJs was larger than the influence of sounds on tactile TOJs, thus suggesting a potential asymmetry between the two modalities.

In general terms, the findings discussed above may point to the idea that changes in the strength of multisensory interactions can be modulated by certain cognitive or top-down factors such as attention (e.g., Canon, 1970, 1971; Warren & Schmitt, 1978) or expectations (e.g., Bertelson, 1998; Welch, 1999).[12] But what is the interpretation of asymmetries between motion signals in different modalities when the potential role of cognitive factors is kept to a minimum? One possibility is that the perceptual system is organized so that input from one modality will receive a higher weighting in the integration process than input from another modality. Along these lines, some researchers have argued that humans may have an inherent bias to attend to vision (Bald, Berrien, Price, & Sprague, 1942; Colavita, 1974; Hohnsbein, Falkenstein, & Hoormann, 1991; Klein, 1977; Posner, Nissen, & Klein, 1976; Spence, Shore, & Klein, 2001).[13] Although this visual dominance account may explain the hierarchy of modalities found in multisensory integration of motion, it performs poorly with findings such as the auditory dominance of vision in the perception of temporal order (e.g., Morein-Zamir, Soto-Faraco, & Kingstone, 2001, 2003; Shams, Kamitani, & Shimojo, 2000; Welch, Warren, & DuttonHurt, 1986; see Shams, Kamitani, & Shimojo, this volume, for a review). Other researchers have argued that modality dominance may

depend on what modality produces the most accurate information for the particular task being performed (e.g., Welch & Warren, 1980). This account highlights the importance of intrinsic processing factors as a possible source of any asymmetries. For instance, in the case of motion, because vision typically provides more accurate directional information than other sensory systems, it would tend to dominate when intersensory conflict occurs.

The other potential source for cross-modal asymmetries, including the asymmetries found in multisensory interactions for moving stimuli, has to do with the stimulus properties themselves. Indeed, if input in one modality is presented at a higher intensity or has a better "quality" of information than input in another modality, the integration process may be biased by the more salient input. In this case, asymmetries would be the consequence of a particular set of stimulus values rather than a built-in feature of the processing system (e.g., Welch & Warren, 1980, 1986). There are many cases in which it is difficult to control for these imbalances in an objective way, because the types of energy used by the different senses may be difficult to compare, and therefore trying to disentangle processing factors and stimulus properties is difficult (see, e.g., Spence et al., 2001).[14]

The multisensory integration of dynamic events in vision and audition is a case in point (Kitagawa & Ichihara, 2002; Soto-Faraco, Spence, & Kingstone, 2002, in press). The visual dominance found in the study of Kitagawa and Ichihara (2002) was attributed to intrinsic processing mechanisms. However, the cues used to generate auditory motion in depth (intensity changes) may have been less effective in conveying the impression of motion than the cues used for visual motion in depth (size change or binocular disparity). Nevertheless, these concerns are at least partially alleviated in studies where the stimuli are equated along some variables, such as the subjective quality of the motion signals (Soto-Faraco, Spence, & Kingstone, in

---

[12]The involvement of attention in cross-modal integration has been brought into question recently (Bertelson, Vroomen, de Gelder, & Driver, 2000; Caclin et al., 2002; Driver, 1996; Spence & Driver, 2000; Vroomen, Bertelson, & de Gelder, 2001). For example, Driver (1996) showed that multisensory integration can serve as the basis for attentional selection, implying that it occurs pre-attentively. It is worth noting that these results may reflect the distinction between different means of manipulating attention: attentional effects seem to be found more readily by manipulating the distribution of attention across modalities (Canon, 1970, 1971; Warren & Schmitt, 1978) than when manipulating the spatial distribution of attention (e.g., Bertelson et al., 2000; Driver, 1996; Spence & Driver, 2000; Vroomen et al., 2001). Regarding cross-modal dynamic capture, no studies have yet addressed a systematic manipulation of attention. Ongoing research in our own laboratory points to the possible existence of attentional modulation in cross-modal dynamic capture (Soto-Faraco et al., 2000). And in agreement with the point above, these experiments manipulated the cross-modal distribution of attention between sensory modalities rather than its spatial distribution.

[13]Some authors have also highlighted the role of reflexive attention in visual dominance by pointing out that the attentional bias toward visual stimuli may be due to intrinsic properties of the visual events that would make them more "attention-grabbing" than other sensory stimuli (see Spence et al., 2001).

---

[14]The potential solutions that have been proposed to address this issue normally involve describing different modality stimuli according to some common metric, such as the decibel scale (e.g., Kohfeld, 1971; Stevens, 1955), detection threshold (Goldstone, 1968), magnitude estimations (e.g., Bolanowski, Zwislocki, & Gescheider, 1991; West, Ward, & Khosla, 2000; Zwislocki & Goodman, 1980), or cross-modal matching (e.g., Baird, 1975; Stevens & Marks, 1980). However, often these methods bear on other kinds of processes such as decision criteria, distribution of attention, response strategies, and expectations (particularly true for those requiring observers to make subjective judgments such as estimations or comparisons).

press) or the psychophysical threshold for the perception of apparent motion (Soto-Faraco, Spence, et al., 2002).

Summary and conclusions

In this chapter we have reviewed previous research on multisensory integration in motion perception and presented recent data of our own. Several studies have shown that static stimulation in one modality can modulate certain aspects of the perception of dynamic information in another modality. Typically, auditory and tactile stimuli can introduce changes in the threshold at which visual apparent motion is experienced (Gilbert, 1939; Hall & Earle, 1954; Hall et al., 1952; Maass, 1938; Zietz & Werner, 1927), although this has not always been the case (Allen & Kolers, 1981; Staal & Donderi, 1983). The trajectory of visual apparent motion (Hall & Earle, 1954; Hall et al., 1952; Sekuler & Sekuler, 1999; Sekuler et al., 1997; Shimojo et al., 2001; Watanabe & Shimojo, 2001) and even its perceived velocity (Manabe & Riquimaroux, 2000) have also been shown to be modulated by static stimulation in vision and touch. Modulations of auditory apparent motion as a function of static stimulation in other modalities have been studied far less. The extant data suggest that cross-modal influences do occur, although their nature remains unclear (Allen & Kolers, 1981; Ohmura, 1987).

Evidence for multisensory integration of information from two moving events has been fragmentary and sometimes open to important methodological questions. Among the more important concerns is the fact that stimuli have often been presented from different spatial locations (e.g., Allen & Kolers, 1981; Kitagawa & Ichihara, 2002; Staal & Donderi, 1983; Zapparoli & Reatto, 1969), thus weakening the chances of multisensory interactions (e.g., Soto-Faraco, Lyons, et al., 2002; Stein & Meredith, 1993). Another potentially important issue concerns the actual role that dynamic attributes (i.e., motion direction) play in studies of dynamic multisensory integration. From the results described here about the critical role of motion (Soto-Faraco, Lyons, et al., 2002; Soto-Faraco, Spence, & Kingstone, 2002, in press), as well as the data from experiments using continuous motion (e.g., Kitagawa & Ichihara, 2002; Meyer & Wuerger, 2001; Soto-Faraco, Spence, & Kingstone, in press), it seems reasonable to conclude that multisensory integration processes for dynamic stimulus information exist, over and above the multisensory integration processes that have been described for static stimulus information.

Given the existence of cross-modal dynamic interactions, another important issue concerns the level of processing at which these interactions occur. Response interference and decisional biases (postperceptual processes) are very likely involved in many of the observed cross-modal interactions between dynamic events (Meyer & Wuerger, 2001). These processes imply the action of general cognitive processes that are not specifically related to motion or to cross-modal stimulation. A contribution of earlier (i.e., perceptual) processes that are related specifically to the integration of motion information during perception has also been suggested. Here we have discussed some of the difficulties in isolating the early components of multisensory interactions and have described one study that attempted to demonstrate the perceptual aspects of multisensory integration of motion by neutralizing the contribution of late postperceptual processes (Soto-Faraco, Spence, & Kingstone, 2002; see also Vroomen & de Gelder, 2003, for another recent example). The data are consistent with the idea that, in agreement with other multisensory phenomena, early integration processes play a significant role in multisensory integration of dynamic information.

Finally, this chapter has addressed the existence and interpretation of modality dominance for dynamic interactions. Certain asymmetries, such as visual motion signals influencing the perception of auditory motion but not vice versa, have been found consistently across a wide range of methodologies (e.g., Allen & Kolers, 1981; Anstis, 1973; Kitagawa & Ichiara, 2001; Soto-Faraco, Spence, & Kingstone, 2002, in press; Staal & Donderi, 1983). We have described data from our own studies suggesting the presence of other asymmetries, including those between audition and touch and between vision and touch. In general, the data on dynamic multisensory integration research indicate that visual input is more influential than input from other sensory modalities, although there are some exceptions. It is important to note, however, that the data do not support a simple visual dominance position in which cross-modal interactions map to a fixed, predetermined pattern. Rather, it appears that a more flexible relation exists between the modalities. Whether this relation is based on the distribution of attention, on the appropriateness of the modality for the particular task, or on a combination of these factors (see Spence et al., 2001; Welch, 1999; Welch & Warren, 1980) is an important matter for future research.

ACKNOWLEDGMENTS Work was supported in part by a Killam postdoctoral fellowship (S.S.-F.) and by grants from the Michael Smith Foundation for Health Research, the National Science and Engineering Research Council of Canada, and the Human Frontier Science Program (A. K.).

REFERENCES

Allen, P. G., & Kolers, P. A. (1981). Sensory specificity of apparent motion. *Journal of Experimental Psychology: Human Perception and Performance, 7,* 1318–1326.

Anstis, S. M. (1973). Hearing with the hands. *Perception, 2,* 337–341.

Aspell, J. E., Bramwell, D. I., & Hurlbert, A. C. (2000). Interactions between visual and auditory movement perception in a direction discrimination task. *Perception, 29* (Suppl), 74.

Baird, J. C. (1975). Psychophysical study of numbers: IV. Generalized preferred state theory. *Psychological Research, 38,* 175–187.

Bald, L., Berrien, F. K., Price, J. B., & Sprague, R. O. (1942). Errors in perceiving the temporal order of auditory and visual stimuli. *Journal of Applied Psychology, 26,* 382–388.

Benussi, V. (1913). Kinematohaptische Erscheinungen (Vorläufige Mitteilung über Scheinbewegungsauffassung aufgrund haptischer Eindrücke) [Kinematohaptic illusion (preliminary report on apparent motion from haptic sensations)]. *Archiv für die Gesamte Psychologie, 29,* 385–388.

Benussi, V. (1914). Kinematohaptische Scheinbewegungen und Auffassungsumformung [Kinematohaptic apparent movement and the change of perception]. *Bericht VI Kongress für Experimentelle Psychologie* (pp. 31–35). Göttingen.

Berrio, V., Lupiánez, J., Spence, C., & Martos, F. (1999). *Audiovisual integration affects perception of apparent motion and momentum.* Poster presented at the First International Multisensory Research Conference: Crossmodal Attention and Multisensory Integration. Oxford, England, October 1–2. Available: http://www.wfubmc.edu/nba/IMRF/99abstracts.html.

Bertelson, P. (1998). Starting from the ventriloquist: The perception of multimodal events. In M. Sabourin, C. Fergus, et al. (Eds.), *Advances in psychological science: Vol. 2. Biological and cognitive aspects* (pp. 419–439). Hove, England: Psychology Press.

Bertelson, P., & Aschersleben, G. (1998). Automatic visual bias of perceived auditory location. *Psychonomic Bulletin and Review, 5,* 482–489.

Bertelson, P., & Radeau, M. (1981). Cross-modal bias and perceptual fusion with auditory-visual spatial discordance. *Perception and Psychophysics, 29,* 578–587.

Bertelson, P., Vroomen, J., de Gelder, B., & Driver, J. (2000). The ventriloquist effect does not depend on the direction of deliberate visual attention. *Perception & Psychophysics, 62,* 321–332.

Bolanowski, S. J., Zwislocki, J. J., & Gescheider, G. A. (1991). Intersensory generality of psychological units. In S. J. Bolanowski and G. A. Gescheider (Eds.), *Ratio scale of psychological magnitude* (pp. 277–293). Hillsdale, NJ: Erlsbaum.

Botvinick, M., & Cohen, J. (1998). Rubber hands "feel" touch that eyes see. *Nature, 391,* 756.

Burtt, H. E. (1917a). Auditory illusions of movement: A preliminary study. *Journal of Experimental Psychology, 2,* 63–75.

Burtt, H. E. (1917b). Tactile illusions of movement. *Journal of Experimental Psychology, 2,* 371–385.

Caclin, A., Soto-Faraco, S., Kingstone, A., & Spence, C. (2002). Tactile "capture" of audition. *Perception & Psychophysics, 64,* 616–630.

Canon, L. K. (1970). Intermodality inconsistency of input and directed attention as determinants of the nature of adaptation. *Journal of Experimental Psychology, 84,* 141–147.

Canon, L. K. (1971). Directed attention and maladaptive "adaptation" to displacement of the visual field. *Journal of Experimental Psychology, 88,* 403–408.

Choe, C. S., Welch, R. B., Gilford, R. M., & Juola, J. F. (1975). The "ventriloquist effect": Visual dominance or response bias? *Perception & Psychophysics, 18,* 55–60.

Colavita, F. B. (1974). Human sensory dominance. *Perception & Psychophysics, 16,* 409–412.

Cornsweet, T. N. (1962). The staircase method in psychophysics. *American Journal of Psychology, 75,* 485–491.

Driver, J. (1996). Enhancement of selective listening by illusory mislocation of speech sounds due to lip-reading. *Nature, 381,* 66–68.

Gazzaniga, M. S. (1987). Perceptual and attentional processes following callosal section in humans. *Neuropsychologia, 25,* 119–133.

Gilbert, G. M. (1939). Dynamic psychophysics and the phi phenomenon. *Archives of Psychology, 237,* 5–43.

Goldstone, S. (1968). Reaction time to onset and termination of lights and sounds. *Perceptual and Motor Skills, 27,* 1023–1029.

Hall, K. R. L., & Earle, A. E. (1954). A further study of the pendulum phenomenon. *Quarterly Journal of Experimental Psychology, 6,* 112–124.

Hall, K. R. L., Earle, A. E., & Crookes, T. G. (1952). A pendulum phenomenon in the visual perception of apparent movement. *Quarterly Journal of Experimental Psychology, 4,* 109–120.

Hay, J. C., Pick, H. L., & Ikeda, K. (1965). Visual capture produced by prism spectacles. *Psychonomic Science, 2,* 215–216.

Hohnsbein, J., Falkenstein, M., & Hoormann, J. (1991). Visual dominance is reflected in reaction times and event-related potentials (ERPs). In B. Blum (Ed.), *Channels in the visual nervous system: Neurophysiology, psychophysics and models* (pp. 315–333). London: Freund.

Howard, I. P., & Templeton, W. B. (1966). *Human spatial orientation.* New York: Wiley.

Hulin, W. S. (1927). An experimental study of apparent tactual movement. *Journal of Experimental Psychology, 10,* 293–320.

Kirman, J. H. (1974). Tactile apparent movement: The effects of interstimulus onset interval and stimulus duration. *Perception & Psychophysics, 15,* 1–6.

Kitagawa, N., & Ichihara, S. (2002). Hearing visual motion in depth. *Nature, 416,* 172–174.

Klein, R. M. (1977). Attention and visual dominance: A chronometric analysis. *Journal of Experimental Psychology: Human Perception and Performance, 3,* 365–378.

Kohfeld, D. (1971). Simple reaction times as a function of stimulus intensity in decibels of light and sound. *Journal of Experimental Psychology, 88,* 251–257.

Kolers, P. A. (1964). The illusion of movement. *Scientific American, 21,* 98–106.

Korte, A. (1915). Kinematoscopische Untersuchungen. *Zeitschrift für Psychologie, 72,* 193–296.

Lakatos, S. (1995). The influence of visual cues on the localisation of circular auditory motion. *Perception, 24,* 457–465.

Lakatos, S., & Shepard, R. N. (1997). Constraints common to apparent motion in visual, tactile and auditory space.

Journal of Experimental Psychology: Human Perception and Performance, 23, 1050–1060.

Maass, H. (1938). Über den Einfluss akustischer Rhythmen auf optische Bewegungsgestaltungen [About the influence of acoustic rhythms on visual motion]. (Sander, F.: Ganzheit und Gestalt. Psychol. Untersuch. VIII). *Archiv für die Gesamte Psychologie, 100,* 424–464.

Manabe, K., & Riquimaroux, H. (2000). Sound controls velocity perception of visual apparent motion. *Journal of the Acoustical Society of Japan, 21,* 171–174.

Mateef, S., Hohnsbein, J., & Noack, T. (1985). Dynamic visual capture: Apparent auditory motion induced by a moving visual target. *Perception, 14,* 721–727.

Meyer, G. F., & Wuerger, M. (2001). Cross-modal integration of auditory and visual motion signals. *NeuroReport, 12,* 2557–2560.

Morein-Zamir, S., Soto-Faraco, S., & Kingstone, A. (2001). Captured vision: Sounds influence the perception of visual temporal order. *Abstracts of the Psychonomic Society, 6,* 623.

Morein-Zamir, S., Soto-Faraco, S., & Kingstone, A. (2003). Auditory capture of vision: Examining temporal ventriloquism. *Cognitive Brain Research, 17,* 154–163.

Nielsen, T. I. (1963). Volition: A new experimental approach. *Scandinavian Journal of Psychology, 4,* 225–230.

Ohmura, H. (1987). Intersensory influences on the perception of apparent movement. *Japanese Psychological Research, 29,* 1–19.

Pavani, F., Spence, C., & Driver, J. (2000). Visual capture of touch: Out-of-the-body experiences with rubber gloves. *Psychological Science, 11,* 353–359.

Pick, H. L., Warren, D. H., & Hay, J. C. (1969). Sensory conflict in judgments of spatial direction. *Perception & Psychophysics, 6,* 203–205.

Posner, M. I., Nissen, M. J., & Klein, R. M. (1976). Visual dominance: An information-processing account of its origins and significance. *Psychological Review, 83,* 157–171.

Radeau, M., & Bertelson, P. (1976). The effect of a textured visual field on modality dominance in a ventriloquism situation. *Perception & Psychophysics, 20,* 227–235.

Radeau, M., & Bertelson, P. (1987). Auditory-visual interaction and the timing of inputs: Thomas (1941) revisited. *Psychological Research, 49,* 17–22.

Rock, I., & Harris, C. S. (1967). Vision and touch. *Scientific American, 216,* 96–104.

Sekuler, A. B., & Sekuler, R. (1999). Collisions between moving visual targets: What controls alternative ways of seeing an ambiguous display? *Perception, 28,* 415–432.

Sekuler, R., Sekuler, A. B., & Lau, R. (1997). Sound alters visual motion perception. *Nature, 385,* 308.

Shams, L., Kamitani, Y., & Shimojo, S. (2000). What you see is what you hear. *Nature, 408,* 788.

Sherrick, C. E. (1976). The antagonisms of hearing and touch. In S. K. Hirsh, D. H. Eldredge, I. J., Hirsh, & S. R. Silverman (Eds.), *Hearing and Davis: Essays honoring Hallowell Davis* (pp. 149–158). St. Louis, MO: Washington University Press.

Sherrick, C. E., & Rogers, R. (1966). Apparent haptic movement. *Perception & Psychophysics, 1,* 175–180.

Shimojo, S., Scheier, C., Nijhawan, R., Shams, L., Kamitani, Y., & Watanabe, K. (2001). Beyond perceptual modality: Auditory effects on visual perception. *Acoustical Science and Technology, 22,* 61–67.

Soto-Faraco, S., Kingstone, A., & Spence, C. (2000). The role of movement and attention in modulating audiovisual and audiotactile "ventriloquism" effects. *Abstracts of the Psychonomic Society, 5,* 40.

Soto-Faraco, S., Lyons, J., Gazzaniga, M. S., Spence, C., & Kingstone, A. (2002). The ventriloquist in motion: Illusory capture of dynamic information across sensory modalities. *Cognitive Brain Research, 14,* 139–146.

Soto-Faraco, S., Spence, C., & Kingstone, A. (2002). *Automatic visual capture of auditory apparent motion.* Manuscript submitted for publication.

Soto-Faraco, S., Spence, C., & Kingstone, A. (in press). *Crossmodal dynamic capture: Congruency effects in the perception of motion across sensory modalities. Journal of Experimental Psychology: Human pereception and performance.* Manuscript submitted for publication.

Soto-Faraco, S., Spence, C., Fairbank, K., Kingstone, A., Hillstrom, A. P., & Shapiro, K. (2002). A crossmodal attentional blink between vision and touch. *Psychonomic Bulletin and Review, 9,* 731–738.

Spence, C., & Driver, J. (2000). Attracting attention to the illusory location of a sound: Reflexive crossmodal orienting and ventriloquism. *NeuroReport: For Rapid Communication of Neuroscience Research, 11,* 2057–2061.

Spence, C., Shore, D. I., & Klein, R. M. (2001). Multisensory prior entry. *Journal of Experimental Psychology: General, 130,* 799–837.

Staal, H. E., & Donderi, D. C. (1983). The effect of sound on visual apparent movement. *American Journal of Psychology, 96,* 95–105.

Stein, B. E., & Meredith, M. A. (1993). *The merging of the senses.* Cambridge, MA: MIT Press.

Stevens, J. C., & Marks, L. E. (1980). Cross-modality matching functions generated by magnitude estimation. *Perception & Psychophysics, 27,* 379–389.

Stevens, S. S. (1955). Decibels of light and sound. *Physics Today, 8,* 12–17.

Vroomen, J., Bertelson, P., & de Gelder, B. (2001). The ventriloquist effect does not depend on the direction of automatic visual attention. *Perception & Psychophysics, 63,* 651–659.

Vroomen, J., & de Gelder, B. (2003). Visual motion influences the contingent auditory motion after-effect. *Psychological Science, 14,* 357–361.

Warren, D. H., & Pick, H. L. (1970). Intermodality relations in localization in blind and sighted people. *Perception & Psychophysics, 8,* 430–432.

Warren, D. H., & Schmitt, T. L. (1978). On the plasticity of visual-proprioceptive bias effects. *Journal of Experimental Psychology: Human Perception and Performance, 4,* 302–310.

Watanabe, K., & Shimojo, S. (2001). When sound affects vision: Effects of auditory grouping on visual motion perception. *Psychological Science, 121,* 109–116.

Welch, R. B. (1999). Meaning, attention, and the "unity assumption" in the intersensory bias of spatial and temporal perceptions. In G. Ascherlseben, T. Bachmann, & J. Musseler (Eds.), *Cognitive contributions to the perception of spatial and temporal events* (pp. 371–387): Amsterdam: Elsevier.

Welch, R. B., DuttonHurt, L. D., & Warren, D. H. (1986). Contributions of audition and vision to temporal rate perception. *Perception & Psychophysics, 39,* 294–300.

Welch, R. B., & Warren, D. H. (1980). Immediate perceptual response to intersensory discrepancy. *Psychological Bulletin, 88,* 638–667.

Welch, R. B., & Warren, D. H. (1986). Intersensory interactions. In K. R. Boff, L. Kaufman, & J. P. Thomas (Eds.), *Handbook of perception and human performance: Vol. 1. Sensory processes and perception* (pp. 25.1–25.36). New York: Wiley.

Wertheimer, M. (1912). Experimentelle Studien über das Sehen von Bewegung. [Experimental studies on the visual perception of movement]. *Zeitschrift für Psychologie, 61,* 161–265.

West, R. L., Ward, L. M., & Khosla, R. (2000). Constrained scaling: The effect of learned psychophysical scales on idiosyncratic response bias. *Perception & Psychophysics, 62,* 137–151.

Wuerger, S. M., Hofbauer, M., & Meyer, G. F. (2002). The integration of auditory and visual motion signals. Manuscript submitted for publication.

Zapparoli, G. C., & Reatto, L. L. (1969). The apparent movement between visual and acoustic stimulus and the problem of intermodal relations. *Acta Psychologica, 29,* 256–267.

Zietz, K., & Werner, H. (1927). Über die dynamische Struktur der Bewegung. Werner's Studien über Strukturgesetze, VIII. [On the dynamic structure of movement. Werner's studies on the laws of structure, VIII]. *Zeitschrift für Psychologie, 105,* 226–249.

Zihl, J., von Cramon, D., & Mai, N. (1983). Selective disturbance of movement vision after bilateral brain damage. *Brain, 106,* 313–340.

Zwislocki, J. J., & Goodman, D. A. (1980). Absolute scaling of sensory magnitudes: A validation. *Perception & Psychophysics, 28,* 28–38.

5 Sweet and Sour Smells: Learned Synesthesia Between the Senses of Taste and Smell

RICHARD J. STEVENSON AND ROBERT A. BOAKES

Introduction

Telephones ring, dogs bark, and computers hum, yet seeing any of these objects when their characteristic sound is absent does not automatically induce a compelling auditory hallucination of that sound. In olfaction, this type of automatic cross-modal hallucination can occur routinely. Certain odors, such as vanilla, are consistently reported as smelling sweet, yet sweetness is normally associated with the stimulation of another sense, that of taste. This phenomenon has been termed odor-taste synesthesia (Stevenson, Boakes, & Prescott, 1998), and its prevalence, reliability, validity, and origins are the focus of this chapter.

Because considerable confusion surrounds use of the terms taste and smell, the following definitions are used here. *Taste* refers to sensations induced primarily by stimulation of receptors located on the surface of the tongue (McLaughlin & Margolskee, 1994). The five basic taste sensations (along with their prototypical stimuli) are sweet (sucrose), salty (sodium chloride), sour (citric acid), bitter (quinine), and umami, or "meaty taste" (monosodium glutamate). On the other hand, odors (*smells*) are detected by receptors on the olfactory epithelium, which is located a short distance back from the bridge of the nose (Buck, 1996). There is a separate piece of olfactory epithelium for each nostril (Lanza & Clerico, 1995). An unusual feature of olfaction is that the receptors can be stimulated by two anatomically distinct routes: either via the nose, by sniffing (orthonasal olfaction), or via the mouth, as volatile chemicals rise up the nasopharynx during eating and drinking (retronasal olfaction; Pierce & Halpern, 1996). There appear to be about 1000 different types of olfactory receptors, with the result that olfactory sensations are far more diverse than the range of sensations produced by the relatively small set of taste receptors.

Occurrence

The most commonly documented form of synesthesia is the illusory perception of written words, numbers, or letters as having particular colors (e.g., Marks, 1975). The prevalence of this kind of synesthesia is low, estimated at approximately 1 in 2000 people (Baron-Cohen, Burt, Smith-Laittan, Harrison, & Bolton, 1996). Equivalent data on the prevalence of odor-taste synesthesia have not been collected, probably because it is such a common effect that it has largely escaped popular and scientific attention.

Based on evidence from several sources, the majority of people appear to experience odor-taste synesthesia. First, *sweet* is one of the most common descriptors applied to odors (Harper, Land, Griffiths, & Bate-Smith, 1968). A large number of odorants that differ widely both chemically and perceptually are commonly described as sweet. Second, in studies in which a large number of participants (100–200) have profiled sets of odors on many dimensions (i.e., rating how similar the odor smells to a large number of descriptors), there is typically more agreement that a given odor is sweet than agreement on its other properties. In a major study of this kind, Dravnieks (1985) found that of 140 participants asked to describe a strawberry odor, 110 reported that it smelled sweet, but only 60 reported that it smelled like strawberries and 99 that it was fruitlike. The many other such examples include amyl acetate, which is widely used as a banana flavoring in confectionery products. Although 76 of 139 participants reported that it had a sweet odor, only 60 of 139 reported the odor as banana-like and 73 of 139 reported it as fruitlike. Such data point to the conclusion that, when smelling an odor, most people can more easily recognize a tastelike quality such as sweetness than more specific qualities such as strawberry- or banana-likeness.

A third source of evidence is research that has examined the similarity between sweet tastes and sweet smells. Such studies have concentrated on a phenomenon termed *sweetness enhancement*. Sweetness enhancement occurs when a sucrose solution containing a sweet-smelling odor is judged to be sweeter than plain sucrose (e.g., Frank & Byram, 1988; Frank, Ducheny, & Mize, 1989). In two experiments requiring such comparisons (Stevenson, Prescott, & Boakes, 1999), we found that all but two of 31 participants experienced a sweetness enhancement effect. Insofar as sweetness enhancement is a direct consequence of odors smelling sweet, these results strengthen the conclusion that it is a very common experience to perceive sweetness when sniffing certain odors.

Reliability

The reliability of color-word (letter or number) synesthesia is impressive. In one case study, Baron-Cohen, Wyke, and Binnie (1987) found that 2.5 months after an initial test, a particular synesthete was able to provide identical color descriptions for the 103 test words. Similar results were obtained with a larger group of color-word synesthetes, who showed 98% accuracy at a retest conducted one hour after the original test. This contrasted with the 19% accuracy of a nonsynesthetic control group. As yet there are no comparable data for assessing the reliability of odor-taste synesthesia. Nevertheless, we can extract data on the reliability of odor sweetness ratings from experiments that we have carried out for other reasons. Because unfamiliar odors are more labile and less discriminable than familiar odors (e.g., Rabin, 1988; Rabin & Cain, 1984), they may also show less test-retest reliability than familiar odors. Consequently, we treat familiar and unfamiliar odors separately here.

In a recent unpublished experiment we presented participants with the familiar odors of banana, mint, and vanilla. Using visual analogue scales, participants rated these odors for their specific quality (e.g., "How mint-like does it smell?"), for sweetness, and for overall intensity (total strength). These ratings were made for five different concentrations of each odorant in a single session. The correlations reported here represent the median from the ten possible correlations for each odor and scale with itself. It may be noted that these are likely to produce lower estimates of reliability than if there had been no variation in concentration. The median Pearson correlations for banana were 0.64 (sweetness), 0.52 (banana-like), and 0.60 (strength); for mint, 0.50 (sweetness), 0.41 (mintlike), and 0.38 (strength); and for vanilla, 0.48 (sweetness), 0.41 (vanilla-like), and

0.48 (strength). Thus, for these familiar odors, reliability for sweetness was better than or equal to reliability for other odor attributes that were unequivocally present.

We have used unfamiliar odors in a different kind of experiment that examined the role of learning in odor perception. Data from one of these experiments can be used to assess the reliability of sweetness ratings over relatively long periods of time (Stevenson, Boakes, & Wilson, 2000b, Experiment 3). Participants completed an odor pretest in which they rated three target odors for sweetness and intensity, on four separate occasions, all within a period of a few minutes. The median correlation on this pretest for sweetness was 0.45 and for overall intensity was 0.58 (based on 18 correlations, six per odor). The same odors were then sniffed one week later in an identical posttest. The median Pearson correlations between pretest and posttest ratings were 0.51 for sweetness and 0.57 for overall intensity (based on 48 correlations, 16 per odor). A month later the same posttest was administered again. The median Pearson correlations between the first and second posttest ratings were 0.49 for sweetness and 0.54 for overall intensity (based on 48 correlations, 16 per odor). Thus, for the unfamiliar odors used in this experiment, test-retest correlations were relatively stable over time periods varying from minutes to months.

Overall, test-retest correlations for sweetness range around 0.5. This level of reliability is similar to that found previously for intensity ratings within days (around 0.5) and between days (around 0.4; Lawless, Thomas, & Johnston, 1995). Thus, although obtained under less than ideal circumstances, the test-retest data from our experiment suggest that the reliability of odor sweetness ratings is comparable with that of other types of ratings in olfaction.

Validity

Describing an odor as sweet does not necessarily indicate that the sensation it produces is the same as that produced by a sweet taste. Because odors are difficult to describe, the use of "sweet" may reflect the lack of any more adequate term to indicate the perceptual element that sweet odors have in common. Furthermore, in English and other languages "sweet" is often used metaphorically. Describing a person as sweet carries implications about that individual's personal characteristics but not about how he or she tastes. To what extent, then, does the sensation that participants label sweet, when they smell an odorant like vanilla, resemble the sensation of sweet generated when the tongue is stimulated by a tastant such as sucrose?

The main evidence for similarity between the sensation of odor sweetness and the sensation of tasted sweetness comes from the phenomenon of sweetness enhancement. Anecdotal evidence suggests that the effect has long been known and widely exploited in commercial settings. However, its scientific study is relatively recent (Frank & Byram, 1988). In such experiments a sweet-smelling odor is added to a sucrose solution and the sweetness of this mixture is evaluated and compared with that of an otherwise equivalent unflavored sucrose solution. To the extent that the sensation evoked by the (retronasal) odor is similar to the sensation evoked by sucrose, three predictions can be made about the perceived sweetness of an odor-sucrose mixture. First, the "sweetness" from the odor and the sucrose should summate, leading to a higher sweetness rating for the sucrose-odor mixture than for sucrose alone. Second, the degree of summation—sweetness enhancement— should be monotonically related to the perceived sweetness of the odor. Third, the reverse effect to enhancement should also obtain, in that sweet-smelling odors should act to reduce the perceived sourness of sour tastants such as citric acid, in the same way that a sweet taste such as sucrose can suppress the sourness of citric acid (Stevenson & Prescott, 1997). Each of these predictions has been confirmed, as detailed below.

A variety of different procedures have produced summation of sweetness ratings when a sweet-smelling odor and sucrose are sampled as a mixture. In the first experiment of this kind, participants rated the sweetness of a sucrose plus strawberry solution as higher than that of sucrose alone (Frank & Byram, 1988). This effect did not appear to be a general consequence of adding any odor to sucrose, because enhancement was not obtained when a peanut butter odor was used instead of strawberry (Frank et al., 1989). Sweetness enhancement has since been obtained with a variety of sweet-smelling odors and with a number of different rating techniques, including category, line scale, and magnitude matching (e.g., Bingham, Birch, de Graaf, Behan, & Perrin, 1990; Cliff & Noble, 1990; Clark & Lawless, 1994; Schifferstein & Verlegh, 1996; Stevenson, 2001a).

A monotonic relationship between the sweetness rating for an odor when sniffed and its ability to enhance the sweetness of a sucrose solution when sipped was found in a study that used a range of odors (Stevenson et al., 1999). In the first experiment, participants were asked to sniff 20 odors and rate how sweet, sour, and strong each smelled and how much they liked or disliked it. They were then presented with the same odors again, this time dissolved in sucrose solution and sampled by mouth. For each solution they rated how sweet, sour, and intense the "taste" was and how much they

liked or disliked it. Regression analyses were then carried out to estimate which sniffed variable (i.e., ratings made when smelling) best predicted the degree of sweetness taste enhancement (i.e., the difference between sucrose alone and sucrose plus odor when tasting). The results were very clear. The best model included two variables, odor sweetness and odor intensity, with intensity acting as a suppressor variable (i.e., when differences in intensity are controlled for, more variance in sweetness enhancement can be accounted for by odor sweetness). Overall, this model could predict 60% of the variability in the magnitude of sweetness enhancement, supporting the claim of a strong relationship between the smelled sweetness of an odor and its ability to enhance the sweetness of a sucrose solution.

In the first experiment of this study the largest sweetness enhancement effect was produced by retronasal caramel odor. In the next experiment we found that this odor also suppressed sourness ratings for a citric acid solution, thus confirming the third of the predictions listed above (Stevenson et al., 1999, Experiment 2). We would like to emphasize that none of the odors used in these experiments produced any oral stimulation. That retronasal odorants of the kind used in such studies produce only nasal stimulation can be readily checked by pinching closed the nose, which prevents volatiles from rising from the mouth via the nasopharynx to the olfactory receptors, thus allowing any true taste component to be readily detectable by the tongue (Sakai, Kobayakawa, Gotow, Saito, & Imada, 2001; Schifferstein & Verlegh, 1996).

Although sweetness enhancement effects have been demonstrated under a range of conditions, they are sensitive to the type of ratings made by participants. When ratings are required for both sweetness and some more specific quality of the solution, such as "fruity" for a strawberry-sucrose solution, the enhancement effect is typically diminished or lost (Clark & Lawless, 1994; Frank, van der Klaauw, & Schifferstein, 1993). However, enhancement is not affected when an additional, inappropriate rating scale is added, such as floral or bitter for a strawberry-sucrose solution (van der Klaauw & Frank, 1996). One explanation for these findings is consistent with our claim of perceptual similarity between odor sweetness and tasted sweetness. This explanation proposes that rating a particular quality involves a decision about exactly what constitutes that quality (van der Klaauw & Frank, 1996). Under conditions in which only sweetness ratings are made, the criterion for sweetness will be more liberal than under conditions in which both sweetness *and* the odor's other primary quality are rated (e.g., sweetness and fruitiness). Presumably, such criterion shifts are limited only to those sensations that typically occur together (e.g., sweetness and fruitiness), as this past history of co-occurrence may reduce the degree to which the two sensations are discriminable. This finding of a criterion shift does not affect the conclusions drawn earlier about the perceptual similarity of odor sweetness and taste sweetness. This is because the key findings were obtained under conditions where such criterion shifts were unlikely, as the same number and type of scales were used within each experiment.

Although sweetness enhancement research supports the assumption of perceptual similarity between tasted and smelled sweetness, these effects could instead reflect the influence of another variable—liking (see Schifferstein & Verlegh, 1996). This brings us to an issue raised at the start of this section, namely, the extent to which describing an odor as sweet is a metaphor for liking it. Does "smelling as sweet as a rose" imply that roses produce the same sensation as sugar, or does it instead imply that the attractiveness of their scent is comparable to that of their visual appearance and symbolism? Liking for an odor can be increased by pairing it with sucrose (Zellner, Rozin, Aron, & Kulish, 1983), sweet-smelling odors tend to be liked (e.g., strawberry, vanilla, caramel), and moderately sweet tastes are generally deemed pleasant by adults, children, and neonates (e.g., Steiner, Glaser, Hawilo, & Berridge, 2001). Although these and other observations suggest a strong link between sweetness and liking, other kinds of evidence indicate that the two attributes can be dissociated in interesting ways.

One source of evidence is the study of alliesthesia, that is, changes in pleasantness depending on internal state. This research has found that, although ratings of liking for sucrose change after it is ingested, ratings of its intensity (i.e., sweetness) remain stable (e.g., Cabanac, 1971). Alliesthesia has also been obtained with odors. After a savory meal, food odors were rated as less pleasant than before the meal, while nonfood odors were unaffected (Duclaux, Feisthauer, & Cabanac, 1973). Three of the four food odors came from savory foods. Although it is unfortunate for the present argument that no sweetness ratings of these odors were obtained, it seems unlikely that the participants would have judged marmite, cheese, and fish to smell sweet. Yet all three odors were liked less after the meal. The only sweet-smelling odor included in the food set was honey, which showed the smallest alliesthetic effect, possibly because of the savory nature of the experimental meal. Clearly, a more direct test based on alliesthesia is still needed for distinguishing between liking for an odor and the perceived sweetness of that odor.

A second type of evidence for a dissociation between liking and odor sweetness comes from research on odor-taste learning (discussed later in this chapter). In all these experiments participants made liking as well as sweetness ratings (and intensity and sourness ratings, too). We found that changes in liking for an odor are more difficult to produce than changes in how it smells (e.g., how sweet), and liking ratings are more variable than sweetness ratings (Stevenson, Boakes, & Prescott, 1998; Stevenson, Prescott, & Boakes, 1995; see also Rozin, Wrzesniewski, & Byrnes, 1998, for a similar conclusion). These findings are difficult to explain if participants are supposed to be making the same kind of judgment for sweetness as they are for liking.

A third kind of evidence comes from changes in ratings of liking and sweetness as stimulus concentration increases. For sweet tastes and smells, liking tends to follow an inverted U function with increasing concentration, but ratings of odor and taste qualities are usually monotonically related to concentration (e.g., Doty, 1975; Kocher & Fisher, 1969).

In summary, with regard to the question of whether the sensation of sweetness generated when an odor is smelled is perceptually similar to the sensation of sweetness generated by sucrose, research on sweetness enhancement provides evidence that odor sweetness is perceptually akin to tasted sweetness, especially in the case of food-related odors. Other evidence also indicates that describing an odor as sweet is not simply a metaphor for liking it.

Nose and mouth, smell and taste

Odors display taste properties but do not elicit auditory or visual sensations. Clearly, the anatomy of the nose and mouth has to be important here. Any account of why an odor can induce a taste sensation must begin by examining when these two senses interact most closely. During eating and drinking, the constituent chemicals of the food and drink can stimulate simultaneously both the tongue (taste) and the olfactory mucosa via the nasopharynx (retronasal smell). We propose that particular combinations of taste and smell (e.g., sugar and strawberry) probably start as relatively discrete sensations (e.g., strawberry smell, sweet taste), but that frequent pairings result in the odor component producing an added taste sensation (e.g., strawberries now smell sweet). Before reviewing our research on this question, we discuss whether from a perceptual as opposed to an anatomical viewpoint there is any distinction between tastes and retronasal odors.

Ordinarily, people do not appear to treat tastes and smells from the mouth as different kinds of sensation

(Lawless, 1996). Rozin (1978) reported that of the ten languages he surveyed—English, Spanish, German, Czech, Hebrew, Hindi, Tamil, Mandarin, French, and Hungarian—none had terms that clearly distinguished the olfactory input to eating and drinking. Thus, at a linguistic level we fail to distinguish between sensations produced by food in the mouth (taste) and those produced by stimulation of olfactory receptors in the nose (smell). Our informal observations suggest that most people are very surprised to find that "taste" has a nasal component, as when, for example, someone discovers tea and coffee to have only an indistinguishable and unpleasant bitter taste if he or she pinches the nose when sipping. In the same way, people rendered anosmic by an accident or by infection but with their taste receptor system intact generally report losing both their sense of smell *and* taste (Deems et al., 1991).

Some psychophysical results have nonetheless been used to argue that taste and retronasal olfactory sensations are perceptually distinct. These results have been obtained from experiments in which participants made intensity judgments of taste and smell alone, and then of the overall combination judged as a mixture. Some such studies have found the judged intensity of the taste-odor combination to be the sum of the intensities of its parts (additivity), prompting the suggestion that the taste and the retronasal odor are perceived as separable components (Hornung & Enns, 1984; Murphy & Cain, 1980; Murphy, Cain, & Bartoshuk, 1977). However, other experiments of this kind have failed to demonstrate additivity, for reasons that are not currently understood (García-Medina, 1981; Hornung & Enns, 1986). It is far from clear what significance can be attached to finding additivity in these experiments. Where perceptual independence of the elements is not in doubt, additivity is again found in some cases, as when participants are asked to judge the combined intensity of auditory and visual stimuli (Ward, 1990), but not in others (Feldman & Baird, 1971). Moreover, in experiments in which the elements are clearly from the same modality, additivity has again been found under some conditions, such as binaural loudness (Algom & Marks, 1984) and pain summation (Algom, Raphaeli, & Cohen-Raz, 1986), but not under others; the most important example here is the failure to find additivity for mixtures of different odors (Cain & Drexler, 1974). In summary, evidence based on intensity judgments seems unlikely to make any definitive contribution toward assessing the perceptual independence of taste and retronasal odor stimuli.

One reason why mixtures of odors and tastes are perceived as just tastes may be a general lack of knowledge about the chemical senses. Young children know that you need eyes to see and ears to hear. Few adults, however, know that you need a nose to taste. The common belief in a single oral sense (flavor or taste) rather than two (taste and smell) could reflect an implicit assumption of a one-to-one correspondence between a sense and a sensory channel. This would imply, erroneously, that, because the nose (including the olfactory sensors it contains) is used for smelling (orthonasal olfaction), it cannot be involved in sensing oral events (retronasal olfaction). Failure to distinguish between oral and nasal sensations may also result partly from stimulation of mechanoreceptors in the mouth during eating and drinking and thus the mislocalization of all sensation to that location (Murphy & Cain, 1980). A possibly related effect is observed with temperature, where touching a spot of skin can result in the mislocalization of felt hotness when heat is concurrently applied to an adjacent area of skin (Green, 1978). Finally, the contrast with ventriloquism should be noted. Whereas in ventriloquism, a voice is falsely attributed to a source (the dummy; Bertelson, 1998), the sensations generated by various sensors in different locations when food or drink is in the mouth are attributed to the correct source.

A further reason why people may experience a single percept located in the mouth rather than two or more percepts in different locations is that they may pay little attention to its component parts. Stevenson (2001a) found that giving participants information about the sensory components of "tastes" had no impact on the magnitude of the sweetness enhancement effect unless these participants were expressly told to attend to the olfactory component and separate out its effects. Similarly, the limited and imprecise vocabulary most of us have to describe olfactory sensations may also affect perception, as many people consistently report inability to imagine smells and flavors (Stevenson & Boakes, 2003). Lack of a precise, descriptive language may make it much harder to reflect on olfactory stimuli in their absence, verbally or perceptually, when compared with visual or auditory events.

Another way of looking at the issue is that people are not confused but are perfectly correct in combining oral and nasal stimulation into a single "taste" sense (Abdi, 2002). From a functional point of view, the main point of our senses is to identify events, not to provide sensations. Events or objects external to our bodies are identified primarily by vision, touch, and audition. In the absence of such input, orthonasal olfaction provides cues as to what might be out there, such as the smell of an unseen fire. Thus, the terms we use for smells are predominantly ones that refer to their usual origin, such as "floral," "fruity," "musty," or "acrid."

Visual identification may employ different systems to assess movement, detect color, or recognize shape. Only sensory neurophysiologists know about such parallel processing. Most of us simply "see," say, a rabbit heading off at high speed (Abdi, 2002). Whether this functional perspective is more appropriate than a psychophysical one, and whatever the underlying reasons might be, the important point here is that in general, people treat odor-taste mixtures as wholes rather than as combinations of discrete perceptual events.

Odor-taste learning

So far we have examined the phenomenon of experiencing the sensation of sweetness when certain odors are smelled as an example of odor-taste synesthesia. In this section we consider a possible theoretical account of its cause. We start by reviewing findings from the use of a conditioning procedure that can produce changes in the way an odor is perceived, so that, for example, it can come to smell sweeter as a result of being paired with sucrose. Then we examine the unusual properties of this type of learning and why these properties appear to reflect the configural encoding of odor-taste combinations that gives rise to odor-taste synesthesia.

Many sweet-smelling odors either have a history of co-occurrence with sweet tastes, as is typically the case for caramel, vanilla, or strawberry, or resemble odors with such a history, as is the case for unfamiliar fruits. This observation led Frank and Byram (1988) to suggest that a person's experience of an odor at the same time as a sweet taste might influence whether the odor was perceived as sweet-smelling. To test this notion we chose two odors, lychee and water chestnut, that pilot work suggested would be unfamiliar to most Australian undergraduates and would be initially perceived as moderately sweet (by virtue of their resemblance to other fruits). The methods employed in our first experiments were time-consuming, occupying several sessions over several days. In the first session participants were given a pretest in which they sniffed and rated on line scales a number of odors, including lychee and water chestnut, for sweetness, sourness, liking, and intensity. The training, or "conditioning," phase that followed consisted of three sessions in which participants sampled sucrose solutions flavored with lychee, for example, and citric acid solutions flavored with water chestnut. (The allocation of flavors—i.e., retronasal odors—to tastes was counterbalanced across participants.) Sampling consisted of sipping and then expectorating the solutions. A discrimination task was given to the participants, both to ensure that they attended to the "tastes" of the solutions and to mask the main aim of the experiment. Also

for the latter reason, many dummy trials were included in the training sessions, exceeding the number of actual training trials. The final session contained a posttest that was identical to the pretest.

We predicted that the perceived sweetness of the odor paired with sucrose would increase from pretest to posttest and that there would likewise be an increase in the perceived sourness of the citric-paired odor. The first two experiments confirmed these predictions. Rated sweetness of the sucrose-paired odor increased by about 12 points on a 100-point scale and rated sourness of the citric-paired odor increased by about 13 points. Complementary changes were also found in that the sucrose-paired odor decreased in sourness and the citric-paired odor decreased in sweetness (Stevenson et al., 1995).

Subsequent experiments confirmed that an increase in the sniffed sweetness of a target odor could also be obtained by adding the target to a sucrose solution and a second odor to water rather than to citric acid. To control for possible demand characteristics, these experiments used blind testing, in that the experimenter did not know which odors had been paired with sucrose. As before, the sucrose-paired odor was judged to smell sweeter by about 12 points from pretest to posttest. No significant change in sweetness or sourness rating was found for the water-paired odor. To date, 12 experiments using variations of this procedure have consistently obtained the basic effect. These results confirm very strongly that the taste properties of an odor can be affected by a history of co-occurrence with a sweet or sour taste.

As noted earlier in this chapter, this research started from speculation about the nature of sweetness enhancement. A connection from these conditioning effects back to sweetness enhancement has recently been made. Prescott (1999) found that flavored sucrose solutions were judged sweeter (i.e., produced a greater enhancement effect) after conditioning, that is, after the target odor had been paired with sucrose.

Finally, before turning to the specific properties of odor-taste learning, we emphasize that changes in sweetness are not the only form of odor-taste synesthesia. In several studies we have observed that odors paired with the sour taste of citric acid can become more sour-smelling (Stevenson et al., 1995, 1998). In addition, we have acquired unpublished data that show that odors paired with the bitter taste of sucrose-octa-acetate come to smell more bitter (Boakes & Stevenson, 2003). Although we have not yet tested for effects involving salt and monosodium glutamate, we would predict that conditioning effects involving these tastes would also be present.

PROPERTIES OF ODOR-TASTE LEARNING: 1. ACQUISITION AND AWARENESS   The first property we investigated was influenced by the work of Baeyens and his colleagues on human evaluative conditioning (Baeyens, Eelen, van den Bergh, & Crombez, 1990). They had reported that dislike for a flavor could be conditioned by having participants drink a mixture of the flavor with a disgusting taste, Tween-20. Particularly interesting was their claim that this conditioned change in liking occurred without awareness. After exposure to a set of flavor, color, and taste mixtures, participants showed no explicit knowledge of which flavor had been mixed with which taste, even though they could identify which color went with which taste (Baeyens et al., 1990). Research on conditioning without awareness has a long history but is short on robust evidence that the phenomenon exists (Boakes, 1989; Lovibond & Shanks, 2002). Consequently, we wished to find out whether explicit knowledge of the odor-taste contingencies employed in our experiments was important for changes in the perceptual properties of odors, as opposed to the affective—or "evaluative"—properties studied by Baeyens et al. (1990). In other words, is odor-taste learning implicit?

We tackled this issue using three methods to assess awareness of (1) the experimental contingencies and (2) the real aim of the experiment (i.e., conditioning rather than "perceptual judgment," which is what participants were initially told). The first and simplest method, used in five experiments (Stevenson et al., 1995, 1998), was simply to ask participants at the end of the experiment what they thought the purpose of the study was. Out of the approximately 180 such participants, including a group of fourth-year psychology students taking a seminar on learning theory, only one person, a first-year undergraduate, ever came close to identifying the true nature of the experimental procedure as a learning task rather than as a perception experiment.

The second method was to ask participants at the end of the experiment to smell each of the target odors and to identify which taste they thought that odor was paired with during training (Stevenson et al., 1995, 1998). Participants who correctly identified which odor went with which taste were classified as aware and were compared, in terms of the size of the learning effect, with participants who were classified as unaware. We did not find any significant differences between aware and unaware participants. However, it should be noted that this conclusion relied on a null result, which could of course just indicate insufficient sensitivity. A further problem with this method for assessing awareness is that it includes in the aware group participants who may have guessed the prior history of an odor on the basis of its perceptual properties. Thus, a participant finding that a particular odor smells sweet may be inclined to select "sweet" as the taste with which it was paired, in the absence of any explicit recall of this odor-sweet combination.

A third type of test asked participants to sample all possible combinations of the odors and tastes used during the preceding training phase and rate each combination for the frequency with which it was encountered during training. Thus, a participant who was given Odor 1 in sucrose and Odor 2 in citric acid during training and who could remember this explicitly should rate the Odor 1-sucrose combination as having occurred more frequently than the Odor 2-sucrose combination. Even when measured by this more sensitive test, the level of contingency awareness was still very low. Most important, there was again no relationship between the magnitude of the conditioning effect and the degree of awareness (Stevenson et al., 1998; but note that the caveat on null results applies here as well).

The low level of awareness in these experiments was perhaps unsurprising, given the measures taken to obscure the purpose of the experiments. As already noted, they included an irrelevant task and many dummy trials. Subsequently, we streamlined the procedure in various ways, including omission of all dummy trials, to reduce the time needed to complete an experiment. Thus, in more recent studies participants attended only two 50-minute sessions, the first including a pretest and initial training and the second including further training followed by a posttest (Stevenson, Boakes, & Wilson, 2000a, 2000b). There appeared to be no obvious disadvantage to this change. Although we did not include any recognition or frequency tests to assess contingency awareness after experiments in which the streamlined procedure was used, informal observations suggested that participants in the modified procedure still had little explicit knowledge about the various odor-taste contingencies they had been exposed to during training.

A second issue we have addressed is whether odor-taste learning is based on successive or simultaneous associations. In theory, participants in these experiments could easily have smelled the odors prior to sipping the solution and consequently, in principle, could have formed a successive association between the odor (prior to sipping) and the taste (during sipping). To check for this possibility we used a training procedure in which one odor was added to a sucrose solution that was sucked through a straw, while a second odor was added to a solution presented in a plastic cup, as in the normal procedure (Stevenson et al., 1998). The straw condition was to prevent the participants from smelling the odor before the solution entered the mouth. After training, participants were asked as usual to sniff and rate the set of odors they had been given in the pretest. From pretest to posttest, rated sweetness for the sucrose-paired odors increased by the same amount in both conditions (Stevenson et al., 1998, Experiment 2). Thus, odor-taste learning can take place when presentation is unambiguously simultaneous, and successive associations do not seem to be important.

We have not directly tested for the effect on acquisition of factors other than the ones just discussed. However, comparisons across experiments do suggest the optimum number of pairings needed to generate odor-taste learning. In our published experiments (Stevenson et al., 1995, 1998, 2000a, 2000b), participants received either eight or nine pairings of taste and odor. These pairings produced changes in rated sweetness of about 12 points on a 100-point scale. A smaller number of pairings in two subsequent experiments produced significant effects that were larger than those observed previously. Stevenson and Case (2003) presented only four odor-taste pairings during training and observed a 20-point change in sweetness ratings, while Prescott, Francis, and Johnstone (2003), using only a single pairing, also obtained a 20-point change. Despite reservations about between-experiment comparisons, these two recent experiments suggest that odor-taste learning can take place rapidly and that a small number of pairings can produce as large an effect size as eight or more pairings.

Properties of Odor-Taste Learning: 2. Retention and Resistance to Interference Several of our experiments were designed to provide direct comparisons between odor-taste learning and more familiar "signal learning" based on associations between successive events (Baeyens et al., 1990). This was done by training participants concurrently on both odor-taste and color-taste combinations. Clearly, color-taste learning is based on successive associations: the color of a drink provides a signal of how it is likely to taste, just as various visual cues create expectancies as to the taste of some food. The task given participants in these experiments was to try to predict the taste of each sample they were given in training. One of the subsequent tests for the effectiveness of training was an expectancy test. In this test participants were asked first to look at and sniff a sample and then to rate what they expected it to taste like, using our standard set of scales for sweetness, sourness, intensity, and liking. This test allows the use of both explicit knowledge—"Red samples always had a sour taste"—and inference from implicit knowledge—"This smells sour, so it probably tastes sour."

One property we looked at using this design was retention over a long period. We had found previously that a delay between training and posttest failed to reduce the effect of odor-taste learning. In the straw experiment we had participants complete a posttest either immediately after the final conditioning session or after a delay of at least 24 hours. The learning effect was somewhat larger in the delay condition, but the difference between the groups just failed to reach significance (Stevenson et al., 1998, Experiment 2). We examined retention over a much longer interval in the odor-color study by giving an initial test immediately after training and then repeating it a month later. Odor-taste learning was again very well retained; the effect after one month was the same size as in the immediate test. There was some indication that color-taste learning was weaker after a month, but in general, the two kinds of learning did not appear to differ greatly with respect to simple retention (Stevenson et al., 2000b).

We reached a different conclusion when we compared the effects of further training on the retention of odor-taste and color-taste learning. In two experiments using within-participant designs that differed in some details, this further training took the form of what we referred to as an extinction procedure. The initial training consisted of eight pairings of two odors (O1 and O2) with citric acid and also eight pairings of two colors (C1 and C2) with citric acid, along with a third odor and a third color that were both paired with sucrose. The extinction procedure consisted of presenting in water one of the previously citric-paired odors (O1) and one of the previously citric-paired colors (C1), each for a total of 12 trials. Thus, in the subsequent tests comparisons between O1 and O2 would reveal the effect of extinction on odor-citric learning, and comparisons between C1 and C2 would reveal the effect of extinction on color-citric learning (Stevenson et al., 2000a, Experiments 3 and 4).

The first major finding was obtained when we gave participants the standard sniffing test in order to assess the perceptual properties of the odors. Once again this revealed the odor-taste effect: relative to pretest ratings, O1 and O2 were both rated sourer, and less sweet, than the sucrose-paired odor. The new finding was that there was no significant difference between O1 and O2. Thus, the extinction procedure had failed to produce lower sourness ratings for O1 than for O2. This result was not entirely a surprise, since Baeyens and his colleagues had claimed that odor-taste evaluative conditioning was also highly resistant to extinction (Baeyens et al., 1990), and, in addition, evidence from recognition memory experiments using odors suggests the same conclusion (Herz & Engen, 1996).

The next test, the expectancy test described earlier, allowed a critical comparison between the effects of extinction on odor-citric and color-citric learning. When participants had to rate the taste they expected for a given color, the extinguished color, C1, was given a lower sourness rating than the control color, C2. Thus, the extinction procedure had interfered with the initial training on color-taste combinations. This effect was not observed for odor-taste learning. The sucrose-paired odor was predicted to taste sweet, and both the citric-paired odors, O1 and O2, were predicted to taste sour, but again, there was no difference between the extinguished odor, O1, and its nonextinguished control, O2.

In order to test an interference condition that seemed likely to be more effective than extinction, we modified the color-taste/odor-taste design by substituting counterconditioning for the extinction procedure used in the two experiments just described. As before, during training, two odors, O1 and O2, were added to a citric acid solution, as were two colors, C1 and C2, while a third odor and third color were added to sucrose. In the second phase of the experiment, one of the previously citric-paired odors, O1, was now added to a sucrose solution, as was one of the colors, C1. Exactly as in the previous experiments, after these two training phases participants were first given the standard sniffing test and then the expectancy test, which involved the full set of odors and colors (Stevenson et al., 2000b).

Samples with the counterconditioned color, C1, were expected to taste sweeter than any other stimulus, indicating that pairing this color with sucrose in the second training phase had changed participants' expectations relative to the control color, C2, which had been paired only with citric acid. For odors, however, no counterconditioning effect was observed in that, relative to the sucrose-paired control odor, both O1 and O2 were rated as predicting a sour taste, and there was no difference between them. A similar result was found on the sniffing test. As in the extinction experiments, there was a significant correlation between the odor sourness ratings participants gave in the two tests. Both the extinction and the counterconditioning experiments suggest that, once odor-taste learning has occurred, it is unusually resistant to further change.

PROPERTIES OF ODOR-TASTE LEARNING: 3. PREEXPOSURE AND TRAINING A property of classical conditioning found across a wide range of preparations using animals is *latent inhibition* or the *stimulus preexposure* effect. This refers to the finding that prior exposure to a stimulus, particularly in the same context, retards conditioning.

Various forms of simultaneous conditioning have shown this property (e.g., Rescorla, 1980). On the other hand, obtaining the stimulus preexposure effect in human conditioning has proved difficult (Lubow & Gewirtz, 1995), for reasons that are not entirely clear but that must include the difficulty of finding stimuli for human adults that are both entirely novel and difficult to describe.

This is less difficult in the case of odors. Exposure to a previously unfamiliar and difficult to describe odor can produce marked perceptual changes. Thus, simply sniffing such an odor a few times can increase its discriminability (Rabin, 1988; Rabin & Cain, 1984). In addition, Lawless and Engen (1977), using pairings of odors and pictures, found evidence of proactive interference but no evidence of retroactive interference. We might therefore also expect preexposure to an odor to affect odor-taste learning.

We have obtained evidence of preexposure effects in odor-taste learning using preexposure to both odors and tastes (Stevenson & Case, 2003). In the preexposure phase participants were presented with two different odors in water (twice each) and solutions of sucrose and citric acid in water (twice each). They were then given each of these odors mixed with a taste, so that one odor was paired with sucrose and the second with citric acid. This conditioning phase also included two additional odors, one paired with citric acid and the other with sucrose. A second session consisted of further conditioning, followed by an expectancy test and then an odor perceptual test. Both tests showed the same pattern of findings. Exposure to the elements prior to exposure to the mixture completely disrupted learning, whereas the control condition yielded the standard odor-taste effect.

The data we obtained indicate that simple exposure to the stimuli prior to the conditioning phase can interfere with odor-taste learning. We have also examined the effects of various kinds of explicit training with odors prior to conditioning. The results to date do not suggest any simple generalization. One question we asked was whether being able to identify the target odor influenced odor-taste learning. In these experiments, participants were exposed solely to an odor. Half the participants learned the odor's name (Label group) and the other half simply sampled it (No-Label group). After a training phase in which the preexposed odor was paired with a taste, no evidence of conditioning was obtained in the No-Label group. However, label learning prevented this proactive interference, as odor-taste conditioning was observed in this group (Boakes & Stevenson, 2003).

We have also explored the effect of giving participants detailed knowledge about tastes and smells. One experiment contained a Knowledge group, which received detailed briefing about the olfactory and taste system, followed by solutions containing tastes (sucrose and citric acid), odors (Odor 1 and Odor 2), and taste-odor mixtures (Odor 1-sucrose and Odor 2-citric acid). Participants in the Knowledge group were required to sip each solution and then pinch and release the nose in order to assess the relevant olfactory and gustatory contribution of each stimulus. This was accompanied by a discussion of what each had experienced. A second, Exposure group received the same stimuli but no explicit training (data from this second group were discussed earlier in this chapter) (Stevenson & Case, 2003). The experiment found no evidence of any training effect. That is, although exposure prevented conditioning, the training procedure exerted no detectable effect.

One reason for this lack of a training effect may be that participants, following training, simply default to a synthetic processing strategy and thus fail to attend to the mixture's components. Prescott (1999) found evidence consistent with this interpretation. After a training phase that included two odor-sucrose mixtures, one including a novel odor and the other a familiar one, participants rated these mixtures either for odor intensity (Integration group) or for odor *and* taste (Separation group). A control group experienced the odors and tastes separately. Only the Integration group showed odor-taste learning, as measured by an increase in odor sweetness from pre- to posttest for the novel odor but not the familiar odor.

In summary, experiments in which participants have various kinds of exposure to a target odor before experiencing an odor-taste mixture containing the odor suggest that (1) simple preexposure to a relatively unfamiliar odor or the use of an already familiar odor can interfere with subsequent odor-taste learning (latent inhibition); (2) this preexposure effect is unaffected by training participants to distinguish between a retronasal odor and a taste in the mouth; and (3) learning to label an initially unfamiliar odor does not interfere with odor-taste learning but does appear to prevent the latent inhibition.

Configural encoding of odor-taste mixtures

In this section we tackle two related issues. First, because the meaning of "configural" can vary substantially, we clarify what we mean by it here. Second, we discuss the extent to which the properties of odor-taste learning can be explained in terms of configural encoding.

DEFINING CONFIGURAL ENCODING   First, we should make it clear that we are not using the term *configural* as it is often understood in the context of visual perception. In that context it usually refers to representations of an object that include information about spatial relationships between its component parts. For example, encoding of a face can contain both feature information—properties of the eyes, nose, and mouth, for example—and configural information about the spatial relationships between these features (e.g., Tanaka & Sengco, 1997). Similarly, in the context of auditory perception, configural encoding can refer to pitch relationships and to temporal relationships in music and speech.

Instead, the meaning we have adopted here corresponds to its use in associative learning theory, where it is defined as the level of representation of an event at which associations can be made with representations of other events occurring at a different time (i.e., successive associations). This can be explained in terms of the kind of example that has proved important for contemporary learning theories based on animal conditioning experiments. What does a rat learn when a simultaneous compound—LT, say, made up of a light (L) and a tone (T)—regularly precedes the delivery of food? The answer given by most influential theories of the past few decades, notably the Rescorla-Wagner model (Rescorla & Wagner, 1972), is based on treating L and T as separate elements: The rat learns that L signals food and that T signals food. Elemental theories of this kind face the problem of explaining how rats—or, based on the same principle, neural nets—can learn "positive patterning" problems of the kind LT→food vs. L→no_food vs. T→no_food, and "negative patterning" problems of the kind L→food vs. T→food vs. LT→no_food. Solution of these problems is assumed to involve an additional representation, a configural one, *lt*, produced by the simultaneous occurrence of the two events. Thus, the answer above is amended: When LT signals food, the rat learns L→food, T→food, and *lt*→food. Such theories assume that the configural representation, *lt*, is less salient than representations of the components, L and T (but see Pearce, 1994; Wagner & Brandon, 2001). General associative learning theories rarely acknowledge that the nature of the specific stimuli employed in a conditioning experiment might affect the way their joint occurrence is represented. We suggest here that, although the configural representation of a compound consisting of a light and a tone might be relatively weak, the configural representation of an odor-taste combination is normally far more salient than the representation of its individual components. The reason why tastes and smells may be treated this way was discussed earlier under Nose and Mouth, Smell and Taste.

Another concept that can be taken from contemporary animal learning theory is that of unitization produced by "within-compound associations" (Hall, 2001). In this process, when an animal encounters a novel and complex object such as a new environment, its representation of the object develops on the basis of associative links between its constituent elements. Thus, when the combination of a retronasal odor and a taste is experienced, an associative link may develop, resulting in an odor-taste "unit." A recent detailed example of such a theory has been applied to latent inhibition and perceptual learning, as well as other learning phenomena (McLaren & Mackintosh, 2000). However, like all such theories, it does not predict the resistance to extinction displayed by odor-taste learning.

An alternative view of configural representation is that certain types of information (e.g., odors and tastes) are simply encoded as one event by virtue of simultaneous occurrence, with minimal attention to the stimulus. In this case, no within-compound associations are required, because there is only one perceptual event. This approach circumvents the extremely difficult problem, inherent to the elementalist account, of adequately defining what constitutes an "element" of experience.

A CONFIGURAL INTERPRETATION Although the central focus of this chapter has been on odor-taste synesthesia, this phenomenon appears to be one facet of a more general odor-learning system. According to this view, the most crucial aspect of odor perception is the process of matching to odor memory (Stevenson, 2001b; Stevenson, 2001c; Stevenson & Boakes, 2003). When a novel odor is smelled for the first time, its neural representation is compared with all previously stored odor memories. The degree to which it activates each of these previous memories corresponds to the qualities that the person experiences when smelling that odor. Over subsequent sniffs of the odor, the activated components of odor memory and the pattern of the particular target odor itself may undergo *unitization,* becoming a *configural* odor memory bound together by within-event associations, or, by the alternative account, becoming a configuration by virtue of encoding this simultaneous pattern of activation. Taking this process as a starting point, the key features of odor-taste synesthesia that we have detailed in this chapter fall readily into place.

During acquisition, an odor-taste compound is experienced in the mouth. The olfactory and taste components are experienced as one perceptual event and are stored as such in odor memory. This process prevents the formation of a predictive relationship between these two events, because the participant does not know that two events have in fact taken place. Thus, learning can occur without awareness. Later, when the odor component is smelled alone in the absence of any taste, the smell is a good match for the odor-taste memory, and it is this memory that is experienced; hence the synesthetic sensation of taste, a process that has been termed *redintegration* (Horowitz & Prytulak, 1969). Under conditions in which a novel odor is experienced several times before being paired with a taste, no learning will take place between the taste and the smell, because the smell will already have been encoded in odor memory. Thus, when the odor-taste compound is experienced, the odor component will be far more readily discriminable, eliminating the conditions necessary for configural encoding. A similar process works in reverse to prevent interference following encoding of an odor-taste memory. When the odor component is experienced alone (i.e., an interference trial), it will not be encoded because it will be *experienced* as an odor-taste compound. It is this memory experience that, if anything, will be relearned, producing apparently larger conditioning effects in the extinguished condition (see Stevenson et al., 2000a). In summary, it is the process of redintegration, the part recovering the whole, that we feel best accounts for odor-taste synesthesia and its properties.

Implications and conclusions

In the preceding sections we have drawn heavily on associative learning theory as a basis for our view of configural learning and their role in odor-taste learning and synesthesia. Although this approach has been very fruitful, it does encourage the conclusion that no counterpart to the effects discussed here exist in the literature on human perception and cognition. Such a view, however, would be mistaken. Several features of odor-taste learning bear a striking resemblance to effects documented using implicit memory procedures. For our purposes here, an implicit memory effect is defined to have occurred when prior experience affects performance (perception) without requiring intentional recollection (Schachter, 1987). There are a number of parallels between odor-taste learning and implicit memory effects; these parallels include the following. First, both show rapid and effortless acquisition (DeSchepper & Treisman, 1996). Second, both can show resistance to interference (e.g., Graf & Schacter, 1987) and persistence (e.g., Sloman, Hayman, Ohta, Law, & Tulving, 1988).

Third, as for odor-taste learning, items processed analytically appear to facilitate explicit memory, whereas items processed configurally facilitate implicit memory (Graf & Schacter, 1989). Fourth, implicit memory can influence performance (or perception) without intent or awareness (Schacter, 1987). Fifth, certain types of implicit memory procedure, particularly those most similar to odor-taste learning in terms of their properties (as above), are often viewed as being perceptual in nature (e.g., Schacter & Church, 1992; Schacter, Cooper, Delaney, Peterson, & Tharan, 1991). In these cases prior experience acts to modify perceptual processes (e.g., enhance discrimination or identification) in a manner that is directly analogous to the view we have taken here.

There are, however, two intriguing differences. First, and perhaps most important, is that to our knowledge, most implicit memory procedures are exclusively unimodal, whereas encodings of odor and taste are clearly cross-modal. Second, most neurological conditions that degrade explicit memory (e.g., Alzheimer's disease) have little impact on many types of implicit memory procedures (e.g., Winograd, Goldstein, Monarch, Peluso, & Goldman, 1999) but typically *do* impair olfactory perception while sparing detection (e.g., in Alzheimer's disease; see Kareken et al., 2001). Notwithstanding these important differences, the general equating of implicit memory effects with perceptual processes and their parallels here provide an important link to contemporary studies of human perception and cognition, as well validating the interpretive framework adopted in this chapter.

The basic question we have sought to address is why some odors come to smell sweet; that is, why do people experience odor-taste synesthesia? Our conclusions are at some variance with those drawn from the other principal form of human synesthesia, color-word synesthesia. For this type of synesthesia, one prominent model suggests a failure to cull connections in the brain that are present during infancy but are lost in non-synesthetic adults (Harrison & Baron-Cohen, 1997; see other chapters in this handbook for alternative accounts). This model accounts for many features of color-word synesthesia. Our work on odors and tastes demonstrates that failure to cull connections cannot be the only mechanism. Although learning-based explanations for other forms of synesthesia have generally not fared well (Harrison & Baron-Cohen, 1997), they do provide a ready explanation for odor-taste synesthesia. Moreover, the ubiquity of this effect in adults automatically argues against any explanation dependent on abnormal brain development. It would appear that the way that we attribute sensation to particular sense domains retains some plasticity, even in normal adults.

For us, one of the most intriguing aspects of the interaction between odors and tastes is the more general implication for odor perception. The experiments on odor-taste learning summarized in this chapter provided the first direct evidence that odor qualities can be acquired. These findings suggest that any model of odor perception based solely on the stimulus properties of the odorant is unlikely to provide a complete account of olfactory perception. In a recent series of studies we have taken this view further by using a similar methodology to explore the effects of experiencing mixtures of odors on subsequent perception of the individual components (Stevenson, 2001b, 2001c, 2001d). This work has supported our view that a routine part of odor processing, as noted earlier, involves the comparison of an odor's representation with a store of odor memories and the encoding of the subsequent pattern of activation as a new configuration. For odor mixtures (e.g., mushroom-cherry), as with mixtures of odors and tastes, the consequence of this process can be observed when a component odor is smelled alone (e.g., mushroom). Just as an odor paired with sucrose gets to smell sweet, an odor previously mixed with a cherry-smelling odor generally gets to smell more cherry-like. In addition to producing changes in odor quality, the experience of odor mixtures can also produce related changes such as an increase in the perceived similarity of the component odors and a reduced ability to discriminate between them (Stevenson, 2001c). These recent findings on odor-odor learning suggest that the processes we claim in this chapter to provide the basis for odor-taste learning are a pervasive feature of olfactory information processing. This would probably not have been so evident were it not for the study of multisensory interactions between taste and smell.

Summary

The perceptual qualities of many odors are consistently described in terms of properties that are appropriate to tastes. Even though there are no equivalent olfactory receptor systems, the sensation of sweetness produced by a sniffed odor appears to be the same as the sensation produced, for example, by an odorless sucrose solution in the mouth. The strongest evidence for this claim comes from studies of the sweetness enhancement effect, in which adding a tasteless odor as a flavorant to a sucrose solution increases the perceived sweetness of the solution. The rated sweetness of an odor when sniffed predicts the extent to which it will produce sweetness enhancement. Consequently, we argue that the taste properties of odors should be regarded as a form of synesthesia. The near universality of this effect, in contrast to the low incidence of other forms of synesthesia, appears to reflect the unusual functional properties of the olfactory system. The key property is that olfactory receptors can be stimulated in a near identical manner by chemicals that enter via the nose—orthonasal odors—giving rise to "smells," and by chemicals entering via the mouth—retronasal odors—that give rise to sensations commonly referred to as "tastes."

The central argument of this chapter is that, as a result of eating and drinking, patterns of retronasal odor stimulation co-occur with oral stimulation, notably of the taste receptors, so that a unitary percept is produced by a process of either within-event associative learning or by simply encoding it as one event. Eating sweet vanilla-flavored ice cream will ensure that the retronasal odor of vanilla becomes associated with sweetness; on some later occasion the smell of vanilla will seem sweet, even if no conscious recollection of eating ice cream comes to mind. Experiments that were successful in providing evidence for such odor-taste learning have also uncovered some unusual properties of this kind of learning. Unlike almost all other forms of human conditioning studied in the laboratory it does not require awareness of the contingencies set up by the procedure; odor-taste learning occurs whether or not participants realize that one odor is always mixed with one taste and other odors with other tastes. The second unusual property, although an apparently general feature of odor memory, is its resistance to interference by later experience. This appears to account for the stability that the taste properties of odors normally display. Whereas other forms of synesthesia tend to be rare curiosities, perceiving many odors as having taste properties seems to be a nearly universal feature of human perception of odors. Consequently, we regard the study of odor-taste learning as an important step toward a better understanding of olfactory perception.

REFERENCES

Abdi, H. (2002). What can psychology and sensory evaluation learn from each other. *Food Quality and Preference, 13*, 1–16.

Algom, D., & Marks, L. E. (1984). Individual differences in loudness processing and loudness scales. *Journal of Experimental Psychology: General, 113*, 571–593.

Algom, D., Raphaeli, N., & Cohen-Raz, L. (1986). Integration of noxious stimulation across separate somatosensory communications systems: A functional theory of pain. *Journal of Experimental Psychology: Human Perception and Performance, 12*, 92–102.

Baeyens, F., Eelen, P., van den Bergh, O., & Crombez, G. (1990). Flavor-flavor and color-flavor conditioning in humans. *Learning and Motivation, 21*, 434–455.

Baron-Cohen, S., Burt, L., Smith-Laittan, F., Harrison, J., & Bolton, P. (1996). Synesthesia: Prevalence and familiarity. *Perception, 25*, 1073–1079.

Baron-Cohen, S., Wyke, M. A., & Binnie, C. (1987). Hearing words and seeing colors: An experimental investigation of a case of synesthesia. *Perception, 16*, 761–767.

Bertelson, P. (1998). Starting from the ventriloquist: The perception of multimodal events. In M. Sabourin, F. I. M. Craik, & M. Robert (Eds.), *Advances in psychological science: Vol. 2. Biological and cognitive aspects* (pp. 419–439). Hove, England: Psychology Press.

Bingham, A. F., Birch, C. G., de Graaf, C., Behan, J. M., & Perrin, R. (1990). Sensory studies with sucrose-maltol mixtures. *Chemical Senses, 15*, 447–456.

Boakes, R. A. (1989). How one might find evidence for conditioning in adult humans. In T. Archer & L.-G. Nilsson (Eds.), *Aversion, avoidance and anxiety: Perspectives on aversively motivated behavior* (pp. 381–402). Hillsdale, NJ: Erlbaum.

Boakes, R. A., & Stevenson, R. J. (2003). [Latent inhibition with odors: But not when they acquire a name.] Unpublished raw data.

Buck, L. B. (1996). Information coding in the vertebrate olfactory system. *Annual Review of Neuroscience, 19*, 517–544.

Cabanac, M. (1971). The physiological role of pleasure. *Science, 173*, 1103–1107.

Cain, W. S. (1979). To know with the nose: Keys to odor and identification. *Science, 203*, 468–470.

Cain, W. S., & Drexler, M. (1974). Scope and evaluation of odor counteraction and masking. *Annals of the New York Academy of Sciences, 237*, 427–439.

Clark, C. C., & Lawless, H. T. (1994). Limiting response alternatives in time-intensity scaling: An examination of the halo dumping effect. *Chemical Senses, 19*, 583–594.

Cliff, M., & Noble, A. C. (1990). Time-intensity evaluation of sweetness and fruitiness and their interaction in a model solution. *Journal of Food Science, 55*, 450–454.

Deems, D. A., Doty, R. L., Settle, R. G., Moore-Gillon, V., Shaman, P., Mester, A. F., et al. (1991). Smell and taste disorders: A study of 750 patients from the University of Pennsylvania Smell and Taste Center. *Archives of Otorhinolaryngology, Head and Neck Surgery, 117*, 519–528.

DeSchepper, B., & Treisman, A. (1996). Visual memory for novel shapes: Implicit coding without attention. *Journal of Experimental Psychology: Learning, Memory and Cognition, 22*, 27–47.

Desor, J. A., & Beauchamp, G. K. (1974). The human capacity to transmit olfactory information. *Perception & Psychophysics, 16*, 551–556.

Doty, R. L. (1975). An examination of relationships between the pleasantness, intensity and concentration of 10 odorous stimuli. *Perception and Psychophysics, 17*, 492–496.

Dravnieks, A. (1985). *Atlas of odor character profiles.* ASTM Data series DS61. Philadelphia: ASTM Publishers.

Duclaux, R., Feisthauer, J., & Cabanac, M. (1973). Effects of eating a meal on the pleasantness of food and non-food odors in man. *Physiology and Behavior, 10*, 1029–1033.

Feldman, J., & Baird, J. C. (1971). Magnitude estimation of multidimensional stimuli. *Perception & Psychophysics, 10*, 418–422.

Frank, R. A., & Byram, J. (1988). Taste-smell interactions are tastant and odorant dependent. *Chemical Senses, 13*, 445–455.

Frank, R. A., Ducheny, K., & Mize, S. J. S. (1989). Strawberry odor, but not red color, enhances the sweetness of sucrose solutions. *Chemical Senses, 14*, 371–377.

Frank, R. A., van der Klaauw, N. J., & Schifferstein, H. N. J. (1993). Both perceptual and conceptual factors influence taste-odor and taste-taste interactions. *Perception & Psychophysics, 54*, 343–354.

Garcia-Medina, M. R. (1981). Flavor-odor taste interactions in solutions of acetic acid and coffee. *Chemical Senses, 6*, 13–22.

Graf, P., & Schacter, D. L. (1987). Selective effects of interference on implicit and explicit memory for new associations. *Journal of Experimental Psychology: Learning, Memory and Cognition, 13*, 45–53.

Graf, P., & Schacter, D. L. (1989). Unitization and grouping mediate dissociations in memory for new associations. *Journal of Experimental Psychology: Learning, Memory and Cognition, 15*, 930–940.

Green, B. G. (1978). Referred thermal sensations: Warmth versus cold. *Sensory Processes, 2*, 220–230.

Hall, G. (2001). Perceptual learning: Association and differentiation. In R. R. Mowrer & S. B. Klein (Eds.), *Handbook of contemporary learning theories* (pp. 367–407). Hillsdale, NJ: Erlbaum.

Harper, R., Land, D. G., Griffiths, N. M., & Bate-Smith, E. C. (1968). Odor qualities: A glossary of usage. *British Journal of Psychology, 59*, 231–252.

Harrison, J. E., & Baron-Cohen, S. (1997). Synaesthesia: A review of psychological theories. In S. Baron-Cohen & J. Harrison (Eds.), *Synaesthesia: Classic and contemporary readings* (pp. 109–122). Oxford, England: Basil Blackwell.

Herz, R. S., & Engen, T. (1996). Odor memory: Review and analysis. *Psychonomic Bulletin and Review, 3*, 300–313.

Hornung, D. E., & Enns, M. P. (1984). The independence and integration of olfaction and taste. *Chemical Senses, 9*, 97–106.

Hornung, D. E., & Enns, M. P. (1986). The contribution of smell and taste to overall intensity: A model. *Perception & Psychophysics, 39*, 385–391.

Horowitz, L. M., & Prytulak, L. S. (1969). Redintegrative memory. *Psychological Review, 76*, 519–531.

Kareken, D. A., Doty, R. L., Moberg, P. J., Mosnik, D., Chen, S. H., Farlow, M. R., & Hutchins, G. D. (2001). Olfactory-evoked regional cerebral blood flow in Alzheimer's disease. *Neuropsychology, 15*, 18–29.

Kocher, E. C., & Fisher, G. L. (1969). Subjective intensity and taste preference. *Perceptual and Motor Skills, 28*, 735–740.

Lanza, D. C., & Clerico, D. M. (1995). Anatomy of the human nasal passages. In R. L. Doty (Ed.), *Handbook of olfaction and gustation* (pp. 53–75). New York: Marcel Dekker.

Lawless, H. T. (1996). Flavor. In M. P. Friedman & E. C. Carterette (Eds.), *Handbook of perception: Vol. 16. Cognitive ecology* (pp. 325–380). San Diego, CA: Academic Press.

Lawless, H. T., & Engen, T. (1977). Associations to odors: Interference, mnemonics and verbal labeling. *Journal of Experimental Psychology: Human Learning and Memory, 3*, 52–59.

Lawless, H. T., Thomas, C. J., & Johnston, M. (1995). Variation in odor thresholds for l-carvone and cineole and correlations with suprathreshold intensity ratings. *Chemical Senses, 20*, 9–17.

Lovibond, P. F., & Shanks, D. R. (2002). The role of awareness in Pavlovian conditioning: Empirical evidence and theoretical implications. *Journal of Experimental Psychology: Animal Behavior Processes, 28*, 3–26.

Lubow, R. E., & Gewirtz, D. (1995). Latent inhibition in humans: Data theory and implications for schizophrenia. *Psychological Bulletin, 117*, 87–103.

Marks, L. E. (1975). On colored-hearing synesthesia: Cross-modal translations of sensory dimensions. *Psychological Bulletin, 82*, 303–331.

McLaren, I. P. L., & Mackintosh, N. J. (2000). An elemental model of associative learning: I. Latent inhibition and perceptual learning. *Animal Learning and Behavior, 28*, 211–246.

McLaughlin, S., & Margolskee, R. F. (1994). The sense of taste: The internal molecular workings of the taste bud help it distinguish the bitter from the sweet. *American Scientist, 82*, 538–545.

Murphy, C., & Cain, W. S. (1980). Taste and olfaction: Independence vs interaction. *Physiology and Behavior, 24*, 601–605.

Murphy, C., Cain, W. S., & Bartoshuk, L. M. (1977). Mutual action of taste and olfaction. *Sensory Processes, 1*, 204–211.

Pearce, J. M. (1994). Similarity and discrimination: A selective review and a connectionist model. *Psychological Review, 101*, 587–607.

Pierce, J., & Halpern, B. (1996). Orthonasal and retronasal odorant identification based upon vapor phase input from common substances. *Chemical Senses, 21*, 529–543.

Prescott, J. (1999). Flavor as a psychological construct: Implications for perceiving and measuring the sensory qualities of foods. *Food Quality and Preference, 10*, 1–8.

Prescott, J., Francis, J., & Johnstone, V. (2003). Effects of different perceptual strategies during exposure to odor/taste mixtures on the properties and interactions of the mixture components. Manuscript submitted for publication.

Rabin, M. D. (1988). Experience facilitates olfactory quality discrimination. *Perception & Psychophysics, 44*, 532–540.

Rabin, M. D., & Cain, W. S. (1984). Odor recognition: Familiarity, identifiability and encoding consistency. *Journal of Experimental Psychology: Learning, Memory and Cognition, 10*, 316–325.

Rescorla, R. A. (1980). Simultaneous and successive associations in sensory preconditioning. *Journal of Experimental Psychology: Animal Behavior Processes, 6*, 207–216.

Rescorla, R. A., & Wagner, A. R. (1972). A theory of Pavlovian conditioning: Variations in the effectiveness of reinforcement and nonreinforcement. In A. H. Black & W. F. Prokasy (Eds.), *Classical conditioning II* (pp. 64–99). New York: Appleton-Century-Crofts.

Rozin, P. (1978). "Taste-smell confusions" and the duality of the olfactory sense. *Perception & Psychophysics, 31*, 397–401.

Rozin, P., Wrzesniewski, A., & Byrnes, D. (1998). The elusiveness of evaluative conditioning. *Learning and Motivation, 29*, 397–415.

Sakai, N., Kobayakaw, T., Gotow, N., Saito, S., & Imada, S. (2001). Enhancement of sweetness ratings of aspartame by a vanilla odor presented either by orthonasal or retronasal routes. *Perceptual and Motor Skills, 92*, 1002–1008.

Schacter, D. L. (1987). Implicit memory: History and current status. *Journal of Experimental Psychology: Learning, Memory and Cognition, 13*, 501–518.

Schacter, D. L., & Church, B. A. (1992). Auditory priming: Implicit and explicit memory for words and voices. *Journal of Experimental Psychology: Learning, Memory and Cognition, 18*, 915–930.

Schacter, D. L., Cooper, L. A., Delaney, S. M., Peterson, M. A., & Tharan, M. (1991). Implicit memory for possible and impossible objects: Constraints on the construction of structural descriptions. *Journal of Experimental Psychology: Learning, Memory and Cognition, 17,* 3–19.

Schifferstein, H. N. J., & Verlegh, P. W. J. (1996). The role of congruency and pleasantness in odor-induced taste enhancement. *Acta Psychologica, 94,* 87–105.

Sloman, S. A., Hayman, C. A. G., Ohta, N., Law, J., & Tulving, E. (1988). Forgetting in primed fragment completion. *Journal of Experimental Psychology: Learning, Memory and Cognition, 14,* 223–239.

Steiner, J. E., Glaser, D., Hawilo, M. E., & Berridge, K. C. (2001). Comparative expression of hedonic impact: Affective reactions to taste by human infants and other primates. *Neuroscience and Biobehavioral Reviews, 25,* 53–74.

Stevenson, R. J. (2001a). Is sweetness taste enhancement cognitively impenetrable? Effects of exposure, training and knowledge. *Appetite, 36,* 241–242.

Stevenson, R. J. (2001b). The acquisition of odor quality. *Quarterly Journal of Experimental Psychology, 54A,* 561–578.

Stevenson, R. J. (2001c). Associative learning and odor quality perception: How sniffing an odor mixture can alter the smell of its parts. *Learning and Motivation, 32,* 154–177.

Stevenson, R. J. (2001d). Perceptual learning with odors: Implications for psychological accounts of odor quality perception. *Psychonomic Bulletin and Review, 8,* 708–712.

Stevenson, R. J., & Boakes, R. A. (2003). A mnemonic theory of odor perception. *Psychological Review, 110,* 340–364.

Stevenson, R. J., Boakes, R. A., & Prescott, J. (1998). Changes in odor sweetness resulting from implicit learning of a simultaneous odor-sweetness association: An example of learned synesthesia. *Learning and Motivation, 29,* 113–132.

Stevenson, R. J., Boakes, R. A., & Wilson, J. P. (2000a). Counter-conditioning following human odor-taste and color-taste learning. *Learning and Motivation, 31,* 114–127.

Stevenson, R. J., Boakes, R. A., & Wilson, J. P. (2000b). Resistance to extinction of conditioned odor perceptions: Evaluative conditioning is not unique. *Journal of Experimental Psychology: Learning, Memory and Cognition, 26,* 423–440.

Stevenson, R. J., & Case, T. I. (2003). Preexposure to the stimulus elements, but not training to detect them, retards human odour-taste learning. *Behavioural Processes, 61,* 13–25.

Stevenson, R. J., & Prescott, J. (1997). Judgments of chemosensory mixtures in memory. *Acta Psychologica, 95,* 195–214.

Stevenson, R. J., Prescott, J., & Boakes, R. A. (1995). The acquisition of taste properties by odors. *Learning and Motivation, 26,* 433–455.

Stevenson, R. J., Prescott, J., & Boakes, R. A. (1999). Confusing tastes and smells: How odors can influence the perception of sweet and sour tastes. *Chemical Senses, 24,* 627–635.

Tanaka, J. W., & Sengco, J. A. (1997). Features and their configuration in face recognition. *Memory and Cognition, 25,* 583–592.

van der Klaauw, N. J., & Frank, R. A. (1996). Scaling component intensities of complex stimuli: The influence of response alternatives. *Environment International, 22,* 21–31.

Wagner, A. R., & Brandon, S. E. (2001). A componential theory of Pavlovian conditioning. In R. R. Mowrer & S. B. Klein (Eds.), *Handbook of contemporary learning theories* (pp. 23–64). Hillsdale, NJ: Erlbaum.

Ward, L. M. (1990). Cross-modal additive conjoint structures and psychophysical scale convergence. *Journal of Experimental Psychology: General, 119,* 161–175.

Winograd, E., Goldstein, F, C, G., Monarch, E. S., Peluso, J. P., & Goldman, W. P. (1999). The mere exposure effect in patients with Alzheimer's disease. *Neuropsychology, 13,* 41–46.

Zellner, D. A., Rozin, P., Aron, M., & Kulish, C. (1983). Conditioned enhancement of human's liking for flavor by pairing with sweetness. *Learning and Motivation, 14,* 338–350.

6 Cross-Modal Interactions in Speeded Classification

LAWRENCE E. MARKS

Introduction

It has become something of a truism to say that the information-processing capacity of humans is limited, that at any given moment in time the nervous system is capable of fully processing only a fraction of the information that is potentially available. Sometimes the multifarious information arrives through a single sensory modality, but more often information arrives simultaneously through several modalities. Because of our limited capacity for processing information, mechanisms of selective attention provide a means to ensure or enhance the processing of some of the incoming stimulus information.

Given this framework, one of the central questions is the following: How selective is attention? How well can we process information about one perceptual dimension or coming from one sensory modality and ignore information in other dimensions or from other modalities? This chapter is concerned with selective attention in the face of cross-modal stimulation. In particular, the chapter focuses on the failure of selective attention that occurs when people are presented with compound or complex stimuli activating different sensory modalities and asked to respond to only one component.

These failures of selective attention are often characterized as "dimensional interactions," a term that originated in research concerned with selective attention to component features or attributes of stimuli presented within a single modality. Dimensional interactions, or failures of selective attention, are readily observed in tasks of speeded classification—tasks that require subjects to classify each of several stimuli as quickly as possible. This chapter begins by outlining the main findings that have been obtained in studies of speeded classification of unimodal stimuli, primarily vision, where most research has been conducted. After reviewing the unimodal findings, the chapter continues with a more detailed analysis of interactions observed in speeded classification of cross-modal stimuli.

Background, methods, and definitions

A research program initiated in the 1960s by Garner and then continued by Garner, his colleagues, and others has sought to elucidate the basic characteristics and principles of selective attention to multidimensionally varying stimuli (e.g., Garner, 1974b; Lockhead, 1972; Melara & Marks, 1990a; Smith & Kemler, 1978). In brief, the program aims at learning how attention affects the perception of stimuli, presented within a single modality, that vary along several stimulus dimensions, either from moment to moment (as they do in the world) or from trial to trial (as they do in most experiments). How well can people attend to particular attributes or features of a stimulus, taken from one stimulus dimension or component, while ignoring attributes or features of other components or dimensions of the same stimulus?

THE PARADIGM OF SPEEDED CLASSIFICATION The traditional paradigm for studying this kind of selective attention is speeded classification. In the speeded classification paradigm, subjects must identify particular characteristics of a stimulus as quickly as possible while ignoring any other, irrelevant characteristics. In the simplest version of the speeded classification paradigm, there is just one relevant dimension (R) and just one irrelevant dimension (I), and each of these dimensions can take on either of two possible values (a or b), making four possible stimuli in all: $R_a I_a$, $R_a I_b$, $R_b I_a$, and $R_b I_b$. So, for example, the stimuli might be auditory, varying along the dimensions of pitch (low or high) and loudness (soft and loud), or the stimuli might be visual, varying along the dimensions of size (small or large) and color (dark or light). The speeded classification paradigm compares subjects' performance on a control or *baseline task* to performance on a *selective attention task*. In the baseline task, the only attributes or features that vary from trial to trial are those relevant to classification on dimension R; attributes or features in the irrelevant dimension I remain constant. Thus, subjects might be asked, for example, to classify auditory stimuli by their pitch, while loudness stays constant, or to classify visual stimuli by their size, while color stays constant. In the selective attention task, not only do the critical attributes or features vary, but so also do other, irrelevant attributes or features. In tasks of selective attention, subjects might classify auditory stimuli according to their pitch, in the face of irrelevant variation in loudness, or classify visual stimuli according to their size, in the face of irrelevant variation in color.

In speeded classification, subjects try to classify each stimulus as quickly as possible, the primary measure of performance typically being response time. Errors sometimes serve as a secondary measure of performance, and these two measures, response times and errors, usually correlate positively. That is, when subjects are slower in responding, they also make more errors. Response times are used more often than errors as a primary measure of performance because response times generally prove more sensitive. A handful of studies, however, have used unspeeded versions of the paradigm, measuring accuracy alone, within more traditional psychophysical paradigms that place no time constraint on responding. This approach has the virtue of making it possible to quantify the results within the framework of signal detection theory (e.g., Kingston & Macmillan, 1995; Macmillan & Ornstein, 1998).

As already stated, research using the speeded classification paradigm originated in studies that were concerned with interactions of dimensions within a single sensory modality. Consider, as an example, the question asked by Garner (1977): Can a person attend to the size of a visual stimulus independent of its color (in Garner's experiment, dark versus light), and can a person attend to the color of a visual stimulus independent of its size? Following the design just described, Garner used two pairs of baseline tasks. One pair of baseline tasks required the subjects to classify the stimuli on the basis of their size (R = size), deciding on each trial whether each stimulus was the small one (R_a) or the large one (R_b), with the color of the stimulus held constant across trials. In one of these baseline tasks the color was dark (I_a) and in another the color was light (I_b). And in a complementary pair of baseline tasks, the subjects classified the stimuli on the basis of their color (R = color), as dark (R_a) or light (R_b), while size (I_a or I_b) remained constant.

To ask about the ability to attend selectively is to ask whether, relative to performance at baseline, performance remains as good in the selective attention task, where values on the irrelevant dimension vary from trial to trial. Note that each baseline task is properly termed *identification*, as there are, in each, two possible

stimuli and two possible responses. By contrast, the selective attention task is one of *classification*, as there are four possible stimuli but only two possible responses. The selective attention task is also sometimes called an *orthogonal task* (Ben-Artzi & Marks, 1995b; Garner, 1974b), because the attributes on the relevant and irrelevant dimensions vary orthogonally, and sometimes called a *filtering task* (Posner, 1964), because it is assumed that in order to classify correctly, subjects must "filter out" variations along an irrelevant dimension. In the case of color and size, as reported by Garner (1977), performance on baseline tasks and performance on selective attention tasks were virtually identical, meaning that subjects can attend fully and selectively to either of these dimensions and ignore irrelevant variation in the other. Garner characterized pairs of dimensions showing this pattern of performance as *separable*.

SEPARABLE AND INTEGRAL DIMENSIONS: GARNER INTERFERENCE   In many instances, subjects cannot attend selectively to one dimension when attributes or features of other, irrelevant dimensions vary from trial to trial. Instead, there is often an incremental cost in terms of processing efficiency—a difference between performance at baseline and performance when values on an irrelevant dimension vary orthogonally. A prototypical example, again from the realm of vision, is found in the component dimensions of color. When the common scheme of classifying color dimensions by hue, saturation, and brightness is used, it turns out that in every case—that is, for every pair of dimensions—hue and saturation, hue and brightness, saturation and brightness—performance requiring selective attention is poorer than performance at baseline (e.g., Garner & Felfoldy, 1970; Melara, Marks, & Potts, 1993; Smith & Kemler, 1978). Classifying color stimuli by their brightness, hue, or saturation is impaired when values on one of the other dimensions vary irrelevantly. It is harder to attend selectively to the brightness of a visual stimulus, for example, when the stimulus also varies unpredictably in its hue or its saturation. These combinations of perceptual dimensions are said to be *integral* (Garner, 1974b).

The difference between performance at baseline and performance on an orthogonal (filtering) task provides a defining characteristic of *separable* versus *integral* combinations of dimensions (e.g., Garner, 1974b; Garner & Felfoldy, 1970). Dimensions have been called *separable* if subjects could attend selectively to either, that is, if performance measured when the irrelevant dimension varies orthogonally is equivalent to performance measured at baseline, as in the case of size and color.

A second characteristic that often distinguishes (but does not define) integral from separable pairs of dimensions is performance, relative to baseline, when values on two dimensions are correlated. Subjects may, for example, be asked to classify stimuli by color, as dark or light, but the dark object may always be high in saturation or large in size, while the light object is always low in saturation or small. In this case, the values on the two dimensions are correlated, and, according to Garner (1974b), the presence of such a correlation should provide some benefit to performance when dimensions are integral but not when they are separable. Indeed, following Garner's prediction, performance on a task where values on two dimensions are correlated is often equivalent to performance at baseline when the dimensions are separable, but superior to performance at baseline when the dimensions are integral. Other investigators, however, have questioned the rationale behind the prediction itself. For example, Ashby and Townsend (1986; see also Ashby & Maddox, 1994) pointed out that even models that assume that dimensions are processed independently (in a statistical sense) can predict improvement in performance when dimensions are correlated. That is, when the dimensions are perceptually separable, performance can be better when stimuli vary along two correlated dimensions, compared with one dimension, because of "probability summation." Consequently, the failure to find improved performance, relative to baseline, with correlated separable dimensions is not so much a defining characteristic of separability as it is a failure of real subjects to perform as well as ideal observers who make use of all of the available information.

The failure to filter out irrelevant variation in an unattended perceptual dimension has come to be called *Garner interference* (Pomerantz, Pristach, & Carson, 1989). In the case of integral dimensions within a single modality, Garner interference has sometimes been attributed to hypothesized characteristics of early sensory processing. In particular, several investigators have proposed that early processing of certain combinations of stimulus dimensions—dimensions that are integral—is holistic, which is to say that at the earliest stages of processing, the dimensions themselves are not fully differentiated one from another (Lockhead, 1972; see also Garner, 1974b; Kemler Nelson, 1989). The early holistic hypothesis makes the following claims: first, integral dimensions are not fully differentiated early in processing; second, consequently, early in processing, attributes on two (or more) integral dimensions are confused; and third, speeded classification taps perception at this early stage of processing. Thus, irrelevant stimulation in an irrelevant dimension increases the time and decreases the accuracy to classify attributes on the relevant dimension (Garner

interference). Separable dimensions, by contrast, are presumably well differentiated even at early stages of processing. And so, with separable dimensions, processing of each dimension proceeds independently of processing of the other dimensions, there is no confusion, and Garner interference is absent.

Working within this framework, several investigators assumed that the best examples of separable dimensions would be cross-modal (Garner, 1974a; Treisman, 1969), which is to say, these investigators implied that subjects would most easily be able to attend to a single perceptual dimension and ignore variations on another dimension when the two dimensions were presented to different sensory modalities. In this regard, Garner (1974a) cited the findings of Tulving and Lindsay (1967), who had subjects make absolute judgments about the brightness of lights and the loudness of sounds, in an unspeeded task, under several stimulus conditions: when the stimulus set consisted of lights alone, varying in luminance; when the set consisted of tones alone, varying in sound pressure; and when the set consisted of all combinations of lights and tones. Tulving and Lindsay found that subjects could classify the stimuli on either modality, largely independently of stimulation on the other. Overall performance, measured in terms of transmitted information, was essentially the same in the presence and in the absence of cross-modal stimulation. As it turns out, this does not hold for tasks of speeded classification. When instructed to respond as quickly as possible, subjects cannot attend selectively to the brightness or lightness of a visual stimulus and disregard a concomitant sound varying in its loudness (Marks, 1987) or pitch (Marks, 1987; Martino & Marks, 1999; Melara, 1989a).

EFFECTS OF STIMULUS CONGRUENCE In addition to Garner interference, results obtained with the method of speeded classification sometimes reveal a second kind of dimensional interaction, one that has been termed a *congruence effect*. Congruence effects refer to patterns of performance in which responses are quicker and more accurate when the stimulus has two or more perceptual attributes that are congruent, attributes that (broadly speaking) match in some way, compared to stimuli whose perceptual attributes are incongruent, that is, stimuli whose attributes mismatch.

An early report of congruence effects came from Clark and Brownell (1975), who asked subjects to make speeded classifications of arrows that pointed up or down when these visual stimuli appeared at different vertical positions within a rectangle. Clark and Brownell found an interaction between the direction the arrow pointed and its spatial position: when the arrow pointed up (or, to describe the stimulus equivalently, when the arrowhead appeared at the top of the shaft), response speed increased when the arrow's position was higher within the rectangle, and when the arrow pointed down (arrowhead at the bottom of the shaft), response speed increased when the arrow's position was lower within the rectangle.

Where Garner interference represents a global decrease in performance across all of the levels of the relevant stimulus in the ensemble, congruence effects represent differences in performance among the various stimuli within the ensemble. In principle, congruence effects could occur in the absence of Garner interference. If so—if performance on a selective attention task were equivalent to performance at baseline—then it would follow that, within the selective attention task, performance with congruent stimulus combinations would show facilitation (superior to performance at baseline), while performance with incongruent combinations would show inhibition (inferior to performance at baseline). Typically, however, when congruent effects do occur, overall performance on the selective attention task is inferior to performance at baseline. That is, Garner interference generally accompanies congruence effects. In reviewing more than 60 studies from Pomerantz's laboratory, Pomerantz et al. (1989) noted that Garner interference and congruence effects usually, though not always, accompanied each other. In general, the magnitude of Garner interference is greater than that of congruence effects. Interestingly, Garner interference may occur without congruence effects, but congruence effects rarely occur without Garner interference (though exceptions occur, as with complex visual shapes: see van Leeuwen & Bakker, 1995; congruence effects without Garner interference are also evident in the results of Patching & Quinlan, 2002). That is, congruence effects almost never show up alone, whereas interference effects may. This is true both of dimensional interactions found with unimodal stimuli and of dimensional interactions found with cross-modal stimuli.

It is useful to consider more fully what is meant by congruence. As Clark and Brownell (1975) wrote, "subjects were faster when the arrow's 'intrusive attribute' (its height) had the same value as its 'criterial attribute' (its direction)" (p. 339). Implicit in this statement is the notion that stimuli are congruent when they "have the same value"—in the case of Clark and Brownell's stimuli, when they had, or indicated, the same relative vertical spatial location. Kornblum, Hasbroucq, and Osman (1990) used the term "dimensional overlap" to describe congruence, and they trace the latter term, and the underlying conceptual framework, to the work of Fitts (e.g., Fitts & Deininger, 1954), who designated congruence as a correspondence between the spatial layout of a set of stimuli and the spatial pattern of the responses.

Over the last three decades, the term "congruence" has been applied by various investigators to many different combinations of stimulus dimensions and perceptual dimensions, sometimes to dimensions within a single modality and sometimes to dimensions in different modalities. In each case, at least by implication, congruence refers to the sharing of relative (or, less often, absolute) values of different stimuli, or of the perceptual attributes of the stimuli. Although in some instances what are shared are values on a common physical dimension (in Clark and Brownell's 1975 study, relative position/direction in the vertical spatial dimension), in other instances what are shared are relative levels along two dimensions that are inferred to bear some kind of normative alignment. Typically the dimensions are polar, in that they have one end-point that is designated as negative, indicating "little" of an attribute, and another that is positive, indicating "much" of the attribute. Pitch, loudness, brightness, saturation, and size are examples.

Two dimensions of the same, or different, modalities are therefore aligned when their negative and positive poles match. For example, Melara and Marks (1990a) asked subjects to classify tones that varied from trial to trial in pitch and loudness, defining the combinations low pitch + low loudness and high pitch + high loudness as congruent, low pitch + high loudness and high pitch + low loudness as incongruent. In this example, congruence implicitly referred to the sharing of relative positions on the two quantitative perceptual dimensions, pitch and loudness. The results of Melara and Marks's study showed congruence effects in speeded classification, in that subjects classified congruent combinations faster than incongruent combinations in the orthogonal, selective attention task. Melara et al. (1993) reported similar findings for vision. Defining colors as congruent in saturation and lightness when both values were relatively low or relatively high and as incongruent when one value was relatively low and the other relatively high, Melara et al. too found congruence effects; subjects classified congruent stimulus combinations of colors more quickly than they classified incongruent combinations.

Although rarely done, it seems feasible to devise relatively simple and straightforward empirical tests for congruence between values on any two dimensions, A and B. Given a pair of stimuli with levels a_1 and a_2 on dimension A, and another pair with levels b_1 and b_2 on dimension B, one could ask subjects which stimulus on *A* "matches" or "goes with" which stimulus on *B*. Presumably, subjects would match, say, an upwardly versus downwardly pointing arrow to a high versus low spatial position, would match the higher-pitched to the louder of two sounds, and would match the more saturated to the lighter of two colors. Just such a paradigm has in fact been deployed in order to determine congruence of cross-modal combinations of stimuli, as discussed in the next section.

Cross-modal selective attention

Failures of separability, evident as Garner interference and effects of congruence, are not limited to multidimensionally varying stimuli of a single modality but frequently arise also when subjects try to attend selectively to attributes or features in one modality within a cross-modal (e.g., auditory-visual, auditory-tactile) display. As already mentioned, with unimodal stimuli it has been proposed that interference effects (and congruence effects) in selective attention tasks reflect the outcome of holistic early perceptual processing, although the adequacy of this account is questionable (see Melara & Marks, 1990a; Melara et al., 1993). With cross-modally varying stimuli, this explanation seems even more dubious. To extend the hypothesis that early perceptual processing is holistic to the cross-modal domain is to imply that in the very early stages of perceptual processing, sensory information is still not fully differentiated with regard to modality; it is to treat cross-modally interacting stimuli as akin to integral stimuli of a single modality, such as colors. Such an explanation seems unlikely, and to the best of my knowledge it lacks supporting evidence. Indeed, as mentioned, there is even some question whether the hypothesis of early holistic processing can adequately explain integral interactions with unimodal stimuli. The hypothesis implies that, early in processing, perceptual differences among stimuli are represented only as quantitative variations in global similarity, not as differences on explicit perceptual dimensions such as pitch, loudness, lightness, or saturation. Studies of selective attention using speeded classification in hearing (Melara & Marks, 1990a) and color vision (Melara et al., 1993) show, to the contrary, that subjects' responses do in fact derive from information on underlying perceptual dimensions, even though the results at the same time reveal integral interactions, such as Garner interference.

But even if failures of separability cannot be attributed to early holistic processing, it is still possible that Garner interference and congruence effects result from some other property of early perceptual processing, and in principle this could be the case with cross-modal stimuli as well as unimodal stimuli. That at least some kinds of cross-modal interactions in selective attention may occur relatively early in processing is suggested by a study of Driver (1996). Driver took advantage of a version of the *ventriloquist effect* (e.g., Bertelson, Vroomen, de Gelder, & Driver, 2000; Radeau & Bertelson, 1977)—the tendency, for example, to perceive speech sounds as arising from the visual location of the speaker's face when the sources of the auditory and visual information are spatially displaced—to show that this type of auditory-visual interaction can affect the discriminability of the speech signal itself. Driver presented two streams of speech at the same location in space (through the same loudspeaker, leading to mutual interference), together with a visible face, spatially displaced, that corresponded to one of the speech streams. Under these circumstances, the face "captured" the perceived auditory location of its corresponding speech stream, and, Driver found, could actually increase its intelligibility.

The improvement in performance, a kind of "unmasking" of an acoustic signal through a cross-modally induced shift in its apparent spatial location (away from that of the second source, which otherwise interferes with intelligibility), is reminiscent of the phenomenon known as "binaural unmasking" in hearing (see Moore, 1997, Chap. 6). In the condition of binaural masking that is most directly analogous to Driver's (1996), a tonal signal that is presented to just one ear is accompanied by a masking noise in that ear selected to make the signal just imperceptible. This imperceptible tone can then be made perceptible, or unmasked, by adding identical noise to the contralateral ear. Adding noise to the contralateral ear causes the apparent location of the noise to shift to the midline, away from the perceived (lateralized) location of tonal signal, which then becomes more detectable.

Like binaural unmasking, the cross-modal interactions reported by Driver (1996) appear to arise relatively early in perceptual processing—at least, they presumably precede processes of speech identification. What, then, of cross-modal interactions in selective attention using Garner's paradigm? The evidence reviewed in the subsequent sections suggests that some of these interactions, many instances of congruence effects in particular, likely do not arise out of interactions in perception but instead from relatively late processes of stimulus recoding and decision.

CROSS-MODAL CONGRUENCE   A simple empirical method, outlined earlier in the chapter, can be used to define congruence relations among various pairs of dimensions taken from different sensory modalities. The method entails presenting subjects with two (or more) levels on a stimulus dimension of modality *A* and two (or more) levels on a dimension of modality *B*, then asking the subjects which stimulus on *A* matches which on *B*. Marks, Hammeal, and Bornstein (1987) used this method to obtain matches between sounds and lights that varied along such dimensions as brightness, pitch, and loudness. Adult subjects were virtually unanimous in matching the brighter of two lights with both the higher-pitched and the louder of two sounds, thereby indicating that the cross-modal combinations dim + low pitch, dim + soft, bright + high pitch, and bright + loud are congruent, whereas dim + high pitch, dim + loud, bright + low pitch, and bright + soft are incongruent. Further, the vast majority of 4-year-old children agreed with adults, as assessed by their cross-modal matches, regarding the congruence of both loudness and brightness (75% of 4-year-olds) and pitch and brightness (90% of 4-year-olds). Congruence between loudness and brightness and between pitch and brightness characterizes perception in young children as well as in adults.

Marks (1974) had previously obtained related results in adults, using larger ensembles of stimuli. In one of his experiments, subjects adjusted the pitch of a tone to match each of several gray patches varying in lightness. The results, analogous to those of Marks et al. (1987), indicated congruence relations between pitch and lightness: low pitch congruent with black and high pitch with white. Subsequently, Marks (1989) reported findings obtained with a similarity scaling method. Subjects judged the degree of similarity between all possible pairs of visual stimuli—varying in luminance—and auditory stimuli—tones varying in sound pressure and frequency; that is, subjects judged the degree of similarity of pairs of lights, pairs of sounds, and cross-modal pairs. The ratings of similarity were then subjected to multidimensional scaling, which yielded a two-dimensional solution in which loudness was represented on one axis, pitch on the other, and brightness as a vector through both, again indicating congruence between both pitch and brightness and between loudness and brightness (see also Wicker, 1968). Figure 6.1 shows the results, being a representation of an abstract perceptual space in which the relative proximity of visual and auditory stimuli reflects the congruence relations of visual brightness to auditory pitch and loudness.

It is noteworthy that the dimension of brightness in vision is congruent with two dimensions in hearing: loudness and pitch. In this regard, it is important to distinguish between two attributes of visual experience that are sometimes loosely grouped together as "brightness": one refers to the brightness of spots of light, or brightness proper, the dimension of visual perception

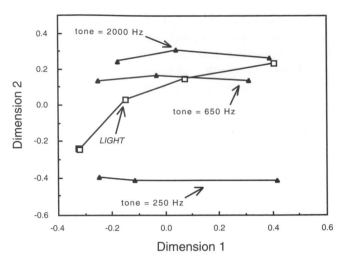

FIGURE 6.1 Spatial representation of similarity relations among auditory and visual stimuli. Multidimensional scaling of similarity judgments of tone-tone, light-light, and light-tone pairs gave a two-dimensional solution. Dimension 1 represents loudness (for each tone frequency, sound pressure is smallest for the data point at the left and greatest for the data point at the right), Dimension 2 represents pitch, and both Dimensions 1 and 2 represent brightness (luminance increases monotonically from the lower left to the upper right). (Data from Marks, 1989.)

whose attributes vary from dim to bright; the other refers to the lightness of surfaces, the dimension of visual perception whose attributes vary from dark to light. The distinction is important in the context of cross-modal interactions because, as already indicated, brightness is congruent with both pitch and loudness (subjects consistently match low-pitched and soft sounds to dim lights, high-pitched and loud sounds to bright lights), whereas lightness is congruent only with pitch and not with loudness (subjects consistently match low- and high-pitched sounds to dark and light colors, respectively, but do not consistently match soft and loud sounds to dark and light colors, either directly or inversely) (Marks, 1974). As we shall see, these differences in cross-modal congruence relations also reveal themselves in selective attention, as assessed through speeded classification.

Note that the dimensions of pitch and loudness in hearing, and lightness and brightness in vision, are by no means exhaustive, even with the simplest of stimuli (pure tones, spot of light, or patches of color). Visual and auditory stimuli may also vary in their duration, their spatial extents, and their spatial locations. Spatial location turns out to be a dimension of particular interest, in part because the verbal labels for the poles of vertical position, "low" and "high," are also the labels typically applied to the negative and positive poles of the dimension of auditory pitch. Thus, one might anticipate congruence between auditory pitch and visual vertical spatial position, as reported for instance by Mudd (1963), based on the use of common labels. While labeling is a plausible explanation of congruence between pitch and position, it is also possible that the application of the labels "low" and "high" to sounds, and the extensive use of this cross-modal correspondence (consider, for instance, the musical staff, which provides a vertical spatial representation of the pitch of notes), is not a mere accident of our linguistic culture. Stumpf (1883), for example, noted that almost every language applies labels for low and high position to frequency of tones. Perhaps the labels "low" and "high" come to designate both positions in space and pitch of sounds because of an intrinsic similarity between these perceptual dimensions (for speculations regarding the source of the linguistic connection, see Marks, 1997). Be this as it may, all of the congruence relations just described readily reveal themselves in tasks of selective attention.

Let me summarize here the very different kinds of congruence relations encountered so far. In Clark and Brownell's (1975) study of visual direction and position, congruence referred to a common (albeit relational) property of a single stimulus dimension (and modality), namely, the vertical dimension of space. In Melara and Marks's (1990a) study of auditory pitch and loudness and in Melara et al.'s (1993) study of visual lightness and saturation, congruence in each case referred to corresponding relative values on two dimensions that lacked any common environmental referent. Again, the congruence in each study was intramodal, but in both studies the relation between the congruent or corresponding dimensions is more abstract than it is in Clark and Brownell's study. Where vertical position and vertical direction are not identical dimensions, they do partake of a common spatial dimension. By contrast, pitch and loudness are not by any means the same dimension (neither are lightness and saturation) and have no common acoustic or optical referent. And in the case of cross-modal congruence relations involving pitch, loudness, lightness, brightness, and spatial position, the correspondences are still more abstract, more figurative, more metaphorical. In fact, it has even been possible to infer the congruence relations between loudness and brightness and between pitch and brightness from ratings given to verbal expressions (Marks, 1982a), and in the case of loudness and brightness, from settings of sound intensities and light intensities made to metaphors taken from poetry (Marks, 1982b).

CROSS-MODAL INTERACTIONS   Cross-modal interactions, especially interactions involving congruence relations,

have been repeatedly reported in tasks of selective attention, as measured by speeded classification. Perhaps the first such finding was provided by Bernstein and Edelstein (1971), who had subjects classify visual stimuli as spatially high or low. As it turned out, the responses were quicker when the visual stimulus was accompanied by a tone that was congruent rather than incongruent in pitch. That is, the response was quicker when the visual stimulus in the low spatial position was accompanied by a tone of low rather than high frequency, and when the visual stimulus in the high spatial position was accompanied by a tone of high rather than low frequency.

Melara and O'Brien (1987) later extended Bernstein and Edelstein's (1971) finding, showing in addition that the mere variation of the stimuli in the irrelevant modality impedes performance (that is, produces Garner interference). Subjects needed on average about 400 ms to classify a tone's pitch as low or high at baseline, where a visual stimulus was always presented simultaneously but in a constant position. Further, the relative position of the visual stimulus did not matter on the baseline task. That is, responses at baseline were no different with congruent and incongruent auditory-visual combinations. In a sense, of course, this is expected, as the low or high position of the visual stimulus, and thus the congruence relation between pitch and position, is itself defined contextually. Presumably, one of the visual stimuli is perceived as low and the other as high only when the subjects are exposed to stimuli in both spatial positions. Because, by definition, the position of the visual stimulus in the baseline task is constant, it is neither low nor high, and hence no congruence relation is established, and no congruence effect occurs in classification performance.

Melara and O'Brien (1987) did find congruence effects in the orthogonal or filtering task, where the response times were about 425 ms when pitch and position matched (low frequency with low position, high frequency with high position) but about 450 ms when the pitch and position mismatched (low frequency with high position, high frequency with low position). The difference of 25 ms constitutes the magnitude of the congruence effect. That response times with both the congruent and the incongruent auditory-visual combinations were greater in the orthogonal task compared to the baseline task constitutes the interference effect. On average, responses in the orthogonal condition took nearly 40 ms longer than did responses in the baseline condition.

A similar pattern of results appeared when subjects classified the position of the visual stimulus while the frequency of the auditory stimulus varied irrelevantly

(Melara & O'Brien, 1987). No congruence effect appeared at baseline (average response times around 360 ms), but a congruence effect did emerge in the orthogonal condition (response times of 385 ms when stimuli matched, 395 ms when they mismatched), as did Garner interference (about 30 ms in size). Thus, both kinds of interaction, congruence effects and Garner interference, were evident when subjects attempted to attend selectively to tones of low and high pitch in the face of visual stimuli varying in up-down position, and vice versa.

In a series of 16 experiments in which the investigators systematically varied both the physical difference between the sound frequencies and the physical difference between the visual positions, Ben-Artzi and Marks (1995b) confirmed Melara and O'Brien's (1987) general findings, and made two other significant observations. First, the size of the physical difference in visual position mattered little to performance, but the size of the physical difference in auditory pitch did matter to the magnitude of both the interference effects and congruence effects. And second, the interference and congruence interactions observed when subjects classified the stimuli according to their pitch were greater than the corresponding interactions observed when the subjects classified the stimuli according to their visual position. A similar trend is evident in the findings of Melara and O'Brien (see also Patching & Quinlan, 2002).

In the studies of Melara and O'Brien (1987), Ben-Artzi and Marks (1995b), and Patching and Quinlan (2002), it is noteworthy that performance on the two dimensions was not equivalent at baseline. Baseline responses were faster when the subjects judged visual position than when the subjects judged pitch. Consequently, the asymmetry in the magnitude of interference and congruence effects observed for the selective attention task could relate to the difference in baseline performance. As Melara and Mounts (1993) have pointed out, when subjects respond more quickly at baseline to one of the stimulus dimensions than to the other, interactions in the selective attention task tend to be asymmetric, being greater when subjects classify the "poorer dimension." Presumably, if, at baseline, levels on dimension A are processed more quickly than levels on dimension B, then when levels on A vary irrelevantly, being processed quickly, the variation in A strongly affects classification of B. But when levels on dimension B vary irrelevantly, being processed slowly, the variation in B less strongly affects classification of A.

The findings just reviewed show that the ability to attend and respond selectively to a visual or auditory stimulus can be modulated by simultaneous stimulation in the other sensory modality, even though the properties of the secondary stimulus are irrelevant to the subject's task. In the examples just considered, the interactions take the form of both interference and congruence effects, the latter looking suspiciously like the possible outcome of application of common verbal labels "low" and "high" to the different stimuli.

But cross-modal interactions—Garner interference and congruence effects—can arise even when the stimuli do not share labels in any obvious fashion. In particular, interactions readily appear in results of speeded classification studies where the dimensions in the different modalities bear what seem to be wholly abstract or figurative correspondence and where the attributes are not typically given the same descriptive labels. Prominent among these are the interactions observed between auditory stimuli that vary in their pitch (low versus high) and visual stimuli that vary in their color (black versus white). Irrelevant variation in stimulation on either one of these modalities can impede performance in classifying stimuli on the other modality—which is to say, pitch and color show Garner interference (Martino & Marks, 1999; Melara, 1989a). And, even more consistently, speeded classification of pitch and color shows congruence effects (Marks, 1987; Martino & Marks, 1999; Melara, 1989a). Subjects respond more quickly and accurately, both while classifying pitch and while classifying color, when presented with the congruent combinations of stimuli, low pitch + black and high pitch + white, than when presented with the incongruent combinations, low pitch + white and high pitch + black.

To summarize the results of several experiments: paradigms of speeded classification have revealed cross-modal interactions in studies using five different combinations of auditory and visual dimensions: (1) pitch and visual position (Ben-Artzi & Marks, 1995b; Bernstein & Edelstein, 1971; Melara & O'Brien, 1987; Patching & Quinlan, 2002); (2) pitch and color (lightness, the perceptual dimension of surfaces varying from black to white) (Marks, 1987; Martino & Marks, 1999; Melara, 1989a); (3) pitch and brightness (the perceptual dimension of lights varying from dim to bright) (Marks, 1987); (4) loudness and brightness (Marks, 1987); and (5) pitch (low vs. high) and shape (rounded vs. angular) (Marks, 1987).

Cross-modal interactions have been observed in speeded classification tasks involving the tactile sense as well. Taking advantage of the phenomenological and psychophysical similarities between the auditory perception of tones and the tactile perception of vibratory stimuli delivered to the skin, Martino and Marks (2000) tested for a possible tactile-visual analogue to pitch-color interactions. These investigators substituted vibrations to the hand for tones to the ears, and tested the ability of subjects to attend selectively, in a speeded classification paradigm, to vibrations varying in frequency and to colors varying in lightness. The results showed both interference and congruence effects, though mostly when subjects classified the vibratory stimuli (as expected, given how much more rapidly the baseline responses were made to the visual compared to the vibrotactile stimuli).

In general, selective attention, as measured by tasks of speeded classification, has revealed congruence effects whenever cross-modal matching tasks, described earlier, show congruence relations—for example, between pitch and brightness, between pitch and lightness, and between loudness and brightness (Marks, 1987). Just as important, however, where no congruence effect is evident in cross-modal matching, as is the case with the dimensions of loudness and lightness (Marks, 1974), speeded classification also showed no congruence-like effects in response time or accuracy (Marks, 1987). In short, where cross-modal congruence effects are evident in perception, they exert effects on selective attention as assessed by speeded classification. With cross-modal dimensions that do not bear a congruence relation, analogous effects are absent from speeded classification.

CONGRUENCE INTERACTIONS, SYNESTHESIA, AND CROSS-MODAL SIMILARITY Many of the interactions observed in speeded classification, but in particular those between auditory pitch and visual lightness, are striking in part because pitch and lightness appear so prominently in the literature on synesthesia. Synesthesia is that curious phenomenon in which, to the relatively small number of individuals who experience the world in their unique fashions, stimulation of one sensory modality regularly and reliably arouses not only the sensory experiences appropriate to that modality but also strong sensory images of another modality, as when sounds induce colors (though the term synesthesia also includes the induction of strong sensory images in other dimensions of the same modality, as when letters of the alphabet induce colors) (Cytowic, 1989; Harrison, 2001; Marks, 1975, 1978, 2000; see also Stevenson & Boakes, Chap. 5, this volume; Dixon, Smilek, Wagar, & Merikle, Chap. 52, this volume; Mattingley & Rich, Chap. 53, this volume). A common form of synesthesia is auditory-visual, the evocation by sounds of shapes and, especially, of colors. And in auditory-visual synesthesia, the color quality that is induced by the auditory stimulus often follows directly from its perceived pitch: the higher the pitch of the sound, the lighter or brighter the induced color (for reviews, see Marks, 1975, 1978, 2000).

Cross-modal congruence relations reveal themselves, therefore, in three domains: in cross-modal matches, and analogous measures of similarity, which may serve to define the congruence relations; in synesthesia; and in tasks of speeded classification. And, as noted already, at least some of these congruence relations are evident in the cross-modal matches of children as young as 4 years (Marks et al., 1987). Pertinent here is the study of Lewkowicz and Turkewitz (1980), who reported loudness-brightness "matching" in one-month-old infants, as quantified by changes in heart rate in response to shifts in stimulus intensities within and across the auditory and visual modalities. Besides providing evidence of cross-modal correspondence soon after birth, there is another particularly intriguing aspect to Lewkowicz and Turkewitz's results: they imply that, in infants, the congruence relation between loudness and brightness is based not on relative or contextual levels of the stimuli but on their absolute levels; that, in infants, there are particular levels of brightness that are perceptually equal to particular levels of loudness. The findings raise the intriguing possibility that absolute cross-modal correspondences exist in infants, in which case we may infer that these correspondences change, over the ensuing years, from being absolute to being predominantly contextual. The development of language, and the availability of verbal labels, may play an important role in the transition from absolute to relative or contextual processing.

All of these findings are compatible with the hypothesis that certain cross-modal congruence relations—relations among such dimensions as pitch, loudness, and brightness—originate in intrinsic similarities between perceptual dimensions in different modalities. Further, these phenomenally experienced cross-modal similarities in turn may derive, at least in part, from common characteristics of the underlying neural codes. Such an account has traditionally been used to explain cross-modal equivalence in the realm of perceived intensity, under the assumption that the perception of intensity—including loudness in hearing and brightness in vision—is encoded in the rate or number of neural impulses. Perhaps because information about neural rate, or periodicity, also plays a major role in coding pitch, neural firing rate may provide a basis for the underlying similarity relation between pitch and brightness, as well as that between loudness and brightness. But a caveat is in order: Even if principles of neural coding can account for the origin of these cross-modal similarities, the contextuality of cross-modal congruence evident after infancy implies that a neural code as simple as firing rate or periodicity does not by itself continue to provide the mechanism underlying congruence interactions in children or, especially, in adults.

Mechanisms underlying congruence interactions

The findings reviewed so far suggest three main principles:

First, in situations in which stimulation in one modality is relevant to the task while stimulation in other modalities is irrelevant, and subjects try to attend selectively to the relevant modality of information, stimulation on irrelevant modalities can interfere with processing relevant information, meaning that stimulation on irrelevant modalities is processed nonetheless. This conclusion is consistent with the widely held view that unattended stimuli are processed at least partially (see Pashler, 1998, for review). Were unattended stimuli not processed at all, congruence interactions would be absent from speeded classification.

Second, the presence of stimulation in an irrelevant modality can notably influence the processing of an attended stimulus if the unattended and attended stimuli bear some kind of congruence relation.

And third, the cross-modal congruence relations themselves are typically determined contextually, at least in adults. Presented with a tone of a given frequency and intensity, perceptual and cognitive systems encode the tone as low or high in pitch, as soft or as loud, relative to other tones. Presented with a light of a given luminance and spatial position, perceptual and cognitive systems encode the light as dim or bright, as spatially low or high, relative to other lights. The assessment of relative pitch, loudness, brightness, or position comes about contextually, from the location of the given stimulus in its perceptual dimension relative to the set of possible levels in that dimension. Thus, it is not surprising that congruence effects are generally evident only in performance measured on selective attention tasks (orthogonal or filtering tasks), where values on both the irrelevant and relevant stimulus dimensions vary from trial to trial, but are generally not evident in performance measured on baseline tasks, where the irrelevant stimulus maintains a constant value throughout the block of trials (e.g., Martino & Marks, 1999; Melara, 1989a; Melara & Marks, 1990a; Melara & O'Brien, 1987). Indeed, the very same auditory stimulus can interact differently with a visual stimulus, depending on the contextual set of stimuli to which the auditory stimulus belongs (Marks, 1987).

What has not yet been addressed is the underlying mechanism. Given the general principles just reviewed, what kinds of mechanism might underlie cross-modal interactions, and in particular congruence effects, assessed through tasks of speeded classification? One possibility, already considered briefly, is early holistic processing, which has been proposed to account for interactions (mainly Garner interference) found with integral dimensions of a single modality, for instance, interactions among lightness or brightness, saturation, and hue (Kemler Nelson, 1989; Lockhead, 1972). According to these accounts, variations in certain stimulus dimensions are processed independently of one another, even early in processing, making it possible to attend selectively, in speeded classification, to the values on any of them without interference from irrelevant variation in another. A prototypical example consists of the separable pair of dimensions: color (lightness) and size. By contrast, variations in other dimensions are processed as an ensemble, making it impossible to attend selectively, in speeded classification, to the values on any one dimension while values on another dimension vary irrelevantly. The prototype here consists of the integral dimensions of color: lightness, saturation, and hue.

For several reasons, it is questionable whether the hypothesis of early holistic processing can account for cross-modal interactions in speeded classification. For one, it seems unlikely that early processing is so syncretic that it fails to provide any information to distinguish modalities. And for another, it is not clear that the early holistic model can even account for integral interactions within individual modalities. The model predicts that information about levels on particular perceptual dimensions, such as pitch and loudness in hearing, or brightness and saturation in vision, arises relatively late in processing. Early in processing, stimuli are undifferentiated except in terms of overall dissimilarity to one another, and no privileged perceptual dimensions yet exist. Stimuli may be represented in a perceptual space lacking meaningful axes or dimensions; these axes emerge later in processing. According to the holistic model, interactions in speeded classification represent processing at an early stage of processing, where percepts are not yet differentiated with respect to the underlying dimensions. Contrary to this prediction, subjects do in fact rely on privileged dimensions in speeded classification of sounds (Melara & Marks, 1990a), lights (Melara et al., 1993; see also Grau & Kemler Nelson, 1988), and even tactile vibrations (Melara & Day, 1992). Furthermore, reliance on privileged dimensions would seem necessary to establish congruence relations; it is difficult to see how congruence could emerge from early holistic processes.

An alternative explanation for cross-modal interactions in speeded classification, and in particular for effects of congruence, postulates some kind of cross-talk between sources of information. Let us consider three possible ways this could occur.

First, concurrent or overlapping stimulation in different modalities might have mutual effects on the resulting perceptual representations. Presenting a tone might increase or decrease the brightness of a light, depending on whether the tone is relatively loud or soft, while the presence of the light might increase or decrease the loudness of the tone, depending on whether the light is dim or bright. Second, the perceptual responses to stimulation in two (or more) modalities might proceed more or less independently, leading to perceptual representations unaffected by cross-modal stimulation, but interactions could occur at a postperceptual stage of processing, perhaps at a stage where information is recoded into a more abstract, and perhaps linguistic or semantic, format. And third, even if or when representations in different modalities are independent of each other, congruence interactions may emerge at a stage of decision making, where the decisions could be made on the basis of either perceptually or postperceptually coded information. Finally, it should go without saying, but will be said nevertheless, that the three mechanisms just sketched are by no means exclusive. It is conceivable that cross-modal stimulation leads to interactions in the resulting perceptual representations, to interactions in postperceptual representations of the perceptual information, and to interactions in decisional processes. Different mechanisms of interaction may operate with different kinds of cross-modal stimuli, and the interactions observed with a particular cross-modal stimulus may reflect the outcome of two or more different mechanisms. Unfortunately, it is not always easy to dissociate the mechanisms that may operate at different stages in processing information. Nevertheless, there are data pertinent to this issue.

CROSS-MODAL CONGRUENCE INTERACTIONS: CHANGES IN PERCEPTUAL REPRESENTATIONS? A few experiments have sought to determine whether cross-modal stimulation induces changes in underlying perceptual representations. When visual and auditory stimuli are presented together, does each affect the other—for example, by the rules of cross-modal congruence? If so, then the louder or higher-pitched a sound, the greater might be the brightness of a concurrent light, and the greater the brightness of the light, the greater might be the loudness and the higher the pitch of the sound. Melara (1989b) addressed this question with respect to the dimensions of auditory pitch and visual lightness.

He posed the following hypothesis: Assume that congruence interactions between pitch and lightness reflect perceptual enhancement in congruent combinations and perceptual inhibition (or smaller enhancement) in incongruent combinations. If so, then the representation of these stimuli (formed by orthogonally combining each of two pitches with each of two equally discriminable lightnesses) in a cross-modal perceptual space should take the form not of a square but of a parallelogram, in which the diagonal distance between congruent stimulus combinations is greater than the diagonal distance between incongruent combinations.

A simple quantitative example can illustrate the point. Let us assume that, with no cross-modal interaction, two sounds have relative pitches of numerical value 2 (low) and 4 (high) and two colors have relative lightnesses of the same numerical values, 2 (dark) and 4 (light). The four possible cross-modal combinations could be represented spatially as the four corners of a square, as shown in the lower part of Figure 6.2. Now, let us assume a perceptual interaction, such that high pitch adds 1 unit of lightness to each color and low pitch subtracts 1 unit, while high lightness adds 1 unit of pitch to each sound and low lightness subtracts 1 unit. It follows that in the congruent combination of high pitch + high lightness, the levels of both lightness and pitch increase to 5, while in the congruent combination of low pitch + low lightness, the levels of both decrease to 1. In the incongruent combination low pitch + high lightness, the level of pitch increases to 3 but lightness decreases to 3, and in the incongruent high pitch + low lightness, the level of pitch decreases to 3 and lightness increases to 3. This prediction is characterized in the upper part of Figure 6.2.

Greater distance in the spatial model represents greater "discriminability" (analogous to d' in signal detection theory), and discriminability should be inversely related to response time. So congruent combinations should be more discriminable than incongruent combinations and therefore be processed more quickly in a selective attention task. The difference in discriminability on the diagonals has been called "mean shift integrality" in models of multidimensional stimulus interaction (e.g., Ashby & Maddox, 1994; Macmillan & Ornstein, 1998).

Melara (1989b) sought to test this model directly by asking subjects to compare the dissimilarities of cross-modal combinations of auditory stimuli varying in pitch and visual stimuli varying in lightness. Analysis of the results by multidimensional scaling failed to support the prediction of mean-integral interaction. The perceptual locations of the visual stimuli remained intact, independent of the level of the auditory stimulus, and the

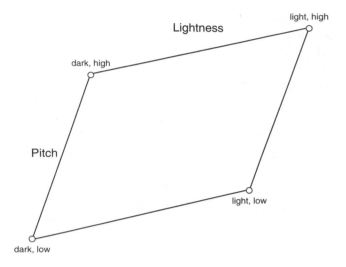

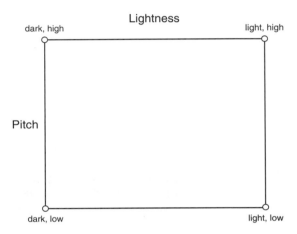

FIGURE 6.2 The upper figure is a spatial representation of similarity relations of auditory pitch and visual lightness, assuming that these dimensions show mean integrality. The diagonal connecting congruent pairs (low pitch + dark, high pitch + light) is greater than the diagonal connecting incongruent pairs (low pitch + light, high pitch + dark), indicating that the perceptual representations are modified with cross-modal presentation. The lower figure is a spatial representation of the similarity relations of pitch and lightness assuming that there is no change in the perceptual representations.

perceptual locations of the auditory stimuli remained intact, independent of the levels of the visual stimuli. Presenting cross-modal combinations of stimuli apparently had no effect on the perceived levels of pitch and lightness. The results of Melara's analyses suggested that pitch and lightness are configured as a square (or rectangle) in cross-modal space, as shown in the lower part of Figure 6.2. This configuration is consistent with "perceptual independence" between the modalities, in which the two diagonals are equal in length, and suggests further that the congruence effects between pitch and lightness, and conceivably also Garner interference, observed in speeded classification may result

from processes that involve failures of decisional separability rather than failures of perceptual separability (Ashby & Maddox, 1994; Ashby & Townsend, 1986; Maddox, 1992). A decisional model is considered later.

A related question was addressed by Stein, London, Wilkinson, and Price (1996), who asked whether presenting a pulse of white noise enhances the brightness of a concurrently presented flash of light. Rather than using different levels of noise, Stein et al. compared ratings of brightness in the presence of noise to ratings of brightness in the absence of noise. With certain spatial arrangements, the ratings of brightness were greater in the presence of the noise, leading the authors to infer a direct enhancement of brightness by loudness. Taken at face value, these results might seem to support a model of perceptual interaction.

Unfortunately, the findings of Stein et al. (1996) could simply reflect a cross-modally generated response bias; that is, subjects may be induced to give larger ratings of brightness in the presence of sound, relative to the ratings they give in the absence of sound, because a cross-modal stimulus affects decisional processes. A subsequent study by Odgaard, Arieh, and Marks (2003) provided experimental support for the latter interpretation. Odgaard et al. found that concurrent pulses of noise could indeed affect ratings of brightness, but the magnitude of the effect depended on the proportion of the total trials containing light + sound as opposed to light alone. Indeed, when noise accompanied the light on only 25% of the trials, the ratings showed essentially no enhancement of brightness by sound.

It is hard to square these findings with the hypothesis that sound automatically modifies the sensory representation of brightness, as such an effect should then occur regardless of the probability of cross-modal association. It is more likely that the noise affected decisional processes, which are well known to depend on probabilities of stimulus presentation (e.g., Tanner, Haller, & Atkinson, 1967). Further, Odgaard et al. (2003) examined performance on a task in which, rather than having subjects rate the brightness of each flash of light, they asked the subjects to compare directly on each trial the brightness of a flash of light accompanied by noise and a flash of light presented alone. Using in different conditions several sets of stimulus intensities, selected so as to control for possible effects of subjects' expectations, Odgaard et al. found no evidence at all in the paired comparisons for noise-generated effects on brightness. The authors concluded that concurrent noise can affect decisional processes involved in the judgment of brightness but leaves the representations of visual brightness unchanged.

The findings of Melara (1989b) and Odgaard et al. (2003) as well as those of Marks, Ben-Artzi, and Lakatos (2003), who examined cross-modal influences on discrimination of pitch, loudness, and brightness, concur in suggesting that the individual components of cross-modal stimuli, or at least stimuli such as tones or noises varying in loudness and pitch and patches of light or color varying in brightness, are processed more or less independently. If so, then the interactions observed on tasks of speeded classification may represent failures of decisional separability rather than failures of perceptual separability. Failure of decisional separability is a formal term for what could be, in this case, the outcome of a relatively late process in which information about the levels on different perceptual dimensions accrues independently in the separate modalities. The outputs encoding information about these dimensions would then combine in a decisional process before a response is made. By this token, congruent combinations of information would reach a criterion level for response more quickly than would incongruent combinations. Such a decisional model is considered later in this chapter.

CROSS-MODAL CONGRUENCE INTERACTIONS: ROLE OF LINGUISTIC PROCESSES? A main question of interest is, of course, what kind of information is transmitted to the decision mechanism? In particular, might the information be semantic or even linguistic? Although congruence effects presumably do not always require the use of explicit common labels (except perhaps in a few cases, such as auditory pitch and visual position, where the attributes in both modalities can be labeled as "low" and "high"), congruence effects could rely on implicit labeling of the perceptual events, even when the labels applied to stimuli in different modalities are not identical. Attributes may be encoded on abstract dimensions, or with abstract features, such as "intensity," that transcend the representations of percepts on individual modalities. Interactions could, therefore, derive from commonality in abstract features. That linguistic processes may be involved in dimensional interactions, both within and between modalities, is consistent with several findings that have applied the speeded classification paradigm to situations in which one component was nonlinguistic, a stimulus producing variations along a perceptual dimension (e.g., a sound varying in frequency or a light varying in luminance), whereas the other component was linguistic (e.g., the words *black* and *white* or the bigrams LO and HI).

Walker and Smith (1984) measured congruence effects in speeded responses to low- versus high-pitched auditory stimuli where these stimuli were accompanied by visually presented words—adjectives whose meanings were cross-modally (metaphorically) related to low or high pitch (e.g., *blunt* versus *sharp*). Response times were smaller when the irrelevant words had meanings that matched rather than mismatched the tones; thus, responses to the low tone were quicker when the word was *blunt* rather than *sharp*, but responses to the high tone were quicker when the word was *sharp* rather than *blunt*.

Melara and Marks (1990b) systematically investigated interactions within and between visual and auditory stimuli whose attributes varied on a dimension that could be labeled "low" or "high." In one experiment, their stimuli consisted of acoustic signals varying linguistically, such as the words *low* and *high*, and perceptually, in their fundamental frequency (pitch). In another experiment, the same acoustic words *low* and *high* were presented through sound sources varying in their vertical position. In a third experiment, the stimuli consisted of visual bigrams LO and HI, presented in different vertical spatial positions. Note that in each of these experiments, the stimuli were unimodal: auditory in the first two and visual in the third. A fourth experiment used cross-modal stimuli: the visual bigrams LO and HI, accompanied by tones that could be low or high in frequency. In all four experiments, regardless of whether the subjects were identifying a linguistic dimension (a word) or a perceptual dimension (pitch or spatial location), and regardless of whether the irrelevant dimension came from the same or different modality, performance revealed both Garner interference and congruence effects.

Thus, similar cross-modal interactions reveal themselves with two classes of stimuli: linguistic stimuli (words that refer semantically to sensory or perceptual attributes) and perceptual stimuli (nonwords that vary along various sensory or perceptual dimensions). (Of course, perceptual qualities of the words also vary, but the stimuli are constructed to minimize any potential confounding of perceptual qualities with semantic referents.) The similarity in patterns of results does not mean, of course, that linguistic processing is necessarily involved in generating the cross-modal interactions observed when stimuli are wholly perceptual. It is conceivable that linguistic processes underlie the cross-modal interactions involving linguistic stimuli but not the interactions involving nonlinguistic (perceptual) stimuli. Nevertheless, the presence of both Garner interference and congruence effects in speeded classification tasks using linguistic stimuli makes it plausible to entertain the hypothesis that linguistic processes, or at least semantic processes, also play a role in generating cross-modal interactions when the stimuli are not linguistic.

Note, however, that even if linguistic processes are involved, and in particular even if implicit or explicit labeling is important, the verbal labels applied to stimuli in different modalities presumably need not be identical. Interference effects and congruence effects arise even with cross-modal combinations of stimuli that do not share obvious verbal labels, as in the case of high versus low pitch and black versus white colors.

Finally, following this line of reasoning, linguistic processes might be involved in interactions found in speeded classification of stimuli within a single modality. Given, for example, the results of Melara and Marks (1990b), who reported interactions between stimuli with referents "low" and "high"—whether these positions were designated linguistically, by words, or perceptually, by presenting visual or auditory stimuli at different spatial positions—it is conceivable that linguistic processes underlie, or at least contribute to, the congruence interactions between spatial direction and position of visual stimuli reported by Clark and Brownell (1975).

Semantic Coding Hypothesis One possible explanation for the findings comes from the *semantic coding hypothesis* (Martino & Marks, 1999). The semantic coding hypothesis constitutes one model of late rather than early cross-modal interaction, and it aims explicitly at explaining congruence effects. According to the hypothesis, congruence interactions arise because stimuli eventually activate abstract representations, possibly semantic or even linguistic ones, whose dimensions or features overlap at least in part across sensory modalities. Representations of stimuli presented in different modalities are generally not identical, of course, because each representation contains distinguishing features of information, for instance, about perceptual qualities that are specific to the modality of origin. Abstract representations of low-pitched sounds overlap those of dim lights, and abstract representations of high-pitched sounds overlap those of bright lights, but in each case the representations are not identical, else they would not make it possible to distinguish what is heard from what is seen.

The overlapping or common properties of these postperceptual representations themselves ultimately derive, in the case of figurative cross-modal relations, from perceptual similarities that themselves require explanation. To be sure, a few cross-modal perceptual similarities seem to emerge directly from experienced association; one example is the similarity between decreasing pitch and increasing size, which may derive from our experience with resonance properties of small and large objects, while another is the association of warmth with orange and red colors and coolness with blue and green colors, which may derive from experience with fire and bodies of water. Neither pitch-size congruence nor color-temperature congruence is evident in children before adolescence (see Marks et al., 1987, and Morgan, Goodson, & Jones, 1975, respectively). But several other cross-modal similarities appear to originate in phenomenal experience itself, being evident in early childhood (e.g., Marks et al., 1987), and even in infancy (Lewkowicz & Turkewitz, 1980). In such examples as loudness and brightness, or pitch and lightness, the similarity in each case may ultimately have its source, in infancy, in commonalities of neural coding mechanisms, although other mechanisms, notably language, may subsequently contribute to congruence in later childhood and adulthood.

Importantly, however, according to the semantic coding hypothesis, even if the similarities derive initially from neural characteristics of perceptual processing, with years of perceptual and linguistic experience, the cross-modal correspondences eventually become accessible to, and indeed dominated by, more abstract, contextual linguistic processes. Consequently, when an adult confronts a cross-modal stimulus, framed within a context that defines relative values on dimensions such as pitch, position, and brightness, through the activation of abstract but overlapping representations, the implicit cross-modal correspondences can influence the speed and accuracy of information processing. This occurs even though the person tries to ignore stimulation on an irrelevant modality.

Decisional Model of Cross-Modal Interactions in Selective Attention The semantic coding hypothesis—the hypothesis that information about the values on different dimensions in the same sensory modality or in different modalities accrues in a common abstract, and perhaps semantic or linguistic, representation—can be instantiated in a decisional model based on principles of signal detection theory (e.g., Ben-Artzi & Marks, 1995a). The model makes two main assumptions. One is an assumption about the way that perceptual information resulting from stimulation on the relevant dimension, R, changes over time, and the other is an assumption about the way that the presence of an irrelevant stimulus dimension, I, influences the accrual of information relative to the locations of the response criteria.

Figure 6.3 gives an example. Consider a task in which subjects classify tones on the basis of their pitch (R) in the presence of irrelevant visual stimuli varying in brightness (I). The model postulates that subjects set two criteria and then make a response only when the

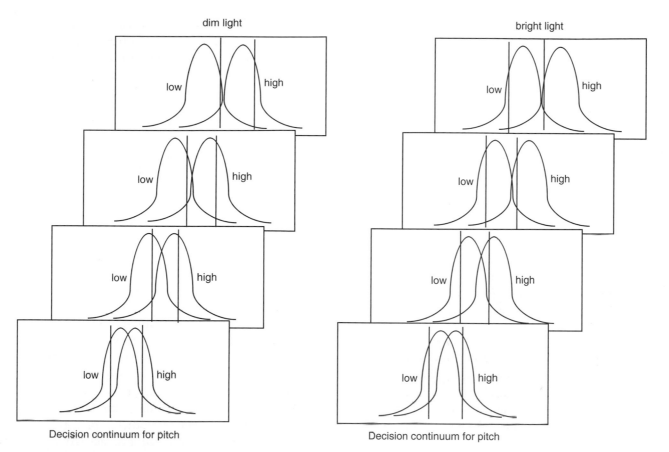

FIGURE 6.3   A decisional model of congruence effects, based on the semantic coding hypothesis. The figure shows how the criteria for responding to low- and high-frequency tones (vertical lines in each panel, criterion for low on the left and criterion for high on the right) depend on the presence of irrelevant dim lights (left panels) and bright lights (right panels). Starting at the bottom, each set of panels shows how the underlying distributions of low-frequency and high-frequency events change over time, while the locations of the criteria depend on the value of the irrelevant visual stimulus.

stimulus information surpasses one criterion or the other. Thus, subjects respond "low" (e.g., by pressing an appropriate button) when the information falls below the lower criterion, C_l, and they respond "high" (by pressing another button) when the information falls above the upper criterion, C_h. The greater the time since the onset of stimulation, the more likely it is that the information will surpass the correct criterion. The representations of the signals are noisy, however, not only because effects of stimulation are always variable but also because of temporal fluctuation. Even though information tends to move over time toward one criterion or another, there are moment-to-moment fluctuations in the level of information.

Each of the overlapping pairs of curves in Figure 6.3 shows hypothetical distributions of perceptual events produced by the two possible acoustic signals at a given point in time after the onset of the cross-modal stimulus. Immediately after a tone is presented, information about its frequency is most ambiguous, and the two

distributions overlap substantially. But with the passage of time, the mean of the distribution produced by the low-frequency tone shifts down, while the mean of the distribution produced by the high-frequency tone shifts up, so the distance between the means increases. The greater the separation between means at any point in time, the easier it is for the subject to decide whether a particular sample comes from the "low" distribution or the "high" distribution. Assuming (simply as a matter of convenience) that the variances of the distributions remain unchanged over time, these variances can be assigned a value of unity, so the difference between the means at any point in time corresponds to the discriminability of the stimuli, as measured in terms such as d'.

The model also assumes, because there is a common representation of information from both the irrelevant dimension, I, and the relevant dimension, R (e.g., by the semantic coding hypothesis), that variation in levels on I affects the processing of information on R. One way to conceptualize the influence of I on R is to assume that, at each moment in time, the information that has accrued regarding the level on I influences the two distributions on R—essentially, shifting both distributions either up or down (to the right or to the left, in Figure 6.3). That is, stimulation on dimension I shifts the two distributions relative to their criteria. A quantitatively equivalent way to conceptualize this same process is to assume that the accrued information on R leaves the distributions in place but shifts the criteria relative to the distributions. The magnitude of the shift increases over time from the onset of the compound stimulus, as evidence increases regarding the level on dimension I.

Thus, although the model assumes the momentary existence of two criteria for responding, the locations of these criteria are not static but shift as the subject accrues information about I—in this case, about the brightness of a light. The locations of the criteria at the start of each trial undoubtedly themselves depend on both long-term and short-term factors (for instance, the stimulus combination presented on the previous trial). Again for simplicity, however, assume that the criteria start, on average, at nominally "neutral" locations. As information accrues regarding the brightness of the light, the criteria for responding "low" and "high" begin to shift, with evidence that the light is dim causing both C_l and C_h to move up (in the figure, to the right) and evidence that the light is bright causing both C_l and C_h to move down (in the figure, to the left). Evidence that the visual stimulus is dim, therefore, makes the criterion for responding "low" become more lax and the criterion for responding "high" more strict. By analogy, evidence that the visual stimulus is bright makes the criterion for responding "high" more lax and the criterion for responding "low" more strict.

As a consequence, on trials in which the light is dim, it takes relatively less time on average for the cumulative evidence that the tone is low-pitched to reach the criterion to respond "low," and relatively more time for the evidence that the tone is high-pitched to reach the criterion to respond "high." When the light is bright, it takes relatively more time for the evidence that the tone is low-pitched to reach the criterion for responding "low," but relatively less time for the evidence that the tone is high-pitched to reach the criterion "high." The overall result is a congruence effect, based on decisional rather than perceptual interactions.

Implicit in this model is the supposition that the presence of an irrelevant stimulus dimension I has no effect on the perceptual representation of the relevant stimulus dimension R—consistent with the findings of Melara (1989b) and Odgaard et al. (2003), discussed earlier. Increasing the pitch of a tone does not increase

the perceived lightness of a color, and increasing the lightness of a color does not increase the perceived pitch of a tone. Presumably, neither does increasing brightness enhance loudness or pitch, nor does increasing loudness or pitch enhance brightness. Even assuming perceptual independence, the model can account for the congruence effects observed in cross-modal selective attention tasks. Additional assumptions would be needed, however, to account also for the Garner interference observed with cross-modal stimulation; interference might result, for instance, from additional variability or noise introduced into the system by the presence of irrelevant variation of stimulation on the second modality, I. Note, however, the possibility that Garner interference could originate earlier in processing, and thus could conceivably represent perceptual interaction.

The evidence at hand speaks against cross-modal effects on perceptual representations as a mechanism of interaction, or at least against cross-modal effects being the mechanism underlying congruence effects, but the evidence is consistent with a decisional mechanism for congruence interactions. On the other hand, the evidence is also consistent with the hypothesis that postperceptual, or at least nonperceptual, representations, for instance, semantic ones, can interact. At this point, it is difficult if not impossible to distinguish between a decisional model and a model postulating mutual enhancement and inhibition in semantic representations of sensory stimuli in different modalities, akin to the interactions considered with respect to perceptual representations (Melara, 1989b) and sketched in the upper portion of Figure 6.2. A model hypothesizing interactions between semantic representations of stimuli in different modalities is compatible with the data, given the proviso that when subjects classify stimuli as quickly as they can, these speeded classifications depend on semantic representations, whereas judgments or comparisons that are not speeded, as in the similarity scaling task of Melara (1989b) and the rating and paired comparison tasks of Odgaard et al. (2003), rely on perceptual representations generated earlier in processing.

The important distinction between sensory-perceptual and decisional aspects of separability, integrality, and dimensional interaction is not easily addressed in many of the selective attention paradigms, especially those that use response time procedures, although Ashby and Maddox (1994) have taken steps toward developing a formal model of response times in speeded classification tasks. Nevertheless, a general conclusion is possible: To the extent that the failures of selective attention commonly observed in speeded classification tasks reflect events that take place relatively late rather than early in processing, events that take place after information has been encoded into an abstract and possibly semantic format, then it is likely that these processes are best formalized in terms of interactions between streams of recoded perceptual information and the decision rules operating on the outputs from these perceptual streams. In principle, the same conclusion could apply to at least some examples of failure of selective attention found to occur within a single modality. So, for example, the congruence effects reported by Clark and Brownell (1975) could involve the activation of abstract, perhaps semantic, representations of spatial direction and position.

Cross-modal interactions: Perceptual congruence and stimulus congruence

Before concluding, it is worth mentioning once again the basic conceptual framework of the speeded classification paradigm as developed by Garner (1974b) and to indicate important examples of similar cross-modal paradigms not heretofore considered in this chapter. By and large, experiments using the speeded classification paradigm aim to answer the broad question, can people attend selectively to information about values of a stimulus that lie on one dimension, independently of variation in the values on other dimensions? Many of the earliest experiments used relatively simple sensory stimuli: patches of color that varied in lightness, saturation, or size; tones that varied in pitch or loudness. So a question asked in these investigations was, can subjects identify colors varying in lightness as quickly when the saturation, or size, varies unpredictably from trial to trial as they can when saturation, or size, remains constant? In all of these studies, the irrelevantly varying dimension is not only irrelevant by instruction (for example, subjects are told to respond to lightness only, and to ignore changes in saturation or size), but also in some sense irrelevant "ecologically," in that both large and small objects in the world present themselves in dark and light colors, so the size of an object generally does not predict its color.

In extending the speeded classification paradigm to the cross-modal domain, many investigations—indeed, essentially all of those reviewed so far in this chapter—have followed a similar tack. That is, in these investigations, subjects tried to attend selectively to a dimension in one modality while ignoring instructionally and ecologically irrelevant variations in another; they tried to attend, for example, to pitch or loudness of a tone accompanied by a light varying irrelevantly in brightness or vertical spatial position. Irrelevant variation in levels on the unattended modality typically affects the speed (and accuracy) of processing on the attended modality,

as revealed in interference and congruence effects, even though the ecological connection between the stimuli presented to the two modalities is tenuous. With congruence effects in particular, where subject are quicker to classify congruent combinations, such as low pitch + dim and high pitch + bright, relative to incongruent combinations, low + bright and high + dim, the congruence relations themselves are figurative or synesthetic. Indeed, the congruence relation is figurative, or at least abstract, in many unimodal cases, for example in the congruence between the auditory dimensions of pitch and loudness, and in the congruence between the visual dimensions of lightness and saturation.

It is not only convenient but perhaps also theoretically significant to distinguish all of these examples of what I shall call *perceptual congruence* from what I call, for lack of a better term, *stimulus congruence*. As already indicated, perceptual congruence may be defined through any of a number of matching paradigms, a simple one being the determination of pairwise similarity relations (Marks et al., 1987), and thus is essentially a psychophysical or perceptual construct. Perceptual congruence is first and foremost a psychological phenomenon.

Stimulus congruence, on the other hand, may be defined in terms of properties of the stimuli themselves. With stimulus congruence there is a dimension or feature of the stimuli, in a single modality or different modalities, that is common to them. Most often the common dimension or feature is, or refers to, locations in space. So, for example, visual, auditory, and tactile stimuli may be defined as spatially congruent (their sources having the same spatial location) or incongruent (having different locations).

A study of the role of cross-modal stimulus congruence was reported by Soto-Faraco, Lyons, Gazzaniga, Spence, and Kingstone (2002). In a series of experiments, these investigators examined interactions between vision and hearing in the perception of dynamic (temporal-spatial displays). The basic task (which emphasized accuracy over speed) was to identify the direction of apparent auditory motion (sounds came from two laterally displaced loudspeakers) given simultaneous, or asynchronous, flashes of lights producing visual apparent movement.

Four of the findings of Soto-Faraco et al. (2002) are especially pertinent here. First, they found a congruence effect, in that accuracy was greater when the direction of visual motion was congruent with the direction of the auditory motion, but this occurred only when the visual and auditory stimuli were synchronous (simultaneous), and not when they were asynchronous (offset by 500 ms). Second, the congruence effect was strongest when the visual and auditory stimuli came from common spatial locations (that is, when the light sources were located at the sites of the loudspeakers): the congruence effects diminished markedly when the auditory stimuli were presented over headphones (and thus no longer completely congruent with the visual stimuli, by the definition above, but only *relatively* congruent). Third, the congruence effects diminished in magnitude when the auditory stimuli were presented through loudspeakers and the visual stimuli were located nearby, but spatially offset from the loudspeakers, even though the trajectories of the visual motion and the auditory motion overlapped. Finally, congruence effects were greatest when the interstimulus interval (ISI) between the auditory and visual stimuli in each pair was small enough to produce phenomenal motion, though residual effects remained even at ISIs as long as 900 ms, where there was presumably no phenomenal motion.

The study of Soto-Faraco et al. (2002) reveals several important characteristics of cross-modal interactions induced by stimulus congruence that differ from the interactions induced by perceptual congruence. Perhaps most important is the dependence of stimulus congruence effects on the absolute values of the stimuli. Visual capture of auditory perceived direction was greatest when the visual and auditory stimuli were not only temporally synchronous but also spatially colocated. Effects were relatively weak when the congruence was only relative, that is, when the auditory and visual stimuli moved in the same direction but had different locations. This finding contrasts with the relativity that pervades the effects of perceptual congruence and thereby suggests that different mechanisms may underpin effects of stimulus congruence (at least the effects of spatial coregistration) and effects of perceptual congruence.

Where, it was argued earlier, the effects of perceptual congruence relations likely arise postperceptually, perhaps even in decisional processes, the effects of spatial stimulus congruence seem more likely to reflect perceptual interactions per se. This hypothesis is consistent with the conclusion of Soto-Faraco et al. (2002), who inferred that, as in the ventriloquism effect observed with static displays, where visual locations tend to capture auditory locations, in dynamic displays, visual apparent movement tends to capture auditory apparent motion when the visual and auditory stimuli are synchronous and spatially colocated. In the case of spatial stimulus congruence, cross-modal interactions likely involve changes in perceptual representations per se.

Although this conclusion is reasonable, it should be mentioned that none of the experiments reported by Soto-Faraco et al. (2002) explicitly eliminated an explanation in terms of decisional processes. A wholly decisional account, however, would require two assumptions: not only that the direction of visual motion affects criteria for responding to direction of auditory motion, but also that the degree of temporal synchrony and the spatial coincidence affect the magnitude of the shifts in criteria. Still, given the pervasiveness of criterion setting in perceptual judgment, it remains possible that both perceptual and decisional processes contribute to spatial congruence effects.

The findings of Soto-Faraco et al. (2002) raise several questions about spatial congruence effects that are still unanswered: How close in space do stimuli have to be for them to be fully congruent? And to what extent might the effects depend on relative rather than absolute spatial congruence? Soto-Faraco et al. did observe small effects of congruence even when the visual and auditory stimuli were not colocated in space; that is, small effects appeared even when the congruence was relational. There is evidence that spatial congruence effects can also depend on the commonality of *perceived* rather than *physical* spatial locations. Pavani, Spence, and Driver (2000) investigated how concurrent flashes of spatially congruent or incongruent light affected speeded identifications of vibrotactile stimulation of two fingers (one held above the other) of the two hands. Responses were much quicker and errors were fewer when the vertical position of the light was congruent rather than incongruent with the vertical position of the tactile stimulus. Further, the congruence effects were greater when the light appeared on side of the stimulated hand rather than on the side of the unstimulated hand. Finally, in an especially clever experimental twist, in all conditions of the experiment the subjects' view of their hands was occluded, but in some conditions the subjects saw a pair of rubber hands, constructed so the subjects would interpret them as their own, and located at the light sources. In the latter conditions, the subjects presumably felt the vibrations localized at the lights, and, accordingly, congruence effects were greatest.

The results of Pavani et al. (2000) suggest that what may sometimes matter to spatial congruence effects is absolute perceived location rather than absolute physical location. To the extent that effects of spatial congruence can rely on perceived as opposed to physical location, it may be necessary to refine the global terminological distinction made in this chapter between perceptual congruence and stimulus congruence. It may turn out that congruence effects involving spatial locations are in some fashion special, that congruence effects involving locations in space involve processing mechanisms that differ, in a fundamental manner, from the mechanisms underlying many or most other congruence effects. This should perhaps not be surprising, given the considerable hardware of the brain devoted to spatial registration of multisensory information. Neurons in several regions of the brain are responsive to spatially aligned stimuli in different modalities (e.g., Stein, Magalhaes-Castro, & Kruger, 1975; Wallace, Meredith, & Stein, 1992; see also Stein, Jiang, & Stanford, Chap. 15, this volume), suggesting that coregistration of multisensory information may play a privileged role in spatial perception.

Finally, it is important to keep in mind that even spatial congruence can be based on relative and not absolute locations—indeed, that the relations constituting spatial congruence can be abstract ones, akin to the figurative relations that play so prominent a role in many other examples of dimensional interaction, within as well as between modalities. Consider again, in this regard, the study of Clark and Brownell (1975). They reported effects of congruence between the relative vertical position of a visual stimulus, an arrow, and the direction that the arrow pointed. These unimodal spatial interactions are presumably based on an abstract spatial relation between the two dimensions—on correspondences between high versus low position and pointing up versus pointing down. An abstract spatial relation likely also underlay the findings of Klein (1977, Experiment 3), who studied the effects of relative spatial congruence in a cross-modal setting. Klein presented subjects with visual and kinesthetic stimuli that were relationally congruent or incongruent—a dot on a screen that could move to the left or right, and leftward or rightward movement of the subject's finger. Subjects made speeded classifications of the direction of visual or kinesthetic movement, with concomitant stimulation in the other modality. Both visual classification and kinesthetic classification showed substantial congruence effects, response times being shorter and errors fewer with congruent stimulus combinations (both stimuli moving left or right) compared to incongruent combinations (one moving in each direction).

It may be tempting to apply a single explanatory scheme to all classes of congruence effects—effects related to perceptual congruence within a single modality (e.g., between lightness and saturation of colors), effects related to spatial congruence within a modality (e.g., between spatial direction and position of visual shapes), effects related to perceptual congruence across modalities (e.g., between pitch and brightness), and effects related to spatial congruence across modalities (e.g., between visual and tactile location). Although decisional processes, operating on information in postperceptual, abstract or semantic, representations of stimuli, can account for many of the findings, it seems improbable that all of these interactions result from a common mechanism. To be sure, there are theoretical approaches to perception, notably Gibson's (e.g., 1979), that are compatible with the notion that perception ultimately rests on the discrimination of amodal properties of stimuli, and so one might be tempted to propose that all congruence effects represent decisions made on the basis of amodal representations of stimulation. But the behavioral characteristics that differentiate many cross-modal effects of perceptual congruence from cross-modal effects of spatial congruence suggest instead a less cohesive and parsimonious but perhaps ultimately more fruitful view: that cross-modal congruence effects, like other forms of interaction observed in selective attention, may reflect processes arising at several levels of transformation and integration of multisensory information.

REFERENCES

Ashby, F. G., & Maddox, W. T. (1994). A response time theory of separability and integrality in speeded classification. *Journal of Mathematics and Psychology, 38*, 423–466.

Ashby, F. G., & Townsend, J. T. (1986). Varieties of perceptual independence. *Psychological Review, 93*, 154–179.

Ben-Artzi, E., & Marks, L. E. (1995a). Congruence effects in classifying auditory stimuli: A review and a model. In B. Scharf & C.-A. Possamaï (Eds.), *Fechner Day 95: Proceedings of the Eleventh Annual Meeting of the International Society for Psychophysics* (pp. 145–150). Vancouver: ISP.

Ben-Artzi, E., & Marks, L. E. (1995b). Visual-auditory interaction in speeded classification: Role of stimulus difference. *Perception & Psychophysics, 57*, 1151–1162.

Bertelson, P., Vroomen, J., de Gelder, B., & Driver, J. (2000). The ventriloquist effect does not depend on the direction of deliberate visual attention. *Perception & Psychophysics, 62*, 321–332.

Bernstein, I. H., & Edelstein, B. A. (1971). Effects of some variations in auditory input upon visual choice reaction time. *Journal of Experimental Psychology, 87*, 241–247.

Clark, H. H., & Brownell, H. H. (1975). Judging up and down. *Journal of Experimental Psychology: Human Perception and Performance, 1*, 339–352.

Cytowic, R. E. (1989). *Synaesthesia: A union of the senses.* Berlin: Springer-Verlag.

Driver, J. (1996). Enhancement of selective listening by illusory mislocalization of speech sounds due to lip-reading. *Nature, 381*, 66–68.

Fitts, P. M., & Deininger, M. L. (1954). S-R compatibility: Correspondence among paired elements within stimulus and response codes. *Journal of Experimental Psychology, 48*, 483–492.

Garner, W. R. (1974a). Attention: The processing of multiple sources of information. In E. C. Carterette & M. P. Friedman (Eds.), *Handbook of perception: Vol. 2. Psychophysical measurement and judgment* (pp. 29–39). New York: Academic Press.

Garner, W. R. (1974b). *The processing of information and structure.* Hillsdale, NJ: Erlbaum.

Garner, W. R. (1977). The effect of absolute size on the separability of the dimensions of size and brightness. *Bulletin of the Psychonomic Society, 9,* 380–382.

Garner, W. R., & Felfoldy, G. L. (1970). Integrality of stimulus dimensions in various types of information processing. *Cognitive Psychology, 1,* 225–241.

Gibson, J. J. (1979). *The ecological approach to visual perception.* Boston: Houghton Mifflin.

Grau, J. W., & Kemler Nelson, D. G. (1988). The distinction between integral and separable dimensions: Evidence for the integrality of pitch and loudness. *Journal of Experimental Psychology: General, 117,* 347–370.

Harrison, J. (2001). *Synaesthesia: The strangest thing.* Oxford, England: Oxford University Press.

Kemler Nelson, D. G. (1989). The nature of occurrence of holistic processing. In B. E. Shepp & S. Ballesteros (Eds.), *Object perception: Structure and process* (pp. 203–233). Hillsdale, NJ: Erlbaum.

Kingston, J., & Macmillan, N. A. (1995). Integrality of nasalization and F_1 in vowels in isolation and before oral and nasal consonants: A detection-theoretic application of the Garner paradigm. *Journal of the Acoustical Society of America, 97,* 1261–1285.

Klein, R. (1977). Attention and visual dominance: A chronometric analysis. *Journal of Experimental Psychology: Human Perception and Performance, 3,* 365–378.

Kornblum, S., Hasbroucq, T., & Osman, A. (1990). Dimensional overlap: Cognitive basis for stimulus-response compatibility. A model and taxonomy. *Psychological Review, 97,* 253–270.

Lewkowicz, D. J., & Turkewitz, G. (1980). Cross-modal equivalence in early infancy: Auditory-visual intensity matching. *Developmental Psychology, 16,* 597–607.

Lockhead, G. R. (1972). Processing dimensional stimuli: A note. *Psychological Review, 79,* 410–419.

Macmillan, N. A., & Ornstein, A. S. (1998). The mean-integral representation of rectangles. *Perception & Psychophysics, 60,* 250–262.

Maddox, W. T. (1992). Perceptual and decisional separability. In F. G. Ashby (Ed.), *Multidimensional models of perception and cognition* (pp. 147–180). Hillsdale, NJ: Erlbaum.

Marks, L. E. (1974). On associations of light and sound: The mediation of brightness, pitch, and loudness. *American Journal of Psycholology, 87,* 173–188.

Marks, L. E. (1975). On colored-hearing synesthesia: Cross-modal translations of sensory dimensions. *Psychological Bulletin, 82,* 303–331.

Marks, L. E. (1978). *The unity of the senses: Interrelations among the modalities.* New York: Academic Press.

Marks, L. E. (1982a). Bright sneezes and dark coughs, loud sunlight and soft moonlight. *Journal of Experimental Psychology: Human Perception and Performance, 8,* 177–193.

Marks, L. E. (1982b). Synesthetic perception and poetic metaphor. *Journal of Experimental Psychology: Human Perception and Performance, 8,* 15–23.

Marks, L. E. (1987). On cross-modal similarity: Auditory-visual interactions in speeded discrimination. *Journal of Experimental Psychology: Human Perception and Performance, 13,* 384–394.

Marks, L. E. (1989). On cross-modal similarity: The perceptual structure of pitch, loudness, and brightness. *Journal of Experimental Psychology: Human Perception and Performance, 15,* 586–602.

Marks, L. E. (1997). Are tones spatial? A response time analysis. In M. Guirao (Ed.), *Procesos sensoriales y cognitivos: Artículos presentados en adhesión al XXV Aniversario del Laboratorio de Investigaciones Sensoriales (LIS) CONICET* (pp. 95–114). Buenos Aires: Ediciones Duncan.

Marks, L. E. (2000). Synesthesia. In E. Cardena, S. J. Lynn, & S. C. Krippner (Eds.), *Varieties of anomalous experience: Phenomenological and scientific foundations* (pp. 121–149). Washington, DC: American Psychological Association.

Marks, L. E., Ben-Artzi, E., & Lakatos, S. (2003). Cross-modal interactions in auditory and visual discrimination. *International Journal of Psychophysiology, 50,* 125–145.

Marks, L. E., Hammeal, R. J., & Bornstein, M. H. (1987). Children's comprehension of cross-modal similarity: Perception and metaphor. *Monographs in Social Research and Child Developments 42*(1, Serial No. 215), 1–91.

Martino, G., & Marks, L. E. (1999). Perceptual and linguistic interactions in speeded classification: Tests of the semantic coding hypothesis. *Perception, 28,* 903–923.

Martino, G., & Marks, L. E. (2000). Cross-modal interaction between vision and touch: The role of synesthetic correspondence. *Perception, 29,* 745–754.

Melara, R. D. (1989a). Dimensional interaction between color and pitch. *Journal of Experimental Psychology: Human Perception and Performance, 15,* 69–79.

Melara, R. D. (1989b). Similarity relations among synesthetic stimuli and their attributes. *Journal of Experimental Psychology: Human Perception and Performance, 15,* 212–231.

Melara, R. D., & Day, D. J. A. (1992). Primacy of dimensions in vibrotactile perception: An evaluation of early holistic models. *Perception & Psychophysics, 52,* 1–17.

Melara, R. D., & Marks, L. E. (1990a). Perceptual primacy of dimensions: Support for a model of dimensional interaction. *Journal of Experimental Psychology: Human Perception and Performance, 16,* 398–414.

Melara, R. D., & Marks, L. E. (1990b). Processes underlying dimensional interactions: Correspondences between linguistic and nonlinguistic dimensions. *Memory and Cognition, 18,* 477–495.

Melara, R. D., Marks, L. E., & Potts, B. C. (1993). Primacy of dimensions in color perception. *Journal of Experimental Psychology: Human Perception and Performance, 19,* 1082–1104.

Melara, R. D., & Mounts, J. R. (1993). Selective attention to Stroop dimensions: Effects of baseline discriminability, response mode, and practice. *Memory and Cognition, 21,* 627–645.

Melara, R. D., & O'Brien, T. P. (1987). Interaction between synesthetically corresponding dimensions. *Journal of Experimental Psychology: General, 116,* 323–336.

Moore, B. C. J. (1997). *An introduction to the psychology of hearing* (4th ed.). New York: Academic Press.

Morgan, G. A., Goodson, F. E., & Jones, T. (1975). Age differences in the associations between felt temperatures and color choices. *American Journal of Psychology, 88,* 125–130.

Mudd, S. A. (1963). Spatial stereotypes of four dimensions of pure tone. *Journal of Experimental Psychology, 66,* 347–352.

Odgaard, E. C., Arieh, Y., & Marks, L. E. (2003). Cross-modal enhancement of perceived brightness: Sensory interaction versus response bias. *Perception & Psychophysics, 65,* 123–132.

Pashler, H. E. (1998). *The psychology of attention.* Cambridge, MA: MIT Press.

Patching, G. R., & Quinlan, P. T. (2002). Garner and congruence effects in the speeded classification of bimodal stimuli.

Journal of Experimental Psychology: Human Perception and Performance, 28, 755–775.

Pavani, F., Spence, C., & Driver, J. (2000). Visual capture of touch: Out-of-the-body experiences with rubber gloves. Psychological Science, 11, 353–359.

Pomerantz, J. R., Pristach, E. A., & Carson, C. E. (1989). Attention and object perception. In B. E. Shepp & S. Ballesteros (Eds.), Object perception: Structure and process (pp. 53–89). Hillsdale, NJ: Erlbaum.

Posner, M. I. (1964). Information reduction in the analysis of sequential tasks. Psychological Review, 71, 491–504.

Radeau, M., & Bertelson, P. (1977). Adaptation to auditory-visual discordance and ventriloquism in semirealistic situations. Perception & Psychophysics, 22, 137–146.

Smith, L. B., & Kemler, D. G. (1978). Levels of experienced dimensionality in children and adults. Cognitive Psychology, 10, 502–532.

Soto-Faraco, S., Lyons, J., Gazzaniga, M., Spence, C., & Kingstone, A. (2002). The ventriloquist in motion: Illusory capture of dynamic information across sensory modalities. Cognitive Brain Research, 14, 139–146.

Stein, B. E., London, N., Wilkinson, L. K., & Price, D. D. (1996). Enhancement of perceived visual intensity by auditory stimuli: A psychophysical analysis. Journal of Cognitive Neuroscience, 8, 497–506.

Stein, B. E., Magalhaes-Castro, B., & Kruger, L. (1975). Superior colliculus: Visuotopic-somatotopic overlap. Science, 189, 224–226.

Stumpf, K. (1883). Tonpsychologie [Psychology of sound]. Leipzig: Hirzel.

Tanner, T. A., Haller, R. W., & Atkinson, R. C. (1967). Signal recognition as influenced by presentation schedule. Perception & Psychophysics, 2, 349–358.

Treisman, A. M. (1969). Strategies and models of selective attention. Psychological Review, 76, 282–299.

Tulving, E., & Lindsay, P. H. (1967). Identification of simultaneously presented simple visual and auditory stimuli. Acta Psychologica, 27, 101–109.

van Leeuwen, C., & Bakker, L. (1995). Stroop can occur without Garner interference: Strategic and mandatory influences in multidimensional stimuli. Perception & Psychophysics, 57, 379–392.

Walker, P., & Smith, W. (1984). Stroop interference based on the synaesthetic qualities of auditory pitch. Perception, 13, 75–81.

Wallace, M. T., Meredith, M. A., & Stein, B. E. (1992). Integration of multiple sensory inputs in cat cortex. Experimental Brain Research, 91, 484–488.

Wicker, F. W. (1968). Mapping the intersensory regions of perceptual space. American Journal of Psychology, 81, 178–188.

7 Multisensory Texture Perception

SUSAN J. LEDERMAN AND ROBERTA L. KLATZKY

Introduction

Most of the scientific research on the perception of material qualities of objects has focused on the perception of texture. By texture, we mean the *microstructure of surfaces* as opposed to the large-scale macrostructure of objects (e.g., form, shape). The surface texture is independent of the macrostructure on which it is superimposed. The material from which objects are constructed also possesses other prominent properties, such as softness or hardness, slipperiness and friction, and thermal qualities such as thermal flow and thermal conductivity. The general issues we raise in this chapter with respect to texture perception pertain as well to these other properties of object materials. However, because there has been relatively little scientific research on these topics to date, we will consider them at the end of the chapter.

The perception of surface texture is a *multidimensional* task; however, the most salient dimensions remain somewhat uncertain (see Hollins, Faldowski, Rao, & Young, 1993; Hollins & Risner, 2000). When we describe the texture of a surface, we may focus on dimensions such as roughness/smoothness, bumpiness, or jaggedness, or perhaps on the degree of element cluster that produces the surface microstructure. The perception of surface texture is also *multisensory*. That is, regardless of the properties to which we attend, we may use any or all of the following modalities during perception: haptics, vision, and audition. (The haptic system uses sensory inputs from mechanoreceptors in the skin, muscles, tendons, and joints, and typically involves voluntary manual exploration of surfaces, objects, and their spatial layout.)

The availability of more than one sensory source may serve a number of different functions. First, when the information obtained via different sensory modalities about a given property is exactly the same, the modalities will provide redundant cues about the targeted property. Second, even if the sensory sources provide concordant information, one modality may provide more accurate or more precise information than another. Alternately or in addition, it may obtain that information faster than another modality. Third, the modalities may actually provide discrepant information about a targeted property. Fourth, the senses may simultaneously provide qualitatively different yet complementary information about a texture. For example, vision provides information about surface properties such as color, lightness, and reflectance, whereas touch provides information about roughness, hardness, slipperiness, and thermal properties.

The following discussion considers relevant empirical findings, theoretical perspectives, and the implications of such fundamental scientific work for the design of multisensory interfaces for teleoperation and virtual environments.

Empirical findings

Empirical studies have addressed two critical questions that pertain to multisensory texture perception. Our presentation of the experimental research findings is organized around these two questions.

1. *How does the perceiver integrate information about surface texture from different sensory modalities?*

The perceiver may choose to ignore information made available through one modality (e.g., Rock & Victor, 1964). Alternatively, the perceiver may integrate the different sensory sources in some form of compromise that is not identical to any one of them. Table 7.1 summarizes the multisensory dominance findings of this and other relevant experiments discussed in this chapter.

Sensory conflict and sensory dominance paradigms offer one experimental approach to the study of multisensory integration. Several studies have employed either artificial or natural discrepancies in the texture information presented simultaneously to the eye and the hand.

We begin with studies that focus on haptics and vision. Lederman and Abbott (1981, Experiment 1) created an artificial discrepancy between the two senses by simultaneously exposing two physically different (i.e., discrepant) black abrasive surfaces to vision and touch. The subjects in this modality discrepancy group were led to believe that they were examining two spatially separated areas on a single surface. Two other modality control groups (vision only, touch only) examined

TABLE 7.1
Summary of qualitative/quantitative intersensory bias/dominance results

Study	Property	Modality		
		V	H	A
Lederman & Abbott (1981)*	Texture (Exp. 1)	V = 50%	H = 50%	N/A
Lederman, Thorne, & Jones (1986)†	Roughness (Exp. 2)	V[H] = 33.2%	H[V] = 73.2%	N/A
	Roughness (Exp. 3)	V[H] = 31.0%	H[V] = 69.0%	N/A
	Roughness (Exp. 6)	V <	H	N/A
	Spatial density (Exp. 1)	V[H] = 76.3%	H[V] = 6.8%	N/A
	Density (Exp. 4)	V[H] = 49.0%	H[V] = 51.0%	N/A
	Spatial density (Exp. 5)	V >	H	N/A
Klatzky, Lederman, & Reed (1987)	Object similarity	Geometry favored when biased to sort by vision	Material favored when biased to sort by haptics	N/A
Klatzky, Lederman, & Matula (1993)	Material properties (texture, hardness, thermal, weight)	Vision always available	Haptics rarely used, when tasks easy; H used on 80% of trials when tasks hard (H only used to judge material)	N/A
	Geometric properties (shape, size, weight)	Vision always available	Haptics never used, regardless of task difficulty (only used to reorient objects to judge size)	N/A
Lederman (1979)*	Roughness (Exp. 3)	N/A	H = 100%	A = 0%
Lederman et al. (2002)*	Roughness	N/A	H = 62%	A = 38%
Guest & Spence (in press)	Roughness	V influenced by incongruent haptic distractors	H uninfluenced by incongruent V distractors	N/A
Jousmaki & Hari (1998)	Skin roughness and moistness	N/A	Bias of A by H not assessed	A biased H
Guest et al. (in press)	Roughness of abrasive surfaces (Exp. 1)	N/A	Bias of A by H not assessed	A biased H
	Roughness and wetness of skin (Exp. 2)	N/A	Bias of A by H not assessed	A biased H
	Roughness and wetness of skin (Exp. 3)	N/A	Bias of A by H not assessed	A biased H

Note: Percent bias of one modality by a second modality was calculated as discussed under Empirical Findings.
Abbreviations: V, vision; H, haptics; A, audition; V[H], visual bias of haptics; H[V], haptic bias of vision.
*These modality bias effects were not independent and must sum to 100.
†These modality bias effects were independent and therefore do not necessarily sum to 100.

either the visual or the tactual standard texture from the discrepant standard stimulus pair.

Subjects were required to select the surface that best matched the "texture" of the standard stimulus from among pairs of identical comparison surfaces. Within each of the three standard modality groups, three subgroups responded using vision only, touch only, or vision and touch together. There were thus nine groups in all. The results indicated that subjects selected a surface pair that lay midway (i.e., 50%)

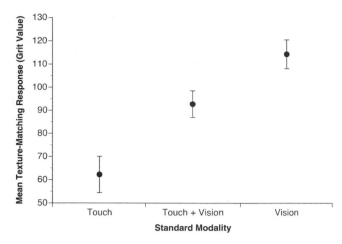

FIGURE 7.1 Mean texture-matching responses (grit value) for unimodal touch, unimodal vision, and bimodal touch plus vision conditions. The standard grit values used in the two unimodal conditions were 60 for touch and 150 for vision. Both were used to create the discrepant texture pair in the bimodal condition. As grit value increases, the particles that produce the abrasive texture become smaller and more densely distributed. (Adapted from Lederman and Abbott, 1981, with permission.)

between the two discrepant stimuli, regardless of the response-matching modality (Fig. 7.1). Because the effect of response modality was not significant, the matching responses are averaged over the three response-modality conditions in the figure. The Lederman and Abbott (1981) study showed that subjects altered their matching response in the bimodal discrepancy condition so that it lay halfway between those of the unimodal controls.

In a series of six experiments, Lederman, Thorne, and Jones (1986) demonstrated that there is in fact no fixed dominance hierarchy among modalities for the perception of textured surfaces, and with this observation underscored the multidimensional nature of texture perception. Changing the dimension that subjects were required to judge produced sizable adjustments in the relative weighting of the haptic and visual inputs. On each trial, subjects were asked to numerically estimate the perceived magnitude of the "spatial density" of raised two-dimensional dot patterns (Experiment 1) or of the "density" of abrasive surfaces (Experiment 4). Subjects examined the surface by touch alone, by vision alone, or by touch and vision together. In the bimodal trials, a pair of surfaces was presented, but unbeknownst to the subject, the two were discrepant. Only after exploration was the subject informed whether to judge how the surface felt (touch in the presence of vision) or looked (vision in the presence of touch). The independent mutual biasing effects of touch and vision

were calculated as follows:

$$\text{Visual bias of haptics } (\% \ V[H]) = \frac{(H_c - V[H])}{(H_c - V_c)} \times 100$$

$$\text{Haptic bias of vision } (\% \ H[V]) = \frac{(V_c - H[V])}{(V_c - H_c)} \times 100$$

where $V[H]$ and $H[V]$ represent the results of the bimodal conditions that indicate the mutual biasing effects of vision on haptics and of haptics on vision, respectively, and V_c and H_c represent the results of the visual and haptic control conditions, respectively.

Felt spatial density judgments were strongly dominated by the concomitant visual inputs (i.e., 76.3%, Experiment 1), while felt density judgments of abrasive surfaces were somewhat less so but still strongly affected by vision (i.e., 49.0%, Experiment 4). (Two reasons for the difference in the magnitude of the visual bias on touch were suggested. The simpler term *density*, which was used subsequently to avoid possible confusion among subjects concerning what they were to judge, may have also de-emphasized the importance of the spatial cues. Alternatively, judging the (spatial) density of abrasive surfaces may have been more difficult than judging the more clearly distinct photoengraved raised-dot surfaces.) The influence of haptic inputs on the independently obtained but corresponding estimates of seen spatial density was very minor, only 7.0% (Experiment 1); for density judgments of abrasive surfaces, haptic dominance was equivalent to visual dominance, 51.0% (Experiment 4), for reasons we suggest later. In sum, subjects weighted touch and vision cues about equally when asked to judge surface texture (Lederman & Abbott, 1981). In contrast, when asked to judge (spatial) density, they tended to weight the visual inputs more strongly. And when asked to judge the roughness of these same surfaces, they weighted the tactual inputs more strongly (Lederman et al., 1986).

The method used to assess the relative contributions of vision and touch to bimodal judgments of discrepant textured surfaces required that the subject believe that the visually and tactually derived information depicted the same surface. Experiments 5 and 6 used a different method known as functional measurement (Anderson, 1974). In this method, subjects are knowingly presented with pairs of stimuli that may or may not be the same. Anderson demonstrated that across a variety of tasks (e.g., weight assessment), information from at least two sources is integrated according to simple additive models. Subjects are presented with pairs of values drawn from two independently manipulated stimulus dimensions. The task requires subjects to provide a combined judgment of pairs of stimuli produced by factorially combining all possible values from the two dimensions.

Lederman et al. (1986) used this paradigm as a converging method for comparing the relative weighting of vision versus haptics in judgments of "spatial density" (Experiment 5) versus "roughness" (Experiment 6). The stimulus pairs were drawn from the same set of two-dimensional raised-dot patterns used in Experiments 1 and 2. When subjects assessed surface roughness bimodally by vision and touch, they treated the two modality inputs as independent. The results of these experiments confirmed the relative dominance of touch by vision for the spatial density task and of vision by touch for the roughness task. The results were best described by a linear averaging model in which subjects averaged the two unimodal control judgments to produce a weighted average judgment in the corresponding bimodal condition. The theoretical details of this model are discussed later in the section titled Modeling Multisensory Texture Perception.

Sensory dominance and intersensory integration have been explored with respect to texture perception using a number of other methodologies. For example, Klatzky, Lederman, and Reed (1987) demonstrated the relatively greater importance of surface texture and hardness for touch than vision using a different experimental paradigm. They custom-designed and constructed a large set of multiattribute artificial objects that varied along four different object dimensions in psychophysically equivalent ways, whether objects were grouped according to their surface texture (three values), hardness (three values), shape (three values), or size (three values). The three different values for each property were combined across all dimensions, producing a set of 81 objects. Each object had one of three textures, one of three hardness values, one of three shape values, and one of three size values. Subjects were required to sort the objects into piles according to their perceived similarity. Objects that were most similar to each other were to be grouped together. Different instruction sets were used to deliberately bias subjects toward favoring their haptically derived or visually derived object representations in their sorting judgments. When biased to process and represent objects in terms of haptic similarity, subjects preferred to sort objects in terms of the available material properties as opposed to the objects' geometric properties. In contrast, when biased to sort on the basis of visual similarity, subjects sorted primarily by shape and secondarily by texture. People tend to be more efficient—more accurate or faster—when accessing precise material variation with their hands than with their eyes, as other research has tended to show (e.g., Heller, 1989; Lederman & Klatzky,

1987; but see also Jones & O'Neil, 1985, discussed later in this chapter under question 2: "How does multisensory integration affect performance?"). Conversely, when biased to process and represent objects using vision, subjects strongly preferred to sort by differences in object shape. This finding too makes sense, because vision is considerably more efficient at processing geometric information (e.g., Klatzky & Lederman, 2003; Lederman & Klatzky, 1987; Walk & Pick, 1981). The results of this study were subsequently confirmed by Lederman, Summers, and Klatzky (1996) with three-dimensional objects.

Collectively, these studies suggest that when multiattribute objects vary in perceptually equivalent ways, subjects will choose to develop representations of these objects more in terms of the objects' variation in material properties (e.g., texture, hardness) than in terms of their geometric properties (e.g., size, shape) when focused on the haptic inputs. Our data indicate that texture plays an important role in both types of representations; however, it appears to be more cognitively salient to haptically than to visually derived representations of the same objects.

Klatzky, Lederman, and Matula (1993) used a different experimental paradigm to address the issue of multisensory texture perception. They considered situations in which people chose to use touch, even though visual exploration was available. In the study, subjects were required to make discriminations between common-object pairs with respect to six targeted perceptual dimensions—four material dimensions (roughness, hardness, thermal properties, and weight) and two geometric dimensions (shape and size). When the discriminations were very easy, subjects chose not to use touch very often, relying solely on vision. The situations in which touch was used for easy judgments tended to involve decisions regarding the material characteristics of objects. When the discriminations were difficult, subjects chose to use touch in addition to vision in about 80% of the trials that required judgments about material properties, including roughness. In contrast, subjects did not use touch to make perceptual discriminations about shape or size. This study indicates that people elect to use tactual information about surface roughness when relatively precise information about the material features of objects is required, even when visual information is available.

Finally, Guest and Spence (2003) have examined visual-tactual integration of texture information in a speeded texture task. Participants were required to make speeded discrimination judgments of the roughness of abraded (pilled) textile samples by one modality (either vision or touch) in the presence of congruent or incongruent information about a textile distracter presented to the other modality (touch or vision, respectively). Visual discrimination of textile roughness was altered by incongruous tactual distracters. However, the reverse did not occur, even when the visual distracters were more discriminable than the tactile targets. Guest and Spence concluded that the asymmetric interference effect implied that ecological validity must play a role, in addition to modality appropriateness. In keeping with Lederman's initial interpretation (1979), which will be discussed in the following section on haptics and audition studies, Guest and Spence argued that the assessment of textile surfaces is better suited to tactual than to visual assessment.

In summary, there appears to be no fixed sensory dominance with respect to the multisensory perception of texture by vision and haptics. Rather, the lability with which one modality dominates the other with respect to order and magnitude is influenced by the selected emphasis on some aspect of surface texture (e.g., texture, roughness, spatial density).

We turn now to studies that have involved haptic and auditory processing. Another potentially valuable source of information about surface texture is the accompanying set of sounds that are generated when one touches a surface. For example, Katz (1989) showed that people are remarkably skilled at identifying different materials using the touch-produced sounds alone.

Lederman (1979) used a natural discrepancy paradigm to investigate whether people can use such sounds alone to evaluate the roughness magnitude of metal gratings. The paradigm also allowed consideration of the relative contributions of haptic and haptically produced sounds to the perception of roughness when both sources of information were simultaneously available. In one experiment (Experiment 3), subjects were required to estimate the magnitude of perceived roughness of rigid, unidimensional gratings that varied in terms of groove width (constant ridge width). For such stimulus surfaces groove width is known to be the primary parameter that affects the haptic perception of roughness by touch (in contrast to ridge width, spatial period, and groove-to-ridge width ratio, which have little or no effect; see, e.g., Lederman, 1974). Subjects participated in each of three modality conditions—haptics only, audition only (sounds generated by experimenter), and haptics plus audition (sounds generated by the subject). The psychophysical functions (perceived roughness magnitude as a function of the groove width of linear engraved gratings, on log-log scales) increased considerably less rapidly for audition alone (particularly for the plates with the narrower grooves) than for either haptics alone or haptics plus audition.

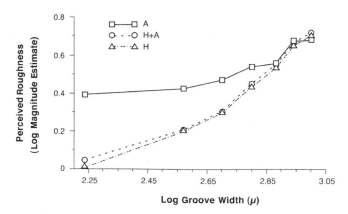

FIGURE 7.2 Perceived roughness magnitude (log magnitude estimates) as a function of log groove width for haptics only (bare finger), audition only, and haptics (bare finger) plus audition conditions. H, haptic only; A, auditory only; H+A, haptic plus auditory. (Adapted from Lederman, 1979, Figure 2, with permission.)

These results indicate that subjects could use the auditory cues generated by gratings, although not as well as they could the haptic cues. Indeed, when both auditory and haptic cues were available, the psychophysical function for roughness was virtually identical to that for haptics alone (Fig. 7.2; see also Table 7.1). That these two functions were identical suggests that in contrast to the results of von Schiller (1932), subjects in Lederman's (1979) experiment ignored the available auditory information when estimating roughness magnitude.

In Lederman's (1979) study, subjects used their bare fingers to explore the textured surfaces. However, people also frequently use intermediate tools to perceive and interact with objects. When judging surface properties haptically with a probe, people must use vibrations as the source of their information, one that is accessible to both hand and ear. Just recently Lederman, Klatzky, Hamilton, and Morgan (2002) used Lederman's (1979) psychophysical paradigm (magnitude estimation) in their investigation of the remote perception of surface texture via a rigid stylus. Different groups of subjects explored the roughness magnitude of spatially jittered, raised two-dimensional dot patterns under one of three different modality conditions: unimodal haptics, unimodal audition (sounds produced by the experimenter), and bimodal haptics plus audition (sounds produced by the subjects). The results indicated that, as with direct contact between hand and surface, exploration with a stylus created a natural perceptual discrepancy between unimodal haptic and auditory estimates of roughness; that is, the two psychophysical control functions (haptics only and audition only) differed. However, unlike the results of the earlier bare finger study, when both sensory sources were simultaneously

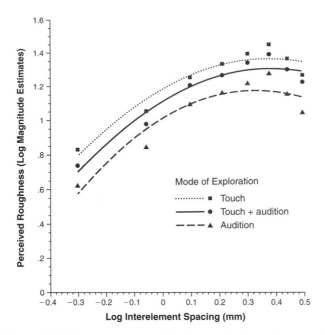

FIGURE 7.3 Log mean normalized magnitude estimates of perceived roughness via a rigid probe as a function of log inter-element spacing for touch only, audition only, and touch plus audition exploration conditions. (Reproduced from Lederman et al., 2002, by permission of the publishers.)

available, subjects chose to use both remote sources of information in their bimodal judgments, weighting the haptic inputs somewhat more (62%) than the auditory inputs (38%) (Fig. 7.3).

Converging evidence that people use auditory information to judge surface roughness remotely via a probe in bimodal touch/audition conditions was reported in a second experiment in this study (Morgan, 2001). Subjects bimodally explored the same raised two-dimensional dot patterns with a rigid probe in each of three sound-amplification level conditions. Their roughness estimates increased systematically as a function of the increasing amplification of the touch-produced sounds produced as the subject explored the surfaces with a rigid probe. The results converge with those reported by Lederman et al. (2002), in that subjects did indeed use the touch-produced sounds to make their remote judgments bimodally, using cues generated with a rigid probe and concomitant touch-produced sounds.

Additional support for the intersensory bias of haptic estimates of surface roughness by concomitant sounds comes from an intriguing phenomenon discovered by Jousmaki and Hari (1998), known as the parchment-skin illusion. As subjects rubbed their hands back and forth together, the sounds were recorded and played back to the subjects through headphones as normal or altered sounds. One parameter was the amplitude of the sound frequencies above 2000 Hz: values included natural level (i.e., identical to the original sounds), amplification to 15 dB above natural level, and attenuation to 15 dB below the natural level. A second parameter was average sound level, which was adjusted relative to a comfortable listening level ("normal"): values included the average sound level adjusted to normal, 20 dB below normal, and 40 dB below normal. Subjects were required to judge skin roughness on a scale from 0 (rough or moist) to 10 (smooth or dry). Subjects judged the skin surface to increase in smoothness/dryness as the values of both parameters were increased. This increase was compared to the feel of parchment paper. The results of this study clearly indicate the bias of touch by audition and a role for sound amplitude in the perception of the roughness of this naturally occurring surface.

Guest, Catmur, Lloyd, and Spence (2002) extended the work of Jousmaki and Hari by investigating the role of haptically produced sounds on the perceived roughness of abrasive surfaces. In contrast to Jousmaki and Hari, they found that in a speeded discrimination task, reducing the high-frequency auditory feedback biased subjects toward judging surfaces by touch as smoother (Experiment 1). Experiment 2 replicated Jousmaki and Hari's hand-rubbing experiment but asked subjects to scale both the wetness and the roughness of their hands. The results for wetness judgments replicated Jousmaki and Hari's findings; however, those for roughness confirmed those obtained by Guest et al. in their Experiment 1. Finally, in Experiment 3, they showed that delaying the auditory feedback for hand rubbing reduced the size of the parchment-skin illusion in Experiment 2. Collectively, the results strongly indicate the influence of concurrent sounds (i.e., auditory frequency) on the tactile assessment of roughness and hand moistness. Gaver (e.g., 1993) has provided additional examples of "textural" properties obtained via sound.

To summarize, as noted with the vision and haptics intersensory bias studies, results of the audition and haptics studies likewise indicate that the relative order and magnitude of sensory dominance is labile. As we later discuss later under Modeling Multisensory Texture Perception, transient or short-term factors may also play a role by influencing the relative perceptual accessibility of the stimulus information available in the given task.

2. *How does multisensory integration affect performance?*

If the perceiver integrates information from more than one modality, do the multiple sources improve, impair,

TABLE 7.2
Relative unimodal and bimodal performance on texture-related tasks

Study	Task	Performance Variables	Outcomes
Lederman & Abbott (1981)	1. "Texture" matching	1. Accuracy	1. H = V = (H+V)
		1. Variability	1. H = V = (H+V)
	2. Rate of growth of perceived "roughness" (magnitude estimation)	2. Exponent of psychophysical power function	2. H = V = (H+V)
		2. Variability	2. H = V = (H+V)
Jones & O'Neil (1985)	1. 2-AFC for relative "roughness" (Exp. 1)	1. Accuracy	1. H = V = (H+V)
		1. Response time	1. V < (H+V) < H
	2. Same/different for relative roughness (Exp. 2)	2. Accuracy	2. H = V = (H+V)
		2. Response time	2. V < (H+V) < H
	3. 2-AFC for relative roughness (Exp. 3)	3. Accuracy	3. H < (H+V) < V
		3. Response time	3. V < (H+V) < H
Heller (1982)	3-AFC for relative "smoothness" (coarse textures)	Accuracy	H = V
			H and V < (H+V)
Heller (1989)	2-AFC relative "smoothness"	Accuracy (coarse stimuli)	H = V
		accuracy (very smooth stimuli)	H > V
Lederman (1979)	Magnitude estimation of roughness (Exp. 1)	Exponent of psychophysical power function	A < H
	Magnitude estimation of roughness (Exp. 2)	Exponent of psychophysical power function	H = (H+A)
Lederman, Klatzky, Hamilton, & Morgan (2002)	Confidence estimation of magnitude estimates of roughness	Confidence ratings	Mean of H and A < (H+A)
Lederman et al. (2003)	Absolute roughness identification	Amount learned (bits)	A < H = (A+H)
		Rate of learning	H = (A+H) < A (but see text for proper interpretation)
		Confidence rating	A < H = (A+H)
Wu, Basdogan, & Srinivasan (1999)	2-AFC relative stiffness	Resolution	H and V < (H+V)

Abbreviations: A, audition only; H, haptic only; V, vision only; 2(3)-AFC, two (three)-alternative forced-choice task. Bimodal conditions are represented in parentheses.

or have no influence on performance (e.g., accuracy, variability, confidence, response time)? For the purpose of comparing unimodal and bimodal performance on texture-related perceptual tasks, Table 7.2 summarizes the results of all experiments in this section. Many of these studies were discussed in the preceding section.

Once again, we begin with studies on vision and haptics. An additional experiment in the Lederman and Abbott study (1981, Experiment 2) assessed the associated relative performance by the two modalities on a texture-matching task. Subjects participated in one of three modality conditions: touch only, vision only, or

haptics plus vision. In this experiment, however, the bimodal condition presented identical pairs of relatively coarse, black abrasive surfaces to both vision and touch. The results indicated virtually identical performance among the two unimodal and one bimodal groups, both in terms of texture-matching accuracy and in terms of response precision (i.e., consistency). Finally, Lederman and Abbott (1981, Experiment 3) compared haptics, vision, and touch plus vision in terms of the rate of growth of the corresponding psychophysical functions for perceived "roughness" magnitude (i.e., the increase in reported roughness magnitude with increased size of the particles that formed the textured surface). Subjects were required to judge the roughness magnitudes of black abrasive surfaces using a magnitude-estimation procedure. The results indicated that there were no differences among the modality conditions in either rate of growth of roughness magnitude or relative precision. In addition, there was no difference in performance among the two unimodal and bimodal conditions with respect to accuracy and precision on the texture-matching task (Experiment 2) and with respect to rate of growth and precision on a magnitude-estimation task (Experiment 3).

Jones and O'Neil (1985) also compared unimodal (vision only, haptics only) and bimodal judgments of surface roughness. Subjects performed two-alternative, forced-choice (Experiments 1 and 3) and same/different (Experiment 2) tasks. In keeping with the earlier results obtained by Lederman and Abbott (1981), subjects tended to be about equally accurate on Experiments 1 and 2, regardless of the modality used during exploration. Moreover, using two sources of information about surface roughness did not improve accuracy compared with either of the unimodal conditions. With respect to speed, vision was faster than touch, with the bimodal condition falling midway between the two unimodal conditions. Thus, vision was more effective than touch with respect to speed of responding, and served to improve unimodal tactual performance, whereas the addition of touch slowed down unimodal visual performance. The relatively greater temporal efficiency of vision is not surprising, because the eye can process a wide spatial area simultaneously without movement, while the hand must move to sample the surface. In Experiment 3, subjects were more accurate and faster using unimodal vision than unimodal haptics, while the bimodal condition lay between the two.

Heller (1982) required his subjects to perform three-alternative, forced-choice relative "smoothness" tasks using a similar range of abrasive surfaces to those used by Lederman and Abbott (1981) and Jones and O'Neil (1985). In Experiment 1, subjects chose the smoothest of three abrasive surfaces, with texture triads created from the set of abrasive surfaces. Subjects participated in three modality conditions: unimodal vision, unimodal haptics, and bimodal haptics plus vision. Although subjects performed very well in all three modality conditions, the bimodal condition resulted in greater accuracy than either of the unimodal haptics or vision conditions, which were not significantly different from each other (Fig. 7.4; see also Table 7.2). The added benefit of the bimodal inputs was considered as well in Experiment 2, which confirmed Heller's

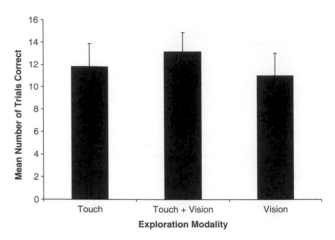

FIGURE 7.4   Mean number of trials correct (out of 16) using vision, touch, and vision plus touch. The value of +1 SEM is shown for each exploration modality condition. (Based on data from Heller, 1982, and used by permission of the author and the Psychonomic Society.)

earlier findings, namely, the equivalent accuracy in the two unimodal conditions and greater accuracy in the bimodal condition.

In summary, unlike either Lederman and Abbott (1981) or Jones and O'Neil (1985), Heller found that performance improved when subjects used bimodal (i.e., vision and haptics) exploration (see Table 7.2). He found no benefit from the auditory cues that were also available, in keeping with an earlier study by Lederman (1979) that will be discussed in detail later in the chapter. Experiment 2 also confirmed that subjects in Experiment 1 did not capitalize on the better visual illumination cues available only in the bimodal condition of that experiment. (In Experiment 1, subjects had been allowed to handle the objects with the gloved, nonexploring hand and thus to move them closer for better viewing.) Therefore, in Experiment 3, Heller extended his examination of the role of vision in bimodal texture judgments, using the same set of surfaces as in Experiment 2. Subjects participated in one of three experimental conditions. One group was required to judge the relative smoothness of abrasive surfaces using available visual and haptic cues to texture, along with sight of their hands. A second group was permitted to use normal haptic texture cues and subjects could see their hands; however, they were denied visual cues to texture. In this condition, subjects manually explored the abrasive surfaces while viewing their hands through a plastic stained glass filter. The visual filter served to eliminate the use of visual texture cues while retaining sight of the moving hand for purposes of visual guidance. If subjects used visual texture cues in their bimodal judgments, then Group 1 should have performed better than Group 2. However, there was no difference in performance, leading Heller to conclude that subjects used sight of their hand movements, not the visual texture cues, to make their bimodal estimates. Group 3 served to confirm that visual judgments of texture were indeed impossible when the surfaces were viewed through the visual filter. In this condition, both the haptic cues to texture and sight of the moving hand were eliminated as potential sources of information.

Heller suggested that the superior bimodal performance on the smoothness discrimination task resulted because the two modalities cooperated with one another, with touch providing the relevant texture information and vision providing complementary information about the hand movements. However, his data do not suggest that subjects used texture inputs from both modalities to derive a compromise judgment about relative smoothness.

In a subsequent paper, Heller (1989) showed that texture perception of relatively coarse abrasive surfaces was essentially equivalent for sighted, late-blind and early-blind subjects. He concluded that visual imagery too was not necessary for texture perception. He used a two-alternative, forced-choice task to compare the accuracy with which subjects picked the smoother of two surfaces using either unimodal haptics or unimodal vision. In a second experiment, Heller required subjects to perform the same two-alternative, forced-choice relative smoothness task; however, pairs were chosen that included new very smooth surfaces in addition to the previous coarser surfaces (similar to those used in his 1982 study). The results confirmed the equivalence of touch and vision for the coarser pairs; however, touch proved to be considerably more accurate than vision for the very smooth pairs (see Table 7.2).

In summary, the studies on relative performance in conditions of unimodal vision, unimodal haptics, and bimodal vision plus haptics (see Table 7.2) have collectively tended to show that haptics and vision are relatively equal in terms of their relative accuracy, variability, and rate of growth of roughness magnitude; not surprisingly, vision is faster. With the exception of Heller (e.g., 1982), most studies have shown no benefit from using both modalities together.

Next we consider studies that have addressed relative performance involving unimanual haptics, unimanual audition, and bimodal haptics plus audition. In the previously described study by Lederman (1979), subjects also estimated the roughness magnitude of linear gratings in two other experiments. In Experiment 1, subjects used only the haptically produced sounds produced by the experimenter. In Experiment 2, subjects used either haptics or haptics plus audition together; in the latter case the sounds were produced by the subject. The stimulus set consisted of gratings that varied in ridge width (groove width was constant). Perceived roughness tended to decline with increasing ridge width regardless of the modality (or modalities) used. Moreover, the unimodal and bimodal haptics conditions were not statistically different from one another. The auditory estimates for the wider-ridge gratings differentiated the plates less than did estimates from the two haptics conditions, suggesting a slight advantage for haptics over audition. Nevertheless, neither modality was particularly effective at differentiating the set of ridge-varying gratings.

Finally, we consider recent data from roughness perception tasks that involved exploring raised two-dimensional dot patterns with a rigid probe as opposed to the bare finger. Confidence estimates were also obtained at the end of the experiment by Lederman et al. (2002, Experiment 1) from subjects in the haptics, audition, and haptics plus audition conditions. The results were suggestive: confidence in the bimodal condition was higher than the mean of the combined unimodal conditions. Because relative performance was not the primary focus of the Lederman et al. (2002) study, Lederman, Klatzky, Martin, and Tong (2003) subsequently addressed this issue directly by comparing performance on a difficult absolute texture (i.e., roughness) identification task with a rigid probe. Subjects were assigned to one of the following three exploration conditions: haptics only, audition only (haptically produced sounds), or haptics plus audition. Subjects learned to associate a man's name with each of the stimulus textures. Feedback was provided after each response. Subjects repeated the stimulus set a total of 14 times. Performance for each modality was assessed in terms of efficiency (i.e., amount learned and rate of learning) and confidence. Unimodal haptics proved to be equivalent to bimodal haptics plus audition, and both were associated with greater learning and higher confidence scores than unimodal audition. The greater learning rate for audition than haptics may seem to indicate that audition is the superior modality for this task, but that is not the case: the result actually occurred because accuracy for audition was lower than haptics at the start, and both modality conditions ultimately reached the same level of accuracy. When the experiment was repeated using an easier texture identification task, the pattern of results was similar; however, subjects were equally confident, regardless of whether either unimodal condition or the bimodal condition was used.

In conclusion, studies comparing haptics and audition in texture perception have shown that when the bare finger is used, the rate of growth in roughness is slower for audition than for haptics, which in turn is equivalent to bimodal haptics plus audition. When touching is remote (i.e., via a rigid probe), if the task is difficult, subjects tend to show an advantage early in learning and are more confident using either haptics alone or bimodal haptics plus audition than using audition alone. When the task is easier, the results are similar, but subjects are equally confident in all three modality conditions.

Modeling multisensory texture perception

To fully understand multisensory texture perception, it is critical that in addition to addressing issues that pertain to intersensory representation, we must also consider those relating to the processes by which those representations are created. In the following section, we describe several theoretical approaches that have been, or could be, adopted.

THE "MODALITY APPROPRIATENESS" HYPOTHESIS This hypothesis offers an early qualitative theoretical approach to the basis of intersensory integration (e.g., Friedes, 1974; Welch & Warren, 1980). According to the general form of the modality appropriateness hypothesis, observers choose to weight the various modality inputs according to their relative unimodal performance capabilities with respect to the given task (form, size, texture, etc.). Several relative performance measures have been considered: accuracy, response time, and precision or variability. Even relative availability of different information sources has been proposed; however, just below we consider whether it is as appropriate a dependent measure as the preceding ones. The modality appropriateness interpretation contrasts with that used in earlier research, which argued for the universal dominance of vision in perception (e.g., Rock & Victor, 1964). According to the modality appropriateness hypothesis, however, vision should strongly dominate touch, which should dominate audition, on spatial tasks, because vision is spatially best and audition is spatially worst (egocentric location, e.g., Hay, Pick, & Ikeda, 1965; object shape and size, e.g., Rock & Victor, 1964; orientation, e.g., Over, 1966). In contrast, audition should strongly dominate vision (with touch in the middle) on temporal tasks, because people perform such tasks best with audition and worst with vision (e.g., Myers, Cotton, & Hilp, 1981; Nazarro & Nazarro, 1970; Welch, DuttonHurt, & Warren, 1986).

As noted earlier, texture perception is a multidimensional task that can rely on intensive spatial or temporal processing (or both), depending on the particular property in question (e.g., roughness/smoothness vs. spatial density of the surface elements) and the proximal stimulus cues used to derive the percept (e.g., spatial deformation vs. vibration). Indeed, we saw that subjects weighted haptic and visual inputs about equally when they were asked to judge the perceived "texture" of abrasive surfaces (Lederman & Abbott, 1981) using a bimodal discrepancy paradigm. Because the term *texture* was deliberately left undefined, subjects could have been performing this task by focusing on different surface properties with vision and touch. For example, subjects might have processed roughness via touch and spatial density via vision. After all, the haptic system is equal to or better than vision at discriminating surface roughness in terms of accuracy and precision (Heller, 1989; Lederman & Abbott, 1981), whereas vision is superior to haptics in processing fine spatial details. This interpretation is supported by the results of the Lederman et al. (1986) study. When subjects were explicitly instructed to judge the spatial density of a discrepant pair of textured surfaces, they weighted the visual cues more strongly; in striking contrast, when asked to judge the roughness of the same surfaces, subjects weighted the haptic cues more strongly.

The results that pertain to the relative weighting of auditory versus haptic information on roughness perception tasks may also lend themselves to a modality appropriateness interpretation, which assumes that people process information in a modality according to the value it possesses, based on long-term experience. For example, Lederman (1979) showed that subjects ignored the touch-produced sounds when using their bare finger to explore. She argued that such sounds are typically of very low amplitude, and therefore are often masked by other extraneous environmental sounds. As these touch-produced sounds are relatively unavailable during common auditory experience, observers may simply choose to ignore them. However, contrary to this interpretation, when texture-related sound cues were generated instead with a rigid probe (Lederman et al., 2002), subjects weighted them more strongly in their judgments of roughness magnitude. That is, they no longer ignored the auditory information, although that would be appropriate to their common experience with that modality. We must note, however, that probe-produced sounds are typically considerably louder than those produced with a bare finger, and therefore would be relatively more accessible. In hindsight, such logic implies that the appropriateness of a modality per se depends to some extent on transient characteristics of the input rather than on its general utility. This was probably not the intent of either

Friedes (1974) or Welch and Warren (1980) when they proposed the modality appropriateness hypothesis.

Here we consider a new interpretation of the results offered by Lederman and her colleagues (Lederman, 1979; Lederman et al., 2002). The factor they addressed, relative cue availability, relates more to transient modality effects than to those due to the long-term characterization of the modality per se (e.g., accuracy, precision, speed of response). Lederman et al. (1996) have recently proposed that long-term appropriateness and current (and therefore short-term) accessibility be treated as independent factors that might both affect the relative cognitive salience of different sources of information. The transient changes in the relative modality weights may be primarily determined by what they have called relative "perceptual accessibility" of information to multiple modalities that may vary across perceptual conditions. When perceptual accessibility of a cue to one modality is considerably higher than to another modality, it could mask more long-term effects of modality appropriateness that favor the latter. This appears to be the case for probe-produced sounds, which, having relatively high amplitude, override a more general tendency to ignore auditory cues produced when feeling textures. A conceptual model that reflects the contribution of these factors is presented in Figure 7.5, using haptics and audition as examples. The stronger weighting of haptics than audition is indicated by the relative thickness of the arrow representing the generation of the haptic weight.

Regardless of how we choose to treat the relative availability of cues to different modalities, the modality appropriateness hypothesis does not allow quantitative predictions about the relative modality weights. Nor does it specify what particular factors affect the process or processes that determine the differential weightings (e.g., long-term modality appropriateness or immediate stimulus attributes).

In summary, many human studies using the perceptual discrepancy paradigm have offered strong behavioral support for the bimodal percept of a single object as involving some compromise (0%–100%) between the two unimodal inputs—for spatial location (e.g., Hay et al., 1965; Pick, Warren, & Hay, 1969), for shape (e.g., Rock & Victor, 1964; Miller, 1972), for size (e.g., Fishkin, Pishkin, & Stahl, 1975; Klein, 1966), for orientation (e.g., Over, 1966; Singer & Day, 1966), and for texture (e.g., Heller, 1989; Lederman & Abbott, 1981; Lederman et al., 1986). This can result in bimodal performance being inferior to performance with a unimodal condition.

However, there is also behavioral evidence of information summation, both within and between the senses (e.g., within vision, Meese & Williams, 2000; for smell and taste, Dalton, Doolittle, Nagata, & Breslin, 2000; for audition & vision, Mulligan & Shaw, 1980). With this

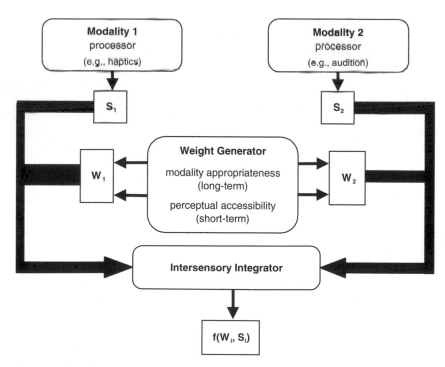

FIGURE 7.5   A conceptual model of intersensory integration. Oval boxes represent processors, square boxes represent outputs, and arrows represent process.

outcome, the bimodal condition results in superior performance relative to either unimodal input.

In addition, there now exists a substantial neurophysiological literature that is relevant to multisensory integration. This work indicates that the responses elicited by simultaneous inputs from two modalities may be greater than the responses elicited by either modality on its own, and may well be significantly greater than the sum of the unimodal responses found within and across many sensory domains (e.g., visual-auditory, auditory-somatosensory, and somatosensory-visual in primate superior colliculus [SC], Wallace, Wilkinson, & Stein, 1996; for cat sc, Meredith & Stein, 1986; see also Calvert, Campbell, & Brammer, 2000, for superadditivity in humans). There is one major difference between discrepancy studies on intersensory texture perception and those on multisensory integration in the SC. The former use models of intersensory discrepancy to monitor changes in perception, whereas the latter do the reverse, namely, they match bimodal inputs in space and/or time. Clearly, much more needs to be done before we can resolve the apparent conflict between the two literatures on multisensory integration. How, for example, can additive models be applied to the superadditive response gains observed in electrophysiology?

LINEAR INTEGRATION MODELS A more quantitative approach to the nature of multisensory texture perception has involved the use of additive and weighted averaging models, although no explicit mechanisms are proposed. The general form of such models is one in which R_V and R_H are associated with different weight parameters to represent the level of compromise between the two modalities, as follows:

$$R_{VH} = w_V R_V + w_H R_H \qquad (1)$$

where R_{VH} is the multisensory judgment of texture, R_V is the corresponding unimodal response using vision alone, and R_H is the corresponding unimodal response using haptics alone; w_V and w_H are the weights associated with the vision-only and touch-only responses. This is a specific version of the conceptual model in Figure 7.5, where the integration function is linear. The results of Experiments 1–4 by Lederman et al. (1986) could be explained in terms of such a general model, with vision being more strongly weighted than touch for judgments of spatial density, and touch being more strongly weighted than vision for judgments of roughness.

Jones and O'Neil (1985: their Equation 2) have derived a *complete dominance* process from the general model just presented, in which less efficiently processed information from one modality is totally ignored. The

following equation is based on their forced-choice task. Hence P replaces the more general R in Equation 1 to represent probability responses:

$$P_{VH} = \max P \qquad (2)$$

where max P is the larger of P_V or P_H. Again, this is a specific version of the conceptual model in Figure 7.5, but in this situation, there is linear averaging where the weight for the lesser of P_V or P_H is set to zero and the weight for the larger is set to 1. The only empirical work that could be viewed as supporting a total dominance model of multisensory roughness perception is by Lederman (1979) and by Heller (1982, Experiment 3). In Lederman's study, when estimating the magnitude of perceived roughness, subjects ignored the sounds produced by touching textured surfaces with their bare fingers and focused solely on the associated haptic cues. In Heller's study, subjects ignored the cues to visual texture in the bimodal condition.

Jones and O'Neil (1985, their Equation 3) also proposed a very simple version of the general model (Equation 1) in which the bimodal response P_{VH} is modeled as the arithmetic mean of the two inputs:

$$P_{VH} = (P_V + P_H)/2 \qquad (3)$$

Again, this is a linear averaging model where the weights are $1/N$, with N corresponding to the number of modalities. The results of all three experiments in the Jones and O'Neil study (1985) are well described by such a model.

Note that Jones and O'Neil derived their models of multisensory integration of texture based on data obtained using a texture discrimination paradigm. Anderson (e.g., 1974) has offered a different experimental paradigm for formally evaluating the integration of two sources, known as the functional measurement approach. The general model used to represent the integration of two information sources is given by:

$$R_{ij} = w_i s_i + w_j s_j \qquad (4)$$

where R_{ij} represents the mean rating scale response to the combination of two stimuli, which may or may not be the same. In a more restrictive variant model, the weights are constrained to sum to 1. A simple empirical test of the averaging model requires subjects to produce a combined judgment of two sensory inputs with a rating scale. As described earlier under Empirical Findings, the sensory inputs are obtained from pairs of stimuli that vary on two dimensions and are presented in all factorial combinations.

Jones and O'Neil (1985) suggested that Anderson's method might also be extended to the study of multisensory integration of roughness by two modalities. In Experiments 5 and 6, Lederman et al. (1986) formally adopted Anderson's empirical test (described earlier) as a complementary method for studying multisensory texture perception. The results converged with those obtained in Experiments 1–4 and provided support for weighted averaging models of bimodal roughness perception and of bimodal spatial density perception. The weights for touch and vision in both tasks summed to 1, thus supporting a weighted averaging model as opposed to an additive model. Notably, however, the relative magnitude of the two weights reversed with perceptual task. That is, the touch weight was larger than the vision weight in the roughness task, but larger for vision than for touch in the spatial density task. The details concerning how the relative weighting between haptics and vision was calculated in the functional measurement analysis are beyond the scope of this chapter but are detailed in Lederman et al. (1986). For summary purposes, we have indicated in Table 7.1 which modality obtained the stronger weighting.

Weighted averaging models quantitatively represent the bimodal response as a compromise between the two modalities; however, they do not specify how the relative weighting that defines the nature of the compromise is derived (for further consideration, see, e.g., Mulligan & Shaw, 1980; Shaw, 1982).

In the remaining subsections, the models are not simple linear models.

MAXIMUM-LIKELIHOOD INTEGRATION MODEL Very recently, Ernst and Banks (2001) hypothesized that the observer determines the modality weights by operating as a maximum-likelihood integrator to minimize uncertainty. Such a process would produce a multisensory response with a variance that is lower than either unimodal estimator, assuming both unimodal estimators are finite. The maximum-likelihood integration model successfully predicted visual dominance of haptics on a task that required subjects to judge the height of a virtual block that was presented visually, haptically, or bimodally. Variances were obtained in the two unimodal conditions and used to predict the bimodal response based on a maximum-likelihood integration solution. Dominance of the haptic system by vision was predicted on the basis of lower visual than haptic variance. The magnitude of visual dominance also declined progressively, with increasing variability in the visual responses that was effected through deliberate experimental manipulation. This model may predict the relatively equal weighting between vision and touch in the multisensory texture discrepancy experiment

conducted by Lederman and Abbott (1981). Note, however, that this model is constrained by the need to use perceptual tasks that permit the calculation of a relative threshold (i.e., just noticeable difference).

OTHER MODELS In addition to weighted averaging models, Massaro and Friedman (1990) have considered a number of alternative models of information integration. Of those, *fuzzy logical* and *connectionist* models offer two additional theoretical approaches to modeling multisensory texture perception. To end this section, we will consider each of them briefly.

Massaro and Friedman (1990) have described the fuzzy logical model as involving three processing operations during pattern recognition tasks: feature evaluation, feature integration, and decision. "Continuously valued features are evaluated, integrated, and matched against prototype descriptions in memory, and an identification decision is made on the basis of the relative goodness of match of the stimulus information with the relevant prototype descriptions" (p. 231). To permit comparison of the extent to which each feature matches a prototype in the feature evaluation stage, fuzzy truth values are used. These may vary between 0 (completely false) and 1 (completely true), and can therefore represent categorical or continuous information. They can also be used to represent different sources of information, as is relevant to our current discussion of multisensory integration. A value of 0.5 indicates a completely ambiguous situation. The second integration stage provides a multiplicative combination of truth values. The final decision stage involves pattern classification and requires the application of a relative-goodness rule (pp. 230–231). Because not all of the perceptual tasks used to study multisensory texture perception to date have involved pattern recognition, the third process may not always be required (e.g., forced-choice and magnitude-estimation tasks); however, relative goodness would presumably be used in tasks such as similarity sorting (Klatzky et al., 1987; Lederman et al., 1996).

Massaro and Friedman (1990) also propose a "two-layer (i.e., input, output) connectionist" approach to modeling information integration that may be usefully applied to the problem of multisensory integration in general and, more specifically, to multisensory texture perception. Each input unit is connected to each output unit (e.g., unique roughness responses). The activation of an output unit is determined by the product of the input activation and the specific weight associated with that input-output connection. The total activation of a specific output unit (i.e., the integration stage) involves the summation of the separate activations to a given output unit passed through a sigmoid-squashing function (Rumelhart, Hinton, & Williams, 1986). The activations at the output layer must then be mapped into a response, usually according to a relative-goodness rule. The decision follows this rule.

Massaro and Cohen (1987) have observed that although the fuzzy logical and connectionist models are expressed in different conceptual frameworks, when there are only two response alternatives, they make similar predictions (for further discussion, see Movellan & McClelland, 2001).

One final group of models involving signal detection theory may prove relevant to issues pertaining to how stimulus inputs are combined. Details are available in Ashby and Townsend (1986), Ashby and Maddox (1994), and Massarro and Friedman (1990).

Other material properties

Although this chapter has focused primarily on the multisensory perception of surface texture, the material used to construct objects and surfaces varies in other ways as well. In this section, therefore, we consider what is known about the multisensory perception of hardness, softness, and stiffness, the only other material properties that have been formally investigated. We know of no work that has addressed the multisensory processing of thermal properties such as temperature or thermal conductivity. Presumably visual cues would play a considerably lesser role under such circumstances, except under conditions of extreme heat, in which the visual cues are informative.

SOFTNESS AND HARDNESS Binns (1937) performed a study in which a number of highly trained and untrained groups of subjects ranked six different grades of wool fibers multiple times, both visually in terms of "fineness" (presumed to be determined by the apparent average diameter of the fibers) and haptically in terms of "softness" (presumed to be determined by the relative softness or evenness of groups of fibers explored by hand). He found that people were remarkably proficient at this task using either modality. Very few mistakes were made; moreover, the visual and haptic judgments correlated very highly both with each other and with the professional standard ranking scale. (Unfortunately, Binns provided no numerical values for the correlations in this paper.)

STIFFNESS In a series of studies, Srinivasan and his colleagues (DiFranco, Beauregard, & Srinivasan, 1997; Srinivasan, Beauregard, & Brock, 1996; Wu, Basdogan, &

Srinivasan, 1999) have investigated the role of cross-modal sources of sensory information pertaining to the perceived stiffness of deformable objects in virtual environments. Srinivasan et al. (1996) pitted vision against kinesthesis in a two-alternative forced-choice task in which subjects were required to choose which of two virtual springs was "stiffer." Subjects felt the stiffness of each spring by pushing a contact knob on a device that provided the subject with force profiles of virtual springs (displayed via a force-reflecting haptic device) while they watched on a computer screen the images that graphically represented the corresponding spring compressions. The discrepancy between the actual deformation of the spring (kinesthetic cue) and the deformation displayed on the computer monitor (visual cues) was varied across trials. Values ranged from zero (i.e., the actual and visual deformation signals were in complete registration) to complete reversal (i.e., the physically softer spring looked like the harder spring, and vice versa). The results indicated that the visual system strongly dominated the kinesthetically sensed position of the hand. The authors concluded that subjects ignored the latter information about spring deformation and based their judgments on the relationship between the visual position information and the indentation force sensed tactually. Although some may argue that perceiving spring tension should not be regarded as a property of texture, the latter term is not so well defined in the literature that we feel justified in omitting this set of provocative studies.

In the next study in this series, DiFranco et al. (1997) considered the influence of auditory cues on the haptic perception of the stiffness of virtual springs. In the first experiment, subjects tapped on virtual surfaces while simultaneously hearing various prerecorded impact sounds that represented compliant and rigid surfaces (e.g., polyfoam, metal). Subjects were asked to rank the virtual surfaces in terms of perceived stiffness. They were unaware that the physical stiffness was uncorrelated with the sounds. The results indicated that in general, when the surface was paired with the sounds associated with tapping more rigid surfaces, it was ranked as being stiffer than when it was paired with sounds associated with tapping more compliant surfaces. In a second experiment, subjects were able to rank-order fairly well the perceived stiffness of five different surfaces in the absence of auditory cues. In a third experiment, a selection of five sounds from Experiment 1 were paired with each of the five haptic stiffness values used in Experiment 2. The results obtained by DiFranco et al. are in keeping with the demonstrated influence of auditory cues on the remote perception of actual surface roughness with a rigid probe (Lederman et al., 2002). The auditory cues influenced subjects' judgments of stiffness, particularly for those experimentally naive subjects who did not participate in Experiment 2 (haptics only). Overall, the influence of auditory cues was somewhat less strong than that of vision. The authors suggest that the reason may be that the visual graphics cues on the monitor provided excellent spatial information about the changing position of the stylus, whereas the sound cues did not.

Continuing their investigation of the multisensory perception of stiffness in a virtual environment, Wu et al. (1999) showed that when only haptic feedback was provided, subjects judged compliant objects that were further away as being softer than those that were presented closer to them. However, the addition of visual-perspective feedback served both to reduce this form of haptic distortion and to improve resolution, thus demonstrating two advantages to representing virtual stiffness bimodally (see Table 7.2).

Practical implications of scientific research on multisensory texture perception

The scientific results from the study of intersensory texture perception are critically important to those who wish to design multisensory systems for a variety of applications, including, for example, teleoperation tasks and virtual environments that can be seen as well as heard and felt.

Srinivasan and his colleagues have highlighted the value of creating cross-modal displays to overcome the current limitations in the haptic display hardware used to deliver force and cutaneous feedback when operating in teleoperator and virtual environments. Potentially exciting medical applications include using multisensory interfaces to display texture and other material properties (hardness/softness, stiffness, thermal properties) during remote dermatological diagnosis, with the properties conveyed to the visual and haptic systems complementing one another. Another powerful application involving the display of surface texture and other material properties includes the use of virtual training systems to teach novice surgeons complex surgical procedures as tissue compliance and texture are important diagnostic predictors. Novice dermatologists could also benefit from learning dermatological diagnosis procedures by working with virtual diseased skin models. And on the business side, e-commerce offers yet another promising application in which the user could explore the properties of fabrics and other products via multisensory interfaces.

REFERENCES

Anderson, N. H. (1974). Algebraic models in perception. In E. Carterette and M. Friedman (Eds.), *Handbook of perception II* (pp. 215–298). New York: Academic Press.

Ashby, F. G., & Maddox, W. T. (1994). A response time theory of separability and integrality in speeded classification. *Journal of Mathematical Psychology, 38,* 423–466.

Ashby, F. G., & Townsend, J. T. (1986). Varieties of perceptual independence. *Psychological Review, 93,* 154–179.

Binns, H. (1937). Visual and tactual "judgment" as illustrated in a practical experiment. *British Journal of Psychology, 27,* 404–410.

Calvert, G. A., Campbell, R., & Brammer, M. J. (2000). Evidence from functional magnetic resonance imaging of crossmodal binding in the human heromodal cortex. *Current Biology, 10,* 649–657.

Dalton, P., Doolittle, N., Nagata, H., & Breslin, P. A. S. (2000). The merging of the senses: Integration of subthreshold taste and smell. *Nature, 3*(5), 431–432.

DiFranco, D. E., Beauregard, G. L., & Srinivasan, M. (1997). The effect of auditory cues on the haptic perception of stiffness in virtual environments. *Proceedings of the ASME Dynamics Systems and Control Division, DSC 61,* 17–22.

Ernst, M. O., & Banks, M. S. (2001). Humans integrate visual and haptic information in a statistically optimal fashion. *Nature, 415,* 429–433.

Fishkin, S. M., Pishkin, V., & Stahl, M. L. (1975). Factors involved in visual capture. *Perceptual and Motor Skills, 40*(2), 427–434.

Friedes, D. (1974). Human information processing and sensory modality: Cross-modal functions, intersensory complexity, memory and deficit. *Psychological Bulletin, 81,* 284–310.

Gaver, W. W. (1993). What in the world do we hear? An ecological approach to auditory source perception. *Ecological Psychology 1*(5), 1–29.

Guest, S., Catmur, C., Lloyd, D., & Spence, C. (2002). Audiotactile interactions in roughness perception. *Experimental Brain Research, 146,* 161–171.

Guest, S., & Spence, C. (2003). Tactile dominance in speeded discrimination of pilled fabric samples. *Experimental Brain Research, 150,* 201–207.

Hay, J. C., Pick, H. L., & Ikeda, K. (1965). Visual capture produced by prism spectacles. *Psychonomic Science, 2*(8), 215–216.

Heller, M. A. (1982). Visual and tactual texture perception: Intersensory cooperation. *Perception & Psychophysics, 31,* 339–344.

Heller, M. A. (1989). Texture perception in sighted and blind observers. *Perception & Psychophysics, 45,* 49–54.

Hollins, M., Faldowski, R., Rao, S., & Young, F. (1993). Perceptual dimensions of tactile surface texture: A multidimensional scaling analysis. *Perception & Psychophysics, 54,* 697–705.

Hollins, M., & Risner, S. R. (2000). Evidence for the duplex theory of tactile texture perception. *Perception & Psychophysics, 62,* 695–716.

Jones, B., & O'Neil, S. (1985). Combining vision and touch in texture perception. *Perception & Psychophysics, 37*(1), 66–72.

Jousmaki, V., & Hari, R. (1998). Parchment-skin illusion: Sound-biased touch. *Current Biology, 8*(6), R190.

Katz, D. (1989). *The world of touch.* Hillsdale, NJ: Erlbaum.

Klatzky, R. L., & Lederman, S. J. (2003). Touch. In I. B. Weiner (Editor-in-Chief), *Handbook of psychology: Vol. 4. Experimental psychology* (A. F. Healy & R. W. Proctor, Volume Eds., pp. 147–176). New York: Wiley.

Klatzky, R. L., Lederman, S. J., & Matula, D. E. (1993). Haptic exploration in the presence of vision. *Journal of Experimental Psychology: Human Perception and Motivation, 19*(4), 726–743.

Klatzky, R. L., Lederman, S. J., & Reed, C. (1987). There's more to touch than meets the eye: Relative salience of object dimensions for touch with and without vision. *Journal of Experimental Psychology: General, 116*(4), 356–369.

Klein, R. (1966). A developmental study of perception under conditions of conflicting sensory cues. *Dissertation Abstracts International, 27,* 2162B–2163B.

Lederman, S. J. (1974). Tactile roughness of grooved surfaces: The touching process and effects of macro- and micro-surface structure, *Perception & Psychophysics, 16*(2), 385–395.

Lederman, S. J. (1979). Auditory texture perception. *Perception, 8,* 93–103.

Lederman, S. J., & Abbott, S. G. (1981). Texture perception: Studies of intersensory organization using a discrepancy paradigm, and visual versus tactual psychophysics. *Journal of Experimental Psychology: Human, 7*(4), 902–915.

Lederman, S. J., & Klatzky, R. L. (1987). Hand movements: A window into haptic object recognition. *Cognitive Psychology, 19*(3), 342–368.

Lederman, S. J., Klatzky, R. L., Hamilton, C., & Morgan, T. (2002). Integrating multimodal information about surface texture via a probe: Relative contributions of haptic and touch-produced sound sources. *Proceedings of the 10th Annual Symposium on Haptic Interfaces for Teleoperators and Virtual Environment Systems* (IEEE VR '02, pp. 97–104).

Lederman, S. J., Klatzky, R. L., Martin, A., & Tong, C. (2003). Relative performance using haptic and/or touch-produced auditory cues in a remote absolute texture identification task. *Proceedings of the 11th Annual Haptics Symposium for Virtual Environment and Teleoperator Systems* (IEEE VR '03, pp. 151–158).

Lederman, S. J., Summers, C., & Klatzky, R. (1996). Cognitive salience of haptic object properties: Role of modality-encoding bias. *Perception, 25*(8), 983–998.

Lederman, S. J., Thorne, G., & Jones, B. (1986). Perception of texture by vision and touch: Multidimensionality and intersensory integration. *Journal of Experimental Psychology: Human, 12*(2), 169–180.

Massaro, D. W., & Cohen, M. M. (1987). Process and connectionist models of pattern recognition. *Proceedings of the Ninth Annual Conference of the Cognitive Science Society* (pp. 258–264). Hillsdale, NJ: Erlbaum.

Massaro, D. W., & Friedman, D. (1990). Models of integration given multiple sources of information. *Psychological Review, 97*(2), 225–252.

Meese, T. S., & Williams, C. B. (2000). Probability summation for multiple patches of luminance modulation. *Vision Research, 40*(16), 2101–2113.

Meredith, M. A., & Stein, B. E. (1986). Spatial factors determine the activity of multisensory neurons in cat superior colliculus. *Brain Research, 365,* 350–354.

Miller, E. A. (1972). Interaction of vision and touch in conflict and nonconflict form perception tasks. *Journal of Experimental Psychology, 96,* 114–123.

Morgan, T. (2001). *Effect of touch-produced auditory cues on modality integration and roughness perception via a rigid probe.* Unpublished bachelor's thesis, Queen's University, Kingston, Ontario, Canada.

Movellan, J. R., & McClelland, J. L. (2001). The Morton-Massaro law of Information integration: Implications for models of perception. *Psychological Review, 108,* 113–148.

Mulligan, R. M., & Shaw, M. L. (1980). Multimodal signal detection: Independent decisions vs. integration. *Perception & Psychophysics, 28*(5), 471–478.

Myers, A. K., Cotton, B., & Hilp, H. A. (1981). Matching the rate of concurrent tone bursts and light flashes as a function of flash surround luminance. *Perception & Psychophysics, 30,* 33–38.

Nazzaro, J. R., & Nazzaro, J. N. (1970). Auditory versus visual learning of temporal patterns. *Journal of Experimental Psychology, 84,* 477–478.

Over, R. (1966). Context and movement as factors influencing haptic illusions. *Aust. Journal of Psychology, 18,* 262–265.

Pick, H. L., Jr., Warren, D. H., & Hay, J. C. (1969). Sensory conflict in judgments of spatial direction. *Perception & Psychophysics, 6,* 203–205.

Rock, I., & Victor, J. (1964). Vision and touch: An experimentally created conflict between the two senses. *Science, 143,* 594–596.

Rumelhart, D., Hinton, G., & Williams, R. J. (1986). Learning internal representations by error propagation. In D. E. Rumelhart & J. L. McClelland (Eds.), *Parallel distributed processing: Vol. 1. Foundations.* Cambridge, MA: MIT Press.

Shaw, M. L. (1982). Attending to multiple sources of information: I. The integration of information in decision making. *Cognitive Psychology, 14,* 353–409.

Singer, G., & Day, R. H. (1966). The effects of spatial judgments on the perceptual aftereffect resulting from transformed vision. *Australian Journal of Psychology, 18,* 63–70.

Srinivasan, M. A., Beauregard, G. L., & Brock, D. L. (1996). The impact of visual information on the haptic perception of stiffness in virtual environments. *Proceedings of the ASME Dynamics Systems and Control Division, DSC 58,* 555–559.

von Schiller, P. (1932). Die Rauhigkeit als intermodale Erscheinung. *Zeitschrift für Psychologic, 127,* 265–289.

Walk, R. D., & Pick, H. L., Jr. (1981). *Intersensory perception and sensory integration.* New York: Plenum Press.

Wallace, M. T., Wilkinson, L. K., & Stein, B. E. (1996). Representation and integration of multiple sensory inputs in primate superior colliculus. *Journal of Neurophysiology, 76,* 1246–1266.

Welch, R. B., DuttonHurt, L. B., & Warren, D. H. (1986). Contributions of audition and vision to temporal rate perception. *Perception & Psychophysics, 39,* 294–300.

Welch, R. B., & Warren, D. H. (1980). Immediate perceptual response to intersensory discrepancy. *Psychological Bulletin, 88,* 638–667.

Wu, W.-C., Basdogan, C., & Srinivasan, M. (1999). Visual, haptic and bimodal perception of size and stiffness in virtual environments. *Proceedings of the ASME Dynamics Systems and Control Division, DSC 67,* 19–26.

8 Cross-Modal Object Recognition

FIONA N. NEWELL

Introduction

Object recognition has traditionally been couched in terms of visual processing. However, in the real world we explore our environment using a variety of modalities, and internal representations of the sensory world are formed by integrating information from different sources. The information arriving through different sensory pathways may be complementary. For object identification, for example, auditory information, such as the moo of a cow, may help to identify the visual entity, the shape of the cow. Furthermore, in order to guide actions and permit interaction with objects, information acquired from the different senses must converge to form a coherent percept.

This chapter reviews the current literature on cross-modal object recognition. Specifically, I consider the nature of the representation underlying each sensory system that facilitates convergence across the senses, and how perception is modified by the interaction of the senses. I will concentrate mainly on the visual and tactile recognition of objects because of my own research interests, although many of the principles of cross-modal—visual and haptic—recognition that I discuss could easily relate to other sensory modalities. The chapter lays out the cortical, behavioral, and experimental correlates of cross-modal recognition. The first section offers some background literature on the neural correlates of cross-modal recognition under conditions of sensory deprivation and multisensory activation. The second section includes a review of the behavioral characteristics of sensory-specific (e.g., visual or tactile) and cross-modal perception. Finally, in the third section I discuss some of our own recent experimental studies on cross-modal recognition of single and multiple objects.

In order to recognize objects, the human visual system is faced with the problem of maintaining object constancy. Specifically, the problem is the following: despite changes in the retinal projection of an object whenever the observer or the object moves, the object representation must remain constant for recognition to occur. In the past, several mechanisms were proposed to allow for object constancy within the visual system. Because our exploration of the environment generally involves more than one modality, however, object constancy could as well be achieved through a multisensory representation of objects. In this way, a change or reduction in information acquired through one sensory modality can be compensated for by information acquired through another modality. Thus, if a cat creeps under a chair and out of sight, it can still be recognized as a cat because of the sound it makes or the way it feels when it rubs against the sitter's feet.

We know very little about how information from different modalities combines to form a single multisensory representation of an object. It might be argued that in order for information to be shared across modalities, the information must be encoded in a similar manner for all modalities—which assumes a functional equivalence among the modalities. That is, although the range and focus of information might be different across the different modalities, the general principles with which information is treated would be the same. For example, vision and haptics can both be seen as image-processing systems, and therefore amenable to similar functional descriptors. However, vision is able to recruit a larger spatial bandwidth in images than the haptics system. Yet as Loomis and others have shown, when the spatial bandwidth of vision is reduced to that of haptics, then letter identification performance is equivalent across both senses (see Loomis, 1990, for a discussion and model). Visual and haptic recognition performance are also more similar when the visual field of view is reduced by placing an aperture over an image of a picture, thus simulating haptic encoding (Loomis, Klatzky, & Lederman, 1991). If both systems are amenable to the same functional processing of image information, then we can extend these properties beyond image resolution and viewing window size. Thus, functional similarities between vision and haptics should be observable using behavioral performance measures. Furthermore, multisensory information about an object must be combined at the cortical level, and should be amenable to measuring using brain imaging techniques such as functional magnetic resonance imaging (fMRI), positron emission tomography (PET), and electrophysiological techniques. These issues are discussed in the following sections.

Neuronal correlates of unimodal and cross-modal recognition

Traditionally, cortical areas have been considered to be functionally separate and generally sensory specific (Felleman & Van Essen, 1991; Penfield & Rasmussen, 1950). However, this view has been challenged in recent years. For example, it has become apparent that the brain does not have a fixed structure but can exhibit what is known as plasticity; that is, neighboring cortical areas can remap in situations of sensory deprivation or as a result of sensory experience. Dramatic examples of the effect of cortical remapping have been described by Ramachandran and others (see Ramachandran, Rogers-Ramachandran, & Stewart, 1992). For example, in one patient with a limb amputation, the somatosensory areas originally associated with areas on the limb were remapped onto face areas. When the patient's face was stimulated, the phenomenological experience was sensation in the phantom limb. This phenomenon challenged the traditional notion that sensory modalities were structurally and functionally separate. Instead, it is now known that cortical areas can be plastic and can, to some extent, reorganize themselves accordingly (see Shimojo & Shams, 2001, for a review).

EVIDENCE OF ACTIVATION IN PRIMARY SENSORY AREAS FOR CROSS-MODAL RECOGNITION Long-held notions of the role of primary sensory areas in perception have come under increasing pressure recently with the mounting evidence for cross-modal plasticity. When information from one sensory modality is deprived, cortical areas that are normally associated with the sensory-specific processing can be recruited by other sensory-specific areas. For example, Sadato et al. (1996) reported a PET study that revealed activation in primary visual areas (i.e., V1) in congenitally and adventitiously blind participants while they were reading Braille letters. No such activation was found in sighted control participants. Sadato et al. argued that in persons who are blind, somatosensory information can be relayed to V1 via the visual association areas during Braille reading. Furthermore, in another study using magnetoencephalography (MEG), evidence for activation of the visual cortex in response to auditory information (i.e., discriminating pitch changes) was found in early blind individuals (Kujala et al., 1995). Conversely, using fMRI, Finney, Fine, and Dobkins (2001) recently reported that visual stimulation promoted activation of auditory primary cortex (as well as higher auditory areas) in early deaf persons but not in hearing individuals. What is not yet fully understood is the extent to which primary visual areas are recruited by other sensory modalities in humans when vision is absent. Rauschecker (1995) reported that visual deprivation in a cat resulted in complete recruitment of the anterior ectosylvian visual area by both the auditory and the somatosensory areas. Very recently, some evidence for a similar reorganization of multisensory brain structures has been reported in humans as well (see Röder & Rösler, chap. 46, this volume).

There is some evidence for cross-modal processing in the primary visual areas of normal individuals (see Schroeder & Foxe, chap. 18, this volume, for a more in-depth review of this literature). For example, Sathian, Zangaladze, Hoffman, and Grafton (1997) have shown using PET that the primary visual area is active during tasks involving the tactile discrimination of oriented gratings, although they argue that this effect may be indirect and probably mediated by visual imagery. More recently, however, this research group has argued that visual primary areas play a much more crucial role in tactile discrimination tasks than was previously considered (Zangaladze, Epstein, Grafton, & Sathian, 1999). Using transcranial magnetic stimulation (TMS), they blocked processing in the occipital cortex of normal individuals and found impaired tactile discrimination of grating orientation. Using more complex stimuli, Deibert, Kraut, Kremen, and Hart (1999) investigated the neural correlates of tactile object recognition using fMRI. They found that visual areas (notably calcarine and extrastriatal areas) were also activated during tactile object recognition (along with somatosensory, motor, and other peripheral areas involved in language perception). Deibert et al. argued that visual activation might suggest the role of spatial processing in tactile object recognition. Their study, however, does not indicate whether visual processing is necessary for tactile object recognition in sighted individuals. It could be that visual activation has a functional role in higher-level tactile object recognition in sighted individuals such that blocking this activity significantly reduces (or wipes out) higher-level tactile object recognition but not, for example, texture recognition. A study involving focal TMS of primary visual areas would go some way toward addressing this issue.

At this point, we might ask what role primary visual areas have in tactile object recognition. Activation in the visual areas in all the studies mentioned above may reflect the generic role of visual imagery in tasks such as orientation discrimination and object recognition. Kosslyn and his colleagues recently reported that tasks involving mental imagery increased activation in primary visual areas, and performance was reduced when activation in these visual areas was blocked (Kosslyn et al., 1999). It may be, therefore, that visual imagery mediates, and perhaps is necessary for, cross-modal tasks such as tactile object discrimination.

Other suggestions about why visual areas are active during tactile tasks include the possibility that it is a result of backprojections from other sensory areas or even polysensory areas (see Calvert, Campbell, & Brammer, 2000). Alternatively, activation of visual areas could be evidence for task-related or stimulus-specific correlations of activation between several sensory areas. For example, if both vision and tactile perception are often involved in orientation detection or in discriminating certain stimuli, then subsequent activation in sensory-irrelevant areas may be due to experience or learned associations. In fact, Laurenti et al. (2002) have shown that sensory-specific stimuli (e.g., a visual checkerboard) will activate the relevant cortical areas (e.g., visual areas) but cause a deactivation in irrelevant cortical areas (e.g., auditory cortex). When both visual and auditory stimuli are presented simultaneously, then increased activation occurs in both respective cortical areas. It would be interesting to test the role of learning in the cross-modal condition: the sensory-specific deactivation effect may disappear and higher activation levels may be observed as a result of the learned association between vision and audition.

Visual activation may also be important for nonvisual processing such as subjective sensations, awareness, or *qualia*. Some researchers argue for a crucial role of primary visual areas in subjective experience (Crick & Koch, 1995; Stoerig & Cowey, 1995), whereas others argue that later visual areas, such as anterior inferotemporal cortex, play more of a role in awareness in object recognition (Bar & Biederman, 1999; Milner, 1997; see Rees, Kreiman, & Koch, 2002, for a review of the neural correlates of consciousness). None of these researchers, however, speculate on whether the visual areas play a role in awareness of object information in other modalities.

Studies of this sort lead to the question of whether information from one sensory domain can be processed by another domain in a functionally relevant way. The findings themselves suggest that information can easily be shared across modalities that have common functional principles. But the question still remains as to whether, for example, visual activation has an effect on our perception of tactile or auditory stimuli. Some recent research has suggested that this may be the case. Kubovy and van Valkenburg (2001), for example, argue that one of the key functions of vision and audition is the formation of edges. If an edge can be temporal as well as spatial (e.g., discontinuities in time or space), then it is likely that both auditory and visual edges can be processed by visual cortical areas and perceived as

such, irrespective of modality. If information from a stimulus is shared across modalities in order to create a percept, then interference effects should occur in perception when different information is presented to each modality. This is indeed what happens: auditory information, for example, can affect our visual percept for low-level stimuli (Shams, Kamitani, & Shimojo, 2002). Shams et al. reported that when a (constant) number of visual flashes is accompanied by a variable number of auditory beeps, the number of perceived visual flashes is related to the number of beeps heard and not to the actual number of flashes.

Cohen et al. (1997) addressed the issue of the functional relevance of visual activation for nonvisual tasks in a recent study. They applied focal TMS to the cortical visual areas of blind individuals and sighted individuals while they conducted a Braille or Roman letter identification task, respectively. TMS selectively impaired recognition in the blind individuals but not in sighted individuals. The authors argued that when visual areas are deprived of visual information, they can be recruited to play a role in tactile perception. Furthermore, they add that these extra areas may account for the superior perceptual performance of tactile and auditory stimuli in blind persons (Wanet-Defalque et al., 1988).

Similarly, Hamilton, Keenan, Catala, and Pascual-Leone (2000) reported a case of a congenitally blind individual who, as an adult, suffered an ischemic stroke, causing bilateral damage to the visual cortex but not to somatosensory areas. The effect of the stroke was that the individual could no longer read Braille, even though this individual was a proficient Braille reader prior to the stroke. Thus, primary visual areas play a crucial role not just in visual processing but also in nonvisual recognition tasks.

Such cortical remapping may depend on a critical time period, or perhaps on the degree of sensory stimulation of the spared senses from the environment. A review of the developmental aspects of cross-modal plasticity is beyond the scope of this chapter, but recent literature related to these particular issues is discussed in Bavelier and Neville (2002) and Sadato, Okada, Honda, and Yonekura (2002). For the purposes of the present argument, it is sufficient to note that there is evidence to support the idea that, at least at the cortical level, different primary sensory areas can be involved in the recognition of an object, which suggests that an object's representation in memory can be multisensory.

EVIDENCE OF ACTIVATION IN HIGHER CORTICAL AREAS FOR CROSS-MODAL RECOGNITION It is evident that primary visual areas are important for the processing of nonvisual stimuli. We might now ask about the role of higher visual areas, such as those involved in the recognition of more complex stimuli than line orientation or gratings, in cross-modal recognition. Are higher visual areas involved in haptic object recognition, for example?

In primates, the perception of the world is subserved by two functionally and anatomically distinct pathways emanating from the primary visual cortex. These pathways are constituted by projections to the temporal lobe, also known as the ventral or "what" pathway, and projections to the parietal lobe, also known as the dorsal or "where" pathway (Ungerleider & Mishkin, 1982; see also Sereno & Maunsell, 1998, for a recent qualification of the role of these pathways). For visual object recognition, neurons in the inferotemporal cortex of macaques respond to complex stimuli such as objects (Tanaka, Saito, Fukada, & Moriya, 1991) and faces (Perrett, Hietanen, Oram, & Benson, 1992; Yamane, Kaji, & Kawano, 1988). It could be suggested that activation of the early visual areas mentioned previously underlies the involvement of the dorsal pathway for the function of vision-for-action (Colby & Duhamel, 1996), but not the visual recognition areas per se.

In humans, an area known as the lateral occipital complex (LOC) within the occipitotemporal part of the cortex has been found to respond to visual objects defined either by motion, texture, and luminance contrast using fMRI techniques (Grill-Spector, Kushnir, Edelman, Itzchak, & Malach, 1998). The evidence suggests that the LOC plays an active role in visual object processing. Other imaging studies, particularly fMRI, have also supported the idea that LOC is involved in object recognition relative to textures or scrambled images (Malach et al., 1995). Given that the LOC area is involved in visual object recognition, we might ask whether it is also involved in multisensory object recognition.

Amedi, Malach, Hender, Peled, and Zohary (2001) conducted a cross-modal object recognition study while measuring cortical activity using fMRI. Participants were presented with four different stimulus conditions, two visual (seeing objects or textures) and two haptic (feeling objects or textures). The object set included objects such as a toy horse, clothes peg, syringe, and fork (18 in total) and the texture set included graded sandpaper and fur (again, 18 in total). Activation for object recognition was therefore compared against activation for textures and rest periods. Apart from the typical sensory-specific activation, the authors found significantly higher activation for object recognition relative to textures in the occipitotemporal areas, and this effect was independent of sensory modality. With respect to the LOC area in particular, activation in response to the haptic objects overlapped that of activation in response to the visual objects. Notably, activation was significantly reduced in this area during control tasks involving imagery, motor control recall, or object naming, suggesting that the activation was specific to recognition. Their data suggest that the LOC area is involved in cross-modal recognition, either by integrating information from the two senses or by representing haptic information about an object in a visual code for recognition.

Amedi et al. did not test for cross-modal activation directly, so the functional role of LOC in cross-modal object recognition is unclear. In a direct test of the neural correlates of cross-modal transfer, Hadjikhani and Roland (1998) measured brain activation using PET while participants performed a within-modality or cross-modality shape matching test. The stimuli consisted of simple elliptical and spherical shapes. In the conditions involving cross-modal transfer, the authors found activation in the relevant sensory areas but also in the claustrum. They suggested that the claustrum may play an important role in cross-modal matching because multisensory cortical projections stem from, and are projected to, the claustrum. Given the differences between the studies, it is unclear to what extent activation in the LOC found in the study by Amedi et al. was due to the familiarity or the complexity of the objects, or whether the neural correlates of cross-modal activation are task dependent.

A recent study has gone some way to addressing these questions. James et al. (2002) reported the effects of haptic priming on visual object recognition by measuring fMRI activation. In their task, participants were first required to learn a set of novel objects, either haptically or visually. The investigators then tested visual recognition for these objects (and a set of neutral, unprimed objects) while participants were being scanned. They reported an increase in activation in visual areas for both haptic and visually primed objects relative to neutral objects. These specific areas were the middle occipital area and the LOC area. James et al. argue that the ventral pathway may very well be a generic object representational subsystem, such that objects that are encoded haptically are then represented in terms of a visual or multisensory code.

If higher visual areas are involved in multisensory object recognition, then we would predict that selective damage of the LOC region (occipitotemporal cortex), or a focal TMS applied to LOC areas, would necessarily result in impaired visual and also haptic object recognition. Patients with visual agnosia (the inability to recognize familiar objects) are not generally impaired on tasks involving the recognition of the function of the object, suggesting that some haptic properties (e.g., to do with action) remain intact. However, haptic, or tactile, *object* agnosia is not often reported in the literature. In one exception, Saetti, De Renzi, and Comper (1999) described an individual with tactile agnosia whose performance was impaired on haptic recognition but was intact for tactile matching and tactile imagery. This patient had sustained damage to the entire right occipital lobe, including the lateral convexity, and damage to the inferolateral part of the left occipital lobe that extended to the posterior temporal cortex. He was also severely impaired on tactile discrimination of orientation. The authors tried to test orientation discrimination in the visual domain, but, unfortunately, the patient reported not being able to see any visual stimulus presented to him. It is interesting to note that the areas assumed to be involved in tactile perception—that is, the parietal lobe and insula—were intact in the left hemisphere of the patient, although tactile agnosia was observed for the right hand also. It might be that this patient had impaired haptic recognition because the visual areas involved in object recognition (i.e., the lateral occipital areas) were damaged. Furthermore, based on the findings from Zangaladze et al. (1999), it could be suggested that his impaired tactile orientation discrimination was due to damage in the visual areas which may, in turn, subserve the cortical route to object recognition (Deibert et al., 1999).

Imaging studies not only can reveal the spatial location of cortical activation, they can also indicate the timing of information consolidation. A reported electroencephalographic (EEG) study showed that theta power, an event-related spectral change that often reflects underlying cognitive processing, increased toward the end of haptic exploration of objects; the EEG study thus revealed the time course of integration (Grunwald et al., 2001). Furthermore, theta power correlated with object complexity. Grunwald et al. argued that the increase in theta power toward the end of object exploration reflected an increase in working memory load required for spatially integrating information into a coherent representational whole. Interestingly, an increase in the power spectrum was also found in visual areas (O2 but not O1) and in the more visual object recognition areas (T3 and T4) as well as somatosensory-related areas during the haptic task. Grunwald et al. do not discuss this particular finding in depth, although it would have been interesting to explore whether activation in these areas was related to imagery by using an appropriate control condition.

Behavioral studies can reveal phenomenological experiences that observations of neural activation alone

might not reveal. For example, neuronal activation would not reveal the nature of the subjective experience in an individual, or whether the person was experiencing an illusory percept or a veridical percept. The next section includes a brief discussion of studies on the behavioral correlates of uni- and cross-modal recognition.

Behavioral correlates of unimodal and cross-modal recognition

VISUAL OBJECT RECOGNITION   An outstanding achievement of human vision is the rapid and seemingly effortless recognition of objects. The problem for the visual system is that recognition has to be achieved despite variation in sensory information about an object. Sources of variation in an object's image on the retina, for example, can include changes in viewpoint, changes in shape with nonrigid movement, or changes in illumination. Figure 8.1 illustrates some of these variations. Yet the visual system must allow for such changes while also maintaining the uniqueness of an object's representation with respect to other, similar objects, such as members of its own category (as in face recognition for example). In other words, vision has to achieve what is known as object constancy. The visual recognition process has been the subject of much recent work by both experimental and theoretical researchers. Reviews of the literature on visual object recognition are

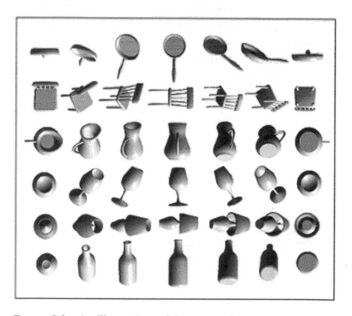

FIGURE 8.1   An illustration of the types of variation in images from one viewpoint on an object to the next. Changes in an object's position in the environment can also change illumination information on the surface of the object. Despite these changes, the visual system must achieve object constancy for efficient recognition to occur.

available in Tarr and Bülthoff (1999), Edelman (1999), and Ullman (1996).

Recent studies on how object constancy is achieved have led some researchers to suggest that objects are represented in memory as image-based collections of multiple views (Tarr & Bülthoff, 1995). Image-based models generally predict, for example, that familiar views are likely to be recognized faster and more accurately than unfamiliar views. Indeed, many studies have provided evidence in support of this prediction (Edelman & Bülthoff, 1992; Humphrey & Khan, 1992; Newell & Findlay, 1997; Tarr & Pinker, 1989). Furthermore, the effects of viewpoint can also depend on inter-item similarity as well as object familiarity (Edelman, 1999; Newell, 1998).

A countervailing argument is that object representations are not necessarily image-based but instead are structural descriptions in which the relations of the parts of an object are specified independently of other shape attributes (Biederman, 1987). Biederman and Gerhardstein (1993) have argued that under certain conditions, changes in viewpoint do not affect recognition performance. They argue that these conditions are generic in real-world object recognition tasks. Their conditions for view-invariant recognition include the following: (1) that the objects be decomposable into parts, or "geons," (2) that the objects have unique structural descriptions, and (3) that the object geons be visible in the image across changes in view. When all conditions are met, then recognition is invariant to viewpoint, according to Biederman and Gerhardstein (1993).

Some recent research has challenged the notion that visual object representations are either image-based or structural and has instead called for a more hybrid model of object recognition that would incorporate both structural and image-based components in an object's representation (Edelman, 1999; Newell, Shepard, Edelman, & Shapiro, 2003). A hybrid model would encapsulate better the fact that human recognition performance is viewpoint sensitive, and the fact that judgments about an object's structure can be readily made.

Most theories of object recognition are couched in terms of visual processing. Indeed, it is normally assumed that any researcher who is interested in human object recognition approaches this research from a visual perspective. Vision is believed to dominate our perception of the world, at least in most circumstances. Yet humans have available a vast array of modalities for interacting with their environment. For example, one other modality through which information about the shape of an object can be obtained is the haptic modality.

HAPTIC OBJECT RECOGNITION The word *haptic* means active touch, and it is the most common way in which we explore our environments using our sense of touch. J. J. Gibson (1962) argued that information acquisition is dependent on our active exploration of our environment. In a now classic experiment, he demonstrated his argument by testing the role of active and passive touch perception in object identification. He used cookie cutters as stimuli. Either participants could haptically explore actively or the objects were placed passively into a participant's hand. Gibson found that actively touching the objects provided better identity performance than passively touching the objects. In a later study based on Gibson's experiment, Heller (1984) found that even when participants were given only 5 seconds for active exploration, performance on the passive learning condition reached equivalency only when participants were allowed relatively long exposure times (more than 30 seconds).

Lederman and Klatzky (1987) found that active touch procedures, or so-called exploratory procedures when participants were actively touching objects, were specific to the demands of the task. In their publication, they illustrate qualitatively different hand movements depending on what information the participant was required to obtain. They argue that each type of exploratory procedure maximized the information specific for that task. For example, participants would typically use an up-down movement of the hand and arm when trying to establish the weight of an object, or would apply a contour-tracing procedure when attempting to identify the object.

Other studies from neuropsychology have further emphasized the role of active touch in perception. Valenza et al. (2001), for example, studied a patient with a right hemisphere infarct who was impaired on tactile object recognition. The patient's haptic exploratory procedures were random and disorganized relative to the stereotyped procedures described by Lederman and Klatzky (1987), resulting in poor recognition performance. However, when the authors guided the patient's hands during exploration, or verbally indicated the appropriate movements, then recognition of the tactile shapes was intact. Similarly, passive shape recognition was also unimpaired. The authors argue that tactile agnosia was affected by the patient's inability to generate efficient exploratory procedures (i.e., tactile apraxia). A counter example is also reported in the literature: Reed, Caselli, and Farah (1996) studied a patient with tactile agnosia who exhibited normal exploratory procedures, which suggests that haptic recognition can be disrupted independently of normal active touch strategies. Exploratory procedures are therefore not sufficient for haptic recognition, although they are perhaps necessary for efficient performance.

CROSS-MODAL OBJECT RECOGNITION   Active exploration of an object in one sense can often complement the perception of an object in another (Klatzky, Lederman, & Matula, 1993). Take, for example, the active manipulation of small (hand-sized) unfamiliar objects. The consequences of such haptic exploration of an object are easily observed by the visual system: as the object is manipulated, different parts of the object can be viewed (see Harman, Humphrey, & Goodale, 1999, for the effects of manipulating a virtual object). Through this process of haptic and visual interaction, a rich, view-independent representation of the object may be created in memory, thus solving the object constancy problem. Moreover, information from other modalities can converge to provide a more complete representation of the object. This might occur when it is impossible for a single modality to perceive all of an object's properties in detail because the information is impoverished or unavailable. For example, for objects that are fixed, the haptic system can provide information about the surfaces of the object that the visual system cannot perceive, such as the back of an object.

Object recognition performance has been extensively studied in the visual system but has received relatively less attention in other modalities. However, the findings from recent studies suggest that both the visual and haptic systems can create a representation of an object that allows common access across these modalities (Reales & Ballesteros, 1999; Easton, Srinivas, & Greene, 1997). For example, Reales and Ballesteros used both implicit (i.e., priming) and explicit experimental paradigms to measure cross-modal recognition of familiar objects. They found evidence for cross-modal priming, suggesting that object representations can be easily shared between the haptic and visual systems (see also Easton, Greene, & Srinivas, 1997).

The efficient interaction between modalities for the purpose of recognizing an object relies on the fact that the same object is being perceived by all senses, and this is generally true in the real world. In cases of ambiguity, or when information sent to the different modalities is discrepant, perception in one sense may dominate perception in other senses. Under many circumstances, visual information overrides information perceived from another modality. This effect is termed "visual capture" (Rock & Victor, 1964). An example of visual capture is when there is a discrepancy between what is perceived by the different senses and the participant's decision is based on visual information only. For example, when participants grasp a square shape that is viewed through

an optical device that distorts its shape to make it appear rectangular, then they see and feel the shape as if it were a rectangle, not a square (Rock & Victor, 1964).

Recent studies, however, have challenged the notion of visual capture and have argued that vision does not necessarily prevail over touch. For example, using mirrors, Heller (1992) put vision and touch information about letters in conflict with each other and found that touch information dominated letter identification most of the time. Other studies have also found that vision does not perceive events independently of touch, as the "capture" idea suggests. Ernst and Banks (2002) proposed that it is the relative reliability of the sensory estimates in the individual modalities that determines the degree to which vision or touch dominates. For example, when judging the roughness of a texture, touch is more reliable and therefore would dominate the combined percept. On the other hand, if the task is to judge the size of an object, such as in Rock and Victor's (1964) study, then vision will win over touch and will be weighted more heavily because it provides the more reliable estimate of size. According to Ernst and Banks, therefore, "visual or haptic capture" occurs naturally, based on the maximal likelihood of the sensory estimates.

Heller, Calcaterra, Green, and Brown (1999) further qualified the conditions of perceptual dominance. In their study on size judgments of visual or haptic perception of blocks, they found that changes in task and attentional allocations affected which sense dominated a perceptual decision, and that size judgment was not always dominated by vision.

That vision is not necessarily the "gold standard" to which all other modalities are adapted was recently demonstrated in a number of studies. For example, Ernst, Banks, and Bülthoff (2000) found that, through feedback, the haptic modality can influence the visual perception of the degree of slant in a stimulus. Atkins, Fiser, and Jacobs (2001) also reported a similar finding on the perception of the depth of a stimulus. They found that cues from both vision and haptics would be combined to discriminate depth when these cues were consistent across modalities, but not when they were inconsistent.

We know very little about how information from different modalities combines to form a single, multisensory representation of an object. Our understanding of how spatial information is shared across modalities (i.e., where an object lies relative to another in a scene) is also quite poor. Some researchers have argued that object representations across vision and haptics are not necessarily combined but are mediated by imagery (Easton, Srinivas, et al., 1997). Imagery may also be involved in haptic object recognition (Klatzky, Lederman, & Matula, 1991), although this may be task dependent. For example, if the haptic recognition task depends on perceiving the substance of the object (e.g., weight or temperature), then no visual translation stage would be necessary (see Lederman, Klatzky, Chataway, & Summers, 1990). However, as Lederman et al. (1990) have argued, more difficult tasks of haptic recognition, such as the recognition of objects depicted as raised line drawings, may indeed require the use of "image mediation."

Nevertheless, as argued earlier, in order for information to be shared across modalities, these different modalities should organize information using common principles, that is, they should be functionally equivalent, and the consequent effects should be observable using experimental procedures. For example, if the visual system is sensitive to changes in the orientation of an object or scene, then we would expect the haptic system to be orientation sensitive also, thus allowing for corresponding surfaces to be combined in memory. In the following section I discuss findings from studies conducted in my laboratory and in collaboration with colleagues at the Max Planck Institute for Biological Cybernetics, Tübingen, on factors affecting cross-modal recognition of objects. In our initial studies we concentrated on the recognition of single objects using vision and haptics. In our more recent studies, we have been interested in the cross-modal recognition of multiple objects, or scenes.

Experimental studies on the cross-modal recognition of objects

CROSS-MODAL RECOGNITION OF SINGLE OBJECTS We recently reported that vision and haptics can often complement each other in forming a representation of a three-dimensional object (Newell, Ernst, Tjan, & Bülthoff, 2001). We were particularly interested to see whether combining the modalities in a recognition test would help solve some of the problems affecting object constancy, particularly the problem of changing viewpoints. In our experiments we measured the effects of viewpoint on visual, haptic, and cross-modal recognition. We used a set of unfamiliar objects made from six identical red Lego bricks, and objects were presented in a fixed position throughout the study. Each object had a different configuration of these bricks; hence, we controlled for differences in size, texture, and color, which may aid recognition performance in one modality only (Fig. 8.2). Participants performed a recognition memory task in all the experiments. First they were required to learn four target objects in a sequential order, either

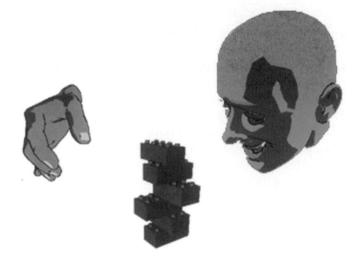

FIGURE 8.2 A typical target object in our haptic and visual object recognition experiments.

visually (for 30 seconds) or haptically (for 1 minute). The objects were placed behind a curtain during the haptic condition, and participants placed their hands underneath the curtain to touch the objects. We gave no explicit instructions on how to learn the objects except that they could not move the objects. There followed a test session in which participants had to recognize and discriminate the four target objects from four similar, nontarget objects. During the test, each target object was presented to the participant in the same orientation as learning (0 degrees), or rotated by 180 degrees, and in the same modality as learning or in the other modality.

Our first basic finding was that within-modality recognition was view dependent. Thus, we replicated the literature on view-dependent effects in visual object recognition while also presenting a new finding on view dependency in haptic object recognition. Although the effects of orientation on tactile perception, such as the mental rotation of abstract forms (e.g., Dellantonio & Spagnolo, 1990), have previously been reported in the literature, to our knowledge the effect of orientation on haptic object recognition was not found prior to our study. More interestingly, we found that the effects of view dependency were reversed when recognition was conducted across modalities. In other words, in the cross-modal condition, recognition was better when there was a change in orientation between learning and test, but only when there was an interchange between the front and the back of the objects (Fig. 8.3). Our findings suggest that both the visual and the haptic system code view-specific representations of objects, but each system has its own preferential "view" of an object: For the visual system, it was the surface of the object facing the observer whereas for the haptic system it was

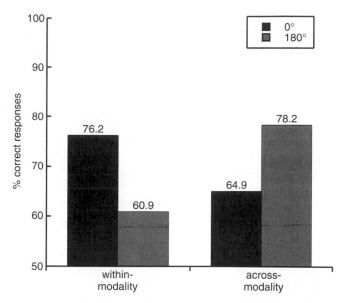

FIGURE 8.3 The results of our single-object recognition experiments across changes in viewpoint involving an interchange of the front and back surfaces. A change in viewpoint caused a decrease in percentage of correct responses within modalities but an increase in percentage of correct responses across modalities. See text.

the surface of the object that the fingers explored more, namely, the back side of the object (with respect to the observer). We surmise that this back surface was preferential for the haptic system mainly because of the position of the hands in relation to the body (Fig. 8.4) and the specific hand-sized objects used in our experiments. Representations of these "best" views can then be easily shared across modalities when they are in correspondence (i.e., when the hands explore a previously viewed surface, and vice versa).

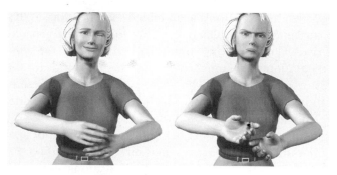

FIGURE 8.4 Haptic recognition of the back of objects may be easier because of the natural position of our hands relative to our bodies, as shown in the individual on the left. If, say, our hands happened to be attached to our bodies as illustrated in the individual on the right, then we might expect different effects on recognition. Anatomical restrictions do not allow us to test this prediction directly. (Illustration courtesy of Marc Ernst and Heinrich Bülthoff.)

Previous studies have also emphasized the contribution of integration of information across the fingers for efficient haptic object recognition (Klatzky, Loomis, Lederman, Wake, & Fujita, 1993). Our study provides further support for this notion and extends it with the finding that the representation of a surface of an object from haptic exploration can be shared with the visual system. For this to happen, though, the same surface should be perceived by both modalities. We might therefore ask what would happen under conditions of free viewing and palpating of an object. We would predict poor cross-modal performance in this case because the "best" surfaces are unlikely to be properly matched and integrated. We recently tested cross-modal recognition of objects under conditions of unconstrained viewing (Ernst, Bülthoff, & Newell, 2003). We used the same stimuli and design as in the Newell et al. (2001) study, but here participants were allowed to freely palpate the objects in the haptic modality. For the visual condition we placed each object into a transparent perspex sphere (the type used for homemade Christmas tree decorations). In this way the participants could freely view each object without actually touching the object. Both within-modal and cross-modal recognition were measured. We found that when viewing or palpation was unconstrained, cross-modal recognition was worse than within-modal recognition (Fig. 8.5). This finding fits with our prediction that efficient cross-modal recognition depends on spatially constraining the surfaces of objects in order to match the best "views" across modalities. In other words, for recognizing objects across changes in viewpoint, spatial integration of the surfaces of the

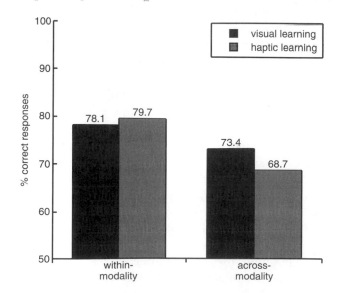

FIGURE 8.5 Effect of unimodal and cross-modal recognition of objects under free "viewing" conditions—that is, the objects were not placed in a fixed position and could be moved for visual or haptic sampling.

objects is the key to efficient cross-modal recognition. We might ask, however, how cross-modal recognition is affected when both modalities are used simultaneously during learning—that is, when the object is actively touched in the presence of vision—relative to the situation in which one modality is used during learning. Here we would predict that bimodal learning would enhance recognition performance because all surfaces are necessarily in correspondence during learning. This is exactly what we found. When objects were learned bimodally, that is, using both haptics and vision simultaneously, recognition performance was almost 10% better than when the objects were learned either visually alone or haptically alone (Ernst et al., 2003).

An interesting study reported by Harman et al. in 1999 suggests a possible parallel to our findings on cross-modal learning. They tested object recognition when participants were allowed either to actively manipulate a virtual object on a screen or to passively view the same sequence of object views. They found that active control improved recognition performance relative to passive viewing. This study shows that visual recognition is enhanced when an object is manipulated, suggesting that vision and haptic perception are complementary in object recognition. Haptic perception per se was not tested in the study by Harman et al. (1999). However, our findings demonstrate that bimodal active learning (i.e., seeing and feeling the object at the same time) can enhance recognition relative to active visual or haptic learning alone.

With respect to our haptic "view" finding, an interesting study has just been published on haptic face recognition. Kilgour and Lederman (2002) tested haptic and cross-modal matching performance of real faces and face masks. They found that visual to haptic face matching was more accurate than haptic to visual face matching, although this result was not found for all face stimuli sets. They argue that the different matching performance across face sets may be due to differences in interface similarity between face sets, but not to a generally poor matching performance by the haptic system. Haptic matching performance was not improved by the addition of vision during learning, leading to the suggestion that a visual code did not easily transfer to haptics for matching purposes. We would like to offer a possible explanation for their cross-modal results. On the basis of our findings, we would argue that during haptic learning, the face stimuli were not presented in an optimal orientation with respect to the observer to allow for efficient cross-modal matching. Kilgour and Lederman do not state explicitly the orientation of the face stimuli with respect to the observer, but we presume the stimuli were facing the observer. We suggest that if the face stimuli were positioned such that they were facing away from the participant, and the participant's hands explored the face from that position (a more natural position for the hands, as argued earlier), then cross-modal performance may have improved. We might even extend this point and suggest that for efficient tactile face recognition in persons who are blind, the person to be recognized should face away from the observer. Clearly, more research is required to test the generalizability of our "haptic view" claim.

CROSS-MODAL RECOGNITION OF MULTIPLE OBJECTS The simultaneous recognition of more than one object, for example a scene of objects, clearly presents a different problem for cross-modal recognition because of the larger spatial scales involved. It is unlikely, for example, that fast scene recognition would involve the type of exploratory hand movements typical for single-object recognition (see Lederman & Klatzky, 1987). Spatial integration for scene recognition involves integrating across objects over a possibly large scale, which could mean larger differences between visual and haptic encoding. There may be a sequential nature to scene exploration within the haptic domain (i.e., the hands moving to one object at a time), which would mean that the spatial structure of the scene would be available only when information about the entire contents of the scene were integrated. Visual scene recognition, on the other hand, does not necessarily involve the same serial processes. In large-scale scenes, however, spatial integration would be required across eye fixations (Henderson & Hollingworth, 1999; Rayner & Pollatsek, 1992). Generally, though, the contents of a scene can be rapidly perceived (see Biederman, Rabinowitz, Glass, & Stacy, 1974). Haptic space, moreover, is limited to peripersonal space, although it does have some flexibility, such as when tools are wielded (see Làdavas, 2002; Làdavas & Farnè, Chap. 50, this volume; Maravita & Driver, Chap. 51, this volume). Furthermore, the representation of haptic space has been found to be distorted—non-Euclidean—compared to the representation of visual space, which is considered to be Euclidean (Kappers & Koenderink, 1999).

If we argue that in order for vision and haptics to communicate, the representation of information in each modality needs to be organized along common principles, then we can ask whether or not spatial memory for haptic scenes is functionally similar to spatial memory for visual scenes. Specifically, our two experimental questions were (1) Is cross-modal scene recognition efficient relative to within-modal recognition? and (2) Is cross-modal recognition affected by changes in the orientation of the scene?

Recent research has shown that visual memory for scenes is sensitive to changes in orientation with respect to the observer (Diwadkar & McNamara, 1997; Simons & Wang, 1998). In the study by Diwadkar and McNamara, participants were first required to study a real scene of six objects for 30 seconds. Their memory for this scene was then tested using images of the target scene from different angles against similar distractor scenes (i.e., novel configurations of the same objects). Diwadkar and McNamara found that scene recognition performance was a function of angular distance to the original view (Experiment 1) or different training views (Experiment 2). Christou and Bülthoff (1999) replicated these findings using virtual displays of room scenes. Simons and Wang (1998) also tested the effects of orientation on the recognition of real scenes of objects placed on a table. They found that 47-degree changes in the orientation of a scene of objects between learning and test significantly reduced recognition performance. Interestingly, scene recognition performance was not just dependent on the retinal projection of the scene, because no effects of orientation were found when the observer could move himself or herself to a new viewing position 47 degrees away from the learning position, again indicating the importance of active perception or extra retinal information in visual recognition (Simons, Wang, & Roddenberry, 2002). However, Wang and Simons (1999) reported in a subsequent study that actively moving the scene did not reduce the effects of orientation to the same extent than if the participant actually moved to a new viewpoint of the scene. These studies, therefore, suggest that visual spatial memory performance is similar to single-object recognition, at least in terms of orientation dependency. But what was not known is how similar haptic spatial memory is to visuospatial memory.

By investigating cross-modal recognition performance we may be able to provide a clearer understanding of the nature of the encoded information within each modality and how this information is shared in order to recognize scenes of objects. In our study we tested observers' ability to recognize the spatial layout of objects in a scene both unimodally (either haptically or visually) and across modalities (Newell, Woods, Mernagh, & Bülthoff, 2003). The stimulus set of objects used included 15 wooden shapes of familiar objects, seven of which were randomly placed on a rotatable platform in any one trial (Fig. 8.6 shows a typical scene). We attempted to provide equal accessibility to object properties across both modalities. We achieved this by allowing participants 10 seconds to view the scene and one minute for haptic exploration during learning. These presentation times were determined in a pilot study. After learning, the position of two of the seven objects was exchanged while the orientation of the individual object was kept constant, and participants had to identify the swapped objects at test. Thus, the same configuration of objects was used between learning and test (i.e., within a trial, the same object positions were occupied between learning and test). We maintained configural information for two reasons: First, at least for visual processing, we did not want participants extracting a global shape of the scene in order to do the task (which may have occurred in the Simons and Wang study). Second, we wanted to be sure that haptic memory was based on touch alone and not on proprioceptive cues such as body movement or body-centered posture due to changes in the global

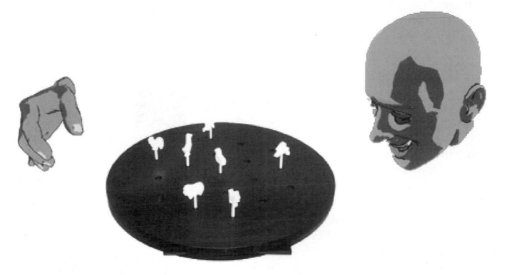

FIGURE 8.6 A typical target scene in our haptic and visual multiple-object recognition experiments.

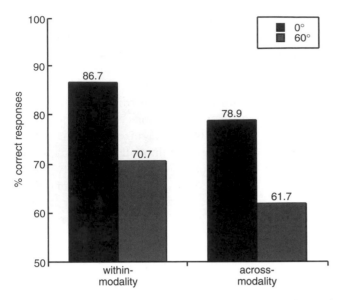

FIGURE 8.7 Effects of orientation during within-modal and cross-modal scene recognition. A cost in recognition performance was also found in the cross-modal condition relative to within-modal recognition.

configuration (Millar, 1999). Testing occurred either within or across modalities and under 0-degrees or 60-degrees rotation of the scene.

We found that recognition performance was impaired by a change in modalities at test. We also found that both within- and cross-modal scene perception was sensitive to the orientation of the scene with respect to the observer (Fig. 8.7). This result indicates that vision and haptics may share a common, orientation-sensitive code for scene perception.

The relative cost in cross-modal recognition suggests a difference in encoding of information between vision and haptics. One possible difference is that visual information can be encoded holistically over large scales, whereas haptic encoding is generally serial. However, we also noticed that some participants recalled the objects' names. We therefore decided to test the role of verbal mediation in cross-modal recognition performance. We repeated our experiment described above, but now required participants to perform a verbal interpolation task (i.e., generate lists of words beginning with a random letter) between learning and test. Again we found that cross-modal recognition was less efficient than within-modal performance. More pertinently, verbal interference produced more errors in all conditions involving haptic perception, relative to the vision-vision condition. Furthermore, the effect of orientation remained for within-modal but not for cross-modal recognition, suggesting a demand on central processes that made the task more difficult (Fig. 8.8).

However, the relatively poor transfer from haptics with verbal interference suggested a modality-encoding bias, with evidence for a role of verbal recoding in haptic perception.

Other studies have also shown an effect of verbal interference in haptic memory tasks. When two sequences of tactile stimuli were presented to the fingers, Mahrer and Miles (2002) reported that matching performance was affected by the presence of a verbal interpolation task during the delay between presentations but not by the presence of a tactile interference task. This result suggests a role for verbal rehearsal in memory for tactile sequences. However, their results also indicate a role for visuospatial processing: when the task required matching the tactile sequence to a visual image of a hand, performance improved. Therefore, tactile memory can exploit both visuospatial and verbal processes for recall purposes. In monkeys, however, matching across modalities is more efficient from vision to haptics than vice versa (DiMattia, Posley, & Fuster, 1990). This may be due to stimulus differences or modality-encoding biases, however, rather than to any differences between verbal and nonverbal capabilities of man and monkey. In any case, our data also indicate a role for both a verbal recoding in haptic learning and a more visuospatial encoding for the purposes of cross-modal recognition. Furthermore, our data suggest that both visual and haptic encoding involve a mapping of spatial relations between objects into, perhaps, a body-centred reference frame (see also Easton & Sholl,

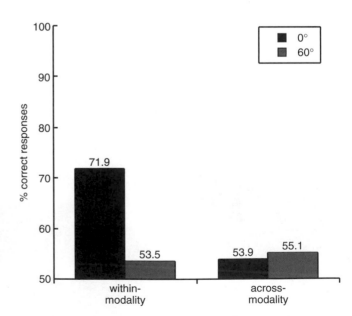

FIGURE 8.8 Effects of a verbal interpolation task between within-modal and cross-modal scene recognition. All conditions except vision-vision condition were affected by the interpolation task.

1995), thus accounting for the effect of orientation within and across modalities.

Taken together, our findings from single-object and multiple-object recognition tasks indicate that orientation dependency is a common characteristic of different sensory systems. For cross-modal recognition, our data suggest that efficient performance is based on equivalent encoding of shapes across modalities. For example, visual and haptic recognition of single objects was view dependent, and efficient cross-modal performance was based on matching across corresponding "views." This finding suggests that it is a common code (i.e., surface-related) coupled with common processing (i.e., view dependence) that allows cross-modal recognition to occur. Thus, when there was a possible discrepancy in representation across modalities, as in scene perception (e.g., Euclidean-based representation for vision versus non-Euclidean representation for haptics), less efficient cross-modal recognition occurred. This reduction in efficiency may be due to a recoding of information in one modality into a format congruent with the other modality. Further investigations of the mechanisms underlying cross-modal recognition are currently in progress.

Conclusions

Our perception of the world is a consequence of our actions on the world. Gibson (1966), for example, argued that we do not simply passively receive information about our world, but instead actively perceive the world through our different senses. Perception is thus a complex process that entails more than the simple detection and measure of sensory stimuli. It is often dependent on the integration of sensory information entering through a number of different channels, and this information in turn is subject to modulation by higher cognitive processes acting at the cortical level. Perception is not, therefore, a fixed concept, as it is significantly modulated by many contextual factors such as multisensory information, past experiences, internal predictions, associations, ongoing motor behavior, spatial relations, and the nature of the task itself.

In this chapter, I have argued for the functional interdependence of haptics and vision at not only the neuronal level but also at the behavioral level in relation to object recognition. When information about events (objects) in the real world is integrated across modalities, more efficient recognition can occur. I propose that in order for such integration to occur, the following conditions must apply: the information should be (1) contextually or task-relevant, (2) spatially congruent, and (3) temporally congruent. It is probably not very

controversial to assert that unattended task-irrelevant information is not integrated into a meaningful representation of an object. This leaves the other two conditions, which I will now attempt to qualify further.

SPATIAL CONSTRAINTS ON CROSS-MODAL INTEGRATION The scale of a spatial layout specific to a task may promote a modality-encoding bias. For example, the range of the visual spatial scale is more extensive than the range of the haptic spatial scale. Nevertheless, even when the space is within the range of haptic processing, the encoding of objects within that space is necessarily serial, whereas encoding may be parallel for vision. In this case, responses may depend on the visual rather than the haptic representation. These encoding differences can be controlled, however. If the visual window is reduced in size or if vision is blurred, then recognition performance is more equivalent across the senses (e.g., Loomis et al., 1991), indicating that encoding opportunities can affect our cross-modal representation of space.

When the spatial characteristics of stimuli are highly similar across the senses, this cross-modal information typically interacts either to enhance the representation or to interfere with the representation. For example, if the target stimulus is preceded by a spatially similar stimulus, then priming effects are generally observed. Reales and Ballestersos (1999) reported a greater effect of cross-modal priming when the same stimulus formats were used between learning and test (i.e., pictures) than when different stimulus formats were used (i.e., objects then pictures). Conversely, if the target stimulus is followed by a spatially similar stimulus from another modality, then the memory for the target can decline. Logie and Marchetti (1991) reported an example of this effect. They have shown that short-term memory of visuospatial information can be disrupted by a subsequent sequence of movements of the arm that are related to the spatial layout in the visual memory task. They argue that it is the spatial nature of the visual task that, during a rehearsal process, is affected by the changes of the spatial position of the arm. Similarly, Kerzel (2001) found that memory for the velocity of a visual stimulus was affected if participants were required to move their arm (unseen) in a velocity slightly deviant from the velocity of the visual stimulus. Thus, if the hand movement was fast, then the remembered velocity of the visual stimulus was slightly faster than its real velocity. The opposite was also true: when the hand movement was slow, the remembered visual velocity was also slow. Kerzel and others argue that the spatial similarities of the stimuli across modalities allow a blending of the information in memory. It might even be said that when spatial similarities are high (i.e., when the information emanates from the same location in space, or when the spatial properties are similar), then the brain has no choice but to integrate this information. However, spatial congruency alone may not be sufficient for integration, because the information probably also must be presented within a limited time window in order for sensory combination to occur.

TEMPORAL CONSTRAINTS ON CROSS-MODAL INTEGRATION
The simultaneous presentation of spatially congruent information promotes integration. This combined percept may be a veridical representation of the world or it may be illusory. For example, Ernst and Banks (2002) found that participants integrate information about the height of an object across vision and haptics in a statistically optimal way. Their model is based on the idea that an observer's use of sensory information is dependent on the estimated reliability of that information from each modality. Simultaneously presented information across modalities, however, can be combined to form an illusory percept. Well-known examples of cross-modal illusions include the McGurk effect (McGurk & McDonald, 1976), the rubber arm illusion (Botvinick & Cohen, 1998), and the "flashing" illusion recently reported by Shams et al. (2002), in which the number of visual flashes perceived is related to the number of beeps heard.

Time delays in sensory presentation may promote interference in the original representation, as in the memory experiments reported by Kerzel (2001), Mahrer and Miles (2002), and Miles and Borthwick (1996). In general, the haptic memory for objects is reported to have the same temporal properties as visual memory. For example, as in vision, there is a fading quality to tactile memory. When participants were asked to recall the location of a tactile stimulus presented on the underside of the forearm of the participant, accuracy decreased with respect to delay between stimulus and recall (see Gilson & Baddeley, 1969; Sullivan & Turvey, 1972). Gilson and Baddeley, however, argued that some aspects of tactile memory are unique; for example, memory decay occurred only after a 15-second retention period (although temporal decay began immediately in the study by Sullivan and Turvey). More recently, Kiphart, Hughes, Simmons, and Cross (1992) conducted a haptic object-matching test and reported that delay intervals of more than 15 seconds caused memory to decay.

We do not know, however, the extent of the time window optimal for integration across the visual and haptic domains. These experiments are not yet reported in the literature, but such findings would be a very important contribution to our understanding of cross-modal combining of information. A recent event-related potential study on the integration of auditory and visual information for object recognition reported the time course of activation of unimodal and cross-modal conditions (Giard & Peronnet, 1999). The authors reported better recognition performance in response to the cross-modal condition than to either of the unimodal conditions. Furthermore, their data suggest that modulation effects due to visual-auditory interaction occur between 40 and 200 ms after stimulus presentation. The question remains, however, whether cross-modal interactions (at least between vision and audition) are possible with delays of more than 200 ms in the presentation times of sensory specific stimuli.

SOME FINAL THOUGHTS   The extent to which spatial and temporal constraints are true for efficient cross-modal recognition is also not fully understood. For example, we might ask to what extent an object that one is feeling and an image that one is seeing have to be spatially congruent to allow for cross-modal integration. Must they be spatially identical before integration can occur? If not, at what point do the senses decide that the objects are not the same? What role does spatial complexity play in sensory integration? Neither do we yet know the precise time course of sensory integration. Clearly, events occurring simultaneously across the senses (provided they are from the same spatial location) are likely to arise from the same source and are therefore correctly integrated. However, a time delay between an event occurring in one modality and an event occurring in another modality could reduce the likelihood of integration. Finally, we might also ask how these factors interact with each other. Although our knowledge of processes underlying multisensory integration at the neuronal level and cross-modal perception at the behavioral level has increased dramatically over the past decade, further research is required to allow us to have a better understanding of the nature of cross-modal recognition. The research field is wide open. We can only look forward to the day when some, if not all, of these outstanding issues will be answered by new research, and indeed by new researchers, in the field.

REFERENCES

Amedi, A., Malach, R., Hendler, T., Peled, S., & Zohary, E. (2001). Visuo-haptic object-related activation in the ventral visual pathway. *Nature Neuroscience, 4,* 324–330.

Atkins, J. E., Fiser, J., & Jacobs, R. A. (2001). Experience-dependent visual cue integration based on consistencies between visual and haptic percepts. *Vision Research, 41,* 449–461.

Baddeley, A. D. (1999). *Essentials of human memory*. Hove, England: Psychology Press.

Bar, M., & Biederman, I. (1999). Localizing the cortical region mediating visual awareness of object identity. *Proceedings of the National Academy of Sciences of the United States of America, 96*, 1790–1793.

Bavelier, D., & Neville, H. J. (2002). Cross-modal plasticity: Where and how? *Nature Reviews in Neuroscience, 3*, 443–452.

Biederman, I. (1987). Recognition by components: A theory of human image understanding. *Psychological Review, 94*, 115–147.

Biederman, I., & Gerhardstein, P. C. (1993). Recognizing depth-rotated objects: Evidence and conditions for three-dimensional viewpoint invariance. *Journal of Experimental Psychology: Human Perception and Performance, 19*, 1162–1182.

Biederman, I., Rabinowitz, J. C., Glass, A. L., & Stacy, E. W. (1974). On the information extracted from a glance at a scene. *Journal of Experimental Psychology, 103*, 597–600.

Botvinick, M., & Cohen, J. (1998). Rubber hands "feel" touch that eyes see. *Nature, 391*, 756.

Calvert, G. A., Campbell, R., & Brammer, M. J. (2000). Evidence from functional magnetic resonance imaging of cross-modal binding in the human heteromodal cortex. *Current Biology, 10*, 649–657.

Christou, C. G., & Bülthoff, H. H. (1999). View dependence in scene recognition after active learning. *Memory and Cognition, 27*, 996–1007.

Cohen, L. G., Celnik, P., Pascual-Leone, A., Corwell, B., Faiz, L., Dambrosia, J., et al. (1997). Functional relevance of cross-modal plasticity in blind humans. *Nature, 389*(6647), 180–183.

Colby, C. L., & Duhamel, J.-R. (1996). Spatial representations for action in parietal cortex. *Cognitive Brain Research, 5*, 105–115.

Crick, F., & Koch, C. (1995). Cortical areas in visual awareness. *Nature, 377*(6547), 294–295.

Deibert, E., Kraut, M., Kremen, S., & Hart, J., Jr. (1999). Neural pathways in tactile object recognition. *Neurology, 52*(7), 1413–1417.

Dellantonio, A., & Spagnolo, F. (1990). Mental rotation of tactual stimuli. *Acta Psychologica, 73*, 245–257.

DiMattia, B. V., Posley, K. A., & Fuster, J. M. (1990). Cross-modal short-term memory of haptic and visual information. *Neuropsychologia, 28*, 17–33.

Diwadkar, V. A., & McNamara, T. P. (1997). Viewpoint dependence in scene recognition. *Psychological Science, 8*, 302–307.

Easton, R. D., Greene, A. J., & Srinivas, K. (1997). Transfer between vision and haptics: Memory for 2-D patterns and 3-D objects. *Psychonomic Bulletin and Review, 4*, 403–410.

Easton, R. D., & Sholl, M. J. (1995). Object-array structure, frames of reference, and retrieval of spatial knowledge. *Journal of Experimental Psychology: Learning, Memory and Cognition, 21*, 483–500.

Easton, R. D., Srinivas, K., & Greene, A. J. (1997). Do vision and haptics share common representations? Implicit and explicit memory within and between modalities. *Journal of Experimental Psychology: Learning, Memory and Cognition, 23*, 153–163.

Edelman, S. (1999). *Representation and recognition in vision*. Cambridge, MA: MIT Press Bradford Books.

Edelman, S., & Bülthoff, H. H. (1992). Orientation dependence in the recognition of familiar and novel views of 3-dimensional objects. *Vision Research, 32*, 2385–2400.

Ernst, M. O., & Banks, M. S. (2002). Humans integrate visual and haptic information in a statistically optimal fashion. *Nature, 415*(6870), 429–433.

Ernst, M. O., Banks, M. S., & Bülthoff, H. H. (2000). Touch can change visual slant perception. *Nature Neuroscience, 3*, 69–73.

Ernst, M. O., Bülthoff, H. H., & Newell, F. N. (2003). *Visual and haptic recognition of actively explored objects*. Manuscript submitted for publication.

Felleman, D. J., & Van Essen, D. C. (1991). Distributed hierarchical processing in the primate cerebral cortex. *Cerebral Cortex, 1*, 1–47.

Finney, E. M., Fine, I., & Dobkins, K. R. (2001). Visual stimuli activate auditory cortex in the deaf. *Nature Neuroscience, 4*, 1171–1173.

Giard, M. H., & Peronnet, F. (1999). Auditory-visual integration during multimodal object recognition in humans: A behavioural and electrophysiological study. *Journal of Cognitive Neuroscience, 11*, 473–490.

Gibson, J. J. (1962). Observations on active touch. *Psychological Review, 69*, 477–491.

Gibson, J. J. (1966). *The senses considered as perceptual systems*. Boston: Houghton Mifflin.

Gilson, E. Q., & Baddeley, A. D. (1969). Tactile short-term memory. *Quarterly Journal of Experimental Psychology, 21*, 180–184.

Grill-Spector, K., Kushnir, T., Edelman, S., Itzchak, Y., & Malach, R. (1998). Cue-invariant activation in object-related areas of the human occipital lobe. *Neuron, 21*, 191–202.

Grunwald, M., Weiss, T., Krause, W., Beyer, L., Rost, R., Gutberlet, I., et al. (2001). Theta power in the EEG of humans during ongoing processing in a haptic object recognition task. *Cognitive Brain Research, 11*, 33–37.

Hadjikhani, N., & Roland, P. E. (1998). Cross-modal transfer of information between the tactile and the visual representations in the human brain: A positron emission tomographic study. *Journal of Neuroscience, 18*, 1072–1084.

Hamilton, R., Keenan, J. P., Catala, M., & Pascual-Leone, A. (2000). Alexia for Braille following bilateral occipital stroke in an early blind woman. *NeuroReport, 11*, 237–240.

Harman, K. L., Humphrey, G. K., & Goodale, M. A. (1999). Active manual control of object views facilitates visual recognition. *Current Biology, 9*, 1315–1318.

Heller, M. A. (1984). Active and passive touch: The influence of exploration time on form recognition. *Journal of General Psychology, 110*, 243–249.

Heller, M. A. (1992). Haptic dominance in form perception: Vision versus proprioception. *Perception, 21*, 655–660.

Heller, M. A., Calcaterra, J. A., Green, S. L., & Brown, L. (1999). Intersensory conflict between vision and touch: The response modality dominates when precise, attention-riveting judgements are required. *Perception & Psychophysics, 61*, 1384–1389.

Henderson, J. M., & Hollingworth, A. (1999). High level scene perception. *Annual Review of Psychology, 50*, 243–271.

Humphrey, G. K., & Khan, S. C. (1992). Recognising novel views of 3-dimensional objects. *Canadian Journal of Psychology, 46*, 170–190.

James, T. W., Humphrey, G. K., Gati, J. S., Servos, P., Menon, R., & Goodale, M. A. (2002). Haptic study of three-dimensional objects activates extrastriate visual areas. *Neuropsychologia, 40*, 1706–1714.

Kappers, A. M. L., & Koenderink, J. J. (1999). Haptic perception of spatial relations. *Perception, 28*, 781–795.

Kerzel, D. (2001). Visual short-term memory is influenced by haptic perception. *Journal of Experimental Psychology: Learning, Memory and Cognition, 27*, 1101–1109.

Kilgour, A. R., & Lederman, S. J. (2002). Face recognition by hand. *Perception & Psychophysics, 64*(3), 339–352.

Kiphart, M. J., Hughes, J. L., Simmons, J. P., & Cross, H. A. (1992). Short-term haptic memory for complex objects. *Bulletin of the Psychonomic Society, 30*, 212–214.

Klatzky, R. L., Lederman, S. J., & Matula, D. E. (1991). Imagined haptic exploration in judgements of object properties. *Journal of Experimental Psychology: Learning, Memory and Cognition, 17*, 314–322.

Klatzky, R. L., Lederman, S. J., & Matula, D. E. (1993). Haptic exploration in the presence of vision. *Journal of Experimental Psychology: Human Perception and Performance, 19*, 726–743.

Klatzky, R. L., Loomis, J. M., Lederman, S. L., Wake, H., & Fujita, N. (1993). Haptic identification of objects and their depictions. *Perception & Psychophysics, 54*, 170–178.

Kosslyn, S. M., Pascual-Leone, A., Felician, O., Camposano, S., Keenan, J. P., Thompson, W. L., et al. (1999). The role of area 17 in visual imagery: Convergent evidence from PET and rTMS. *Science, 284*(5411), 167–170.

Kubovy, M., & van Valkenburg, D. (2001). Auditory and visual objects. *Cognition, 80*, 97–126.

Kujala, T., Huotilainen, M., Sinkkonen, J., Ahonen, A. I., Alho, K., Hamalainen, M. S., et al. (1995). Visual cortex activation in blind humans during sound discrimination. *Neuroscience Letters, 183*, 143–146.

Làdavas, E. (2002). Functional and dynamic properties of visual peripersonal space. *Trends in Cognitive Sciences, 6*, 17–22.

Laurenti, P. J., Burdette, J. H., Wallace, M. T., Yen, Y.-F., Field, A. S., & Stein, B. E. (2002). Deactivation of sensory-specific cortex by cross-modal stimuli. *Journal of Cognitive Neuroscience, 14*, 420–429.

Lederman, S. J., & Klatzky, R. L. (1987). Hand movements: A window into haptic object recognition. *Cognitive Psychology, 19*, 342–368.

Lederman, S. J., Klatzky, R. L., Chataway, C., & Summers, C. D. (1990). Visual mediation and the haptic recognition of two dimensional pictures of common objects. *Perception & Psychophysics, 47*, 54–64.

Logie, R. H., & Marchetti, C. (1991). Visuo-spatial working memory: Visual, spatial or central executive? In R. H. Logie & M. Denis (Eds.), *Mental images and human cognition*. Amsterdam: Elsevier.

Logothetis, N. K., Pauls, J., Bülthoff, H. H., & Poggio, T. (1994). View-dependent object recognition by monkeys. *Current Biology, 4*, 401–414.

Loomis, J. M. (1990). A model of character recognition and legibility. *Journal of Experimental Psychology: Human Perception and Performance, 16*, 106–120.

Loomis, J. M., Klatzky, R. L., & Lederman, S. J. (1991). Similarity of tactual and visual picture recognition with limited field of view. *Perception, 20*, 167–177.

Mahrer, P., & Miles, C. (2002). Recognition memory for tactile sequences. *Memory, 10*, 7–20.

Malach, R., Reppas, J. B., Benson, R. R., Kwong, K. K., Jiang, H., Kennedy, W. A., et al. (1995). Object-related activity revealed by functional magnetic resonance imaging in human occipital cortex. *Proceedings of the National Academy of Sciences, USA, 92*, 8135–8139.

McGurk, H., & MacDonald, J. (1976). Hearing lips and seeing voices. *Nature, 264*, 746–748.

Miles, C., & Borthwick, H. (1996). Tactile memory revisited. *Memory, 4*, 655–668.

Millar, S. (1999). Memory in touch. *Psicothema, 11*, 747–767.

Milner, A. D. (1997). Vision without knowledge. *Philosophical Transactions of the Royal Society of London, Series B, 352*, 1249–1256.

Newell, F. N. (1998). Stimulus context and view dependence in object recognition. *Perception, 27*, 47–68.

Newell, F. N., Ernst, M. O., Tjan, B. S., & Bülthoff, H. H. (2001). Viewpoint dependence in visual and haptic object recognition. *Psychological Science, 12*, 37–42.

Newell, F. N., & Findlay, J. M. (1997). The effect of depth rotation on object identification. *Perception, 26*, 1231–1257.

Newell, F. N., Shepard, D., Edelman, S., & Shapiro, K. (2003). *The interaction of shape- and location-based priming in object categorisation: Evidence for a hybrid "what+where" representation stage.* Manuscript submitted for publication.

Newell, F. N., Woods, A., Mernagh, M., & Bülthoff, H. H. (2003). *Visual and haptic recognition of scenes.* Manuscript submitted for publication.

Penfield, W., & Rasmussen, T. (1950). *The cerebral cortex of man: A clinical study of localisation of function.* New York: Macmillan.

Perrett, D. I., Hietanen, J. K., Oram, M. W., & Benson, P. J. (1992). Organization and functions of cells responsive to faces in the temporal cortex. *Philosophical Transactions of the Royal Society of London, Series B, 335*, 23–30.

Ramachandran, V. S., Rogers-Ramachandran, D., & Stewart, M. (1992). Perceptual correlates of massive cortical reorganization. *Science, 258*(5085), 1159–1160.

Rauschecker, J. P. (1995). Compensatory plasticity and sensory substitution in the cerebral cortex. *Trends in Neurosciences, 18*, 36–43.

Rayner, K., & Pollatsek, A. (1992). Eye-movements and scene perception. *Canadian Journal of Psychology, 46*, 342–376.

Reales, J. M., & Ballesteros, S. (1999). Implicit and explicit memory for visual and haptic objects: Cross-modal priming depends on structural descriptions. *Journal of Experimental Psychology: Learning, Memory and Cognition, 25*, 644–663.

Reed, C. L., Caselli, R. J., & Farah, M. J. (1996). Tactile agnosia: Underlying impairment and implications for normal tactile object recognition. *Brain, 119*, 875–888.

Rees, G., Kreiman, G., & Koch, C. (2002). Neural correlates of consciousness in humans. *Nature Review of Neuroscience, 3*, 261–270.

Rock, I., & Victor, J. (1964). Vision and touch: An experimentally created conflict between the two senses. *Science, 143*, 595–569.

Sadato, N., Okada, T., Honda, M., & Yonekura, Y. (2002). Critical period for cross-modal plasticity in blind humans: A functional MRI study. *Neuroimage, 16*, 389–400.

Sadato, N., Pascual-Leone, A., Grafman, J., Ibanez, V., Deiber, M. P., Dold, G., et al. (1996). Activation of the primary visual cortex by Braille reading in blind subjects. *Nature, 380*(6574), 526–528.

Saetti, M. C., De Renzi, E., & Comper, M. (1999). Tactile morphagnosia secondary to spatial deficits. *Neuropsychologia, 37*, 1087–1100.

Sathian, K., Zangaladze, A., Hoffman, J. M., & Grafton, S. T. (1997). Feeling with the mind's eye. *NeuroReport, 8*, 3877–3881.

Sereno, A. B., & Maunsell, J. H. R. (1998). Shape selectivity in primate lateral intraparietal cortex. *Nature, 395*, 500–503.

Shams, L., Kamitani, Y., & Shimojo, S. (2002). Visual illusion induced by sound. *Cognitive Brain Research, 14*(1), 147–152.

Shimojo, S., & Shams, L. (2001). Sensory modalities are not separate modalities: Plasticity and interactions. *Current Opinion in Neurobiology, 11,* 505–509.

Simons, D. J., & Wang, R. F. (1998). Perceiving real-world viewpoint changes. *Psychological Science, 9,* 315–320.

Simons, D. J., Wang, R. F., & Roddenberry, D. (2002). Object recognition is mediated by extraretinal information. *Perception & Psychophysics, 64*(4), 521–530.

Stoerig, P., & Cowey, A. (1995). Visual perception and phenomenal consciousness. *Behavioral Brain Research, 71,* 147–156.

Sullivan, E. V., & Turvey, M. T. (1972). Short-term retention of tactile stimulation. *Quarterly Journal of Experimental Psychology, 24,* 253–261.

Tanaka, K., Saito, H., Fukada, Y., & Moriya, M. (1991). Coding visual images of objects in the inferotemporal cortex of the macaque monkey. *Journal of Neurophysiology, 66,* 170–189.

Tarr, M. J., & Bülthoff, H. H. (1995). Is human object recognition better described by geon structural descriptions or by multiple views? Comment on Biederman and Gerhardstein (1993). *Journal of Experimental Psychology: Human Perception and Performance, 21,* 1494–1505.

Tarr, M. J., & Bülthoff, H. H. (1999). [Eds.] *Object recognition in man, monkey and machine* [Special issue]. *Cognition, 67*(1–2).

Tarr, M. J., & Pinker, S. (1989). Mental rotation and orientation dependence in shape recognition. *Cognitive Psychology, 21,* 233–282.

Ullman, S. (1996). *High-level vision: Object recognition and visual cognition.* Cambridge, MA: MIT Press.

Ungerleider, L. G., & Mishkin, M. (1982). Two cortical visual systems. In D. J. Ingle, M. A. Goodale, & R. J. W. Mansfield (Eds.), *Analysis of visual behaviour* (pp. 549–586). Cambridge, MA: MIT Press.

Valenza, N., Ptak, R., Zimine, I., Badan, M., Lazeyras, F., & Schnider, A. (2001). Dissociated active and passive tactile shape recognition: A case study of pure tactile apraxia. *Brain, 124,* 2287–2298.

Wanet-Defalque, M. C., Veraart, C., De Volder, A. G., Metz, R., Michel, C., Dooms, G., et al. (1988). High metabolic activity in the visual cortex of early blind human subjects. *Brain Research, 446,* 369–373.

Wang, R. F., & Simons, D. J. (1999). Active and passive scene recognition across views. *Cognition, 70,* 191–210.

Yamane, S., Kaji, S., & Kawano, K. (1988). What facial features activate face neurons in inferotemporal cortex of monkeys? *Experimental Brain Research, 73,* 209–214.

Zangaladze, A., Epstein, C. M., Grafton, S. T., & Sathian, K. (1999). Involvement of visual cortex in tactile discrimination of orientation. *Nature, 401,* 587–590.

9 Perceptual Effects of Cross-Modal Stimulation: Ventriloquism and the Freezing Phenomenon

JEAN VROOMEN AND BEATRICE DE GELDER

Introduction

For readers of a book on multimodal perception, it probably comes as no surprise that most events in real life consist of perceptual inputs in more than one modality and that sensory modalities may influence each other. For example, seeing a speaker provides not only auditory information, conveyed in what is said, but also visual information, conveyed through the movements of the lips, face, and body, as well as visual cues about the origin of the sound. Most handbooks on cognitive psychology pay comparatively little attention to this multimodal state of affairs, and the different senses—seeing, hearing, smell, taste, touch—are treated as distinct and separate modules with little or no interaction. It is becoming increasingly clear, however, that when the different senses receive correlated input about the same external object or event, information is often combined by the perceptual system to yield a multimodally determined percept.

An important issue is to characterize such multisensory interactions and their cross-modal effects. There are at least three different notions at stake here. One is that information is processed in a hierarchical and strictly *feed-forward* fashion. In this view, information from different sensory modalities converges in a multimodal representation in a feed-forward way. For example, in the fuzzy logic model of perception (Massaro, 1998), degrees of support for different alternatives from each modality—say, audition and vision—are determined and then combined to give an overall degree of support. Information is propagated in a strictly feed-forward fashion so that higher-order multimodal representations do not affect lower-order sensory-specific representations. There is thus no cross-talk between the sensory modalities such that, say, vision affects early processing stages of audition or vice versa. Cross-modal interactions in feed-forward models take place only at or beyond multimodal stages. An alternative possibility is

that multimodal representations send *feedback* to primary sensory levels (e.g., Driver & Spence, 2000). In this view, higher-order multimodal levels can affect sensory levels. Vision might thus affect audition, but only via multimodal representations. Alternatively, it may also be the case that cross-modal interactions take place without multimodal representations. For example, it may be that the senses access each other directly from their sensory-specific systems (e.g., Ettlinger & Wilson, 1990). Vision might then affect audition without the involvement of a multimodal representation (see, e.g., Falchier, Clavagnier, Barone, & Kennedy, 2002, for recent neuroanatomical evidence showing that there are projections from primary auditory cortex to the visual area V1).

The role of feedback in sensory processing has been debated for a long time (e.g., the interactive activation model of reading by Rumelhart and McClelland, 1982). However, as far as cross-modal effects are concerned, there is at present no clear empirical evidence that allows distinguishing among feed-forward, feedback, and direct-access models. Feed-forward models predict that early sensory processing levels should be autonomous and unaffected by higher-order processing levels, whereas feedback or direct-access models would, in principle, allow that vision affects auditory processes, or vice versa. Although this theoretical distinction seems straightforward, empirical demonstration in favor of one or another alternative has proved difficult to obtain. One of the main problems is to find measures that are sufficiently unambiguous and that can be taken as pure indices of an auditory or visual sensory process.

Among the minimal requirements for stating that a cross-modal effect has perceptual consequences at early sensory stages, the phenomenon should at least be (1) robust, (2) not explainable as a strategic effect, and (3) not occurring at response-related processing stages. If one assumes stagewise processing, with sensation coming before attention (e.g. the "late selection" view of attention), one might also want to argue that (4) cross-modal effects should be pre-attentive. If these minimal criteria are met, it becomes at least likely that cross-modal interactions occur at early perceptual processing stages, and thus that models that allow access to primary processing levels (i.e., feedback or direct-access models) better describe the phenomenon. In our work on cross-modal perception, we investigated the extent to which such minimal criteria apply to some cases of audiovisual perception. One case concerns a situation in which vision affects the localization of a sound (the ventriloquism effect), the other a situation in which an abrupt sound affects visual processing of a rapidly presented visual stimulus (the freezing phenomenon). In Chapter 36 of this volume, we describe the case of cross-modal interactions in affect perception. Each of these phenomena we consider to be based on cross-modal interactions affecting early levels of perception.

Vision affecting sound localization: The ventriloquism effect

Presenting synchronous auditory and visual information in slightly separate locations creates the illusion that the sound is coming from the direction of the visual stimulus. Although the effect is smaller, shifting of the visual percept in the direction of the sound has, at least in some studies, also been observed (Bertelson & Radeau, 1981). The auditory shift is usually measured by asking subjects to localize the sound by pointing or by fixating the eyes on the apparent location of the sound. When localization responses are compared with a control condition (e.g., a condition in which the sound is presented in isolation without a visual stimulus), a shift of a few degrees in the direction of the visual stimulus is usually observed. Such an effect, produced by audiovisual spatial conflict, is called the *ventriloquism effect,* because one of the most spectacular everyday examples is the illusion created by performing ventriloquists that the speech they produce without visible facial movements comes from a puppet they agitate in synchrony with the speech.

A standard explanation of the ventriloquism effect is the following: when auditory and visual stimuli occur in close temporal and spatial proximity, the perceptual system assumes that a single event has occurred. The perceptual system then tries to reduce the conflict between the location of the visual and auditory data, because there is an a priori constraint that an object or event can have only one location (e.g., Bedford, 1999). Shifting the auditory location in the direction of the visual event rather than the other way around would seem to be ecologically useful, because spatial resolution in the visual modality is better than in the auditory one.

However, there are also other, more trivial explanations of the ventriloquism effect. One alternative is similar to Stroop task interference: when two conflicting stimuli are presented together, such as when the word blue is written in red ink, there is competition at the level of response selection rather than at a perceptual level per se. Stroop-like response competition may also be at play in the ventriloquism effect. In that case, there would be no real attraction between sound and vision, but the ventriloquist illusion would be derived from the fact that subjects sometimes point to the visual stimulus instead of the sound by mistake. Strategic or cognitive factors may also play a role. For example, a subject may wonder why sounds and lights are presented from different locations, and then adopt a postperceptual response strategy that satisfies the experimenter's ideas of the task (Bertelson, 1999). Of course, these possibilities are not exclusive, and the experimenter should find ways to check or circumvent them.

In our research, we dealt with these and other aspects of the ventriloquist situation in the hope of showing that the apparent location of a sound is indeed shifted at a perceptual level of auditory space perception. More specifically, we asked whether a ventriloquism effect can be observed (1) when subjects are explicitly trained to ignore the visual distracter; (2) when cognitive strategies of the subject to respond in a particular way can be excluded; (3) when the visual distracter is not attended, either endogenously or exogenously; and (4) when the visual distracter is not seen consciously. We also asked (5) whether the ventriloquism effect as such is possibly a pre-attentive phenomenon.

1. A visual distracter cannot be ignored In a typical ventriloquism situation, subjects are asked to locate a sound while ignoring a visual distracter. Typically, subjects remain unaware of how well they perform during the experiment and how well they succeed in obeying instructions. In one of our experiments, though, we asked whether it is possible to train subjects explicitly to ignore the visual distracter (Vroomen, Bertelson, & de Gelder, 1998). If despite training it is impossible to ignore the visual distracter, this speaks to the robustness of the effect. Subjects were trained to discriminate among sequences of tones that emanated either from a central location only or from alternating locations, in which case two speakers located next to a computer screen emitted the tones. With no visual input, this same/different location task was very easy, because the difference between the central and lateral locations was clearly noticeable. However, the task was much more difficult when, in synchrony with the tones, light flashes were alternated left and right on a computer screen. This condition created the strong impression that sounds from the central location now alternated between left and right, presumably because the light flashes attracted the apparent location of the sounds. We then tried to train subjects to discriminate centrally presented but ventriloquized sounds from sounds that alternated physically between the left and right. Subjects were instructed to ignore the lights as much as possible (but without closing their eyes), and they received corrective feedback after each trial. The results were that the larger the separation between the lights, the more false alarms occurred (subjects responded "alternating sound" to a centrally presented ventriloquized sound), presumably because the farther apart the lights were, the farther apart was the perceived location of the sounds. Moreover, although feedback was provided after each trial, performance did not improve in the course of the experiment. Instructions and feedback thus could not overcome the effect of the visual distracter on sound localization, which indicates that the ventriloquism effect is indeed very robust.

2. A ventriloquism effect is obtained even when cognitive strategies can be excluded When subjects are asked to point to the location of auditory stimuli while ignoring spatially discrepant visual distracters, they may be aware of the spatial discrepancy and adjust their response accordingly. The visual bias one obtains may then reflect postperceptual decisions rather than genuine perceptual effects. However, contamination by strategies can be prevented when ventriloquism effects are studied via a *staircase procedure* or as an *aftereffect*.

Bertelson and Aschersleben (1998) were the first to apply the staircase procedure in the ventriloquism situation. The advantage of a staircase procedure is that it is not transparent, and the effects are therefore more likely to reflect genuine perceptual processes. In the staircase procedure used by Bertelson and Aschersleben, subjects had to judge the apparent origin of a stereophonically controlled sound as left or right of a median reference point. Unknown to the subjects, the location of the sound was changed as a function of their judgment, following the principle of the psychophysical staircase. After a "left" judgment, the next sound on the same staircase was moved one step to the right, and vice versa. A staircase started with sounds coming from an extreme left or an extreme right position. At that stage, correct responses were generally given on each successive trial, so that the target sounds moved progressively toward the center. Then, at some point, *response reversals* (responses different from the preceding one on the same staircase) began to occur. Thereafter, the subjects were no longer certain about the location of the sound.

The location at which these response reversals began to occur was the dependent variable. In the study by Bertelson and Aschersleben, sounds were delivered together with a visual distracter, a light-emitting diode (LED) flash, in a central location. When the LED flash was synchronized with the sound, response reversal occurred earlier than when the light was desynchronized from the sound. Apparently, the synchronized LED flashes attracted the apparent location of the sound toward its central location, so that response reversal occurred earlier on the staircase. Similar results have now been reported by Caclin, Soto-Faraco, Kingstone, and Spence (2002) showing that a centrally located tactile stimulus attracts a peripheral sound toward the middle. It is important to note that there is no way subjects can figure out a response strategy that might lead to this result, because once response reversal begins to occur, subjects no longer know whether a sound belongs to a left or a right staircase. A conscious response strategy in this situation is thus extremely unlikely to account for the effect.

Conscious strategies are also unlikely to play a role when the effect of presenting auditory and visual stimuli at separate locations is measured as an aftereffect. The aftereffect is a shift in the apparent location of *unimodally* presented acoustic stimuli consequent on exposure to synchronous but spatially disparate auditory-visual stimulus pairs. Initial studies used prisms to shift the relative locations of visual and auditory stimuli (Canon, 1970; Radeau & Bertelson, 1974). Participants localized acoustic targets before and after a period of adaptation. During the adaptation phase, there was a mismatch between the spatial locations of acoustic and visual stimuli. Typically, between pre- and posttest a shift of about 1–4 degrees was found in the direction of the visual attractor. Presumably, the spatial conflict between auditory and visual data during the adaptation phase was resolved by recalibration of the perceptual system, and this alteration lasted long enough to be detected as aftereffects. It should be noted that aftereffects are measured by comparing *unimodal* pointing to a sound before and after an adaptation phase. Stroop-like response competition between the auditory target and visual distractor during the test situation thus plays no role, because the test sound is presented without a visual distracter. Moreover, aftereffects are usually obtained when the spatial discrepancy between auditory and visual stimuli is so small that subjects do not even notice the separation (Frissen, Bertelson, Vroomen, & de Gelder, 2003; Radeau & Bertelson, 1974; Vroomen et al., 2003; Woods & Recanzone, Chap. 3, this volume). Aftereffects can therefore be interpreted as true perceptual recalibration effects (e.g., Radeau, 1994).

3. Attention toward the visual distracter is not needed to obtain a ventriloquism effect A relevant question is whether attention plays a role in the ventriloquism effect. One could argue, as Treisman and Gelade (1980) have done in feature-integration theory for the visual modality, that focused attention might be the glue that combines features across modalities. Could it be, then, that when a sound and visual distracter are attended, an integrated cross-modal event is perceived, but when they are unattended, two separate events are perceived that do not interact? If so, one might predict that a visual distracter would have a stronger effect on the apparent location of a sound when it is focused upon.

We considered the possibility that ventriloquism indeed requires or is modulated by this kind of focused attention (Bertelson, Vroomen, de Gelder, & Driver, 2000). The subjects' task was to localize trains of tones while monitoring visual events on a computer screen. On experimental trials, a bright square appeared on the left or the right of the screen in exact synchrony with the tones. No square appeared on control trials. The attentional manipulation consisted of having subjects monitor either the center of the display, in which case the attractor square was in the visual periphery, or the lateral square itself for occasional occurrences of a catch stimulus (a very small diamond that could only be detected when in the fovea). The attentional hypothesis predicts that the attraction of the apparent location of the sound by the square would be stronger with attention focused on the attractor square than with attention focused on the center. In fact, though, equal degrees of attraction were obtained in the two attention conditions. Focused attention thus did not modulate the ventriloquist effect.

However, the effect of attention might have been small and overruled by the bottom-up information from the laterally presented visual square. What would happen when the bottom-up information was more ambiguous? Would an effect of attention then appear? In a second experiment, we used bilateral squares that were flashed in synchrony with the sound so as to provide competing visual attractors. When the two squares were of equal size, auditory localization was unaffected by which side participants monitored for visual targets, but when one square was larger than the other, auditory localization was reliably attracted toward the bigger square, again regardless of where visual monitoring was required. This led to the conclusion that the ventriloquism effect largely reflects automatic sensory interactions, with little or no role for focused attention.

In discussing how attention might influence ventriloquism, though, one must distinguish several senses in which the term *attention* is used. One may attend to one sensory modality rather than another regardless of location (Spence & Driver, 1997a), or one may attend to one particular location rather than another regardless of modality. Furthermore, in the literature on spatial attention, two different means of the allocation of attention are generally distinguished. First, there is an *endogenous* process by which attention can be moved voluntarily. Second, there is an automatic or *exogenous* mechanism by which attention is reoriented automatically to stimuli in the environment with some special features. The study by Bertelson, Vroomen, et al. (2000) manipulated endogenous attention by asking subjects to focus on one or the other location. Yet it may have been the case that the visual distracter received a certain amount of exogenous attention independent of where the subject was focusing. For that reason, one might ask whether capture of exogenous attention by the visual distracter is essential to affect the perceived location of a sound.

To investigate this possibility, we tried to create a situation in which exogenous attention was captured in one direction, whereas the apparent location of a sound was ventriloquized in the other direction (Vroomen, Bertelson, & de Gelder, 2001a). Our choice was influenced by earlier data showing that attention can be captured by a visual item differing substantially in one or several attributes (e.g., color, form, orientation, shape) from a set of identical items among which it is displayed (e.g., Treisman & Gelade, 1980). The unique item is sometimes called the *singleton,* and its influence on attention is referred to as the singleton effect. If ventriloquism is mediated by exogenous attention, presenting a sound in synchrony with a display that contains a singleton should shift the apparent location of the sound toward the singleton. Consequently, finding a singleton that would not shift the location of a sound in its direction would provide evidence that exogenous attention can be dissociated from ventriloquism.

We used a psychophysical staircase procedure as in Bertelson and Aschersleben (1998). The occurrence of visual bias was examined by presenting a display in synchrony with the sound. We tried to shift the apparent location of the sound in the opposite direction of the singleton by using a display that consisted of four horizontally aligned squares: two big squares on one side, and a big square and a small square (the singleton) on the other side (Fig. 9.1). The singleton was either in the far left or in the far right position. A visual bias dependent on the position of the singleton should manifest itself at the level of the locations at which reversals begin to occur on the staircases for the two visual displays. If, for instance, the apparent location of the sound were attracted toward the singleton, reversals

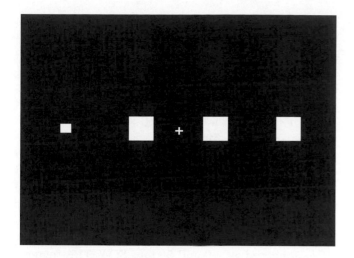

FIGURE 9.1 An example of one of the displays used by Vroomen, Bertelson, and de Gelder (2001a). Subjects saw four squares, one (the singleton) smaller than the others. When the display was flashed on a computer screen, subjects heard a stereophonically controlled sound whose location had to be judged as left or right of the median fixation cross. The results showed that the apparent location of the sound was shifted in the direction of the two big squares, and not toward the singleton. On control trials, it was found that the singleton attracted visual attention. The direction in which a sound was ventriloquized was thus dissociated from where exogenous attention was captured.

would first occur at locations more to the left for the display with the singleton on the right than for the display with the singleton on the left.

The results of this experiment were very straightforward. The apparent origin of the sound was not shifted toward the singleton but in the opposite direction, toward the two big squares. Apparently, the two big squares on one side of the display were attracting the apparent origin of the sound more strongly than the small and big square at the other side. Thus, the attractor size effect that we previously obtained (Bertelson, Vroomen, de Gelder, & Driver, 2000) occurred with the present visual display as well. This result thus suggested that attraction of a sound was not mediated through exogenous attention capture. However, before that conclusion could be drawn, it was necessary to check that the visual display had the capacity to attract attention toward the singleton. We therefore ran a control experiment in which the principle was to measure the attention-attracting capacity of the small square through its effect on the discrimination of targets presented elsewhere in the display. In the singleton condition, participants were shown the previously used display with the three big squares and the small one. A target letter X or O, calling for a choice reaction, was displayed in the most peripheral big square opposite

the singleton. In the control condition, the display consisted of four equally sized big squares. Discrimination performance was worse in the singleton condition than in the control condition, thus showing that attention was attracted away from the target letter and toward the singleton. Nevertheless, one might still argue that a singleton in the sound localization task did not capture attention because subjects were paying attention to audition, not vision. In a third experiment, we therefore randomized sound localization trials with visual X/O discrimination trials so that subjects did not know in advance which task they had to perform. When subjects saw an X or an O, they pressed as fast as possible a corresponding key; otherwise, when no letter was detected, they decided whether the sound had come from the left or right of the central reference. With this mixed design, results were still exactly as before: attention was attracted toward the singleton while the sound was shifted away from the singleton. Strategic differences between an auditory and a visual task were thus unlikely to explain the result. Rather, we demonstrated a dissociation between ventriloquism and exogenous attention: the apparent location of the sound was shifted toward the two big squares (or the "center of gravity" of the visual display), while the singleton attracted exogenous attention. The findings from the studies concerning the role of exogenous attention together with those of the earlier one showing the independence of ventriloquism from the direction of endogenous attention (Bertelson, Vroomen, et al., 2000) thus support the conclusion that ventriloquism is not affected by the direction of attention.

4. The ventriloquism effect is still obtained when the visual distracter is not seen consciously The conclusion that attention is not needed to obtain a ventriloquism effect is further corroborated by our work on patients with unilateral visual neglect (Bertelson, Pavani, Ladavas, Vroomen, & de Gelder, 2000). The neglect syndrome is usually interpreted as an attentional deficit and reflected in a reduced capacity to report stimuli in the contralateral side (usually the left). Previously, it had been reported that ventriloquism could improve the attentional deficit. Soroker, Calamaro, and Myslobodsky (1995) showed that inferior identification of syllables delivered through a loudspeaker on the left (auditory neglect) could be improved when the same stimuli on the left were administered in the presence of a fictitious loudspeaker on the right. The authors attributed this improvement to a ventriloquism effect, even though their setting was very different from the usual ventriloquism situation. That is, their visual stimulus was stationary, whereas typically the onset and offset of an auditory and visual stimulus are synchronized. The effect was therefore probably mediated by higher-order knowledge about the fact that sounds can be delivered through loudspeakers.

In our research, we used the more typical ventriloquism situation (a light and a sound presented simultaneously) and asked whether a visual stimulus that remains undetected because it is presented in the neglected field nevertheless shifts the apparent location of the sound toward its location. This may occur because although perceptual awareness is compromised in neglect, much perceptual processing can still proceed unconsciously for the affected side. Our results were clear: patients with left visual neglect consistently failed to detect a stimulus presented in their left visual field; nevertheless, their pointing to a sound was shifted in the direction of the visual stimulus. This is thus another demonstration that ventriloquism is not dependent on attention or even awareness of the visual distracter.

5. The ventriloquism effect is a pre-attentive phenomenon
The previous studies led us to conclude that cross-modal interactions take place without the need of attention. This stage is presumably one concerned with the initial analysis of the spatial scene (Bertelson, 1994). The presumption receives additional support from the findings by Driver (1996) in which the visual bias of auditory location was measured in the classic "cocktail party" situation through its effect in facilitating the focusing of attention on one of two simultaneous spoken messages. Subjects found the shadowing task easier when the apparent location of the target sound was attracted away from the distracter by a moving face. This result thus implies that focused attention operates on a representation of the external scene that has already been spatially reorganized by cross-modal interactions.

We asked whether a similar cross-modal reorganization of external space occurs when exogenous rather than focused attention is at stake (Vroomen, Bertelson, & de Gelder, 2001b). To do so, we used the orthogonal cross-modal cuing task introduced by Spence and Driver (1997b). In this task, participants are asked to judge the elevation (up vs. down, regardless of whether it is on the left or right of fixation) of peripheral targets in either audition, vision, or touch following an uninformative cue in either one of these modalities. In general, cuing effects (i.e., faster responses when the cue is on the same side as the target) have been found across all modalities, except that visual cues do not affect responses to auditory targets (Driver & Spence, 1998; but see McDonald, Teder-Sälejärvi, Heraldez, & Hillyard, 2001; Spence, 2001). This then opens an intriguing possibility: What happens with an auditory cue whose veridical location is in the center but whose apparent location is ventriloquized toward a simultaneous light in the periphery? Can such a ventriloquized cue affect responses to auditory targets? The ventriloquized cue consisted of a tone presented from an invisible central speaker synchronized with a visual cue presented on the left or right. Depending on the stimulus onset asynchrony (SOA)—100, 300, or 500 ms—a target sound (white noise bursts) was delivered with equal probabilities from one of the four target speakers. Subjects made a speeded decision about whether the target had been delivered through one of the upper speakers or one of the lower speakers. Results showed that visual cues had no effect on auditory target detection (see also Spence & Driver, 1997b). More important, ventriloquized cues had no cuing effect at 100 ms SOA, but the facilitatory effect appeared at 300 and 500 ms SOA. This suggests that a ventriloquized cue directed auditory exogenous attention to the perceived rather than the physical auditory location, implying that the cross-modal interaction between vision and audition reorganized space on which auditory exogenous attention operates. Spence and Driver (2000) reported similar cuing effects (with a somewhat different time course) in their study of ventriloquized cues in the vertical dimension. They showed that a visual cue presented above or below fixation led to a vertical shift of auditory attention when it was paired with a tone presented at fixation. Attentional capture can thus be directed to the apparent location of a ventriloquized sound, suggesting that cross-modal integration precedes or at least co-occurs with reflexive shifts of covert attention.

To summarize the case of ventriloquism, the apparent location of a sound can be shifted in the direction of a visual stimulus that is synchronized with the sound. It is unlikely that this robust effect can be explained solely by voluntary response strategies, as it is obtained with a psychophysical staircase procedure and can be observed as an aftereffect. The effect is even obtained when the visual distracter is not seen consciously, as in patients with hemineglect. Moreover, the ventriloquism effect does not require attention because it is not affected by whether a visual distracter is focused on or not, and the direction of ventriloquism can be dissociated from where visual attention is captured. In fact, the ventriloquism effect may be a pre-attentive phenomenon, because auditory attention can be captured at the ventriloquized location of a sound. Taken together, these observations indicate that the ventriloquism effect is perceptually "real."

Sound affecting vision: The freezing phenomenon

Recently we described a case of sound affecting vision (Vroomen & de Gelder, 2000). The basic phenomenon can be described as follows: when subjects are shown a rapidly changing visual display, an abrupt sound may "freeze" the display with which the sound is synchronized. Perceptually, the display appears brighter or appears to be shown for a longer period of time. We described this phenomenon against the background of scene analysis.

Scene analysis refers to the concept that information reaching the sense organs is parsed into objects and events. In vision, scene analysis succeeds despite partial occlusion of one object by the other, the presence of shadows extending across object boundaries, and deformations of the retinal image produced by moving objects. Vision is not the only modality in which object segregation occurs. Auditory object segregation has also been demonstrated (Bregman, 1990). It occurs, for instance, when a sequence of alternating high- and low-frequency tones is played at a certain rate. When the frequency difference between the tones is small, or when the tones are played at a slow rate, listeners are able to follow the entire sequence of tones. But at bigger frequency differences or higher rates, the sequence splits into two streams, one high and one low in pitch. Although it is possible to shift attention between the two streams, it is difficult to report the order of the tones in the entire sequence. Auditory stream segregation, like apparent motion in vision, appears to follow Korte's third law (Korte, 1915). When the difference in frequency between the tones increases, stream segregation occurs at longer SOAs.

Bregman (1990) described a number of *Gestalt* principles for auditory scene analysis in which he stressed the resemblance between audition and vision, since principles of perceptual organization such as similarity (in volume, timbre, spatial location), good continuation, and common fate seem to play similar roles in the two modalities. Such a correspondence between principles of visual and auditory organization raises the question of whether the perceptual system utilizes information from one sensory modality to organize the perceptual array in the other modality. In other words, is scene analysis itself a cross-modal phenomenon?

Previously, O'Leary and Rhodes (1984) showed that perceptual segmentation in one modality could influence the concomitant segmentation in another modality. They used a display of six dots, three high and three low. The dots were displayed one by one, alternating between the high and low positions and moving from left to right. At slow rates, a single dot appeared to move up and down, while at faster rates two dots were seen as moving horizontally, one above the other. A sequence that was perceived as two dots caused a concurrent auditory sequence to be perceived as two tones as well

at a rate that would yield a single perceptual object when the accompanying visual sequence was perceived as a single object. The number of objects seen thus influenced the number of objects heard. They also found the opposite influence from audition to vision. Segmentation in one modality thus affected segmentation in the other modality. To us, though, it was not clear whether the cross-modal effect was truly perceptual, or whether it occurred because participants deliberately changed their interpretation of the sounds and dots. It is well known that there is a broad range of rates and tones at which listeners can hear, at will, one or two streams (van Noorden, 1975). O'Leary and Rhodes presented ambiguous sequences, and this raises the possibility that a cross-modal influence was found because perceivers changed their *interpretation* of the sounds and dots, but the *perception* may have been the same. For example, participants under the impression of hearing two streams instead of one may have inferred that in vision there should also be two streams instead of one. Such a conscious strategy would explain the observations of the cross-modal influence without the need for a direct perceptual link between audition and vision.

We pursued this question in a study that led us to observe the freezing phenomenon. We first tried to determine whether the freezing of the display to which an abrupt tone is synchronized is a perceptually genuine effect or not. Previously, Stein, London, Wilkinson, & Price (1996) had shown, with normal subjects, that a sound enhances the perceived visual intensity of a stimulus. The latter seemed to be a close analogue of the freezing phenomenon we wanted to create. However, Stein et al. used a somewhat indirect measure of visual intensity (a visual analogue scale; participants judged the intensity of a light by rotating a dial), and they could not find an enhancement by a sound when the visual stimulus was presented subthreshold. It was therefore unclear whether their effect was truly perceptual rather than postperceptual. In our experiments, we tried to avoid this difficulty by using a more direct estimate of visual persistence by measuring speeded performance on a detection task. Participants saw a 4 × 4 matrix of flickering dots that was created by rapidly presenting four different displays, each containing four dots in quasi-random positions (Fig. 9.2). Each display on its own was difficult to see, because it was shown only briefly and was immediately followed by a mask. One of the four displays contained a target to be detected. The target consisted of four dots that made up a diamond in the upper left, upper right, lower left, or lower right corner of the matrix. The task of the participants was to detect the position of the diamond as fast and as accurately as possible. We investigated whether the detectability of

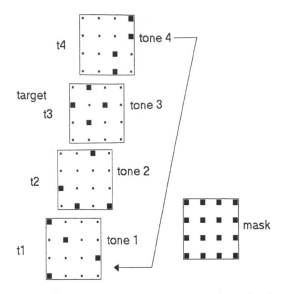

FIGURE 9.2 A simplified representation of a stimulus sequence used in Vroomen and de Gelder (2000). Big squares represent the dots shown at time t; small squares were actually not presented to the viewers but are in the figure to show the position of the dots within the 4 × 4 matrix. The four-dot displays were shown for 97 ms each. Each display was immediately followed by a mask (the full matrix of 16 dots) for 97 ms, followed by a dark blank screen for 60 ms. The target display (in this example, the diamond in the upper left corner whose position had to be detected) was presented at t_3. The sequence of the four-dot displays was repeated without interruption until a response was given. Tones (97 ms in duration) were synchronized with the onset of the four-dot displays. Results showed that when a tone was presented at t_3 that segregated, target detection was enhanced, presumably because the visibility of the target display was increased. When a segregating tone was presented at t_2, target detection became worse because the visual distracter at t_2 caused more interference. There was no enhancement when the tone at t_3 did not segregate. The visibility of a display was thus increased when synchronized with an abrupt tone.

the target could be improved by the presentation of an abrupt sound together with the target. The tones were delivered through a loudspeaker under the monitor. Participants in the experimental condition heard a high tone at the target display and a low tone at the other four-dot displays (the distracters). In the control condition, participants heard only low tones. The idea was that the high tone in the sequence of tones segregated from the low tones, and that under the experimental circumstances it would increase the detectability of the target display. The results indeed showed that the target was detected more easily when presentation of the target was synchronized with presentation of the high tone. Subjects were faster and more accurate when a high tone was presented at target onset. Did the high tone simply act as a warning signal, giving subjects

information about when to expect the target? In a second experiment we controlled for this possibility and synchronized the high tone with a distracter display that immediately preceded presentation of the target. Participants were informed about the temporal relation between high tone and target display and thus knew that the target would be presented immediately after the high tone. Yet, although the participants were now also given a cue about when to expect the target their performance actually worsened. As reported by the participants, it is probable that the high tone contributed to higher visibility of the distracter display with which it was synchronized, thereby increasing interference.

However, the most important result was that we could show that the perceptual organization of the tone sequence determined the cross-modal enhancement. Our introspective observation was that visual detection was improved only when the high tone was segregated from the tone sequence. In our next experiment we prevented segregation of the high tone by making it part of the beginning of the well-known tune "Frère Jacques." When subjects heard repetitively a low-middle-high-low tone sequence while seeing the target on the third high tone, there was no enhancement of the visual display. Thus, the perceptual organization of the tone in the sequence increased the visibility of the target display rather than the high tone per se, showing that cross-modal interactions can occur at the level of scene analysis.

How to qualify the nature of cross-modal interactions?

We have argued that ventriloquism and the freezing phenomenon are two examples of intersensory interactions with consequences at perceptual processing levels (see also Vroomen & de Gelder, 2003, for audiovisual interactions between moving stimuli). They may therefore be likely candidates for showing that cross-modal interactions can affect primary sensory levels. There is now also some preliminary neurophysiological evidence showing that brain areas that are usually considered to be unimodal can be affected by input from different modalities. For example, with functional magnetic resonance imaging, Calvert, Campbell, and Brammer (2000) found that lipreading could affect primary auditory cortex. In a similar vein, Macaluso, Frith, and Driver (2000) showed that a tactile cue could enhance neural responses to a visual target in visual cortex. Giard and Peronnet (1999) also reported that tones synchronized with a visual stimulus affected event-related potentials (ERPs) in visual cortex. Pourtois, de Gelder, Vroomen, Rossion, and Crommelink (2000) found early modulation of auditory

ERPs when facial expressions of emotions were presented with auditory sentence fragments, the prosodic content of which was congruent with or incongruent with the face. When the face-voice pairs were congruent, there was a bigger auditory N1 component at around 110 ms than when they were incongruent. All these findings are in accordance with the idea that there is feedback from multimodal levels to unimodal levels of perception or with the notion that sensory modalities access each other directly.

Such cross-talk between primary sensory areas may also be related to the fact that the subjective experience of cross-modal interaction affects the target modality. In the McGurk effect (McGurk & MacDonald, 1976), visual information provided by lipreading changes the way a sound is *heard*. In the ventriloquism situation, when a sound is presented with a spatially conflicting light, the location of the *sound* is changed. With emotions, when a fearful voice is shown with a happy face, the voice *sounds* happier (de Gelder & Vroomen, 2000). There are other examples of such qualitative changes: For example, when a single flash of light is accompanied by multiple beeps, the light is *seen* as multiple flashes (Shams, Kamitani, & Shimojo, 2000). These multimodally determined percepts thus have the unimodal qualia of the sensory input from the primary modality, and this may be due to the existence of backprojections to the primary sensory areas.

Yet this is not to say that a percept resulting from cross-modal interactions is, in all its relevant aspects, equivalent to its unimodal counterpart. For example, is a ventriloquized sound in all its perceptual and neurophysiological relevant dimensions the same as a sound played from the direction from where the ventriloquized sound was perceived? For McGurk-like stimulus combinations (i.e., hearing /ba/ and seeing /ga/), the auditory component can be dissociated from the perceived component, as the contrast effect in selective speech adaptation is driven mainly by the auditory stimulus, and not by the perceived aspect of the audiovisual stimulus combination (Roberts & Summerfield, 1981; but see Bertelson, Vroomen, & de Gelder, 2003). For other cross-modal phenomena such as ventriloquism, a number of intriguing questions remain about the extent to which the illusory percept is distinguishable, or not, from its veridical counterpart.

REFERENCES

Bedford, F. L. (1999). Keeping perception accurate. *Trends in Cognitive Sciences, 2*, 4–11.

Bertelson, P. (1994). The cognitive architecture behind auditory-visual interaction in scene analysis and speech identification. *Cahiers de Psychologie Cognitive, 13*, 69–75.

Bertelson, P. (1999). Ventriloquism: A case of cross-modal perceptual grouping. In G. Aschersleben, T. Bachmann, & J. Müssler (Eds.), *Cognitive contributions to the perception of spatial and temporal events* (pp. 347–362). Amsterdam: Elsevier.

Bertelson, P., & Aschersleben, G. (1998). Automatic visual bias of auditory location. *Psychonomic Bulletin and Review, 5*, 482–489.

Bertelson, P., Pavani, F., Ladavas, E., Vroomen, J., & de Gelder, B. (2000). Ventriloquism in patients with unilateral visual neglect. *Neuropsychologia, 38*, 1634–1642.

Bertelson, P., & Radeau, M. (1981). Cross-modal bias and perceptual fusion with auditory-visual spatial discordance. *Perception & Psychophysics, 29*, 578–584.

Bertelson, P., Vroomen, J., & de Gelder, B. (2003). Visual recalibration of auditory speech identification. *Psychological Science*.

Bertelson, P., Vroomen, J., de Gelder, B., & Driver, J. (2000). The ventriloquist effect does not depend on the direction of deliberate visual attention. *Perception & Psychophysics, 62*, 321–332.

Bregman, A. S. (1990). *Auditory scene analysis*. Cambridge, MA: MIT Press.

Caclin, A., Soto-Faraco, S., Kingstone, A., & Spence, C. (2002). Tactile "capture" of audition. *Perception & Psychophysics, 64*, 616–630.

Calvert, G. A., Campbell, R., & Brammer, M. J. (2000). Evidence from functional magnetic resonance imaging of cross-modal binding in the human heteromodal cortex. *Current Biology, 10*, 649–657.

Canon, L. K. (1970). Intermodality inconsistency of input and directed attention as determinants of the nature of adaptation. *Journal of Experimental Psychology, 84*, 141–147.

de Gelder, B., & Vroomen, J. (2000). The perception of emotions by ear and by eye. *Cognition and Emotion, 14*, 289–311.

Driver, J. (1996). Enhancement of selective listening by illusory mislocalization of speech sounds due to lip-reading. *Nature, 381*, 66–68.

Driver, J., & Spence, C. (1998). Attention and the cross-modal construction of space. *Trends in Cognitive Sciences, 2*, 254–262.

Driver, J., & Spence, C. (2000). Multisensory perception: Beyond modularity and convergence. *Current Biology, 10*, 731–735.

Ettlinger, G., & Wilson, W. A. (1990). Cross-modal performance: Behavioural processes, phylogenetic considerations and neural mechanisms. *Behavioural Brain Research, 40*, 169–192.

Falchier, A., Renaud, L., Barone, P., & Kennedy, H. (2001). Extensive projections from the primary auditory cortex and polysensory area STP to peripheral area V1 in the macaque. *The Journal of Neuroscience, 27*, 511–521.

Falchier, A., Clavagnier, S., Barone, P., & Kennedy, H. (2002). Anatomical evidence of multimodal integration in primate striate cortex. *The Journal of Neuroscience, 22*, 5749–5759.

Frissen, I., Bertelson, P., Vroomen, J., & de Gelder, B. (2003). The aftereffects of ventriloquism: Are they sound frequency specific? *Acta Psychologica, 113*, 315–327.

Giard, M. H., & Peronnet, F. (1999). Auditory-visual integration during multimodal object recognition in humans: A behavioural and electrophysiological study. *Journal of Cognitive Neuroscience, 11*, 473–490.

Korte, A. (1915). Kinematoscopische Untersuchungen [Kinematoscopic research]. *Zeitschrift für Psychologie der Sinnesorgane, 72*, 193–296.

Macaluso, E., Frith, C., & Driver, J. (2000). Modulation of human visual cortex by cross-modal spatial attention. *Science, 289*, 1206–1208.

Massaro, D. W. (1998). *Perceiving talking faces: From speech perception to a behavioral principle.* Cambridge: MA: MIT Press.

McDonald, J. J., Teder-Sälejärvi, W. A., Heraldez, D., & Hillyard, S. A. (2001). Electrophysiological evidence for the "missing link" in cross-modal attention. *Canadian Journal of Psychology, 55*, 143–151.

McGurk, H., & MacDonald, J. (1976). Hearing lips and seeing voices. *Nature, 264*, 746–748.

O'Leary, A., & Rhodes, G. (1984). Cross-modal effects on visual and auditory object perception. *Perception & Psychophysics, 35*, 565–569.

Pourtois, G., de Gelder, B., Vroomen, J., Rossion, B., & Crommelink, M. (2000). The time-course of intermodal binding between seeing and hearing affective information. *NeuroReport, 11*, 1329–1333.

Radeau, M. (1994). Auditory-visual spatial interaction and modularity. *Cahiers de Psychologie Cognitive, 13*, 3–51.

Radeau, M., & Bertelson, P. (1974). The after-effects of ventriloquism. *The Quarterly Journal of Experimental Psychology, 26*, 63–71.

Roberts, M., & Summerfield, Q. (1981). Audiovisual presentation demonstrates that selective attention to speech is purely auditory. *Perception & Psychophysics, 30*, 309–314.

Rumelhart, D., & McClelland, J. (1982). An interactive activation model of context effects in letter perception: Part 2. The contextual enhancement effect and some tests and extensions of the model. *Psychological Review, 89*, 60–94.

Shams, L., Kamitani, Y., & Shimojo, S. (2000). What you see is what you hear. *Nature, 408*, 708.

Soroker, N., Calamaro, N., & Myslobodsky, M. S. (1995). Ventriloquism reinstates responsiveness to auditory stimuli in the "ignored" space in patients with hemispatial neglect. *Journal of Clinical and Experimental Neuropsychology, 17*, 243–255.

Spence, C. (2001). Cross-modal attentional capture: A controversy resolved? In C. Folk & B. Gibson (Eds.), *Attention, distraction and action: Multiple perspectives on attentional capture* (pp. 231–262). Amsterdam: Elsevier.

Spence, C., & Driver, J. (1997a). On measuring selective attention to a specific sensory modality. *Perception & Psychophysics, 59*, 389–403.

Spence, C., & Driver, J. (1997b). Audiovisual links in exogenous covert spatial attention. *Perception & Psychophysics, 59*, 1–22.

Spence, C., & Driver, J. (2000). Attracting attention to the illusory location of a sound: Reflexive cross-modal orienting and ventriloquism. *NeuroReport, 11*, 2057–2061.

Stein, B. E., London, N., Wilkinson, L. K., & Price, D. D. (1996). Enhancement of perceived visual intensity by auditory stimuli: A psychophysical analysis. *Journal of Cognitive Neuroscience, 8*, 497–506.

Treisman, A. M., & Gelade, G. (1980). A feature-integration theory of attention. *Cognitive Psychology, 5*, 109–137.

van Noorden, L. P. A. S. (1975). *Temporal coherence in the perception of tone sequences.* Unpublished doctoral dissertation, Technische Hogeschool Eindhoven, The Netherlands.

Vroomen, J., Bertelson, P., & de Gelder, B. (1998). A visual influence in the discrimination of auditory location. *Proceedings of the International Conference on Auditory-Visual Speech Processing (AVSP '98)* (pp. 131–135). Terrigal-Sydney, Australia: Causal Productions.

Vroomen, J., Bertelson, P., & de Gelder, B. (2001a). The ventriloquist effect does not depend on the direction of automatic visual attention. *Perception & Psychophysics, 63*, 651–659.

Vroomen, J., Bertelson, P., & de Gelder, B. (2001b). Directing spatial attention towards the illusory location of a ventriloquized sound. *Acta Psychologica, 108*, 21–33.

Vroomen, J., Bertelson, P., Frissen, I., & de Gelder, B. (2003). *A spatial gradient in the ventriloquism after-effect.* Unpublished manuscript.

Vroomen, J., & de Gelder, B. (2000). Sound enhances visual perception: Cross-modal effects of auditory organisation on vision. *Journal of Experimental Psychology: Human Perception and Performance, 26*, 1583–1590.

Vroomen, J., & de Gelder, B. (2003). Visual motion influences the contingent auditory motion aftereffect. *Psychological Science, 14*, 357–361.

II IS SPEECH A SPECIAL CASE OF MULTISENSORY INTEGRATION?

10 From Multisensory Integration to Talking Heads and Language Learning

DOMINIC W. MASSARO

Introduction

In this handbook of multisensory processes, we learn that perceptual and behavioral outcomes are influenced by simultaneous inputs from several senses. In this chapter, we present theoretical and empirical research on speech perception by eye and ear, and address the question of whether speech is a special case of multisensory processing. Our conclusion is that speech perception is indeed an ideal or prototypical situation in which information from the face and voice is seamlessly processed to impose meaning in face-to-face communication.

Scientists are often intrigued by questions whose answers foreground some striking phenomena. One question about language is whether speech perception is uniquely specialized for processing multisensory information or whether it is simply a prototypical instance of cross-modal processing that occurs in many domains of pattern recognition. Speech is clearly special, at least in the sense that (as of now) only we big-mouthed, biped creatures can talk. Although some chimpanzees have demonstrated remarkable speech perception and understanding of spoken language, they seem to have physiological and anatomical constraints that preclude them from assuming bona fide interlocutor status (Lieberman, 2000; Savage-Rumbaugh, Shanker, & Taylor, 1998). An important item of debate, of course, is whether they also have neurological, cognitive, or linguistic constraints that will prove an impenetrable barrier for language use (Arbib, 2002). We begin with a short description of the idea that speech is special.

Speech is special

Noam Chomsky (1980) envisioned language ability as dependent on an independent language organ (or module), analogous to other organs such as the digestive system. This organ follows an independent course of development in the first years of life and allows the child to achieve a language competence that cannot be elucidated in terms of traditional learning theory. This mental organ, responsible for the human language faculty and language competence, matures and develops with experience, but the mature system does not simply mirror this experience. The language user inherits rule systems of highly specific structure. This innate knowledge allows us to acquire the rules of the language, which cannot be induced from normal language experience because (advocates argue) of the paucity of the language input. The data of language experience are so limited that no process of induction, abstraction, generalization, analogy, or association could account for our observed language competence. Somehow, the universal grammar given by our biological endowment allows the child to learn to use language appropriately without learning many of the formal intricacies of the language. Developmental psychologists, however, are finding that infants are exposed to a rich sample of their mother tongue and are highly influenced by this experience (e.g., Saffran, Johnson, Aslin, & Newport, 1999). Moreover, the frequency and ordering of speech inputs have immediate and strong influences on perceptual processing, and these influences are similar for speech and nonspeech (Aslin, Saffran, & Newport, 1998; Gomez & Gerken, 2000). Linguists are also documenting that the child's language input is not as sparse as the nativists had argued (Pullum & Scholz, 2002).

Although speech has not had a spokesperson as charismatic and as influential as Chomsky, a similar description is given for speech perception. In addition, advocates of the special nature of speech are encouraged by Fodor's (1983) influential proposal of the modularity of mind. Some of our magnificent capabilities result from a set of innate and independent input systems, such as vision, hearing, and language (Fodor, 1983, 2000). Speech-is-special theorists now assume that a specialized biological speech module is responsible for speech perception (Liberman & Mattingly, 1985; Mattingly & Studdert-Kennedy, 1991; Trout, 2001). Given the environmental information, the speech module analyzes this information in terms of possible articulatory sequences of speech segments. The perceiver of speech uses his or her own speech-motor system to achieve speech recognition.

In some ways, it is ironic that multisensory processing should serve as a touchstone for advocates that speech is special, and for articulatory mediation of speech perception. It all began with the McGurk's discovery (McGurk & MacDonald, 1976), which has gained widespread attention in many circles of psychological inquiry and cognitive science. The classic McGurk effect involves the situation in which an auditory /ba/ is paired with a visible /ga/ and the perceiver reports *hearing* /da/. The reverse pairing, an auditory /ga/ and visual /ba/, tends to produce a perceptual judgment of *hearing* /bga/. It was apparently unimaginable at the time that this type of cross-modal influence could occur in other domains. However, as discussed in several chapters in this handbook, multisensory integration is the rule rather than the exception (see Lederman & Klatzky, Chap. 7, this volume; Làdavas & Farnè, Chap. 50, this volume). As an example, both sound and sight contribute to our localization of an event in space, and the visual input can distort our experience, such as when we hear the puppet's voice coming from the puppet rather than the ventriloquist. This similarity to other domains dictates a more general account of sensory fusion and modality-specific experience rather than one unique to speech perception.

It should be noted, however, that the perceiver might have a unimodal experience even though multisensory integration contributed to the experience. This is clearly a nonintuitive outcome, and one requiring explanation. Speech information from the auditory and visual modalities provides a situation in which the brain combines both sources of information to create an interpretation that is easily mistaken for an auditory one. An exactly analogous outcome is found when our perceived taste is influenced by smell, as in the pleasurable taste of coffee accompanied by smell. If the nose is pinched, the taste becomes either indistinguishable or bitter (see Stevenson & Boakes, Chap. 5, this volume). For spoken language, we believe we hear speech, because perhaps audition is the most informative modality for spoken language. A caveat, therefore, is that we cannot trust a modality-specific experience as implying that only that modality played a role.

We present a short review of existing theories of speech perception before turning to relevant empirical evidence. The powerful influence that visible speech has in face-to-face communication speaks to both traditional and current theoretical accounts. The influence of several sources of information from several modalities provides a new challenge for theoretical accounts of speech perception. Most theories were developed to account for the perception of unimodal auditory speech, and it is not always obvious how they would account for the positive contribution of visible speech.

Theories of speech perception

PSYCHOACOUSTIC ACCOUNTS   One class of theory seems to be either contradicted or at least placed outside the domain of bimodal speech perception. Psychoacoustic accounts of speech perception are grounded in the idea that speech is nothing more than a complex auditory signal and its processing can be understood by the psychophysics of complex sounds, without any reference to language-specific processes. This chapter reinforces the conclusion that a psychoacoustic account of speech perception is not sufficient because speech perception is not strictly a function of auditory information. Advocates of the psychoacoustic account have modified their stance accordingly and now acknowledge the influence of visible speech (e.g., Diehl & Kluender, 1987). They have not specified, however, how visible speech makes its contribution, but it would appear that visible speech would somehow have to be secondary to audible speech. If psychoacoustic theorists propose that visible speech need not be secondary in their framework, then we might ask what is uniquely psychoacoustic about it.

MOTOR THEORY   The motor theory assumes that the perceiver uses the sensory input to best determine the set of articulatory gestures that produced this input (Liberman & Mattingly, 1985; Mattingly & Studdert-Kennedy, 1991). The main motivation and support for this theory is that phoneme perception is putatively more easily predicted on the basis of articulation than in terms of acoustic cues. Speech scientists learned that there did not appear to be a one-to-one correspondence between a set of acoustic properties and a phonetic segment. On the other hand, the phonetic segment could be more adequately described in terms of articulation. The best-known example is the difference between /di/ and /du/. The onset of these two syllables has very different acoustic properties in each case but similar articulatory gestures, which involves a constriction of the tongue against the alveolar ridge of the hard palate. The syllables with different vowels differ in their sound even at onset because the consonant and vowel are co-articulated. Thus, motor theory appeared to solve the mapping problem from stimulus to percept by viewing articulation as mediating representation.

According to motor theory, the inadequate auditory input is assessed in terms of the articulation, and it is only natural that visible speech could contribute to this process. The motor theory is consistent with a contribution of visible speech because visible speech can be considered to be an integral part of the sensory input, reflecting the talker's articulatory gestures. In a related proposal, Robert-Ribes, Schwartz, and Escudier (1995) advocate an amodal motor representation to account for the integration of audible and visible speech. The motor theory has not been sufficiently formalized, however, to account for the vast set of empirical findings on the integration of audible and visible speech.

The motor theory found new life in Fodor's notion of modularity, in which an input system operates in an encapsulated manner. Speech perception is viewed as a module with its own unique set of processes and information. The phonetic module has been succinctly described by Liberman (1996, p. 29) as "a distinct system that uses its own kind of signal processing and its own primitives to form a specifically phonetic way of acting and perceiving." This statement seems to imply that not only the information but also the information processing should be qualitatively different in the speech domain than in other domains of perceptual and cognitive functioning. However, that this expectation does not hold up to experimental tests. For example, perceiving emotion from the face and voice follows the same processing algorithm as speech perception.

It is very difficult to determine the representation medium in which integration occurs. There is no reason, however, to postulate a motor representation for integration. Integration occurs in a variety of other domains, such as object recognition, that involve no analogous motor medium.

DIRECT PERCEPTION   In contrast to the motor theory, and consistent with our view, the direct perception theory assumes that speech perception is not special (Fowler, 1996, Chap. 12, this volume). Thus, although gestures are the objects of speech perception, the speech-motor system does not play a role. Furthermore, speech perception is just one of many different perceptual domains in which direct perception occurs. According to direct perception theory, persons directly perceive the causes of sensory input. In spoken language, the cause of an audible-visible speech percept is the vocal tract activity of the talker. Accordingly, it is reasoned that visible speech should influence speech perception because it also reveals the vocal tract activity of the talker. Speech perceivers therefore obtain direct information from integrated perceptual systems from the flow of stimulation provided by the talker (Best, 1993).

The observed influence of visible speech is easily predicted by this theory because visible speech represents another source of stimulation, providing direct information about the gestural actions of the talker. However, we know of no convincing evidence for the gesture as the primary object of speech perception (see Massaro, 1998b, Chap. 11). For now, it seems most parsimonious to assume that the objects of speech perception are relatively abstract symbols (Nearey, 1992).

On the basis of this short review of extant theories of speech perception, it is apparent that they are stated in verbal rather than quantitative form. Although no one can deny that a qualitative fact is more informative than a quantitative one, qualitative theories do not seem to be sufficiently precise to be distinguishable from one another. Very different theories can make similar predictions. Some quantitative refinement of the theories is usually necessary to create a chance for falsification and strong inference (Platt, 1964; Popper, 1959). Therefore, our strategy has been to quantify and test a family of specific models that represent the extant theories and also other reasonable alternatives (Massaro, 1987b, 1998b).

PATTERN RECOGNITION   We envision speech perception as a prototypical instance of pattern recognition. The term *pattern recognition* describes what is commonly meant by recognition, identification, or categorization. Although these terms have different meanings, they are all concerned with roughly the same phenomenon. Recognition means re-cognizing something we experienced previously. Identification involves mapping a unique stimulus into a unique response. Categorization means placing several noticeably different stimuli into the same class. For example, a child perceives a dog, recognizes it as a dog she has seen before, identifies it as Fido, and categorizes it as a dog. Recognition, identification, and categorization appear to be central to perceptual and cognitive functioning (Quinn, 2002). They entail the same fundamental processes to allow a person, given some input, to settle on one of a set of alternative interpretations. Pattern recognition has been found to be fundamental in such different domains as depth perception, playing chess, examining radiographs, and reading text (Quinn, 2002). It involves similar operations regardless of the specific nature of the patterns, the sensory inputs, and the underlying brain structures, and is thus equally appropriate for an informative description of speech perception.

There is a growing consensus that speech perception should be viewed as an instance of a general form of pattern recognition (e.g., Nearey, 1997). To understand speech perception, the researcher need only describe how pattern recognition works in this domain.

Questions include the ecological and functional properties of audible and visible speech, as well as other influences such as top-down constraints on what can occur when and where—that is, those sources of information that influence speech perception. Although there are a variety of frameworks to describe pattern recognition, their similarities far exceed their differences. Reading about one framework will certainly prepare the reader to better understand other frameworks. In this chapter, I will describe speech perception within a specific framework, one that is representative of a prototypical framework for pattern recognition. Central to this framework is the natural ease of cross-modal perception, particularly the value of visible speech when it is presented with auditory speech.

Data without theory are considered by some to be meaningless. As noted earlier, any meaningful theory is most likely to be quantitative and our bias is an empirical and theoretical framework of pattern recognition. Our work has evolved over the last three decades with what we believe to be substantial progress. Various types of model-fitting strategies have been employed in a variety of experimental tests. These model tests have been highly informative about how cross-modal spoken language is perceived and understood. We begin with an experimental study of the processing of unimodal and bimodal speech.

A paradigm for psychological inquiry

We are attracted to bimodal speech perception as a paradigm for psychological inquiry, for several reasons (Massaro & Cohen, 1983). It offers a compelling example of how processing information from one modality (vision) appears to influence our experience in another modality (audition). Second, it provides a unique situation in which multiple modalities appear to be combined or integrated in a natural manner. Third, experimental manipulation of these two sources of information is easily carried out in pattern recognition tasks. Finally, conceptualizing speech as cross-modal has the potential for valuable applications for individuals with hearing loss, persons with language challenges, learners of a new language, and for other domains of language learning.

The study of speech perception by ear and eye has been and continues to be a powerful paradigm for uncovering fundamental properties of the information sources in speech and how speech is perceived and understood. Our general framework documents the value of a combined experimental and theoretical approach. The research has contributed to our understanding of the characteristics used in speech perception, how

speech is perceived and recognized, and the fundamental psychological processes that occur in speech perception and pattern recognition in a variety of other domains.

We believe that our empirical work would be inadequate and perhaps invalid without the corresponding theoretical framework. Thus, the work continues to address both empirical and theoretical issues. At the empirical level, experiments have been carried out to determine how visible speech is used alone and with auditory speech for a broad range of individuals and across a wide variation of situational domains. At the theoretical level, the assumptions and predictions of several models have been analyzed, contrasted, and tested. In addition, a general framework for inquiry and a universal principle of behavior have been proposed, as described in the next section.

Demonstration experiment: Varying the ambiguity of the speech modalities

Most experiments of multimodal speech perception have been carried out in the context of the McGurk effect (McGurk & MacDonald, 1976), a striking demonstration of how visual speech can influence the perceiver's perceptual experience. It has been well over two decades since this effect was first described. The classic McGurk effect involves a situation in which an auditory /ba/ is paired with a visible /ga/ and the perceiver reports hearing /da/. The reverse pairing, an auditory /ga/ and visual /ba/, tends to produce a perceptual judgment of /bga/. Most studies of the McGurk effect, however, use just a few experimental conditions in which the auditory and visual sources of information are made to mismatch. Investigators also sometimes fail to test the unimodal conditions separately, so there is no independent index of the perception of the single modalities. The data analysis is also usually compromised because investigators analyze the data with respect to whether or not there was a McGurk effect, which often is simply taken to mean whether the auditory speech was inaccurately perceived. Investigators also tend to make too few observations under each of the stimulus conditions, which precludes an analysis of individual behavior and limits the analyses to group averages. A better understanding of the McGurk effect will occur when we have a better account of speech perception more generally. Our approach involves enhancing the database and testing formal models of the perceptual process.

An important manipulation is to systematically vary the ambiguity of each of the sources of information in terms of how much it resembles each syllable. Synthetic

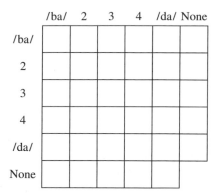

	/ba/	2	3	4	/da/	None
/ba/						
2						
3						
4						
/da/						
None						

FIGURE 10.1 Expansion of a typical factorial design to include auditory and visual conditions presented alone. The five levels along the auditory and visible continua represent auditory and visible speech syllables varying in equal physical steps between /ba/ and /da/.

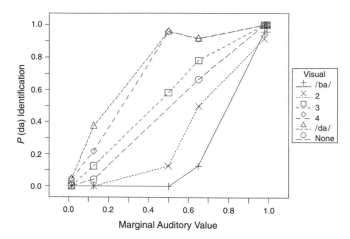

FIGURE 10.2 The points give the observed proportion of /da/ identifications in the unimodal and factorial auditory-visual conditions as a function of the five levels of synthetic auditory and visual speech varying between /ba/ and /da/. The columns of points are placed at a value corresponding to the marginal probability of a /da/ judgment for each auditory level on the independent variable. The auditory-alone conditions are given by the open circles. The unimodal visual condition is plotted at 0.5 (completely neutral) on the auditory scale. Results are for participant 9.

speech (or at least a systematic modification of natural speech) is necessary to implement this manipulation. In a previous experimental task, we used synthetic speech to cross five levels of audible speech varying between /ba/ and /da/ with five levels of visible speech varying between the same alternatives. We also included the unimodal test stimuli to implement the expanded factorial design, as shown in Figure 10.1.

PROTOTYPICAL METHOD   The properties of the auditory stimulus were varied to give an auditory continuum between the syllables /ba/ and /da/. In analogous fashion, properties of our animated face were varied to give a continuum between visual /ba/ and /da/. Five levels of audible speech varying between /ba/ and /da/ were crossed with five levels of visible speech varying between the same alternatives. In addition, the audible and visible speech were presented alone, for a total of 25 + 5 + 5 = 35 independent stimulus conditions. Six random sequences were determined by sampling the 35 conditions without replacement, giving six different blocks of 35 trials. An experimental session consisted of these six blocks, preceded by six practice trials, and with a short break between sessions. There were four sessions of testing, for a total of 840 test trials ($35 \times 6 \times 4$). Thus, there were 24 observations for each of the 35 unique experimental conditions. Participants were instructed to listen to and watch the speaker, and to identify the syllable as /ba/ or /da/. This experimental design was used with 82 participants, and the results of this study have served as a database for testing models of pattern recognition (Massaro, 1998b).

PROTOTYPICAL RESULTS   We call these results prototypical because they are highly representative of many different experiments of this type. The mean observed proportion of /da/ identifications was computed for each of the 82 participants for the 35 unimodal and bimodal conditions. Although it is not feasible to present the results of each of the participants, we will show the outcomes for five different individuals. For this tutorial, we begin with the results for a single participant who can be considered typical of the others in this task.

The points in Figure 10.2 give the observed proportion of /da/ responses for the auditory-alone, the bimodal, and the visual-alone conditions as a function of the five levels of the synthetic auditory and visual speech varying between /ba/ and /da/. Although this plot of the results might seem somewhat intimidating at first glance, a graphical analysis of this kind can facilitate understanding dramatically. It should be noted that the columns of points are spread unevenly along the x-axis, because they are placed at a value corresponding to the marginal probability of a /da/ judgment for each auditory level of the independent variable. This spacing reflects the relative influence of adjacent levels of the auditory condition.

The unimodal auditory curve (indicated by the open circles) shows that the auditory speech had a large influence on the judgments. More generally, the degree of influence of this modality when presented alone would be indicated by the steepness of the response function. The unimodal visual condition is plotted at 0.5 (which is considered to be completely neutral) on the auditory scale. The influence of the visual speech when presented alone is indexed by the vertical spread among the five levels of the visual condition.

The other points give performance for the bimodal conditions. This graphical analysis shows that both the auditory and the visual sources of information had a strong impact on the identification judgments. The likelihood of a /da/ identification increased as the auditory speech changed from /ba/ to /da/, and analogously for the visible speech. The curves across changes in the auditory variable are relatively steep and also spread out from one another with changes in the visual variable. By these criteria, both sources had a large influence in the bimodal conditions.

Finally, the auditory and visual effects were not additive in the bimodal condition, as demonstrated by a significant auditory-visual interaction. The interaction is indexed by the change in the spread among the curves across changes in the auditory variable. This vertical spread between the curves is about four times greater in the middle than at the end of the auditory continuum. It means that the influence of one source of information is greatest when the other source is neutral or ambiguous. We now address how the two sources of information are used in perception.

EVALUATION OF HOW TWO SOURCES ARE USED   Of course, an important question is how the two sources of information are used in perceptual recognition. An analysis of several results informs this question. Figure 10.3 gives the results for another participant in the task. Three points are circled in the figure to highlight the conditions in which the second level of auditory information is paired with the fifth (/da/) level of visual information. When presented alone, $P(/da/ \mid A_2)$ is about 0.25, whereas $P(/da/ \mid V_5)$ is about 0.8. When these two stimuli occur together, $P(/da/ \mid A_2 V_5)$ is about 0.6. This subset of results is consistent with just about any theoretical explanation, for example, one in which only a single source of information is used on a given trial. Similarly, a simple averaging of the audible and visible speech predicts this outcome.

Other observations, however, allow us to reject these alternatives. Figure 10.4 gives the results for yet another participant in the task. Three points are circled in the figure to highlight the conditions in which the second level of auditory information is paired with the second level of visual information. Recall that in this forced-choice task, $P(/ba/)$ is equal to $1 - P(/da/)$. When presented alone, $P(/ba/ \mid A_3)$ and $P(/ba/ \mid V_1)$ are both about 0.75. When these two stimuli occur together, $P(/ba/ \mid A_3 V_1)$ is about 9. This so-called superadditive result (the bimodal response is more extreme than

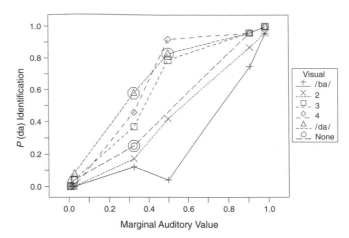

FIGURE 10.3   The points give the observed proportion of /da/ identifications in the unimodal and factorial auditory-visual conditions as a function of the five levels of synthetic auditory and visual speech varying between /ba/ and /da/. The columns of points are placed at a value corresponding to the marginal probability of a /da/ judgment for each auditory level on the independent variable. The auditory-alone conditions are given by the open circles. The unimodal visual condition is plotted at 0.5 (completely neutral) on the auditory scale. Results are for participant 41. The lines are drawn through the observed points. The three large-circled points $A_2 V_5$ give two unimodal conditions and the corresponding bimodal condition. The relationship among the three points can be explained by the use of a single modality, a weighted averaging of the two sources, or a multiplicative integration of the two sources.

either unimodal response proportion) does not seem to be easily explained by either the use of a single modality or a simple averaging of the two sources. In order to evaluate theoretical alternatives, however, formal models must be proposed and tested against all of the results, not just selected conditions. We now formalize two competing models and test them against the results.

TESTS OF COMPETING MODELS   To explain pattern recognition, representations in memory are an essential component. The current stimulus input has to be compared to the pattern recognizer's memory of previous patterns. One type of memory is a set of summary descriptions of the meaningful patterns. These summary descriptions are called prototypes, and they contain a description of features of the pattern. The features of the prototype correspond to the ideal values that an exemplar should have if it is a member of that category. To recognize a speech segment, the evaluation process assesses the input information relative to the prototypes in memory.

Given this general theoretical framework, we consider whether or not integration of auditory and visual speech occurs. It might seem obvious that integration

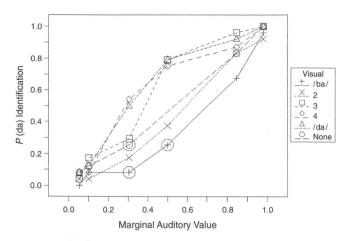

FIGURE 10.4 The points give the observed proportion of /da/ identifications in the unimodal and factorial auditory-visual conditions as a function of the five levels of synthetic auditory and visual speech varying between /ba/ and /da/. The columns of points are placed at a value corresponding to the marginal probability of a /da/ judgment for each auditory level on the independent variable. The auditory-alone conditions are given by the open circles. The unimodal visual condition is plotted at 0.5 (completely neutral) on the auditory scale. Results are for participant 25. The lines are drawn through the observed points. The three large-circled points A_3V_1 give two unimodal conditions and the corresponding bimodal condition. The relationship among the three points *cannot* be explained by the use of a single modality or a weighted averaging of the two sources, but it can be described by a multiplicative integration of the two sources.

occurred in our experiment because there were strong effects of both auditory and visual speech. In fact, this outcome is logically possible even if integration did not occur. Most experiments using the McGurk effect paradigm were not able to demonstrate conclusively that integration occurred. It is possible, for example, that only the visual speech was used and simply dominated the judgments on some of the trials. This type of nonintegration is the simpler account of pattern recognition, and we begin with a formalization of this type of model.

Nonintegration models of bimodal speech perception

According to nonintegration models, any perceptual experience results from only a single sensory influence. Thus the pattern recognition of any cross-modal event is determined by only one of the modalities, even though the influential modality might vary. Although this class of models involves a variety of alternatives that are worthy of formulation and empirical testing (see Massaro, 1998b), we will formulate and test just one for illustrative purposes.

SINGLE-CHANNEL MODEL Although there are multiple inputs, it is possible that only one of them is used. This idea is in the tradition of selective attention theories according to which only a single channel of information can be processed at any one time (Pashler, 1998). According to the single-channel model, only one of the two sources of information determines the response on any given trial. Given a unimodal stimulus, it is assumed that the response is determined by the presented modality. A unimodal auditory stimulus will be identified as /da/ with probability a_i, and, analogously, the unimodal visual stimulus will be identified as /da/ with probability v_j. The value i simply indexes the ith level along the auditory continuum and j indexes the level of the visual input.

Given that only one of the auditory and visual inputs can be used on any bimodal trial, it is assumed that the auditory modality is selected with some bias probability p, and the visual modality with bias $1 - p$. If only one modality is used, it is reasonable to assume that it will be processed exactly as it is on unimodal trials. In this case, for a given bimodal stimulus, the auditory information will be identified as /da/ with probability a_i, and the visual information with probability v_j. Thus, the predicted probability of a /da/ response given the ith level of the auditory stimulus, a_i, and the jth level of the visual stimulus, v_j, is

$$P(/\mathrm{da}/ \mid A_iV_j) = pa_i + \{(1 - p)v_j\} \qquad (1)$$

Equation 1 predicts that a /da/ response can come about in two ways: (1) the auditory input is selected and is identified as /da/, or (2) the visual input is selected and is identified as /da/. This formalization of the single-channel model assumes a fixed p across all conditions, an a_i value that varies with the auditory information, and a v_j value that varies with the visual information.

We can assess the predictive power of the single-channel model and other models using the 5×5 expanded factorial design. The points in Figure 10.5 gives the proportion of /da/ identifications for another prototypical participant in the task. Figure 10.5 also shows the predictions of the single-channel model, as represented by Equation 1. Equation 1 is a linear function and it predicts a set of parallel functions with this type of plot. The equation and graph illustrate how a constant increase in a_i and v_j leads to a constant increase in $P(/\mathrm{da}/)$. The mismatch between the observations and predictions illustrates that this model appears to be inadequate. Even so, a formal test is required. Before we present this test of the single-channel model, it is necessary to discuss estimation of the free parameters in a model.

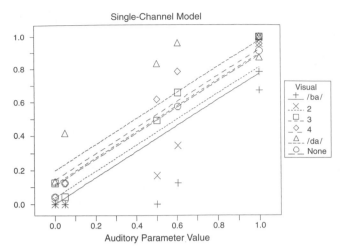

FIGURE 10.5 The points give the observed proportion of /da/ identifications in the unimodal and factorial auditory-visual conditions as a function of the five levels of synthetic auditory and visual speech varying between /ba/ and /da/. The columns of points are placed at a value corresponding to the marginal probability of a /da/ judgment for each auditory level on the independent variable. The auditory-alone conditions are given by the open circles. The unimodal visual condition is plotted at 0.5 (completely neutral) on the auditory scale. Results are for participant 7. The lines give the predictions of the single-channel model, with an RMSD of 0.115.

Testing a model's predictions

We cannot expect a model's predictions of behavior to be exact or even very accurate without first taking into account what results are being predicted. As an example, we cannot know exactly how often a given person will identify one of the visible speech syllables as a particular alternative. As can be seen in a comparison of Figures 10.2, 10.3, and 10.4, individual participants give similar but not identical results for the same experiment. We can know that one syllable might be more likely to be identified as /ba/, but we cannot predict ahead of time the actual probability of a /ba/ response by an individual participant. This uncertainty would preclude the quantitative test of models if we were not able to determine (estimate) the values of free parameters.

FREE PARAMETERS AND THEIR ESTIMATION   When applied to empirical data, most computational or quantitative descriptions have a set of free parameters. A free parameter in a model is a variable whose values cannot be exactly predicted in advance. We do not know what these values are, and we must use the observed results given to find them. The actual performance of the participant is used to set the value of this variable. This process is called parameter estimation.

In parameter estimation, we use our observations of behavior to estimate the values of the free parameters of the model being tested. Because we want to give every model its best shot, the goal is to find the values of the parameters that maximize how accurately the model is able to account for the results. The optimal parameter values can be found with an iterative search algorithm to find those parameter values that minimize the differences between the predicted and observed results. The parameters and parameter space must be specified for the search. In the single-channel model, for example, the parameters are p, a_i, and v_j. These values are probabilities and thus must be between 0 and 1.

Equation 1 predicts $P(/da/)$ for each of the 35 conditions in the expanded factorial experiment. The single-channel model does not predict in advance how often the syllable in each modality will be identified as /ba/ or /da/. According to the model, there can be a unique value of a_i for each unique level of audible speech. Similarly, there can be a unique value of v_j for each level of visual speech. We also do not know the value of p on bimodal trials, which requires another free parameter. For unimodal trials, we assume that the presented modality is always used. We have 35 equations with 11 free parameters: the p value, the five a_i values, and the five v_j values. Finding values for these 11 unknowns allows us to predict the 35 observations.

RMSD MEASURE OF GOODNESS OF FIT   A measure that is often used to maximize the goodness of fit is the root mean squared deviation (RMSD) between the predicted and observed values. The best fit is that which gives the minimal RMSD. The RMSD is computed by (1) squaring the difference between each predicted and observed value, (2) summing across all conditions, (3) taking the mean, and (4) taking the square root of this mean. (Squaring the differences makes all differences positive and also magnifies large deviations compared to small ones.) The RMSD can be thought of as a standard deviation of the differences between the 35 predicted and observed values. The RMSD would increase as the differences increase. In general, the smaller the RMSD value, the better the fit of the model.

The quantitative predictions of the model are determined by using any minimization routine such as the program STEPIT (Chandler, 1969). The model is represented to the program in terms of a set of prediction equations and a set of unknown parameters. By iteratively adjusting the parameters of the model, the program maximizes the accuracy of the predictions by minimizing the RMSD. The outcome is a set of parameter values which, when put into the model, come closest to predicting the observed results.

DATABASE AND MODEL TESTS   The results for the present model tests come from the results from 82 participants, with 24 observations from each participant under each of the 35 conditions (Massaro, 1998b). The model fit was carried out separately on each participant's results. We have learned that individuals differ from one another, and that averaging the results across individuals can be hazardous. The free parameters of a model should be capable of handling the individual differences. Fitting a model to single individuals should permit the model to describe individual participants while also accounting for between-participant differences, insofar as they can be captured by the differences among the 11 parameters.

The observations and predictions of the single-channel model for a representative participant are given in Figure 10.5. The data points in the figure are the observations, and the lines correspond to the model predictions. We use lines for the predictions so that one can see the form of a model's predictions. The distance between the observed points and these predictions gives a graphical measure of goodness of fit. The predictions of the single-channel model do not capture the trends in the data. The predictions are a set of parallel lines, whereas the observations resemble an American football, wide in the middle and narrowing at the ends.

The RMSD is also used to evaluate the goodness of fit of a model both in absolute terms and in comparison to other models. Of course, the smaller the RMSD, the better the fit of a model. The RMSD for the fit of the single-channel model for the participant shown in Figure 10.5 was 0.15. The RMSDs for the fit of the single-channel model across all 82 participants averaged 0.097. We now formalize an integration model, called the fuzzy logical model of perception.

The fuzzy logical model of perception

The fuzzy logical model of perception (FLMP) is shown in Figure 10.6. Let us consider the case in which the perceiver is watching the face and listening to the speaker. Although both the visible and the audible speech signals are processed, each source is evaluated independently of the other source. The evaluation process consists in determining how much that source supports various alternatives. The integration process combines these sources and outputs how much their combination supports the various alternatives. The perceptual outcome for the perceiver will be a function of the relative degree of support among the competing alternatives.

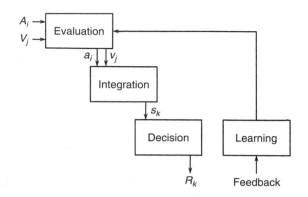

FIGURE 10.6   Schematic representation of the three processes involved in perceptual recognition. The three processes are shown left to right in time to illustrate their necessarily successive but overlapping processing. These processes make use of prototypes stored in long-term memory. The sources of information are represented by uppercase letters. Auditory information is represented by A_i and visual information by V_j. The evaluation process transforms these sources of information into psychological values (indicated by lowercase letters a_i and v_j). These sources are then integrated to give an overall degree of support, s_k, for each speech alternative k. The decision operation maps the outputs of integration into some response alternative, R_k. The response can take the form of a discrete decision or a rating of the degree to which the alternative is likely. The learning process receives feedback, which is assumed to tune the prototypical values of the features used by the evaluation process.

More generally, multiple sources of information contribute to the identification and interpretation of the language input. The assumptions central to the model are (1) each source of information is evaluated to give the continuous degree to which that source specifies various alternatives, (2) the sources of information are evaluated independently of one another, (3) the sources are integrated multiplicatively to provide an overall degree of support for each alternative, and (4) perceptual identification and interpretation follows the relative degree of support among the alternatives. The quantitative predictions of the FLMP have been derived and formalized in a number of different publications (e.g., Massaro, 1987a, 1998). In a two-alternative task with /ba/ and /da/ alternatives, the degree of auditory support for /da/ can be represented by a_i, and the support for /ba/ by $(1 - a_i)$. Similarly, the degree of visual support for /da/ can be represented by v_j, and the support for /ba/ by $(1 - v_j)$. The probability of a response to the unimodal stimulus is simply equal to its feature value. The predicted probability of a /da/ response given an auditory input, $P(/\text{da}/ \mid A_i)$, is equal to

$$P(/\text{da}/ \mid A_i) = \frac{a_i}{a_i + (1 - a_i)} = a_i \qquad (2)$$

Similarly, the predicted probability of a /da/ response given a visual input, $P(/\text{da}/ \mid V_j)$, is equal to

$$P(/\text{da}/ \mid V_j) = \frac{v_j}{v_j + (1 - v_j)} = v_j \qquad (3)$$

For bimodal trials, the predicted probability of a /da/ response given auditory and visual inputs, $P(/\text{da}/ \mid A_iV_j)$, is equal to

$$P(/\text{da}/ \mid A_iV_j) = \frac{a_iv_j}{a_iv_j + (1 - a_i)(1 - v_j)} \qquad (4)$$

Equations 2–4 assume independence between the auditory and visual sources of information. Independence of sources at the evaluation stage is motivated by the principle of category-conditional independence (Massaro, 1998b; Massaro & Stork, 1998). Given that it is not possible to predict the evaluation of one source on the basis of the evaluation of another, the independent evaluation of both sources is necessary to make an optimal category judgment. Although the sources are kept separate at evaluation, they are integrated to achieve perception, recognition, and interpretation. The FLMP assumes multiplicative integration, which yields a measure of total support for a given category identification. This operation, implemented in the model, allows the combination of two imperfect sources of information to yield better performance than would be possible using either source by itself. However, the output of integration is an absolute measure of support; it must be relativized, which is effected through a decision stage, which divides the support for one category by the summed support for all categories.

UNDERLYING NEURAL MECHANISM   A natural question is, what is the neural mechanism postulated by the integration algorithm specified in the FLMP? An important set of observations from single-cell recordings in the cat could be interpreted in terms integration of the form specified by the FLMP (Stein & Meredith, 1993; see also Stein, Jiang, & Stanford, Chap. 15, this volume; Meredith, Chap. 21, this volume). A single hissing sound or a light spot can activate neurons in the superior colliculus. A much more vigorous response is produced, however, when both signals are simultaneously presented from the same location. This result parallels the outcomes we have observed in unimodal and bimodal speech perception.

As shown elsewhere, the FLMP is mathematically equivalent to Bayes' theorem (Massaro, 1998b, Chap. 4). Anastasio and Patton (Chap. 16, this volume) propose that the brain can implement a computation analogous to Bayes' rule, and that the response of a neuron in the superior colliculus is proportional to the posterior probability that a target is present in its receptive fields, given its sensory input. The authors also assume that the visual and auditory inputs are conditionally independent, given the target. This implies that the visibility of the target indicates nothing about the audibility of the target, and vice versa. This assumption corresponds to our assumption of category-conditional independence. They show that the target-present posterior probability computed from the impulses from the auditory and visual neurons is higher given the sensory inputs of two modalities than it is given the input of only one modality. In addition, when only one modality is activated, the target-present posterior probability computed from the impulses from the auditory and visual neurons is less than the modality-specific posterior probability from the activated modality.

In light of the value of neurons that evaluate input from several modalities, Anatasio and Patton ask why not all neurons have this property. The answer is that inputs from two modalities can actually produce more uncertainty than an input from just one of the modalities. This situation occurs when one of the inputs has very little resolution, which can degrade their joint occurrence. We have observed similar results, particularly in the perception of emotion, in which adding information from the voice and information from the face can actually decrease accurate identification relative to achieved with information from the face alone.

Bernstein, Auer, and Moore (Chap. 13, this volume) distinguish whether speech perception is best described by convergence or by an association of modality-specific speech representations. These two alternatives bear some similarity to two of the three alternatives that I have proposed as possible mechanisms for the joint influence of audible and visible speech (Massaro, 1998b; 1999). These alternatives are shown in Figure 10.7. Bernstein et al. claim that the FLMP might be interpreted as claiming convergent integration. In my

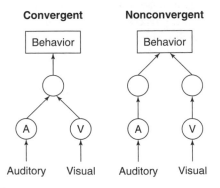

FIGURE 10.7   Neural representations of convergent integration and nonconvergent integration.

discussion of these alternatives (Massaro, 1999), I indicated that "convergent integration offers a potential implementation of the FLMP" but did not mean to imply that I favored this type of integration over nonconvergent integration. In fact, I observed that nonconvergent integration "was most consistent with the findings," findings that we review later in this chapter under the heading The Relationship Between Identification and Discrimination.

When considering the important relationship between psychological models like the FLMP and underlying neural mechanisms, we must keep in mind that information-processing algorithms will not be easily observable in the underlying hardware. As I have stated elsewhere, "Only biology is found in living systems, not algorithms . . . a biological explanation cannot represent and therefore replace the algorithm. Biology is only biology. Similarly, we do not expect to find our law of pattern recognition in the brain. We expect to observe only chemical and electrical activity, not the algorithm itself. Of course, this activity can be interpreted in different ways" (Massaro, 1998b, p. 105).

Before addressing the issue of neural mechanism, a couple of attributes of the FLMP should be emphasized. The FLMP takes a strong stance on the question of discrete versus continuous information processing (Massaro, 1989, 1996). Information input to a stage or output from a stage is continuous rather than discrete. Furthermore, the transmission of information from one stage to the next is assumed to occur continuously rather than discretely. The three processes shown in Figure 10.6 are offset to emphasize their temporal overlap. Evaluated information is passed continuously to integration while additional evaluation is taking place. Although it is logically the case that some evaluation must occur before integration can proceed, the processes are assumed to overlap in time. Similarly, integrated information is continuously made available to the decision process.

It is important to emphasize that information transmitted from one stage to another does not obliterate the information from the earlier stage. Thus, evaluation maintains its information even while simultaneously passing it forward to the integration process. There is evidence that information can be maintained in memory at multiple levels and in various forms. As observed by Mesulam (1998) in a review of the neural underpinnings of sensation to cognition, "[in the] transfer of information . . . , several (synaptic) levels remain active as the pertinent information is conveyed from one node to the other" (Mesulam, 1998, p. 1041). This parallel storage of information does not negate the sequential stage model in Figure 10.6. What is important to

remember is that transfer of information from one stage to another does not require that the information be lost from the earlier stage. Integrating auditory and visual speech does not necessarily compromise or modify the information at the evaluation stage. Thus, given that multiple representations can exist in parallel, there may be both convergence and association operative in the perception of auditory-visual speech. There appears to be strong neural evidence for two types of processes: (i) "the establishment, by local neuronal groups, of convergent cross-modal associations related to a target event; and (ii) the formation of a directory pointing to the distributed sources of information" (Mesulam, 1998, p. 1024). These can be interpreted to correspond to convergent and nonconvergent integration (association), respectively. We believe that the FLMP algorithm can be implemented by both of these neural mechanisms. It might be the case that auditory-visual speech processing follows only nonconvergent integration, but there are other domains such as localizing an event given sound and sight that follow convergent integration (see Anastasio & Patton, Chap. 16, this volume; Meredith, Chap. 21, this volume).

We do not really know how well the single-channel model performs without contrasting it with other models. We favor the FLMP, which is an integration model. The FLMP was fitted to these same results, using Equations 2–4 with ten free parameters. Like the single-channel model, the FLMP also requires five a_i and five v_j values. In the FLMP, however, these are not probabilities but fuzzy truth values between 0 and 1 indicating the degree to which the information supports the alternative /da/ (see Equations 2–4). The RMSD for the fit of the FLMP for the participant shown in Figure 10.8 was 0.051, and the RMSDs for the fit of the FLMP for the 82 individual participants averaged 0.051.

As in all areas of scientific inquiry, it is important to replicate this task under a broader set of conditions. These basic findings hold up under a variety of experimental conditions (Massaro, 1998b, Chap. 6). In one case participants were given just two alternatives, and in the other the same participants were allowed an open-ended set of alternatives. When tested against the results, the FLMP gives a good description of performance, even with the constraint that the same parameter values are used to describe performance when the number of response alternatives is varied (see Massaro, 1998b, pp. 265–268).

We have explored alternative methods of model testing. The first involves the match between the goodness of fit of a model and a benchmark measure that indexes what the goodness of fit should be if indeed the model was correct. Because of sampling variability, we cannot

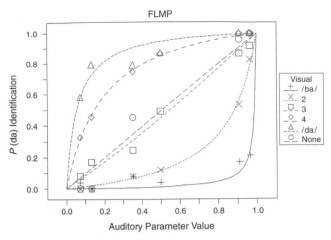

FIGURE 10.8 The points give the observed proportion of /da/ identifications in the unimodal and factorial auditory-visual conditions as a function of the five levels of synthetic auditory and visual speech varying between /ba/ and /da/. The columns of points are placed at a value corresponding to the marginal probability of a /da/ judgment for each auditory level on the independent variable. The auditory-alone conditions are given by the open circles. The unimodal visual condition is plotted at 0.5 (completely neutral) on the auditory scale. Results are for participant 30. The lines give the predictions of the FLMP, with an RMSD of 0.051.

expect a model to give a perfect description of the results. Second, we have used a model selection procedure, Bayes' factor, suggested by Myung and Pitt (1997; Massaro, Cohen, Campbell, & Rodriguez, 2001). The advantage of the FLMP over the single-channel model and other competing models holds up under these alternative procedures of model testing (Massaro, 1998b, Chap. 10; Massaro et al., 2001). Thus, the validity of the FLMP holds up under even more demanding methods of model selection.

As in all things, there is no holy grail of model evaluation for scientific inquiry. As elegantly concluded by Myung and Pitt (1997), the use of judgment is central to model selection. Extending their advice, we propose that investigators should make use of as many techniques as feasible to provide converging evidence for the selection of one model over another. More specifically, both RMSD and Bayes' factor can be used as independent metrics of model selection. Inconsistent outcomes should provide a strong caveat about the validity of selecting one model over another, in the same way that conflicting sources of information create an ambiguous speech event for the perceiver.

BROADENING THE DOMAIN OF INQUIRY We have broadened our domain of inquiry in several directions. The first direction involves the development of a framework for understanding individual differences. One of the

first impressions a researcher obtains is how differently individuals perform on the same experimental task. This variability is not surprising once we consider that each of us has unique life histories and genetics. With the FLMP framework, however, we are able to make a distinction between *information* and *information processing*. The sources of information from the auditory and visual channels make contact with the perceiver at the evaluation stage of processing. The reduction in uncertainty effected by each source is defined as information. In the fit of the FLMP, for example, the parameter values (a_i's and v_j's) indicating the degree of support for each alternative from each modality correspond to information. These parameter values represent how informative each source of information is. Information processing refers to how the sources of information are processed. In the FLMP, this processing is described by the evaluation, integration, and decision stages.

Once individual variability is accounted for, by estimating free parameters in the fit of the model, we are able to provide a convincing description of how the information is processed and mapped into a response. Although we cannot predict a priori how /ba/-like a particular audible or visible speech syllable is for a given individual, we can predict how these two sources of information are integrated and a decision is made. In addition, the model does take a stand on the evaluation process in the sense that it is assumed that the auditory and visual sources of information are evaluated independently of one another.

Our research has made important progress by analyzing the results of individual participants rather than averaging the data. As is well known, it is possible that the average results of an experiment do not reflect the results of any individual making up that average. Our research has adapted the sophisticated methodology developed in psychophysics and the theory of signal detection to provide a framework for the study of individual participants (Massaro, 1998b).

Given this framework, we have explored a broad variety of dimensions of individual variability in terms of the distinction between information and information processing. These include (1) life span variability, (2) language variability, (3) sensory impairment, (4) brain trauma, (5) personality, (6) sex differences, and (7) experience and learning. The methodology of a set of cross-linguistic experiments allowed us to separate information differences from information-processing differences. Earlier cross-linguistic results had led investigators to conclude that the *processing* of bimodal speech differed for Japanese and English speakers. Although the results of experiments with native English, Spanish, Japanese, and Dutch speakers showed substantial differences in performance across the different languages (Massaro, Cohen, Gesi, & Heredia, 1993; Massaro, Cohen, & Smeele, 1995), application of the FLMP indicated that these differences could be completely accounted for by information differences, with no differences in information processing. The information in a speech segment made available by the evaluation process naturally differs for speakers of different languages, whereas the information processing appears to be invariant. The differences that are observed are primarily the different speech categories used by the different linguistic groups, which can be attributed to differences in the phonemic repertoires, phonetic realizations of the syllables, and phonotactic constraints in these different languages. In addition, speakers of different languages are similarly influenced by visible speech, with its contribution larger to the extent the other source is ambiguous. The details of these judgments are nicely captured in the predictions of the FLMP.

A second direction of our research concerns ecological variability, which refers to different perceptual and cognitive situations involving pattern recognition and to variations in the task itself. Generally, we have asked to what extent the processes uncovered in bimodal speech perception generalize across (1) sensory modalities, (2) environmental domains, (3) test items, (4) behavioral measures, (5) instructions, and (6) tasks.

Pursuing the question of whether our model of pattern recognition is valid across different domains, we examined how emotion is perceived, given the facial and vocal cues of a speaker (Massaro, 1998b; Massaro & Egan, 1996). Three levels of facial affect were presented using a computer-generated face. Three levels of vocal affect were obtained by recording the voice of a male amateur actor who spoke a semantically neutral word in different simulated emotional states. These two independent variables were presented to participants of the experiment in all possible permutations, i.e., visual cues alone, vocal cues alone and visual and vocal cues together, which gave a total set of 15 stimuli. The participants were asked to judge the emotion of the stimuli in a two-alternative forced-choice task (either HAPPY or ANGRY).

The results indicate that participants evaluated and integrated information from both modalities to perceive emotion. The influence of one modality was greater to the extent that the other was ambiguous (neutral). The FLMP fitted the judgments significantly better than an additive model, which weakens theories based on an additive combination of modalities, categorical perception, and influence from only a single modality. Similar results have been found in other laboratories (see de Gelder, Vroomen, & Pourtois,

Chap. 36, this volume). The perception of emotion appears to be well described by our theoretical framework. Analogous to speech perception, we find a synergistic relationship between the face and the voice. Messages communicated by both of the modalities are usually more informative than messages communicated by either one alone (Massaro, 1998b).

A UNIVERSAL PRINCIPLE In the course of our research, we have developed a universal principle of perceptual cognitive performance to explain pattern recognition (Campbell, Schwarzer, & Massaro, 2001; Massaro, 1998b; Massaro et al., 2001). Animals are influenced by multiple sources of information in a diverse set of situations. In multisensory texture perception, for example, there appears to be no fixed sensory dominance by vision or haptics, and the bimodal presentation yields higher accuracy than either of the unimodal conditions (see Lederman & Klatzky, Chap. 7, this volume). In many cases, these sources of information are ambiguous and any particular source alone does not usually specify completely the appropriate interpretation. According to the FLMP, the perceiver evaluates these multiple sources of information in parallel and determines the degree to which each source supports various interpretations. The sources are then integrated to derive the overall support for each alternative interpretation. Finally, the relative support for each alternative determines the perceptual judgment. Parenthetically, it should be emphasized that these processes are not necessarily conscious or under deliberate control.

ADVANTAGES OF BIMODAL SPEECH PERCEPTION There are several reasons why the use of auditory and visual information together is so successful and why it holds so much promise for educational applications such as language tutoring. These reasons include (1) the robustness of visual speech, (2) the complementarity of auditory and visual speech, and (3) the optimal integration of these two sources of information.

Empirical findings show that speech-reading, or the ability to obtain speech information from the face, is robust. Perceivers are fairly good at speech-reading even when they are not looking directly at the speaker's lips. Furthermore, accuracy is not dramatically reduced when the facial image is blurred (because of poor vision, for example), when the face is viewed from above, below, or in profile, or when there is a large distance between the speaker and the viewer (Jordan & Sergeant, 2000; Massaro, 1998a; see also Munhall & Vatikiotis-Bateson, Chap. 11, this volume). These findings indicate that speech-reading is highly functional in a variety of nonoptimal situations.

Another example of the robustness of the influence of visible speech is that people naturally integrate visible speech with audible speech even when the temporal occurrence of the two sources is displaced by about a $\frac{1}{5}$ of a second. Given that light and sound travel at different speeds and that the dynamics of their corresponding sensory systems also differ, a cross-modal integration must be relatively immune to small temporal asynchronies. To assess the robustness of the integration process across relatively small temporal asynchronies, the relative onset time of the audible and visible sources was systematically varied (Massaro & Cohen, 1993). In the first experiment, bimodal syllables composed of the auditory and visible syllables /ba/ and /da/ were presented at five different onset asynchronies. The second experiment replicated the same procedure but with the vowels /i/ and /u/. The results indicated that perceivers integrated the two sources at asynchronies of 200 ms or less.

More recently, two experiments were carried out to study whether integration would be disrupted by differences in the temporal arrival of the two sources of information (Massaro, Cohen, & Smeele, 1996). Synthetic visible speech and natural and synthetic auditory speech were used to create the syllables /ba/, /va/, /tha/, and /da/. An expanded factorial design was used to present all possible combinations of the auditory and visual syllables, as well as the unimodal syllables. The tests of formal models made it possible to determine when integration of audible and visible speech did occur. The FLMP, an additive model, and an auditory dominance model were tested. The FLMP gave the best description of the results when the temporal arrival of the two sources of information was within 250 ms. Results indicated that integration was not severely disrupted with asynchronies of 250 ms or less. These results are in agreement with similar experiments reviewed by Munhall and Vatikiotis-Bateson (Chap. 11, this volume). The findings support the conclusion that integration of auditory and visual speech is a robust process and is not easily precluded by offsetting the temporal occurrence of the two sources of information.

Complementarity of auditory and visual information simply means that one of the sources is more informative in those cases in which the other is weaker. Because of this, a speech distinction is differentially supported by the two sources of information. That is, two segments that are robustly conveyed in one modality are relatively ambiguous in the other modality. For example, the difference between /ba/ and /da/ is easy to see but relatively difficult to hear. On the other hand, the difference between /ba/ and /pa/ is relatively easy to hear but very difficult to discriminate visually. The fact that two sources of information are complementary makes their combined use much more informative than would be the case if the two sources were noncomplementary or redundant (Massaro, 1998b, Chap. 14).

The final characteristic is that perceivers combine or integrate the auditory and visual sources of information in an optimally efficient manner (Massaro, 1987b; Massaro & Stork, 1998). There are many possible ways to treat two sources of information: use only the most informative source, average the two sources together, or integrate them in such a fashion that both sources are used but the less ambiguous source has the greater influence. Perceivers in fact integrate the information available from each modality to perform as efficiently as possible.

One might question why perceivers integrate several sources of information when just one of them might be sufficient. Most of us do reasonably well in communicating over the telephone, for example. Part of the answer might be grounded in our ontogeny. Integration might be so natural for adults even when information from just one sense would be sufficient because, during development, there was much less information from each sense, and therefore integration was all the more critical for accurate performance (see Lewkowicz & Kraebel, Chap. 41, this volume).

Additional tests of the fuzzy logical model of perception

Perceivers who are hard of hearing obviously have less auditory information, but we can also ask whether they differ in terms of information processing. We can ask whether the integration process works the same way regardless of the degree of hearing loss. By comparing individuals using hearing aids to those with cochlear implants, we can also address information and information-processing questions in terms of the nature of the assistive device. For example, it is possible that integration of the two modalities is more difficult with cochlear implants than with hearing aids. It should be noted that addressing this question does not depend on controlling for individual characteristics such as the level of hearing loss, when it occurred, how long it has persisted, when the hearing aid or implant was received, and so on. Given our distinction between information and information processing within the FLMP framework, we can address the nature of information processing across the inevitable differences that will necessarily exist among the individuals in the study.

STUDY OF CHILDREN WITH HEARING LOSS   Erber (1972) tested three populations of children (adolescents and

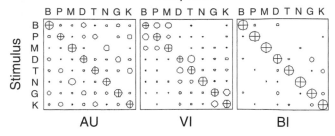

Response

Figure 10.9 Confusion matrix for children with severely impaired (SI) hearing. The area of the circle is proportional to response probability. The results should be interpreted as both the observations and the predictions of the FLMP because they were essentially equivalent to one another; small differences are not noticeable in this type of plot.

young teenagers): normal hearing (NH), severely impaired (SI), and profoundly deaf (PD). All of the children with hearing loss had sustained the loss before the acquisition of speech and language. They also had extensive experience with hearing aids, had at least four years of experience with the oral method of cross-modal speech perception, and used their hearing-assisted devices during the test. None of the children with normal hearing had any training in speech-reading. The test consisted of a videotape of the eight consonants /b, d, g, k, m, n, p, t/ spoken in a bisyllabic context /aCa/, where C refers to one of the eight consonants. It is important to note that the speaker's face was intensely illuminated so that the inside of the oral cavity was visible. The test was presented under auditory, visual, and bimodal conditions.

The results for the SI group under the three presentation conditions are shown in Figure 10.9 in the form of confusion matrices. These data are not as overwhelming as they might seem at first glance. The confusion matrix provides for each of the eight stimuli the proportions of each of the eight possible responses. Although the SI group made many errors on the auditory speech, participants revealed a tremendous performance in the bimodal condition relative to either of the unimodal conditions.

The FLMP was applied to the results of all three groups and gave an excellent description of the confusion errors of all three groups of children. The predicted values are not plotted in Figure 10.9 because they would not be noticeably different from the observed. Or equivalently, one can say that the predictions are also plotted but they are perceptually identical to the observations. Erber's results also reveal a strong complementarity between the audible and visible modalities in speech, which is discussed more fully in Massaro (1998b, Chap. 14).

STUDY OF ADULTS WITH HEARING LOSS   Many individuals with hearing aids (HAs) or cochlear implants (CIs) are able to understand auditory speech. In a substantial number of cases, however, neither device provides a sufficiently rich information source. We also know too well that visible speech does not transmit the complete linguistic message. The synergy between two (degraded) channels, however, offers the potential for a robust communication environment for these individuals with one of these two assistive devices. Solid evidence for this conclusion comes from a study by Agelfors (1996). She studied persons with HAs and CIs in several speech tests under auditory, visual, and bimodal presentations. One test involved the identification of 16 Swedish consonants presented in an /aCa/ context preceded by a carrier phase. The 16 syllables were /p, b, m, t, d, n, g, ng, f, v, s, sh, r, l, j/. A videotape was made with four repetitions of each syllable presented in a random order. The auditory level was adjusted by each participant to provide a comfortable "listening" level. The loudspeaker was turned off for the visual presentation.

Massaro & Cohen (1999) evaluated these results in the context of the FLMP and other competing models. According to the FLMP, there should be a superadditive effect of the bimodal presentation relative to the unimodal conditions. The superadditivity results from both complementarity and an optimal integration algorithm (Massaro, 1998b, Chap. 14). The FLMP analysis of Agelfors's study addresses an interesting question. Does bimodal presentation give the same synergy advantage for HA and CI? Perhaps integration does not occur as optimally with CI relative to HA, for example. To address this question, we can ask whether the synergy of bimodal speech perception predicted by the FLMP holds for both of these subgroups. For the HA group, there were 12 participants with better hearing (HA+) and three with poorer hearing (HA−). For the CI group, there were eight participants with better auditory recognition (CI+) and seven with poorer auditory recognition (CI−).

Given the experimental design, a confusion matrix gives the results to be predicted. The confusion matrix provides for each of the 16 stimuli the proportions of each of the 16 possible responses. A modality-analysis FLMP can be tested against this confusion matrix by estimating the amount of support that a modality-specific syllable presentation provides for each of the 16 consonants. Thus, $16 \times 16 = 256$ parameters are necessary to describe the auditory information and the same number to describe the visual, for a total of 512. Given the three confusion matrices in each condition, there is a total of $3 \times 256 = 768$ independent data points. Thus, the ratio of data points to free parameters is 3:2.

The results showed that all individuals performed more accurately in the bimodal condition relative to the unimodal conditions; that is, superadditivity was obtained. Furthermore, the FLMP gave a good description of performance of each of the four subgroups. The single-channel model with an additional weight parameter was also tested and performed much more poorly than the FLMP in that its RMSD was about six to eight times larger than the RMSD for the FLMP. To reduce the number of free parameters in the model tests, we also tested the models by describing the auditory and visual speech in terms of features.

FEATURE ANALYSIS IMPLEMENTATION The model test we have presented in the previous section makes no assumptions about the psychophysical properties of the test items. A unique parameter is estimated for each possible pairing. For example, a unique parameter is estimated to represent the amount of support a visual /b/ provides for the response alternative /d/. A description of the features of the speech segments can save a large number of free parameters, because it is assumed that a given feature in a given modality has the same impact regardless of what segment it is in. Following the tradition begun with Miller and Nicely (1955), we can define each segment by five features: voicing, nasality, place, frication, and duration. The feature values for one modality are assumed to be independent of the feature values for another modality. For example, we would expect that voicing and nasality would have informative feature values for auditory speech and relatively neutral feature values for visible speech. The place feature, on the other hand, would give relatively informative values for visible speech.

In this implementation, each of the test syllables is described by the conjunction of five features for unimodal speech and the conjunction of ten features for bimodal speech. Even though each feature is defined as a discrete category or its complement (e.g., voiced or voiceless), its influence in the perception of visible speech is represented by a continuous value between 0 and 1. The parameter value for the feature indicates the amount of influence that feature has. Therefore, if the /ma/ and /na/ prototypes are each expected to have a nasal feature and the calculated parameter value for this feature is 0.90 then the nasal feature is highly functional in the expected direction. Alternatively, if the calculated parameter value for the nasal feature is 0.50, then the interpretation would be that the nasal feature is not functional at all. Because of the definition of negation as 1 minus the feature value, a feature value of 0.5 would give the same degree of support for a segment that has the feature as it would for a viseme that does not have the feature. If the calculated parameter value is 0.20, however, then the nasal feature is functional but opposite of the expected direction. Finally, it should be noted that the features are not marked in this formulation: absence of nasality is as informative as presence of nasality. Thus, if a nasal stimulus supports non-nasal response alternatives to degree 0.9, then a non-nasal stimulus also supports a non-nasal alternative to degree 0.9.

The overall match of the feature set to the prototype was calculated by combining the features according to the FLMP. These assumptions dictate that (1) the features are the sources of information that are evaluated independently of one another, (2) the features are integrated multiplicatively (conjoined) to give the overall degree of support for a viseme alternative, and (3) the stimulus is categorized according to the relative goodness decision rule. Thus, this implementation parallels modality-analysis FLMP in all aspects except for the featural description of the stimulus and response alternatives. The single-channel model was also implemented with this same featural description. The FLMP and the single-channel model were tested against the confusion matrices by estimating the amount of information in each feature and the featural correspondence between the stimulus and response prototypes. Thus, five parameters are necessary to describe the auditory information and the same number to describe the visual information. The single-channel model requires an additional weight parameter. The fit of the FLMP to the four different groups gave an average RMSD about half of that given for the fit of the single-channel model.

The Relationship between Identification and Discrimination One of the themes of research from the speech-is-special perspective concerns how speech perception differs from prototypical perception. As an example, two stimuli that differ in two ways are easier to discriminate than if they differ in just one of the two ways. Advocates of the speech-is-special persuasion have claimed to provide evidence that this is not always the case in speech (see Fowler, Chap. 12, this volume). Let us consider two speech categories, /ba/ and /da/, cued by auditory and visual speech. A visual /ba/ paired with an auditory /da/ might give a similar degree of overall support for the category /da/ as an auditory /ba/ paired with a visual /da/. The speech-is-special claim is that these two items should be difficult to discriminate from one another. However, the research that has been cited as support for this outcome has a number of theoretical and methodological limitations (Massaro, 1987a, 1998b) similar to those impeding claims for categorical perception. Basically, these studies are simply another variant of categorical perception in disguise, and are vulnerable to a host of criticisms (Massaro, 1998a).

To illustrate that speech is not special, it is worthwhile to review a test (Massaro & Ferguson, 1993). Participants performed both a perceptual identification task and a same-different discrimination task. There were three levels (/ba/, neutral, /da/) of visual speech and two levels (/ba/, /da/) of auditory speech. This design gives $2 \times 3 = 6$ unique bimodal syllables for the identification task. In the identification task, participants identified these syllables as /ba/ or /da/. For the same-different task discrimination task, two of the bimodal syllables were presented successively, and the task was to indicate whether the two syllables differed on either the auditory or visual channels. There were 20 types of discrimination trials: six "same" trials, six trials with auditory different, four trials with visual different, and four trials with both auditory and visual different.

The predictions of the FLMP were derived for both tasks, and the observed results of both tasks were described with the same set of parameter values. The predictions for the identification task were derived in the standard manner. At the evaluation stage, truth values (of fuzzy logic) are assigned to the auditory and visual sources of information indicating the degree of support for each of the response alternatives /ba/ and /da/. The truth values lie between zero and 1, with zero being no support, 1 being full support, and 0.5 being completely ambiguous. Integration computes the overall support for each alternative. The decision operation in the identification task determines the support for the /da/ alternative relative to the sum of support for each of the /ba/ and /da/ alternatives, and translates relative support into a probability.

Given the FLMP's prediction for the identification task, its prediction for a same-different task can also be derived. Participants are instructed to respond "different" if a difference is perceived along either or both modalities. Within the framework of fuzzy logic, this discrimination task is a disjunction task. The perceived difference along the visual dimension is given by the difference in their truth values assigned at the evaluation stage, and analogously for the auditory dimension. The perceived difference given two bimodal speech syllables can be derived from the assumption of a multiplicative conjunction rule for integration in combination with DeMorgan's law. It is also assumed that the participant computes the degree of sameness from the degree of difference, using the fuzzy logic definition of negation. The participant is required to select a response of "same" or "different" in the discrimination task, and the actual "same" or "different" response is derived from

the relative goodness rule used in the decision operation. The predictions of the FLMP were determined for both the identification and discrimination tasks. There were six unique syllables in identification, and there were 14 types of different trials and six types of same trials. These 26 independent observations were predicted with just five free parameters, corresponding to the three levels of the visual factor and the two levels of the auditory factor. Values of the five parameters were estimated to give the optimal predictions of the observed results, with the goodness of fit based on the RMSD between predicted and observed values. The model was fitted to the average results (pooled across the 20 participants). The best fit of the FLMP to the average results gave an RMSD of 0.0805, a good fit considering that 26 data points were being predicted with just five free parameters. Figure 10.10 plots the observed versus the predicted outcomes of the FLMP for these 26 observations.

As noted, the application of the FLMP to the results carries the assumption that the output of the evaluation stage is identical in both the identification and discrimination tasks. This assumption captures the proposal that integration of the audible and visible sources does not modify or eliminate their representations given by

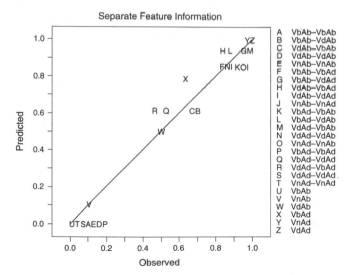

FIGURE 10.10 Observed and predicted probability of a /da/ identification in the identification task and observed and predicted probability of a different judgment in the discrimination task, as a function of the different test events. The points are given by letters: the letters A through T give the discrimination performance, and the letters U through Z give identification. The conditions are listed on the right of the graph. For example, A corresponds to a visual /ba/ auditory /ba/ followed by a visual /ba/ auditory /ba/. Predictions are of the FLMP, which assumes maintenance of separate auditory and visual feature information at the evaluation stage.

the feature evaluation stage. If it did, then the model could not have accurately predicted the results with the same parameter values for identification and discrimination. According to the application of the model, the only difference between the two tasks is how the truth values provided by evaluation are combined. They are conjoined in the identification task and disjoined in the discrimination task.

To further test the assumption that the feature values produced by evaluation are maintained throughout integration and decision, we formulated an alternative model carrying the opposite assumption, and tested it against the same data. This speech-is-special model assumes that auditory and visual sources are blended into a single representation, without separate access to the auditory and visual representations. According to this model, the only representation that remains after a bimodal syllable is presented is the overall degree of support for the response alternatives. What is important for this model is that the overall degree of support for /da/ is functional independently of how much the auditory and visual modalities individually contributed to that support. It is possible to have two bimodal syllables made up of different auditory and visual components but with the same overall degree of support for /da/. For example, a visual /ba/ paired with an auditory /da/ might give a similar degree of overall support for /da/ as an auditory /ba/ paired with a visual /da/. The FLMP predicts that these two bimodal syllables could be discriminated from one another. On the other hand, the speech-is-special model predicts that only the output of integration is available and, therefore, these two different bimodal syllables could not be discriminated from one another. Figure 10.11 plots the observed versus the predicted outcomes for this model for these 26 observations. When formulated, this speech-is-special model gave a significantly poorer ($P < 0.001$) description of the results, with an RMSD of 0.1764.

These results substantiate the claim that information at evaluation maintains its integrity, and can be used independently of the output of integration and decision. Thus, it is inappropriate to believe that perceivers are limited to the output of integration and decision. Perceivers can also use information at the level of evaluation when appropriate. A related result consistent with this conclusion is the observed difference between the detection of temporal asynchrony between auditory and visual speech and the interval over which integration occurs. An observer can detect asynchrony at relatively short asynchronies whereas integration can occur across much longer asynchronies (Massaro & Cohen, 1993; Massaro et al., 1996).

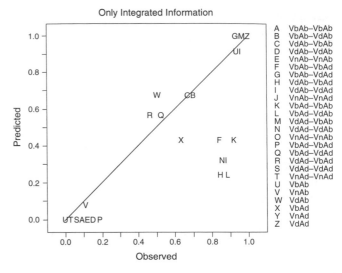

FIGURE 10.11 Observed and predicted probability of a /da/ identification in the identification task and the observed and predicted probability of a different judgment in the discrimination task, as a function of the different test events. The points are given by letters: the letters A through T give the discrimination performance, and the letters U through Z give identification. The conditions are listed on the right of the graph. For example, A corresponds to a visual /ba/ auditory /ba/ followed by a visual /ba/ auditory /ba/. Predictions are of the speech-is-special model, which assumes no maintenance of separate auditory and visual feature information.

Fowler (Chap. 12, this volume) reviews other experiments exploring the relationship between identification and discrimination given conflicting and cooperating cues. Her gesture theory interpretation of the results from unimodal auditory speech experiments are the opposite of what we concluded from the auditory-visual speech perception experiments. It is possible that unimodal versus cross-modal conditions are responsible for the different conclusions (Massaro, 1987b, p. 110). More important, however, is the possibility that participants in the discrimination task were actually basing their judgments on the categorizations of the speech stimuli. In this case, observed discrimination of stimuli with cooperating cues would be poorer relative to stimuli with conflicting cues because the integrated percepts would be much more similar with conflicting cues than cooperating cues. Most important, however, is that quantitative model tests of the gesture theory were not carried out in the unimodal auditory speech experiments. Insofar as Fowler's gesture theory would predict the same outcome as the speech-is-special formulation, we can reject this theory in favor of the FLMP for the auditory-visual experiments.

The results of the identification/discrimination task suggest that observers appear to maintain access to information at evaluation even though integration has occurred. Furthermore, the integration process does not modify the representation corresponding to evaluation. When a perceptual identification judgment that reflects the influence of both audible and visible speech is presented, it is often concluded that a new representation has somehow supplanted the separate auditory and visual codes. However, we learned that we can tap into these separate codes with the appropriate type of psychophysical task. This result is similar to the finding that observers can report the degree to which a syllable was presented even though they categorically labeled it as one syllable or another (Massaro, 1987a). If we grant that the integration of audible and visible speech produced a new representation, then we see that multiple representations can be held in parallel. On the one hand, this result should not be surprising, because a system is more flexible when it has multiple representations of the events in progress and can draw on the different representations when necessary. On the other hand, we might question the assumption of representation altogether and view the perceiver as simply using the information available to act appropriately in respect to the demands of the current situation (O'Regan & Noe, 2001; Dennett, 1991).

One might question why we have been so concerned about current theories of speech and language when the emphasis here is on multisensory fusion or integration. The reason is that the theoretical framework we accept has important ramifications about how we can understand how information from several senses can be combined in speech perception. If indeed speech is special and categorically perceived, then it precludes many reasonable kinds of cross-modal integration (Massaro, 1987b, 1998b).

Learning in the FLMP   Figure 10.6 illustrates how learning is conceptualized within the model by specifying exactly how the feature values used at evaluation change with experience. Learning in the FLMP can be described by the following algorithm (Friedman, Massaro, Kitzis, & Cohen, 1995; Kitzis, Kelley, Berg, Massaro, & Friedman, 1999). The initial feature value representing the support for an alternative is initially set to 0.5 (since 0.5 is neutral in fuzzy logic). A learning trial consists of a feature (such as closed lips at onset) occurring in a test item followed by informative feedback (such as the syllable /ba/). After each trial, the feature values would be updated according to the feedback, as illustrated in Figure 10.6. Thus, the perceiver uses the feedback to modify the prototype representations, and these in turn become better tuned to the informative characteristics of the patterns being identified. This algorithm is

highly similar to many contemporary views of language acquisition (Best, 1993; Best, McRoberts, Goodell, 2001; Werker & Logan, 1985).

LEARNING SPEECH-READING   Because vision is important for understanding spoken language, a significant question is to what extent skill in speech-reading can be learned. In addition, it is important to determine whether the FLMP can describe speech perception at several levels of skill. Following the strategy of earlier training studies (e.g., Walden, Prosek, Montgomery, Scherr, & Jones, 1977), a long-term training paradigm in speech-reading was used to test the FLMP across changes in experience and learning (Massaro, Cohen, & Gesi, 1993). The experiment provided tests of the FLMP at several different levels of speech-reading skill. Participants were taught to speech-read 22 initial consonants in three different vowel contexts. Training involved a variety of discrimination and identification lessons with the consonant-vowel syllables. Throughout their training, participants were repeatedly tested on their recognition of syllables, words, and sentences. The test items were presented visually, auditorily, and bimodally, and presented at normal rate or three times normal rate. Participants improved in their speech-reading ability across all three types of test items. Figure 10.12 gives their individual performance on the syllables across seven sessions. The results are plotted in terms of correct viseme classifications, which group similar visible consonants together. As can be seen in the figure, all six participants improved over training.

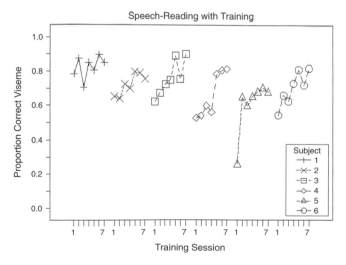

FIGURE 10.12   Proportion of correct viseme recognition of the initial consonant in the visible presentation of consonant-vowel syllables as a function of the seven sessions of training in speech-reading for each of six participants.

Replicating previous results (Walden et al., 1977), the present study illustrates that substantial gains in speech-reading performance are possible.

The FLMP was tested against the results at both the beginning and end of practice. According to the model, a participant would have better information after training than before. To implement this gain in information, we simply assume more informative feature values before and after training. However, the audible and visible sources should be combined in the same manner regardless of training level. Consistent with these assumptions, the FLMP gave a good description of performance at both levels of speech-reading skill. Thus, the FLMP was able to account for the gains in bimodal speech perception as the participants improved their speech-reading and listening abilities. This success suggests that the FLMP and its distinction between information and information processing would provide a valuable framework for the study of language learning.

We have seen that speech-reading can be taught, and one important consideration is the best method for instruction. Different models predict different outcomes for training participants to speech-read in unimodal versus bimodal paradigms. In the unimodal paradigm, visible speech is presented alone, followed by feedback, whereas visible speech is paired with auditory speech in the bimodal paradigm. The single-channel model predicts that unimodal learning would be better, the FLMP predicts no difference, and an extension of the less-is-more hypothesis predicts that bimodal learning would be better. The results of two recent experiments show that participants learn the same amount during unimodal and bimodal learning, supporting the FLMP (Geraci & Massaro, 2002).

Language Learning The FLMP paradigm offers a potentially useful framework for the assessment and training of individuals with language delay due to various factors, such as difficulty hearing, autism, or specific language impairment (Massaro, Cohen, & Beskow, 2000). An important assumption is that while information may vary from one perceptual situation to the next, the manner of combining this information, called information processing, is invariant. With our algorithm, we thus propose an invariant law of pattern recognition describing how continuously perceived (fuzzy) information is processed to achieve perception of a category.

Insofar as speech-reading is highly functional in a variety of situations, a visible speech technology could be of great practical value in many spheres of communication. We have developed a synthetic talking face, called Baldi, to achieve control over the visible speech and accompanying facial movements to study those visible aspects that are informative. Our talking head can be heard, communicates paralinguistic as well as linguistic information, and is controlled by a text-to-speech system or can be aligned with natural speech. Baldi, the animated talking agent, has innovative features, and testing has shown him to be an effective speech and language tutor. The special features include skin transparency controls that reveal the vocal cavity, so that the lips, tongue, and teeth can show how sounds are formed for better inspection, and the head can be rotated at any angle, moved near and far, or displayed in cross section (Cohen, Beskow, & Massaro, 1998). Finally, the visual enunciation of speech can be paused, slowed, or replayed.

The positive research findings and our technology encourage the use of cross-modal environments for persons with hearing loss. Ling (1976), however, reports that clinical experience seems to show that "children taught exclusively through a multisensory approach generally make less use of residual audition" (p. 51). For these reasons, speech-language professionals might use bimodal training less often than would be beneficial. We have carried out two recent studies to evaluate the multisensory instruction of speech perception and production. Our working hypothesis is that speech perception and production will be better (and learned more easily) if bimodal input is used than if either source of information is presented alone.

Although there is a long history of using visible cues in speech training for individuals with hearing loss, these cues have usually been abstract or symbolic rather than direct representations of the vocal tract and articulators. Our goal is to create an articulatory simulation that is as accurate as possible, and to assess whether this information can guide speech production. We know from children born without sight that the ear alone can guide language learning. Our question is whether the eye can do the same, or at least the eye supplemented with degraded auditory information from the ear.

SPEECH TUTORING FOR CHILDREN WITH HEARING LOSS One of the original goals for the application of our technology was to use Baldi as a language and speech tutor for deaf and hard-of-hearing children. Baldi's technology seems ideally suited for improving the perception and production of English speech segments. Baldi can speak slowly, illustrate articulation by making his skin transparent to reveal the tongue, teeth, and palate, and show supplementary articulatory features such as vibration of the neck to show voicing and air expulsion to show frication. Massaro and Light (in press-b) implemented these features in a set for

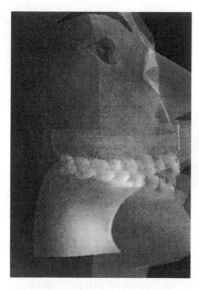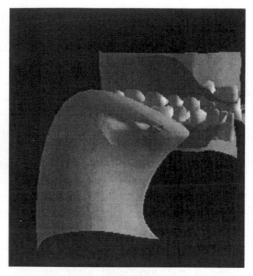

FIGURE 10.13   Two of the four presentation conditions. Shown are a side view of Baldi's whole face, in which his skin is made transparent, and a side view of Baldi's tongue, teeth, and palate.

language exercises. Seven students with hearing loss between the ages of 8 and 13 years were trained for 6 hours across 21 weeks on eight categories of segments (four voiced vs. voiceless distinctions, three consonant cluster distinctions, and one fricative vs. affricate distinction). Training included practice at the segment and the word level.

The student was trained on how to produce the target segments by illustrating various relevant aspects of the articulation (De Filippo & Sims, 1995; Ling, 1976; Massaro et al., in press). A variety of views and illustrations were used, as shown in Figure 10.13. For example, a side view of Baldi with transparent skin was used during voiced versus voiceless training along with the supplementary features such as vibration of the neck and air expulsion to visibly indicate the difference between voiceless and voiced contrasts (e.g., /f/ vs. /v/). For consonant cluster training, internal views of the oral cavity were important to show place features of the tongue during production. Slowing down Baldi's speech emphasized the articulatory sequence involved in producing a consonant cluster. Four different internal views of the oral cavity were shown: a view from the back of Baldi's head looking in, a sagittal view of Baldi's mouth alone (static and dynamic), a side view of Baldi's whole face where his skin was transparent, and a frontal view of Baldi's face with transparent skin. Each view gave the student a unique perspective of the activity, which took place during production.

During all training lessons, the students were instructed on how to produce the segments, they were required to produce the segment in isolation as well as in words, and they heard their productions by a playback feature. No feedback was given during the training stage, but "good job" cartoons were given as reinforcement.

Perception improved for each of the seven children. Figure 10.14 shows that perceptual identification accuracy improved for each of the eight types of distinctions. There was also significant improvement in the production of these same segments. The students' productions of words containing these segments were recorded and presented to native English-speaking college students. These judges were asked to rate the intelligibility of a word against the target text, which was simultaneously presented on the computer monitor. Intelligibility was rated on a scale from 1 to 5 (1 = unintelligible, 2 = ambiguous, 3 = distinguishable, 4 = unambiguous, 5 = good/clear pronunciation). Figure 10.15 shows the judges' ratings transformed to a scale ranging from 0 to 1. According to these ratings, the children's speech production improved for each of the eight categories of segments. Speech production also generalized to new

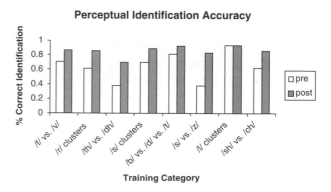

FIGURE 10.14   Percentage of correct identifications during pretest and posttest for each of the eight training categories.

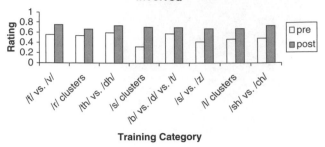

Production Ratings as a Function of Category Involved

FIGURE 10.15 Intelligibility ratings of the pretest and posttest word productions for each of the eight training categories.

words not included in our training lessons. Finally, speech production deteriorated somewhat after six weeks without training, indicating that the training method rather than some other experience was responsible for the improvement that was found.

OTHER APPLICATIONS This pedagogy also has promise to teach second language learners to perceive and produce spoken words, the skills needed for ordinary communication in everyday contexts. In addition, the same application can be used to carry out accent training for students across a wide range of second language competency. For example, beginning students would focus on perception and production of segments, words, and short phrases, whereas advanced students might focus on accent neutralization. This spectrum of training is particularly important because training a second language is a labor-intensive task, traditionally involving significant one-on-one interaction with a teacher.

There is recent evidence that speech tutoring using the Baldi technology is effective for teaching the perception and production of non-native phonetic contrasts to college students (Massaro & Light, 2003). Japanese speakers were trained to identify and produce American English /r/ and /l/ over a three week period. Three minimal word pairs were used in identification and production training (r/light, r/lip, and grew/glue). The results indicated varying difficulty with respect to word pair involved in training (r/light being the easiest to perceive and grew/glue showing the most difficulty). Most important, learning occurred for these words, which also generalized to the production of new words.

In addition to speech tutoring, Baldi is featured in a Language Wizard/Player for teaching new vocabulary items to hard-of-hearing and autistic children (Bosseler & Massaro, in press; Massaro & Light, in press-a). To ensure that the program itself was responsible for the learning, we used a within-student multiple baseline design

where certain words were continuously being tested while other words were being tested and trained. Knowledge of the words remained negligible without training, and learning occurred fairly quickly for all words once training began. Finally, knowledge of the trained words did not degrade after training, generalized to new images and outside of the learning situation, and was retained at least four weeks after training ended.

Retrospective

Speech perception has been studied extensively in recent decades, and we have learned that people use many sources of information in perceiving and understanding speech. Utilizing a general framework of pattern recognition, we have described the important contribution of visible information in the speaker's face and how it is combined with auditory speech. Speech perception is usually successful because perceivers optimally integrate several sources of information. In addition, audible and visible speech are complementary in that one source of information is more informative when the other source is less so. These properties are well described by a fuzzy logical model of perception, a process model mathematically equivalent to Bayes' theorem. The FLMP has also proved to provide a good description of performance in a wide variety of other domains of pattern recognition. For example, it describes how cues from both the face and the voice are evaluated and integrated to perceive emotion. The FLMP is also consistent with findings in neuroscience and provides an algorithmic description of two different neural mechanisms of multisensory processing. Our empirical and theoretical research encouraged us to apply our findings to facilitate language learning. In sum, the study of multisensory processing not only has uncovered fundamental facts about how we perceive and act in a world of many sensory inputs, it has also led to a pedagogy and a technology that are useful for language learning.

REFERENCES

Agelfors, E. (1996). A comparison between patients using cochlear implants and hearing aids: Part I. Results on speech tests. Royal Institute of Technology, Speech, Music and Hearing. *KTH Quarterly Progress and Status Report* (TMH-APSR 1), 63–75.

Arbib, M. A. (2002). The mirror system, imitation, and the evolution of language. In K. Dautenhahn & C. L. Nehaniv (Eds.), *Imitation in animals and artefacts* (pp. 229–280). Cambridge, MA: MIT Press.

Aslin, R. N., Saffran, J. R., & Newport, E. L. (1998). Computation of conditional probability statistics by 8-month-old infants. *Psychological Science, 9,* 321–324.

Best, C. (1993). Emergence of language-specific constraints in perception of non-native speech: A window on early phonological development. In B. de Boysson-Bardies & S. de Schonen (Eds.), *Developmental neurocognition: Speech and face processing in the first year of life* (pp. 289–304). Norwell, MA: Kluwer Academic Publishers.

Best, C., McRoberts, G., & Goodell, E. (2001). Discrimination of non-native consonant contrasts varying in perceptual assimilation to the listener's native phonological system. *Journal of the Acoustical Society of America, 109*(2), 775–795.

Bosseler, A., & Massaro, D. W. (in press). Development and evaluation of a computer-animated tutor for vocabulary and language learning for children with autism. *Journal of Autism and Developmental Disorders.*

Campbell, C. S., Schwarzer, G., & Massaro, D. W. (2001). Face perception: An information processing perspective. In M. J. Wenger & J. T. Townsend (Eds.), *Computational, geometric, and process perspectives on facial cognition: Contexts and challenges* (pp. 285–345). Mahwah, NJ: Erlbaum.

Chandler, J. P. (1969). Subroutine STEPIT finds local minima of a smooth function of several parameters. *Behavioral Science, 14,* 81–82.

Chomsky, N. (1980). *Rules and representations.* Oxford, England: Blackwell.

Cohen, M. M., Beskow, J., & Massaro, D. W. (1998). Recent developments in facial animation: An inside view. *Proceedings of the International Conference on Auditory-Visual Speech Processing—AVSP '98* (pp. 201–206). Terrigal-Sydney, Australia: Causal Productions.

Diehl, R. L., & Kluender, K. R. (1987). On the categorization of speech sounds. In S. Harnad (Ed.), *Categorical perception* (pp. 226–253). Cambridge, England: Cambridge University Press.

Dennett, D. C. (1991). *Consciousness explained.* Boston: Little, Brown.

De Filippo, C. L., & Sims, D. G. (1995). Linking visual and kinesthetic imagery in lipreading instruction. *Journal of Speech and Hearing Research, 38,* 244–256.

Erber, N. P. (1972). Auditory, visual, and auditory-visual recognition of consonants by children with normal and impaired hearing. *Journal of Speech and Hearing Research, 15,* 413–422.

Fodor, J. A. (1983). *Modularity of mind.* Cambridge, MA: MIT Press/Bradford Books.

Fodor, J. A. (2000). *The mind doesn't work that way: The scope and limits of computational psychology.* Cambridge, MA: MIT Press.

Fowler, C. A. (1996). Listeners do hear sounds, not tongues. *Journal of the Acoustical Society of America, 99,* 1730–1741.

Friedman, D., Massaro, D. W., Kitzis, S. N., & Cohen, M. M. (1995). A comparison of learning models. *Journal of Mathematical Psychology, 39,* 164–178.

Geraci, K., & Massaro, D. W. (2002). *Teaching speechreading: Is unimodal or bimodal training more effective?* Unpublished manuscript.

Gomez, R. L., & Gerken, L. (2000). Infant artificial language learning and language acquisition. *Trends in Cognitive Sciences, 4,* 178–186.

Jordan, T., & Sergeant, P. (2000). Effects of distance on visual and audiovisual speech recognition. *Language and Speech, 43,* 107–124.

Kitzis, S. N., Kelley, H., Berg, E., Massaro, D. W., & Friedman, D. (1999). Broadening the tests of learning models. *Journal of Mathematical Psychology, 42,* 327–355.

Liberman, A. M. (1996). *Speech: A special code.* Cambridge, MA: MIT Press.

Liberman, A. M., & Mattingly, I. G. (1985). The motor theory of speech perception revised. *Cognition, 21,* 1–36.

Lieberman, P. (2000). *Human language and our reptilian brain: The subcortical bases of speech, syntax, and thought.* Cambridge, MA: Harvard University Press.

Ling, D. (1976). *Speech and the hearing-impaired child: Theory and practice.* Washington, DC: Alexander Graham Bell.

Massaro, D. W. (1987a). Categorical partition: A fuzzy logical model of categorization behavior. In S. Harnad (Ed.), *Categorical perception.* Hillsdale, NJ: Erlbaum.

Massaro, D. W. (1987b). *Speech perception by ear and eye: A paradigm for psychological inquiry.* Hillsdale, NJ: Erlbaum.

Massaro, D. W. (1989). Multiple book review of *Speech perception by ear and eye: A paradigm for psychological inquiry,* by D. W. Massaro. *Behavioral and Brain Sciences, 12,* 741–794.

Massaro, D. W. (1996). Integration of multiple sources of information in language processing. In T. Inui & J. L. McClelland (Eds.), *Attention and performance XVI: Information integration in perception and communication* (pp. 397–432). Cambridge, MA: MIT Press.

Massaro, D. W. (1998a). Categorical perception: Important Phenomenon or Lasting Myth? *Proceedings of the International Congress of Spoken Language Processing.* Sydney, Australia: Causal Productions.

Massaro, D. W. (1998b). *Perceiving talking faces: From speech perception to a behavioral principle.* Cambridge, MA: MIT Press.

Massaro, D. W. (1999). Speechreading: Illusion or window into pattern recognition? *Trends in Cognitive Sciences, 3,* 310–317.

Massaro, D. W., Bosseler, A., & Light, J. (2003, August). *Development and evaluation of a computer-animated tutor for language and vocabulary learning.* Paper presented at the 15th International Congress of Phonetic Sciences (ICPhS '03), Barcelona, Spain.

Massaro, D. W., & Cohen, M. M. (1983). Categorical or continuous speech perception: A new test. *Speech Communication, 2,* 15–35.

Massaro, D. W., & Cohen, M. M. (1993). Perceiving asynchronous bimodal speech in consonant-vowel and vowel syllables. *Speech Communication, 13,* 127–134.

Massaro, D. W., & Cohen, M. M. (1999). Speech perception in perceivers with hearing loss: Synergy of multiple modalities. *Journal of Speech, Language, and Hearing Research, 42,* 21–41.

Massaro, D. W., Cohen, M. M., & Beskow, J. (2000). Developing and evaluating conversational agents. In J. Cassell, J. Sullivan, S. Prevost, & E. Churchill (Eds.), *Embodied conversational agents.* Cambridge, MA: MIT Press.

Massaro, D. W., Cohen, M. M., Campbell, C. S., & Rodriguez, T. (2001). Bayes' factor of model selection validates FLMP. *Psychonomic Bulletin and Review, 8,* 1–17.

Massaro, D. W., Cohen, M. M., & Gesi, A. T. (1993). Long-term training, transfer, and retention in learning to lipread. *Perception & Psychophysics, 53*(5), 549–562.

Massaro, D. W., Cohen, M. M., Gesi, A., & Heredia, R. (1993). Bimodal speech perception: An examination across languages. *Journal of Phonetics, 21,* 445–478.

Massaro, D. W., Cohen, M. M., & Smeele, P. M. T. (1995). Cross-linguistic comparisons in the integration of visual and auditory speech. *Memory and Cognition, 23,* 113–131.

Massaro, D. W., Cohen, M. M., & Smeele, P. M. T. (1996). Perception of asynchronous and conflicting visual and auditory speech. *Journal of the Acoustical Society of America, 100,* 1777–1786.

Massaro, D. W., Cohen, M. M., Tabain, M., Beskow, J., & Clark, R. (in press). Animated speech: Research progress and applications. In Vatikiotis-Bateson, E., Perrier, P., & Bailly, G. (Eds.), *Advances in audio-visual speech processing.* Cambridge: MIT Press.

Massaro, D. W., & Egan, P. B. (1996). Perceiving affect from the face and the voice. *Psychonomic Bulletin & Review, 3,* 215–221.

Massaro, D. W., & Ferguson, E. L. (1993). Cognitive style and perception: The relationship between category width and speech perception, categorization and discrimination. *American Journal of Psychology, 103,* 25–49.

Massaro, D. W., & Light, J. (2003, September). *Read my tongue movements: Bimodal learning to perceive and produce non-native speech /r/ and /l/.* Presented at Eurospeech 2003—Switzerland (Interspeech), 8th European Conference on Speech Communication and Technology, Geneva, Switzerland.

Massaro, D. W., & Light, J. (in press-a). Improving the vocabulary of children with hearing loss. *Volta Review.*

Massaro, D. W., & Light, J. (in press-b). Using visible speech for training perception and production of speech for hard of hearing individuals. *Journal of Speech, Language, and Hearing Research.*

Massaro, D. W., & Stork, D. G. (1998). Speech recognition and sensory integration. *American Scientist, 86,* 236–244.

Mattingly. I. G., & Studdert-Kennedy, M. (Eds.). (1991). *Modularity and the motor theory of speech perception.* Hillsdale, NJ: Erlbaum.

McGurk, H., & MacDonald, J. (1976). Hearing lips and seeing voices. *Nature, 264,* 746–748.

Mesulam, M. M. (1998). From sensation to cognition. *Brain, 121,* 1013–1052.

Miller, G. A., & Nicely, P. E. (1955). An analysis of perceptual confusions among some English consonants. *Journal of the Acoustical Society of America, 27,* 338–352.

Myung, I. J., & Pitt, M. A. (1997). Applying Occam's razor in modeling cognition: A Bayesian approach. *Psychonomic Bulletin & Review, 4,* 79–95.

Nearey, T. M. (1992). Context effects in a double-weak theory of speech perception. [Special Issue: Festschrift for John J. Ohala]. *Language & Speech, 35,* 153–171.

Nearey, T. (1997). Speech perception as pattern recognition. *Journal of the Acoustical Society of America, 101,* 3241–3254.

O'Regan, J. K., & Noe, A. (2001). A sensorimotor account of vision and visual consciousness. *Behavioral and Brain Sciences, 24,* 939–1031.

Pashler, H. E. (1998). *The psychology of attention.* Cambridge, MA: MIT Press.

Platt, J. R. (1964). Strong inference. *Science, 146,* 347–353.

Popper, K. R. (1959). *The logic of scientific discovery.* New York: Basic Books.

Pullum, G. K., & Scholz, B. C. (2002). Empirical assessment of stimulus poverty arguments [Special issue]. *The Linguistic Review, 19*(1–2), 9–50.

Quinn, P. C. (2002). Early categorization: A new synthesis. In U. Goswami (Ed.), *Blackwell handbook of childhood cognitive development* (pp. 84–101). Malden, MA: Blackwell.

Robert-Ribes, J., Schwartz, J.-L., & Escudier, P. (1995). A comparison of models for fusion of the auditory and visual sensors in speech perception. *Artificial Intelligence Review, 9,* 323–346.

Saffran, J. R., Johnson, E. K., Aslin, R. N., & Newport, E. L. (1999). Statistical learning of tone sequences by human infants and adults. *Cognition, 70,* 27–52.

Savage-Rumbaugh, S., Shanker, S. G., & Taylor, T. J. (1998). *Apes, language, and the human mind.* New York: Oxford University Press.

Smeele, P. M. T., Massaro, D. W., Cohen, M. M., & Sittig, A. C. (1998). Laterality in visual speech perception. *Journal of Experimental Psychology: Human Perception and Performance, 24,* 1232–1242.

Stein, B. E., & Meredith, M. A. (1993). *The merging of the senses.* Cambridge, MA: MIT Press.

Trout, J. D. (2001). The biological basis of speech: What to infer from talking to the animals. *Psychological Review, 108,* 523–549.

Walden, B., Prosek, R., Montgomery, A., Scherr, C. K., & Jones, C. J. (1977). Effects of training on the visual recognition of consonants. *Journal of Speech and Hearing Research, 20,* 130–145.

Werker, J., & Logan, J. (1985). Cross-language evidence for three factors in speech perception. *Perception & Psychophysics, 37*(1), 35–44.

11 Spatial and Temporal Constraints on Audiovisual Speech Perception

KEVIN G. MUNHALL AND ERIC VATIKIOTIS-BATESON

Introduction

Grasping the full meaning of a message during face-to-face conversation requires the perception of diverse auditory and visual information. When people listen to someone speaking, their processing of the utterances extends beyond the linguistic analysis of the words to include the perception of visible speech movements, facial expression, body posture, manual gestures, and the tone and timing of the voice. This extensive audiovisual information is produced in parallel by the talker and must be processed and integrated by the listener in order to understand the talker's full intent. Thus, human communication in its most natural form is cross-modal and multidimensional. In this chapter we focus on one part of this complex sensory processing, the audiovisual perception of speech.

It has been known for many years that the information for speech is both auditory and visual. With the exception of some rare individuals who can identify most of what is said from speech-reading alone (e.g., Bernstein, Demorest, & Tucker, 2000), most people are quite limited in their ability to identify speech from visual-only signals. A more pervasive phenomenon is the ability of visual speech to enhance the intelligibility of auditory speech in noise. When a talker's face is visible in a noisy environment, the intelligibility of the auditory speech is significantly better than auditory-alone speech perception (Sumby & Pollack, 1954). Visible speech can even alter the perception of perfectly audible speech sounds when the visual speech stimuli are mismatched with the auditory speech, as demonstrated by the McGurk effect (McGurk & MacDonald, 1976).

In this chapter we address the audiovisual integration of information for speech. We first summarize the spatial and temporal features of normal speech communication and the conditions that characterize face-to-face communication. Next we discuss the spatial and temporal limits of audiovisual speech integration. Finally, we summarize our production-based animation projects that provide audiovisual stimulus control for the examination of speech production and perception as coordinated processes.

Before we consider the existing data, we present the different experimental tasks that are used in visual and audiovisual speech perception research. Data from three different types of tasks are discussed in this chapter: speech-reading, speech-in-noise perception tasks, and McGurk effect tasks. Speech-reading in its strictest definition involves visual-only (silent) speech presentation, as would be the case when a person watches television with the sound turned off. "Speech-reading" is also used to refer to the speech perception of individuals with profound hearing impairments. However, the use of the term in this context can be misleading because in many cases, the visual signals of speech are being used to augment residual hearing. In such cases, speech perception is more akin to understanding speech in noise than to silent speech-reading, because the visual speech complements a weak or distorted auditory signal. The final audiovisual task concerns the audiovisual illusion known as the *McGurk effect* (McGurk & MacDonald, 1976). In this task a visual consonant is dubbed onto a different auditory consonant and the incongruent visual stimulus modifies the auditory percept. For example, when a visual *g* is dubbed onto an auditory *b*, subjects frequently hear a different consonant, such as *d* or *th*. Of course, subjects would clearly perceive the /b/ if they closed their eyes.

Although these three tasks clearly involve related information and similar information-processing skills, they are not equivalent. All of the tasks exhibit considerable individual differences that are not strongly correlated within subjects (Munhall, 2002; Watson, Qui, Chamberlain, & Li, 1996; cf. MacLeod & Summerfield, 1987). In particular, performance on silent speech-reading does not correlate with performance on either perceiving sentences in noise or McGurk effect tasks.

Heightened performance on speech-reading correlates with a range of cognitive and perceptual abilities that are not necessarily related to speech (Rönnberg et al., 1999; cf. Summerfield, 1992). There are other indications that the three visual tasks employ different perceptual and cognitive components. Speech-reading abilities are very limited in the general population.[1] The visual enhancement of the perception of speech in noise, on the other hand, is a more general and widespread phenomenon. There are also hints that the McGurk effect should be distinguished from the perception of congruent audiovisual speech (Jordan & Sergeant, 2000). For instance, the two tasks show different thresholds for the influence of degraded visual information (cf. Massaro, 1998).

A second task factor additionally complicates the literature on audiovisual speech—the stimulus corpus. In some tasks, such as in most McGurk effect studies, subjects choose answers from a small set of nonsense syllables. At the other extreme, subjects identify words in sentences, with the words drawn from the full corpus of the language. Experiments that use tasks from different parts of this range invoke different strategies from the subjects and require different parts of the linguistic system. Not surprisingly, individual differences on audiovisual recognition of nonsense syllables do not correlate with individual differences on audiovisual perception of sentence materials (Grant & Seitz, 1998).

Unfortunately, the issue of task differences in audiovisual speech perception cannot be resolved without obtaining data from direct comparisons. Thus, for the purpose of this chapter, we review data from all three tasks together, taking care to indicate the experimental tasks in each case and to warn that the conclusions may not generalize across tasks.

The conditions for audiovisual speech

Face-to-face conversation is one of the oldest and still the most pervasive modes of human communication; therefore, the circumstances of normal conversation define the standard conditions for audiovisual speech perception. The primary visual information for speech comes from visible movements of the eyes, mouth, and head, and people are able to use these visible movements to retrieve crucial information from unfamiliar speakers across a range of conditions. The size and location of these visual targets and the characteristics of their movements are factors that determine the spatial resolution required for visual speech. Fortunately, these factors do not vary greatly across differences in age, sex, and physiognomy. For example, Figure 11.1 shows horizontal lip width and the distance between the external margins of the eyes as a function of age and sex. As is evident from the figure, there is only a modest growth curve for these measures after age 6, and only a small sex difference.

A more important determinant of the range of visual angles subtended by these facial features during conversation is viewing distance. Interpersonal distance in conversation varies with a number of factors, such as culture and intimacy. In North American culture, intimate conversational distances may be less than a meter, but more public or formal distances may exceed 3–5 meters (e.g., Hall, 1966). At these viewing distances, features such as the width of the mouth can subtend less than half a degree of visual angle, which would greatly reduce the visibility of the fine details of oral shape and movement.

Temporally, speech is produced relatively slowly, at syllable rates that are usually within a narrow band of 3–6 Hz. Greenberg's (1999) analysis of a large database of spontaneous speech showed that the average syllable duration was approximately 200 ms (5 Hz). Although there was considerable variability in the measured syllable durations, only 15% exceeded 300 ms (<3.3 Hz). Within the 3–6 Hz range, speaking rates vary as a function of many factors, such as emotion, social formality, fatigue, and precision of articulation. Languages also differ in speed of production as a result of factors such as linguistic rhythm and syllable structure constraints (Vatikiotis-Bateson & Kelso, 1993).

Although the range of typical speaking rates is relatively narrow, the extremes of speaking rate can be considerably faster or slower. For example, novelty acts such as "the world's fastest talker" produce speech at rates exceeding 600 words per minute (less than 100 ms per syllable).[2] At the slow end of the speech range, naturally produced syllables can be as long as 500 ms or more due to emphasis (Greenberg, 1999). Artificially prolonged speech, as employed in some stuttering therapies, can

---

[1]Performance on speech-reading tests is actually quite variable. Summerfield (1992) reviews a set of studies with individual subject speech-reading accuracies varying from 1% to 93% words correct. A number of factors influence these scores including talker characteristics, talker speaking style, subject experience with speech-reading, corpus and task. However, when speech-reading is measured with an open-set task where the talker produces the material in a natural, casual speech manner, most untrained individuals will find the task daunting.

---

[2]As of 2001, the world's fastest talker was Steve Woodmore of England, who produced speech at a rate of 637 words per minute.

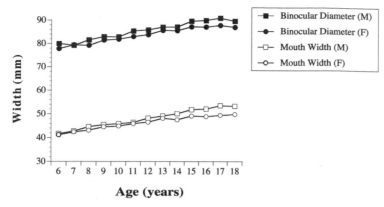

FIGURE 11.1   Horizontal size of face features as a function of age and sex.

produce even slower rates; however, naturalness and sometimes intelligibility suffer.

The human voice has a dynamic range of acoustic energy of about 60 dB and can reach maximum amplitudes of approximately 100 dB. Standard conversational speech occurs at sound pressure levels (SPL) of 75–80 dB. Fundamental frequencies of voicing average approximately 120 Hz for males and 220 Hz for females. For example, Fitch and Holbrook (1970) reported that the average speaking fundamental frequency for 100 males was 116.65 Hz and for 100 females was 217 Hz. (See Baken, 1987, for a review of other studies of voicing characteristics.) Speech has a complex frequency spectrum with multiple energy peaks. Although information may be provided by frequencies as high as 10 kHz, most of the energy is distributed well below 6 kHz. This can be seen in Figure 11.2, which shows the long-term average spectrum of speech, with a peak of energy at 500 Hz.

In summary, face-to-face conversation involves a visual stimulus that varies at the syllable rate of the speech (4–5 Hz for English) and has visual features that subtend 5–10 degrees of visual angle at an interpersonal distance of 1 meter. The acoustics of speech involve

information in a broad band ranging from 100 Hz to 10 kHz, with a spectral energy peak at approximately 500 Hz.

Image characteristics

Visual information processing for speech is influenced by the quality of the visual image as well as by information-processing strategies. The studies reviewed in this section summarize what is known about the influence of image characteristics on speech perception.

One indication of the spatial resolution requirements of visual speech perception can be found in studies that manipulate viewing distance. Jordan and Sergeant (2000) manipulated distance from 1 to 30 meters in an audiovisual task in which subjects perceived consonant-vowel syllables. Some of the syllables were congruent (i.e., auditory and visual stimuli matched), while other stimuli were incongruent (the McGurk effect: visual and auditory stimuli did not match). Vision improved performance with congruent auditory speech at all distances and influenced incongruent auditory speech up to 20 meters. The use of modern display systems allows image size to be manipulated independently of viewing distance. Jordan and Sergeant (1998) displayed a talking head at 100%, 20%, 10%, 5%, and 2.5% of full size. They found no influence of reduction in image size on visual speech or incongruent audiovisual speech until the talking face was less than 10% of full size. For congruent audiovisual speech, only small reductions in performance were observed at the smallest image size (2.5% of full size).

The same results may not hold for visual-only speech perception. In a study of viewing distance during silent speech-reading, Erber (1971) presented stimuli over a range of distances. Two live (not videotaped) talkers spoke common nouns at 5, 10, 20, 40, 70, and 100 feet

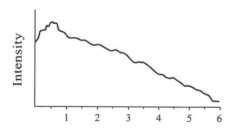

FIGURE 11.2   Long-term average spectrum of speech. (Adapted from Kent, R. D., & Read, C. [1992]. *The Acoustic analysis of speech.* San Diego, CA: Singular.)

from the six profoundly deaf children who served as subjects. Unlike the audiovisual speech tested by Jordan and Sergeant (2000), performance showed a linear decline with distance.[3] At a distance of 5 feet, performance averaged about 75% correct, while at 100 feet, accuracy was only 11%. In a replication involving manipulations of viewing angle and illumination, Erber (1974) found the same rate of decline in accuracy over a 6- to 24-foot range of viewing distances. On the other hand, Neely (1956) found no effect on speech-reading of viewing distances ranging from 3 to 9 feet, and Small and Infante (1988) found no effects of distances ranging from 3 to 18 feet.

Both distance and image size manipulations reduce the visible information for the observer, and audiovisual speech is not greatly affected by these manipulations. Visual speech perception has also been shown to be quite robust when image quality is directly degraded. In one of the first studies of this kind, Brooke and Templeton (1990) manipulated the quantization level of a display showing the mouth region during articulation of English vowels. Varying the quantization level across a range of display resolutions (from 8×8 to 128×128 pixels), Brooke and Templeton found that performance on a silent speech-reading task decreased only after the spatial resolution was reduced to 16×16 or 8×8 pixels. Similar methods have been used by MacDonald, Andersen, and Bachmann (2000) to study the McGurk effect, and by Campbell and Massaro (1997) and Vitkovich and Barber (1996) to study speech-reading. MacDonald et al. (2000) found that the McGurk effect persisted to some degree even at low spatial resolution. Campbell and Massaro found similar effects for speech-reading. Vitkovich and Barber found no effect of pixel density manipulation but did observe changes in performance when the gray-scale resolution (number of gray levels) of the images was drastically reduced.

Quantization techniques such as those used in these studies introduce spurious high-frequency information at the quantization boundaries. Recently, we (Munhall, Kroos, Jozan, & Vatikiotis-Bateson, in press) conducted a series of studies to evaluate this issue with other techniques. Using video images produced with one-octave band-pass filters, we tested the influence of different spatial scales on audiovisual speech perception.

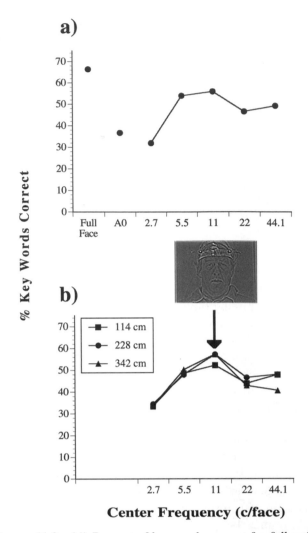

FIGURE 11.3 (A) Percent of key words correct for full unfiltered video (Full), auditory only (A0), and five band-pass spatial-frequency-filtered video conditions. (B) Data when the videos are viewed at three different viewing distances.

Specifically, we tested the visual enhancement of intelligibility of the Central Institute for the Deaf Everyday Sentences in noise for five spatial frequency bands with center frequencies of 2.7, 5.5, 11, 22, and 44.1 cycles per face.[4] Our results indicated that there is a peak gain in intelligibility in a speech-in-noise task for the band with center frequency of 11 cycles per face, but that the bands lower (center frequency of 5.5 cycles per face) and higher (center frequency of 22 and 44.1 cycles per face) than this band also significantly enhanced intelligibility over the auditory-only condition (Fig. 11.3A). As can be seen in Fig. 11.3B, this pattern is not affected by

---

[3]It should be noted that Jordan and Sergeant used a closed-set phoneme identification task, while Erber's task used sentence material. This factor may contribute to the observed differences. However, Massaro (1998) also found greater degradation with reduced image size for speech-reading nonsense syllables.

---

[4]Rate of change of contrast in object (face) coordinates.

viewing distance. When subjects viewed the stimuli from three distances (114, 228, and 342 cm), the intelligibility curves showed the same peak at 11 cycles per face and were largely similar overall. This peak in accuracy corresponds with peak sensitivity values found for static face identification and facial expression discrimination (e.g., Näsänen, 1999).

It is clear from these band-pass data that information is spread across the spatial frequency spectrum and that significant speech information is available in the low spatial frequency bands. What is not clear from these data, however, is the degree to which the information in the various bands is redundant. That performance does not reach the level of the unfiltered face in any one spatial frequency band suggests that perceivers require information from more than one frequency band or that the optimal bandwidth is broader than one octave (Näsänen, 1999). One way to test this is to look at low-pass filtered stimuli and identify the cutoff frequency at which performance reaches an asymptote. The quantization data that exist are similar to low-pass filtering in that each quantization level includes all of the lower spatial frequencies. Data from Campbell and Massaro (1997) and MacDonald et al. (2000) show a monotonic increase in performance with each increase in level of quantization. Although the slope of this function decreases markedly for higher levels of quantization, it raises the possibility that the higher-frequency bands carry some unique information that aids speechreading and audiovisual speech.

A direct low-pass approach, however, is preferred over quantization approaches (e.g., Campbell & Massaro, 1997; MacDonald et al., 2000), because spurious high-frequency information is introduced by the boundaries of the quantization blocks. In order to examine this without the artifacts introduced by quantization, we recently created a dataset by low-pass filtering video recordings of a talker saying sentences. These stimuli were presented with the acoustics mixed with noise, and subjects were required to identify the words in an open-set task. The cutoff frequencies were 1.8, 3.7, 7.3, 15, 29, and 59 cycles per face.

As shown in Figure 11.4, intelligibility reached an asymptote at 7.3 cycles per face, with no significant differences between any of the conditions above this cutoff. In addition, perception performance for this condition and all cutoff frequencies above this condition was equal to the unfiltered face condition. Of note, the 7.3 cycles per face cutoff corresponds to the upper boundary of the one-octave filter centered on 5.5 cycles per face (see Fig. 11.3). These results provide strong evidence that relatively low spatial frequencies are sufficient for audiovisual speech perception.

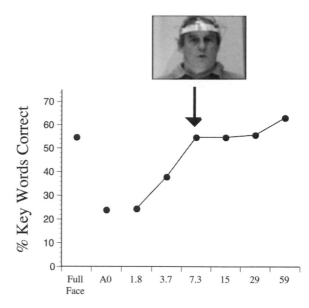

FIGURE 11.4   Percent key words correct for full unfiltered video (Full Face), auditory only (A0), and six low-pass spatial frequency filtered video conditions. The filtered conditions are labeled with their filter cutoff frequency.

Studies of varied illumination of the face and other optical distortions that reduce the visible details of the face reinforce this conclusion. When the frontal illumination level of the face was varied, Erber (1974) found only modest decrements in speech-reading intelligibility. When facial luminance decreased from 30 to 0.03 foot-lamberts, performance decreased only 13%. Thomas (1964, cited in Erber, 1974) found no significant decrease in speech-reading until the illumination level was about 0.5 foot-candles. In studies of optical blurring of visual speech, only small effects have been reported. Using convex lenses, Thorn and Thorn (1989) tested the speech-reading of sentences across a range of different blur conditions. Their subjects showed little influence for up to 4 diopters of blur. Erber (1979) produced optical distortion by placing a sheet of rough-surfaced Plexiglas between the subjects and talkers. Varying the distance between the Plexiglas and stimulus from 2 to 60 cm caused an increase in blurring of the talking face and a sharp decrease in the visual intelligibility of the spoken words. However, even at the greatest visual blurring (60 cm distance between Plexiglas and stimulus), the presence of the visual stimulus enhanced auditory perception. (For a similar approach see Fixmer & Hawkins, 1998.)

Another way to approach the question of visual resolution requirements for speech perception is to examine the pattern of gaze during audiovisual speech. Because acuity varies across the retina, foveation on one facial location will mean that only lower-resolution information will be available elsewhere on the face. Thus, if high-resolution information is a requirement for visual speech perception, subjects' gaze locations could directly reveal the locations of this information.

A small number of studies have examined eye movements and gaze location during audiovisual and visual speech perception. Vatikiotis-Bateson, Eigsti, Yano, and Munhall (1998) studied eye movements while subjects watched a talker speaking short monologues. The results showed that subjects divided their gaze between the mouth and eyes, with less than 40% of the fixations in the mouth region. When noise was added to the audio signal, the percentage of fixations in the mouth region increased to approximately 60% for the highest noise level. In addition to the noise manipulation, Vatikiotis-Bateson et al. (1998) varied the size of the image from life size to approximately five times larger. Surprisingly, no difference in gaze pattern was observed as a function of image size. This finding suggests either that gaze in this context is determined by stereotypic information-gathering routines or that information was sufficient across the different gaze locations and image sizes.

Lansing and McConkie (1999) examined the influence of task on gaze patterns during silent speech-reading of sentences and found a slightly different pattern. When subjects were directed to discriminate between statements and questions, 39.5% of the gaze fixations were within an upper facial (eyes) region. However, when the task was to identify which words were spoken, only 14.4% of the fixations were in this region. The task specificity of the gaze distribution indicates that subjects have different overt strategies, but it does not reveal whether the strategies alter the accuracy of visual speech information processing. This issue was addressed directly in a recent study by Paré, Richler, ten Hove, and Munhall (2001).

Paré et al. (2001) examined the distribution of gaze during the McGurk effect. This study involved a more fine-grained analysis of gaze and the perception of individual sounds. The results showed once again that the eye and mouth regions dominate the gaze patterns. Approximately 60% of the fixations at the time of the consonant release were on the mouth; however, the strength of the McGurk effect was not influenced by where in the face region subjects fixated. More important, Paré et al. demonstrated that the McGurk effect did not disappear when subjects directed their gaze well beyond the facial region. Thus, high-acuity foveal vision does not seem to be a requirement for visual speech perception.

These results have a certain commonsense appeal. In natural face-to-face communication, the demands of conversation and social interaction will produce gaze fixations on various facial features as well as many locations beyond the face and beyond the talker. Insofar as visual acuity varies across the visual field, these fixations will introduce varying levels of spatial frequency filtering to the visible correlates of speech production. Both our spatial filtering and gaze studies suggest that visual speech processing is robust under these conditions (see also Massaro, 1998).

SPATIAL DISTRIBUTION OF SPEECH INFORMATION   Although they are only part of the visual speech signal, most of what is known about visible speech derives from the study of the movements of the lips and jaw. The jaw's motion during speech is mostly confined to translation and rotation in the midsagittal plane (Vatikiotis-Bateson & Ostry, 1995): as the jaw rotates open, the condyle translates down and forward (Ostry & Munhall, 1994). Unlike in mastication, there is little motion in the other degrees of freedom (Ostry, Vatikiotis-Bateson, & Gribble, 1997). The magnitude of jaw movement varies with the individual and with the speaking style, but average speech movements are consistently smaller than jaw movements during mastication (Ostry & Munhall, 1994). The peak velocity of jaw movement varies linearly with movement amplitude, with overall speaking rate constraining movement range (Nelson, 1983).

Movement of the lips traditionally is described as having two phonetically relevant degrees of freedom, rounding and opening. Statistical studies of the principal components of static lip shape (Linker, 1982) and lip movements (Ramsay, Munhall, Gracco, & Ostry, 1996) have revealed a small number of modes of variation. For example, in Linker's data the vowels of English could be distinguished on the basis of a single measure, horizontal opening, while the vowels of Finnish, Swedish, and French required three factors.

The opening motions of the lips are on average relatively small (<1 cm), with upper lip movements being characteristically smaller than lower lip movements (see Smith, 1992, for a review of speech articulation). Rounding movements for the lips are also quite small, with peak rounding frequently less than 5 mm from the neutral position (Daniloff & Moll, 1968). As for jaw movements, the relationship between the peak instantaneous velocity and the movement amplitude is largely linear (e.g., Vatikiotis-Bateson & Kelso, 1993).

Visible speech information comes from more than lip and jaw movements. Speech is produced by changing the shape of the vocal tract. This internal articulation produces a range of visible effects; the whole face moves and changes shape during articulation. This full facial motion contains both redundant and independent information from lip articulation. When kinematics are measured from locations across the face, such as the lower face, cheeks, and periorally on the vermilion borders of the lips, the motions of the perioral markers are highly predictable (92%–99%) from the motions of the more peripheral markers on the cheeks and lower face (Vatikiotis-Bateson, Munhall, Hirayama, Kasahara, & Yehia, 1996). This result indicates that audiovisual speech information is distributed over much wider regions of the face than just the vicinity of the mouth (Vatikiotis-Bateson et al., 1998). This larger distribution of information may reflect the physical influence of the jaw, whose cycle of opening and closing deforms the facial surface and contributes to the changes in oral aperture size.

Despite the high degree to which lip behavior can be recovered from more remote regions on the face, both the perioral and the remote facial locations contain independent speech information. Initially this was demonstrated by comparing the recovery of acoustic root mean square (RMS) amplitude from various combinations of the facial marker motion data (Vatikiotis-Bateson & Yehia, 1996). In particular, when the markers used to transduce the three-dimensional (3D) facial motion were divided into perioral and more peripheral (cheek and lower face) sets, the R^2 values for both sets were quite high (about 80%). However, the R^2 values for the RMS amplitude recovered from the complete marker set were consistently much higher (>90%; see below for a detailed discussion of kinematic-acoustic correlations).

TEMPORAL CHARACTERISTICS OF SPEECH MOVEMENTS   The timing of speech movements corresponds with the syllable rate reported in the previous section. In a study of jaw motion during oral reading, Ohala (1975) found that the primary spectral peak of the movements was around 4 Hz. Muller and MacLeod (1982) and Munhall and Vatikiotis-Bateson (1998) reported similar ranges for lip movement frequencies. Several studies have revealed that disruption of the visual display of these facial movements impairs audiovisual speech perception. For example, Vitkovich and Barber (1994) manipulated the frame rate of video speech by dropping frames. When the frame rate went below about 17 Hz, audiovisual intelligibility was reduced. Temporal manipulations have also been shown to interfere with speech-reading. In a study by Campbell and colleagues (Campbell, Harvey, Troscianko, Massaro, & Cohen, 1996), a dynamic visual noise mask whose contrast fluctuated was laid over the video images. When the contrast of the visual noise fluctuated at a frequency of 20 Hz, performance went down.

The level at which these relatively crude temporal manipulations interfere with speech perception is not clear. A large literature on movements, ranging from eye movements to limb movements to speech motion, shows a similarity in velocity profiles. All of these diverse movements exhibit smooth acceleration and deceleration, with peak velocities occurring approximately midway through the movements (e.g., Morasso, 1981). Whether the perceptual system is sensitive to such kinematic fine structure requires more detailed study.

AUDIOVISUAL SYNCHRONY   Under natural conditions, there is little variation in the relative timing of signals in the visual and auditory modalities. The difference in the speed of transmission of light and sound can lead to auditory delays, but within the range of normal conversational distances the auditory delays are negligible. For example, at a distance of 30 feet, sound reaching a perceiver will be delayed 88 ms relative to the visual signal. However, in modern telecommunications, audiovisual asynchronies frequently occur, and these timing disturbances lead to decrements in perceptual performance and acceptability ratings.

Experimental manipulations of synchrony have been carried out to examine audiovisual integration of speech. A series of studies have attempted to find the threshold for detection of desynchrony. Dixon and Spitz (1980) had subjects move the sound and video out of synchrony until they could perceive the asynchrony. When the stimuli were audiovisual recordings of a man reading prose, the mean desynchrony at detection was 257.9 ms when the voice was delayed with respect to the video, and 131.1 ms when the voice was advanced with respect to the video. In a second condition, subjects varied the timing of an audiovisual recording of a hammer striking a nail. Detection thresholds were shorter for this event (187.5 ms for auditory delay and 74.8 ms for auditory advance), but the same pattern of asynchrony was evident. For both stimuli, longer auditory delays than auditory advances were needed before subjects detected the desynchrony.

A similar pattern of results was reported by Munhall, Gribble, Sacco, and Ward (1996), who used the McGurk effect to test sensitivity to asynchrony. They found that the auditory stimuli had to be advanced by 60 ms or delayed by 240 ms with respect to the visual stimuli before the strength of the McGurk effect was reliably different from the synchronous presentation.

In a study of the perception of speech in noise, Pandey, Kunov, and Abel (1986) delayed the auditory speech signal across a 300 ms range. For subjects who had little speech-reading experience, the auditory signal was delayed 120 ms before their performance differed from the synchronous presentation and 300 ms before the audiovisual condition was equal to the visual-only condition. A second group of subjects with some speech-reading experience were tested at a higher signal-to-noise ratio and showed a similar pattern of results. The auditory signal was delayed 80 ms before their performance differed from the synchronous presentation and 240 ms before the audiovisual condition was equal to the visual-only condition.

McGrath and Summerfield (1985) studied the effects of auditory delay when the audio signal was a measure of vocal fold contact area (electroglottograph). This signal primarily contains information about the fundamental frequency of voicing and by itself is unintelligible. The auditory signal was delayed by 20, 40, 80, and 160 ms. Only at the 160 ms delay did performance decrease significantly.

These studies and others (e.g., Campbell & Dodd, 1980; Koenig, 1965, cited in Pandey et al., 1986, Massaro & Cohen, 1993; Massaro, Cohen, & Smeele, 1996; Smeele, Sittig, & van Heuven, 1992; Summerfield, 1992; Tillmann, Pompino-Marschall, & Porzig, 1984) suggest that the perceptual system needs only loose temporal association between the visual and auditory modalities. This temporal "sloppiness" is surprising because of the strong statistical relationship between visual speech movements and the simultaneous acoustics.

Audiovisual speech production

In recent years, we have made substantial progress in characterizing the dependencies that exist between measures of vocal tract, facial, and acoustic behavior during production of audiovisual speech. The main results of this research program are summarized briefly here.

In a complex production study for speakers of Japanese and English, measures of the midsagittal vocal tract (tongue, lips, and jaw) were compared with measures of the three-dimensional face and with the spectral acoustics. As a first step, we examined the statistical structure of the data from each data source. Using a simple linear decomposition technique, *principal components analysis* (PCA), we found that the dimensionality of events within each measurement domain could be reduced substantially (for details, see Yehia, Rubin, & Vatikiotis-Bateson, 1998). For example, more than 99% of the 3D face motion measured with 18 position markers could be recovered from just seven principal components. The same was true of vocal tract measures and the spectral components of the acoustics. This is shown in Figure 11.5. This is consistent with the finding that there is a great deal of redundancy in the visual speech signal.

A second major finding was that the events in one domain could be reliably estimated from measures made in other domains. Having observed that vertical

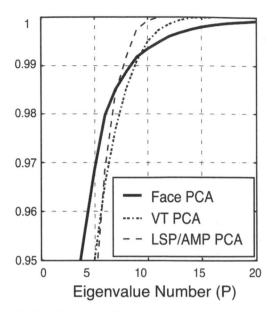

FIGURE 11.5 Dimensionality of events shown as a cumulative percentage of the variance recovered for PCA decomposition of a single subject's time-varying data within each measurement domain: motions of the face and vocal tract (VT), and the combined correlation of frequency (LSP) and amplitude (AMP) for the speech acoustics.

jaw position, the primary contributor to mouth opening, was the largest component of the PCA for both the vocal tract and face domains, we were not surprised to discover that 90%–95% of the face position data could be recovered from vocal tract components. This is shown in Figure 11.6, where the correlation of data in different measurement domains is computed using *singular value decomposition* (SVD). The resulting eigenvectors are ranked and their contribution to estimating the behavior is summed to show the small number needed to characterize the correspondence. Also plotted are the within-domain PCA results (eigenvalues) for comparison purposes. Similar results have been obtained recently by other groups using these and slightly different techniques for different languages (Badin, Bailly, Reveret, Baciu, Segebarth, & Savariaux, in press) and tasks (Jiang, Alwan, Keating, Auer, & Bernstein, in press).

This work has also revealed that face motion during speech can be reliably estimated from the spectral acoustics, and vice versa. Although linear techniques account for only about 70% of the variance in these estimations, the introduction of simple nonlinear estimation techniques has allowed recovery of up to 100% of the face motion for individual sentences from the speech acoustics (Yehia, Kuratate, & Vatikiotis-Bateson, 1999). The degree of recovery depends on factors such as training set size, the complexity of the estimation

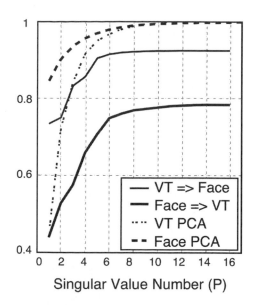

FIGURE 11.6 Cross-domain correlation results based on singular value decomposition (SVD) are shown as estimation percentages for face from vocal tract (VT) motion (VT → Face) and VT from face (Face → VT).

TABLE 11.1

Reliability of estimating f_0 from head motion, and vice versa

Direction of Estimation	Subject E.V.B.		Subject T.K.	
	Mean	(SD)	Mean	(SD)
Head motion > f_0	0.88	(0.09)	0.73	(0.13)
f_0 > head motion	0.50	(0.19)	0.25	(0.19)

Note: Table shows the reliability of estimating f_0 from head motion and vice versa for an English speaker (E.V.B.) and a Japanese speaker (T.K.). The dimensionality of head motion can be reduced from six (three rotations, three translations) to three factors (accounting for 99% of the variance). This is sufficient for reliable estimations of f_0 from head motion, but the reverse estimation is ill-posed and results in substantially weaker results.

Data from Yehia et al. (2002).

algorithm, and whether or not the analyzed speech samples were excised from the same speaking sequence (Vatikiotis-Bateson & Yehia, in press).

The motions of the head during speech are also highly correlated with the speech acoustics, specifically the fundamental frequency (f_0) of the vocal folds. Vocal fold vibration is the primary source of vocal tract excitation resulting in vowels, sonorants such as /r/ and /l/, and voiced consonants such as /b, d, g/. Fluctuations in f_0 give speech its melodic quality and specific patterns of fluctuation along with changes of intensity (RMS amplitude) and duration comprise the prosody of speech. Speech prosody conveys linguistic information about utterance structure as well as paralinguistic information about the speaker's mood, sincerity, and intent. Correlations between f_0 and rigid body head motion—the rotations and translations of the head about the three coordinate axes—have been consistently high, accounting for 80%–90% of the variance during sentence production by Japanese and English speakers (Yehia, Kuratate, & Vatikiotis-Bateson, in press) (Table 11.1).

Are these correspondences between measurement domains really so surprising? We think not, insofar as the vocal tract acts as a common source for both speech acoustics and phonetically relevant events on the face. Physiological support for this notion is provided by the ability to estimate vocal tract, facial, and even acoustic signals accurately from measured electromyographic (EMG) activity of the orofacial muscles

(Vatikiotis-Bateson & Yehia, 1996; Yared, Yehia, Vatikiotis-Bateson, & Aguirre, 2002).

Production-based animation

The linear and nonlinear dependencies observed analytically during speech production between signals measured in different domains means that phonetic information is redundantly specified in the audible and visible components. This does not mean that *all* speech information is multimodally redundant. There are undoubtedly independent components of the acoustics not represented in the visible motions of the face or head. There is also no guarantee that the redundancies revealed by statistical analysis of production are relevant to audiovisual speech perception. The extent to which perceivers have access to and take advantage of these structures must be demonstrated.

One way to do that is to construct multimodal stimuli from measured production data and evaluate them perceptually. To this end, two animation systems have been devised in which both static and time-varying measurements are used to generate cosmetically and behaviorally realistic talking heads. One system, developed at ATR Laboratories in Japan, uses measured or estimated face motions to reconfigure a 3D face (3D mesh plus video texture map) whose deformation characteristics have been derived statistically from a set of static postures (for details, see Kuratate, Yehia, & Vatikiotis-Bateson, 1998). The animation process is schematized in Figure 11.7.

The second system also incorporates a 3D face, but its deformation is constrained by physical models of the skin and musculoskeletal structures. This model is "driven" either in a feed-forward manner by muscle EMG signals previously recorded (for details see Lucero & Munhall, 1999) or in an inverse manner by estimating muscle signals from recorded face motion (Pitermann &

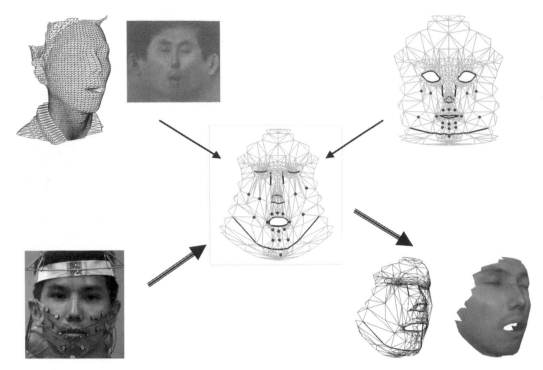

FIGURE 11.7   Schematic overview of kinematics-based animation. Static 3D head scans for nine expressive postures (example shown in upper left) are fitted with a generic face mesh (upper right) in order to compute the geometric deformation parameters for a speaker's face. The resulting mean face (middle) is then parameterized frame by frame by the time-varying position of marker positions recorded during speech production (lower left). The video texture map is attached to deformed mesh for each frame (lower right) and animated.

Munhall, 2001). Because the time-varying output of both models is derived from signals measured during speech production, audio synchronization is not an issue, and the audio signal can be modified or replaced by synthesized speech signals.

Conclusion

In this chapter we have summarized data showing some of the spatial and temporal conditions that influence speech perception. The overall impression from this work is that audiovisual speech is a coarsely coded signal: neither high-temporal-frequency nor high-spatial-frequency information seems necessary for perceptual success. The rich information in the low-frequency portion of the spectrum of speech signals presumably accounts for the robustness of audiovisual speech perception. This low-frequency character of speech fits with the variable visual conditions of face-to-face conversation, in which conversational distances and social gaze patterns reduce the visual resolution of visible speech. It also matches the temporal rates of articulation.

The process by which this low-frequency visual and auditory information is linked during perception, however, is still unclear. One possibility is that there is a common temporal signature in both modalities

because they result from the same speech movements. The slow changes in the acoustics reflect the opening and closing of the vocal tract, and these patterns directly correspond to the visual kinematics (see also Greenberg & Arai, 2001; Munhall et al., 1996; Remez, Fellowes, Pisoni, Goh, & Rubin, 1998). To test whether these dynamic patterns are important for audiovisual integration, we need to control both the visual and auditory dynamics. The production-based animation that we and others are developing permits such direct manipulations of visual and auditory kinematics. Future progress in understanding natural conversation will depend on these simulations.

ACKNOWLEDGMENTS   This work was funded by grants from the NIDCD (grant DC-05774), NSERC, and CRL Keihanna Info-Communications Research Laboratories, and by the Telecommunications Advancement Organization of Japan.

REFERENCES

Badin, P., Bailly, G., Reveret, L., Baciu, M., Segebarth, C., & Savariaux, C. (in press). Three-dimensional linear articulatory modeling of tongue, lips and face, based on MRI and video images. *Journal of Phonetics.*

Baken, R. J. (1987). *Clinical measurement of speech and voice.* Boston: College-Hill.

Bernstein, L. E., Demorest, M. E., & Tucker, P. E. (2000). Speech perception without hearing. *Perception & Psychophysics, 62,* 233–252.

Brooke, N. M., & Templeton, P. D. (1990). Visual speech intelligibility of digitally processed facial images. *Proceedings of the Institute of Acoustics, 12,* 483–490.

Campbell, R., & Dodd, B. (1980). Hearing by eye. *Quarterly Journal of Experimental Psychology, 32,* 85–99.

Campbell, C., & Massaro, D. (1997). Perception of visible speech: Influence of spatial quantization. *Perception, 26,* 129–146.

Campbell, R., Harvey, M., Troscianko, T., Massaro, D., & Cohen, M. (1996). *Form and movement in speechreading: Effects of static and dynamic noise masks on speechreading faces and point-light displays.* Paper presented at WIGLS, Delaware.

Daniloff, R. G., & Moll, K. L. (1968). Coarticulation of lip rounding. *Journal of Speech and Hearing Research, 11,* 707–721.

Dixon, N., & Spitz, L. (1980). The detection of audiovisual desynchrony. *Perception, 9,* 719–721.

Erber, N. P. (1971). Effects of distance on the visual reception of speech. *Journal of Speech and Hearing Research, 14,* 848–857.

Erber, N. P. (1974). Effects of angle, distance, and illumination on visual reception of speech by profoundly deaf children. *Journal of Speech and Hearing Research, 17,* 99–112.

Erber, N. P. (1979). Auditory-visual perception of speech with reduced optical clarity. *Journal of Speech and Hearing Research, 22,* 212–223.

Fitch, J. L., & Holbrook, A. (1970). Modal vocal fundamental frequency of young adults. *Archives of Otolaryngology, 92,* 379–382.

Fixmer, E., & Hawkins, S. (1998). The influence of quality of information on the McGurk effect. Paper presented at the International Conference on Auditory-Visual Speech Processing—AVSP '98, Terrigal, Australia.

Grant, K. W., & Seitz, P. F. (1998). Measures of auditory-visual integration in nonsense syllables and sentences, *Journal of the Acoustical Society of America, 104,* 2438–2450.

Greenberg, S. (1999). Speaking in shorthand: A syllable-centric perspective for understanding pronunciation variation. *Speech Communication, 29,* 159–176.

Greenberg, S., & Arai, T. (2001). The relation between speech intelligibility and the complex modulation spectrum. *Proceedings of the 7th European Conference on Speech Communication and Technology (Eurospeech-2001).* Aalborg, Denmark.

Hall, E. T. (1966). *The hidden dimension.* New York: Doubleday.

Jiang, J., Alwan, A., Keating, P. A., Auer Jr., E. T., & Bernstein, L. E. (in press). On the relationship between face movements, tongue movements and speech acoustics. *EURASIP Special Issue: Joint Audio-Visual Speech Processing.*

Jordan, T., & Sergeant, P. (1998). Effects of facial image size on visual and audiovisual speech recognition. In R. Campbell, B. Dodd, & D. Burnham (Eds.), *Hearing by eye: II. Advances in the psychology of speechreading and auditory-visual speech* (pp. 155–176). London: Psychology Press.

Jordan, T., & Sergeant, P. (2000). Effects of distance on visual and audiovisual speech recognition. *Language and Speech, 43,* 107–124.

Kent, R. D., & Read, C. (1992). *The acoustic analysis of speech.* San Diego, CA: Singular.

Kuratate, T., Yehia, H., & Vatikiotis-Bateson, E. (1998). Kinematics-based synthesis of realistic talking faces. In D. Burnham, J. Robert-Ribes, & E. Vatikiotis-Bateson (Eds.), *International Conference on Auditory-Visual Speech Processing (AVSP '98)* (pp. 185–190). Terrigal-Sydney, Australia: Causal Productions.

Lansing, C. R., & McConkie, G. W. (1999). Attention to facial regions in segmental and prosodic visual speech perception tasks. *Journal of Speech, Language, and Hearing Research, 42,* 526–538.

Linker, W. (1982). Articulatory and acoustic correlates of labial activity in vowels: A cross-linguistic study. *UCLA Working Papers in Phonetics, 56,* 1–154.

Lucero, J. C., & Munhall, K. G. (1999). A model of facial biomechanics for speech production. *Journal of the Acoustical Society of America, 106,* 2834–2842.

MacLeod, A., & Summerfield, Q. (1987). Quantifying the contribution of vision to speech perception in noise. *British Journal of Audiology, 12,* 131–141.

Massaro, D. W. (1998). *Perceiving talking faces: From speech perception to a behavioral principle.* Cambridge, MA: MIT Press.

Massaro, D. W., & Cohen, M. M. (1993). Perceiving asynchronous bimodal speech in consonant-vowel and vowel syllables. *Speech Communication, 13,* 127–134.

Massaro, D., Cohen, M. M., & Smeele, P. M. (1996). Perception of asynchronous and conflicting visual and auditory speech. *Journal of the Acoustical Society of America, 100,* 1777–1786.

MacDonald, J., Andersen, S., & Bachmann, T. (2000). Hearing by eye: How much spatial degradation can be tolerated? *Perception, 29,* 1155–1168.

McGrath, M., & Summerfield, Q. (1985). Intermodal timing relations and audio-visual speech recognition by normal-hearing adults. *Journal of the Acoustical Society of America, 77*(2), 678–684.

McGurk, H., & MacDonald, J. (1976). Hearing lips and seeing voices. *Nature, 264,* 746–748.

Morasso, P. (1981). Spatial control of arm movements. *Experimental Brain Research, 42,* 223–227.

Muller, E. M., & MacLeod, G. (1982). *Perioral biomechanics and its relation to labial motor control.* Paper presented at a meeting of the Acoustical Society of America, Chicago.

Munhall, K. G. (2002). Unpublished raw data.

Munhall, K. G., Gribble, P., Sacco, L., & Ward, M. (1996). Temporal constraints on the McGurk effect. *Perception & Psychophysics, 58,* 351–362.

Munhall, K. G., Kroos, C., Jozan, G., & Vatikiotis-Bateson, E. (in press). Spatial frequency requirements for audiovisual speech perception. *Perception and Psychophysics.*

Munhall, K. G., & Vatikiotis-Bateson, E. (1998). The moving face during speech communication. In *Hearing by eye: Part 2. The psychology of speechreading and audiovisual speech* (pp. 123–136). London: Taylor & Francis.

Näsänen, R. (1999). Spatial frequency bandwidth used in the recognition of facial images. *Vision Research, 39,* 3824–3833.

Neely, K. K. (1956). Effect of visual factors on the intelligibility of speech. *Journal of the Acoustical Society of America, 28,* 1275–1277.

Nelson, W. L. (1983). Physical principles for economies of skilled movements. *Biological Cybernetics, 46,* 135–147.

Ohala, J. J. (1975). The temporal regulation of speech. In G. Fant & M. A. A. Tatham (Eds.), *Auditory analysis and perception of speech.* London: Academic Press.

Ostry, D. J., & Munhall, K. G. (1994). Control of jaw orientation and position in mastication and speech. *Journal of Neurophysiology, 71*, 1528–1545.

Ostry, D. J., Vatikiotis-Bateson, E., Gribble, P. L. (1997). An examination of the degrees of freedom of human jaw motion in speech. *Journal of Speech, Language and Hearing Research, 40*, 1341–1351.

Pandey, C. P., Kunov, H., & Abel, M. S. (1986). Disruptive effects of auditory signal delay on speech perception with lip-reading. *The Journal of Auditory Research, 26*, 27–41.

Paré, M., Richler, R., ten Hove, M., & Munhall, K. G. (2001). *Gaze behavior in audiovisual speech perception: The influence of ocular fixations on the McGurk effect.* Manuscript submitted for publication.

Pitermann, M., & Munhall, K. G. (2001). An inverse dynamics approach to facial animation. *Journal of the Acoustical Society of America, 110*, 1570–1580.

Ramsay, J. O., Munhall, K. G., Gracco, G. L., & Ostry, D. J. (1996). Functional data analyses of lip motion. *Journal of the Acoustical Society of America, 99*, 3718–3727.

Remez, R., Fellowes, J., Pisoni, D., Goh, W., & Rubin, P. (1998). Multimodal perceptual organization of speech: Evidence from tone analogs of spoken utterances. *Speech Communication, 26*, 65–73.

Rönnberg, J., Andersson, J., Samuelsson, S., Soderfeldt, B., Lyxell, B., & Risberg, J. (1999). A speechreading expert: The case of MM. *Journal of Speech, Language and Hearing Research, 42*, 5–20.

Small, L. H., & Infante, A. A. (1988). Effects of training and visual distance on speechreading performance. *Perceptual and Motor Skills, 66*, 415–418.

Smeele, P. M. T., Sittig, A. C., & van Heuven, V. J. (1992). Intelligibility of audio-visually desynchronized speech: Asymmetrical effect of phoneme position. *Proceedings of the International Conference on Spoken Language Processing* (pp. 65–68), Banff, Canada.

Smith, A. (1992). The control of orofacial movements in speech. *Critical Reviews in Oral Biology and Medicine, 3*, 233–267.

Sumby, W. H., & Pollack, I. (1954). Visual contribution to speech intelligibility in noise. *Journal of the Acoustical Society of America, 26*, 212–215.

Summerfield, Q. (1992). Lipreading and audio-visual speech perception. *Philosophical Transactions of the Royal Society of London. Series B: Biological Sciences, 335*, 71–78.

Thorn, F., & Thorn, S. (1989). Speechreading with reduced vision: A problem of aging. *Journal of the Optical Society of America, 6*, 491–499.

Tillmann, H. G., Pompino-Marschall, B., & Porzig, H. (1984). Zum Einfluß visuell dargeborener Sprechbewegungen auf die Wahrnehmung der akustisch kodierten Artikulation. *Forschungsberichte des Instituts für Phonetik und Sprachliche Dommunikation der Universität Munchen, 19*, 318–338.

Vatikiotis-Bateson, E., Eigsti, I.-M., Yano, S., & Munhall, K. G. (1998). Eye movement of perceivers during audiovisual speech perception. *Perception & Psychophysics, 60*(6), 926–940.

Vatikiotis-Bateson, E., & Kelso, J. A. S. (1993). Rhythm type and articulatory dynamics in English, French and Japanese. *Journal of Phonetics, 21*, 231–265.

Vatikiotis-Bateson, E., Munhall, K. G., Hirayama, M., Kasahara, Y., & Yehia, H. (1996). Physiology-based synthesis of audiovisual speech. *4th Speech Production Seminar: Models and data* (pp. 241–244). Autrans, France.

Vatikiotis-Bateson, E., & Ostry, D. J. (1995). An analysis of the dimensionality of jaw motion in speech. *Journal of Phonetics, 23*, 101–117.

Vatikiotis-Bateson, E., & Yehia, H. (1996). Physiological modeling of facial motion during speech. *Transactions of the Technical Committee, Psychological and Physiological Acoustics, H-96-65*, 1–8.

Vatikiotis-Bateson, E., & Yehia, H. C. (2001). Speaking mode variability in multimodal speech production. *IEEE Transactions in Neural Networks.*

Vitkovich, M., & Barber, P. (1994). Effects of video frame rate on subjects' ability to shadow one of two competing verbal passages. *Journal of Speech and Hearing Research, 37*, 1204–1210.

Vitkovich, M., & Barber, P. (1996). Visible speech as a function of image quality: Effects of display parameters on lipreading ability. *Applied Cognitive Psychology, 10*, 121–140.

Watson, C. S., Qui, W. W., Chamberlain, M., & Li, X. (1996). Auditory and visual speech perception: Confirmation of a modality-independent source of individual differences in speech recognition. *Journal of the Acoustical Society of America, 100*, 1153–1162.

Yared, G. F. G., Yehia, H. C., Vatikiotis-Bateson, E., & Aguirre, L. A. (2002). Facial motion synthesis during speech from physiological signals. *Proceedings of the XIV Congresso Brasileiro de Automatica (CBA 2002)*, Natal, Brazil.

Yehia, H. C., Kuratate, T., & Vatikiotis-Bateson, E. (1999). Using speech acoustics to drive facial motion. *Proceedings of the 14th International Congress of Phonetic Sciences* (Vol. 1, pp. 631–634), San Francisco.

Yehia, H. C., Kuratate, T., & Vatikitotis-Bateson, E. (2002). Linking facial animation, head motion and speech acoustics. *Journal of Phonetics, 30*, 555–568.

Yehia, H. C., Rubin, P. E., & Vatikiotis-Bateson, E. (1998). Quantitative association of vocal-tract and facial behavior. *Speech Communication, 26*, 23–44.

12 Speech as a Supramodal or Amodal Phenomenon

CAROL A. FOWLER

Introduction

Speech perceivers are informational omnivores. Although the acoustic medium provides necessary and sometimes sufficient information for phonetic perception, listeners use other sources as well. The surface of the speaking face provides surprising amounts of phonetic information (e.g., Yehia & Vatikiotis-Bateson, 1998), at least some of which observers use when it is available. In noisy settings, perceivers who can see the face of a speaker achieve more accurate percepts than those who cannot (e.g., Sumby & Pollack, 1954). Moreover, given appropriate dubbings of acoustic syllables or words onto visible facial gestures for other syllables or words, perceivers integrate information from the two modalities (the *McGurk effect;* e.g., Brancazio, in press; Massaro, 1998; McGurk & MacDonald, 1976). For example, acoustic *ma* dubbed onto visible *da* is identified predominantly as *na,* an outcome that integrates visible information for place of articulation with acoustic information for manner and voicing. This outcome can be phenomenally striking; people hear one syllable with their eyes open and a different one with their eyes closed.

Another perceptual system that provides useful information about speech is the haptic system. Some individuals who are deaf and blind have learned to talk by placing their hands on the face of (and, in Helen Keller's case, sometimes in the mouth of) a speaker (Lash, 1980; Chomsky, 1986). Moreover, naive normally seeing and hearing individuals show a haptic version of the McGurk effect. With hands in surgical gloves placed over the mouth and jaw of a speaker as the speaker mouths *ga,* perceivers increase identifications as *ga* of syllables along an acoustic continuum ranging from *ba* to *ga* (Fowler & Dekle, 1991).

How should we understand speech perception such that phonetic perception can be achieved in all of these ways?

An analogous question arises when we consider speech production as perceptually guided action. We can first consider speech production guided by the perception of one's own speech. When speakers' own acoustic signals are fed back transformed in some way, their speech is affected. For example, in the Lombard effect, speakers increase their vocal amplitude in the presence of noise (e.g., Lane & Tranel, 1971). When feedback about vowel production is transformed acoustically, speakers change the way they produce vowels as if in compensation (Houde & Jordan, 1998). Hommel, Müsseler, Aschersleben, and Prinz (in press) raise the more general question, how can percepts communicate with action plans? Aren't they coded in different ways, percepts as representations of features of the stimulus input and action plans as some kind of motoric specification? How should we understand speech production and speech perception such that perceived speech can affect produced speech?

Finally, a related question arises when we consider speech as a communicative activity taking place between people. In cooperative conversations, speakers may converge in their dialects, vocal intensity, speaking rate, and rate of pausing (see Giles, Coupland, & Coupland, 1991, for a review). More generally, listeners perceive the phonological message that talkers meant to convey. Speakers talk by producing actions of vocal tract articulators. Ultimately their speech action plan must be to produce those actions. For their part, listeners receive acoustic speech signals, signals that have acoustic, not motoric, features. How can speakers communicate with listeners? How can we understand speaking and listening such that a perceived dialect can affect a produced one, and so, more fundamentally, that a listener can perceive a talker's phonological message? Each of these questions is addressed in this chapter.

Cross-modal speech perception

I consider four approaches to an understanding of cross-modal speech perception. Of these, three invoke the need for a "common currency," that is, a common kind of representation or percept that can be achieved by the different modalities. Effectively, in these approaches, information integrates across the perceptual modalities, because it is information about a common object or common event. Likewise, perceptual information can affect action because perception and action planning share a common currency. The fourth approach is quite different. It proposes integration by fiat. Information acquired cross-modally integrates because templates for speech percepts in the head associate compatible features acquired by different sensory modalities. Perceived information can communicate with action planning for unspecified reasons.

One approach, derived from Meltzoff and Moore's (1997) AIM (active intermodal mapping) hypothesis, suggests that speech perceivers achieve a supramodal representation of a speaker's utterance—a representation, that is, that somehow transcends the sensory modalities from which it derives. It is the supramodal nature of the representation that allows integration of information derived from different perceptual modalities. A supramodal representation of speech that is compatible with the supramodal representations proposed by Meltzoff and Moore is of vocal tract organs and their actions.

Two other approaches share one idea about speech perception but disagree on another. According to both the motor theory of speech perception (Liberman & Mattingly, 1985, 1989; Liberman & Whalen, 2000) and the direct-realist theory (Best, 1994; Fowler, 1986, 1994), speech perceivers perceive the linguistically significant actions ("gestures") of the vocal tract that occur during speech. Gestural percepts are achieved regardless of the perceptual modality that provides information about them. This proposal is compatible with the extension of AIM to speech, as just proposed.

In the motor theory, these gestural percepts are effectively representations of gestures that are generated in a module of the brain specialized to extract them from perceptual information. These gestural representations, like the supramodal representation of an AIM hypothesis, provide a common currency that allows information to be integrated across, for example, the acoustic and optical modalities (and to be integrated across sensory modalities and motor production systems). I will refer to these representations as amodal, because they are motoric rather than perceptual in nature.

In direct-realist theories of perception (e.g., Gibson, 1979), perception is not mediated by representations. Rather, perceptual systems universally use structure in media that stimulate the sense organs (e.g., patterning in reflected light for vision and patterning in air for hearing) to perceive the world of distal objects and events directly. Information is integrated across the perceptual modalities because it is information about a common object or event. Speech perceivers perceive

gestures because that is what information for a speech event, whether it is acoustic, optical, haptic, or proprioceptive, is about. In this case perception is amodal, because it is direct perception of events in the world.

In all of these accounts integration occurs because the representations or the percepts are uniformly of distal properties of the world, not of the proximal stimulation that the sense organs intercept. However, the fourth account of integration discussed in this chapter does not invoke the idea of common currency. Instead, speech percepts achieved auditorily are cued by acoustic features and those achieved optically are cued by visible speech gestures (e.g., Massaro, 1998). The information integrates despite the fact that acoustic features are features of the proximal stimulus, while optical features are properties of the distal event—even in the absence of a common currency—because possible speech percepts are represented mentally associated with both the acoustic cues and the visible gestures that provide information about them. In the following discussion, I elaborate on each of these four theoretical ideas.

SPEECH PERCEPTION AS SUPRAMODAL   Meltzoff and Moore (1997, 1999) proposed their AIM hypothesis to explain the remarkable propensity and ability of newborns to imitate facial gestures. Infants do not necessarily imitate accurately right away. They typically get the organ—tongue or lips—right immediately, but they may not get the gesture right. However, they keep trying and keep refining their own gestures to approximate more closely those of their model over many repeated attempts.

Within hours of being born, infants will imitate a tongue protrusion gesture by an adult (Meltzoff & Moore, 1977). (Imitations are identified as such by coders of videotapes of the infants who are blind to the particular gesture that an infant saw. They use pre-established criteria to classify the infants' facial gestures.) It has been found that tongue gestures by infants are more likely to occur when the adult model is producing or has just produced a tongue gesture rather than a lip gesture. In contrast, lip gestures by infants are more common in response to modeled lip gestures than to tongue gestures. How do the infants do it? As Meltzoff and Moore (1997) point out, the infants can see the model's gesture, but not their own. They can proprioceptively feel their tongue, say, and any gesture that they produce with it, but they cannot feel the model's tongue or its gesture. Accordingly, they must have some way of relating information acquired by different sensory modalities.

Meltzoff and Moore (1997, 1999) propose that perceivers, including young infants, establish "supramodal representations" of bodily organs and their interrelations (e.g., a tongue protruded between teeth). These representations in some way transcend the sensory modalities, providing a single framework within which information acquired from different perceptual modalities can be compared and contrasted. The representations transcend the modalities by representing the distal world of objects (e.g., tongues) and events (e.g., protrusion gestures) rather than the proximal world of sensory stimulation. That is, given optical proximal stimulation caused by a tongue protrusion gesture, the infants represent not a reflected-light structure but a protruding tongue. Given proprioceptive proximal stimulation caused by their own tongue and its action, they represent not proprioceptive "raw feels" but a tongue in action. Because both modalities yield these representations of distal events, components of the events perceived in different modalities (e.g., tongues) can be compared and identified as equivalent.

Vocal imitation, which infants also show from a young age (by 12 weeks of age in Kuhl & Meltzoff, 1996), Meltzoff and Moore suggest is based essentially on intramodal comparisons. This may appear to pose less of a challenge to understand than the cross-modal imitation of facial gestures. However, vocal imitation and infant speech perception more generally pose some very interesting challenges to theorists. It is likely true that vocal imitation depends most heavily on intramodal comparisons. (However, Kuhl and Meltzoff's model was visible to the imitating infants.) Nevertheless, even in that case the infant solves a rather large problem. There is no way that an infant can come close to reproducing the acoustic signal of an adult model, even setting aside the fact that 12-week-old infants are unskilled speakers. This is because an infant has a tiny vocal tract and an adult has a large one. Accordingly, the fundamental frequencies of infant vocalizations and the formant frequencies of the vowel-like sounds they produce at 12 weeks are much higher in frequency than those of an adult. Infants could not imitate by achieving an acoustic match to adult vowels even if they were skilled enough to produce the same vocalic gestures as an adult. On what basis does the infant detect correspondences between its productions and those of other speakers? Even intramodal comparisons require establishment of a common currency that allows abstract equivalences in events to be detected.

In any case, infant speech perception itself is not unimodal (just as infants' perception generally is cross-modal; e.g., Bahrick, 1987; Bahrick & Watson, 1985; Spelke, 1979). In research by Kuhl and Meltzoff (1982, 1988; MacKain, Studdert-Kennedy, Spieker, & Stern, 1983), infants looked at two films showing a speaker producing the vowel they heard being produced. In the films, which were presented side by side, one speaker

mouthed /i/ and the other mouthed /a/. If the acoustic vowel was /a/, infants looked longer at the visible /a/ than at the visible /i/; they looked longer at the visible /i/ if the acoustic vowel was /i/ rather than /a/. Kuhl and Meltzoff (1988) report replicating the finding with the vowels /i/ and /u/.

Compatibly, Rosenblum, Schmuckler, and Johnson (1997) reported finding a McGurk effect in 5-month-old infants. They used a procedure in which discrimination is assessed with a looking-time habituation procedure. As long as infants watched a video display, they heard a sound being produced. When they looked away, the sound stopped. In such circumstances, when the same sound is repeated over trials, once the infants detect the contingency between their looking and the presentation of a sound, they look for a long time initially, but over trials their looking time decreases. For infants in experimental conditions, following habituation to the first sound (indexed by a criterion decrease in looking time), a new sound accompanies the video display. If the infant discriminates the sound, looking time increases again; if he or she does not, looking time remains at a low level or decreases further. Infants in a control condition receive the same sound before and after habituation. Rosenblum et al. used a face mouthing /va/ as the video display and, during habituation, a /va/ acoustic syllable. After habituation, infants in the experimental group received (on alternate trials) video /va/ accompanied by audio /ba/ or video /va/ accompanied by audio /da/. (Adults hear the first pairing as /va/ but the second as /da/.) In the experiment, infants increased their looking time (relative to no-shift control infants) only when the acoustic signal was /da/. A subsequent experiment, in which an unmoving face accompanied the same acoustic syllables as in the first experiment, yielded a different pattern of looking-time changes. In the presence of an unmoving face, adults should hear the prehabituation syllable as /va/ and the posthabituation syllables as /ba/ and /da/. In this experiment, infants' looking times increased relative to the no-shift condition only on /ba/ trials. Accordingly, the experimenters inferred that the result pattern in the first experiment was not due to acoustic /ba/ sounding less different from /va/ than acoustic /da/. Rather, infants experienced cross-modal integration such that video /va/-audio /va/ and video /va/-audio /ba/ sound the same, just as they do for adult listener-viewers.

These findings raise questions very much like those posed for infants who imitate visible facial gestures. In Kuhl's research, how do infants know which facial speech gestures match which acoustic vowel? In the research of Rosenblum et al., how are optical and acoustic speech displays perceived such that the infants experience cross-modal integration? There has to be a way to compare information acquired in two different perceptual modalities.

Meltzoff and Kuhl (1994; cf. Meltzoff, Kuhl, & Moore, 1991) propose that the basis for infants' cross-modal integrations is a learning process in which infants come to associate vocal gestures and their auditory outcomes during cooing and babbling when they both see and hear speech. These associations permit integration of audiovisual information such as that provided by Kuhl and Meltzoff (1982) and Rosenblum et al. (1997). It may also serve imitation of speech, as observed by Kuhl and Meltzoff (1996). Given a (normalized) acoustic signal produced by a model speaker, infants can use the associations to determine which gestures will generate the equivalent infant vocalization.

This proposal is not analogous to the proposal that Meltzoff and Moore (1997, 1999) developed to explain infants' cross-modal identification of facial gesture equivalences. A proposal analogous to the AIM hypothesis would be that cross-modal speech perception implies establishment of supramodal representations of what it looks like and sounds like to produce a particular sequence of gestures. What would such a representation be like? Meltzoff and Moore propose that supramodal representations supporting facial gesture imitation are representations of real-world—that is, distal—objects (organs) and events (gestures). That is what unites the perceptual input from different sensory modalities. We need an idea like that of Meltzoff and Moore for speech perception. The real-world events of phonetic speech production are, as they are for facial-gesture production and perception, actions of organs of the vocal tract. Facial gestures and speech gestures are alike in this respect. They differ in two ways. Speech actions cause patterning, and not only in the optic array and, for the speaker, proprioceptively; they also structure the air. Moreover, and relatedly, they are linguistically significant vocal tract actions; we refer to them as *phonetic gestures*. If infants (and adults) perceive phonetic gestures from both acoustic information (e.g., Fowler, 1986) and optical information about them, the ability of infants to detect which of two visible faces is mouthing the vowel they hear is understandable.

Supramodally represented speech gestures can also be invoked to account for the findings of Rosenblum et al. (1997). It is understandable that infants as well as adults integrate optical and acoustic information for speech if both modalities yield supramodal, distal percepts—that is, percepts of the speaker's phonetic gestures. In that way, gestures specified by one modality may be compared and, if the information warrants it, identified with those specified by another.

Note that if infants perceive phonetic gestures, we can understand not only their audiovisual speech skills but perhaps their vocal imitation skill as well. Gesture perception provides an abstract equivalence of the sort that infants must achieve in order to compare their own vowels with those of an adult. Infants who perceive acoustic /u/ as a high back gesture of the tongue coupled to a protrusion gesture of the lips when an adult produces it can attempt to generate those gestures in their own vocal tract based on proprioceptive information. Likewise, infants can detect the match between the gestures of /u/ that they hear and the visible lip protrusion of a videotaped speaker producing /u/.

Do infants perceive phonetic gestures (see Lewkowicz and Kraebel, Chap. 41, this volume)? The experimental data are not in yet, but we do know that infants integrate information about speech cross-modally. We also know that they learn to produce speech by perceiving it spoken by others and by themselves. They must get gestural information from what they see and hear if perception guides their learning to talk. I will also suggest next that there is considerable evidence for gesture perception by adults.

EVIDENCE FOR PHONETIC GESTURE PERCEPTION The idea that listeners to speech perceive linguistically significant actions of the vocal tract is central to the account of cross-modal speech perception that this chapter has offered so far. It is justified in the AIM-derived account by the need for a common currency that allows perceptual information to be integrated cross-modally. It is justified in this and other ways by the two accounts to be presented next. Nonetheless, the idea is considered radical in the field of speech research.

Here I summarize some of the evidence that gestures are perceived. The review is brief and incomplete; the point here is to justify the idea.

Equivalence of cross-modal information This evidence has already been described. It includes the evidence that infants and adults integrate speech cross-modally and that they imitate speech. As Meltzoff and Moore (1997) propose for facial gestures, there must be a common currency for percepts achieved by different sensory modalities to be compared. The obvious domain is that of distal events—in speech, phonetic gestures.

The rapidity of imitation Luce (1986) points out that there is canonically a 100 to 150 ms difference in latencies to comparable simple and choice response tasks. Simple tasks are those in which participants make speeded responses when they detect an event. The response does not vary with the event. In choice tasks, different responses are made to different events, so the participant needs to do more than detect the occurrence of an event to choose his or her response. With appropriately chosen speech tasks, however, the difference in latencies can be very much smaller than the canonical difference, and both sets of latencies are in the range of canonical simple response times.

Both Kozhevnikov and colleagues (Kozhevnikov & Chistovich, 1965) and Porter and colleagues (Porter & Castellanos, 1980; Porter & Lubker, 1980) have obtained this outcome. Porter and Lubker had participants "shadow" a model speaker who produced an extended /a/ vowel followed at an unpredictable interval by a consonant-vowel (CV) syllable. In the simple task, participants produced the extended vowel with the model and switched to a designated syllable (/ba/) when the model produced a CV. In the choice task, participants produced the extended vowel with the model, and when the model shifted to a CV, the participant shifted to the same CV. In that experiment, choice task times exceeded simple task times by only 50 ms. In a recent replication of our own (Fowler, Brown, Sabadini, & Weihing, 2003), the difference was 26 ms. In both experiments, responses were very fast and more characteristic of canonical simple than choice latencies. Kozhevnikov et al., Porter et al., and Fowler et al. all interpreted the findings as demonstrating gesture perception. If speech perceivers perceive the speaker's gestures, then, in the choice condition, the percept provides instructions for the required response.

The disposition to imitate   Infants (e.g., Meltzoff & Moore, 1977) and adults (e.g., McHugo, Lanzetta, Sullivan, Masters, & Englis, 1985) are disposed to imitate others' facial gestures, and infants (Kuhl & Meltzoff, 1996) and adults (Goldinger, 1998) imitate others' speech. In infancy, imitation may have the function of helping children to acquire culturally appropriate behavior. But the tendency persists into adulthood. The persistence of imitation may occur because perception generally provides instructions for action. In speech, instructions for producing gestures are perceived gestures.

Conflicting and cooperating cues   Generally, if two stimuli differ in two ways acoustically, they are easier to discriminate than if they differ in just one of two ways. This is not always the case in speech, however. Fitch, Halwes, Erickson, and Liberman (1980) synthesized stimuli ranging from *slit* to *split* by varying two acoustic cues. A silent interval between the offset of the initial /s/ and the onset of /l/ was varied in duration. In addition, labial formant transitions either followed the silence or were absent. Both a silent interval and labial transitions provide information for /p/. Fitch et al. first found a trading relation between the cues. That is, silence of a

long enough duration was sufficient, in the absence of transitions, to yield a *split* percept, but less silence was needed if transitions were present. Some amount of silence could be traded for transitions. Next, Fitch et al. had participants discriminate pairs of the syllables in which pair members differed in either of three ways. In the first way, the syllables differed only in the silence duration; transitions were either present or absent in both members of a pair. In the two other conditions, pair members differed in both cues. In the "cooperating cues" condition, one member of a pair had a longer silent interval than the other, and it had transitions, whereas the other did not. That is, either both cues signaled /p/ or both signaled its absence. In the "conflicting cues" condition, pair members differed in the same two ways as in the cooperating condition, but one cue was swapped between pair members. Now the pair member with the longer silence lacked transitions whereas the other pair member had them. The striking finding was that listeners did discriminate cooperating pairs better than one-cue-different pairs, but they discriminated the conflicting pairs *worse* than one-cue-different pairs. Even though conflicting pairs differed in the same way as one-cue pairs and differed in one more way as well, discrimination performance was worse than in the one-cue condition. This finding was very surprising on acoustic grounds but is expected in gesture theory. In the cooperating condition, one pair member was a clear *split* and the other a clear *slit*. In the conflicting condition, often both members of a pair sounded like *split* or both like *slit*. It is not the acoustic quality of the cues that matters; rather, it is what they inform the listener about the presence or absence of a labial speech gesture. This finding has been replicated by Best, Morrongiello, and Robson (1981) using a *say-stay* continuum. Using a /sa/-/spa/ continuum, Nittrouer and Crowther (2001) have replicated the findings only in part. Five-year-olds discriminated one-cue-different pairs better than two-cue conflicting pairs; 7-year-olds showed no difference, and adults showed the opposite pattern. However, all three age groups discriminated cooperating cues pairs better than conflicting cues pairs (with the findings for 7-year-olds just marginally significant, $P = 0.10$).

Parsing the speech signal   Speech is coarticulated so that information about different consonants and vowels is conveyed by the same acoustic structure. For example, formant transitions provide information about both a consonantal and a vocalic gesture. In this way, gestures can have converging effects on the same acoustic dimensions. A good example is provided by fundamental frequency (f_0). Generally, the f_0 contour provides information about intonation (speech melody). However, it also shows declination, an early to late decrease in f_0 along a stretch of speech. In addition, high vowels are associated with higher f_0 values than low vowels, and voiceless obstruents cause a high falling tone on a following vowel. Research has shown that listeners "parse" effects of distinct gestures from f_0. That is, for /i/ and /a/ vowels to have the same pitch, /i/ has to be higher in f_0 than /a/ (e.g., Fowler & Brown, 1997). Listeners use the f_0 that a high vocalic gesture should have caused as information for vowel height, not vowel pitch or intonation (Reinholt Peterson, 1986). Declination is also parsed from intontation (Pierrehumbert, 1979; Silverman, 1987), as are the effects of stop consonant devoicing (e.g., Pardo & Fowler, 1997). There are similar findings with regard to segmental information for coarticulated consonants and vowels (e.g., Fowler & Smith, 1986). That is, speech perceivers parse the acoustic signal along gestural lines.

The two remaining accounts of cross-modal perception share with the earlier AIM-derived account a claim that listeners to speech perceive gestures.

SPEECH PERCEPTION AS AMODAL: 1. THE MOTOR THEORY
The motor theory of speech perception (e.g., Liberman,

1982; Liberman & Mattingly, 1985) offers an account of cross-modal speech perception that is similar to the account I derived above as an extension of AIM. The motor theory was developed to account for evidence suggesting a closer correspondence between speech percepts and articulation than between speech perception and the mediating acoustic speech signal. Two findings spurred development of the theory in the 1950s. Liberman and colleagues found that intelligible stop consonants (e.g., /b/, /d/, /g/, /p/, /t/, and /k/ in English) in CV or VC syllables could be synthesized in either of two ways, each way providing one of two prominent acoustic signatures of a stop consonant. One way, in CVs, was to provide the formant transitions into the following vowel appropriate to the consonant in the context of the vowel. The transitions are produced after release of the consonant as the vocal tract opens up for the vowel. The other way was to place the stop burst that occurs at release of the consonantal constriction just before a set of steady-state formants for the vowel.

One critical finding (Liberman, Delattre, Cooper, & Gerstman, 1954) was that the second formant transitions of synthetic syllables are acoustically quite different. As shown in Figure 12.1A, that for /di/ is a high rise in frequency, while that for /du/ is a low fall.

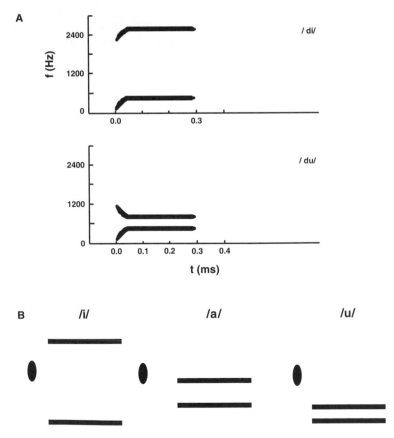

FIGURE 12.1 Schematic display of synthetic syllables /di/ and /du/ (*A*), with consonants specified by their formant transitions, and of /pi/, /ka/, and /pu/ (*B*), with consonants specified by stop bursts.

Isolated from the vowel, the transitions are audibly quite different. However, they are produced by the same gesture, a constriction of the tongue tip against the alveolar ridge of the palate. The acoustic differences arise from coarticulation, that is, from speakers overlapping temporally successive consonants and vowels. While the tongue tip constriction is being produced, the body of the tongue is conforming itself for the following vowel, as are the lips if the vowel is /u/. Therefore, after release of the tongue tip constriction, the vocal tract opens up into different vowels in the two syllables, and the formant transitions as well as the steady-state values of the formants are different. In this finding, two markedly different acoustic cues for /d/ caused by the same gesture (coarticulating with different ones) sound the same. The percept tracks articulation.

The second finding (Liberman, Delattre, & Cooper, 1952) was complementary. Here, the same stop burst placed before /i/ or /u/ was identified as /p/, but when placed before /a/, it was identified as /k/ (Fig. 12.1B). Now the same bit of acoustic signal that, because of coarticulation with the following vowel had to be produced by different constriction gestures before /a/ than before /i/ or /u/, sounded different to listeners. Again, listeners tracked gestures.

The logic by which these findings led Liberman and colleagues to develop the motor theory of speech perception is shown in Figures 12.2A and B. In the case of synthetic /di/ and /du/ the same oral constriction gesture gives rise, because of coarticulation, to different critical formant transitions; however, the consonants perceived, like the gestures, are invariant. In the case of synthetic /pi/, /ka/, and /pu/, different oral constriction gestures give rise, because of coarticulation, to the same acoustic stop burst; the consonants perceived, like the constriction gestures, are different.

In its final or near-final form, the motor theory (e.g., Liberman & Mattingly, 1985) proposed that gesture perception occurs in a module of the brain specialized for both speech production and speech perception. Coarticulation in speech is necessary, in the view of motor theorists, because consonants and vowels have to be sequenced very fast in order not to exceed the memory span of listeners during an utterance; however, if the segments were produced discretely, without coarticulation, the rate at which they occur would exceed the temporal resolving power of the ear. Coarticulation eliminates the discreteness of speech elements, but it creates a new problem. The relation between the acoustic signal and the segments that listeners must recover to identify words is very complex. The phonetic module evolved to deal with that complexity.

Coarticulation and perception of coarticulation are capabilities that had to coevolve, because neither would be useful without the other. According to the motor theory, the phonetic module is a single specialization of the brain that serves both capabilities, and it is this that underlies our perception of gestures rather than acoustic speech signals in the theory. The phonetic module uses its competence to generate coarticulated speech and to

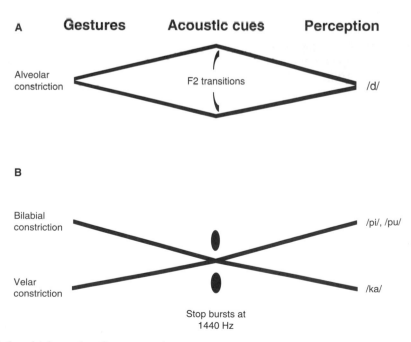

FIGURE 12.2   The logic by which results of perceptual experiments using the stimuli of Figure 12.1 led Liberman to develop his motor theory of speech perception.

recover the speakers' "intended" gestures. (Liberman and Mattingly argued that actual gestures of the vocal tract were not the same as intended gestures, because of coarticulation.)

A gestural percept might be called "amodal" rather than supramodal if the word "modality" refers just to perceptual systems. The percept is motoric in the theory. Otherwise, however, the motor theory's account of cross-modal speech perception is not very different from the account derived as an extension of Meltzoff and Moore's AIM. The gestural percept provides a common currency in which information about gestures derived acoustically, haptically, proprioceptively, and optically can converge.

In Liberman's motor theory, as in the extension of AIM, cross-modal speech perception is achieved by a percept that, in some way, is not tied to any perceptual modality. In the AIM account, the percept achieves that by being about distal properties of an event, not about the proximal stimulation itself. In the motor theory, the percept is not quite about distal properties, because it is of intended gestures rather than actual ones. However, it is similar in not being tied to any perceptual modality. In the motor theory, the percept is a motor percept.

The motor theory makes three central claims. It claims that listeners perceive (intended) speech gestures, that perception is achieved by a module of the brain dedicated to speech production and perception, and that perceptual speech processing recruits the speech motor system and its motor competence. The first claim is common to all three views presented here, and evidence for it has been offered earlier.

Behavioral evidence that has been interpreted as evidence for a dedicated speech processing system is provided by duplex perception. In one version of this finding (e.g., Mann & Liberman, 1983), listeners are presented with synthetic syllables identified as /da/ and /ga/. These syllables can be synthesized so that they are identical except for the third formant transition, which falls for /da/ and rises for /ga/. If the part of the syllable that is the same for /da/ and /ga/ (called the base) is presented to one ear and the distinguishing transition is presented to the other, listeners integrate the information across the ears and hear /da/ or /ga/, depending on the transition. However, at the same time, they also hear the transition as a pitch rise or fall. The finding that part of the signal is heard in two different ways at the same time has been interpreted to suggest that two different perceptual systems are responsible for the two percepts. One, a phonetic processor, integrates the base and transition and yields a phonetic percept, /da/ or /ga/. The other yields a "homomorphic" percept (Liberman & Mattingly,

1989), that is, a percept having the same form as the acoustic signal. Presumably this is an auditory processor.

This interpretation has been challenged on a variety of grounds (e.g., Fowler & Rosenblum, 1990; Pastore, Schmuckler, Rosenblum, & Szczesiul, 1983). I will not review those challenges here. Rather, I note that the motor theoretical interpretation of duplex perception would be strengthened by evidence favoring the third claim of the theory, that there is motor system or motor competence involvement in perceiving speech. This is because theorists do not claim motor involvement in auditory perception generally. If evidence favors motor involvement in speech perception, this would constitute grounds that speech perception is achieved by a different perceptual system than the auditory system, one perhaps dedicated to speech perception.

In fact, evidence for motor involvement in speech perception is weak. However, apparently this is because such evidence has rarely been sought, not because many tests have yielded negative outcomes. I have found three kinds of behavioral data and some suggestive neuropsychological data.

Following a seminal study by Eimas and Corbit (1973), many researchers studied the effects of "selective adaptation" on speech perception. Listeners heard repeated presentations of a syllable at one end of an acoustic continuum, say, /pa/, and then identified members of, say, a /pa/ to /ba/ continuum. The consequence of listeners hearing repeated /pa/ syllables was a reduction in the number of syllables in the ambiguous region of the continuum that listeners identified as /pa/. Eimas and Corbit suggested that phonetic feature detectors (a detector for voicelessness in the example) were being fatigued by the repetitions, so that ambiguous stimuli were more likely to be associated with more activity in the unfatigued voicing feature detector than in the voicelessness detector. This account was challenged (e.g., by Diehl, Kluender, & Parker, 1985). For our purposes, the interpretation is less important than the finding by Cooper (in studies summarized in Cooper, 1979) that repeated presentations of a syllable such as /pi/ had weak but consistent influences on production of the same syllable or another syllable sharing one or more of its features. In the example, voice onset times of produced /pi/s and /ti/s were reduced after adaptation by perceived /pi/s.

Bell-Berti, Raphael, Sawusch, and Pisoni (1978) provided a different kind of evidence for a motor theory. The vowels /i/, /ɪ/, /e/, and /ɛ/ all occur in English. The differences among the vowels can be described in two ways. On the one hand, they decrease in "height" in the series as listed above. On the other hand, /i/ and

/e/ are described as tense vowels; /ɪ/ and /ɛ/ are their lax counterparts. Within the tense vowel pair and the lax pair, vowels differ in height. Bell-Berti et al. found that speakers differed in how they produced the vowels in the series. In four speakers, activity of the genioglossus muscle (a muscle of the tongue affecting tongue height) gradually decreased in the series of four vowels listed above, suggesting progressively lower tongue heights. In contrast, six of the speakers showed comparable levels of activity for /i/ and /e/ that were much higher than activity levels for the two lax vowels. This suggested use of a tense-lax differentiation of the vowels.

Remarkably, on a test of perception, the ten participants partitioned into the same two groups. Listeners identified vowels along an /i/ to /ɪ/ continuum under two conditions. In one, the vowels along the continuum were equally likely to occur. In the other, anchoring, condition the vowel at the /i/ end of the continuum occurred four times as frequently as the other continuum members. This tends to decrease /i/ identifications. Participants who showed progressively decreasing levels of genioglossus activity in their production of the four vowels showed much larger effects of anchoring than the six speakers who produced /e/ with more genioglossus activity, and presumably a higher tongue, than /ɪ/. The authors speculated that the difference occurred because, for the second group of listeners, /i/ and /ɪ/ are not adjacent vowels, whereas they are for members of the first group. Whatever the appropriate account, it is telling that the participants grouped in the same way as talkers that they did as listeners. This provides some evidence suggesting that speech percepts are mediated by information about production of speech.

A final behavioral finding is provided by Kerzel and Bekkering (2000). These investigators looked for compatibility effects in speech production. They presented a face visibly mouthing /bʌ/ or /dʌ/. At a variable interval after that, they presented either of two symbols that participants had learned to associate with the spoken responses /ba/ and /da/. They found an effect of the irrelevant visible speech gesture on latencies to produce the syllables cued by the symbols such that /ba/ responses were faster when the face mouthed /bʌ/ than when it mouthed /dʌ/. Likewise, /da/ responses were facilitated by visible /dʌ/. Kerzel and Bekkering argued that these effects had to be due to stimulus (visible gesture)-response compatibility, not stimulus-stimulus (that is, visible gesture-visible symbol) compatibility, because the symbols (## and &&) bear an arbitrary relation to the visible gestures, whereas the responses do not. Their interpretation was that the visible gestures activated the speech production system and facilitated compatible speech actions, an account

consistent with the motor theory. It has yet to be shown that acoustic speech syllables, rather than visible speech gestures, have the same effect.

There is a little recent neuropsychological evidence providing support for a motor theory of speech perception. Calvert et al. (1997) reported that auditory cortical areas activate when individuals view silent speech or speechlike movements. Moreover, the region of auditory cortex that activated for silent lipreading and for acoustic speech perception were the same. More recently the same group of investigators (MacSweeney et al., 2000) replicated the findings using procedures that ensured that fMRI scanner noise was not the source of the auditory cortical activation.

Using transcranial magnetic stimulation of the motor cortex, Aravind, Sundara, and Chen (2000) recorded motor-evoked potentials in the orbicularis oris muscle of the lips under a variety of audiovisual conditions. Participants listened to acoustic /ba/, they watched visible /ba/, and they watched and listened to audiovisual /ba/. In addition, they watched visible /ta/, as well as audio /ba/ dubbed onto video /ta/. Under the conditions of this dubbing, most people report hearing /da/. In all conditions in which participants perceived a labial consonant, orbicularis oris activity numerically or significantly exceeded that during a baseline condition in which participants saw a motionless face. Lip activity did not exceed baseline in conditions, including the McGurk dubbing condition, in which the percept was a nonlabial consonant.

There is considerable evidence that listeners perceive phonetic gestures and some evidence favoring the motor theory's account that the motor system is involved in perception. This theory explains cross-modal speech perception quite naturally by claiming that all information about gestures is integrated into a motor percept.

SPEECH PERCEPTION AS AMODAL: 2. DIRECT REALISM In both the motor theory and the AIM extension, percepts are achieved in the head. They can be integrated when they are achieved via different sensory modalities because the percepts have distal (or, in the motor theory, almost distal) reference. In speech perception, they are about the gestures of the vocal tract that the speaker used to produce the acoustic speech signal.

In direct realism (e.g., Gibson, 1966, 1979), perceivers do not represent the world, they perceive it. In this account, information extracted about events across different sensory modalities integrates because it is about the same event. It is not that a perceptual representation has distal reference. Rather, perception is of the distal event itself, and distal things are amodal.

In the direct-realist theory of speech perception (Best, 1995; Fowler, 1986), relevant distal events are linguistically significant actions of the vocal tract, that is, phonetic gestures. In contrast to the motor theoretical idea that coarticulation prevents intended gestures from being actual, in the direct-realist view, coarticulation is nondestructive and intended gestures are actual (Fowler & Saltzman, 1993). Despite considerable coarticulatory overlap of /b/ production by surrounding vowels, for example, speakers always get their lips closed, and that is /b/'s constriction gesture (cf. Fowler & Saltzman, 1993).

In direct-realist accounts generally, perception serves a universal function across perceptual modalities. Its very important function is to allow perceiver/actors to know the world. Perception serves its function in just one general way. Structure in informational media (e.g., light for vision, acoustic signals for hearing) is caused by properties of environmental events. Moreover, distinctive properties of events structure the media distinctively and so provide information for their causal source. Perceivers/actors intercept structure in media during their exploratory and performatory actions. The structure, imparted to the sensory modalities, is used perceptually, not as something to be perceived itself but as information for its causal source in the environment.

In this theory, then, as in the previous two, perception is generally of distal properties of the world, not of proximal stimulation. It is this aspect of the theory that underlies its claim, applied to speech, that listeners perceive phonetic gestures. In contrast to AIM, perceived gestures are not mediated by representations in a direct-realist account. In contrast both to AIM and the motor theory, percepts are not representations that are about something distal (or nearly distal in the motor theory), they are distal themselves.

It is also this aspect of the theory that allows it to account for cross-modal speech perception. Speakers cause structure in acoustic signals that constitutes information about gestures. They also cause structure in the light that constitutes information for gestures. If a hand is placed on the face as someone speaks, then the speech also structures the skin on the hand, which provides haptic information for gestures. Because all of the modalities for which speaking generates information use proximal stimulation as information for its causal source in the world, all of them acquire information about gestures, and this is how cross-modal information can integrate.

OTHER ACCOUNTS: NO COMMON CURRENCY The AIM-derived account, the motor theory, and direct realism have much in common in invoking distal speech properties as the common currency that permits cross-modal integration of information. I will summarize just one alternative account of cross-modal speech perception, that offered by Massaro's Fuzzy Logical Model of Perception (FLMP; e.g., Massaro, 1987, 1998). In the theory, speech perceivers have prototypes of CV syllables in their heads. Associated with the prototype are acoustic features and optical gestural descriptions. Audiovisual speech information integrates because of the mutual attachment of acoustic and visible speech information to common prototypes.

When a speech event is both viewed and heard, properties of the event (acoustic cues and visible gesture information) are extracted perceptually. Fuzzy logical values (between 0 and 1) are assigned to each feature of every prototype, with the number reflecting the strength of the evidence that the feature is present in the stimulation. The fuzzy logical numbers for the features of each prototype are multiplied to generate one number per prototype, reflecting its degree of match to the stimulation. The prototype reflecting the best match to the input is chosen as the percept. Because both optical information and acoustic information are associated with prototypes for CVs, both contribute to CV perception.

The FLMP accounts well for findings of audiovisual speech perception. The model can simulate human speech perception data admirably. Although in its current form it does not account for other kinds of cross-modal speech perception that occur, it could by the addition of, say, haptic speech features or proprioceptive ones.

I find the FLMP account unsatisfactory in relation to the other three accounts I have offered, in part because it does not confront the problem of common currency that is necessary to provide not just a simulation of but an explanation of cross-modal speech perception.

In the three gestural accounts that I have offered, proponents identified a need for cross-modal information to be in a common code or currency in order to integrate. This is, for example, a fundamental idea in Meltzoff and Moore's AIM hypothesis that allows it to explain how infants can relate facial gestural information acquired cross-modally. All of the accounts I have offered draw the conclusion that the common currency is gestural. In contrast, in FLMP there is no common currency. The theory proposes that information acquired auditorily is proximal (acoustic cues), whereas information acquired optically is distal (e.g., lip closure for /ba/). Information integrates across the modalities not, therefore, because it is commensurate cross-modally but because optical features for a syllable and acoustic features for the same syllable are attached to the same prototype. However, the theory is less explanatory than any of the other three described earlier. This is because there is no explanation of how the proximal acoustic cues and distal gestures becomes attached to a prototype or why a set of acoustic and optical features amounts to a particular CV. Why are the auditorily extracted properties proximal and the optical ones distal? Pairings of compatible acoustic and gestural cues (that is, cues for the same CV) in memory might be explained by invoking experiences of both seeing and hearing speech (but see Fowler & Dekle, 1991, for a challenge to that account). However, why does any pairing amount to a particular CV whose "name," say, is /di/ or /du/? Where do the names come from, and why do the two syllables in the example have the same C in their names? The answer cannot be found in the acoustic cues (the critical F2 rises for /di/ but falls for /du/) or in the facial gestures (/d/ in /du/ looks more like /g/ in /gu/ than it looks like /d/ in /di/). All of these questions have answers if there is a common currency underlying the integration of auditorily extracted and visually extracted information about speech. They appear not to in the FLMP account.

Common currency and perceptually guided speaking

The discussion so far has been about cross-modal speech perception and how ideas of supramodal representations or common currencies appear to provide the means by which information can be integrated cross-modally. My topic, however, is not speech perception as a supramodal or amodal phenomenon, but speech itself as a supramodal or amodal phenomenon. It is not commonplace, and perhaps is not good usage, to refer to the motor system as a mode, and indeed, I excluded it as such in referring to the motor theory's representations as amodal. However, it is instructive to look at some issues that arise in accounting for perceptually guided action; they appear strictly analogous to those that arise in accounting for cross-modal perception.

Hommel et al. (2001) ask how percepts can communicate with action plans. If there are perceptual codes that are sets of perceptual features and action plans that are motor commands, the two codes cannot communicate, and actions cannot be perceptually guided. But, of course, they are. Hommel et al. propose that there are codes, and that their common currency is featural. The features are those of the distal environment in which the perceptually guided action occurs. A common code is quite analogous to a supramodal representation. An alternative idea is that the common

currency is the distal event itself, not the represented features of that event. It is the event that the talker generates and that the listener perceives cross-modally.

One example of perceptually guided action in speech is the imitation of speech that both infants (Kuhl & Meltzoff, 1996) and adults (Goldinger, 1998) exhibit. How can the speech of a talker guide an imitative response? It can if there is a common currency shared by percepts and preparations for action. Again, we invoke speech gestures. If listeners perceive gestures and plan to produce gestures, an imitative response should be the most straightforward way in which perception can guide action. The instances of convergences in dialect, speaking rate, and vocal intensity cited in the introduction to this chapter are other examples of perceptually guided imitation.

There are other examples of perceptually guided action as well. Houde and Jordan (1998) transformed the formant frequencies of vowels produced by participants so that participants heard fed-back vowels different from the ones they had produced. Just as in cases of adaptation to prisms, this led to compensatory changes in articulation to make the acoustic feedback more appropriate to the vowel that the speaker had intended to say. The fed-back vowel, perceived as the gestures that would have produced it, affected the gestures that the speakers went on to produce.

Common currency and communication

As Liberman understood well there is another critical need for a common currency in speech that a conclusion that listeners perceive phonetic gestures addresses. Liberman and colleagues (e.g., Liberman & Whalen, 2000) referred to a "parity" requirement in speech communication. This, in Liberman and Whalen's article, had three core aspects, the first two of which derived from the fact that speech is a between-person activity. Listeners and talkers have to "agree" on what public actions of a speaker count as producing language forms. (As Liberman and Whalen put it, /ba/ counts, a sniff does not.) In addition, for utterances to do their intended work, listeners have to perceive the language forms that speakers say. In these two ideas of parity, listeners and talkers require a common currency, both in the sense of sharing what the currency is and in the more local sense of listeners recovering the specific forms constituting a speaker's utterance. The third aspect of parity, for Liberman and Whalen, is the necessary coevolution of coarticulation and the ability to perceive coarticulated speech.

The idea of common currency (parity, in the theorizing of Liberman) is absent from nongestural theories of speech perception (e.g., Diehl & Kluender, 1989; Kluender, 1994; Nearey, 1997) but is needed for multiple reasons, not only to explain information integration across the perceptual modalities or perceptually guided action. Liberman and Whalen point out that it is required to explain how speech can communicate. What counts as something phonetic is the same for talkers and listeners. More locally, for communication to take place, generally, listeners have to perceive with sufficient accuracy the language forms produced by the talker. There has to be parity or common currency now between talker and listener.

Conclusion

Speakers and listeners receive multimodal information about language forms. They use the information they receive in all of the modalities that provide information. Their doing so requires a common currency across the sensory modalities. The common currency might be the supramodal representation of Meltzoff and Moore (1997, 1999) or it might, more directly, be the distal object of perception. This same common currency is required to understand how perceptually guided action can occur and how communication can occur between talkers and listeners.

REFERENCES

Aravind, N. K., Sundara, M., & Chen, R. (2000). Effects of auditory and visual stimuli on motor facilitation of speech muscles [Abstract]. *Journal of the Acoustical Society of America, 107,* 2887.

Bahrick, L. (1987). Infants' intermodal perception of two levels of temporal structure in natural events. *Infant Behavior and Development, 10,* 387–416.

Bahrick, L., & Watson, J. S. (1985). Detection of intermodal proprioceptive-visual contingency as a potential basis of self-perception in infancy. *Developmental Psychology, 21,* 963–973.

Bell-Berti, F., Raphael, L. R., Sawusch, J. R., & Pisoni, D. B. (1978). Some relationships between speech production and perception. *Phonetica, 36,* 373–383.

Best, C. (1994). The emergence of native-language phonological influences in infants: A perceptual assimilation model. In J. Goodman & H. Nusbaum (Eds.), *The development of speech perception: The transition from speech sounds to spoken words* (pp. 167–224). Cambridge, MA: MIT Press.

Best, C. T. (1995). A direct realist perspective on cross-language speech perception. In W. Strange & J. J. Jenkins (Eds.), *Cross-language speech perception* (pp. 171–204). Timonium, MD: York Press.

Best, C., Morrongiello, B., & Robson, R. (1981). Perceptual equivalence of acoustic cues in speech and nonspeech perception. *Perception & Psychophysics, 29,* 191–211.

Brancazio, L. (2001). Lexical influences in audiovisual speech perception. *Journal of Experimental Psychology: Human Perception and Performance.*

Calvert, G., Bullmore, E. T., Brammer, M. J., Campbell, R., Williams, S. C., McGuire, P. K., et al. (1997). Activation of auditory cortex during silent lipreading. *Science, 276,* 593–596.

Chomsky, C. (1986). Analytic study of the Tadoma method: Language abilities of three deaf-blind subjects. *Journal of Speech and Hearing Research, 29,* 332–347.

Cooper, W. (1979). *Speech perception and production: Studies in selective adaptation.* Norwood, NJ: Ablex.

Diehl, R., & Kluender, K. (1989). On the objects of speech perception. *Ecological Psychology, 1,* 121–144.

Diehl, R., Kluender, K., & Parker, E. (1985). Are selective adaptation effects and contrast effects really distinct? *Journal of Experimental Psychology: Human Perception and Performance, 11,* 209–220.

Eimas, P., & Corbit, J. (1973). Selective adaptation of feature detectors. *Cognitive Psychology, 4,* 99–109.

Fitch, H., Halwes, T., Erickson, D. M., & Liberman, A. M. (1980). Perceptual equivalence of two acoustic cues for stop-consonant manner. *Perception & Psychophysics, 27,* 343–350.

Fowler, C. (1986). An event approach to the study of speech perception from a direct-realist perspective. *Journal of Phonetics, 14,* 3–28.

Fowler, C. (1994). Speech perception: Direct realist theory. In *Encyclopedia of language and linguistics* (Vol. 8, pp. 4199–4203). Oxford, England: Pergamon Press.

Fowler, C., & Brown, J. (1997). Intrinsic f0 differences in spoken and sung vowels and their perception by listeners. *Perception & Psychophysics, 59,* 729–738.

Fowler, C., Brown, J., Sabadin, L., & Weihing, J. (2003). Rapid access to speech gestures in perception: Evidence from choice and simple response time tasks. *Journal of Memory and Language, 49,* 396–413.

Fowler, C. A., & Dekle, D. J. (1991). Listening with eye and hand: Crossmodal contributions to speech perception. *Journal of Experimental Psychology: Human Perception and Performance, 17,* 816–828.

Fowler, C., & Smith, M. (1986). Speech perception as vector analysis: An approach to the problems of segmentation and invariance. In J. Perkell & D. Klatt (Eds.), *Invariance and variability of speech processes* (pp. 123–136). Hillsdale, NJ: Erlbaum.

Fowler, C. A., & Rosenblum, L. D. (1990). Duplex perception: A comparison of monosyllables and slamming doors. *Journal of Experimental Psychology: Human Perception and Performance, 16,* 742–754.

Fowler, C. A., & Saltzman, E. (1993). Coordination and coarticulation in speech production. *Language and Speech, 36,* 171–195.

Gibson, J. J. (1966). *The senses considered as perceptual systems.* Boston, MA: Houghton Mifflin.

Gibson, J. J. (1979). *The ecological approach to visual perception. Boston:* Houghton Mifflin.

Giles, H., Coupland N., & Coupland, J. (1991). Accommodation theory: Communication, context, and consequence. In H. Giles, J. Coupland, & N. Coupland (Eds.), *Contexts of accommodation: Developments in applied sociolinguistics* (pp. 1–68). Cambridge, England: Cambridge University Press.

Goldinger, S. D. (1998). Echoes of echoes? An episodic theory of lexical access. *Psychological Review, 105,* 251–279.

Hommel, B., Müsseler, J., Aschersleben, G., & Prinz, W. (2001). The theory of event coding TEC: A framework for perception and action planning. *Behavioral and Brain Sciences, 24,* 849–937.

Houde, J. F., & Jordan, M. I. (1998). Sensorimotor adaptation in speech production. *Science, 227,* 1213–1216.

Kerzel, D., & Bekkering, H. (2000). Motor activation from visible speech: Evidence from stimulus-response compatibility. *Journal of Experimental Psychology: Human Perception and Performance, 26,* 634–647.

Kluender, K. (1994). Speech perception as a tractable problem in cognitive science. In M. A. Gernsbacher (Ed.), *Handbook of psycholinguistics* (pp. 173–217). San Diego, CA: Academic Press.

Kozhevnikov, V., & Chistovich, L. (1965). *Speech: Articulation and perception.* Washington, DC: Joint Publications Research Service.

Kuhl, P., & Meltzoff, A. (1982). The bimodal perception of speech in infancy. *Science, 218,* 1138–1141.

Kuhl, P., & Meltzoff, A. (1988). Speech as an intermodal object of perception. In A. Yonas (Ed.), *Perceptual development in infancy. The Minnesota Symposia on Child Psychology, 20,* 235–266. Hillsdale, NJ: Erlbaum.

Kuhl, P., & Meltzoff, A. (1996). Infant vocalizations in response to speech: Vocal imitation and developmental change. *Journal of the Acoustical Society of America, 100,* 2425–2438.

Lane, H., & Tranel, B. (1971). The Lombard sign and the role of hearing in speech. *Journal of Speech and Hearing Research, 14,* 677–709.

Lash, J. (1980). *Helen and teacher.* Reading, MA: Addison-Wesley.

Liberman, A. M. (1982). On finding that speech is special. *American Psychologist, 37,* 148–167.

Liberman, A. M., Delattre, P., & Cooper, F. S. (1952). The role of selected stimulus variables in the perception of the unvoiced-stop consonants. *American Journal of Psychology, 65,* 497–516.

Liberman, A. M., Delattre, P., Cooper, F. S., & Gerstman, L. (1954). The role of consonant-vowel transitions in the perception of the stop and nasal consonants. *Psychological Monographs: General and Applied, 68,* 1–13.

Liberman, A. M., & Mattingly, I. (1985). The motor theory revised. *Cognition, 21,* 1–36.

Liberman, A. M., & Mattingly, I. (1989). A specialization for speech perception. *Science, 243,* 489–494.

Liberman, A. M., & Whalen, D. H. (2000). On the relation of speech to language. *Trends in Cognitive Sciences, 4,* 187–196.

Luce, R. D. (1986). *Response times.* New York: Oxford University Press.

MacKain, K., Studdert-Kennedy, M., Spieker, S., & Stern, D. (1983). Infant intermodal speech perception is a left hemisphere function. *Science, 219,* 1347–1349.

MacSweeney, M., Amaro, E., Calvert, G., Campbell, R., David, A. S., McGuire, P. et al. (2000). Silent speech reading in the absence of scanner noise: An event-related fMRI study. *NeuroReport, 11,* 1729–1733.

Mann, V., & Liberman, A. (1983). Some differences between phonetic and auditory modes of perception. *Cognition, 14,* 211–235.

Massaro, D. (1987). *Speech perception by ear and eye: A paradigm for psychological inquiry.* Hillsdale, NJ: Erlbaum.

Massaro, D. (1998). *Perceiving talking faces.* Cambridge, MA: MIT Press.

McGurk, H., & MacDonald, J. (1976). Hearing lips and seeing voices. *Nature, 264,* 746–748.

McHugo, G., Lanzetta, J., Sullivan, D., Masters, R., & Englis, B. (1985). Emotional reactions to a political leader's expressive displays. *Journal of Personality and Social Psychology, 49,* 1513–1529.

Meltzoff, A., & Kuhl, P. (1994). Faces and speech: Intermodal processing of biologically relevant signals in infants and adults. In D. Lewkowicz & R. Licklikr (Eds). The development of inter sensory perception: Comparative perspective (pp 335–369). Hillsdale, NJ: Lawrence Erlbaum and Associates.

Meltzoff, A., Kuhl, P., & Moore, M. (1991). Perception, representation, and the control of action in newborns and young infants. In M. J. S. Weiss & R. Zelazo (Eds.), *Newborn attention: Biological constraints and the influence of experience* (pp. 377–411). Norwood, NJ: Ablex.

Meltzoff, A., & Moore, M. (1977). Imitation of facial and manual gestures by human neonates. *Science, 198,* 75–78.

Meltzoff, A., & Moore, M. K. (1997). Explaining facial imitation: A theoretical model. *Early Development and Parenting, 6,* 179–192.

Meltzoff, A., & Moore, K. (1999). Persons and representation: Why infant imitation is important for theories of human development. In J. Nadel & G. Butterworth (Eds.), *Imitation in infancy* (pp. 9–35). Cambridge: Cambridge University Press.

Nearey, T. (1997). Speech perception as pattern recognition. *Journal of the Acoustical Society of America, 101,* 3241–3254.

Nittrouer, S., & Crowther, C. (2001). Coherence in children's speech perception. *Journal of the Acoustical Society of America, 110,* 2129–2140.

Pardo, J., & Fowler, C. A. (1997). Perceiving the causes of coarticulatory acoustic variation: Consonant voicing and vowel pitch. *Perception & Psychophysics, 59,* 1141–1152.

Pastore, R., Schmuckler, M., Rosenblum, L., & Szczesiul, R. (1983). Duplex perception for musical stimuli CHK. *Perception & Psychophysics, 33,* 469–474.

Pierrehumbert, J. (1979). The perception of fundamental frequency. *Journal of the Acoustical Society of America, 66,* 363–369.

Porter, R., & Castellanos, F. X. (1980). Speech production measures of speech perception: Rapid shadowing of VCV syllables. *Journal of the Acoustical Society of America, 67,* 1349–1356.

Porter, R., & Lubker, J. (1980). Rapid reproduction of vowel-vowel sequences: Evidence for a fast and direct acoustic-motoric linkage. *Journal of Speech and Hearing Research, 23,* 593–602.

Reinholt Peterson, N. (1986). Perceptual compensation for segmentally-conditioned fundamental-frequency perturbations. *Phonetica, 43,* 31–42.

Rosenblum, L. D., Schmuckler, M., & Johnson, J. A. (1997). The McGurk effect in infants. *Perception & Psychophysics, 59,* 347–357.

Silverman, K. (1987). *The structure and processing of fundamental frequency contours.* Unpublished doctoral dissertation, Cambridge University.

Spelke, E. (1979). Perceiving bimodally specified events in infancy. *Developmental Psychology, 15,* 626–636.

Sumby, W. H., & Pollack, I. (1954). Visual contributions to speech intelligibility in noise. *Journal of the Acoustical Society of America, 26,* 212–215.

Yehia, H., & Vatikiotis-Bateson, E. (1998). Quantitative association of vocal tract and facial behavior. *Speech Communication, 26,* 23–44.

13 Audiovisual Speech Binding: Convergence or Association?

LYNNE E. BERNSTEIN, EDWARD T. AUER, JR., AND JEAN K. MOORE

Introduction

Over the past several decades, behavioral studies in experimental psychology have revealed several intriguing audiovisual (AV) speech perception effects. Under noisy acoustic conditions, being able to see a talker results in substantial gains to comprehending speech, with gains estimated to be equivalent to raising the acoustic signal-to-noise ratio by approximately 11 dB (MacLeod & Summerfield, 1987; Sumby & Pollack, 1954).[1] When speech is severely degraded by filtering out various frequency bands, being able to see the talker results in significant restoration of speech information (Grant & Walden, 1996). Extremely minimal auditory speech information can combine with visible speech information to produce superadditive levels of performance. For example, if an acoustic signal encoding only the voice fundamental frequency is presented, word recognition is impossible. But the combination of the talker's face and voice fundamental frequency results in dramatic enhancements over lipreading alone (e.g., 30% words correct with lipreading alone versus 80% words correct when the fundamental frequency is added; Boothroyd, Hnath-Chisolm, Hanin, & Kishon-Rabin, 1988; Breeuwer & Plomp, 1985; Kishon-Rabin, Boothroyd, & Hanin, 1996).

The AV effect that has been of greatest interest, and for which a substantial perception literature now exists, is obtained with a variety of incongruent (mismatched) pairings of auditory and visual spoken syllables (e.g., Green & Kuhl, 1989; Massaro, 1987; Massaro, Cohen, & Smeele, 1996; Munhall, Gribble, Sacco, & Ward, 1996; Saldana & Rosenblum, 1994; Sekiyama, 1997; Walker, Bruce, & O'Malley, 1995). When incongruent AV stimuli are presented, frequently the speech stimulus that is perceived is not equivalent to what is perceived in the absence of the visual stimulus (Green, 1998; McGurk & MacDonald, 1976). An example of this so-called *McGurk effect* occurs when an auditory /ba/ is dubbed to a visual /ga/, and listeners report hearing /da/. In addition to the blend effect just cited, combination percepts arise, such as /bga/ in response to auditory /ga/ and visual /ba/. Other effects have been obtained with incongruent syllables, several of which are described later in this chapter.

The speech perception literature offers several alternative perceptual theories to account for AV effects. Conveniently, recent developments in functional brain imaging and recordings of cortical event-related potentials (ERPs) and fields afford the opportunity to investigate whether there is support for perceptual theories at the level of neural implementation. For example, theoretical accounts suggesting that AV speech integration is early, at a subsegmental (subphonemic) level, could be taken to imply that auditory and visual speech information combines in the central nervous system (CNS) at early levels of the cortical synaptic hierarchy and/or at early latencies. That is, the linguistic level at which perceptual effects are theorized to occur can suggest the relevant level of CNS processing. Alternatively, the brain mechanisms responsible for speech processing are complex and nonlinear, and the expectation that the translation between perceptual theory and neural implementation could be simple is likely to be overly optimistic (see Friston et al., 1996; Picton, Alain, Otten, Ritter, & Achim, 2000). In addition, considerable leeway is afforded by perceptual theories in the translation to possible theories of neural implementations. This chapter outlines AV speech perception research and theories, adopting a fundamental explanatory distinction that has parallels at the level of plausible neural mechanisms for binding auditory and visual speech information. The chapter also outlines those plausible mechanisms. The goal of the chapter is to provide a

[1]Estimating the functional enhancement in the signal-to-noise ratio (S/N) depends on the speech materials (syllables, words, sentences), the talker, and the noise characteristics. Although Sumby and Pollack (1954) are often cited to indicate a functional enhancement in the range of 15–20 dB S/N, careful examination of the figures shows that for the largest set of words used (256) for values less than −12 dB S/N, the curve is essentially flat. This suggests that the best enhancement under these conditions for these materials is likely close to −11 dB S/N (MacLeod & Summerfield, 1987). With more negative S/N values the performance levels are very close to lipreading alone.

particular integrated view of the perceptual and neural levels of explanation.

Convergence versus association

The combining of auditory and visual speech information is usually referred to in the speech perception literature as *AV integration.* AV integration frequently (although not always) denotes transformation of auditory and visual information into a common format or metric. At the neural level, the term *convergence* (as used here) refers to the processing of auditory and visual speech information by cortical neurons that respond to both auditory and visual speech stimulation. Convergence has been demonstrated in multisensory superior colliculus neurons that respond to stimulation concerning spatial location (Stein & Meredith, 1993). Integration by transformation to a common metric is a possible perceptual explanation for AV speech effects, and convergence is a possible neural mechanism that could support the transformation of auditory and visual speech information to a common format.

Convergence as a mechanism for combining diverse noninvariant information is, however, problematic. Outside of the context of speech perception research, the problem of how diverse information is combined is frequently referred to as the *binding* problem (Treisman, 1996; von der Malsburg, 1995; Zeki, 2001). Significantly, within that broad domain of inquiry into how the brain produces coherent thought, perception, and action, there are questions concerning whether convergence could be a binding mechanism for complex, noninvariant information (e.g., Grey, 1999; Mesulam, 1994, 1998; Singer, 1998). The concerns expressed in the literature raise the possibility that convergence is also not a plausible explanation for AV speech binding. This chapter considers whether AV speech perception can be explained by neuronal convergence and raises the alternative possibility that AV speech binding results from an association of modality-specific speech representations.

The chapter is organized as follows. First, perceptual studies and theories that imply neural convergence of AV speech information are described. The theories are referred to collectively as *common format* theories. Second, perceptual studies and theories that are not compatible with the common format view or that imply that speech information is maintained in modality-specific representations are discussed. These alternative views are collectively referred to as *modality-specific* theory. According to the modality-specific view, auditory and visual speech information is perceptually processed by modality-specific networks and then associated. In order for the modality-specific view to be correct, there must be evidence that in addition to auditory-only speech perception, there is effective visual-only speech perception, and some evidence for that is briefly presented. A short section also discusses the correspondence between acoustic and optical speech signals that could be used by an associative mechanism. The balance of the chapter discusses processing pathways and neural mechanisms that are likely relevant to AV speech perception, given the contending common format and modality-specific perceptual theories. Our discussion of neural implementations relies in part on Mesulam's (1994, 1998) theory about transmodal cortical gateways, which are proposed as the sites that complete networks among modality-specific representations, and between perceptual and conceptual knowledge.

A final preliminary note: We think that the study of AV speech perception primarily concerns the binding of speech *information,* as opposed to the *modulation* of response intensity. It is true that AV stimulation can result in changes in perceived intensity (Stein, London, Wilkinson, & Price, 1996). Also, using speech stimuli, the detectability of acoustic speech signals in noise has been shown to be sensitive to the presentation of the talker's face (Grant & Seitz, 2000). But we think that such effects are not specific to speech processing and are likely the result of mechanisms that are distinct from speech pattern processing. Therefore, in this chapter we focus primarily on speech information processing.

Common format audiovisual speech perception

Speech perception research traditionally is concerned with discovering relationships between signal-based linguistic (phonetic) stimulus attributes and resulting perceptions (e.g., Fowler, 1986; Liberman & Whalen, 2000; Massaro, 1987, 1998; Nearey, 1997; Stevens, 2002). Speech perception theories generally envision a hierarchical process in which subsegmental features such as voicing, manner, place, and nasality[2] are first extracted

---

[2]The features referred to here are frequently categorized in terms of speech articulation distinctions but can also be categorized in terms of acoustic signal attributes. In this chapter, for convenience, the articulatory taxonomy is used. The voicing feature, for example, distinguishes between /b/ and /p/ or /d/ and /t/, and involves the onset time of vocal fold vibration. The manner feature distinguishes between, for example, /d/ and /l/ or /d/ and /r/, and involves the degree of closure in the vocal tract. The place feature distinguishes, for example, between /b/ and d/ or /d/ and /g/, and involves the point of closure in the vocal tract. The nasality feature distinguishes between /n/ and /d/ or /m/ and /b/, and involves the raising or lowering of the velum.

from speech signals, then combined into segments (the consonants and vowels), which are combined into word patterns. Experiments using the McGurk effect have led to the conclusion that auditory and visual speech interact at the level of the speech features. AV speech effects are described as alterations in the perception of speech features (e.g., Fowler, 1986; Green, 1998; Schwartz, Robert-Ribes, & Escudier, 1998; Summerfield, 1987). Furthermore, experiments using McGurk stimuli are frequently seen as strong evidence that a common format representation is achieved prior to segment identification. In fact, this inference seems uncontroversial to some theorists (Schwartz, et al., 1998). Several versions of common format theory have been proposed, but each involves the claim that modality-specific stimulus information is transformed into amodal feature or segment representations. Thus, modality-specific processing is hypothesized to terminate very early. The speech segments, the combinatoric units used to form words, no longer comprise modality-specific perceptual information. Beyond the stage of extracting subsegmental, feature information, speech pattern representations are in a common format.

EMPIRICAL EVIDENCE CONSISTENT WITH COMMON FORMAT THEORY This section outlines some of the McGurk results that provide apparent intuitive validity to the theory that auditory and visual speech bind through transformation to a common format. For example, Green and Kuhl (1989) presented an acoustic continuum of stimuli from /ibi/ to /ipi/, with each acoustic stimulus dubbed to a video of a talker saying /igi/. The voicing category boundary is known to vary with the place of articulation: the boundary for the acoustic /ibi/ to /ipi/ is earlier than for /idi/ to /iti/. Perceivers heard the AV stimuli as a continuum from /idi/ to /iti/. Importantly, the category identification boundary between /idi/ and /iti/ was displaced relative to the /ibi/-/ipi/ boundary, in the direction consistent with that for an acoustic /idi/-/iti/ continuum. The result was interpreted as showing that "the auditory and visual information are combined by the time a phonetic decision is made" (Green, 1998, p. 6; see also Green & Norrix, 2001), that is, at a subsegmental level. Using acoustic stimuli, perception of the voicing feature has also been shown to be influenced by speaking rate. Green and Miller (1985) showed that the voicing boundary for an acoustic /bi/ to /pi/ continuum was appropriately shifted when the acoustic stimuli were dubbed to either a fast or slow visual token of /bi/ or /pi/, suggesting that the visual information influenced the phonetic category identification. Green and Norrix (1997) showed that manipulations of the acoustic phonetic cues to

place of articulation (/b/ vs. /g/), specifically, the release bursts (broad-band energy at consonant onset), aspiration (broad-band energy generated at the larynx), and voiced formant transitions (vocal tract resonances), had systematic effects when auditory stimuli were dubbed to visual stimuli, again suggesting that speech information combines at a fine-grained, subsegmental level.

Support for common format theory has also been derived from research in which the visual stimulus was manipulated. For example, Rosenblum and Saldana (1996) combined point-light speech stimuli with acoustic speech stimuli. In their experiment, the critical AV stimulus was an acoustic /ba/ paired with moving dot patterns made by videorecording reflectors affixed to the talker's face, lips, teeth, and tongue as he said /va/. The dynamic dot patterns significantly influenced perception toward perceiving /va/, although not as effectively as did the full video /va/. This result was seen as evidence that the speech motion information combined with speech acoustics. Green, Kuhl, Meltzoff, and Stevens (1991) mismatched talker gender between the auditory and visual stimuli and obtained McGurk effects of comparable magnitude to ones obtained when the talker's gender was matched, another result compatible with the view that modality-specific information is transformed early in processing. Across many experiments, Massaro (1987, 1998) has shown that with a schematized synthetic talking face used to create continua of visual speech stimuli, graded influences on AV perception can be obtained, once again implicating subsegmental AV interactions. All of the types of effects described in this section thus seem consistent with the possibility that modality-specific speech information is transformed at an early processing level into a common amodal format.

COMMON FORMAT THEORIES Several different common format and modality-specific theories for how AV speech combines were proposed in a seminal essay by Summerfield (1987). Summerfield's first proposed common format theory was that vision contributes a categorical and discrete readout of the place-of-articulation speech feature, and hearing contributes a categorical and discrete readout of the voicing and nasality features. This theory suggests that the perceptual system somehow knows which modality is more reliable for each type of evidence. The theory was deemed invalid, however, because the McGurk effect does not show that perceivers categorically identify a subset of articulatory features within a particular modality and ignore evidence from the other modality. For example, the typical perceivers' report of /bga/ on being presented with auditory /ga/ (alveolar place) and visual /ba/ (bilabial place) cannot be explained as attention to only the more reliable modality for place information (both place-of-articulation features are perceived).

The acoustic transfer function of the vocal tract was proposed by Summerfield as another possible but more abstract common format. The acoustic transfer function represents the resonant frequencies of the vocal tract that result from the kinematics of the lips, tongue, jaw, velum, and larynx (Stevens, 1998). Auditory and visual perception were suggested as possibly involving recovery of the transfer function: auditory perception is sensitive to the frequency distribution of sound, which is a direct result of the vocal tract transfer function; perceivers can see some evidence of the shape of the vocal tract, and hypothetically, that evidence could be used to calculate the transfer function. The visual and auditory estimates of the transfer function would be in a common format in which the information could combine. However, Summerfield did not suggest any evidence that visual information is transformed into the acoustic vocal tract transfer function.

Summerfield also described a common format metric based on speech articulation dynamics. To develop the concept, he asked the reader to imagine the talker vocalizing in a monotone with a lowered velum while oscillating his lips sinusoidally. This action would result in an overall modulation of the signal amplitude, which would correspond with the visible opening and closing of the lips. Furthermore, other types of correspondences should occur between acoustic and optical signals. For example, qualitative changes in state such as closures versus opening, quantitative effects such as rate of movement, and articulatory changes in direction should have acoustic and optical aspects. These changes should occur at roughly equivalent times. Summerfield suggested that a modality-free representation might entail kinematic descriptors such as displacement and its time derivatives. Alternatively, kinematics might be used to derive representations of the dynamics required for speech articulation motor control. Then AV speech perception would involve integrating auditory and visual "evidence of articulatory dynamics."

The hypothesis of a common articulatory format has received enthusiastic support among some speech perception theorists. Fowler's (1986) direct-realist theory (following Gibson, 1966, 1979) of AV speech perception is that articulatory gestures are perceived via hearing and vision, and that auditory and visual speech information are integrated because both are information about a common object or event. According to her view, perception is the detection of stimulus attributes. The sensory/perceptual systems measure what is physi-

cally specified in stimulation. It is hypothesized that articulatory gestures are specified in the acoustic signals, in addition to being evident in the optical signals. Perception of speech is not specialized: the same mechanisms responsible for speech perception are responsible for nonspeech perception of objects or events. Fowler (Chap. 12, this volume) suggests that there are either amodal/supramodal representations of the speech articulatory gestures that somehow transcend the sensory modalities and exist as mental representations, or that perception detects structure (articulatory gestures) directly across modalities (see Green & Norrix, 2001; Rosenblum & Gordon, 2001; Stoffregen & Bardy, 2001).

What is known as the *motor theory* of speech perception also employs an articulatory explanation for AV speech perception (Liberman & Mattingly, 1985; Liberman & Whalen, 2000). The main explanatory mechanism for motor theory is a specialized processing module that interprets perceptual speech information in terms of the talker's articulatory gestures. The speech information can be auditory or visual. The specialized module is also responsible for speech production. That is, the common format comprises not only auditory and visual perception but also production.

Massaro (1987, 1998; see also Chap. 10, this volume) has proposed a mathematically explicit information-processing model (the fuzzy logic model of perception) that is consistent with a common format view. His model incorporates independent modality-specific feature evaluation, integration, and decision. Feature evaluation is conceptualized as a process in which sensory/perceptual systems compare modality-specific stimulus features with ideal features that make up category prototypes in memory. Feature evaluation is continuous, and feature values are the information that varies with the stimulus. Features are evaluated independently, so that the value of one feature cannot affect the value of another. Feature values combine multiplicatively. As a result, the larger values (stronger features) have greater effects. This aspect of the model is somewhat reminiscent of Summerfield's (1987) first common format, for which categorical evidence from each modality is used as a function of its reliability. The selection of a particular perceptual category, the response decision, follows integration using a decision rule that weights the evidence for each alternative category against the evidence for all the relevant alternative categories. The integration process is generic across speech and nonspeech stimuli. Although the theory explicitly posits extraction of modality-specific features, and therefore might seem to be a candidate modality-specific theory, Massaro has explicitly favored neural convergence as the implementation mechanism for feature integration (Massaro, 1999, p. 314). That preference and the integration of subsegmental features followed by abstract phoneme representations qualify the model for inclusion in the common format category of theories (Schwartz et al., 1998).

Modality-specific audiovisual speech perception

There is a body of AV speech perception research that is not consistent with any common format theory but could be accounted for within a modality-specific view of speech perception. According to the version of modality-specific theory that we favor, auditory and visual speech processing result in separate modality-specific representations. Stimulus information is never transformed into a common format. Perceptual representations are linked or associated. The meanings of words can be accessed via modality-specific spoken word representations. Also, the linguistic hierarchy of structural units (segments, syllables, words) does not necessarily correspond to discrete neural processing stages or cortical areas.

EMPIRICAL EVIDENCE CONSISTENT WITH MODALITY-SPECIFIC THEORY Although strong support for common format theory has been obtained with McGurk stimuli, evidence for a modality-specific view has also been obtained with McGurk stimuli. For example, the auditory selective adaptation effect has been shown to be immune to visual speech stimuli, an indication that auditory and visual stimuli do not interact at the level of unisensory auditory processing. Specifically, auditory selective adaptation is demonstrated using an acoustic continuum of speech stimuli, for example, from /b/ to /g/. A stimulus on one end of the acoustic continuum is repeatedly presented, followed by randomized presentation of the other members of the continuum. What typically results with auditory adapters for an auditory continuum is that the category boundary moves toward the adapter. That is, listeners identify more of the continuum as being the category that was not adapted. Saldana and Rosenblum (1994) tested a /va/ to /ba/ acoustic continuum. Audiovisual stimuli were created by dubbing each acoustic stimulus with an optical /va/ stimulus. The AV combination of stimuli produced the perception of /va/. The question was whether the AV stimulus (i.e., auditory /ba/ and visual /va/) as an adapter would have the same effect as the auditory-only /va/ stimulus. The answer was that it did not. Instead, there was no difference between the AV adapter and the auditory /ba/ adapter. Thus, the visual part of the stimulus had no adaptation effect. Recently, Shigeno (2002) replicated this result with different

stimuli. Given that auditory selective adaptation is thought to occur at the level of the auditory patterns, not at an abstract linguistic level, these results suggest that auditory speech pattern processing is not affected by visual speech.

Evidence of top-down, cognitive influences on AV speech categorization suggest that binding occurs later than speech feature processing. Walker et al. (1995) presented McGurk stimuli to perceivers who were familiar or unfamiliar with the recorded talkers. The perceivers who were familiar with the talkers were significantly less susceptible to the McGurk effect. Early bottom-up speech feature processing should be immune to higher-level knowledge such as talker familiarity. Thus, the defeat of the McGurk effect by previous experience of the talker is difficult to explain if features bind early during bottom-up perceptual processing.

A related set of observations come from studies of Japanese listeners. Sekiyama and Tohkura (1997) have shown that the McGurk effect is significantly weaker in Japanese than in American perceivers. Nevertheless, and critically, the Japanese results indicate sensitivity to visual speech information. Sekiyama (1997, p. 76) states:

When the stimuli . . . were composed of conflicting auditory and visual syllables, the Japanese subjects often reported incompatibility between what they heard and what they saw, instead of showing the McGurk effect. . . . This implies that the visual information is processed to the extent that the audiovisual discrepancy is detected most of the time. It suggests that, for clear speech, the Japanese use a type of processing in which visual information is not integrated with the auditory information even when they extract some lip-read information from the face of the talker.

These findings suggest that separate modality-specific representations are maintained by Japanese perceivers, and that AV binding is therefore not obligatory nor early.

Studies that used long stimulus onset asynchronies (SOAs) between auditory and visual stimuli also support later, possibly postperceptual AV interaction, because perceptual integration typically breaks down with desynchrony (e.g., Bertelson & Aschersleben, 1997). Temporal and spatial overlap of auditory and visual stimuli appear to be important to convergence (e.g., Calvert, 2001; Meredith, Nemitz, & Stein, 1987). When AV interactions persist in spite of long SOAs, their source could be due to response biases or to memory effects, not to early perceptual ones. One study involving SOAs reported a strong McGurk effect when a visual stimulus preceded an auditory stimulus by 180 ms (Munhall et al., 1996). A shorter SOA in the opposite direction (60 ms) produced a comparable McGurk effect. Another study reported that McGurk effects persisted at SOAs in both directions of approximately 250 ms and even greater (Massaro et al., 1996). Postperceptual bias or memory effects rather than perceptual effects might account for these findings. The same possibility might hold for a study that used connected speech stimuli and asked participants to adjust the audio signals so that they coincided with the visual signals (Dixon & Spitz, 1980). The audio signals lagged the visual signals by more than 250 ms before the perceivers noticed the discrepancy. The temporal dynamics needed for these judgments would seem to require memory mechanisms that maintain durable modality-specific information, followed by top-down detection of information mismatch. If auditory and visual speech information combined at a subsegmental level, perceivers might be expected to merely perceive unintelligible gibberish resulting from misaligned feature information from vision and hearing.

Whereas the results in this section do not prove that the modality-specific view is correct, they do pose problems for the common format view. The failure of visual speech to selectively adapt an auditory speech continuum delays possible AV interaction to a level beyond auditory speech stimulus processing. Evidence that familiarity with the talker can defeat the McGurk effect suggests that top-down processing is involved. Results observed with Japanese adults suggest that the McGurk effect is sensitive to language and cultural effects, such that it can be defeated even though the perceivers are sensitive to the visual information. Finally, long SOAs that do not defeat AV interactions suggest that phonetic information is maintained in some type of relatively durable store that allows perceivers to detect asynchrony at long lags but nevertheless recover the appropriate alignment of the information. All of these effects imply processing mechanisms that go beyond early transformation of AV speech to a common subsegmental format.

VISUAL SPEECH PERCEPTION One requirement for a modality-specific theory to be true is that the visual pathway must operate effectively in parallel with the auditory pathway in processing speech information. However, visual speech stimuli have been characterized as inadequate to support successful speech communication. Kuhl and Meltzoff summarized this view succinctly, saying "much of speech misses the eye" (1988, p. 241). It is true that visual speech information is impoverished relative to auditory speech information presented under good listening conditions. For example, lipreaders cannot usually discriminate /ba/ from /pa/, because they cannot see the vocal fold vibration that is used to discriminate the two. However, the distinction needed is that between quality of the speech information and the perceptual resources available to process the information. The evidence is that perceivers do have visual speech processing resources, although not all perceivers are equally capable.

Everyday experience working among deaf adults at Gallaudet University, where hearing impairment is a requirement for undergraduate enrollment and lipreading is an effective mode of speech perception, led Bernstein et al. (2000) to investigate lipreading ability in a study of 72 deaf and 96 hearing adults. Normative perceptual data on visual speech perception and spoken word recognition were obtained. Participants lipread consonant-vowel nonsense syllables, and words in isolation and in sentences. The results showed that relatively high levels of visual speech perception and spoken word recognition were obtained by deaf participants, most of whom had congenital profound hearing impairments. The mean scores for words correct with one of the sentence sets were 47% for the deaf and 28% for the hearing participants. The upper quartile scores for both groups provided an estimate of the upper levels of visual speech perception capability under conditions of normal hearing versus deafness. The top 19 hearing lipreaders scored between 42% and 75% words correct on a sentence set for which the top 12 deaf lipreaders scored between 68% and 85% words correct. The high scores achieved by some congenitally deaf adults suggest that they relied on an extensive visual-only processing pathway. Although somewhat less accurate, the more accurate hearing adults also demonstrated the existence of an effective visual route to spoken language comprehension.

Other studies carried out by our group suggest that the impoverishment of visual speech stimuli can be overcome in part because the combinations of segments that make up the words in the language often result in patterns that do not require complete information to be recognized. For example, the word *bought* could be accurately identified despite the fact that the phonemes /b, p, m/ are highly visually similar, because English does not have the words *mought* and *pought*. This issue is explored in detail in Auer and Bernstein (1997). It was investigated further by Mattys, Bernstein, and Auer (2002), who showed that accuracy for lipreading words varied as a function of the number of words predicted to be visually similar to the stimulus word. Given that word recognition is generally assumed to be achieved via competition in the mental lexicon among similar word forms, these results supported the view that the visual stimulus form was relevant at the level of word recognition. Similar results were obtained in a study by Auer (2002).

In summary, various results suggest that humans can process speech visually at a reasonably accurate level, given the limitations on the available information. Setting aside the question of what accounts for individual variation in the ability to process visual speech information, the results for lipreading are consistent with the existence of a visual speech processing pathway.

MODALITY-SPECIFIC THEORIES   Summerfield (1987) briefly outlined two possible theories for modality specific AV speech perception. Following a suggestion that auditory speech recognition could be based on a direct mapping between slices of acoustic spectral patterns and networks that represent words (Klatt, 1979), Summerfield proposed an analogous direct mapping for auditory and visual speech information. The visual information might be represented in a format as simple as the digitized two-dimensional frontal images of a talker's mouth. Both acoustic and optical representations would be mapped directly, via a network, to word patterns stored in long-term memory. But Summerfield rejected this model, because it did not provide a process for dealing with the variability in either auditory or visual speech information that can arise from a variety of sources, such as talker differences and viewing angles. His solution to the noninvariance problem was to transform the visual information into front-face projections of stored vocal tract templates and transform the auditory information into the internal configuration of articulators. This solution, however, seems closer to a common format than to a modality-specific implementation, inasmuch as both auditory and visual information is transformed into articulatory representations.

Braida (1991) proposed a formal mathematical modality-specific model, referred to as a *prelabeling* model. In this model, information is never transformed across modalities. Braida's example of how the model works is that "visual observation of the rate of lip opening might be combined with auditorily estimated 'attack' characteristics and these combined with visual and auditory estimates of duration to produce a four-dimensional vector that characterizes the speech sound" (p. 652). This vector is then mapped to a category label. Braida modeled several sets of published speech data. The prelabeling model accounted quite well for empirical data. Although Braida did not model McGurk effects, he asserted that the prelabeling model could be used to do so in exactly the same manner as it was used for congruent AV stimuli. At the heart of Braida's model is the concept that bimodal speech perception optimizes the use of modality-specific information.

Although the literature has tended to interpret AV speech perception effects in terms of common format theories, the modality-specific theories described here show that skepticism has existed for quite some time concerning the common format view as an explanation for AV binding.

MODELING AUDIOVISUAL SPEECH STIMULUS CORRESPONDENCE   A different approach to understanding AV speech perception has recently been taken in studies that examine speech signals. Common format theories are consistent with the impression that the qualia of auditory and visual speech stimuli are so diverse as to require transformation into a common abstract format in order to bind together. However, the biomechanical speech articulation processes that produce acoustic signals also produce optical signals, and this common origin has justified studies of the relationship between acoustic and optical speech signals (e.g., Yehia, Kuratate, & Vatikiotis-Bateson, 1999; Yehia, Rubin, & Vatikiotis-Bateson, 1998). These studies have involved the application of computational methods to quantify relationships between high-dimensional data sets. Multilinear regression (Bertsimas & Tsitsiklis, 1997) is one such method. Multilinear regression fits a linear combination of the components of a multichannel signal, $\mathbf{X}$, to a single-channel signal y_j and results in a residual error vector; $y_j = a_1 x_1 + a_2 x_2 + \cdots + a_1 x_1 + e$, where x_i ($i = 1, 2, \ldots, I$) is one channel of the multichannel signal $\mathbf{X}$, a is the weighting coefficient, and b is the residual vector. In multilinear regression, the objective is to minimize the root mean square error $\|e\|_2$, using $a = \mathrm{argmin}\,\{\|\mathbf{X}^T a - y^T\|_2\}$. This optimization problem has a standard solution $a = (\mathbf{X}\mathbf{X}^T)^{-1}\,\mathbf{X}y_j^T$. The matrix y^T represents one set of signals and the matrix $\mathbf{X}^T$ represents the other set of signals. Multilinear regression is optimized in the sense of producing the maximum correlation between predicted and obtained data streams (Bertsimas & Tsitsiklis, 1997).

Our group applied this approach to acoustic and optical signals that were recorded simultaneously while talkers produced syllables or sentences (Jiang, Alwan, Keating, Auer, & Bernstein, 2002). The optical data were the positions in three dimensions over time of retroreflectors glued on to the talker's face. The motion data represent what can be seen in speech.[3] The acoustic data were transformed into root mean square energy and line spectral pairs to represent what can be heard. In Jiang et al., the correspondence between data

---

[3]During visual speech perception, the movements of the tongue are intermittently visible through the open mouth. The tongue movements are also highly correlated with movements of the jaw and face that are captured by the optical data.

streams achieved by multilinear regression was tested by calculating the Pearson correlation between one data set and the other data set, after weighting by the optimized transformation matrix. For example, this method was applied to a database of consonant-vowel nonsense syllables with 23 different initial consonants and three different vowels (/a, i, u/) spoken by four talkers, who repeated each syllable in random order four times. One set of Pearson correlations obtained for the evaluation of the goodness of the correspondence between the acoustic and optical data ranged between 0.74 and 0.82, depending on the talker. These results showed that there are predictable relationships between the physical acoustic and optical signals. The fact that a successful transformation can be computed to convert between acoustic and optical signals shows that a process *could* be applied to one modality of speech representation to transform it into another modality representation, as suggested by common format theory. Alternatively, the multilinear approach can be viewed as evidence that a systematic correspondence exists between acoustic and optical speech signals. A speech-perceiving brain could observe, represent, and bind corresponding representations via associations. Long-term perceptual experience could result in cortical networks that represent associations between corresponding auditory and visual speech representations. In the latter scenario, there would be no necessity to re-represent information in a common format.

SUMMARY OF PERCEPTUAL RESULTS AND THEORIES
Research on AV speech perception has disclosed phenomena that seem consistent with the possibility that perceptual processing transforms low-level speech information into a common format, and research has also disclosed phenomena that seem consistent with the possibility that modality-specific speech representations are maintained to a relatively high level of processing. Although speech perception researchers have undertaken many clever and insightful experiments in their attempts to determine whether a common format or a modality-specific view is more correct, ultimately AV speech binding cannot be understood in the absence of knowledge about how the CNS implements speech perception, both unimodal and audiovisual. This is the issue to which we now turn.

Neural implementation of audiovisual speech perception

This section describes the neuroanatomy and function of the synaptic levels of the bottom-up auditory and visual pathways of the CNS that likely support speech processing. The section builds on Mesulam's theory of CNS function, which is a modality-specific theory (Mesulam, 1994, 1998). Mesulam presents a functional as opposed to a structural or architectonic (e.g., Brodmann, 1908) description of the CNS. He identifies five major functional subtypes of the cortical synaptic hierarchy: primary sensorimotor, unimodal association, heteromodal association, paralimbic, and limbic. We focus here on only that portion of the CNS that processes bottom-up perceptual speech information from the sensory periphery, that is, primary sensory, unimodal association, and heteromodal association cortex. Among heteromodal association cortices are what Mesulam refers to as *transmodal gateways*. These gateways create linkages among modality-specific representations. That is, Mesulam proposes an associative alternative to binding by convergence.

Primary sensory areas are the obligatory initial cortical levels of processing for modality-specific sensory information. The flow of information from the sensory periphery, at the cortical level, follows a path from primary sensory to unimodal association areas and also from unimodal association areas to other unimodal association areas. Reciprocal connections in the pathway allow later synaptic levels to exert feedback (modulatory) influences on earlier levels. Crucially, according to Mesulam (1998), a principle of bottom-up sensory processing is that the fidelity of the information in sensory channels is protected from interaction with or contamination by information from other sensory channels through approximately four cortical synaptic levels of bottom-up processing. The implication of this arrangement is that the auditory and visual speech information that undergoes binding depends, at least in part, on the extent of analysis that takes place while modality-specific information is protected from interaction with other sources of information.

Stimulus information processing becomes more specialized in the bottom-up direction. Early processing areas are sensitive to relatively elementary stimulus attributes, and later processing areas (unimodal association) are more specialized for composite stimulus information. Mesulam (1998) attributes the vast areas of cerebral neocortex reserved for modality-specific association processing to the preservation of fidelity of sensory information (see Kaas, 1999). This principal of functional neuroanatomy predicts that the human CNS has the potential to perform elaborated analysis of modality-specific perceptual information separately for auditory versus visual speech stimuli. Transmodal areas at the fifth and sixth synaptic levels, including heteromodal, paralimbic, and limbic areas, are responsible for multimodal interaction and also for top-down influences on unimodal areas. For example, the comprehension of spoken words (understanding their meanings) involves Wernicke's area, a transmodal area that completes the relationship between the forms of words and the semantic networks that code meaning.

THE AUDITORY SPEECH PATHWAY: SYNAPTIC AND FUNCTIONAL LEVELS   The lowest cortical processing level for auditory stimuli occurs in the primary or core auditory cortex. In the human brain, this core area lies in the transverse temporal gyrus (Heschl's gyrus) on the upper surface of the temporal lobe, and was designated *area 41* (Fig. 13.1; Color Plate 1) by Brodmann (1908). It is equivalent to the core area of auditory cortex identified in various species of monkeys and termed *KA (auditory koniocortex;* Galaburda & Pandya, 1983; Pandya & Sanides, 1973) or A1 (Hackett, Stepniewska, & Kaas, 1998a; Morel, Garraghty, & Kaas, 1993; Morel & Kaas, 1992). Both human and monkey core regions are the only portion of the auditory cortex to receive dense input from the principal (ventral, parvocellular) division of the medial geniculate, which is the main thalamic relay for ascending auditory information (Fig. 13.1, solid blue line) (Hashikawa, Molinari, Rausell, & Jones, 1995; Morel et al., 1993; Pandya & Rosene, 1993; Rauschecker, Tian, Pons, & Mishkin, 1997).

A second synaptic level can be identified by the projection from the core auditory cortex to an auditory belt region (Aitkin, Kudo, & Irvine, 1988; Galaburda & Pandya, 1983; Hackett et al., 1998a). Belt cortex surrounds the core rostrally, laterally, and posteriorly and was termed *area 42* (Fig. 13.1) in both human and simian cortex by Brodmann (1908). In addition to transcortical input from the core, the belt area receives thalamic input from the ancillary nuclei of the medial geniculate and from the medial pulvinar (Aitkin et al., 1988; Burton & Jones, 1976; Hackett, Stepniewska, & Kaas, 1998b; Luethke, Krubitzer, & Kaas, 1989; Rauschecker, Tian, & Hauser 1995). However, this thalamic input apparently does not suffice to mediate responses to auditory stimuli, as destruction of core cortex abolishes responses in the belt area (Rauschecker et al., 1995). This is in accord with Mesulam's theory that within each sensory system, the primary or core area provides "an obligatory portal for the entry of sensory information into the cortical circuitry" (Mesulam, 1998, p. 1015).

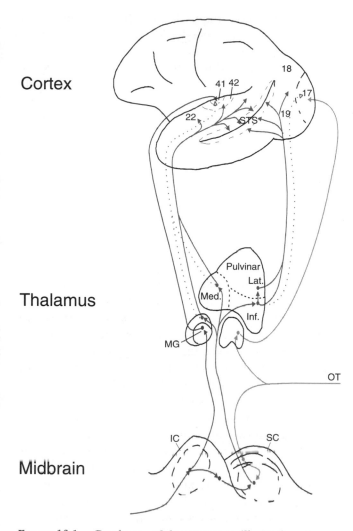

FIGURE 13.1.   Cerebrum of the macaque, illustrating sensory pathways revealed by tract tracing studies in monkeys.

Shown in green, visual input from the retina by way of the optic tract (OT) innervates the primary visual nucleus of the thalamus, the lateral geniculate (LG). The lateral geniculate in turn densely innervates the primary visual cortex (area 17). A collateral pathway from the optic tract goes to the superficial layers of the superior colliculus (SC) in the midbrain, and from there to the deeper layers of the superior colliculus.

Shown in blue, the auditory pathway ascends through the brainstem to the central nucleus of the inferior colliculus (IC). From this midbrain center, axons project to the primary auditory nucleus of the thalamus, the medial geniculate (MG). The medial geniculate in turn innervates the primary or core auditory cortex (area 41). A collateral branch of the auditory pathway extends to the external region of the inferior colliculus, and from there to the deep layers of the adjacent superior colliculus.

Shown in red, individual neurons in the deep superior colliculus that receive convergent visual and auditory information project to nonprimary thalamic nuclei, including the medial, lateral, and inferior pulvinar and the ancillary nuclei of the medial geniculate. From those nuclei, two types of projections are formed to sensory cortex. Shown in solid red lines, the lateral and inferior pulvinar nuclei project to layer 4 of higher levels of visual cortex (areas 18 and 19), while the

medial pulvinar and ancillary medial geniculate nuclei project to higher-level auditory cortex (areas 42 and 22). Shown in dotted red lines, the same pathways form tangential axons in layer 1 of primary visual cortex (area 17) and core auditory cortex (area 41). (See Color Plate 1.)

A third synaptic level consists of an extensive parabelt area that surrounds the core/belt and extends over the lateral surface of the superior temporal gyrus. This large area was designated *area 22* (Fig. 13.1) by Brodmann (1908). Tracer studies in monkeys have shown projections from belt auditory cortex to the parabelt (Hackett et al., 1998a; Luethke et al., 1989; Morel & Kaas, 1992; Morel et al., 1993). Thalamic input to the parabelt, like that of the belt region, comes only from the ancillary geniculate nuclei and the medial pulvinar (Burton & Jones, 1976; Hackett et al., 1998b).

A fourth synaptic level has also been defined in auditory cortex by projections that pass from the parabelt to the superior temporal sulcus (Fig. 13.1) (Kaas & Hackett, 2000; Ettlinger & Wilson, 1990; Seltzer & Pandya, 1978, 1994). It is interesting to note that the superior temporal sulcus is the fourth level in a chain of projections from the primary visual and somatosensory cortical areas, as well as the primary auditory cortex (Jones & Powell, 1970), and thus is a region in which modality-specific information might interact.

Auditory processing in the core consists of coding of elementary auditory stimulus features. Electrophysiological recording studies in monkeys have shown that core cortex has a precise tonotopic organization, that is, an orderly representation of best frequencies (Morel & Kaas, 1992; Morel et al., 1993). A similar tonotopic organization has been demonstrated in the human primary auditory area by magnetoencephalography (Elberling, Bak, Kofoed, Lebech, & Saermark, 1982; Pantev et al., 1988), by positron emission tomography (PET; Lauter, Herscovitch, Formby, & Raichle, 1985), and by functional magnetic resonance imaging (fMRI; Wessinger, Buonocore, Kussmaul, & Mangun, 1997). However, information processing in the core is not limited to analysis of pitch. Overlying but independent functional maps for sharpness of frequency tuning, intensity tuning and sensitivity, response latency, and binaural interaction have been demonstrated by unit recordings in monkey core cortex (Recanzone, Schreiner, Sutter, Beitel, & Merzenich, 1999). Results of functional imaging studies support the generalization that the core does not respond differentially to speech versus nonspeech stimuli (Binder et al., 2000; Celsis et al., 1999; Huckins, Turner, Doherty, Fonte, & Szeverenyi, 1998; Scott, Blank, Rosen, & Wise, 2000).

Belt neurons are more difficult to characterize by best frequencies (Imig, Ruggero, Kitzes, Javel, & Brugge, 1977; Merzenich & Brugge, 1973), but selective responses to complex stimuli, including species-specific calls, have been demonstrated in this area (Rauschecker et al., 1995; Wang, Merzenich, Beitel, & Schreiner, 1995). This accords with Mesulam's theory

that at the second synaptic level, "sectors of unimodal association areas encode basic features of sensation such as colour, motion, form and pitch" (Mesulam, 1998, p. 1013). In addition, the belt area also seems not to be specialized functionally in terms of the speech versus nonspeech distinction in humans (e.g., Binder et al., 2000; Steinschneider, Volkov, Noh, Garell, & Howard, 1999; Wise et al., 2001).

Human functional studies suggest a hierarchical processing of auditory stimuli similar to the neuroanatomical sequence of early to later synaptic levels indicated by the connectional studies in monkeys. Electrodes placed on the surface of the human temporal lobe during surgery have shown transcortical passage of excitation from Heschl's gyrus laterally into the superior temporal gyrus (Howard et al., 2000; Liégeois-Chauvel, Musolino, Badier, Marquis, & Chauvel, 1994). Functional imaging studies demonstrate activation by auditory stimuli spreading across the core and belt in the superior temporal plane, across the lateral surface of the parabelt to the superior temporal sulcus, and in some cases into the middle temporal gyrus (Binder et al., 2000; Huckins, et al., 1998; Price et al., 1996; Rosen, Scott, Lang, & Wise, 2001; Scott et al., 2000; Zatorre, Meyer, Gjedde, & Evans, 1996).

More detailed investigations of the functions of specific cortical locations activated by speech have been sought. Binder et al. (2000), using fMRI, showed that tone stimuli activated the early areas of the auditory pathway, that is, the core and belt areas on the superior temporal plane. Passive listening to words, pseudowords, and text passages resulted in spread of activation into the parabelt on the lateral surface of the superior temporal gyrus. Word classification produced activity in areas beyond the parabelt, including the superior temporal sulcus, middle temporal gyrus, and temporoparietal cortex (Wernicke's area), with greater activity in the language-dominant hemisphere. These results suggest that the parabelt is more specialized than the core/belt for the complexity of stimulus features and that the fourth and higher synaptic levels appear to perform preferential processing of meaningful speech. Scott et al. (2000) carried out a PET study designed to "separate the left temporal lobe system responsible for the speech-specific processing of familiar, intelligible words from more general auditory processing" (p. 2400). Even when the speech stimuli were spectrally rotated, so that they were unintelligible but contained similar spectral and temporal variation to speech, left hemisphere activation was obtained in the lateral and anterior parabelt and in the posterior superior temporal sulcus. A functional transition from posterior to anterior in the left superior temporal sulcus was identified in response to increased speech intelligibility. The authors interpreted their results as evidence for phonetic processing in the left parabelt, with processing by the posterior superior temporal sulcus more related to short-term memory for sound sequences. Taken together, the evidence to date from human functional studies seems to indicate that areas that preferentially process speech are first encountered at the third or fourth auditory synaptic levels.

THE VISUAL SPEECH PATHWAY: SYNAPTIC AND FUNCTIONAL LEVELS   Regardless of where visual speech information becomes associated with auditory speech information, without doubt it enters the cortex via the primary visual area, V1, which is at the first synaptic level of the visual pathway and is the exclusive recipient of projections from the magnocellular and parvocellular layers of the lateral geniculate nucleus (Felleman & Van Essen, 1991). V1 receives approximately 90% of visual inputs to cortex. Like the auditory core, which codes fine-grained auditory features, V1 has a fine-grained retinotopic mapping, and its neurons are sensitive to orientation, movement, binocular disparity, length, spatial frequency, wavelength, and luminance.

Unimodal association areas, such as V2, V4, and V5, are monosynaptically connected with V1 at the second synaptic level (Mesulam, 1998). These areas are more specialized than V1. For example, V5 (MT) is specialized for motion (Watson et al., 1993). However, these areas do not code complex objects such as faces. Visual speech-specific processing is not predicted for the first two synaptic levels, although it is possible that enhancement in processing for features of visual speech information could occur, particularly under conditions of deafness. For example, attention to visible speech motion might lead to enhanced peripheral sensitivity for motion, as appears to be the case for attention to sign language (Bavelier et al., 2001).

At the third and fourth synaptic levels of the visual system, unimodal visual association areas include the fusiform, inferior temporal, and middle temporal gyri. The area defined as the lateral occipital complex, located on the lateral bank of the fusiform gyrus extending ventrally and dorsally, appears to have a strong role in processing information about object shape or structure independent of the particular visual cues to structure and not to be differentially activated by types of visual objects (Grill-Spector, Kourtzi, & Kanwisher, 2001). Differential activations are observed due to complex objects versus faces (Halgren et al., 1999; Nobre, Allison, & McCarthy, 1994; Puce, Allison, Asgari, Gore, & McCarthy, 1996). Face processing at the level of the fusiform face area seems to be concerned with the general category of faces, with detecting faces and perceiving faces but not recognizing specific faces (Tong, Nakayama, Moscovitch, Weinrib, & Kanwisher, 2000). Recognition of specific faces relies on connections through transmodal areas to stored semantic knowledge (Daffner et al., 2000; Halgren et al., 1999).

Studies of humans viewing eye and mouth movements disclose some activation areas overlapping with ones from viewing of static faces, along with some additional areas of activation. Puce, Allison, Bentin, Gore, and McCarthy (1998, Fig. 7) summarize a number of studies. Moving eyes and mouths activated a bilateral region centered in the posterior superior temporal sulcus, 0.5 to 1.5 cm anterior and inferior to a region activated by hand and body movement (Bonda, Petrides, Ostry, & Evans, 1996). Puce et al. (1998) suggest that the area responsive to mouth movements might receive its information directly from the motion-processing area, such that nonspeech mouth movements are processed no earlier than the third synaptic level. It is not known whether or not there are many category-specific visual areas such as the face area in the human ventral visual pathway (Grill-Spector et al., 2001; Kanwisher, 2000). If the modality-specific theory is correct, then visual speech stimuli are processed in areas that differentially respond to visual speech.

Relatively few functional imaging results have been obtained for the visual speech pathway (see Auer, Bernstein, & Singh, 2003; Bernstein et al., 2002, 2003; Calvert, 2001; Calvert et al., 1997, 1999; Campbell et al., 2001; Ludman et al., 2000; MacSweeney et al., 2001, 2002; Sekiyama & Sugita, in press; Surguladze et al., 2001). Studies have involved relatively few participants, although they have included both deaf and hearing adults. Stimuli have been spoken numbers, isolated words, and sentences. Control conditions have included still faces and nonspeech mouth movements. Many different cortical locations have been reported to be activated during lipreading relative to control conditions, including V1, V5/MT, inferior temporal gyrus, middle temporal gyrus, superior temporal gyrus, superior temporal sulcus, angular gyrus, and the auditory core, as well as frontal areas such as the inferior frontal gyrus and middle frontal gyrus. The results are generally consistent with the existence of an extensive visual pathway for speech stimulus processing, one that involves primary sensory- and motion-processing areas, and association cortices in the vicinity of regions responsible for visual object or face processing.

As yet, however, isolation of levels of visual speech processing has not been accomplished. The talking face is a complex stimulus, and isolation of the cortical areas that process information that is specific to speech has only begun (Bernstein et al., 2003; Calvert et al., 1997;

Campbell et al., 2001). Visual speech-processing studies have for the most part focused on only the grossest contrasts, such as speech versus still face. Cortical areas for which there is some evidence of preference for visual speech include regions of the left superior temporal gyrus, left superior temporal sulcus, left middle temporal gyrus, right middle temporal gyrus, and bilateral inferior temporal gyrus (Bernstein et al., 2003; Calvert et al., 1997; Campbell et al., 2001; MacSweeney et al., 2002). Of course, isolation of areas that might be specialized for visual speech requires not only controls for nonspeech stimulus attributes of the face but also controls for auditory speech attributes. To our knowledge, this work remains to be done.

MULTISENSORY INPUT TO CORTEX FROM THE BRAINSTEM Mesulam (1998) has argued that the absence of interconnections linking unimodal areas is one of the most important principles of the primate cerebral cortex:

This is particularly interesting since many of these unimodal association areas receive monosynaptic feedback projections from heteromodal cortices which are responsive to both auditory and visual stimuli. The sensory-petal (or feedback) projections from heteromodal cortices therefore appear to display a highly selective arrangement that actively protects the fidelity of sensory tuning during the first four synaptic levels of sensory-fugal [feed-forward] processing. (p. 1023)

(See Recanzone, 1998, who discusses the lack of connections between unimodal cortices, and Jones & Powell, 1970.)

It is necessary to note, however, that there is anatomical evidence for AV interactions in the brainstem that can be relayed to cortex and influence processing there. As mentioned earlier, AV interaction occurs in the deep layers of the superior colliculus, where visual and auditory inputs converge on individual neurons. These multisensory cells are highly sensitive to temporal and spatial overlap of AV stimuli (Stein & Meredith, 1993) and form pathways to the forebrain that could influence activity at the cortical level (see Fig. 13.1).

The ascending projections from the deep layers of the superior colliculus have been demonstrated by restricted injection of neuronal tracers into the deep layers of the superior colliculus of the macaque monkey (Benevento & Fallon, 1974). These ascending brainstem pathways do not provide input to the main sensory nuclei of the thalamus. Instead, they project to ancillary and multisensory thalamic nuclei, namely, the lateral, inferior, and medial divisions of the pulvinar and the satellite nuclei of the medial geniculate complex . From these nuclei, projections arise to both auditory and visual cortices. The medial pulvinar and satellite nuclei of the medial geniculate project broadly but sparsely to the entire auditory cortex (Hashikawa et al., 1995), while axons from the lateral and inferior pulvinar project to the visual cortex of the occipital lobe (Rezak & Benevento, 1979). Crucially, a similar pattern of projection is seen in both the visual and auditory cortices. In both areas, the thalamic axons end in small patches in layer 4, the thalamocortical input layer, in all higher level cortex (Fig. 13.1, solid red lines). However, within the core cortical areas (area 41 of auditory cortex and area 17 of visual cortex), the thalamic axons form *only* tangential axons in layer 1 (Fig. 13.1, dotted red lines). These layer 1 axons cross and contact large numbers of apical dendritic tufts of deeper lying pyramidal cells, and have been shown to powerfully bias the response of neurons in deeper layers of the cortex (Cauller & Connors, 1994). They thus create a transcortical modulatory system that can potentially influence the excitability of the core areas. Through this system, multisensory input from the brainstem can affect cortical activity *level* whenever AV stimuli are present. However, the content of this brainstem input is primarily related to temporal and spatial stimulus attributes, and thus seems unlikely to provide specific speech pattern information. Its role is thus more likely to be one of modulation of information than one of information processing per se.

TEMPORAL CONSTRAINTS Genuine AV speech information processing effects might be distinguished from more generic AV effects by observing temporal dynamics. For example, Calvert et al. (1999) reported enhanced activation levels in the auditory core and V1 with speech, which was interpreted as possibly due to cortical back-projections. However, latency data unavailable with fMRI might have shown that the enhancements were too early to be attributed to cortical feedback involving information processing, instead deriving from perhaps subcortical AV interactions. Temporal constraints can be learned from event-related potentials obtained using electrophysiological or magnetoencephalographic recordings. Several studies that have used arbitrary, simple nonspeech AV stimuli have also shown early latency, less than 100 ms, electrophysiological effects (Giard & Peronnet, 1999; Saron et al., 2001; Shams et al., 2001). But some subsequent research has shown that apparent early interactions of information could be due to more global effects such as expectation or attention that could contribute to activations in the direction of bottom-up processing (Teder-Salejarvi et al., 2002).

Processing times through the auditory and visual pathways set constraints on when cortically processed information could possibly interact. The first volley of stimulus-driven activity into the auditory core occurs around 11–20 ms post-stimulus onset (Steinschneider et al., 1999; Yvert, Crouzeix, Bertrand, Seither-Preisler, & Pantev, 2001), and the auditory speech percept appears to develop within 150–200 ms post-stimulus onset (Naatanen, 2001). In comparison, intra-cortical recordings in V1/V2 have shown the earliest stimulus-driven response to be at approximately 56–60 ms (Foxe & Simpson, 2002; Krolak-Salmon et al., 2001). Given this early discrepancy in latencies across auditory and visual primary cortices, and given that transcortical processing also requires time, interactions between auditory and visual speech information would seem predicted for latencies beyond 100 or 150 ms post-stimulus onset.

Recently, Ponton, Bernstein, Auer, and Wagner (2003) reported an ERP study that supports this prediction. Although early (100 ms) enhanced responses were obtained with AV speech versus unimodal speech stimuli, those enhancements were similar, whether the AV stimuli were congruent (matched) or incongruent (McGurk type). However, later responses (>200 ms) were found to be sensitive to whether the stimuli were congruent or not. This result was consistent with the modality-specific theory in that speech information processing appears to have occurred at the later latency. These results support the need for combining data on localization with data on latency to narrow in on those AV effects that are specific to speech information processing.

Common format neural implementation

From our perspective, in order for a common format theory to be true at the level of CNS implementation, the single critical component would be convergence of auditory and visual subsegmental speech information onto multisensory neurons. A common format theory would not be satisfied by convergence of phonetic information into a common area but not onto common neurons, or if levels of processing subsequent to the common area were sensitive to modality-specific phonetic information. Convergence must transform modality-specific subsegmental information into a common format at the segmental level. Proving convergence requires showing that there are multisensory neurons that preferentially respond to auditory and visual subsegmental linguistic information, and that these neurons are in the pathway that supports AV speech perception.

Previously, we discussed the theory that there is a common speech production-perception articulatory format (Liberman & Mattingly, 1985; Liberman &

Whalen, 2000). One possibility that has been raised is that so-called *mirror neurons* (Rizzolatti & Arbib, 1998), which have been found in the frontal cortex of monkeys, might implement the production-perception articulatory format and even a common AV format. Mirror neurons respond both to the monkey performing specific actions and to its observing those actions. Sundara, Namasivayam, and Chen (2001) presented auditory-only, visual-only, and AV syllables to human participants. During the presentations, electromyographic recordings were made from the orbicularis oris muscle, used to articulate /b/. Transcranial magnetic stimulation (TMS) was performed during the experiment at the optimal location for eliciting motor-evoked potentials from the orbicularis oris muscle. Comparisons were made between the TMS stimulation and the motor-evoked potentials during speech perception. The *only* conditions with significantly increased motor-evoked potentials in comparison with the TMS-induced baseline were the visual /ba/ and the AV /ba/ (not the auditory /ba/). Crucially, visual /ba/ activation was greater than visual /ta/, for which the orbicularis oris is not a key articulator muscle. The conclusion was that the "OEM [observation-execution matching] system may be modality specific and is not involved in the perception of simple sound stimuli" (p. 1344). Pending further similar studies, these results discourage the notion that a neural implementation of common format perception theory exists at the level of the OEM system.

Direct-realist theory (Fowler, 1986), also reviewed earlier, proposes that perception of speech makes use of no special mechanisms different from perception of nonspeech and that what is perceived is speech articulation. Thus, the neural implementation for this theory needs to contend with detecting articulatory patterns in visual and auditory stimuli and representing those patterns in a common format. To our knowledge, the problem of representing acoustic patterns as articulation has not been studied at the level of the CNS (with the exception of the study of the OEM system). Also, there has not, to our knowledge, been research directly comparing AV speech versus nonspeech object perception. However, across two separate studies by Calvert and colleagues, similar paradigms were used with spoken sentences versus reversing checkerboards, and noise bursts produced different activity, with the result that speech and nonspeech AV combinations were processed at different locations, suggesting that at least the notion of common speech and nonspeech processing of AV objects appears not to be true (Calvert, 2001).

Feature integration information-processing theories of AV speech perception seem most compatible with the notion of convergence onto multisensory neurons. Massaro (1999) has explicitly favored neural convergence as the implementation mechanism for feature integration.

A study by Calvert, Campbell, and Brammer (2000) provided some evidence supporting neural convergence compatible with Massaro's (1999) view. In the study by Calvert et al., participants were imaged while being presented with auditory, visual, or AV spoken sentence stimuli. The AV stimuli were either congruent or incongruent. The goal of the experiment was to test whether "the principle of crossmodal binding by convergence onto multisensory neurons form a general physiological basis for intersensory synthesis that also extends to humans" (p. 650). Evidence for convergence was defined as areas that respond both to auditory and visual speech and also to AV speech, in particular, with superadditivity for congruent and subadditivity for incongruent stimuli. The sole area that fulfilled these criteria consisted of eight voxels in the left ventral bank of the superior temporal sulcus ($x = -49$, $y = -50$, $z = 9$; coordinate system of Talairach & Tournoux, 1988). By relaxing the criteria concerning subadditivity, additional areas were obtained: two were in the STS ($x = 48$, $y = -55$, $z = 20$, and $x = -53$, $y = -48$, $z = 9$). These results were interpreted to "clearly support the hypothesis that crossmodal binding of sensory inputs in man can be achieved by convergence onto multisensory cells localized in heteromodal cortex" (p. 655).

However, the study did not provide direct evidence that the superadditivity was due to convergence of phonetic information per se. As noted earlier, this proof might be difficult to achieve without using temporal data. In addition, studies of auditory speech processing have reported more anterior locations that might be hypothesized to be specialized for subsegmental feature processing. In Binder et al. (2000), all of the relevant speech versus nonspeech contrasts resulted in activation at the midlateral superior temporal gyrus and adjacent superior temporal sulcus. Twenty-three activation peaks were listed (Binder et al., 2000, Table 2), and every one was anterior and inferior to the peaks for AV activation in Calvert et al. (2000). In the study by Scott et al. (2000), which contrasted speech conditions versus reversed spectra noise-vocoded speech, the closest peak to the ones reported in Calvert et al. (transformed from MNI space to Talairach coordinates; Brett, 1999; Talairach & Tournoux, 1988), was anterior and inferior ($x = -63$, $y = -36$, $z = 2$).

MacSweeney et al. (2002) isolated superior temporal sulcus activity during silent lipreading versus a control condition in which the talker performed closed-mouth gurning gestures. This control condition, which arguably could contribute to localizing specifically visual phonetic processing, resulted in superior temporal sulcus activity more anterior to that isolated in Calvert et al. (2000). Thus, results suggest that if phonetic processing occurs in the superior temporal sulcus, it is in a distinct location from the superior temporal sulcus multisensory processing area reported by Calvert et al. On the other hand, the superior temporal sulcus is activated by nonspeech eye and mouth movements (Puce et al., 1998) close (e.g., $x = -47$, $y = -50$, $z = 2$) to the locations reported in Calvert et al. Voice-selective areas have also been localized nearby (e.g., $x = -62$, $y = -40$, $z = 10$; Belin, Zatorre, Lafaille, Ahad, & Pike, 2000), together raising the possibility that natural speech stimuli contribute information other than phonetic features that might contribute to the appearance of segmental AV effects interpretable as due to convergence.

Although some evidence has been presented that is consistent with there being multisensory convergence of AV subsegmental information as the neural implementation for perceptual common format theory, that evidence is necessarily preliminary. Much more work is needed to prove that subsegmental features are processed by multisensory convergence.

Modality-specific neural implementation

In order for a modality-specific theory to be true at the level of CNS implementation, there must be mechanisms that associate modality-specific speech information processed to the level of linguistic units. The research reviewed earlier in this chapter on the auditory and visual speech pathways is consistent with the possibility that there is extensive processing of modality-specific speech information. The issue then is how the modality-specific auditory information and visual information are brought into contact.

Figure 13.2 sketches a proposed functional neuroanatomy for the modality-specific view of AV speech perception. Primary sensory areas visual (V1) and auditory (core), and early unimodal association visual (e.g., V2, V4, V5) and auditory (belt, parabelt) are labeled in terms of neuroanatomy. Later unimodal association, transmodal (Mesulam, 1998), and higher-level areas are labeled in functional terms only. At the level labeled *later unimodal association,* the speech units are listed as feature, segment, syllable, and word. It is not known whether these hierarchically related linguistic units correspond only to the structure of representations or whether they correspond to discrete cortical processing levels. Our earlier discussion of the speech pathways shows that work has only begun to determine the status

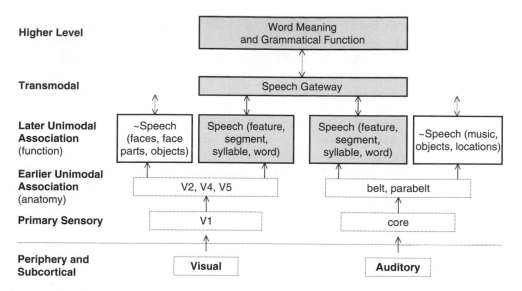

Higher Level	Word Meaning and Grammatical Function			
Transmodal		Speech Gateway		
Later Unimodal Association (function)	~Speech (faces, face parts, objects)	Speech (feature, segment, syllable, word)	Speech (feature, segment, syllable, word)	~Speech (music, objects, locations)
Earlier Unimodal Association (anatomy)	V2, V4, V5		belt, parabelt	
Primary Sensory	V1		core	
Periphery and Subcortical	Visual		Auditory	

FIGURE 13.2   Modality-specific model of AV speech perception from a functional neuroanatomical perspective (see text).

of linguistic units versus cortical processing areas. In Figure 13.2, the later association level is thought to be concerned only with modality-specific speech patterns. The next level is the transmodal speech gateway. This level is instrumental in completing the association between the modality-specific associations.

Transmodal areas are not, according to Mesulam (1998), areas where information converges onto a common amodal/supramodal format or representation. Transmodal areas are "not necessarily centres where convergent knowledge resides, but critical gateways (or hubs, sluices, nexuses) for accessing the relevant distributed information" (Mesulam, 1998, p. 1024). The inputs to heteromodal association areas from unimodal association areas might maintain their modality specificity while being interspersed among different modality-specific neurons, or might converge on multisensory neurons. However, Mesulam (1994, 1998) points out the following primary objections to convergence: (1) if a single cortical area were needed to represent all of the information relevant to a complex percept, then the brain would have to solve the problem of directing all of the information to that location for re-representation; and (2) convergence of the type in (1) would lead to contamination of the original perceptual information. These problems are solved if there are cortical areas that act as transmodal gateways for completing association networks or creating look-up directories. Heteromodal association, paralimbic, and limbic cortices are theoretically at the same synaptic levels and are all considered to be transmodal areas. The superior temporal sulcus could be the heteromodal association area responsible for transmodal binding of AV speech (Calvert

et al., 2000). Alternatively, Wernicke's area could bind modality-specific stimulus representations with representations in long-term lexical memory, or with semantic networks (Mesulam, 1998). The possibility has also been raised that subcortical relay stations, possibly the insula or claustrum, are responsible for associating multimodal representations (Ettlinger & Wilson, 1990), and some evidence for AV speech has been published in support of this view (Olson, Gatenby, & Gore, 2002).

The general notion that an alternative to convergence is needed for binding diverse thoughts, actions, and perceptual information was suggested in our introduction. A substantial theoretical literature is emerging with multiple arguments for associative mechanisms to support binding (Grey, 1999; Singer, 1998; Treisman, 1996; von der Malsburg, 1995, 1999; Zeki, 2001). For example, Singer (1998) makes the point that convergence onto particular sets of neurons in a feed-forward architecture is useful for rapid processing of frequently occurring invariant combinations of stimulus attributes, but such convergence is costly in terms of the number of neurons needed and is not well-suited to dealing with diverse and noninvariant stimulus information. Singer's solution is association of neurons into functionally coherent, dynamically created assemblies that as a whole represent particular stimulus content. One suggestion that has gained extensive attention, and whose status is being actively investigated is that neuronal assemblies are bound via neural coherence (correlation of responses across cortical areas), or alternatively that binding results in coherence (e.g., Basar-Eroglu, Struber, Schurmann, Stadler, & Basar, 1996; Grey, 1999; Singer, 1998; Varela, Lachaux, Rodriguez, & Martinerie, 2001).

Research on AV speech perception has yet to exploit the methodologies involved in studying neural synchrony. Evidence in favor of a modality-specific theory could derive from observing synchrony between cortical areas known to process modality-specific stimulus information. There are results showing synchrony effects resulting from nonspeech multimodal processing (Miltner, Braun, Arnold, Witte, & Taub, 1999).

Another argument in favor of an associative binding mechanism is that even within the visual modality, it is a problematic solution to the binding of diverse types of information. Moutoussi and Zeki (1997) have observed,

To all of us, intuitively much of the most appealing solution [to the binding problem] was an anatomical convergence, a strategy by which the results of operations performed in all the specialized visual areas would be relayed to one area or a set of areas—which would then act as the master integrator and, perhaps, even perceptive areas. Apart from the logical difficulty of who would then perceive the image provided by the master areas(s) . . . , there is a more practical difficulty— the failure to observe an area or a set of areas that receive outputs from all the antecedent visual areas. Thus the convergent anatomical strategy is not the brain's chosen method of bringing this integration about. (pp. 1412–1413)

At this time, a fair statement would be that there is more detailed theoretical rationale for expecting that AV speech perception relies on modality-specific neural processing and association of modality specific representations than there are empirical data. The facts that (1) the theoretical rationale is strong, (2) what is known about the auditory and visual speech pathways is consistent with a modality-specific view, and (3) some of the AV speech perceptual results to date (reviewed earlier) are consistent with modality-specific theory (and inconsistent with common format theory) argue for experimental studies to investigate the modality-specific theory.

Testing theories of neural implementation

Arguably, the ideal conditions for studying neural implementations of AV speech perception theories would involve direct cortical recordings of multiple neurons in networks, in order to test for modality-specific associative mechanisms, temporal dynamics, and level of information representation. Modality-specific theory would be supported by finding both unimodal networks that preferentially process modality-specific phonetic stimulus information and associations among networks, possibly in terms of synchronizing activity. Common format theory would be supported by finding multisensory neurons that transform modality-specific subsegmental information into amodal or abstract subsegmental or segmental representations. Knowledge about processing latencies and locations, along with knowledge about

neuroanatomical constraints, is needed to determine whether common format or modality-specific theory is correct. The ideal experimental conditions can be approximated by combining high spatial resolution (e.g., fMRI) and high temporal resolution (e.g., EEG, MEG) measuring techniques.

As important as experimental techniques, highly explicit hypotheses concerning neural implementations of perceptual models need to be developed. As pointed out earlier, most perceptual theories have not included explicit suggestions for neural implementations. From our perspective, perhaps the most important issue needing attention is how to determine that cortical activity following AV stimulation reflects speech information processing as opposed to modulation. Modality-specific and common format theories are about speech information, but effects that arise in the presence of speech stimuli need not be specific to speech attributes. For example, natural AV speech stimuli afford attributes related to talker identity, sex, race, age, attractiveness, and so on, all of which could induce effects that could be erroneously ascribed to speech information. In order to test theories about speech information processing, speech information processing effects must be isolated from other effects.

Experiments involving novel stimulus combinations or learning could be particularly important for AV speech research. For modality-specific theory, long-term perceptual experience is hypothesized to result in associations that represent the normal correspondence between auditory and visual speech information. During processing of atypical auditory and visual stimulus combinations, bottom-up information would result in a mismatch with the stored network, including the associative connections. Therefore, responses to typical versus atypical stimulus combinations should differ, and we have obtained some evidence that this is the case (Ponton et al., 2003). In addition, modality-specific theory predicts that repeated pairings of auditory and visual speech stimuli should lead to changes in associations. Common format theories appear not to offer mechanisms for representing correspondence between different kinds of modality-specific information. It is unclear to us how or whether learning might be involved in convergent processing.

Summary and conclusions

This chapter has outlined two views of AV speech perception. Common format theories of AV speech perception hypothesize that in order for auditory and visual speech information to integrate, the information must converge at the level of subsegmental features.

The modality-specific view hypothesizes that perceptual systems process speech information in a manner that is linguistically relevant and modality-specific. Modality-specific information associates rather than converges.

Preference for the modality-specific theory was expressed here based on theoretical considerations and on emerging evidence for parallel visual and auditory speech pathways. The modality-specific view finds support in knowledge about the functional neuroanatomy of the CNS. From this perspective, modality-specific cortical pathways process sensory information through several synaptic levels prior to reaching transmodal gateways. Theoretical considerations suggest that convergence is an inadequate solution for the problem of binding noninvariant AV speech information. Studies of the correspondences among naturally produced acoustic and optical speech signals suggest that relationships exist in the stimuli that could be observed by a speech-perceiving brain to establish associative networks. Synchrony among modality-specific areas could fulfill the binding function for which convergence is hypothesized by common format theories. Much work remains to determine whether AV speech perception is explained along the lines we prefer or along the lines of a common format theory. The goal of this chapter has been to suggest some alternative and hopefully productive approaches to the AV speech perception problem.

REFERENCES

Aitkin, L. M., Kudo, M., & Irvine, D. R. (1988). Connections of the primary auditory cortex in the common marmoset, *Callithrix jacchus jacchus. Journal of Comparative Neurology, 269*, 235–248.

Auer, E. T., Jr. (2002). The influence of the lexicon on speech read word recognition: Contrasting segmental and lexical distinctiveness. *Psychonomic Bulletin and Review, 9*, 341–347.

Auer, E. T., Jr., & Bernstein, L. E. (1997). Speechreading and the structure of the lexicon: Computationally modeling the effects of reduced phonetic distinctiveness on lexical uniqueness. *Journal of the Acoustical Society of America 102*, 3704–3710.

Auer, E. T., Jr., Bernstein, L. E., & Singh, M. (2003). Cortical correlates of lexical competitor set-size: An fMRI study of visual spoken word recognition. *Meeting of the Cognitive Neuroscience Society* (p. 136).

Basar-Eroglu, C., Struber, D., Schurmann, M., Stadler, M., & Basar, E. (1996). Gamma-band responses in the brain: A short review of psychophysiological correlates and functional significance. *International Journal of Psychophysiology, 24*, 101–112.

Bavelier, D., Brozinsky, C., Tomann, A., Mitchell, T., Neville, H., & Liu, G. (2001). Impact of early deafness and early exposure to sign language on the cerebral organization for motion processing. *Journal of Neuroscience, 21*, 8931–8942.

Belin, P., Zatorre, R. J., Lafaille, P., Ahad, P., & Pike, B. (2000). Voice-selective areas in human auditory cortex. *Nature, 403*, 309–312.

Benevento, L. A., & Fallon, J. H. (1974). The ascending projections of the superior colliculus in the rhesus monkey (*Macaca mulatta*). *Journal of Comparative Neurology, 160*, 339–362.

Bernstein, L. E., Auer, E. T., Jr., Moore, J. K., Ponton, C. W., Don, M., & Singh, M. (2002). Visual speech perception without primary auditory cortex activation. *NeuroReport, 13*, 311–315.

Bernstein, L. E., Auer, E. T., Zhou, Y., & Singh, M. (2003). Cortical specialization for visual speech versus non-speech face movements in color video and point lights. *Meeting of the Cognitive Neuroscience Society* (p. 173).

Bernstein, L. E., Demorest, M. E., & Tucker, P. E. (2000). Speech perception without hearing. *Perception & Psychophysics, 62*, 233–252.

Bertelson, P., & Aschersleben, G. (1997). Automatic visual bias of perceived auditory location. *Psychonomic Bulletin and Review, 5*, 482–489.

Bertsimas, D., & Tsitsiklis, J. N. (1997). *Introduction to linear optimization.* Belmont, MA: Athena Scientific.

Binder, J. R., Frost, J. A., Hammeke, T. A., Bellgowan, P. S., Springer, J. A., Kaufman, J. N., et al. (2000). Human temporal lobe activation by speech and nonspeech sounds. *Cerebral Cortex, 10*, 512–528.

Bonda, E., Petrides, M., Ostry, D., & Evans, A. (1996). Specific involvement of human parietal systems and the amygdala in the perception of biological motion, *Journal of Neuroscience, 16*, 3737–3744.

Boothroyd, A., Hnath-Chisolm, T., Hanin, L., & Kishon-Rabin, L. (1988). Voice fundamental frequency as an auditory supplement to the speechreading of sentences. *Ear and Hearing, 9*, 306–312.

Braida, L. D. (1991). Crossmodal integration in the identification of consonant segments. *Quarterly Journal of Experimental Psychology. A, Human Experimental Psychology, 43A*, 647–677.

Breeuwer, M., & Plomp, R. (1985). Speechreading supplemented with formant-frequency information from voiced speech. *Journal of the Acoustical Society of America, 77*, 314–317.

Brodmann, K. (1908). Beitrage zur histologischen Lokalisation der Grosshirnrinde: VI Mitteilung. Die Cortexgliederung des Menschen. *Journal of Psychological Neurology, 10*, 231–246.

Burton, H., & Jones, E. G. (1976). The posterior thalamic region and its cortical projection in New World and Old World monkeys. *Journal of Comparative Neurology, 168*, 249–301.

Calvert, G. A. (2001). Crossmodal processing in the human brain: Insights from functional neuroimaging studies. *Cerebral Cortex, 11*, 1110–1123.

Calvert, G. A., Brammer, M. J., Bullmore, E. T., Campbell, R., Iversen, S. D., & David, A. S. (1999). Response amplification in sensory-specific cortices during crossmodal binding. *NeuroReport, 10*, 2619–2623.

Calvert, G. A., Bullmore, E. T., Brammer, M. J., Campbell, R., Williams, S. C., McGuire, P. K., et al. (1997). Activation of auditory cortex during silent lipreading. *Science, 276*, 593–596.

Calvert, G. A., Campbell, R., & Brammer, M. J. (2000). Evidence from functional magnetic resonance imaging of crossmodal binding in the human heteromodal cortex. *Current Biology, 10*, 649–657.

Campbell, R., MacSweeney, M., Surguladze, S., Calvert, G., McGuire, P., Suckling, J., et al. (2001). Cortical substrates for the perception of face actions: An fMRI study of the specificity of activation for seen speech and for meaningless lower-face acts (gurning). *Brain Research. Cognitive Brain Research, 12,* 233–243.

Cauller, L. J., & Connors, B. W. (1994). Synaptic physiology of horizontal afferents to layer I in slices of rat SI neocortex. *Journal of Neuroscience, 14,* 751–762.

Celsis, P., Boulanouar, K., Doyon, B., Ranjeva, J. P., Berry, I., Nespoulous, J. L., et al. (1999). Differential fMRI responses in the left posterior superior temporal gyrus and left supramarginal gyrus to habituation and change detection in syllables and tones. *Neuroimage, 9,* 135–144.

Daffner, K. R., Scinto, L. F. M., Calvo, V., Faust, R., Mesulam, M. M., West, C. W., et al. (2000). The influence of stimulus deviance on electrophysiologic and behavioral responses to novel events. *Journal of Cognitive Neuroscience, 12,* 393–406.

Dixon, N. F., & Spitz, L. (1980). The detection of auditory visual desynchrony. *Perception, 9,* 719–721.

Elberling, C., Bak, C., Kofoed, B., Lebech, J., & Saermark, K. (1982). Auditory magnetic fields from the human cerebral cortex: Location and strength of an equivalent current dipole. *Acta Neurologica Scandinavica, 65,* 553–569.

Ettlinger, G., & Wilson, W. A. (1990). Cross-modal performance: Behavioural processes, phylogenetic considerations and neural mechanisms. *Behavioural Brain Research, 40,* 169–192.

Felleman, D. J., & Van Essen, D. C. (1991). Distributed hierarchical processing in the primate cerebral cortex. *Cerebral Cortex, 1,* 1–47.

Fowler, C. A. (1986). An event approach to the study of speech perception from a direct-realist perspective. *Journal of Phonetics, 14,* 3–28.

Foxe, J. J., & Simpson, G. V. (2002). Flow of activation from V1 to frontal cortex in humans: A framework for defining "early" visual processing. *Experimental Brain Research, 142,* 139–150.

Friston, K. J., Price, C. J., Fletcher, P., Moore, C., Frackowiak, R. S., & Dolan, R. J. (1996). The trouble with cognitive subtraction. *Neuroimage, 4,* 97–104.

Galaburda, A. M., & Pandya, D. N. (1983). The intrinsic architectonic and connectional organization of the superior temporal region of the rhesus monkey. *Journal of Comparative Neurology, 221,* 169–184.

Giard, M. H., & Peronnet, F. (1999). Auditory-visual integration during multimodal object recognition in humans: A behavioral and electrophysiological study. *Journal of Cognitive Neuroscience, 11,* 473–490.

Gibson, J. J. (1966). *The senses considered as perceptual systems.* Boston: Houghton Mifflin.

Gibson, J. J. (1979). *The ecological approach to visual perception.* Boston: Houghton Mifflin.

Grant, K. W., & Seitz, P. F. (2000). The use of visible speech cues for improving auditory detection of spoken sentences. *Journal of the Acoustical Society of America, 108,* 1197–1208.

Grant, K. W., & Walden, B. E. (1996). Evaluating the articulation index for auditory-visual consonant recognition. *Journal of the Acoustical Society of America, 100,* 2415–2424.

Green, K. P. (1998). The use of auditory and visual information during phonetic processing: Implications for theories of speech perception. In R. Campbell, B. Dodd, & D. Burnham (Eds.), *Hearing by eye: Part II. Advances in the psychology of speechreading and auditory-visual speech* (pp. 3–25). East Sussex, England: Psychology Press.

Green, K. P., & Kuhl, P. K. (1989). The role of visual information in the processing of place and manner features in speech perception. *Perception & Psychophysics, 45,* 34–42.

Green, K. P., Kuhl, P. K., Meltzoff, A. N., & Stevens, E. B. (1991). Integrating speech information across talkers, gender, and sensory modality: Female faces and male voices in the McGurk effect. *Perception & Psychophysics, 50,* 524–536.

Green, K. P., & Miller, J. L. (1985). On the role of visual rate information in phonetic perception. *Perception & Psychophysics, 38,* 269–276.

Green, K. P., & Norrix, L. W. (1997). Acoustic cues to place of articulation and the McGurk effect: The role of release bursts, aspiration, and formant transitions. *Journal of Speech, Language and Hearing Research, 40,* 646–665.

Green, K. P., & Norrix, L. W. (2001). Perception of /r/ and /l/ in a stop cluster: Evidence of cross-modal context effects. *Journal of Experimental Psychology: Human Perception and Performance, 27,* 166–177.

Gray, C. M. (1999). The temporal correlation hypothesis of visual feature integration: Still alive and well. *Neuron, 24,* 31–47.

Grill-Spector, K., Kourtzi, Z., & Kanwisher, N. (2001). The lateral occipital complex and its role in object recognition. *Vision Research, 41,* 1409–1422.

Hackett, T. A., Stepniewska, I., & Kaas, J. H. (1998a). Subdivisions of auditory cortex and ipsilateral cortical connections of the parabelt auditory cortex in macaque monkeys. *Journal of Comparative Neurology, 394,* 475–495.

Hackett, T. A., Stepniewska, I., & Kaas, J. H. (1998b). Thalamocortical connections of the parabelt auditory cortex in macaque monkeys. *Journal of Comparative Neurology, 400,* 271–286.

Halgren, E., Dale, A. M., Sereno, M. I., Tootell, R. B., Marinkovic, K., & Rosen, B. R. (1999). Location of human face-selective cortex with respect to retinotopic areas. *Human Brain Mapping, 7,* 29–37.

Hashikawa, T., Molinari, M., Rausell, E., & Jones, E. G. (1995). Patchy and laminar terminations of medial geniculate axons in monkey auditory cortex. *Journal of Comparative Neurology, 362,* 195–208.

Howard, M. A., Volkov, I. O., Mirsky, R., Garell, P. C., Noh, M. D., Granner, M., et al. (2000). Auditory cortex on the human posterior superior temporal gyrus. *Journal of Comparative Neurology, 416,* 79–92.

Huckins, S. C., Turner, C. W., Doherty, K. A., Fonte, M. M., & Szeverenyi, N. M. (1998). Functional magnetic resonance imaging measures of blood flow patterns in the human auditory cortex in response to sound. *Journal of Speech, Language and Hearing Research, 41,* 538–548.

Imig, T. J., Ruggero, M. A., Kitzes, L. M., Javel, E., & Brugge, J. F. (1977). Organization of auditory cortex in the owl monkey (*Aotus trivirgatus*). *Journal of Comparative Neurology, 171,* 111–128.

Jiang, J., Alwan, A., Keating, P., Auer, E. T., & Bernstein, L. E. (2002). On the relationship between face movements, tongue movements, and speech acoustics. *EURASIP Journal on Applied Signal Processing: Special issue on Joint Audio-Visual Speech Processing, 2002,* 1174–1188.

Jones, E. G., & Powell, T. P. S. (1970). An anatomical study of converging sensory pathways within the cerebral cortex of the monkey. *Brain, 93,* 793–820.

Kaas, J. H. (1999). The transformation of association cortex into sensory cortex. *Brain Research Bulletin, 50,* 425.

Kaas, J. H., & Hackett, T. A. (2000). Subdivisions of auditory cortex and processing streams in primates. *Proceedings of the National Academy of Sciences, USA, 97,* 11793–11799.

Kanwisher, N. (2000). Domain specificity in face perception. *Nature Neuroscience, 3,* 759–763.

Kishon-Rabin, L., Boothroyd, A., & Hanin, L. (1996). Speechreading enhancement: A comparison of spatial-tactile display of voice fundamental frequency (F0) with auditory F0. *Journal of the Acoustical Society of America, 100,* 593–602.

Klatt, D. (1979). Speech perception: A model of acoustic-phonetic analysis and lexical access. *Journal of Phonetics, 7,* 279–312.

Krolak-Salmon, P., Henaff, M. A., Tallon-Baudry, C., Yvert, B., Fischer, C., Vighetto, A., et al. (2001). How fast can the human lateral geniculate nucleus and visual striate cortex see? *Society of Neuroscience Abstracts, 27,* 913.

Kuhl, P. K., & Meltzoff, A. N. (1988). Speech as an intermodal object of perception. In A. Yonas (Ed.), *Perceptual development in infancy. The Minnesota Symposia on Child Psychology, 20,* 235–266. Hillsdale, NJ: Erlbaum.

Lauter, J. L., Herscovitch, P., Formby, C., & Raichle, M. E. (1985). Tonotopic organization in human auditory cortex revealed by positron emission tomography. *Hearing Research, 20,* 199–205.

Liberman, A. M., & Mattingly, I. G. (1985). The motor theory of speech perception revised. *Cognition, 21,* 1–36.

Liberman, A. M., & Whalen, D. H. (2000). On the relation of speech to language. *Trends in Cognitive Sciences, 4,* 187–196.

Liégeois-Chauvel, C., Musolino, A., Badier, J. M., Marquis, P., & Chauvel, P. (1994). Evoked potentials recorded from the auditory cortex in man: Evaluation and topography of the middle latency components. *Electroencephalography and Clinical Neurophysiology, 92,* 204–214.

Ludman, C. N., Summerfield, A. Q., Hall, D., Elliott, M., Foster, J., Hykin, J. L., et al. (2000). Lip-reading ability and patterns of cortical activation studied using fMRI. *British Journal of Audiology, 34,* 225–230.

Luethke, L. E., Krubitzer, L. A., & Kaas, J. H. (1989). Connections of primary auditory cortex in the New World monkey, *Saguinus. Journal of Comparative Neurology, 285,* 487–513.

MacLeod, A., & Summerfield, Q. (1987). Quantifying the contribution of vision to speech perception in noise. *British Journal of Audiology, 21,* 131–141.

MacSweeney, M., Calvert, G. A., Campbell, R., McGuire, P. K., David, A. S., Williams, S. C., et al. (2002). Speechreading circuits in people born deaf. *Neuropsychologia, 40,* 801–807.

MacSweeney, M., Campbell, R., Calvert, G. A., McGuire, P. K., David, A. S., Suckling, J., et al. (2001). Dispersed activation in the left temporal cortex for speech-reading in congenitally deaf people. *Proceedings of the Royal Society of London. Series B, Biological Sciences, 268,* 451–457.

Massaro, D. W. (1987). *Speech perception by ear and eye: A paradigm for psychological inquiry.* Hillsdale, NJ: Erlbaum.

Massaro, D. W. (1998). *Perceiving talking faces: From speech perception to a behavioral principle.* Cambridge, MA: MIT Press.

Massaro, D. W. (1999). Speechreading: Illusion or window into pattern recognition? *Trends in Cognitive Sciences, 3,* 310–317.

Massaro, D. W., Cohen, M. M., & Smeele, P. M. (1996). Perception of asynchronous and conflicting visual and auditory speech. *Journal of the Acoustical Society of America, 100,* 1777–1786.

Mattys, S. L., Bernstein, L. E., & Auer, E. T., Jr. (2002). Stimulus-based lexical distinctiveness as a general word-recognition mechanism. *Perception & Psychophysics, 64,* 667–679.

McGurk, H., & MacDonald, J. (1976). Hearing lips and seeing voices. *Nature, 264,* 746–748.

Meredith, M. A., Nemitz, J. W., & Stein, B. E. (1987). Determinants of multisensory integration in superior colliculus neurons. I. Temporal factors. *Journal of Neuroscience, 7,* 3215–3229.

Merzenich, M. M., & Brugge, J. F. (1973). Representation of the cochlear partition of the superior temporal plane of the macaque monkey. *Brain Research, 50,* 275–296.

Mesulam, M. M., (1994). Neurocognitive networks and selectively distributed processing. *Revue Neurologique, 150,* 564–569.

Mesulam, M. M. (1998). From sensation to cognition. *Brain, 121*(Pt. 6), 1013–1052.

Miltner, W. H., Braun, C., Arnold, M., Witte, H., & Taub, E. (1999). Coherence of gamma-band EEG activity as a basis for associative learning. *Nature, 397,* 434–436.

Morel, A., Garraghty, P. E., & Kaas, J. H. (1993). Tonotopic organization, architectonic fields, and connections of auditory cortex in macaque monkeys. *Journal of Comparative Neurology, 335,* 437–459.

Morel, A., & Kaas, J. H. (1992). Subdivisions and connections of auditory cortex in owl monkeys. *Journal of Comparative Neurology, 318,* 27–63.

Moutoussis, K., & Zeki, S. (1997). Functional segregation and temporal hierarchy of the visual perceptive system. *Proceedings of the Royal Society of London. B, 267,* 1404–1407.

Munhall, K. G., Gribble, P., Sacco, L., & Ward, M. (1996). Temporal constraints on the McGurk effect. *Perception & Psychophysics, 58,* 351–362.

Naatanen, R. (2001). The perception of speech sounds by the human brain as reflected by the mismatch negativity (MMN) and its magnetic equivalent (MMNm). *Psychophysiology, 38,* 1–21.

Nearey, T. M. (1997). Speech perception as pattern recognition. *Journal of the Acoustical Society of America, 101,* 3241–3254.

Nobre, A. C., Allison, T., & McCarthy, G. (1994). Word recognition in the human inferior temporal lobe. *Nature, 372,* 260–263.

Olson, I. R., Gatenby, J. C., & Gore, J. C. (2002). A comparison of bound and unbound audio-visual information processing the human cerebral cortex. *Cognitive Brain Research, 14,* 129–138.

Pandya, D. N., & Rosene, D. L. (1993). Laminar termination patterns of thalamic, callosal, and association afferents in the primary auditory area of the rhesus monkey. *Experimental Neurology, 119,* 220–234.

Pandya, D. N., & Sanides, F. (1973). Architectonic parcellation of the temporal operculum in rhesus monkey and its projection pattern. *Zeitschrift für Anatomiische Entwicklungsgeschichte, 139,* 127–161.

Pantev, C., Hoke, M., Lehnertz, K., Lutkenhoner, B., Anogianakis, G., & Wittkowski, W. (1988). Tonotopic organization of the human auditory cortex revealed by transient auditory evoked magnetic fields. *Electroencephalography and Clinical Neurophysiology, 69,* 160–170.

Picton, T. W., Alain, C., Otten, L., Ritter, W., & Achim, A. (2000). Mismatch negativity: Different water in the same river. *Audiology and Neurootology, 5,* 111–139.

Ponton, C. W., Bernstein, L. E., Auer, E. T., & Wagner, M. (2003). Temporal dynamics of cortical activation in audio-visual speech processing. *Meeting of the Cognitive Neuroscience Society.*

Price, C. J., Wise, R. J., Warburton, E. A., Moore, C. J., Howard, D., Patterson, K., et al.(1996). Hearing and saying: The functional neuro-anatomy of auditory word processing. *Brain, 119* (Pt. 3), 919–931.

Puce, A., Allison, T., Asgari, M., Gore, J. C., & McCarthy, G. (1996). Differential sensitivity of human visual cortex to faces, letterstrings, and textures: A functional magnetic resonance imaging study. *Journal of Neuroscience, 16,* 5205–5215.

Puce, A., Allison, T., Bentin, S., Gore, J. C., & McCarthy, G. (1998). Temporal cortex activation in humans viewing eye and mouth movements. *Journal of Neuroscience, 18,* 2188–2199.

Rauschecker, J. P., Tian, B., & Hauser, M. (1995). Processing of complex sounds in the macaque nonprimary auditory cortex. *Science, 268,* 111–114.

Rauschecker, J. P., Tian, B., Pons, T., & Mishkin, M. (1997). Serial and parallel processing in rhesus monkey auditory cortex. *Journal of Comparative Neurology, 382,* 89–103.

Recanzone, G. H. (1998). Rapidly induced auditory plasticity: The ventriloquism aftereffect. *Proceedings of the National Academy of Sciences, USA, 95,* 869–875.

Recanzone, G. H., Schreiner, C. E., Sutter, M. L., Beitel, R. E., & Merzenich, M. M. (1999). Functional organization of spectral receptive fields in the primary auditory cortex of the owl monkey. *Journal of Comparative Neurology, 415,* 460–481.

Rezak, M., & Benevento, L. A. (1979). A comparison of the organization of the projections of the dorsal lateral geniculate nucleus, the inferior pulvinar and adjacent lateral pulvinar to primary visual cortex (area 17) in the macaque monkey. *Brain Research, 167,* 19–40.

Rizzolatti, G., & Arbib, M. A. (1998). Language within our grasp. *Trends in Neuroscience, 21,* 188–194.

Rosen, S., Scott, S. K., Lang, H., & Wise, R. J. S. (2001). Cortical regions associated with intelligible speech. *Meeting of the Eighth Annual Meeting of the Cognitive Neuroscience Society* (pp. 00–00).

Rosenblum, L. D., & Gordon, M. S. (2001). The generality of specificity: Some lessons from audiovisual speech. *Behavioural Brain Science, 24,* 239–240.

Rosenblum, L. D., & Saldana, H. M. (1996). An audiovisual test of kinematic primitives for visual speech perception. *Journal of Experimental Psychology: Human Perception and Performance, 22,* 318–331.

Saldana, H. M., & Rosenblum, L. D. (1994). Selective adaptation in speech perception using a compelling audiovisual adaptor. *Journal of the Acoustical Society of America, 95,* 3658–3661.

Saron, C. D., Molholm, S., Ritter, W., Murray, M. M., Schroeder, C. E., & Foxe, J. J. (2001). Possible auditory activation of visual cortex in a simple reaction time task: A high density ERP study. *Society for Neuroscience Abstracts, 27,* 1795.

Schwartz, J.-L., Robert-Ribes, J., & Escudier, P. (1998). Ten years after Summerfield: A taxonomy of models for audio-visual fusion in speech perception. In R. Campbell, B. Dodd, & D. Burnham (Eds.), *Hearing by eye: Part II. The psychology of speechreading and auditory-visual speech* (pp. 85–108). East Sussex, England: Psychology Press.

Scott, S. K., Blank, C. C., Rosen, S., & Wise, R. J. (2000). Identification of a pathway for intelligible speech in the left temporal lobe. *Brain, 123*(Pt. 12), 2400–2406.

Sekiyama, K. (1997). Cultural and linguistic factors in audio-visual speech processing: The McGurk effect in Chinese subjects. *Perception & Psychophysics, 59,* 73–80.

Sekiyama, K., & Sugita, Y. (in press). Auditory-visual speech perception examined by functional MRI and reaction time.

Sekiyama, K., & Tohkura, Y. (1991). McGurk effect in non-English listeners: Few visual effects for Japanese subjects hearing Japanese syllables of high auditory intelligibility. *Journal of the Acoustical Society of America, 90,* 1797–1805.

Seltzer, B., & Pandya, D. N. (1978). Afferent cortical connections and architectonics of the superior temporal sulcus and surrounding cortex in the rhesus monkey. *Brain Research, 149,* 1–24.

Seltzer, B., & Pandya, D. N. (1994). Parietal, temporal, and occipital projections to cortex of the superior temporal sulcus in the rhesus monkey: A retrograde tracer study. *Journal of Comparative Neurology, 343,* 445–463.

Shams, L., Kamitani, Y., Thompson, S., & Shimojo, S. (2001). Sound alters visual evoked potentials in humans. *NeuroReport, 12,* 3849–3852.

Shigeno, S. (2002). Anchoring effects in audiovisual speech perception. *Journal of the Acoustical Society of America, 111,* 2853–2861.

Singer, W. (1998). Consciousness and the structure of neuronal representations. *Philosophical Transactions of the Royal Society of London. Series B, Biological Science, 353,* 1829–1840.

Stein, B. E., London, N., Wilkinson, L. K., & Price, D. D. (1996). Enhancement of perceived visual intensity by auditory stimuli: A psychophysical analysis. *Journal of Cognitive Neuroscience, 8,* 497–506.

Stein, B. E., & Meredith, M. A. (1993). *The merging of the senses.* Cambridge, MA: MIT Press.

Steinschneider, M., Volkov, I. O., Noh, M. D., Garell, P. C., & Howard, M. A., III (1999). Temporal encoding of the voice onset time phonetic parameter by field potentials recorded directly from human auditory cortex. *Journal of Neurophysiology, 82,* 2346–2357.

Stevens, K. N. (1998). *Acoustic phonetics.* Cambridge, MA: MIT Press.

Stevens, K. N. (2002). Toward a model for lexical access based on acoustic landmarks and distinctive features. *Journal of the Acoustical Society of America, 111,* 1872–1891.

Stoffregen, T. A., & Bardy, B. G. (2001). On specification and the senses. *Behavioural Brain Science, 24,* 195–213.

Sumby, W. H., & Pollack, I. (1954). Visual contribution to speech intelligibility in noise. *Journal of the Acoustical Society of America, 26,* 212–215.

Summerfield, Q. (1987). Some preliminaries to a comprehensive account of audio-visual speech perception. In B. Dodd & R. Campbell (Eds.), *Hearing by eye: The psychology of lip-reading* (pp. 3–52). London: Erlbaum.

Sundara, M., Namasivayam, A. K., & Chen, R. (2001). Observation-execution matching system for speech: A magnetic stimulation study. *NeuroReport, 12,* 1341–1344.

Surguladze, S. A., Calvert, G. A., Brammer, M. J., Campbell, R., Bullmore, E. T., Giampietro, V., et al. (2001). Audio-visual speech perception in schizophrenia: An fMRI study. *Psychiatry Research: Neuroimaging, 106,* 1–14.

Talairach, J., & Tournoux, P. (1988). *Co-planar stereotaxic atlas of the human brain.* New York: Thieme.

Teder-Salejarvi, W. A., McDonald, J. J., Di Russo, F., & Hillyard, S. A. (2002). An analysis of audio-visual cross-modal integration by means of event-related potential (ERP) recordings. *Brain Research: Cognitive Brain Research, 14,* 106–114.

Tong, F., Nakayama, K., Moscovitch, M., Weinrib, O., & Kanwisher, N. (2000). Response properties of the human fusiform face area. *Cognitive Neuropsychology, 17,* 257–279.

Treisman, A. (1996). The binding problem. *Current Opinion in Neurobiology, 6,* 171–178.

Varela, F., Lachaux, J. P., Rodriguez, E., & Martinerie, J. (2001). The brainweb: Phase synchronization and large-scale integration. *Nature Review of Neuroscience, 2,* 229–239.

von der Malsburg, C. (1995). Binding in models of perception and brain function. *Current Opinion in Neurobiology, 5,* 520–526.

von der Malsburg, C. (1999). The what and why of binding: The modeler's perspective. *Neuron, 24,* 95–104.

Walker, S., Bruce, V., & O'Malley, C. (1995). Facial identity and facial speech processing: Familiar faces and voices in the McGurk effect. *Perception & Psychophysics, 57,* 1124–1133.

Wang, X., Merzenich, M. M., Beitel, R., & Schreiner, C. E. (1995). Representation of a species-specific vocalization in the primary auditory cortex of the common marmoset: Temporal and spectral characteristics. *Journal of Neurophysiology, 74,* 2685–2706.

Watson, J. D., Myers, R., Frackowiak, R. S., Hajnal, J. V., Woods, R. P., Mazziotta, J. C., et al. (1993). Area V5 of the human brain: Evidence from a combined study using positron emission tomography and magnetic resonance imaging. *Cerebral Cortex, 3,* 79–94.

Wessinger, C. M., Buonocore, M. H., Kussmaul, C. L., & Mangun, R. (1997). Tonotopy in human auditory cortex examined with functional magnetic resonance imaging. *Human Brain Mapping, 5,* 18–25.

Wise, R. J., Scott, S. K., Blank, S. C., Mummery, C. J., Murphy, K., & Warburton, E. A. (2001). Separate neural subsystems within "Wernicke's area." *Brain, 124,* 83–95.

Yehia, H., Kuratate, T., & Vatikiotis-Bateson, E. (1999). Using speech acoustics to drive facial motion. *Proceedings of ICPhS 1999.*

Yehia, H., Rubin, P., & Vatikiotis-Bateson, E. (1998). Quantitative association of vocal-tract and facial behavior. *Speech and Communication, 26,* 23–43.

Yvert, B., Crouzeix, A., Bertrand, O., Seither-Preisler, A., & Pantev, C. (2001). Multiple supratemporal sources of magnetic and electric auditory evoked middle latency components in humans. *Cerebral Cortex, 11,* 411–423.

Zatorre, R. J., Meyer, E., Gjedde, A., & Evans, A. C. (1996). PET studies of phonetic processing of speech: Review, replication, and reanalysis. *Cerebral Cortex, 6,* 21–30.

Zeki, S. (2001). Localization and globalization in conscious vision. *Annual Review of Neuroscience, 24,* 57–86.

14 Multisensory Animal Communication

SARAH R. PARTAN

Introduction

Animals communicate by emitting and exchanging a wide variety of signals. Many of these signals are unisensory, in that they are received by one sensory system in the perceiving animal. These unisensory signals can be highly effective, as the glorious visual display of the male peacock's tail feathers illustrates. However, in many cases animals do more than just emit a signal in one channel: they simultaneously emit signals in multiple channels. For example, male red jungle fowl display by spreading their colorful wing feathers and simultaneously running a foot through the feathers, creating a staccato auditory signal that accompanies the visual display (Fig. 14.1; Kruijt, 1962). This type of display can be called a *multisensory signal*, because information travels through multiple sensory channels. Since sensory systems are characteristics of perceivers, we can more formally define multisensory signals as signals that can be received simultaneously via more than one sensory system of a perceiver.

Multisensory signals are very common in natural animal behavior. Like unisensory signals, multisensory signals are used to convey various messages in a variety of situations. An animal's choice of signal channel depends on both the biotic and the abiotic environment in which it lives. Mole rats, for example, live underground, so in addition to tactile and olfactory signals, they make copious use of vibratory signals that capitalize on their subterranean environment. By contrast, most birds use visual and acoustic signals that travel well through air. Marler (1959) and Endler (1992) list qualities of each sensory channel independently that make them well-suited for use in particular environments, and Rosenthal and Ryan (2000) have compared the visual and the acoustic modalities in particular. In some cases one sensory system is used in combination with another more frequently than the reverse. In penguins, for example, vocalizations are always associated with particular postures, but not all postures are associated with vocalizations (Jouventin, 1982).

The immediate biotic environment influences the choice of channel in a number of ways. A relatively quiet channel with the fewest competitors is best for effective communication. For example, many sympatric species share "acoustic space" by calling either at a different frequency (pitch) or at a different time of day than their neighbors. Recent evidence suggests that chimpanzees (*Pan troglodytes*) may be able to choose which channel to use (vocal or visual) depending on the attentional state of their audience (i.e., whether or not the audience can see them; Hostetter, Cantero, & Hopkins, 2001). Other influences of receivers on signaler behavior have been discussed by Guilford and Dawkins (1991) and by Rowe (1999).

If unisensory communication signals are effective, why add sensory channels and emit multisensory signals? In theory, if components are redundant (having the same meaning), the message has a higher chance of successful transmission despite a noisy communication channel; this benefit is often referred to as insurance (Rand & Williams, 1970; Wilson, 1975) or error reduction (Wiley, 1983). If components are nonredundant (having different meanings), the display may carry additional information per unit time (e.g., Johnstone, 1995), or its meaning may be modified by the co-occurrence of the multiple channels (Hughes, 1996; Marler, 1967). In practice, what do multiple channels add to the communication event? In this chapter I discuss how multisensory signals enhance animal communication with examples from animals in a wide variety of taxa. Although I do not directly address multicomponent single-channel signals here, much of the following discussion is relevant to the literature on multiple visual signals (e.g., Zucker, 1994; Zuk, Ligon, & Thornhill, 1992) and on complex pheromone blends (e.g., Borden, Chong, & Lindgren, 1990; Johnston, Chiang, & Tung, 1994).

I first provide a brief overview of descriptive observational work documenting multisensory communication in animals. Because the literature on multisensory communication is highly varied in respect to species, methods, and outcomes, I present a framework for classifying multisensory signals in order to help organize types of signals and outcomes that occur in nature (see Partan & Marler, 1999). Most of this chapter is devoted

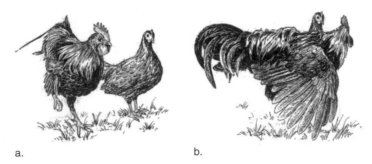

a.   b.

FIGURE 14.1   Courtship display of male Burmese red jungle fowl (after Kruijt, 1962). (*A*) Male circles around female. (*B*) Male stretches out his wing and runs his raised foot through the primary feathers of the wing, creating a staccato sound that accompanies the visual display. (Adapted with permission from Kruijt, J. P. [1962]. On the evolutionary derivation of wing display in Burmese red jungle fowl and other gallinaceous birds. *Symposia of the Zoological Society of London, 8*, 25–35. © 1962 The Zoological Society of London.)

to developing this classification system in detail. The classification is based on the relationship among the signal components. To assess this relationship, I rely on experimental studies that examine the behavioral consequences of signaling in one channel versus signaling in multiple channels and consider what, if any, additional information is provided by the additional channels. To understand how multisensory signals are used in communication we must measure the responses of animals to both the unisensory and multisensory conditions.

Multisensory processes are important for behavior at many levels and in myriad realms. The chapter concludes with a brief review of many other ways, in addition to communication, that multisensory processes play a role in animal lives.

Descriptive observations of multisensory communication

Early ethologists observed and described multisensory signals in a variety of animals. Tinbergen (1959) described in detail the visual and vocal behaviors of gulls (family Laridae), and Lehrman (1965) described the visual bow and vocal "coo" of the ring dove (*Streptopelia risoria*) during the intricate interactions between the sexes during courtship. Von Trumler (1959) described and illustrated vocalizations and associated facial movements of equids. Beach (1951) reviewed the sensory channels used during reproductive behavior in many species and concluded that some species rely largely on one sensory channel during courtship (most often either the chemical or the visual channel), whereas other species, including many mammals, require multisensory stimulation (with various combinations of chemical, visual, auditory, and tactile stimuli).

Cichlid fish (*Cichlasoma centrarchus*) produce sounds during aggressive interactions; visual correlates of the

sounds have been documented by Schwarz (1974). Myrberg (1980) reviewed the use of various sensory systems for recognition in fishes, and pointed out that visual and chemical senses, including olfaction and gustation, have complex interdependencies in mediating fish behavior.

In many cases a very specific multisensory signal has been described, such as the "jump-yip" display of the black-tailed prairie dog (*Cynomys ludovicianus;* Smith, Smith, DeVilla, & Oppenheimer, 1976), involving a sudden thrust of the front of the body into the air accompanied by a distinctive vocalization, or the "tail-flagging" of California ground squirrels (*Spermophilus beecheyi;* Hennessy, Owings, Rowe, Coss, & Leger, 1981), in which the ground squirrels wave their tails in a circular motion while emitting a variety of vocalizations. The female African robin chat (*Cossypha heuglini*) intricately coordinates her wing beats with her vocalizations while singing (Todt, Hultsch, & Duvall, 1981). Male courtship in the Count Raggi Bird-of-Paradise (*Paradisaea raggiana*) includes a high-intensity display with vigorous wing beating and vocalizing (Fig. 14.2; Frith, 1982).

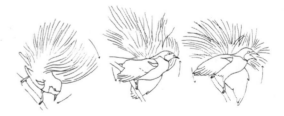

FIGURE 14.2   High-intensity display by male Bird-of-Paradise (after Frith, 1982). Three panels depict the wing-beating phase of the display, from a series of stills drawn from film. The wing-beat phase includes three to six vigorous wing beats, accompanied by loud, repeated *wok-wok-wok* calls. (Reproduced with permission from Frith, C. B. [1982]. Displays of Count Raggi's Bird-of-Paradise *Paradisaea raggiana* and congeneric species. *Emu, 81*, 193–201. © 1982 *Birds of Australia*.)

Wiley (1973) describes the remarkable audiovisual strut display of the male sage grouse (*Centrocercus urophasianus*). This display combines a vivid visual stimulus of brightly contrasting neck plumage revealing the esophageal sac rising and falling with several acoustic stimuli, including a loud explosion of air from the compressed and released sac.

Other multisensory signals that have been described include composite visual and olfactory signals in scent marking by reptiles (Alberts, 1989; Duvall, Graves, & Carpenter, 1987), ungulates (Estes, 1969), canids (Bekoff, 1979), and primates (Jolly, 1966); composite visual and vocal signals in primate communication (e.g., van Hooff, 1962; Marler, 1965; Green, 1975; Partan, 2002a); and composite visual, vocal, and olfactory signals in the sexual behavior of primates (Bielert, 1982; Goldfoot, 1982). Holldobler (1999) has reviewed multisensory communication in ants, including chemical, vibratory, and tactile signals, and Uetz and Roberts (2002) have reviewed multisensory communication in spiders, primarily that involving the visual and vibratory channels.

The classification of multisensory signals

It is apparent from the studies cited in the preceding paragraphs that animals frequently use multisensory signals. In an effort to organize and classify these signals, I will examine in more detail a number of experimental studies that directly address how the combination of channels influences the communication process.

One semantic issue that arises when classifying signals is what exactly to consider a signal. Researchers studying communication have often distinguished between signals and cues. Typically differentiated, *signals* are used specifically for communication, such as the song of a songbird or the eyebrow flash of a baboon. In contrast, simple *cues* are provided by the mere presence of an animal, such as visual or olfactory traits emanating from the body, and are not designed specifically for communication (assuming, although this is controversial, that we can determine for what purpose a trait evolved). This distinction becomes problematic when one considers the inherently multisensory nature of many communication signals. For example, crickets communicate by stridulating, which involves rubbing the legs together to produce a sound. But as a consequence, stridulation also produces a visual image of moving legs. Is the visual cue part of the signal itself? For the purpose of classification of signal types, I consider any detectable behavior of an individual to be part of the communication signal, because these behaviors are all accessible to the perceiver and have the potential to influence their behavior.

A related question is whether to consider the composite multisensory signal to be the signal unit, or whether the component parts should be considered signals themselves. This may depend on whether or not the composite signal is naturally divisible into its component parts (Marler, 1961), how consistently the components are found together, and whether or not they carry the same message (Smith, 1977). Leger (1993) discussed whether concurrent behaviors produced by the signaler should be considered composite signals or context. He suggested that if two signals occur independently, then they can each be considered contextual to the other, whereas if they are not independent, then they are a composite signal. Here I consider any signaler behaviors that co-occur in time to be components of the composite or multichannel signal, regardless of whether or not they can also occur independently. This stance is consistent with the above definition of signal, because in the multisensory case, the perceiver would perceive all components at once. Further discussion of context can be found in papers collected in a special issue of *Journal of Comparative Psychology* (see Greene, Owings, Hart, & Klimley, 2002; Partan & Marler, 2002).

Traditionally, animal communication signals are classified by the sensory channel involved (visual, auditory, chemical, etc.). However, this classification method is impractical for a discussion of multisensory signals. Another method classifies signals by the presumed function or message of the signal (aggression, affiliation, mating, etc.), but this method does not tell us whether or not the signal is multisensory. I organize multisensory signals by the *relationship* among the components. The major division is between signals with redundant or nonredundant components, following Partan and Marler (1999; Fig. 14.3). Theoretical support for this distinction can be found in work such as that by Johnstone (1996), discussed later in the final section of this chapter on function.

To determine whether a multisensory signal contains redundant or nonredundant components, it is necessary to assess the receiver's response to each signal component on its own (unisensory condition) as well as the response to the composite (multisensory) signal. The responses can then be compared to determine whether the responses to each component are equivalent or whether one exceeds or influences the others. This research task can be undertaken using observational methods if the signal components naturally occur separately from the composite case. If the components do not naturally occur alone, the study must use experimental methods to tease apart the channels.

Krebs and Dawkins (1984) suggested that competition should favor the evolution of redundant signals, because

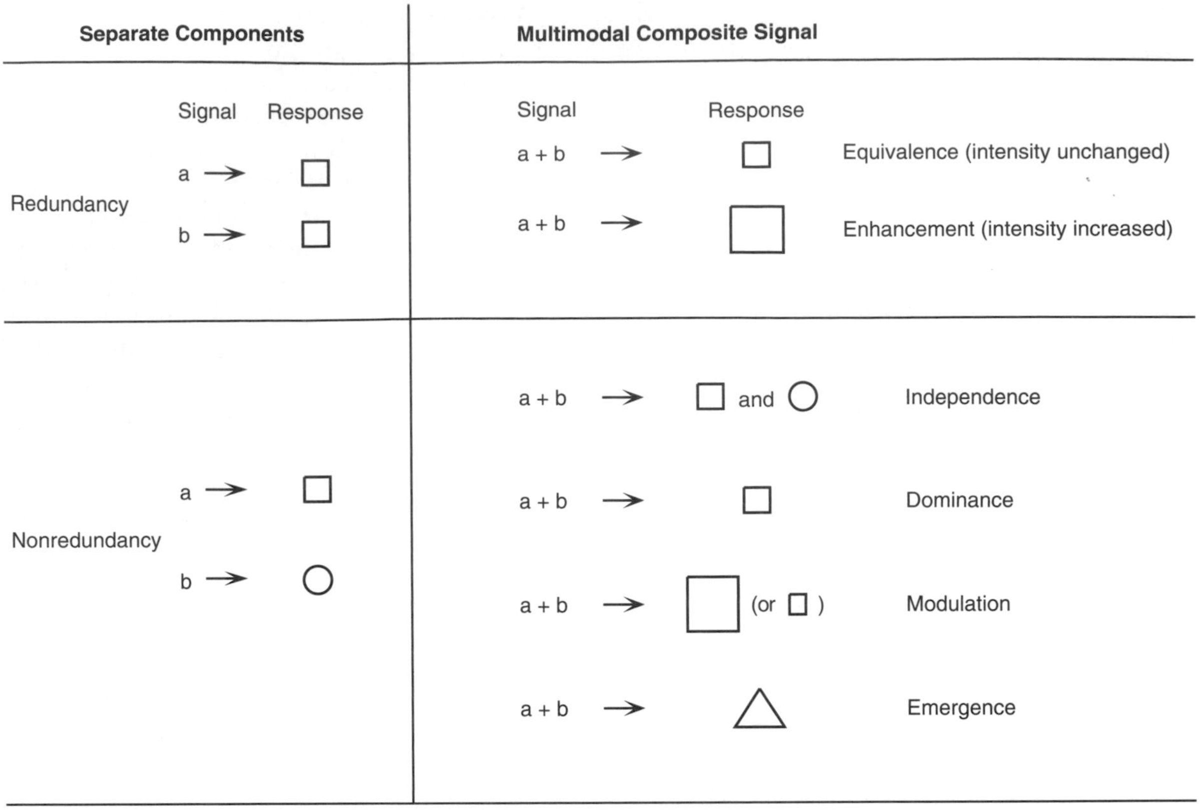

Separate Components			Multimodal Composite Signal		

	Signal	Response	Signal	Response	
Redundancy	a →	☐	a + b →	☐	Equivalence (intensity unchanged)
	b →	☐	a + b →	☐ (larger)	Enhancement (intensity increased)

			a + b →	☐ and ○	Independence
Nonredundancy	a →	☐	a + b →	☐	Dominance
	b →	○	a + b →	☐ (or ☐)	Modulation
			a + b →	△	Emergence

FIGURE 14.3   Classification of multisensory signals. Each signal is made up of components a and b. Geometric shapes symbolize responses to the signals. On the left are the responses to the components tested separately. On the right are the responses to the multisensory signal when tested as a whole. Two types of redundancy are shown in the upper half and four types of nonredundancy in the lower half. The size of the geometric shape indicates intensity of response. Different shapes indicate qualitatively different responses. (Reproduced with permission from Partan, S., & Marler, P. [1999]. Communication goes multimodal. *Science, 283*, 1272–1273. © 1999 American Association for the Advancement of Science.)

they are most effective at "advertising" one's message. Rowe (1999) reviewed receivers' influences on multi-component signals. Based on the literature on divided attention (e.g., Miller, 1982), she argued that multisensory signals (as well as multicomponent unisensory signals, such as a display with multiple visual components) should be redundant, rather than carrying multiple messages, because receivers would not be as efficient at recognizing signals if they carried different messages. Increased efficacy of signal transmission is certainly a benefit of redundant signals. However, there are also benefits to nonredundant signals, such as carrying more information per unit time, and examples of both redundant and nonredundant signals will be discussed in the next two sections.

Redundant multisensory signals

Redundant signals—signals with components that have the same meaning—are common in the animal kingdom (Krebs & Dawkins, 1984; Wilson, 1975).

Redundant signals provide the signaler with insurance that the signal will get through even in the face of biotic or abiotic noise in the channel (Rand & Williams, 1970; Wilson, 1975). For example, in noisy surroundings, human speakers can be understood more easily if they can be seen as well as heard (Sumby & Pollack, 1954). In some cases a channel that is normally relied on may become unavailable, in which case it is prudent to have a backup system. For example, wolf spiders (*Schizocosa* spp.) rely heavily on vibratory communication from the male to the female for successful courtship (Uetz & Stratton, 1982). However, if the transmission of vibrations is limited, as can happen in leaf litter habitats where the substrate is interrupted, then visual cues become important (Scheffer, Uetz, & Stratton, 1996).

Young birds in the nest rely on multisensory begging displays to elicit parental feeding. Studies of magpie nestlings (Redondo & Castro, 1992) and of reed warbler chicks (Kilner, Noble, & Davies, 1999) indicate that the various components of these displays, consisting of visually gaping beaks and characteristic postures combined with vocal begging calls, are largely redundant.

EQUIVALENCE   When multisensory signals are classified in terms of the responses they elicit from other animals, redundant signals can be subclassified into two types: those that produce responses equivalent to the response to each unisensory component, and those whose response exceeds the response to the unisensory components. These subclassifications can be considered *equivalence* and *enhancement*, respectively (see Fig. 14.3; Partan & Marler, 1999). An example of equivalence can be found in the dance communication of honeybees (*Apis mellifera*). A mechanical model honeybee constructed by Michelsen, Andersen, Storm, Kirchner, and Lindauer (1992) waggled and produced both vibratory cues and sound that together recruited other bees to a food source. The acoustic and vibratory components, tested separately, were found to carry redundant information about distance to and direction of food sources. Another example of equivalence is found in the male moth *Cycnia tenera,* which gives ultrasonic vocalizations coupled with pheromonal courtship signals (Conner, 1987). When tested separately, each component produced equivalent responses from a female moth. When tested together, there was no additive quality; rather, the response to the multisensory signal was equivalent to the responses to the unisensory components.

ENHANCEMENT   Enhanced responses to redundant multisensory signals are more common in animal systems than equivalent responses. In fact, some argue that enhanced responses are the rule. Seitz (1940) studied the aggressive responses of cichlid fish (*Astatotilapia strigigena,* now classified as *Haplochromis*) to dummy models that varied in a number of visual signal components (e.g., color, movement, size, orientation). He found that the response to the composite signal equaled the sum of the responses to each of the components. His work has been referred to as the "law of heterogeneous summation" (Lorenz, 1981), and the principle has been supported by a number of other studies. Heiligenberg (1976) replicated Seitz's finding by studying aggressive behavior in fishes (*Haplochromis burton*) using various combinations of visual characteristics (body orientation, black eye bars, orange body spots). The theory has been extended to the multisensory case, for example by Soffie and Zayan (1977), who presented domestic cattle (Friesian-Dutch heifers) with models that varied in visual appearance and movement and also were variably accompanied by audio playbacks of recorded calls. The responses of the cows to the audiovisual playbacks followed Seitz's summation law. Psychophysical studies

of signal detection in noise also support the idea of a simple sum of the two components. For example, Brown and Hopkins (1966) found that simultaneously presenting audio and visual stimuli to human subjects resulted in increased detection consistent with an additive model of sensory action.

Work by Bower (1966) has often been cited as an example of heterogeneous summation in perception in human infants. Bower presented infants with visual stimuli consisting of a circle with a cross and two black spots in the center. He presented four cases: the whole stimulus together, the circle alone, the cross alone, and the spots alone. He did find summation at very young ages (8, 10, and 12 weeks), but by 20 weeks of age the results were more complex. When infants were trained on the whole stimulus first, the whole took on *Gestalt* qualities such that the response to the whole was greater than the sum of the responses to the parts. When they were trained on the parts first, however, the response to the whole was *less* by a third than the sum of the responses to the parts. This latter result was not explained, but it seems plausible that once the infant determined that each component provided redundant information, then the situation became a case of equivalence, in which any component or the whole provided equal information. In that case, each component could have elicited the same response, so their sum would be three times as large as the response to the compound, which in fact it was.

Immelmann (1980) remarked that although multiple stimuli often facilitate one another, causing an enhanced response, in fact strict additive summation may not be the rule. He suggested the term "reciprocal stimulus enhancement" (1980, p. 39) instead. Some authors use the word *summation* without actually meaning an exact mathematical sum. For example, Aydin and Pearce (1997) used visual and audiovisual stimuli in a learning task with pigeons. They considered response summation to be *any* significant increase in response above the level of the unitary stimuli; using this definition, they found summation with the audiovisual stimuli, but not the multicomponent visual stimuli.

For consistency with the earlier works, here I consider summation to be a mathematical addition of the responses measured. The broader term *enhancement* thus covers several possible options: the response to the multisensory signal can be enhanced slightly above the level shown to the unisensory ones, it can be enhanced to the degree that it sums mathematically to the total of the unisensory inputs (summation), or it can be enhanced even further so that it is a "multiplicative" effect, above the sum of the components (Fig. 14.4; see Partan, 2002b, for further discussion of terminology). This terminology is consistent with literature in the

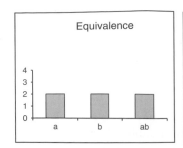 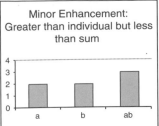 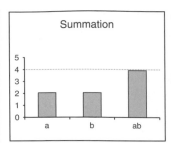 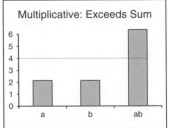

FIGURE 14.4 Graphs show idealized responses to redundant signal components a and b, and to the redundant multisensory signal ab. Equivalence of responses is shown on the left and three types of enhancement are shown on the right: minor enhancement, summation, and multiplicative enhancement (after Partan, 2002b).

neural field that considers multisensory "response enhancement" to be any significant increase in response to a multisensory stimulus above the most effective unimodal case (Meredith & Stein, 1983; Stein, Meredith, & Wallace, 1993). Although the three types of enhancement can be measured in neurons, it is harder to obtain behavioral measurements of response in natural communication systems that allow us to distinguish among these responses. Therefore I do not distinguish among the types of enhancement in the discussion that follows, instead using the term enhancement as a broad category covering all three cases.

Because redundancy can be used to correct errors of signal detection or identification, a receiver may give an enhanced response to a redundant multisensory signal due to the increased assurance about signal meaning provided by the redundancy. For example, both visual and olfactory cues from gravid female goby fishes (*Bathygobius soporator*) elicit courtship in males, but a combination of visual and olfactory stimuli elicited more courtship than did either component on its own (Tavolga, 1956). *Aphaenogaster* ants (*A. cockerelli* or *A. albisetosus*) recruit help for carrying prey items by emitting unisensory chemical signals (Holldobler, 1995, 1999; Markl & Holldobler, 1978). If the prey item is very large, the ants also stridulate, producing a substrate-borne vibratory signal. This stridulation has a small effect on recruitment when emitted alone. When the chemical and vibratory signals are emitted together, the response is enhanced.

Territory-holding male robins (*Erithacus rubecula*) were presented with stuffed models of intruding robins by Chantry and Workman (1984). Two conditions were used: silent models or models accompanied by broadcast song. The silent models were not nearly as effective at eliciting aggressive responses as were the singing models, indicating that the multisensory stimuli elicited stronger responses than the unisensory ones. Chantry and Workman (1984) suggested that the two components are redundant and that their combination allows

the birds to be more accurate in their assessment of intruders on the territory.

Enhancement with redundant stimuli was also found in a study of how visual and auditory cues elicit alarm calling in chickens (*Gallus domesticus;* Evans & Marler, 1991). Male chickens typically give more aerial alarm calls in response to raptors when in the presence of a conspecific female than when alone (Gyger, Karakashian, & Marler, 1986). Evans and Marler (1991) showed that a video image of a hen facilitated a cockerel's alarm calling just as well as the live hen did. They then separated the visual track of the hen video from the audio track. The hen's visual image alone and the hen's sounds alone each elicited the same amount of alarm calling from a cockerel. When the audio track was played together with the hen's visual image, the amount of alarm calling by the cockerel was increased above that produced in the presence of either unimodal stimulus.

Video and audio playbacks have also been conducted with aggressive interactions in black-capped chickadees (*Parus atricapillus;* Baker, Tracy, & Miyasato, 1996). Video stimuli of an aggressive bird combined with the audio track of the "gargle" vocalization elicited stronger avoidance responses in subjects than did either the video or the audio stimuli alone, providing another example of enhancement.

Nonredundant multisensory signals

Multisensory signals may be made up of components that have different meanings or, operationally, cause qualitatively different responses. These signals are considered nonredundant signals. For example, Partan (1998, 2001) studied the responses of rhesus macaques (*Macaca mulatta*) to silent and vocal expressions given by their companions in a naturalistic habitat. Two conditions were studied: silent visual displays and visual displays that included simultaneous vocalizations (Fig. 14.5; Color Plate 2). In aggressive interactions, visual threat signals (such as staring, slapping the ground,

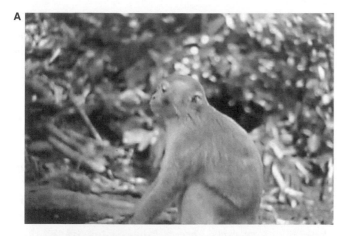

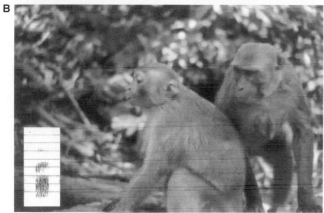

FIGURE 14.5 (A) Silent threat expression by juvenile female rhesus macaque, *Macaca mulatta* (Z63), including a *stare*, *raised eyebrows*, and *ears back*. (B) Vocal threat by same female a moment later, including identical visual components with added *bark*. Inset in *B* shows spectrogram of typical bark, with bars from 1 to 8 kHz. Images were digitized from videotape by the author. Monkeys were filmed with permission from the University of Puerto Rico and the Caribbean Primate Research Center. (See Color Plate 2.)

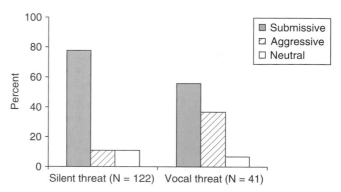

FIGURE 14.6 Responses to threats given by rhesus monkeys. Figure shows proportion of unimodal (silent) and multisensory (vocal) threats by the signaler that were followed by submissive, aggressive, or neutral behavior by the recipient. Submissive responses included *scream, grimace, gaze aversion, lean-away, retreat*; aggressive responses included: *bark, pant-threat, open-mouth, stare, head-lower, lunge,* and *chase*; neutral responses included *sit, look-at, ignore, walk-by*. Overall, silent threats were followed by submissive responses, while vocal threats were followed by aggressive as well as submissive responses (from Partan, 2001).

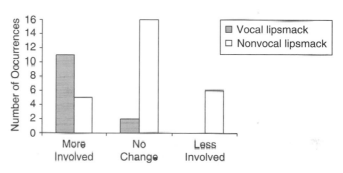

FIGURE 14.7 Outcome after affiliative signals given by rhesus monkeys. Number of vocal and nonvocal *lipsmacks* that were followed by an increase or decrease in involvement between the actor and recipient. Vocal lipsmacks included a *girney* vocalization. More involved: the two animals moved toward each other and/or began to groom; less involved: they moved away and/or stopped grooming; no change: as implied (from Partan, 2001).

lunging, and opening the mouth) elicited fear and submission from recipients, while multisensory visual-vocal threats (including the visual signal components mentioned above, plus a vocal bark) resulted in aggressive responses as often as submissive ones (Fig. 14.6). This finding suggests that the vocal component was not redundant with the visual one. In affiliative (friendly) interactions, rhesus monkeys can produce lipsmacks that may be accompanied by a quiet vocalization (called a "girn" or "girney"). When lipsmacks were accompanied by girneys, the actor and recipient more often approached each other and began to groom than if the lipsmack was given alone (Fig. 14.7). In both aggressive and affiliative contexts, therefore, the multisensory signal was followed by a different outcome than the unisensory visual-only case. (The vocal-only condition was not observed because it was not possible to eliminate the visual channel when animals were interacting naturally in the field. Audio and video playback experiments, which allow the presentation of the audio track separately as well as in combination with the video track, will provide more data on this point.)

There are four possible logical outcomes when nonredundant components are combined into a multisensory signal: independence, dominance, modulation, and emergence (see Fig. 14.3; Partan & Marler, 1999). To categorize the signals, one needs to know the responses of the animal not only to the multisensory signal, but also to both unisensory components.

INDEPENDENCE Independence occurs when the response to the multisensory signal includes the responses to each of the unisensory components (see Fig. 14.3). Each signal component is then working independently, and the multisensory signal is just a co-occurrence of the unisensory parts. In the Caribbean stew *callaloo*, the different ingredients are said to "walk with each other," each carrying its own flavor and none overwhelming the others (LeGrace Benson, Arts of Haiti Research Project, cited in Vesperi, 2001). Similarly, the components of independent multisensory signals are not independent in time, but each has its own impact on the observer.

In this situation it is possible for each signal component to carry a different *type* of information. For example, on detecting a predator, an animal might emit referential vocalizations regarding the identity of the predator while simultaneously emitting visual signals that indicate the location of the predator (such as gaze direction) or its own emotional response to the event (via affective signals from the face or body; see Marler, 1992).

An example of independent signal components is found in the visual and vocal courtship displays of male Barbary doves (*Streptopelia risoria*). Fusani, Hutchison, and Hutchison (1997) made a detailed study of the temporal patterning of the visual bow and the vocal bow-call. They suggested that the visual component of the bowing pattern conveys information on sex, while the simultaneous vocal bow-call plays a different role, signaling individual identity.

Courtship behavior of male jumping spiders, *Maevia inclemens*, may also exemplify independence. These spiders have elaborate visual courtship displays that produce vibratory concomitants (Clark, 1994; Clark & Uetz, 1993). By presenting the components separately and together, Clark (1993, personal communication, March 1995) has suggested that the vibratory component functions as a general panspecific attractant, while the visual component serves for species identification. Both functions, attraction and species recognition, are apparent in the combined bimodal signal.

In a tropical wandering spider, *Cupiennius salei*, Rovner and Barth (1981) suggested that pheromonal signal components indicate female presence; males respond with general undirected courtship behavior. Concomitant vibratory signals from females then signal female location, and males continue to court but now head in the proper direction. These pheromonal and vibratory components can be considered independent. In laboratory studies of maternal responses to infant rats and mice, olfactory cues also indicate the presence of the animal (in this case, the infant), and only in the presence of the appropriate olfactory cue will the mother respond to vocal cues as directional information for finding the pup (Smotherman, Bell, Starzec, Elias, & Zachman, 1974).

Another example of independence is found in feral horses. Rubenstein and Hack (1992) report that olfactory cues from the horses send information about identity (familiarity), while acoustic squeals carry information about status. Although the horses typically follow a sequence in which they first sniff one another and then vocalize, it can be argued that the signal components are in fact simultaneously multisensory, because olfactory cues have a longer time frame than acoustic cues, so they will still be present while the animals are vocalizing.

When the components of multicomponent signals are independent, each part may have its own target audience. For example, a juvenile rhesus monkey (*Macaca mulatta*) was observed with its mouth open in a play gape while gently wrestling with another juvenile. When it noticed the human observer, it laid its ears back in threat toward the observer while still maintaining the play gape with its peer (personal observation). Von Seibt and Wickler (1977) discussed visual signals given during vocal duetting in territorial birds. They suggested that the visual component is directed toward the mate (who can see the signaler) as appeasement so that the mate will not react to the aggressive vocal component being broadcast to a neighbor (who may not be able to see the signaler because of intervening vegetation).

DOMINANCE When the response to the multisensory signal contains only one of the responses to the components, this component can be said to be dominant relative to the other (see Fig. 14.3). For example, dogs sometimes combine visual signal components for soliciting play, such as a paw lift, with auditory aggressive components, such as a growl (Bekoff, 1972). In these cases the visual play component is dominant, taking precedence over the auditory component, and the receiver responds with play behavior.

Video and audio playbacks of conspecifics were presented to young domestic chickens to see if images of conspecifics were attractive to the chicks (Clarke & Jones, 2001). The chicks were strongly attracted to video images played alone; audio sounds played alone were not attractive. The multichannel audiovisual stimulus produced an attraction equal to the visual-only condition, suggesting that visual stimuli are dominant in this situation.

Researchers studying human communication and deception have occasionally found that one channel is dominant. For example, DePaulo, Rosenthal, Eisenstat, Rogers, and Finkelstein (1978) found support for the "video primacy effect," in which subjects rely more on visual than on audio cues when interpreting multichannel communication signals. When the channels were highly discrepant, however, subjects switched to reliance on audio cues. When outright deception was involved, Zuckerman, Amidon, Bishop, and Pomerantz (1982) found that tone of voice was more important than the face for detecting the deception. Other studies have shown variability in the importance of different features depending on the situation (Ekman, Friesen, O'Sullivan, & Scherer, 1980; Noller, 1985). Recent work on the perception of emotion indicates that the face may be more important than the voice in judging emotion (reviewed in de Gelder & Vroomen, 2000).

MODULATION Modulation occurs when one component influences the effect of another component (see Fig. 14.3). The response to the bimodal signal is of the same type as the response to only one of the components, but it is changed in degree. For example, Motley (1993) found that in some types of conversations among humans, visual facial expression cues have no meaning if viewed independently, but when combined with verbal signals the facial expressions take on meaning and add to the conversation. Modulation is distinguished from enhancement because with modulation, the unichannel components have different effects individually, whereas enhancement is a form of redundancy in which each component has the same effect individually.

Wolf spiders, *Schizocosa ocreata*, do not pay attention to vibrations made by young crickets (as potential prey) when they cannot see them (Persons & Uetz, 1996). If the spiders can see the crickets without having access to vibratory information, however, they are strongly attracted. When both visual and vibratory cues are available, the spiders spend significantly more time watching the crickets than they do in the visual-only condition (Persons & Uetz, 1996). In this example, the vibratory component has a modulatory effect on the visual component, causing an increased response.

Male ring-tailed lemurs (*Lemur catta*) display toward each other with visual tail flicks and olfactory signals from glandular secretions with which the tail is often anointed. Mertl (1976) isolated the two channels and found that the olfactory channel alone had no detectable effect on receiver behavior, but the visual channel had a great effect. When she allowed the transmission of olfactory cues along with visual information, the olfactory condition (whether both or only one individual could smell the other) influenced behaviors such as ear position that may play a role in ritualized displays of threat. She concluded that olfactory information modified the reactions to the visual information.

Visual, chemical, and acoustic factors may simultaneously affect sexual behavior of teleost fishes. Tavolga (1956) did a number of experiments with gobiid fishes (*Bathygobius soporator*), manipulating the fishes' access to information from each of the sensory channels. In some male fishes, olfactory stimuli alone were sufficient to elicit full courtship behavior; in these ("type A") animals, the addition of visual information merely helped to orient the behavior toward the recipient. In other males (types B and C), olfactory stimuli elicited little or no courtship behavior; with these fishes the addition of visual information to the olfactory signal elicited a prolonged, vigorous courtship. Tavolga (1956) also studied responses of gravid females to male courtship signals. The females did not respond to chemical cues or to visual stimuli on their own. They did, however, respond to acoustic stimuli of the male courtship grunts, and in these cases the addition of the visual stimulus helped the female orient her behavior toward the male.

Escape responses of tadpoles to chemical, visual, and tactile cues from fish predators have been studied by Stauffer and Semlitsch (1993). They tested each channel independently and in combination with all others. Neither visual nor tactile cues alone evoked much response, but chemical cues did; furthermore, the combination of tactile with chemical cues increased the response above that found to chemical cues alone. They suggested that the tactile cues provided additional information about the specific location or direction of movement of the fish. This is an example of tactile cues modulating (increasing) the response to the chemical cues.

Modulation can also occur after learning, if a signal in one channel affects the salience of other associated signals or cues. Garter snakes (*Thamnophis radix*) can distinguish between bits of fish and earthworm food items presented in the laboratory, most likely by using chemical cues (Terrick, Mumme, & Burghardt, 1995). When ingested fish bits are followed by induced illness but earthworm bits are not, the snakes immediately learn to avoid the fish. If the fish bits are presented on forceps with aposematic (warning) colors (yellow and black), the snakes have a much stronger avoidance response than if they are presented on nonaposematic forceps (green). The aversion response to the aposematic fish does not carry over to the earthworms: even if the worms are placed on yellow and black forceps, the snakes still eat them. The implication from this work is that the visual information from the aposematic color enhances the learning of other cues associated with the object (such as scent; Terrick et al., 1995).

In a study of blind mole rats using chemical cues from urine to identify intruders (Heth & Todrank, 1995), olfactory cues from scent alone had no effect until the rat had a chance to physically contact the urine; this tactile contact (presumably involving the vomeronasal organ) enhanced the avoidance of the chemical cue, and subsequent olfactory-alone trials produced strong avoidance of the urine.

An example in which the modulating component decreases the effect of the first component is found in snapping shrimp, *Alpheus heterochaelis* (Hughes, 1996). Snapping shrimp obtain size information about competitors via visual cues and sex information via chemical cues. Hughes (1996) found that the shrimp respond aggressively to visual cues alone, such as an open chela, or claw, but do not respond noticeably to chemical cues alone. When the two cues are combined and the chemical cue is from a female, the aggressive response from the males is significantly reduced.

EMERGENCE   The final possibility, emergence (see Fig. 14.3), occurs when the response to the multisensory signal is new, qualitatively different from the response to either of the unisensory components. An example of emergence is the McGurk effect in human speech (McGurk & MacDonald, 1976), in which a new phoneme is heard by subjects who observe mismatched audio and visual stimuli. Human speech, a classic example of a multisensory communication signal, is discussed elsewhere in this book (e.g., Massaro, Chap. 10).

A nonhuman example of emergence might be found in aversive responses by domestic chicks to unpalatable prey items. Toxic insects often advertise their toxicity by means of warning signals that are easy for predators (such as birds) to identify, such as bright colors or strong odors (e.g., Rothschild, Moore, & Brown, 1984). Using artificial prey items, Rowe and Guilford (1996) found that pyrazine odor alone produced no response from the chicks. Similarly, red or yellow coloration alone produced no response, but when pyrazine odor was combined with red or yellow color, a strong aversive response emerged.

Other major multisensory processes in an animal's natural behavior

In addition to their role in communication, multisensory processes are important factors for animal behavior at all four of Tinbergen's (1963) levels of biological

explanation: development, mechanism, function, and evolutionary history.

DEVELOPMENT AND LEARNING   Even before birth, multisensory stimuli from the environment have important effects on successful development, as shown in precocial birds (Lickliter & Bahrick, Chap. 40, this volume). For example, if bobwhite quail chicks (*Colinus virginianus*) are deprived of normal tactile and vestibular input during incubation, their subsequent sensory development is delayed (Lickliter & Lewkowicz, 1995). After birth, multisensory input involving visual, olfactory, and auditory cues is important for successful imprinting of the young onto the parent in species with parental care (e.g., domestic chicks; Bolhuis, 1999).

Compound stimuli have long been used in studies of associative learning in animals, beginning with, in the modern era, Pavlov's work on overshadowing and blocking (for discussion see Davis, 1974; Rosenzweig, 1983). In these early learning studies, an animal could be trained to respond to one cue (such as a light), after which a second cue (such as a tone) was added that might interfere with the response to the first cue. Various results were obtained depending on whether the compound cue was presented at the start or the end of the study. In most natural circumstances, however, we learn about associations among stimuli in the environment by using all of our senses simultaneously, so that multisensory learning is the rule from the start. In some cases one cue can even facilitate the learning of other associated cues, as described by Guilford and Dawkins (1991). For example, laboratory-reared and tutored nightingales (*Luscinia megarhynchos*) learned more songs when the tutor songs were paired with a simultaneous visual stimulus (a flashing stroboscopic light) than when the songs were not accompanied by the light (Hultsch, Schleuss, & Todt, 1999). In rats, food aversions to odor can be potentiated by pairing the odor with a strong taste (e.g., Kaye, Mackintosh, Rothschild, & Moore, 1989; von Kluge & Brush, 1992). What determines whether multiple stimuli will interfere with learning, as in blocking or overshadowing (see, e.g., Roper & Marples, 1997), or will facilitate or potentiate learning is an open question.

Theoretical differences abound in the conception of the nature of the compound stimulus in learning: whether it is simply the sum of the component parts, or whether it is has emergent properties as a unique stimulus. Kehoe and Gormezano (1980) provide a review of the main learning theorists who have debated this issue, including Hull, Weiss, and Rescorla and Wagner. They conclude that there is ample evidence to support both perspectives, such that a compound stimulus is both responded to as a unique, functionally distinct entity *and* this response is lawfully related to the reactions to the component parts. Rosenzweig (1983) also discussed this question and suggested similarly that the contradictory evidence from prior studies may be resolved if we postulate that a multisensory stimulus is processed both by modality-specific channels and by an integrated mechanism. Rowe (1999) reviewed this issue as well and suggested that most of the evidence supports the idea that the whole has emergent qualities. It appears that both situations exist in learning about compound stimuli, perhaps analogous to the multiple ways that multisensory signals are used during communication.

MECHANISM   At a physiological level, multisensory integration is an integral component of neural responses to the environment, as is discussed throughout this book (for other reviews, see Bullock, 1983; Calvert, 2001; Horridge, 1983; King & Calvert, 2001; Stein & Meredith, 1993).

At a behavioral level, mechanisms involving natural multisensory integration include attention and perception as well as communication. The simultaneous coincidence of multisensory stimuli has a profound impact on perception. For example, auditory cues presented simultaneously with visual stimuli can influence our perception of several visual characteristics: intensity, as Stein, London, Wilkinson, and Price (1996) showed using lights of differing intensities that were perceived to be brighter when paired with a low broad-band sound than when alone; motion, as Sekuler, Sekuler, and Lau (1997) showed with moving disks on a computer screen that were perceived to either bounce apart or move through one another depending on whether or not a sound was played at the point of coincidence of the two disks; and even visual illusions, as Shams, Kamitani, and Shimojo (2000) found by playing multiple sounds in concert with a single light flash, producing the illusion of multiple flashes.

In some instances, unisensory information (in one channel only) is not sufficient for a response; multisensory information is needed. Bahrick and Lickliter (2000) showed that human infants could discriminate rhythms presented bimodally (visually and audibly) but not unimodally. Cardé and Baker (1984) reported that male oriental fruit moths (*Grapholitha molesta*) need the visual presence of the female in combination with her pheromones before they will perform their most intricate courtship displays, and they need an additional tactile stimulus of a touch on the abdomen before they will copulate.

Cue-conflict work has been done with the perception of visual and magnetic environmental cues used for migration in birds. Although the picture is complex (see Able, 1993, for a review), it appears that many birds use magnetic cues and visual information from sunsets and polarized light more readily than they use the stars. These different sources of information may provide redundancy for the birds, in which case many cues can be observed and assessed for consistency.

Cross-modal perception is a specialized research area that focuses on the ability to transfer information across sensory channels (see reviews in Freides, 1974; Marks, 1978; Rosenzweig, 1983; Campbell & Snowdon, 2001). For example, in a cross-modal matching task a subject is presented with a stimulus in one sensory channel, such as vision, and subsequently asked to match it to the same stimulus presented in a second channel, such as touch. In addition to adult humans, infants (reviewed in Lewkowicz, 2000; Lewkowicz & Lickliter, 1994) and a variety of other species can successfully match items across channels (apes: Davenport, Rogers, & Russell, 1973; monkeys: Cowey & Weiskrantz, 1975; dolphins: Pack & Herman, 1995; Harley, Roitblat, & Nachtigall, 1996).

FUNCTION AND EVOLUTIONARY HISTORY   The function of multisensory processes in animal behavior has been discussed largely in terms of multiple cues used for communication. Baptista (1978) and Beletsky (1983) suggest that different song types (in male Cuban grassquits and female red-winged blackbirds, respectively) help to clarify ambiguous visual displays. Todt and Fiebelkorn (1979) listed a number of reasons for morning warblers to add a visual component to an auditory signal: to attract attention, to increase locatability, to decrease habituation to the auditory component, and to allow an estimate of distance based on the phase mismatch of simultaneously produced audio and visual components as distance from the signaler increases. Wickler (1978) also discussed the importance of the disassociation of fast-traveling visual signals from their somewhat slower acoustic counterparts; he observed that this can be a particularly troublesome issue for duetting birds who use repeated, rhythmic long-distance auditory and visual signals. For this reason, audiovisual composites may work better at close range. Guilford and Dawkins (1991) suggested that multisensory signal components may serve to enhance the "memorability" of their partner components.

Modelers studying sexual selection have discussed the function and evolution of signaling with multiple components, including multicomponent unisensory signals as well as multisensory signals. Schluter and Price (1993) and Iwasa and Pomiankowski (1994) described handicap models of sexual selection using more than one male trait for females to assess during mate choice. Handicap models assume the male trait is costly, so that a male must honestly be in good condition to be able to advertise that he is in good condition. Schluter and Price (1993) modeled female preference for both one and two male traits and found that if females have two traits from which to choose, they should rely on the trait with the greatest honesty (the best predictor of quality) × detectability (this means that if detectability is sufficiently high, it can compensate for low honesty). Iwasa and Pomiankowski (1994) suggested that multiple preferences may evolve as long as the cost of assessment is not too high.

Johnstone (1995, 1996) presented game theory models of mate choice with multiple display traits. He contrasted two main hypotheses, the "multiple-messages" hypothesis and the "redundant-signal" hypothesis (called "backup signal" in Johnstone, 1996). By multiple messages he means that different components of a display give information about different aspects of a signaler, similar to the "independence" category of nonredundant signals discussed above. His redundant-signal category (Johnstone, 1995) means that each component contains only partial information on a condition, so that a female would have a better picture if she assessed multiple components. This use of the term redundant differs from mine; I use redundant to mean that each component sends the same information. However, Johnstone (1996) defines "backup signals" as multiple components about a single aspect of the signaler's condition, which is closer to my use of the term redundant. Johnstone found that the multiple-messages hypothesis is viable (1995), and he found that multiple displays are evolutionarily stable if the costs of signaling accelerate strongly with increasing signal strength (1996).

In addition to the multiple-message and redundant-signal hypotheses, Moller, Saino, Taramino, Galeotti, and Ferrario (1998) discuss the "unreliable-signal" hypothesis, in which signal components do not carry good information about signaler condition. They collected data on barn swallow tail length (a constant morphological trait) and song rate (a flexible behavioral trait), and found that both traits predict paternity. Females can apparently change their preference for the behavioral trait depending on the quality shown in the morphological trait.

The evolutionary history of multisensory processes has been discussed by Shulter and Weatherhead (1990), who analyzed data from previous researchers on the plumage color and song traits of 56 species of wood warblers. The data support the proposal that these traits, used for sexual selection, evolved in concert rather than in opposition to each other.

Conclusion

To understand the role of multisensory communication in the lives of animals, it is necessary not only to parse the compound stimuli into their component parts and examine how they function individually, but also to assess the entire suite of simultaneous components to determine how these signals function as a whole. A classification scheme was described in this chapter (based on Partan & Marler, 1999) for categorizing these signals on the basis of the relationship between the component parts and the whole. The signals are classified into redundant and nonredundant categories, with redundant signals being either equivalent or enhanced and nonredundant ones being independent, dominant, modulatory, or emergent. The categories presented here may be useful for classifying single-channel multicomponent signals as well. All relationships observed behaviorally have also been described at the neural level when cellular responses to multisensory stimuli are assessed (e.g., Meredith & Stein, 1983; Stein & Meredith, 1990). These emerging parallels between behavior and physiology are a rich area for further research.

REFERENCES

Able, K. P. (1993). Orientation cues used by migratory birds: A review of cue-conflict experiments. *Trends in Ecology and Evolution (TREE), 8*(10), 367–371.

Alberts, A. C. (1989). Ultraviolet visual sensitivity in desert iguanas: Implications for pheromone detection. *Animal Behaviour, 38*, 129–137.

Aydin, A., & Pearce, J. M. (1997). Some determinants of response summation. *Animal Learning and Behavior, 25*, 108–121.

Bahrick, L. E., & Lickliter, R. (2000). Intersensory redundancy guides attentional selectivity and perceptual learning in infancy. *Developmental Psychology, 36*, 190–201.

Baker, M. C., Tracy, T. T., & Miyasato, L. E. (1996). Gargle vocalizations of black-capped chickadees: Test of repertoire and video stimuli. *Animal Behaviour, 52*, 1171–1175.

Baptista, L. F. (1978). Territorial, courtship and duet songs of the Cuban Grassquit (*Tiaris canora*). *Journal of Ornithology, 119,* 91–101.

Beach, F. A. (1951). Instinctive behavior: Reproductive activities. In S. S. Stevens (Ed.), *Handbook of experimental psychology* (pp. 387–434). New York: Wiley.

Bekoff, M. (1972). The development of social interaction, play, and metacommunication in mammals: An ethological perspective. *Quarterly Review of Biology, 47*(4), 412–434.

Bekoff, M. (1979). Ground scratching by male domestic dogs: A composite signal. *Journal of Mammalogy, 60*(4), 847–848.

Beletsky, L. D. (1983). Aggressive and pair-bond maintenance songs of female red-winged blackbirds (*Agelatus phoeniceus*). *Zeitschrift für Tierpsychologie, 62*(1), 47–54.

Bielert, C. (1982). Experimental examinations of baboon (*Papio ursinus*) sex stimuli. In C. T. Snowdon, C. H. Brown, &

M. R. Petersen (Eds.), *Primate communication* (pp. 373–395). Cambridge, England, Cambridge University Press.

Bolhuis, J. J. (1999). Early learning and the development of filial preferences in the chick. *Behavioural Brain Research, 98,* 245–252.

Borden, J. H., Chong, L. J., & Lindgren, B. S. (1990). Redundancy in the semiochemical message required to induce attack on lodgepole pines by the mountain pine beetle, *Dendroctonus ponderosae* Hopkins (Coleoptera: Scolytidae). *Canadian Entomologist, 122,* 769–777.

Bower, T. G. R. (1966). Heterogeneous summation in human infants. *Animal Behaviour, 14,* 395–398.

Brown, A. E., & Hopkins, H. K. (1966). Interaction of the auditory and visual sensory modalities. *Journal of the Acoustical Society of America, 41,* 1–6.

Bullock, T. H. (1983). Perspectives on the neuroethology of sensory convergences. In E. Horn (Ed.), *Multimodal convergences in sensory systems* (Vol. 28, pp. 385–395). Stuttgart: Gustav Fischer Verlag.

Calvert, G. A. (2001). Crossmodal processing in the human brain: Insights from functional neuroimaging studies. *Cerebral Cortex, 11*(12), 1110–1123.

Campbell, M. W., & Snowdon, C. T. (2001). Social knowledge: A new domain for testing cross-modal perception and the origins of language. In C. Cavé, I. Guaïtella, & S. Santi (Eds.), *Oralité et gestualité: Interactions et comportements multimodaux dans la communication* (pp. 79–82). Paris: L'Harmattan.

Cardé, R. T., & Baker, T. C, (1984). Sexual communication with pheromones. In W. J. Bell & R. T. Cardé (Eds.), *Chemical ecology of insects* (pp. 367–379). New York: Chapman and Hall,

Chantrey, D. F., & Workman, L. (1984). Song and plumage effects on aggressive display by the Euopean robin, *Erithacus rubecula. Ibis, 126,* 366–371.

Clark, D. L. (1993). *The sights and sounds of courtship in the dimorphic jumping spider (Maevia inclemens).* Presented at the annual meeting of the Animal Behavior Society, Davis, CA.

Clark, D. L. (1994). Sequence analysis of courtship behavior in the dimorphic jumping spider, *Maevia inclemens. Journal of Arachnology, 22,* 94–107.

Clark, D. L., & Uetz, G. W. (1993). Signal efficacy and the evolution of male dimorphism in the jumping spider, *Maevia inclemens. Proceedings of the National Academy of Sciences, USA, 90,* 11954–11957.

Clarke, C. H., & Jones, R. B. (2001). Domestic chicks' runway responses to video images of conspecifics. *Applied Animal Behaviour Science, 70,* 285–295.

Conner, W. E. (1987). Ultrasound: Its role in the courtship of the arctiid moth, *Cycnia tenera. Experientia, 43,* 1029–1031.

Cowey, A., & Weiskrantz, L. (1975). Demonstration of cross-modal matching in rhesus monkeys, *Macaca mulatta. Neuropsychologia, 13,* 117–120.

Davenport, R. K., Rogers, C. M., & Russell, I. S. (1973). Cross modal perception in apes. *Neuropsychologia, 11,* 21–28.

Davis, R. T. (1974). Monkeys as perceivers. In L. A. Rosenblum (Ed.), *Primate behavior: Developments in field and lab research* (Vol. 3, pp. 210–220). New York: Academic Press.

de Gelder, B., & Vroomen, J. (2000). The perception of emotion by ear and by eye. *Cognition and Emotion, 14*(3), 289–311.

DePaulo, B. M., Rosenthal, R., Eisenstat, R. A., Rogers, P. L., & Finkelstein, S. (1978). Decoding discrepant nonverbal cues. *Journal of Personality and Social Psychology, 36*(3), 313–323.

Duvall, D., Graves, B. M., & Carpenter, G. C. (1987). Visual and chemical composite signaling effects of *Sceloporus* lizard fecal boli. *Copeia, 1987*(4), 1028–1031.

Ekman, P., Friesen, K., O'Sullivan, M., & Scherer, K. (1980). Relative importance of face, body, and speech in judgements of personality and affect. *Journal of Personality and Social Psychology, 38,* 270–277.

Endler, J. A. (1992). Signals, signal conditions, and the direction of evolution. *American Naturalist, 139,* S125–S153.

Estes, R. D. (1969). Territorial behavior of the wildebeest (*Connochaetes taurinus* Burchell, 1823). *Zeitschrift für Tierpsychologie, 26,* 284–370.

Evans, C. S., & Marler, P. (1991). On the use of video images as social stimuli in birds: Audience effects on alarm calling. *Animal Behaviour, 41,* 17–26.

Freides, D. (1974). Human information processing and sensory modality: Cross-modal functions, information complexity, memory, and deficit. *Psychological Bulletin, 81*(5), 284–310.

Frith, C. B. (1982). Displays of Count Raggi's Bird-of-Paradise *Paradisaea raggiana* and congeneric species. *Emu, 81,* 193–201.

Fusani, L., Hutchison, R. E., & Hutchison, J. B. (1997). Vocal-postural co-ordination of a sexually dimorphic display in a monomorphic species: The Barbary dove. *Behaviour, 134,* 321–335.

Goldfoot, D. A. (1982). Multiple channels of sexual communication in rhesus monkeys: Role of olfactory cues. In C. T. Snowden, C. H. Brown, & M. R. Peterson (Eds.), *Primate communication* (pp. 413–428). Cambridge, England: Cambridge University Press.

Green, S. (1975). Variation of vocal pattern with social situation in the Japanese monkey (*Macaca fuscata*): A field study. In L. A. Rosenblum (Ed.), *Primate behavior* (Vol. 4, pp. 1–102). New York: Academic Press.

Greene, C. M., Owings, D. H., Hart, L. A., & Klimley, A. P. (2002). Foreword. Revisiting the *Umwelt:* Environments of animal communication. *Journal of Comparative Psychology, 116,* 115.

Guilford, T., & Dawkins, M. S. (1991). Receiver psychology and the evolution of animal signals. *Animal Behaviour, 42,* 1–14.

Gyger, M., Karakashian, S. J., & Marler, P. (1986). Avian alarm calling: Is there an audience effect? *Animal Behaviour, 34*(5), 1570–1572.

Harley, H. E., Roiblat, H. L., & Nachtigall, P. E. (1996). Object representation in the bottlenose dolphin (*Tursiops truncatus*): Integration of visual and echoic information. *Journal of Experimental Psychology: Animal Behavior Processes, 22*(2), 164–174.

Heiligenberg, W. (1976). The interaction of stimulus patterns controlling aggressiveness in the cichlid fish *Haplochromis burton. Animal Behaviour, 24,* 452–458.

Hennessy, D. F., Owings, D. H., Rowe, M. P., Coss, R. G., & Leger, D. W. (1981). The information afforded by a variable signal: Constraints on snake-elicited tail flagging by California ground squirrels. *Behaviour, 78,* 188–226.

Heth, G., & Todrank, J. (1995). Assessing chemosensory perception in subterranean mole rats: Different responses to smelling versus touching odorous stimuli. *Animal Behaviour, 49,* 1009–1015.

Holldobler, B. (1995). The chemistry of social regulation: Multicomponent signals in ant societies. *Proceedings of the National Academy of Sciences, USA, 92,* 19–22.

Holldobler, B. (1999). Multimodal signals in ant communication. *Journal of Comparative Physiology, A: Sensory, Neural, and Behavioral Physiology, 184,* 129–141.

Horridge, G. A. (1983). Neuron function and behaviour: Which explains which? In E. Horn (Ed.), *Multimodal convergences in sensory systems* (Vol. 28, pp. 369–383). Stuttgart: Gustav Fischer Verlag.

Hostetter, A. B., Cantero, M., & Hopkins, W. D. (2001). Differential use of vocal and gestural communication by chimpanzees (*Pan troglodytes*) in response to the attentional status of a human (*Homo sapiens*). *Journal of Comparative Psychology, 115*(4), 337–343.

Hughes, M. (1996). The function of concurrent signals: Visual and chemical communication in snapping shrimp. *Animal Behaviour, 52,* 247–257.

Hultsch, H., Schleuss, F., & Todt, D. (1999). Auditory-visual stimulus pairing enhances perceptual learning in a songbird. *Animal Behaviour, 58,* 143–149.

Immelmann, K. (1980). *Introduction to ethology* (E. Klinghammer, Trans.). New York: Plenum Press.

Iwasa, Y., & Pomiankowski, A. (1994). The evolution of mate preferences for multiple sexual ornaments. *Evolution, 48,* 853–867.

Johnston, R. E., Chiang, G., & Tung, C. (1994). The information in scent over-marks of golden hamsters. *Animal Behaviour, 48,* 323–330.

Johnstone, R. A. (1995). Honest advertisement of multiple qualities using multiple signals. *Journal of Theoretical Biology, 177,* 87–94.

Johnstone, R. A. (1996). Multiple displays in animal communication: "Back up signals" and "multiple messages." *Philosophical Transactions of the Royal Society of London: Series B, Biological Sciences, 351,* 329–338.

Jolly, A. (1966). *Lemur behavior.* Chicago: University of Chicago Press.

Jouventin, P. (1982). Visual and vocal signals in penguins: Their evolution and adaptive characters. *Advances in Ethology, 24.*

Kaye, H., Mackintosh, N. J., Rothschild, M., & Moore, B. P. (1989). Odour of pyrazine potentiates an association between environmental cues and unpalatable taste. *Animal Behaviour, 37,* 563–568.

Kehoe, E. J., & Gormezano, I. (1980). Configuration and combination laws in conditioning with compound stimuli. *Psychological Bulletin, 87*(2), 351–378.

Kilner, R. M., Noble, D. G., & Davies, N. B. (1999). Signals of need in parent-offspring communication and their exploitation by the common cuckoo. *Nature, 397,* 667–672.

King, A. J., & Calvert, G. A. (2001). Multisensory integration: Perceptual grouping by eye and ear. *Current Biology, 11*(8), 322–325.

Krebs, J. R., & Dawkins, R. (1984). Animal signals: Mindreading and manipulation. In J. R. Krebs & N. B. Davies (Eds.), *Behavioural ecology: An evolutionary approach* (2nd ed., pp. 380–402). Sunderland, MA: Sinauer.

Kruijt, J. P. (1962). On the evolutionary derivation of wing display in Burmese red jungle fowl and other gallinaceous birds. *Symposia of the Zoological Society of London, 8,* 25–35.

Leger, D. W. (1993). Contextual sources of information and responses to animal communication signals. *Psychological Bulletin, 113,* 295–304.

Lehrman, D. S. (1965). Interaction between internal and external environments in the regulation of the reproductive cycle of the ring dove. In F. A. Beach (Ed.), *Sex and behavior* (pp. 355–380). New York: Wiley.

Lewkowicz, D. J. (2000). The development of intersensory temporal perception: An epigenetic systems/limitations view. *Psychological Bulletin, 126*(2), 281–308.

Lewkowicz, D. J., & Lickliter, R. (1994). *The development of intersensory perception: Comparative perspectives.* Hillsdale, NJ: Erlbaum.

Lickliter, R., & Lewkowicz, D. J. (1995). Intersensory experience and early perceptual development: Attenuated prenatal sensory stimulation affects postnatal auditory and visual responsiveness in bobwhite quail chicks (*Colinus verginianus*). *Developmental Psychology, 31,* 609–618.

Lorenz, K. (1981). *The foundations of ethology,* New York: Springer-Verlag.

Markl, H., & Holldobler, B. (1978). Recruitment and food-retrieving behavior in *Novomessor* (Formicidae, Hymenoptera): II. Vibration signals. *Behavioral Ecology and Sociobiology, 4,* 183–216.

Marks, L. E. (1978). Multimodal perception. In E. C. Carterette & M. P. Friedman (Eds.), *Handbook of perception: Vol. VIII. Perceptual coding* (pp. 321–339). New York: Academic Press.

Marler, P. (1959). Developments in the study of animal communication. In P. R. Bell (Ed.), *Darwin's biological work: Some aspects reconsidered* (pp. 150–206). Cambridge, England: Cambridge University Press.

Marler, P. (1961). The logical analysis of animal communication. *Journal of Theoretical Biology, 1,* 295–317.

Marler, P. (1965). Communication in monkeys and apes. In I. DeVore (Ed.), *Primate behavior: Field studies of monkeys and apes* (pp. 544–584). New York: Holt, Rinehart, & Winston.

Marler, P. (1967). Animal communication signals. *Science, 157,* 769–774.

Marler, P. (1992). Functions of arousal and emotion in primate communication: A semiotic approach. In T. Nishida, W. C. McGrew, P. Marler, M. Pickford, & F. B. deWaal (Eds.), *Topics in primatology* (Vol. 1, pp. 225–233). Tokyo: University of Tokyo Press.

McGurk, H., & MacDonald, J. (1976). Hearing lips and seeing voices. *Nature, 264*(5588), 746–748.

Meredith, M. A., & Stein, B. E. (1983). Interactions among converging sensory inputs in the superior colliculus. *Science, 221*(4612), 389–391.

Mertl, A. S. (1976). Olfactory and visual cues in social interactions of *Lemur catta. Folia Primatologica, 26,* 151–161.

Michelsen, A., Andersen, B. B., Storm, J., Kirchner, W. H., & Lindauer, M. (1992). How honeybees perceive communication dances, studied by means of a mechanical model. *Behavioral Ecology and Sociobiology, 30*(3–4), 143–150.

Miller, J. (1982). Divided attention: Evidence for coactivation with redundant signals. *Cognitive Psychology, 14,* 247–279.

Moller, A. P., Saino, N., Taramino, G., Galeotti, P., & Ferrario, S., (1998). Paternity and multiple signaling: Effects of a secondary sexual character and song on paternity in the barn swallow. *American Naturalist, 151,* 236–242.

Motley, M. T. (1993). Facial affect and verbal context in conversation, *Human Communication Research, 20*(1), 3–40.

Myrberg, A. A., Jr. (1980). Sensory mediation of social recognition processes in fishes. In J. E. Bardach, J. J. Magnuson, R. C. May, & J. M. Reinhart (Eds.), *Fish behavior and its use in the capture and culture of fishes* (ICLARM Conference Proceedings 5, pp. 146–178). Manila, Philippines: International Center for Living Aquatic Resources Management.

Noller, P. (1985). Video primacy: A further look. *Journal of Nonverbal Behavior, 9*(1), 28–47.

Pack, A. A., & Herman, L. M. (1995). Sensory integration in the bottlenosed dolphin: Immediate recognition of complex shapes across the senses of echolocation and vision. *Journal of the Acoustical Society of America, 98,* 722–733.

Partan, S. R. (1998). *Multimodal communication: The integration of visual and vocal signals by rhesus macaques.* Unpublished doctoral dissertation, University of California, Davis.

Partan, S. R. (2001). Categorization of natural multimodal communication signals. In C. Cavé, I. Guaïtella, & S. Santi (Eds.), *Oralité et gestualité: Interactions et comportements multimodaux dans la communication* (pp. 92–95). Paris: L'Harmattan.

Partan, S. R. (2002a). Single and multichannel signal composition: Facial expressions and vocalizations of rhesus macaques (*Macaca mulatta*). *Behaviour, 139*(8), 993–1028.

Partan, S. R. (2002b). *Multisensory response enhancement and Seitz's law of heterogeneous summation.* Presented at the International Multisensory Research Forum 3rd Annual Conference, Geneva.

Partan, S., & Marler, P. (1999). Communication goes multimodal. *Science, 283*(5406), 1272–1273.

Partan, S., & Marler, P. (2002). The *Umwelt* and its relevance to animal communication: Introduction to special issue. *Journal of Comparative Psychology, 116,* 116–119.

Persons, M. H., & Uetz, G. W. (1996). The influence of sensory information on patch residence time in wolf spiders. *Animal Behaviour, 51,* 1285–1293.

Rand, A. S., & Williams, E. E. (1970). An estimation of redundancy and information content of anole dewlaps. *American Naturalist, 104*(935), 99–103.

Redondo, T., and Castro, F. (1992). Signalling of nutritional need by magpie nestlings. *Ethology, 92,* 193–204.

Roper, T. J., & Marples, N. M. (1997). Odour and colour as cues for taste-avoidance learning in domestic chicks. *Animal Behaviour, 53,* 1241–1250.

Rosenthal, G. G., & Ryan, M. J. (2000). Visual and acoustic communication in non-human animals: A comparison. *Journal of Bioscience, 25,* 285–290.

Rosenzweig, M. R. (1983). Learning and multimodal convergence. In E. Horn (Ed.), *Multimodal convergences in sensory systems* (Vol. 28, pp. 303–324). Stuttgart: Gustav Fischer Verlag.

Rothschild, M., Moore, B. P., & Brown, W. V. (1984). Pyrazines as warning odour components in the Monarch butterfly, *Danaus plexippus*, and in moths of the genera *Zygaena* and *Amata* (Lepidoptera). *Biological Journal of the Linnean Society, 23,* 375–380.

Rovner, J. S., & Barth, F. G. (1981). Vibratory communication through living plants by a tropical wandering spider. *Science, 214,* 464–466.

Rowe, C. (1999). Receiver psychology and the evolution of multicomponent signals. *Animal Behaviour, 58,* 921–931.

Rowe, C., & Guilford, T. (1996). Hidden colour aversions in domestic chicks triggered by pyrazine odours of insect warning displays. *Nature, 383,* 520–522.

Rubenstein, D. I., & Hack, M. A. (1992). Horse signals: The sounds and scents of fury. *Evolution and Ecology, 6,* 254–260.

Scheffer, S. J., Uetz, G. W., & Stratton, G. E. (1996). Sexual selection, male morphology, and the efficacy of courtship signalling in two wolf spiders (Aranae: Lycosidae). *Behavioral Ecology and Sociobiology, 38,* 17–23.

Schluter, D., & Price, T. (1993). Honesty, perception and population divergence in sexually selected traits. *Proceedings of the Royal Society of London. Series B, 253,* 117–122.

Schwarz, A. (1974). Sound production and associated behaviour in a cichlid fish, *Cichlasoma centrarchus. Zeitschrift für Tierpsychologie, 35,* 147–156.

Seitz, A. (1940). Die Paarbildung bei einigen Cichliden: I. *Zeitschrift für Tierpsychologie, 4,* 40–84.

Sekuler, R., Sekuler, A. B., & Lau, R. (1997). Sound alters visual motion perception. *Nature, 385,* 308.

Shams, L., Kamitani, Y., & Shimojo, S. (2000). Illusions: What you see is what you hear. *Nature, 408,* 788.

Shulter, D., & Weatherhead, P. J. (1990). Targets of sexual selection: Song and plumage of Wood Warblers. *Evolution, 44*(8), 1967–1977.

Smith, W. J. (1977). *The behavior of communicating: An ethological approach.* Cambridge, MA: Harvard University Press.

Smith, W. J., Smith, S. L., DeVilla, J. G., & Oppenheimer, E. C. (1976). The jump-yip display of the black-tailed prairie dog *Cynomys ludovicianus. Animal Behaviour, 24,* 609–621.

Smotherman, W. P., Bell, R. W., Starzec, J., Elias, J., & Zachman, T. A. (1974). Maternal responses to infant vocalizations and olfactory cues in rats and mice. *Behavioral Biology, 12,* 55–66.

Soffie, M., & Zayan, R. (1977). Responsiveness to "social" releasers in cattle: I. A study of the differential and additive effects of visual and sound stimuli, with special reference to the law of heterogeneous summation. *Behavioural Processes, 2,* 75–97.

Stauffer, H.-P., & Semlitsch, R. D. (1993). Effects of visual, chemical and tactile cues of fish on the behavioral responses of tadpoles. *Animal Behaviour, 46,* 355–364.

Stein, B. E., London, N., Wilkinson, L. K., & Price, D. D. (1996). Enhancement of perceived visual intensity by auditory stimuli: A psychophysical analysis. *Journal of Cognitive Neuroscience, 8*(6), 497–506.

Stein, B. E., & Meredith, M. A. (1990). Multisensory integration: Neural and behavioral solutions for dealing with stimuli from different sensory modalities. *Annals of the New York Academy of Sciences, 608,* 51–70.

Stein, B. E., & Meredith, M. A. (1993). *The merging of the senses,* Cambridge, MA: MIT Press.

Stein, B. E., Meredith, M. A., & Wallace, M. T. (1993). The visually responsive neuron and beyond: Multisensory integration in cat and monkey. *Progress in Brain Research, 95,* 79–90.

Sumby, W. H., & Pollack, I. (1954). Visual contribution to speech intelligibility in noise. *Journal of the Acoustical Society of America, 26,* 212–215.

Tavolga, W. N. (1956). Visual, chemical and sound stimuli as cues in the sex discriminatory behavior of the gobiid fish *Bathygobius soporator. Zoologica, 41*(2), 49–65.

Terrick, T. D., Mumme, R. L., & Burghardt, G. M. (1995). Aposematic coloration enhances chemosensory recognition of noxious prey in the garter snake *Thamnophis radix. Animal Behaviour, 49,* 857–866.

Tinbergen, N. (1959). Comparative studies of the behaviour of gulls (Laridae): A progress report. *Behaviour, 15,* 1–70.

Tinbergen, N. (1963). On aims and methods of ethology. *Zeitschrift für Tierpsychologie, 20,* 410–433.

Todt, D., & Fiebelkorn, A. (1979). Display, timing and function of wing movements accompanying antiphonal duets of *Cichladusa guttata. Behaviour, 72,* 82–106.

Todt, D., Hultsch, H., & Duvall, F. P., II. (1981). Behavioural significance and social function of vocal and non-vocal displays in the monogamous duet-singer *Cossypha heuglini* H. *Zoologische Beitrage, 27,* 421–448.

Uetz, G. W., & Roberts, J. A. (2002). Multisensory cues and mulitmodal communication in spiders: Insights from video/audio playback studies. *Brain, Behavior and Evolution, 59,* 222–230.

Uetz, G. W., & Stratton, G. E. (1982). Acoustic communication in spiders. In P. N. Witt & J. S. Rovner (Eds.), *Spider communication: Mechanisms and ecological significance* (pp. 123–159). Princeton, NJ: Princeton University Press.

van Hooff, J. A. R. A. M. (1962). Facial expressions in higher primates. *Symposia of the Zoological Society of London, 8,* 97–125.

Vesperi, M. (2001). *Cultural encounter in Cuba: The Eleggua Project.* Presented at the New College Faculty Lecture Series, Sarasota, FL.

von Kluge, S., & Brush, F. R. (1992). Conditioned taste and taste-potentiated odor aversions in the Syracuse high- and low-avoidance (SHA/Bru and SLA/Bru) strains of rats (*Rattus norvegicus*). *Journal of Comparative Psychology, 106,* 248–253.

von Seibt, U., & Wickler, W. (1977). Duettieren als Revier-Anzeige bei Vögeln. *Zeitschrift für Tierpsychologie, 43,* 180–187.

von Trumler, E. (1959). Das "Rossigkeitsgesicht" und ähnliches Ausdrucksverhalten bei Einhufern. *Zeitschrift für Tierpsychologie, 16*(4), 478–488.

Wickler, W. (1978). A special constraint on the evolution of composite signals. *Zeitschrift für Tierpsychologie, 48,* 345–348.

Wiley, R. H. (1973). The strut display of male sage grouse: A "fixed" action pattern. *Behaviour, 47,* 129–152.

Wiley, R. H. (1983). The evolution of communication: Information and manipulation. In T. R. Halliday & P. J. B. Slater (Eds.), *Animal behaviour 2: Communication* (pp. 156–189). New York: Freeman.

Wilson, E. O. (1975). *Sociobiology.* Cambridge, MA: Belknap Press of Harvard University Press.

Zucker, N. (1994). A dual status-signalling system: A matter of redundancy or differing roles? *Animal Behaviour, 47,* 15–22.

Zuckerman, M., Amidon, M. D., Bishop, S. E., & Pomerantz, S. D. (1982). Face and tone of voice in the communication of deception. *Journal of Personality and Social Psychology, 43*(2), 347–357.

Zuk, M., Ligon, J. D., & Thornhill, R. (1992). Effects of experimental manipulation of male secondary sex characters on female mate preference in red jungle fowl. *Animal Behaviour, 44,* 999–1006.

III THE NEURAL MECHANISMS UNDERLYING THE INTEGRATION OF CROSS-MODAL CUES

15 Multisensory Integration in Single Neurons of the Midbrain

BARRY E. STEIN, WAN JIANG, AND TERRENCE R. STANFORD

Introduction

Many of the chapters in this handbook discuss what has been learned about how interactions among the different senses affect perception and overt behavior. Although these chapters often use different combinations of sensory modalities (e.g., visual and auditory versus gustatory and olfactory) and different model species to explore multisensory integration, most touch on the same basic observation: cross-modal stimuli activate neural mechanisms that could not be predicted by thinking of the senses as totally independent of one another. Indeed, there is a growing awareness that the brain normally engages in an ongoing synthesis of streams of information that are being carried over the different sensory channels.

The fundamental nature of this property of the vertebrate brain and the potent effects it has on perception and behavior have been the subjects of a rich history of observation, introspection, and speculation, beginning with the earliest philosophers of science. This long interest in multisensory phenomena, coupled with a comparatively recent upsurge in the number of scientific studies exploring them, has resulted in compelling evidence that the information processed by each of the sensory modalities—visual, auditory, somatosensory, vestibular, olfactory, and gustatory—is highly susceptible to influences from the other senses. Even some of the seemingly exotic sensory systems of species less often examined in this context, such as the infrared system of pit vipers that is used for detecting other animals' heat signatures (Hartline, Kass, & Loop, 1978), the chemical and vibratory sensors in the crayfish claw that the animal uses for identifying and obtaining food (Hatt & Bauer, 1980), or the pheromone inputs to the flight motor neurons that are used by moths to locate mates (Olberg & Willis, 1990; Fig. 15.1), share this susceptibility. The pooling of information across sensory modalities appears to be a primordial organizational scheme (see Stein & Meredith, 1993) that has been retained even as organisms have become progressively more complex.

Despite the considerable vigor and breadth of scientific efforts to detail and understand multisensory integration, however, interactions have not yet been demonstrated among every possible combination of senses: not in studies of human subjects, in which perception is most frequently of primary interest, and certainly not in studies among nonhuman species, where most physiological studies have been conducted and where there is a rich diversity and specialization of sensory systems. Thus, it would be premature to state that multisensory integration is characteristic of all sensory modalities or that it takes place among every combination of them. Nevertheless, until it is shown otherwise, it appears to be a reasonable assumption.

Perhaps as impressive as the ubiquitous nature of multisensory integration is its potency. When multiple sensory cues are provided by the same event, they are usually in close temporal and spatial proximity, and their integration can be of substantial value in enhancing the detection, identification, and orientation to that event (see, e.g., Jiang, Jiang, & Stein, 2000; Stein, Meredith, Huneycutt, & McDade, 1989; Wilkinson, Meredith, & Stein, 1996). They also substantially increase the speed of reactions to these events (see Bernstein, Clark, & Edelstein, 1969; Corneil & Munoz, 1996; Engelken & Stevens, 1989; Frens, Van Opstal, & Van der Willigen, 1995; Gielen, Schmidt, & Van den Heuvel, 1983; Goldring, Dorris, Corneil, Ballantyne, & Munoz, 1996; Harrington & Peck, 1998; Hughes, Reuter-Lorenz, Nozawa, & Fendrich, 1994; Lee, Chung, Kim, & Park, 1991; Perrott, Saberi, Brown, & Strybel, 1990; Zahn, Abel, & Dell'Osso, 1978; see also Marks, Chap. 6, this volume, and Van Opstal & Munoz, Chap. 23, this volume).

Nevertheless, the action of the neural mechanisms that integrate information from multiple sensory systems generally goes unnoticed by the perceiver. There is, after all, nothing particularly noteworthy about the experience. It evokes no signature sensation and is quite commonplace. However, when there are slight discrepancies in the timing or location of cross-modal cues that appear to be derived from the same event, the

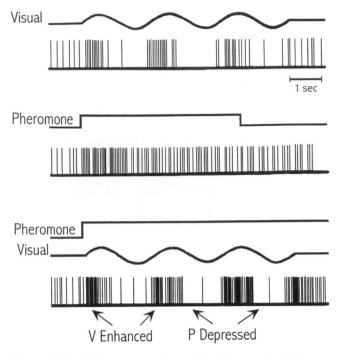

Visual

1 sec

Pheromone

Pheromone

Visual

V Enhanced   P Depressed

FIGURE 15.1 Multisensory integration in a moth interneuron. This neuron responded to a moving visual stimulus (V, top) and to a pheromone (P, middle). The oscillogram at the top illustrates that the movement of a visual stimulus in one direction elicited more impulses than movement in the other. The pheromone elicited a long train of impulses. However, when the two stimuli were combined, the neuron's directional tuning was significantly enhanced, and the long continuous discharge train elicited by the pheromone was no longer apparent. (Reproduced with permission from Stein, B. E., & Meredith, M. A. [1991]. *The merging of the senses.* Cambridge, MA: MIT Press. Modified from Olberg & Willis, 1990.)

result is often a cross-modal illusion. Many such illusions have been documented, and many are quite compelling (see, e.g., Shams, Kamitani, & Shimojo, Chap. 2, this volume). These perceptual experiences are not commonplace and do cause one to take notice. They are sometimes amusing, as when a skilled ventriloquist gives the impression that a dummy is speaking (see Woods & Recanzone, Chap. 3, this volume). But at other times they can have a decidedly negative component. What first comes to mind is the effect of watching a film that has been shot from the pilot's seat of a small plane flying rapidly over mountains and into canyons. The visual experience results in vestibular disruptions that, in turn, cause gastrointestinal changes that only patrons of amusement park rides could find amusing. The results of this relatively harmless experience pale in comparison with those that could result from the visual-vestibular illusions that pilots experience and to which they must accommodate in order to avoid making potentially disastrous decisions during take-off and other

movements that significantly affect the vestibular and proprioceptive systems (see Lackner & DiZio, Chap. 25, this volume).

What should by evident from the foregoing chapters in this handbook is that sensory events are never experienced in isolation, and thus there is always the opportunity to modify the signals initiated by external stimuli and the perceptions to which they give rise. A unimodal (i.e., modality-specific) stimulus in the external environment normally initiates distinct signals in those receptors that are tuned to it, but these signals are no longer immutable when they reach the brain. They may be incorporated into the stream of ongoing neural activity that is subject to modification from a variety of intrinsic sources, some of which result from activation of interoceptors and others of which are not sensory in the traditional use of the term (e.g., attention and expectation); moreover, these modality-specific signals can be coupled with inputs from other exteroceptors. The particular mix of this central stream of signals can change from moment to moment. Thus, there is little evidence to support the common conviction that, for example, the visual percept of an object is invariant as long as the visual environment is unchanged. On the other hand, there is at least one component of the sensory experience that is likely to be immutable, or at least highly resistant to the influences of other sensory stimuli, and that is its subjective impression. For each sensory modality has evolved a unique subjective impression, or *quale.* Hue is specific to the visual system, tickle and itch to the somatosensory system, pitch to the auditory systems, and so on. As a result, whether the visual cortex is activated by a natural visual stimulus, by mechanical distortion of the eye, or by direct electrical stimulation of visual centers in the brain itself, the resulting sensation is visual, one whose essential quality is unambiguous.

The lack of ambiguity may seem paradoxical. For if the brain integrates information from different sensory modalities, how can any sensory stimulus give rise to a unique subjective impression? The answer may lie in the dual nature with which the brain represents and deals with sensory information. Many areas of the brain have become specialized to process information on a sense-by-sense basis. These areas do not receive direct projections from more than a single sensory modality, or, if they do, such seemingly "inappropriate" inputs are comparatively few in number. Most prominent among such areas are the nuclei along the primary sensory projection pathways, such as the projection from the retina to the thalamic nucleus for vision (the lateral geniculate nucleus) and from there to primary visual cortex (V1), or the projection from the skin through its relay nucleus in the spinal cord to the thalamic nucleus for somesthesis (the ventrobasal complex) and from there to primary somatosensory cortex (S1). The primary sensory nuclei are recipients of heavy inputs from the peripheral sensory organs and are among the best-studied areas of the central nervous system (CNS). Direct electrical stimulation of the primary sensory cortices has been conducted in awake patients during neurosurgical procedures and has been found to produce modality-specific sensations appropriate for each area (Brindley & Lewin, 1968; Cushing, 1909; Dobelle & Mladejovsky, 1974; Penfield & Boldrey, 1937; Penfield & Rasmussen, 1952). It is also likely that, when activated by natural environmental stimuli, these areas are the sources of modality-specific subjective impressions. Although the prevailing view is that these regions are unaffected by other sensory inputs, a growing body of evidence indicates that their exclusivity may have been overestimated and that even these areas of the nervous system can be affected by information from other sensory modalities (see, in this volume, Schroeder & Foxe, Chap. 18; Cohen & Anderson, Chap. 29; Calvert & Lewis, Chap. 30; Fort & Giard, Chap. 31). Just how functionally significant this cross-modal influence normally is and how this "nonappropriate" information is relayed to these regions are issues of active exploration.

In contrast to presumptive modality-specific regions, many nuclei outside the primary projection pathways are known to receive substantial inputs from multiple sensory modalities. These areas contain mixtures of neurons, some of which are targeted by inputs from only a single sensory modality but many of which receive converging inputs from multiple modalities and thus are rendered multisensory. In some ways multisensory neurons are the functional polar opposites of their modality-specific counterparts wherever they are found, for they are specialized for pooling rather than segregating modality-specific information and probably have no significant role in producing the qualia mentioned earlier. Multisensory areas are found at various levels in the neuraxis and are involved in many different behavioral, perceptual, and emotive processes. One of the best-known sites of multisensory convergence is in a midbrain structure, the superior colliculus (SC), a structure that has served as a model for understanding multisensory integration from anatomical, physiological, and behavioral perspectives.

The superior colliculus: A model of multisensory integration

The SC appears as a bump (actually, a pair of bumps) on the surface of the midbrain (Fig. 15.2), and is involved in initiating and controlling orientation behaviors (Casagrande, Harting, Hall, & Diamond, 1972; Schneider, 1967; Sprague & Meikle, 1965; see also Stein & Meredith, 1991). It serves this role principally by controlling shifts of gaze (i.e., eye and head movement) to contralateral targets (Goldberg & Wurtz, 1972; Sparks, 1986; Stein, Goldberg, & Clamann, 1976;

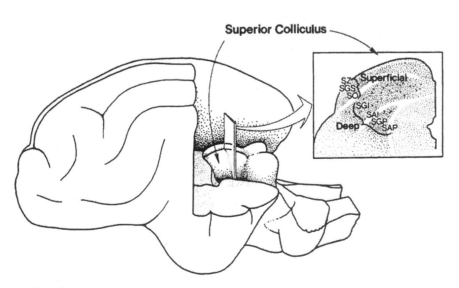

FIGURE 15.2   Location and laminar pattern of the cat superior colliculus (SC). In this schematic the posterior region of the cat's cerebral cortex is removed to reveal the SC in the midbrain. A coronal section (upper right) shows its laminar organization. (Reproduced with permission from Stein, B. E., & Meredith, M. A. [1991]. *The merging of the senses.* Cambridge, MA: MIT Press.)

but see also Dean, Redgrave, & Westby, 1989; Redgrave, Odekunle, & Dean, 1986). It is also involved in coordinated movement of the limbs, whiskers, and mouth that best position the animal to both evaluate and respond to stimuli of interest. These movements are effected through its projections to neurons in the brainstem and spinal cord that are in more direct contact with the muscles (see Grantyn & Grantyn, 1982; Guitton & Munoz, 1991; McHaffie, Kao, & Stein, 1989; Moschovakis & Karabelas, 1985; Munoz & Guitton, 1991; Munoz, Guitton, & Pelisson, 1991; Redgrave et al., 1986; Redgrave, Mitchell, & Dean, 1987; Stuphorn, Bauswein, & Hoffmann, 2000).

SENSORY REPRESENTATIONS IN THE SC   The SC receives the information it needs to initiate and properly guide these movements from sensory systems dealing with extrapersonal (i.e., the visual, auditory systems) and personal (the somatosensory system) space (see Stein & Meredith, 1993). This information is derived from a host of structures, most of which contain only modality-specific neurons. Some of these structures are located in lower regions of the neuraxis; others are in the thalamus and/or cortex (see Edwards, Ginsburgh, Henkel, & Stein, 1979; Huerta & Harting, 1984). They converge on SC neurons in a variety of different patterns, some from structures with matching sensory representations (e.g., visual inputs from the retina and visual cortex can converge on the same SC neuron) and others from structures having different modality-specific neurons (e.g., visual inputs from the retina and auditory inputs from the inferior colliculus). In the latter case the target neuron in the SC is rendered multisensory. These convergence patterns can be quite complicated and include matched ascending and descending projections from multiple sensory modalities (e.g., Wallace, Meredith, & Stein, 1993). All possible varieties of sensory neurons have been noted in the SC, including the three possible modality-specific neuronal types and all multisensory categories. However, while bimodal neurons abound in this structure, trimodal neurons are far less common (Meredith & Stein, 1986; Stein, Goldberg, et al., 1976; Wallace & Stein, 1996).

Despite the complexity and variation among afferent convergence patterns, all sensory inputs to the SC are distributed in the same general maplike fashion. This creates a striking overlap in the representations of visual, auditory, and somatosensory space (see Stein & Meredith, 1993). Anatomical and electrophysiological mapping studies have detailed these representations in a variety of species, but the electrophysiological studies are particularly instructive in the current context. Most of these studies follow a given pattern: an animal is

positioned so that its eyes, ears, and head are facing directly forward, and electrode penetrations are made vertically through the SC in a gridlike pattern in an effort to sample neurons across the length and breadth of the structure. The results have been similar in all species. Neurons within a given electrode penetration have their receptive fields at the same relative locations in visual, auditory, or body space, and these receptive fields shift systematically as neurons are sampled at different locations across the structure. In mammals, neurons in rostral aspects of the structure have their receptive fields in central visual and auditory space and forward on the body (i.e., the face), whereas those at progressively more caudal locations have their receptive fields in increasingly more peripheral regions of visual-auditory space, and increasingly further caudal on the body. Thus, the horizontal meridian of the visual-auditory-somatosensory map runs from rostral to caudal in the structure. The vertical meridian is roughly perpendicular to the horizontal meridian, so that neurons in medial aspects of the structure have their receptive fields in upper space and neurons in progressively more lateral regions have their receptive fields in increasingly more inferior locations. Consequently, a somatosensory neuron rostral and medial in the structure will have its receptive field on the upper face. Nonmammals have a similar maplike representation, though it may be angled with respect to the mammalian plan (e.g., Stein & Gaither, 1981). Receptive field correspondence for different mammalian species is shown in Figure 15.3.

MULTISENSORY NEURONS HAVE MULTIPLE OVERLAPPING RECEPTIVE FIELDS   Regardless of species, the parallel distribution of the converging inputs to the structure yields multisensory neurons whose different receptive fields are in spatial register with one another (see Fig. 15.3). A visual-auditory neuron lateral and caudal in the structure, for example, will have its visual and auditory receptive fields overlapping one another in upper peripheral space (see, e.g., Meredith & Stein, 1996). The sensory representations are in topographic alignment with the motor representation that is involved in moving the eyes, ear, head, and limbs. Perhaps because of the very close relationship that has evolved between the sensory and motor representations in the SC, the sensory maps have taken on a different organization scheme than that found in modality-specific structures. In the latter cases the individual maps are organized with reference to a single sensory organ: the visual map is referred to the retina, the auditory map to the head, and the somatosensory map to the body. In contrast, in monkeys and cats the visual, auditory, and

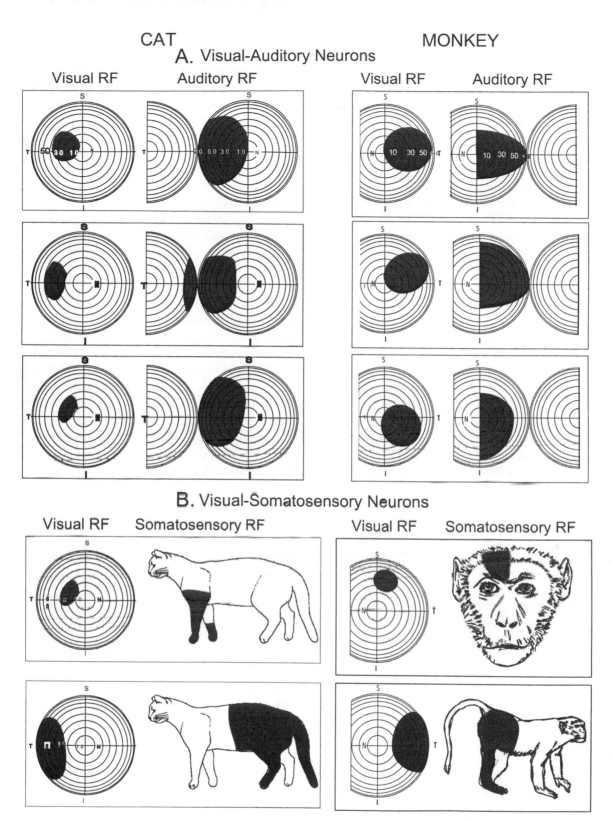

CAT   MONKEY
A. Visual-Auditory Neurons

Visual RF   Auditory RF   Visual RF   Auditory RF

B. Visual-Somatosensory Neurons

Visual RF   Somatosensory RF   Visual RF   Somatosensory RF

FIGURE 15.3   The different sensory receptive fields (RFs) of the same multisensory SC neurons overlap one another. (A) The spatial coincidence between each neuron's visual-auditory RFs is shown in six representative cases, three from cat (left) and three from rhesus monkey (right). Each RF is shown in gray on a circular schematic of visual and auditory space. Each concentric circle in the schematics represents 10 degrees. Note that peripheral visual receptive fields are coupled with peripheral auditory RFs, superior visual RFs are coupled with superior auditory RFs, and so on. (B) A similar scheme is apparent in visual-somatosensory neurons: central visual RFs are linked to frontal (i.e., face) somatosensory RFs, and so on. (Adapted with permission from Jiang, W., et al. [2001]. Two cortical areas mediate multisensory integration in superior colliculus neurons. *Journal of Neurophysiology, 85,* 506–522; Wallace, M. T., et al. [1996]. Representation and integration of multiple sensory inputs in primate superior colliculus. *Journal of Neurophysiology, 76,* 1246–1266.)

somatosensory representations in the SC have been transformed (in part) from their own peculiar modality-specific frames of reference to one that is common: a "motor" frame of reference (Sparks & Nelson, 1987). This transformation may not be complete in every neuron, and some intermediate stages of transformation have been noted among SC neurons. Nevertheless, the locations of the nonvisual receptive fields of SC neurons are strongly influenced by the direction of gaze. This ensures that, regardless of the relative eye, head, and body positions, a visual, auditory, or somatosensory cue will activate the same general site in the SC—one that represents the position of the stimulus with respect to the current line of sight (Groh & Sparks, 1996; Hartline, Vimal, King, Kurylo, & Northmore, 1995; Jay & Sparks, 1987; Yao & Peck, 1997). The result is that the locus of activity in the SC is always appropriate for producing the particular shift of gaze necessary to look directly at the target. In general terms, the site of activity in the motor map of the SC is the determinant of both the size and direction of a shift in gaze.

This is a system that is elegant in its apparent simplicity and whose efficiency is illustrated by the following example. A predator watches and listens for prey in a thicket. All its senses are alerted; its eyes and ears are perfectly aligned and directed forward. It hears a rustle 20 degrees to the right and shifts its line of sight to that location to see if there is a possible meal in the offing. The auditory cue evokes activity that is centered at a site caudal in the left SC. This is the locus of the sensory map that represents space 20 degrees to the right. This is also the site at which motor-related neurons code 20-degree contralateral gaze shifts because motor-related SC neurons (some of which are also sensory) are arranged in the same topographic fashion as their sensory counterparts in this circumstance. Thus, the general motor topography of the SC is familiar. Neurons located in the rostral (front) SC are engaged in coding comparatively small contralateral shifts of gaze. Neurons located at more caudal positions code increasingly larger contralateral gaze shifts. In contrast, movements to upper and lower space are coded by neurons along the mediolateral aspect of the SC.

Now we can consider the circumstance in which, instead of looking directly ahead, the predator's eyes shifted 10 degrees to the left just before the sound emanated from the thicket, while its head and ears did not move. If the maps in the SC were static, the same rustling sound would produce activity at the same site in the SC, and the resultant gaze shift would be 10 degrees short of the target. To be effective, the auditory cue must activate a different site in the auditory map, one that will result in a 30-degree rightward gaze shift, and

indeed this is in large part what happens. The "problem" has been solved by transforming the auditory information from its "natural" head-centered coordinate frame to a common frame of reference based on the visuomotor system. The use of an eye-centered frame of reference requires that the auditory map be dynamic, a solution that is also used by the somatosensory system. Its natural body-centered frame of reference is transformed to the same eye-centered frame of reference. A simple rule of thumb is that, for purposes of gaze control, the sensory maps in the SC largely represent stimulus position with respect to the current gaze position rather than with respect to its position in "sensory space," as is the case in the primary projection nuclei.

The caveat "largely" in the preceding description is due to observations that this coordinate transformation is not always complete and may not take place in every SC neuron. Nevertheless, the transformation appears to be sufficient to maintain a high degree of cross-modal receptive field register among many neurons, even when the peripheral sensory organs move with respect to one another. This is a critical issue for multisensory integration, for, as we will see, among the primary factors that determine the nature of multisensory interactions are the spatial relationships of the various external stimuli and how they relate to the receptive fields of multisensory neurons.

Physiological consequences of multisensory integration: Response enhancement and response depression

Although maintaining multisensory neurons in the brain allows different sensory systems to have access to the same circuits and thereby reduces the need to replicate such circuits in any given multisensory area, the principal benefit of maintaining such neurons is their ability to integrate information derived from different sources (i.e., different senses). For there to be a true synthesis, the response to a multisensory stimulus must differ from all of those elicited by its modality-specific components. Thus, multisensory integration is defined operationally as a statistically significant difference between the number of impulses that are evoked by a cross-modal combination of stimuli and the number of impulses evoked by the most effective of these stimuli individually (Meredith & Stein, 1983). Most multisensory neurons have been shown to be capable of exhibiting such integrated responses, with the most frequent integrated response being an enhanced one (Fig. 15.4). In experiments in monkeys, cats, and rodents, the magnitude of a multisensory enhancement (i.e., the multisensory index) can vary and sometimes exceeds the

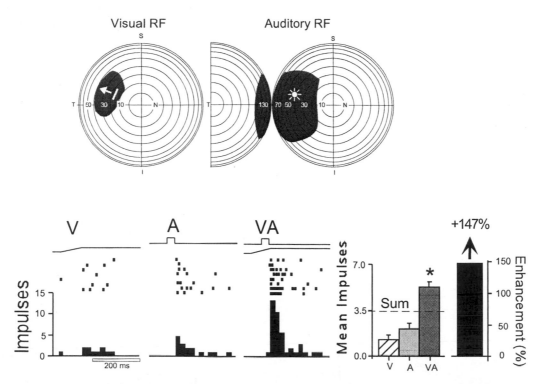

FIGURE 15.4 Spatially coincident stimuli give rise to response enhancement. The top panels show the individual receptive fields (RFs) of this visual-auditory neuron from cat SC as gray-shaded areas on the diagrams of visual-auditory space. The position of each modality-specific stimulus is shown by an icon within the RF. The visual stimulus (V) was a moving bar of light whose direction of movement is indicated by the arrow. The auditory stimulus (A) was a broad-band noise burst delivered from a stationary speaker. The bottom panels contain rasters and histograms illustrating the neuron's response to the modality-specific (visual alone, auditory alone) and multisensory (visual and auditory combined) stimuli, as well as bar graphs summarizing the mean responses and the index of multisensory enhancement. The spatially coincident visual-auditory pairing of stimuli resulted in a 147% response enhancement, well above the best modality-specific response and above the arithmetic sum of the two modality-specific responses (dashed line, t-test, $P < 0.05$).

The percent response enhancement and depression are calculated by the following formula: Enhancement (Depression) = $[(CM - SM_{max})/SM_{max}]$, where CM is the mean number of impulses evoked by the cross-modal stimulus combination and SM_{max} is the mean number of impulses evoked by the best or, "dominant" modality-specific, stimulus.

arithmetic sum of the individual modality-specific responses (Figs. 15.4 and 15.5). Some neurons also show response depression, an effect that is sometimes so powerful that, for example, an auditory stimulus can suppress even a robust visual response (Fig. 15.6; see also Jiang, Wallace, Jiang, Vaughan, & Stein, 2001; Kadunce, Vaughan, Wallace, Benedek, & Stein, 1997; King & Palmer, 1985; Meredith & Stein, 1983, 1986; Wallace & Stein, 1996).

These differing multisensory responses can be evoked with the same stimuli by varying their spatial relationships in ways that make intuitive sense, because any given event that provides multiple sensory cues and thus is more readily detected and identified does so from the same spatial location. The combined excitatory inputs have been shown to produce a synergistic interaction (as long as the stimuli occur close to one another in time; see Meredith, Nemitz, & Stein, 1987) in the same multisensory neurons (Figs. 15.4 and 15.5), which results in an enhanced neural response. On the other hand, cues derived from different events provide inputs from different spatial locations. In such cases, if one of the stimuli falls within the receptive field of a given multisensory neuron, the other stimulus is likely to fall outside the receptive field of that same multisensory neuron. This often results in no interaction between their inputs, and thus no enhancement in the neural signal. But if that extrareceptive field stimulus falls into an inhibitory region bordering the neuron's receptive field, its input can depress the excitatory effects of the other input on this neuron, thereby decreasing or eliminating the neural signal (Fig. 15.6; see also Kadunce et al., 1997; Meredith & Stein, 1996). These possibilities indicate the importance of maintaining receptive field overlap in multisensory neurons even if the various peripheral sensory organs happen to be misaligned. Otherwise the ability to use multiple sensory cues to increase the neural signals used to detect, locate, and identify events would vary depending on the relative positions of the eyes, ears, and body.

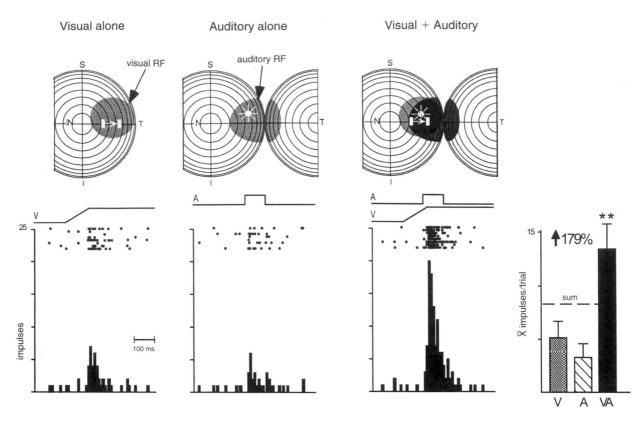

Visual alone   **Auditory alone**   **Visual + Auditory**

FIGURE 15.5   An example of multisensory response enhancement that was obtained from an SC neuron in the SC of the rhesus monkey. Conventions are the same as in Figure 15.4. The top panels show the visual and auditory RFs of this visual-auditory neuron. In the lower panels are the rasters, peristimulus time histograms, and bar graphs illustrating the results obtained in response to the modality-specific and multisensory stimuli. The number of impulses in the multisensory response significantly ($P < 0.01$) exceeded the number evoked by the most effective modality-specific stimulus (visual), and also exceeded the number predicted by simple summation of the visual and auditory responses. (Reproduced with permission from Wallace, M. T., Wilkinson, L. K., & Stein, B. E. [1996]. Representation and integration of multiple sensory inputs in primate superior colliculus. *Journal of Neurophysiology, 76,* 1246–1266.)

Mechanisms underlying SC multisensory integration

As discussed earlier, multisensory integration is operationally determined at the neural level when the response (i.e., number of impulses) elicited by the presentation of stimuli from different sensory modalities is statistically different from the response evoked by the most effective of those stimuli presented individually. Defined in this way, multisensory integration is a measure of the relative efficacy of multisensory versus modality-specific stimulation, and, in principle, corresponds to the potential benefit of combining the influences of cross-modal cues. If the sensory stimuli are imagined to compete for both attention and access to the motor machinery that generates reactions to attended stimuli, then the potential consequence of multisensory enhancement is clear: an increased likelihood of detecting or initiating a response to the source of the multisensory signal.

Although the index of multisensory integration has obvious functional implications, it does not speak directly to the independent issue of neural mechanism. The first question to ask in this regard is, what operation does a multisensory neuron perform on its two (or more) modality-specific inputs to yield the multisensory response? To address this question, we would want to determine whether a simple rule (e.g., addition, multiplication) or set of rules governs the way in which a multisensory neuron transforms its inputs into outputs. The literature is filled with examples of neurons from other brain areas that synthesize information from different input sources and create a novel product at their output. Binaural neurons in the superior olivary complex (SOC), so-called space-specific neurons in the owl inferior colliculus, and simple cells of primary visual cortex (V1) are just a few examples. Both SOC neurons and V1 neurons display forms of input summation. Thus, the interaural time delay (ITD) sensitivity of an SOC neuron to a complex stimulus composed of multiple frequencies

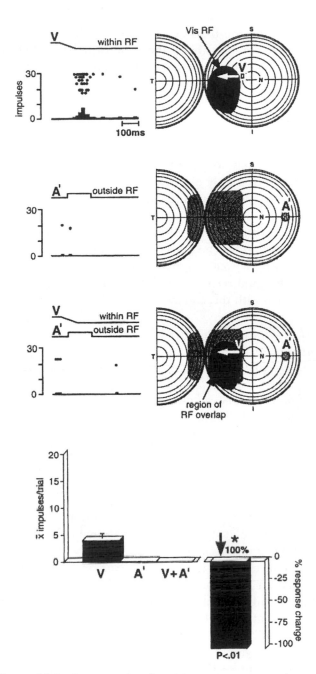

FIGURE 15.6 An example of multisensory response depression that was obtained from a visual-auditory neuron of cat SC. At top, the visual stimulus (a moving bar of light, V) evoked a train of impulses when presented within the neuron's visual RF. Presentation of an auditory stimulus (A') at a fixed position outside the neuron's auditory RF evoked no response (second row). Nevertheless, pairing the visual and the auditory stimuli eliminated the visual response (third row), thereby indicating the presence of a suppressive region bordering the auditory RF. The bar graph at bottom shows the mean responses obtained in each condition (left) and the multisensory index (right; see also the formula in Fig. 15.4), along with the percent response decrement induced by this multisensory stimulus combination. (Adapted with permission from Kadunce, D. C., et al. [1997]. Mechanisms of within-modality and cross-modality suppression in the superior colliculus. *Journal of Neurophysiology, 78,* 2834–2847.)

can be approximated by a linear sum of the individual frequency-specific ITD functions (Yin & Chan, 1990). In combining frequency channels, the SOC neuron encodes information about the azimuthal (i.e., how far to the left or right) location of naturally occurring stimuli, which are often rich in frequency content. Similarly, simple cells in V1 show linearity in the form of spatial summation across the classical receptive field (Carandini, Heeger, & Movshon, 1997; Hubel & Weisel, 1962; Movshon, Thompson, & Tolhurst, 1978), a mechanism that contributes to their ability to represent the edges that help define objects within the visual scene. In contrast, recent data suggest that to specify location in auditory space, a neuron in the owl's inferior colliculus *multiplies* its tuning functions for the binaural cues of interaural time and interaural intensity difference (Pena & Konishi, 2001).

These examples illustrate that different neural populations employ different combinatorial rules. Presumably, different rules reflect different computational goals and require different types of neural machinery for their implementation. Until recently, we knew little about the rules by which SC multisensory neurons combined their modality-specific influences. However, experiments designed to address this question have begun to shed some light on this issue. In a set of experiments, Quessy, Sweatt, Stein, and Stanford (2000) sought to determine if a multisensory neuron simply "adds up" the influences of its modality-specific inputs to produce its multisensory product. To do so, the responsiveness of each multisensory neuron was tested for a wide range of visual-auditory stimulus combinations. For any given visual-auditory stimulus pairing, the response to their concurrent presentation was compared with a response predicted by simple summation of the responses to the visual and auditory stimuli presented individually. When a statistical test was applied to determine whether the magnitude of the multisensory response was significantly greater than (superadditive) or less than (subadditive) the additive prediction, the majority of interactions were found to be neither. Rather, as shown in Figure 15.7A, most responses to combined stimuli were statistically indistinguishable from the additive prediction.

The results suggested that summation of modality-specific influences can account for the majority of multisensory interactions, a finding that indicated that, to a first approximation, multisensory neurons behave linearly. Nevertheless, the frequency with which superadditive and subadditive interactions occurred was not trivial. Further analysis revealed that response magnitude was a powerful predictor of which of these integrative modes would be engaged. As shown in Figure 15.7B,

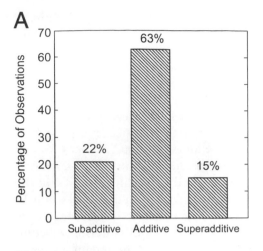

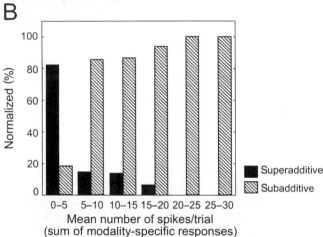

FIGURE 15.7 (A) The relative incidence of subaddi-
tive, additive, and superadditive multisensory interactions for neurons
recorded in SC of the cat. (B) Shown are the relative proportions of superadditive and subadditive multisensory interactions, plotted as a function of the efficacy of the modality-
specific stimulus components. The arithmetic sum of the
responses to the individually presented modality-specific stimuli was used as an index of stimulus effectiveness. At low levels
of modality-specific stimulus effectiveness, significant deviations exceeded additivity, whereas at higher levels subadditivity
predominated.

the overwhelming majority of significantly superadditive
interactions occurred when the modality-specific stimuli
were weakly effective. On the other hand, the most
extremely subadditive interactions occurred in cases in
which the individual modality-specific stimulus components were comparatively effective. This relationship
indicates that these interactions occur at the opposing
ends of the response range, and so may be attributable to
the nonlinear relationships between membrane potential and firing frequency that correspond to neuronal
threshold and saturation.

In summary, it seems that a simple integrative rule
may underlie multisensory integration in the SC.

However, on the basis of a single study, it may be premature to consider this as the final word. Nevertheless,
it is worth pointing out that simple summation is wholly
consistent with the notion that multisensory integration
serves to increase stimulus salience insofar as stimulus
salience is related to the vigor of activity that the stimulus induces. In this regard, it is also interesting to note
that two weakly effective modality-specific stimuli are
the most likely to produce a superadditive response,
whereas two highly effective stimuli are most likely to
yield a response that is less than additive. Whether by
design or coincidence, the functional consequence is
that proportionately, multisensory integration is most
advantageous for the detection of multisensory sources
composed of weak modality-specific stimuli. Indeed,
the behavioral results described in the next section are
consistent with this conclusion.

Behavioral consequences of multisensory integration: Response enhancement and response depression

For multisensory SC neurons to effect behavior, their
synthesized information must ultimately reach the
musculature used in orientation behaviors. This is
accomplished most directly via the predorsal bundle, a
collection of nerve fibers that leaves the SC and de-
scends to the brainstem and spinal cord. Most multisensory neurons send axons out of the SC and reach these
targets via the predorsal bundle (Meredith & Stein,
1985; Wallace et al., 1993), and presumably, enhancing
or degrading the activity of multisensory SC neurons
should be closely linked to enhancing or degrading the
probability (or vigor) of overt orientation behaviors. In
the present context that assumption would lead us to
expect that the rules governing multisensory integration in individual SC neurons also apply to overt orientation behavior. To examine this possibility, cats were
trained to orient to visual or auditory stimuli, or both,
using several different training and testing paradigms
(see Stein, Huneycutt, & Meredith, 1988; Stein et al.,
1989; Wilkinson et al., 1996).

The training-testing device was a darkened enclosure
housed in a sound-attenuating chamber. Within the enclosure was a semicircular hoop, or perimetry device,
on which were mounted light-emitting diodes (LEDs)
and small speakers (Fig. 15.8). These potential targets
for orientation movements were separated from one another by 15 degrees. In each of the training and testing
paradigms an animal was required to first learn to stand
at the start position and direct its gaze to a point directly
ahead at 0 degrees. After learning the fixation task, the
animal then learned that while it fixated directly ahead,

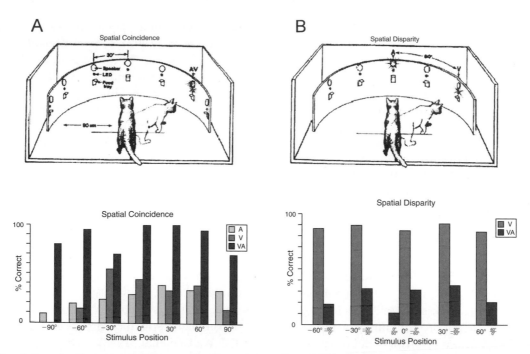

FIGURE 15.8   Spatially coincident visual-auditory stimuli result in enhanced multisensory orientation, whereas when these stimuli are spatially disparate, the result was depressed multisensory orientation. An array of speakers (large circles) and LEDs (smaller circles) were located in vertical pairs above a food tray at each of seven regularly spaced (30-degree) intervals in a perimetry device. In the spatially coincident paradigm (*A*), an animal was required to orient to and move directly toward a low-intensity visual (V) or an auditory (A) stimulus to receive a food reward. During testing, a low-intensity stimulus was presented either alone or in combination with the other sensory stimulus at the same location (VA). The animal's ability to detect and approach the correct position was enhanced by combined-modality stimuli at every location tested (bottom left). In the spatially *disparate* paradigm (*B*), the animal was trained to approach a visual stimulus (V) but to ignore an auditory stimulus (A). During testing, the visual stimulus was presented alone or in combination with an auditory stimulus that was 60 degrees out of register with it (e.g., V at 0 degrees, A at +60 degrees). The intensity of the visual stimulus was such that a high percentage of correct responses were elicited to it alone. However, when this visual stimulus was combined with a spatially disparate auditory stimulus, orientation to the visual stimulus was depressed. (Adapted with permission from Stein, B. E., et al. [1989]. Behavioral indices of multisensory integration: Orientation to visual cues is affected by auditory stimuli. *Journal of Cognitive Neuroscience, 1,* 12–24.)

a stimulus would occur somewhere in the perimetry. Its task was to immediately break fixation, orient, and directly approach the stimulus in order to obtain a food reward (Stein et al., 1988, 1989). In one paradigm the target was a visual stimulus (a dimly illuminating LED) and the animal learned that although an auditory stimulus (a brief, low-intensity broad-band sound) would be presented periodically, it was "neutral." Responses to it never produced a reward, and the animals rapidly learned to "ignore" it. To examine whether the combination of the visual target stimulus and the neutral auditory stimulus would have an impact on orientation, orientation performance to the visual stimulus alone was compared with orientation performance to the visual-auditory stimulus combination. The visual-auditory stimuli were spatially coincident, but their location varied from trial to trial.

Because the visual stimulus was dim, it was difficult to detect, and performance was rather poor. However, the combination of the visual and the neutral auditory

stimuli markedly enhanced correct performance, regardless of their location in the perimetry device (Fig. 15.8*A*). A similar result was obtained when animals learned that both stimuli were potential targets (see Jiang et al., 2000). On the other hand, in a separate paradigm in which the visual and the (neutral) auditory stimuli were spatially disparate, the animals' performance was significantly worse than when the visual stimulus was presented alone (Fig. 15.8*B*). In this circumstance the presence of the seemingly neutral auditory stimulus degraded orientation to the visual target even though the intensity of the visual stimulus was set at a level that was sufficiently high to elicit correct responses on nearly all trials. These behavioral results are strikingly parallel to the results obtained in studies of multisensory SC neurons. They are also in keeping with the concept that cross-modal stimuli produce shifts of attention (Spence & Driver, 1997). Possible "exogenous" shifts of attention would be a likely result of the modulation of the salience of the visual stimulus by the auditory stimulus and would be expressed behaviorally via SC output signals to the brainstem and spinal cord that move the peripheral sensory organs.

Modality-specific neurons in cortex send converging inputs to individual SC neurons

As noted earlier, the SC receives inputs from a variety of structures (see also Edwards et al., 1979; Huerta & Harting, 1984; Stein & Meredith, 1991). Although most of these structures contain modality-specific neurons, there is a substantial input to the SC from association cortex (see, e.g., Baizer, Desimone, & Ungerleider, 1993; Barnes & Pandya, 1992; Fries, 1984; Goldman & Nauta, 1976; Harting, Feig, & Van Lieshout, 1997; Kuypers & Lawrence, 1967; McHaffie, Kruger, Clemo, & Stein, 1988; Meredith & Clemo, 1989; Schmahmann & Pandya, 1989; Segal & Beckstead, 1984; Stein, Spencer, & Edwards, 1983), a region containing a mixture of modality-specific and multisensory neurons (Bruce, Desimone, & Gross, 1986; Colby & Duhamel, 1991; Duhamel, Colby, & Goldberg, 1998; Hikosaka, Iwai, Saito, & Tanaka, 1988; Hyvarinen & Shelepin, 1979; Jiang, Lepore, Ptito, & Guillemot, 1994a, 1994b; Toldi & Feher, 1984; Van Essen, Felleman, DeYoe, Olavarria, & Knierim, 1990; Wallace, Meredith, & Stein, 1992). Thus, the multisensory properties of SC neurons may derive from two very different input patterns: they may be created at the SC neuron itself, because it is a primary site for the convergence of modality-specific inputs, or they may reflect the convergence and integration of cross-modal sensory inputs that takes place in one or more of the input sources of the SC (a third possibility is a mixture of these two).

In order to explore these possibilities, we chose to examine one of the association cortical areas in cat known to have a particularly high incidence of multisensory neurons and a robust projection to the SC. This cortical region, the anterior ectosylvian sulcus (AES), consists of three subregions: a somatosensory region referred to as SIV (Clemo & Stein, 1982), an auditory region referred to as FAES (Clarey & Irvine, 1986), and a visual region referred to as AEV (Mucke, Norita, Benedek, & Creutzfeldt, 1982; Olson & Graybiel, 1987). In addition to the scattered multisensory neurons that are present within these largely modality-specific regions, there are many multisensory neurons clustered at the borders between them (Clemo, Meredith, Wallace, & Stein, 1991; Stein et al., 1993; Wallace et al., 1992; but see Jiang et al., 1994a).

Orthodromic and antidromic stimulation techniques demonstrated that multisensory neurons in the AES do not project to the SC, and that only its modality-specific neurons send their projections to this target structure (Wallace et al., 1993). These modality-specific projections converge on SC neurons in a reliable fashion in order to create the sensory profile of a particular SC neuron. Thus, for example, somatosensory-visual neurons generally receive input from SIV and AEV, but not from FAES. Furthermore, these corticotectal inputs are topographically matched, so that, for example, the ascending and descending visual projections to an SC neuron have similar receptive fields and a visual input (e.g., central receptive field) from AEV is matched with an auditory input (also a central receptive field) from FAES. Based on orthodromic latencies, many of these corticotectal projections appear to be monosynaptic, and most of the SC neurons contacted by AES corticotectal projections in turn, project into the predorsal bundle, so that multisensory signals are heavily represented in the structure's output instructions to the brainstem and spinal cord (Meredith, Wallace, & Stein, 1992; Wallace et al., 1993).

Multisensory integration in cortex is similar to multisensory integration in the superior colliculus

Although multisensory neurons in the AES and SC appear to form separate circuits, they share many of the same organizational features and exhibit many similarities in their response properties. Multisensory AES neurons show the same spatial register among their receptive fields as do SC neurons (Wallace et al., 1992). This appears to be a general feature of the brain and is found among multiple sensory representations in the midbrains of mammals, reptiles, and birds (Drager & Hubel, 1976; Hartline, Kass, & Loop, 1978; Knudsen, 1982; Middlebrooks & Knudsen, 1984; Stein & Gaither, 1981; Stein, Magalhaes-Castro, & Kruger, 1976) and in multisensory cortical regions of cat and rhesus monkey (Bruce, Desimone, & Gross, 1981; Duhamel et al., 1989; Hyvarinen & Shelepin, 1979; Stein et al., 1993; Wallace et al., 1992; Watanabe & Iwai, 1991). However, unlike other brain areas, the cross-modal overlap in AES is achieved in the absence of consistent modality-specific topographies. There is no apparent spatiotopic auditory representation in FAES (Clarey & Irvine, 1986) and no apparent visuotopic representations in AEV (Mucke et al., 1982; Olson & Graybiel, 1987). Thus, the spatial organization of multisensory receptive fields in AES appears to deviate from the overall representational schemes that characterize this region. Presumably, this is a reflection of the importance of cross-modal receptive field overlap for multisensory integration, as the functional impact of overlapping receptive fields is as important a determinant of multisensory integration in AES as it is in SC. Thus, AES neurons also exhibit multisensory response enhancement to spatially coincident cross-modal stimuli and multisensory response depression to spatially disparate cross-modal stimuli (Wallace et al., 1992). In addition, the magnitude of multisensory interactions in AES neurons is greatest when their responses are weakest to the individual components of a cross-modal stimulus pair, just as it is in SC neurons. These parallels in multisensory information processing suggest that a common mode has been established for integrating multisensory information in very different brain regions. Perhaps this serves as a means of achieving coherence in those brain regions responsible for programming the immediate orientation responses to external events and those brain regions involved in the higher-order processes that lead to the emotive, perceptual, and cognitive components of a multisensory experience.

Conspiring with cortex to make multisensory integration possible

Given the apparent independence of the multisensory integration that is taking place in cortex (i.e., AES) and the SC, it was not immediately clear what purpose could be served by the converging modality-specific corticotectal inputs from the AES. The SC receives robust inputs from a wide variety of subcortical visual, auditory, and somatosensory structures, and it seemed unlikely that the corticotectal inputs were providing the only means by which most SC neurons could become multisensory. It seemed more likely that both subcortical and cortical structures provided converging multisensory information to the same SC neurons (see Clemo & Stein, 1984; Wallace et al., 1993), a sort of parallelism in the convergence patterns of the many different afferent projection systems. To examine this possibility, as well as to assess the functional role of corticotectal inputs in multisensory integration, experiments were designed in which the response properties of SC neurons could be assessed in the presence and absence of these corticotectal influences. Initially this was accomplished by using a cooling probe that could be placed directly on the cortex (or the overlying dura) in an acute experiment to temporarily lower AES temperature to a level below that necessary for neurons to remain active (see Clemo & Stein, 1986; Ogasawara, McHaffie, & Stein, 1984; Wallace & Stein, 1994). A more flexible technique was then used in which hollow coils, through which coolant could be circulated (see Lomber, Payne, & Horel, 1999), were implanted within the AES of a chronic preparation (Jiang et al., 2001). Cooling coils were also implanted in a neighboring area of cortex (the rostral aspect of the lateral suprasylvian sulcus, rLS). The rLS was chosen because it, too, has a robust input to the multisensory region of the SC (see Stein et al., 1983) and, like AES, contains a mixture of modality-specific and multisensory neurons (see Irvine & Huebner 1979; Toldi & Feher, 1984; Toldi, Rojik, & Feher, 1981; Wallace et al., 1993; Yaka, Yinon, & Wollberg, 1999). Both techniques permitted the examination of SC responses before, during, and after cryogenic blockage of cortical influences.

A small number of multisensory SC neurons reacted to cortical deactivation by becoming unresponsive to stimuli in one or both (or, in the case of trimodal neurons, all three) sensory modalities. In this condition, even sensory stimuli that previously were highly effective would fail to evoke activity from many of these neurons. Yet several minutes after the cortex was rewarmed, these neurons once again responded to these stimuli, and did so at their predeactivation levels. In some cases this temporary loss of responsiveness resulted from deactivation of AES alone or rLS alone, and in others it happened only during simultaneous deactivation of AES and rLS. But regardless of the cortex (or cortices) involved, these observations suggested that the primary sensory input for some SC neurons is relayed through cortex.

However, this was not the case in the large majority of SC neurons. There was no significant effect of cortical deactivation on their level of responses to modality-specific stimuli. These neurons received multiple sensory inputs from sources other than AES and rLS. What was striking, and quite revealing, however, was that during cortical deactivation these neurons lost their ability to synthesize the multiple sensory inputs they were receiving. Instead, their responses to the spatially coincident cross-modal combination of stimuli were no better than their responses to the most effective of its modality-specific constituents (Fig. 15.9). Yet once the cortex was reactivated, their multisensory synthesizing capabilities returned. Obviously, these neurons did not depend on cortex to be multisensory; they continued to respond to each modality-specific cue during cortical deactivation, and generally these responses were not different from control levels. Their multisensory character was retained, presumably as a result of converging ascending (or, at least, non-AES/rLS) inputs. But while these afferents conferred on these neurons the ability to respond to cross-modal cues, they did not render them able to synthesize multisensory information and thereby produce an enhanced response. This required AES/rLS influences.

Apparently, these two regions of association cortex have developed the ability to use neurons in a distant structure (i.e., the SC) to integrate cross-modal

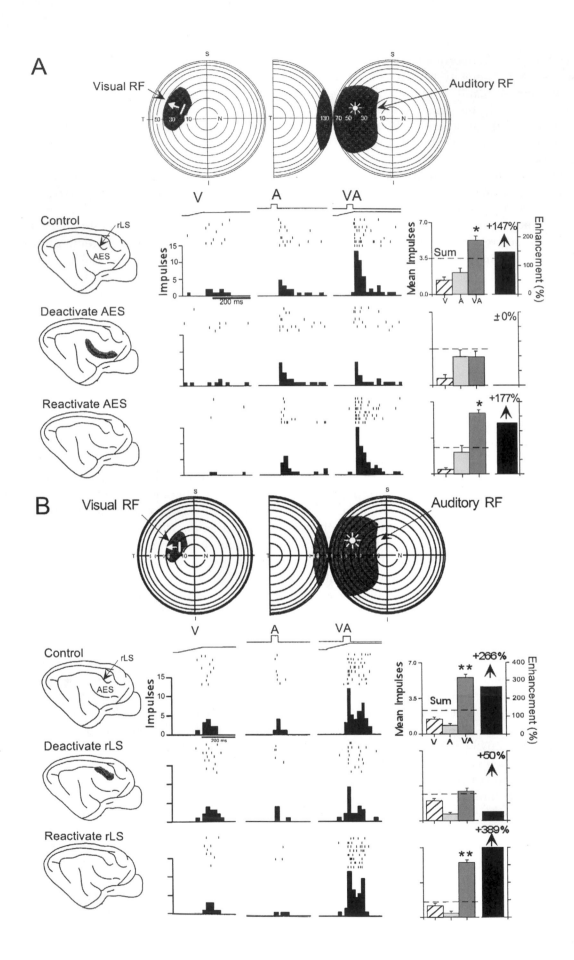

information. These observations, coupled with those showing that multisensory neurons in SC and AES integrate cross-modal information in similar fashion, suggest that there are at least two parallel cortical multisensory operations going on that are important to the synthesis of information from different sensory channels, one on-site and one off-site. In the former case, cortical neurons integrate multisensory information and distribute that product to other cortical targets (see Scannell, Blakemore, & Young, 1995, for AES-cortical interconnections), presumably to facilitate higher-order functions (e.g., perception). In the latter case, the integrated multisensory SC product is due to the action of descending inputs from these cortices working in concert with other afferents and the target neurons in the SC.

Influences of AES and rLS on SC-mediated orientation behavior

The physiological studies discussed in the preceding section suggest that AES and rLS "gate" multisensory integration in SC neurons. Based on these data, it seemed likely that AES and rLS would also prove to be essential for mediating the multisensory integration underlying the enhanced and degraded multisensory orientation behavior that is believed to depend on the SC. To examine this possibility, experiments were conducted using the same perimetry apparatus and similar training and testing paradigms as were used in earlier behavioral studies. The difference was that during the testing period, the cortex was now deactivated on some trials, and performance on the task was compared with that observed during the interleaved control trials (no cortical deactivation).

After an animal learned to orient to visual stimuli at different locations in the perimetry device, the intensity of the LED targets was operationally chosen to be such that the animal's correct performance was marginal (e.g., <50%). Just as noted earlier, animals performed at a strikingly higher level when the visual stimulus was coupled with a neutral auditory stimulus at the same location, and at a markedly lower level when the visual target and auditory stimulus were at different locations. In the first experimental series, cannulas were implanted in several cortical areas, including AES and primary visual and auditory cortices (areas 17/18, AI), as well as the caudal aspect of the lateral suprasylvian cortex, a region of extraprimary cortex (primarily visual) just to the rear of rLS that has a substantial direct projection to the multisensory regions of the SC. Lidocaine could be injected into each cannula to deactivate a local region of cortex (see Wilkinson et al., 1996).

In this study, multisensory orientation behaviors were affected by lidocaine injections in only one cortical area, AES, and the results of AES deactivation were quite specific: there was little or no effect on modality-specific (visual) orientation, but the enhanced performance induced by coupling spatially coincident visual and auditory stimuli was eliminated, and the depression induced by coupling the spatially disparate visual and auditory stimuli was degraded. More recently, the role of AES in multisensory behavior was reexamined using the cryogenic deactivation technique that was used in studies of single SC neurons (Jiang et al., 2001). In addition, the role of rLS in these behaviors was also examined. Indwelling cooling coils were implanted in both AES and rLS in order to selectively deactivate either or both of these regions. The results showed that deactivation of either AES or rLS had the same effect on behavior: there was little change in modality-specific orientation behavior, but the response enhancement seen with spatially coincident cross-modal stimuli was lost, and the response depression seen with spatially disparate cross-modal stimuli was degraded (Fig. 15.10; see also Jiang et al., 2002).

The specific perceptual and/or behavioral roles of AES and rLS are not known. However, given the striking physiological-behavioral parallels produced by AES and/or rLS deactivation on SC neurons and multisensory orientation behavior, the loss of orientation behavior may have reflected disruption of the functional integrity of the AES/rLS-SC circuitry. If so, the same result should be obtained with damage to the SC. To examine this possibility, ibotenic acid lesions of the SC were made in cats that were trained in the same paradigms and same apparatus described above. After a recovery period, the animals' modality-specific and multisensory orientation behaviors were tested. Despite the lack of damage to AES and rLS, the animals lost their ability to integrate the cross-modal cues to enhance orientation responses. In contrast, there were no changes

FIGURE 15.9 An example in which the multisensory response enhancement of a cat SC neuron was dependent on influences from AES (*top*) or rLS (*bottom*). In both examples, deactivation of the relevant cortex eliminated enhanced multisensory responses without eliminating responses to the individual modality-specific stimuli. (Adapted with permission from Jiang, W., et al. [2001]. Two cortical areas mediate multisensory integration in superior colliculus neurons. *Journal of Neurophysiology, 85*, 506–522.)

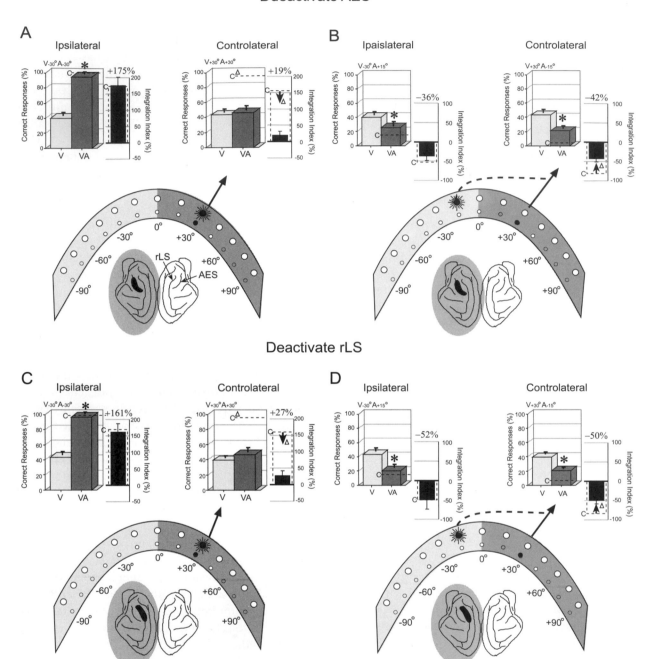

FIGURE 15.10   Deactivation of either AES (*A–B*) or rLS (*C–D*) in behaving cats eliminated the response enhancement normally induced by contralateral spatially coincident visual-auditory stimuli (V plus A at +30 degrees; compare controls (dotted lines) and deactivated conditions in *A* and *C*) and significantly ameliorated the depressive effects of these stimuli when they were spatially disparate (V at +30 degrees, A at −15 degrees; compare controls (dotted lines) and deactivated conditions in *B* and *D*). The bar graphs summarize the results, and in each diagram the dark bar to the right illustrates the percent change of multisensory response from the modality-specific (visual) response (dotted empty bar: control). The arrows above the dark bars indicate the direction of change in the deactivated condition from the control. All tests illustrated here were conducted at 30 degrees to the right of fixation but reflect the changes that were noted at each of the three contralateral locations tested (15, 30, and 45 degrees). Ipsilateral multisensory response enhancement and response depression were not degraded (left panels). The deactivated cortical area is indicated by a black overlay on the schematic of the brain. (**: *t-test* between multisensory and visual responses, *p* < 0.05; Δ: *t-test* between deactivated and comparable control data, *p* < 0.05.)

in responses to modality-specific cues (Burnett, Stein, & Wallace, 2000).

These observations indicate that by establishing dominion over the multisensory integrative capabilities of SC neurons, AES and rLS have also come to exert substantial control over an animal's attentive and orientation responses to cross-modal cues. But the apparent equality of the disruptive effects of rLS and AES deactivation on this task was unexpected. The results of physiological studies strongly suggested that AES would play a more important role in SC-mediated behaviors than would rLS. Approximately 78% of the SC neurons exhibiting multisensory integration that were studied by Jiang et al. (2001) lost their multisensory response enhancement during deactivation of AES, but only 45% of these neurons did so when rLS was deactivated (in many cases a neuron's multisensory capabilities were affected by influences from both AES and rLS). Thus, these observations suggest that disrupting multisensory integration in even a large minority of SC neurons can have potent consequences on the ability to react properly to external events.

The behavioral results showed that there was one exception to the spatial "rule" of multisensory integration derived from studies of single SC neurons (i.e., that coincident visual-auditory stimuli produced response enhancement and disparate visual-auditory stimuli produce response depression), and it was particularly instructive. In both the Wilkinson et al. (1996) and the Jiang et al. (2002) studies, it was found that when the visual target was in the more peripheral regions of space (e.g., at 30 degrees or 45 degrees), the auditory stimulus produced a depression in orientation to the visual target only when it was central to that visual target. When the auditory stimulus was peripheral to the visual target (i.e., at 75 degrees or 90 degrees), it actually enhanced performance. This seemingly odd result is actually consistent with physiological observations that there is an asymmetry in the SC visual-auditory receptive fields that represent peripheral space. The auditory receptive fields have larger excitatory regions (Jiang and Stein, 2003; Kadunce et al., 1997; Meredith & Stein, 1996; Middlebrooks & Knudsen, 1984; Wallace, Wilkinson, & Stein, 1996) than their visual counterparts, with lateral borders that can extend far beyond those of their corresponding visual receptive fields. This visual-auditory receptive field discrepancy is far smaller at their medial borders. The asymmetric extension of the lateral border of auditory receptive fields is a reflection of the fact that the representation of auditory space extends well beyond that of the representation of visual space (the visual field stops at approximately 100 degrees, but auditory space continues around the head). As a result, a visual stimulus

45 degrees into peripheral visual space may be enhanced by an auditory stimulus at 90 degrees because both stimuli fall into their respective excitatory receptive fields of the same multisensory neurons. Their synergistic interaction enhances the activity of each of these neurons, which in turn enhances the impact of this group of neurons on their downstream targets and the probability of evoking overt behavior. In contrast, if the auditory cue is central to the visual target (e.g., auditory at 0 degrees, visual at 45 degrees), it is likely to fall beyond the medial border of the auditory receptive fields of those multisensory neurons that are excited by that visual stimulus. It is also likely that the auditory stimulus will fall into the auditory inhibitory region that borders many of these multisensory neurons (Jiang and Stein, 2003; Kadunce et al., 1997; Meredith & Stein, 1996). The result would be depression of the visually evoked SC activity and a lowered probability of evoking overt SC-mediated responses.

This explanation is based on the "sensory" properties of the SC and does not preclude an explanation based on a parallel "motor" process. Nor are these explanations mutually exclusive. Neurons in the SC that fire in association with orientation movements have movement fields that differ in size, depending on the areas of space the neurons sample and the movements (e.g., gaze shifts) in which they are engaged. For example, those neurons involved in gaze shifts to central visual or auditory targets have smaller movement fields than those used to acquire more eccentric targets. Consequently, having the disparate auditory and visual stimuli in central regions of sensory space could create two separate and distinct competing sites of sensory and motor activity. Given that the specifics of any overt response are believed to depend on the "vector averaging" of the movement fields of the SC neurons activated by an event (see Lee, Rohrer, & Sparks, 1987; Ottes, Van Gisbergen, & Eggermont, 1986; Van Gisbergen, Van Opstal, & Tax, 1987) this situation would produce orientation to a "phantom" target between the two physical stimuli. Such errors were, in fact, among those noted in this particular paradigm. In contrast, because of the very large peripheral auditory receptive fields, the same auditory stimulus in the peripheral disparate condition would produce a rather large area of excitation that would include, and thereby enhance, the more focal excitation produced by the visual target. The result would be an enhanced likelihood of an orientation response to that visual target.

Summary and concluding remarks

Physiological experiments have shown that many SC neurons receive converging inputs from the visual, auditory, and somatosensory modalities, thereby producing a variety of bimodal and, less frequently, trimodal neurons. These multisensory neurons have the ability to integrate the inputs from these different senses and thus can respond to stimuli in ways that differ from their modality-specific neighbors': their responses can be substantially enhanced or degraded by the combinations of cues provided by external events. Whether multisensory integration in any given SC neuron in any given circumstance will result in enhancement or depression has proved to be predictable based largely on the spatial relationships among the stimuli present. Because of the overlap among the modality-specific receptive fields (e.g., visual and auditory) of individual multisensory neurons, the multiple sensory stimuli derived from a given event fall into the excitatory receptive fields of the same neurons, a pooling of excitatory effects that leads to an augmented response. On the other hand, when stimuli are derived from different events, they are likely to be spatially separate and excite different populations of neurons, thus eliminating the possibility of pooling excitatory influences in the SC. In fact, spatially disparate stimuli may yield combinations of excitatory (falling within a receptive field) and inhibitory (falling within an inhibitory region bordering a receptive field) inputs to the same SC neurons, thereby degrading their overall responding. The neural synergy shown by spatially concordant cues and the antagonism displayed by spatially disparate cues each makes sense from a behavioral perspective. Indeed, they have their behavioral counterparts in the increased (concordant stimuli) or decreased (disparate stimuli) probability of evoking an overt orientation response. This is not surprising, given the well-known role of the SC in the generation such behaviors.

Multisensory integration is sure to take place in some form in neurons in the nonmammalian homologue of the SC (the optic tectum) of species possessing less well-developed cortices (e.g., amphibians, reptiles). However, it remains to be determined whether, as in cats, this integration depends on the establishment of an intimate relationship between cortical and midbrain neurons. The necessity of this cortical-midbrain circuit for multisensory integration may seem like a cumbersome organizational scheme, but it has a distinct advantage. The cortex is exceedingly sensitive to environmental influences, perhaps more so than any subcortical sensory structure. It can react rapidly based on experience to alter its circuitry and the properties of its neurons in ways that are adaptive to an animal's particular environment, a way of fine-tuning neuronal circuits to best fit its future needs (see, e.g., Buonomano & Merzenich, 1998; Rauschecker, 1995, 1999). While the circuitry and response properties of SC neurons are certainly influenced by experience (see, e.g., King et al., 1988; Knudsen &

Brainard, 1991; Kujala, Alho, Paavilainen, Summala, & Naatanen, 1992), many of the experience-based changes in response properties appear to be derived from corticotectal influences and are lost when cortex is removed (Wickelgren & Sterling, 1969).

It is interesting to note the marked developmental parallels in the properties of cortical and SC neurons. During the same maturational stage at which the information-processing characteristics of cortical neurons are crafted as a result of an individual's experience, neurons in the SC are first developing their capability to synthesize multisensory information (Wallace, McHaffie, & Stein, 1997). It appears as if the cortex renders SC neurons capable of multisensory integration only after the cortex has sufficient experience with the environment in which such integration is likely to take place (see Jiang & Stein, 2001; Wallace & Stein, 2000). (These issues are dealt with in far more detail in Chapter 39, this volume, by Wallace.) Though these ideas remain speculative at this point, there is intuitive appeal to the idea that cortex ensures that SC multisensory integration, and the behaviors that depend on that integration, are appropriate for a given situation. This ensures that the information provided by cross-modal stimuli can be used to maximum advantage and that there is a tight correspondence between the neural processes leading to perceptual awareness (cortex) and those that are necessary for rapid attentive and orientation responses (midbrain).

REFERENCES

Baizer, J. S., Desimone, R., & Ungerleider, L. G. (1993). Comparison of subcortical connections of inferior temporal and posterior parietal cortex in monkeys. *Visual Neuroscience, 10,* 59–72.

Barnes, C. L., & Pandya, D. N. (1992). Efferent cortical connections of multimodal cortex of the superior temporal sulcus in the rhesus monkey. *Journal of Comparative Neurology, 318,* 222–244.

Bernstein, I. H., Clark, M. H., & Edelstein, G. H. (1969). Effects of an auditory signal on visual reaction time. *Journal of Experimental Psychology, 80,* 567–569.

Brindley, G. S., & Lewin, W. S. (1968). The sensations produced by electrical stimulation of the visual cortex. *Journal of Physiology, 196,* 479–493.

Bruce, C., Desimone, R., & Gross, C. G. (1981). Visual properties of neurons in a polysensory area in superior temporal sulcus of the macaque. *Journal of Neurophysiology, 46,* 369–384.

Bruce, C. J., Desimone, R., & Gross, C. G. (1986). Both striate cortex and superior colliculus contribute to visual properties of neurons in superior temporal polysensory area of macaque monkey. *Journal of Neurophysiology, 55,* 1057–1075.

Buonomano, D. V., & Merzenich, M. M. (1998). Cortical plasticity: From synapse to maps. *Annual Review of Neuroscience, 21,* 149–186.

Burnett, L. R., Stein, B. E., & Wallace, M. T. (2000). Ibotenic acid lesions of the superior colliculus (SC) disrupt multisensory orientation behaviors. *Society of Neuroscience Abstracts, 26,* 1220.

Carandini, M., Heeger, D. J., & Movshon, J. A. (1997). Linearity and normalization in simple cells of the macaque primary visual cortex. *Journal of Neuroscience, 17,* 8621–8644.

Casagrande, V. A., Harting, J. K., Hall, W. C., & Diamond, I. T. (1972). Superior colliculus of the tree shrew: A structural and functional subdivision into superficial and deep layers. *Science, 177,* 444–447.

Clarey, J. C., & Irvine, D. R. F. (1986). Auditory response properties of neurons in the anterior ectosylvian sulcus of the cat. *Brain Research, 386,* 12–19.

Clemo, H. R., Meredith, M. A., Wallace, M. T., & Stein, B. E. (1991). Is the cortex of cat anterior ectosylvian sulcus a polysensory area? *Society of Neuroscience Abstracts, 17,* 1585.

Clemo, H. R., & Stein, B. E. (1982). Somatosensory cortex: A "new" somatotopic representation. *Brain Research, 235,* 162–168.

Clemo, H. R., & Stein, B. E. (1984). Topographic organization of somatosensory corticotectal influences in cat. *Journal of Neurophysiology, 51,* 843–858.

Clemo, H. R., & Stein, B. E. (1986). Effects of cooling somatosensory cortex on response properties of tactile cells in the superior colliculus. *Journal of Neurophysiology, 55,* 1352–1368.

Colby, C. L., & Duhamel, J. R. (1991). Heterogeneity of extrastriate visual areas and multiple parietal areas in the macaque monkey. *Neuropsychologia, 29,* 517–537.

Corneil, B., & Munoz, D. (1996). The influence of auditory and visual distractors on human gaze shifts. *Journal of Neuroscience, 16,* 8193–8207.

Cushing, C. (1909). A note upon the faradic stimulation of the post-central gyrus in conscious patients. *Brain, 32,* 44–53.

Dean, P., Redgrave, P., & Westby, G. W. M. (1989). Event or emergency? Two response systems in mammalian superior colliculus. *Trends in Neurosciences, 12,* 137–147.

Dobelle W. H., & Mladejovsky, M. G. (1974). Phosphenes produced by electrical stimulation of human occipital cortex, and their application to the development of a prosthesis for the blind. *Journal of Physiology, 243,* 553–576.

Drager, U. C., & Hubel, D. H. (1976). Topography of visual and somatosensory projections in mouse superior colliculus. *Journal of Neurophysiology, 39,* 91–101.

Duhamel, J. R., Colby, C. L., & Goldberg, M. E. (1998). Ventral intraparietal area of the macaque: Congruent visual and somatic response properties. *Journal of Neurophysiology, 79,* 126–136.

Edwards, S. B., Ginsburgh, C. L., Henkel, C. K., & Stein, B. E. (1979). Sources of subcortical projections to the superior colliculus in the cat. *Journal of Comparative Neurology, 184,* 309–330.

Engelken, E. J., & Stevens, K. W. (1989). Saccadic eye movements in response to visual, auditory, and bisensory stimuli. *Aviation, Space and Environmental Medicine, 60,* 762–768.

Frens, M. A., Van Opstal, A. J., & Van der Willigen, R. F. (1995). Spatial and temporal factors determine auditory-visual interactions in human saccadic eye movements. *Perception & Psychophysics, 57,* 802–816.

Fries, W. (1984). Cortical projections to the superior colliculus in the macaque monkey: A retrograde study using horseradish peroxidase. *Journal of Comparative Neurology, 230,* 55–76.

Gielen, S. C. A. M., Schmidt, R. A., & Van den Heuvel, P. J. M. (1983). On the nature of intersensory facilitation of reaction time. *Perception & Psychophysics, 34,* 161–168.

Goldberg, M. E., & Wurtz, R. H. (1972). Activity of superior colliculus in behaving monkey: II. Effect of attention on neuronal responses. *Journal of Neurophysiology, 35,* 560–574.

Goldman, P. S., & Nauta, W. H. J. (1976). Autoradiographic demonstration of a projection from prefrontal association cortex to the superior colliculus in the rhesus monkey. *Brain Research, 116,* 145–149.

Goldring, J. E., Dorris, M. C., Corneil, B. D., Ballantyne, P. A., & Munoz, D. P. (1996). Combined eye-head gaze shifts to visual and auditory targets in humans. *Experimental Brain Research, 111,* 68–78.

Grantyn, A., & Grantyn, R. (1982). Axonal patterns and sites of termination of cat superior colliculus neurons projecting in the tecto-bulbo-spinal tract. *Experimental Brain Research, 46,* 243–265.

Groh, J. M., & Sparks, D. L. (1996). Saccades to somatosensory targets: III. eye-position-dependent somatosensory activity in primate superior colliculus. *Journal of Neurophysiology, 75,* 439–453.

Guitton, D., & Munoz, D. P. (1991). Control of orienting gaze shifts by the tectoreticulospinal system in the head-free cat: I. Identification, localization, and effects of behavior on sensory processes. *Journal of Neurophysiology, 66,* 1605–1623.

Harrington, L. K., & Peck, C. K. (1998). Spatial disparity affects visual-auditory interactions in human sensorimotor processing. *Experimental Brain Research, 122,* 247–252.

Harting, J. K., Feig, S., & Van Lieshout, D. P. (1997). Cortical somatosensory and trigeminal inputs to the cat superior colliculus: Light and electron microscopic analyses. *Journal of Comparative Neurology, 388,* 313–326.

Hartline, P. H., Kass, L., & Loop, M. S. (1978). Merging of modalities in the optic tectum: Infrared and visual integration in rattlesnakes. *Science, 199,* 1225–1229.

Hartline, P. H., Vimal, R. L., King, A. J., Kurylo, D. D., & Northmore, D. P. (1995). Effects of eye position on auditory localization and neural representation of space in superior colliculus of cats. *Experimental Brain Research, 104,* 402–408.

Hatt, H., & Bauer, U. (1980). Single unit analysis of mechano- and chemosensitive neurones in the crayfish claw. *Neuroscience Letters, 17,* 203–207.

Hikosaka, K., Iwai, E., Saito, H.-A., & Tanaka, K. (1988). Polysensory properties of neurons in the anterior bank of the caudal superior temporal sulcus of the macaque monkey. *Journal of Neurophysiology, 60,* 1615–1637.

Hubel, D. H., & Wiesel, T. N. (1962). Receptive fields, binocular interaction and functional architecture in the cat's visual cortex. *Journal of Physiology, 160,* 106–154.

Huerta, M. F., & Harting, J. K. (1984). The mammalian superior colliculus: Studies of its morphology and connections. In H. Vanegas (Ed.), *Comparative neurology of the optic tectum* (pp. 687–773). New York: Plenum Press.

Hughes, H. C., Reuter-Lorenz, P. A., Nozawa, G., & Fendrich, R. (1994). Visual-auditory interactions in sensorimotor processing: Saccades versus manual responses. *Journal of Experimental Psychology: Human Perception and Performance, 20,* 131–153.

Hyvarinen, J., & Shelepin, Y. (1979). Distribution of visual and somatic functions in the parietal associative area 7 of the monkey. *Brain Research, 169,* 561–564.

Irvine, D. R., & Huebner, H. (1979). Acoustic response characteristics of neurons on nonspecific areas of cat cerebral cortex. *Journal of Neurophysiology, 42*, 107–122.

Jay, M. F., & Sparks, D. L. (1987). Sensorimotor integration in the primate superior colliculus: II. Coordinates of auditory signals. *Journal of Neurophysiology, 57*, 35–55.

Jiang, W., Jiang, H., & Stein, B. E. (2002). Two corticotectal areas facilitate multisensory orientation behavior. *Journal of Cognitive Neuroscience, 14*, 1240–1255.

Jiang, H., Lepore, F., Ptito, M., & Guillemot, J.-P. (1994a). Sensory modality distribution in the anterior ectosylvian cortex (AEC). *Experimental Brain Research, 97*, 404–414.

Jiang, H., Lepore, F., Ptito, M., & Guillemot, J.-P. (1994b). Sensory interactions in the anterior ectosylvian cortex of cats. *Experimental Brain Research, 101*, 385–396.

Jiang, W., & Stein, B. E. (2001). Multisensory maturation in cat superior colliculus after early ablation of anterior ectosylvian and rostral lateral suprasylvian cortex. *Society of Neuroscience Abstracts, 31*, 511.5.

Jiang, W., & Stein, B. E. (2003). Cortex controls multisensory depression in superior colliculus. *Journal of Neurophysiology, 90*, 2123–2135.

Jiang, W., Wallace, M. T., Jiang, H., Vaughan, J. W., & Stein, B. E. (2001). Two cortical areas mediate multisensory integration in superior colliculus neurons. *Journal of Neurophysiology, 85*, 506–522.

Kadunce, D. C., Vaughan, J. W., Wallace, M. T., Benedek, G., & Stein, B. E. (1997). Mechanisms of within-modality and cross-modality suppression in the superior colliculus. *Journal of Neurophysiology, 78*, 2834–2847.

King, A. J., Hutchings, M. E., Moore, D. R., & Blakemore, C. (1988). Developmental plasticity in the visual and auditory representations in the mammalian superior colliculus. *Nature, 332*, 73–76.

King, A. J., & Palmer, A. R. (1985). Integration of visual and auditory information in bimodal neurones in the guinea-pig superior colliculus. *Experimental Brain Research, 60*, 492–500.

Knudsen, E. I. (1982). Auditory and visual maps of space in the optic tectum of the owl. *Journal of Neuroscience, 2*, 1177–1194.

Knudsen, E. I., & Brainard, M. S. (1991). Visual instruction of the neural map of auditory space in the developing optic tectum. *Science, 253*, 85–87.

Kujala, T., Alho, K., Paavilainen, P., Summala, H., & Naatanen, R. (1992). Neural plasticity in processing of sound location by the early blind: An event-related potential study, *Electroencephraphy and Clinical Neurophysiology, 84*, 469–472.

Kuypers, H. G. J. M., & Lawrence, D. G. (1967). Cortical projections to the red nucleus and the brain stem in the rhesus monkey. *Brain Research, 4*, 151–188.

Lee, C., Rohrer, W., & Sparks, D. L. (1987). Effects of focal inactivation of superior colliculus on saccades: Support for the hypothesis of vector averaging of neuronal population response. *Society of Neuroscience Abstracts, 13*, 394.

Lee, C. S., Chung, S., Kim, J., & Park, J. (1991). Auditory facilitation of visually guided saccades. *Society of Neuroscience Abstracts, 17*, 862.

Lomber, S. G., Payne, B. R., & Horel, J. A. (1999). The cryoloop: An adaptable reversible cooling deactivation method for behavioral or electrophysiological assessment of neural function. *Journal of Neuroscience Methods, 86*, 179–194.

McHaffie, J. G., Kao, C.-Q., & Stein, B. E. (1989). Nociceptive neurons in rat superior colliculus: Response properties, topography, and functional implications. *Journal of Neurophysiology, 62*, 510–525.

McHaffie, J. G., Kruger, L., Clemo, H. R., & Stein, B. E. (1988). Corticothalamic and corticotectal somatosensory projections from the anterior ectosylvian sulcus (SIV cortex) in neonatal cats: An anatomical demonstration with HRP and ^{3}H-leucine. *Journal of Comparative Neurology, 274*, 115–126.

Meredith, M. A., & Clemo, H. R. (1989). Auditory cortical projection from the anterior ectosylvian sulcus (Field AES) to the superior colliculus in the cat: An anatomical and electrophysiological study. *Journal of Comparative Neurology, 289*, 687–707.

Meredith, M. A., Nemitz, J. W., & Stein, B. E. (1987). Determinants of multisensory integration in superior colliculus neurons: I. Temporal factors. *Journal of Neuroscience, 10*, 3215–3229.

Meredith, M. A., & Stein, B. E. (1983). Interactions among converging sensory inputs in the superior colliculus. *Science, 221*, 289–291.

Meredith, M. A., & Stein, B. E. (1985). Descending efferents from the superior colliculus relay integrated multisensory information. *Science, 227*, 657–659.

Meredith, M. A., & Stein, B. E. (1986). Visual, auditory, and somatosensory convergence on cells in superior colliculus results in multisensory integration. *Journal of Neurophysiology, 56*, 640–662.

Meredith, M. A., & Stein, B. E. (1996). Spatial determinants of multisensory integration in cat superior colliculus neurons. *Journal of Neurophysiology, 75*, 1843–1857.

Meredith, M. A., Wallace, M. T., & Stein, B. E. (1992). Visual, auditory and somatosensory convergence in output neurons of the cat superior colliculus: Multisensory properties of the tecto-reticulo-spinal projection. *Experimental Brain Research, 88*, 181–186.

Middlebrooks, J. C., & Knudsen, E. I. (1984). A neural code for auditory space in the cat's superior colliculus. *Journal of Neuroscience, 4*, 2621–2634.

Moschovakis, A. K., & Karabelas, A. B. (1985). Observations on the somatodendritic morphology and axonal trajectory of intracellularly HRP-labeled efferent neurons located in the deeper layers of the superior colliculus of the cat. *Journal of Comparative Neurology, 239*, 276–308.

Movshon, J. A., Thompson, I. D., & Tolhurst, D. J. (1978). Spatial summation in the receptive fields of simple cells in the cat's striate cortex. *Journal of Physiology, 283*, 53–77.

Mucke, L., Norita, M., Benedek, G., & Creutzfeldt, O. (1982). Physiologic and anatomic investigation of a visual cortical area situated in the ventral bank of the anterior ectosylvian sulcus of the cat. *Experimental Brain Research, 46*, 1–11.

Munoz, D. P., & Guitton, D. (1991). Control of orienting gaze shifts by the tectoreticulospinal system in the head-free cat: II. Sustained discharges during motor preparation and fixation. *Journal of Neurophysiology, 66*, 1624–1641.

Munoz, D. P., Guitton, D., & Pelisson, D. (1991). Control of orienting gaze shifts by the tectoreticulospinal system in the head-free cat: III. Spatiotemporal characteristics of phasic motor discharges. *Journal of Neurophysiology, 66*, 1642–1666.

Nozawa, G., Reuter-Lorenz, P. A., & Hughes, H. C. (1994). Parallel and serial processes in the human oculomotor system: Bimodal integration and express saccades. *Biological Cybernetics, 72,* 19–34.

Ogasawara, K., McHaffie, J. G., & Stein, B. E. (1984). Two visual systems in cat. *Journal of Neurophysiology, 52,* 1226–1245.

Olberg, R. M., & Willis, M. A. (1990). Pheromone-modulated optomotor response in male gypsy moths, *Lymantria dispar:* I. Direction selective visual interneurons in the ventral nerve cord. *Journal of Comparative Physiology, 167,* 707–714.

Olson, C. R., & Graybiel, A. M. (1987). Ectosylvian visual area of the cat: Location, retinotopic organization, and connections. *Journal of Comparative Neurology, 261,* 277–294.

Ottes, F. P., Van Gisbergen, J. A. M., & Eggermont, J. (1986). Visuomotor fields of the superior colliculus: A quantitative model. *Vision Research, 26,* 857–873.

Pena, J. L., & Konishi, M. (2001). Auditory spatial receptive fields created by multiplication. *Science, 292,* 249–252.

Penfield, W., & Boldrey, E. (1937). Somatic motor and sensory representation in the cerebral cortex of man as studied by electrical stimulation. *Brain, 60,* 389–443.

Penfield, W., & Rasmussen, T. (1952). *The cerebral cortex of man.* New York: Macmillan.

Perrott, D. R., Saberi, K., Brown, K., & Strybel, T. A. (1990). Auditory psychomotor coordination and visual search performance. *Perception & Psychophysics, 48,* 214–226.

Quessy, S., Sweatt, A., Stein, B. E., & Stanford, T. R. (2000). The influence of stimulus intensity and timing on the responses of neurons in the superior colliculus: Comparison to a model's prediction. *Society of Neuroscience Abstracts, 26,* 1221.

Rauschecker, J. P. (1995). Compensatory plasticity and sensory substitution in the cerebral cortex. *Trends in Neurosciences, 18,* 36–43.

Rauschecker, J. P. (1999). Auditory cortical plasticity: A comparison with other sensory systems. *Trends in Neurosciences, 22,* 74–80.

Redgrave, P., Mitchell, I. J., & Dean, P. (1987). Descending projections from superior colliculus in rat: A study using orthograde transport of wheat germ-agglutinin conjugated horseradish peroxidase. *Experimental Brain Research, 68,* 147–167.

Redgrave, P., Odekunle, A., & Dean, P. (1986). Tectal cells of origin of predorsal bundle in rat: Location and segregation from ipsilateral descending pathway. *Experimental Brain Research, 63,* 279–293.

Scannell, J. W., Blakemore, C., & Young, M. P. (1995). Analysis of connectivity in the cat cerebral cortex. *Journal of Neuroscience, 15,* 1463–1483.

Schmahmann, J. D., & Pandya, D. N. (1989). Anatomical investigation of projections to the basis pontis from posterior parietal association cortices in rhesus monkey. *Journal of Comparative Neurology, 289,* 53–73.

Schneider, G. E. (1967). Contrasing visuomotor function of tectum and cortex in the golden hamster. *Psychologische Forschungen, 31,* 52–62.

Segal, R. L., & Beckstead, R. M. (1984). The lateral suprasylvian corticotectal projection in cats. *Journal of Comparative Neurology, 225,* 259–275.

Sparks, D. L. (1986). Translation of sensory signals into commands for control of saccadic eye movements: Role of primate superior colliculus. *Physiology Reviews, 66,* 118–171.

Sparks, D. L., & Nelson, J. S. (1987). Sensory and motor maps in the mammalian superior colliculus. *Trends in Neurosciences, 10,* 312–317.

Spence, C., & Driver, J. (1997). Audiovisual links in oxogenous covert spatial orienting. *Perception & Psychophysics, 59,* 1–22.

Sprague, J. M., & Meikle, T. H., Jr. (1965). The role of the superior colliculus in visually guided behavior. *Experimental Neurology, 11,* 115–146.

Stein, B. E., & Gaither, N. (1981). Sensory representation in reptilian optic tectum: Some comparisons with mammals. *Journal of Comparative Neurology, 202,* 69–87.

Stein, B. E., Goldberg, S. J., & Clamann, H. P. (1976). The control of eye movements by the superior colliculus in the alert cat. *Brain Research, 118,* 469–474.

Stein, B. E., Huneycutt, W. S., & Meredith, M. A. (1988). Neurons and behavior: The same rules of multisensory integration apply. *Brain Research, 448,* 355–358.

Stein, B. E., Magalhaes-Castro, B., & Kruger, L. (1976). Relationship between visual and tactile representation in cat superior colliculus. *Journal of Neurophysiology, 39,* 401–419.

Stein, B. E., & Meredith, M. A. (1991). Functional organization of the superior colliculus. In A. G. Leventhal (Ed.), *The neural bases of visual function* (pp. 85–110). Hampshire, England: Macmillan.

Stein, B. E., & Meredith, M. A. (1993). *The merging of the senses.* Cambridge, MA: MIT Press.

Stein, B. E., Meredith, M. A., Huneycutt, W. S., & McDade, L. (1989). Behavioral indices of multisensory integration: Orientation to visual cues is affected by auditory stimuli. *Journal of Cognitive Neuroscience, 1,* 12–24.

Stein, B. E., Meredith, M. A., & Wallace, M. T. (1993). Nonvisual responses of visually-responsive neurons. In T. P. Hicks, S. Molotchnikoff, & T. Ono (Eds.), *Progress in brain research: The visually responsive neurons: From basic neurophysiology to behavior* (pp. 79–90). Amsterdam: Elsevier.

Stein, B. E., Spencer, R. F., & Edwards, S. B. (1983). Corticotectal and corticothalamic efferent projections of SIV somatosensory cortex in cat. *Journal of Neurophysiology, 50,* 896–909.

Stuphorn, V., Bauswein, E., & Hoffmann, E. P. (2000). Neurons in the primate superior colliculus coding for arm movement in gaze-related coordinates. *Journal of Neurophysiology, 83,* 1283–1299.

Toldi, J., & Feher, O. (1984). Acoustic sensitivity and bimodal properties of cells in the anterior suprasylvian gyrus of the cat. *Experimental Brain Research, 55,* 180–183.

Toldi, J., Rojik, I., & Feher, O. (1981). Two different polysensory systems in the suprasylvian gyrus of the cat: An electrophysiological and autoreadiographic study. *Neuroscience, 6,* 2539–2545.

Van Essen, D. C., Felleman, D. J., DeYoe, J., Olavarria, J., & Knierim, J. (1990). Organisation of extrastriate visual cortex in the macaque monkey. *Cold Spring Harbor Symposia on Quantitative Biology, 55,* 679–696.

Van Gisbergen, J. A. M., Van Opstal, A. J., & Tax, A. A. M. (1987). Collicular ensemble coding of saccades based on vector summation. *Neuroscience, 21,* 541–555.

Wallace, M. T., McHaffie, J. G., & Stein, B. E. (1997). Visual response properties and visuotopic representation in the newborn monkty superior colliculus. *Journal of Neurophysiology, 78,* 2732–2741.

Wallace, M. T., Meredith, M. A., & Stein, B. E. (1992). The integration of multiple sensory inputs in cat cortex. *Experimental Brain Research, 91,* 484–488.

Wallace, M. T., Meredith, M. A., & Stein, B. E. (1993). Converging influences from visual, auditory, and somatosensory cortices onto output neurons of the superior colliculus. *Journal of Neurophysiology, 69*, 1797–1809.

Wallace, M. T., & Stein, B. E. (1994). Cross-modal synthesis in the midbrain depends on input from cortex. *Journal of Neurophysiology, 71*, 429–432.

Wallace, M. T., & Stein, B. E. (1996). Sensory organization of the superior colliculus in cat and monkey. *Progress in Brain Research, 112*, 301–311.

Wallace, M. T., & Stein, B. E. (2000). The role of experience in the development of multisensory integration. *Society of Neuroscience Abstracts, 26*, 1220.

Wallace, M. T., Wilkinson, L. K., & Stein, B. E. (1996). Representation and integration of multiple sensory inputs in primate superior colliculus. *Journal of Neurophysiology, 76*, 1246–1266.

Watanabe, J., & Iwai, E. (1991). Neuronal activity in visual, auditory and polysensory areas of the monkey temporal cortex during visual fixation task. *Brain Research Bulletin, 26*, 583–592.

Wickelgren, B. G., & Sterling, P. (1969). Influence of visual cortex on receptive fields in the superior colliculus of the cat. *Journal of Neurophysiology, 32*, 16–23.

Wilkinson, L. K., Meredith, M. A., & Stein, B. E. (1996). The role of anterior ectosylvian cortex in cross-modality orientation and approach behavior. *Experimental Brain Research, 112*, 1–10.

Yaka, R., Yinon, U., & Wollberg, Z. (1999). Auditory activation of cortical visual areas in cats after early visual deprivation. *European Journal of Neuroscience, 11*, 1301–1312.

Yao, L., & Peck, C. K. (1997). Saccadic eye movements to visual and auditory targets. *Experimental Brain Research, 115*, 25–34.

Yin, T. C., & Chan, J. C. (1990). Interaural time sensitivity in medial superior olive of cat. *Journal of Neurophysiology, 64*, 465–488.

Zahn, J. R., Abel, L. A., & Dell'Osso, L. F. (1978). Audio-ocular response characteristics. *Sensory Processes, 2*, 32–37.

16 Analysis and Modeling of Multisensory Enhancement in the Deep Superior Colliculus

THOMAS J. ANASTASIO AND PAUL E. PATTON

Introduction

When you want to get your friend's attention at a distance you don't just wave your arms. You don't just shout her name, either, but you do both at the same time. Why? Because you know that your friend will be more likely to detect you if you try to alert more than one of her senses to your presence. Many areas of her brain are involved in detecting and orienting toward you. A pivotal region is located in the midbrain and comprises the deep layers of the superior colliculus.

The deep superior colliculus (DSC) is neurophysiologically and connectionally distinct from the superficial colliculus and comprises the cytoarchitectually distinct intermediate and deep layers (Sparks & Hartwich-Young, 1989). The DSC integrates multisensory input and initiates orienting movements toward the source of stimulation (Stein & Meredith, 1993). Various brain regions involved in visual, auditory, and somatosensory processing provide input to the DSC (Cadusseau & Roger, 1985; Edwards, Ginsburgh, Henkel, & Stein, 1979; Harting, Updyke, & Van Lieshout, 1992; Sparks & Hartwich-Young, 1989). Depending on species, orienting movements produced by the DSC can include saccadic eye movements, head movements, and even whole body movements (monkey: Freedman, Stanford, & Sparks, 1996; Robinson, 1972; Schiller & Stryker, 1972; Stryker & Schiller, 1975; cat: Guitton, Crommelinck, & Roucoux, 1980; Harris, 1980; Paré, Crommelinck, & Guitton, 1994; Roucoux, Guitton, & Crommelinck, 1980; rodent: Sahibzada, Dean, & Redgrave, 1986; toad: Ewert, 1970).

The DSC is organized topographically, so that neurons that are neighbors in the DSC have receptive field centers that are neighbors in the environment (auditory: Middlebrooks & Knudsen, 1984; visual: Meredith & Stein, 1990; somatosensory: Meredith, Clemo, & Stein, 1991). Sensory maps for different modalities are roughly in register in the DSC. Central to analysis of multisensory integration in the DSC is the fact that individual neurons can receive input of more than one sensory modality (Meredith & Stein, 1983, 1985, 1986b; Meredith, Wallace, & Stein, 1992; Stein & Arigbede, 1972; Stein, Magalhaes-Castro, & Kruger, 1976; Wallace, Meredith, & Stein, 1998; Wallace & Stein, 1996; Wallace, Wilkinson, & Stein, 1996). A multisensory DSC neuron has a receptive field for each sensory modality it receives, and these receptive fields overlap (Gordon, 1973; Kadunce, Vaughan, Wallace, & Stein, 2001; Meredith & Stein, 1996; Wickelgren, 1971). Thus, multisensory integration in the DSC can take place on individual neurons.

Multisensory integration in the DSC is of two basic types: enhancement and depression (King & Palmer, 1985; Meredith & Stein, 1983, 1986a, 1986b; Wallace et al., 1996, 1998). They are defined as the augmentation and diminution, respectively, of the response of a neuron to a stimulus of one modality by the presentation of a second stimulus of a different modality. Multisensory interactions depend on the spatial and temporal relationships between the stimuli (Kadunce et al., 2001; Meredith, Nemitz, & Stein, 1987; Meredith & Stein, 1986a, 1996). Stimuli that occur at the same time and place may produce enhancement, while stimuli that occur at different times or places may produce depression. Multisensory depression may result from competitive interactions occurring within the DSC (Findlay & Walker, 1999; Munoz & Istvan, 1998). Multisensory enhancement (MSE) may improve the ability of an organism to detect targets in the environment (Stein, Huneycutt, & Meredith, 1988; Stein, Meredith, Huneycutt, & McDade, 1989; Wilkinson, Meredith, & Stein, 1996). This chapter describes the analysis and modeling of MSE.

Percent MSE ($\%MSE$) has been quantified using the following formula (Meredith & Stein, 1986b):

$$\%MSE = \left(\frac{CM - MS_{Max}}{MS_{Max}} \right) \times 100\% \qquad (1)$$

where *CM* is the number of neural impulses evoked by cross-modal stimulation and MS_{Max} is the number of impulses evoked when the more effective of two modality-specific stimuli is presented alone. Percent MSE can range upward of 1000% (Meredith & Stein, 1986b), but it is dependent on the magnitudes of the modality-specific responses. By the property known as inverse effectiveness, smaller modality-specific responses are associated with larger *%MSE* (Meredith & Stein, 1986b; Wallace & Stein, 1994). Despite the enhanced responsiveness provided by MSE, not all DSC neurons are multisensory. About 46% of DSC neurons in cat and 73% in monkey are unimodal, receiving sensory input of only one modality (Wallace & Stein, 1996). These findings raise intriguing questions.

Neurons in the DSC do more than simply respond to the larger of their cross-modal inputs. They exhibit MSE, which produces enhanced responses that may even be larger than the sum of their responses to the two modality-specific inputs presented alone. What, then, is the functional role of MSE? If an enhanced response is important for signal processing in the DSC, then why is MSE magnitude-dependent? If MSE enhances the responsiveness of DSC neurons, then why are not all DSC neurons multisensory? This chapter introduces our analytical and modeling research, based on probability and information theory, that attempts to answer these questions. Our model, based on Bayes' rule, suggests a functional role for MSE and provides a possible explanation for inverse effectiveness (Anastasio, Patton, & Belkacem-Boussaid, 2000). An experimentally testable prediction can be derived from the Bayes' rule model, which we will illustrate. We also present an information theoretic analysis of the model that offers a possible explanation for why some DSC neurons are multisensory but others are not (Patton, Belkacem-Boussaid, & Anastasio, 2002). This modeling work opens up a new perspective on the phenomenon of MSE.

Bayes' rule model of multisensory enhancement

The job of the DSC is to detect the sources of sensory stimulation in the environment and make them the targets of orienting movements (Sparks & Hartwich-Young, 1989; Stein & Meredith, 1993; Wurtz & Goldberg, 1989). The DSC, like the brain in general, obtains information about the environment from the sensory systems. Being neural, the sensory systems are inherently noisy, and the input they provide is to some extent uncertain. For this reason the sensory systems cannot provide a deterministic, yes/no signal to an individual DSC neuron concerning whether or not a target has appeared in its receptive field. Instead, we postulate that an individual DSC neuron computes the conditional probability that a target is present in its receptive field, given its uncertain sensory input. We model the computation of this probability using Bayes' rule (Appelbaum, 1996; Duda, Hart, & Stork, 2001; Helstrom, 1984).

The Bayes' rule model of MSE is schematized in Figure 16.1. The figure shows a multisensory DSC neuron that receives visual and auditory input, but the model generalizes to any other input combination. The Bayes' rule model is valid for any number of stimulus modalities. To introduce the idea, we begin with the simplest case, that of a unimodal DSC neuron that receives a single, modality-specific input.

BAYES' RULE FOR A UNIMODAL NEURON   We start by assuming that a DSC neuron simply detects the presence or absence of a target, without regard for target identity. Indeed, the identity of a target may be determined only after an orienting movement, initiated by the DSC, has been made toward it. It is possible that target detection in the DSC can be influenced by different expectations for targets in specific regions of the environment. However, the function of the DSC is to detect and initiate orienting movements toward targets, defined broadly as stimulus sources in the environment, while

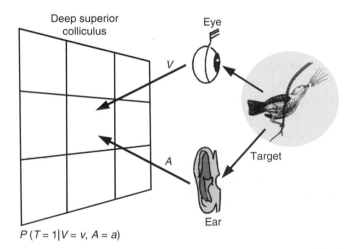

$P(T = 1 | V = v, A = a)$

FIGURE 16.1   Schematic diagram illustrating multisensory integration in the deep superior colliculus (DSC). DSC neurons, represented as blocks on a grid, are organized topographically according to the location in space of their receptive fields. Individual DSC neurons can receive sensory input of more than one modality, and their receptive fields for the different modalities overlap. The binary random variable *T* represents the target. $P(T = 1 | V = v, A = a)$ is the bimodal probability that the target is present, given cross-modal sensory inputs *V* and *A* (Equation 5). The bird image is from Stein and Meredith (1993).

the detailed examination and identification of targets is left to other brain areas.

We model the target as binary random variable T, where $T = 1$ when the target is present and $T = 0$ when the target is absent. The expectation, or prior probability, that a target will be present in the receptive field of a DSC neuron is $P(T = 1)$. The target prior is a function of the environment and of the size and location of the receptive field of each individual DSC neuron. To simplify the initial presentation of the model, we assume that the target prior is the same for all DSC neurons. We further assume that the target is more often absent than present in the receptive field or fields of any DSC neuron, and we arbitrarily assign $P(T = 1) = 0.1$ and $P(T = 0) = 0.9$ for any given DSC neuron. This simply means that, in the absence of any sensory input from the environment, we expect there is a 10% chance that a target is currently present within the receptive field of the DSC neuron in question. Bayes' rule specifies how the expectation of a target can be modified on the basis of sensory input from the environment.

We postulate that an individual DSC neuron computes the conditional probability that a target is present in its receptive field, given its uncertain sensory input. We can consider a unimodal DSC neuron that receives only visual input V. This conditional probability can be computed using the unimodal Bayes' rule model, as follows:

$$P(T = 1 \mid V = v) = \frac{P(V = v \mid T = 1)P(T = 1)}{P(V = v)} \quad (2)$$

Bayes' rule specifies how prior probability $P(T = 1)$ can be modified by sensory input to produce the conditional probability $P(T = 1 \mid V = v)$. The conditional probability $P(T = 1 \mid V = v)$ is the probability that the target is present $(T = 1)$, given that the visual input variable V takes the specific value v ($V = v$). In the context of Bayes' rule, $P(T = 1 \mid V = v)$ is called the posterior probability, because it is the probability of T determined from the prior probability after the input is taken into consideration. The sensory input modifies the prior according to the ratio $P(V = v \mid T = 1)/P(V = v)$. The conditional probability $P(V = v \mid T = 1)$ is the probability of observing some particular visual input $V = v$, given that the target is present. In the context of Bayes' rule, $P(V = v \mid T = 1)$ is called the target-present likelihood that $V = v$. The unconditional probability $P(V = v)$ is the probability of observing visual input $V = v$ whether the target is present or absent. It can be computed using the principle of total probability as:

$$P(V = v) = P(V = v \mid T = 1)P(T = 1)$$
$$+ P(V = v \mid T = 0)P(T = 0) \quad (3)$$

where $P(V = v \mid T = 0)$ is the target-absent likelihood that $V = v$, and $P(T = 0)$ is the target-absent prior. Because the likelihoods and priors are properties of the visual system and the environment, it is likely that the brain can represent them. We propose that the brain can implement a computation analogous to Bayes' rule, and that the response of a DSC neuron is proportional to the posterior probability that a target is present in its receptive field, given its sensory input.

In order to evaluate the unimodal Bayes' rule model in the case of a modality-specific visual input, it is necessary to define the likelihood distributions for V. We model V as a discrete random variable that represents the number of impulses received by a DSC neuron from a visual neuron in one unit of time. The time unit of 250 ms is chosen to roughly match neurophysiological data (Meredith & Stein, 1986b), but the length of the time unit is not critical to the model. We assume that the likelihoods of V are Poisson distributed. Although Bayes' rule is valid for any type of likelihood distribution, the Poisson distribution provides a good first approximation to the numbers of impulses per unit time observed in the spontaneous and driven activity of single neurons (Lestienne, 1996; Munemori, Hara, Kimura, & Sato, 1984; Rieke, Warland, & van Stevenick, 1997; Turcott et al., 1994). The Poisson distribution is parsimonious because it is specified by only one parameter: the mean λ. The Poisson density function for discrete random variable V with mean λ is defined as (Appelbaum, 1996; Helstrom, 1984):

$$P(V = v) = \frac{\lambda^v e^{-\lambda}}{v!} \quad (4)$$

We model the likelihoods of V using two separate Poisson distributions, where the mean λ is higher for the target-present likelihood than for the target-absent likelihood. The target-absent likelihood represents the spontaneous activity of V, while the target-present likelihood represents the activity of V as it is being driven by the sensory attributes of various targets. We make the realistic assumption that the mean number of impulses per unit time will be higher under driven than under spontaneous conditions.

Example likelihood distributions of V are shown in Figure 16.2A. The target-absent (spontaneous) likelihood of V ($P(V = v \mid T = 0)$) has mean $\lambda = 5$, while the target-present (driven) likelihood of V ($P(V = v \mid T = 1)$) has mean $\lambda = 8$. There is overlap between the spontaneous and driven likelihoods of V. Equation 3 shows that the unconditional probability of V is the sum of the likelihoods of V weighted by the priors of T. Since $P(T = 1) < P(T = 0)$, the unconditional probability $P(V = v)$ is roughly equal to the spontaneous likelihood

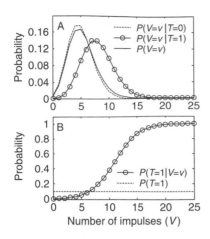

FIGURE 16.2 (A) Sensory input likelihood distributions. Binary random variable T denotes the target. The prior probability is 0.9 that the target is absent ($P(T = 0) = 0.9$) and 0.1 that it is present ($P(T = 1) = 0.1$). Discrete random variable V represents the number of impulses arriving at a DSC neuron from a visual input neuron in a unit time interval (250 ms). It varies over the range from 0 to 25 impulses per unit time. The spontaneous likelihood of V ($P(V = v \mid T = 0)$, dashed line) is given by a Poisson distribution (Equation 4) with mean $\lambda = 5$. The driven likelihood of V ($P(V = v \mid T = 1)$, line with circles) is given by a Poisson distribution with mean $\lambda = 8$. The unconditional likelihood of V ($P(V = v)$, line with no symbols) is computed from the target prior and input likelihood distributions using Equation 3. (B) The unimodal target-present posterior probability, given modality-specific input V. The unimodal target posterior ($P(T = 1 \mid V = v)$, line with circles) is computed using Equation 2 with prior and likelihood distributions as defined in A. Also shown for comparison is the target-present prior probability ($P(T = 1)$, dashed line).

$P(V = v \mid T = 0)$. With the priors of T and the likelihoods of V now defined, the unimodal Bayes' rule model for a single modality-specific input (Equation 2) can be evaluated.

We evaluate the unimodal Bayes' rule model in the case of a single modality-specific input by taking values of v in the range from 0 to 25 impulses per unit time. For each value of v, the driven likelihood $P(V = v \mid T = 1)$ and the unconditional probability $P(V = v)$ are read off the curves previously defined (Fig. 16.2A). The posterior probability $P(T = 1 \mid V = v)$ is computed using Equation 2 and plotted in Figure 16.2B. The prior probability $P(T = 1) = 0.1$ is also plotted for comparison. For the Poisson means chosen, the posterior probability exceeds the prior probability when $v \geqslant 7$. The reason the transition occurs there is that, when $v \geqslant 7$, the driven likelihood of V exceeds the unconditional probability of V (Fig. 16.2A). This provides a graphic illustration of how Bayes' rule uses modality-specific sensory input to modify the target-present prior in order to compute the unimodal posterior probability that a target is present.

As mentioned earlier, the unconditional probability distribution of V is similar to the spontaneous likelihood of V (Fig. 16.2A). This allows the following rough description of the computation being performed by Bayes' rule. As the visual input v increases, it changes from being most likely spontaneous to most likely driven by the target. Correspondingly, the target changes from probably absent to probably present. Thus, Bayes' rule essentially evaluates any sensory input according to its spontaneous and driven likelihoods to determine how it should modify the prior in forming the posterior probability of the target. We suggest that the sigmoid curve describing the target-present posterior probability given modality-specific input V (Fig. 16.2B) is proportional to the response of a unimodal DSC neuron.

BAYES' RULE FOR A MULTISENSORY NEURON The Bayes' rule model can be extended to a bimodal case involving visual input V and auditory input A. We model A as a discrete random variable that represents the number of impulses received by a DSC neuron from an auditory neuron in unit time. As for V, we model the likelihoods of A using two separate Poisson distributions, where the mean λ is higher for the target-present likelihood than for the target-absent likelihood. The posterior probability of the target in the bimodal case can be computed as in the unimodal case, but now the input is the conjunction of V and A. The bimodal target-present posterior can be computed using the bimodal Bayes' rule model as follows:

$$P(T = 1 \mid V = v, A = a)$$
$$= \frac{P(V = v, A = a \mid T = 1)P(T = 1)}{P(V = v, A = a)} \tag{5}$$

To simplify the analysis, we assume that V and A are conditionally independent given the target. This implies that the visibility of the target indicates nothing about the audibility of the target, and vice versa. This assumption corresponds to experimental paradigms in which the sensory attributes of targets are manipulated independently of one another (King & Palmer, 1985; Meredith & Stein, 1986a, 1986b; Meredith et al., 1987; Wallace et al., 1996, 1998). Bayes' rule is valid whether the inputs are conditionally independent or not. Assuming that they are independent, the joint likelihoods of V and A can be computed as the products of the corresponding individual likelihoods of V and A. For the target-present case:

$$P(V = v, A = a \mid T = 1)$$
$$= P(V = v \mid T = 1)P(A = a \mid T = 1) \tag{6}$$

On the same assumption, the unconditional probability of V and A can be computed directly from the individual likelihoods using the principle of total probability:

$$P(V = v, A = a)$$
$$= P(V = v \mid T = 1)P(A = a \mid T = 1)P(T = 1)$$
$$+ P(V = v \mid T = 0)P(A = a \mid T = 0)P(T = 0) \quad (7)$$

The Bayes' rule model in the bimodal case can be evaluated after the likelihoods of A have been defined. We suggest that the response of a bimodal DSC neuron is proportional to the posterior probability that a target is present in its receptive fields, given its cross-modal input.

We begin by considering a hypothetical case in which both V and A have the same likelihood distributions. This simplifies comparison between the bimodal and unimodal versions of the Bayes' rule model. We set the spontaneous means for both V and A to $\lambda = 5$, and the driven means for both V and A to $\lambda = 8$. We evaluate the bimodal Bayes' rule model in the cross-modal case (Equation 5) by taking values of v and a as they increase over the range from 0 to 25 impulses per unit time. To further simplify the comparison, we consider a hypothetical cross-modal case in which v and a are equal. The results are qualitatively similar when v and a are unequal, as long as they both increase together. For each value of v and a, the individual likelihoods can be read off the corresponding Poisson distributions as defined, and the joint conditional likelihoods and unconditional probabilities can be computed using Equations 6 and 7. The bimodal posterior probability $P(T = 1 \mid V = v, A = a)$ in the cross-modal case (v and a, where $v = a$) is then calculated using Equation 5, and the results are plotted in Figure 16.3A. The unimodal posterior probability $P(T = 1 \mid V = v)$ for modality-specific input v, computed using Equation 2, is shown for comparison.

The bimodal and unimodal probabilities (Fig. 16.3A) are similar in that they both rise sigmoidally from 0 to 1, indicating that the target changes from probably absent to probably present as the input increases. However, the bimodal curve rises faster than the unimodal curve. This indicates, over a broad range of input levels, that the target-present posterior probability is higher given sensory inputs of two modalities than it is given input of only one modality. This difference results because a DSC neuron receives more evidence that the target is present in the bimodal than in the unimodal case. Although later informational analysis will place limits on this intuitive picture, the comparison between the bimodal and unimodal cases illustrates the potential usefulness of cross-modal input for computing target-present posterior probabilities.

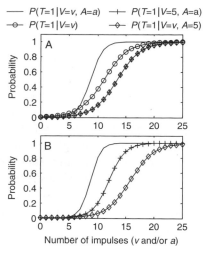

FIGURE 16.3 (A) Bimodal target-present posterior probabilities computed in modality-specific and cross-modal cases. The likelihoods of visual (V) and auditory (A) input are modeled using Poisson distributions (Equation 4). The target prior probability distribution is defined in Figure 16.2. The spontaneous and driven likelihood means are set to $\lambda = 5$ and $\lambda = 8$, respectively, for both V and A. The bimodal target posterior for the cross-modal case, where both modalities are driven by the stimulus (both driven; $P(T = 1 \mid V = v, A = a)$, line with no symbols), is computed using Equation 5. Also shown is the bimodal target posterior for the modality-specific case, where one modality is held fixed at the spontaneous mean while the other is driven by the stimulus (spontaneous-driven; $P(T = 1 \mid V = 5, A = a)$, line with diamonds; $P(T = 1 \mid V = v, A = 5)$, line with crosses; note that these two lines coincide). The unimodal target posterior in the modality-specific case ($P(T = 1 \mid V = v)$, line with circles) from Figure 16.2B is replotted here for comparison. (B) Bimodal target-present posterior probability computed for a cross-modal case in which the driven means of the two input likelihood distributions (Equation 4) are unequal. The spontaneous likelihood mean is set to $\lambda = 5$ for both V and A. The driven likelihood mean is set to $\lambda = 10$ for V and $\lambda = 8$ for A. The target prior probability distribution is defined in Figure 16.2. The cross-modal ($P(T = 1 \mid V = v, A = a)$, line with no symbols) and the two modality-specific ($P(T = 1 \mid V = 5, A = a)$, line with diamonds; $P(T = 1 \mid V = v, A = 5)$, line with crosses) bimodal posterior probability curves are computed using Equation 5.

In order to explore MSE using the Bayes' rule model, we must consider bimodal posterior probabilities not only when both input modalities are driven by sensory stimulation but also when only one input is driven while the other is spontaneous. In the cross-modal case already considered, both v and a vary together over the range. To model the modality-specific case, in which sensory stimulation of only one modality is available, we allow v or a to vary over the range while we fix the other input at the mean of its spontaneous likelihood distribution. Modality-specific bimodal posterior probabilities are computed for an example in which both V and A have the same spontaneous and driven likelihood means of $\lambda = 5$ and $\lambda = 8$, respectively. The resulting bimodal posterior probabilities in the modality-specific case are plotted in Figure 16.3A. Because the likelihoods for V and A are the same, the modality-specific bimodal posteriors with V driven and A spontaneous ($P(T = 1 \mid V = v, A = 5)$) and with A driven and V spontaneous ($P(T = 1 \mid V = 5, A = a)$) are identical. The cross-modal bimodal posterior ($P(T = 1 \mid V = v, A = a)$), and the modality-specific unimodal posterior ($P(T = 1 \mid V = v)$) are also shown in Figure 16.3A. A comparison among these probability curves illustrates the difference between modality-specific unimodal, modality-specific bimodal, and cross-modal bimodal target-present posterior probabilities.

As previously noted, the cross-modal bimodal posterior is greater than the modality-specific unimodal posterior probability over a broad range of input. In contrast, the modality-specific bimodal posterior is less than the modality-specific unimodal posterior probability over the same input range. The relationship among these posterior probabilities makes intuitive sense. When the target drives both inputs, then the evidence on both input channels agrees, and the cross-modal bimodal posterior can be greater than the modality-specific unimodal posterior. Conversely, when the target drives one input but not the other, then the evidence supplied by the two input channels is discrepant, and the modality-specific bimodal posterior can be less than the modality-specific unimodal posterior. For the same reasons, there is a broad range of input over which the bimodal posterior is higher under cross-modal than under modality-specific conditions. This difference corresponds to MSE.

In general, the statistical properties of individual inputs to a multisensory DSC neuron will differ. To illustrate the effect on bimodal posteriors of having different likelihoods for V and A, we increase the driven mean for V from $\lambda = 8$ to $\lambda = 10$. The other likelihood means are kept as they were in the previous example. Note that now the difference between the spontaneous and driven means is larger for V than for A. The bimodal posteriors for the case of different driven means is qualitatively similar to the previous case of equal driven means, except that the two modality-specific probability curves differ. The cross-modal and the two modality-specific bimodal posteriors are computed using Equation 5 and plotted in Figure 16.3B.

The modality-specific bimodal probability curve with V driven and A spontaneous ($P(T = 1 \mid V = v, A = 5)$) rises faster than the modality-specific bimodal posterior probability curve with A driven and V spontaneous ($P(T = 1 \mid V = 5, A = a)$). This is a consequence of the fact that the separation between the spontaneous and

driven likelihood means is larger for V than for A. The cross-modal bimodal posterior probability curve ($P(T = 1 \mid V = v, A = a)$) rises faster than either of the modality-specific curves. There are input levels for which the cross-modal probability is almost one while the modality-specific probabilities are almost zero. If these bimodal posterior probabilities are regarded as proportional to the responses of multisensory DSC neurons, then the predominance of the cross-modal posterior over the modality-specific posteriors corresponds to MSE.

The bimodal posterior probability curves in Figure 16.3B can be used to simulate the results of a neurophysiological experiment on multisensory DSC neurons. The experiment involves recording the responses of a multisensory DSC neuron to visual and auditory input delivered separately or together (King & Palmer, 1985; Meredith & Stein, 1986a, 1986b; Meredith et al., 1987; Wallace et al., 1996, 1998). The stimuli are delivered at each of three different levels that, presented separately, evoke minimal, suboptimal, or optimal responses (Meredith & Stein, 1986b). Values of the V and A inputs are chosen that give bimodal posterior probabilities corresponding to minimal (near 0), suboptimal (near 0.5), or optimal (near 1) responses in the modality-specific cases, and the cross-modal posterior probabilities are computed using the same values. The %MSE is calculated using Equation 1, where the cross-modal posterior is substituted for CM and the larger of the two modality-specific posterior probabilities is substituted for MS_{Max}. The results are presented as a bar graph (Fig. 16.4) to facilitate comparison with

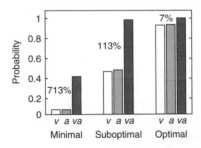

FIGURE 16.4 Graph comparing the modality-specific with the corresponding cross-modal posterior probabilities at three different sensory input levels for the bimodal Bayes' rule model. Target prior and input likelihood distributions are defined in Figures 16.2 and 16.3, respectively. Cross-modal target posteriors (Equation 5) are computed when v and a are both driven (va, black bars; minimal: $v = 8$, $a = 9$; suboptimal: $v = 12$, $a = 15$; optimal: $v = 16$, $a = 21$). Modality-specific target posteriors (Equation 5) are computed when one input takes the driven value (v, white bars; a, gray bars) but the other is fixed at the spontaneous mean $\lambda = 5$. Percentage enhancements (Equation 1) are shown for each of the three input levels.

experimental data. The simulation results using the Bayes' rule model are in qualitative agreement with the experimental data and capture the main features of MSE as observed in the DSC.

The Bayes' rule simulation reproduces both MSE and inverse effectiveness, and in so doing provides a functional interpretation of MSE. That interpretation follows directly from our hypothesis: that the function of a DSC neuron is to compute the probability that a target is present in its receptive fields, given its sensory input. Figure 16.4 illustrates the bimodal Bayes' rule computation for a multisensory DSC neuron receiving visual and auditory input. In the optimal case, either visual or auditory input on its own provides strong evidence of a target, and the target-present posterior probability is already high for modality-specific input. Sensory input of another modality, providing a cross-modal input, cannot greatly increase the already high modality-specific posterior probability. In contrast, in the minimal case, visual or auditory input on its own provides very weak evidence of a target, and the target-present posterior is low for modality-specific input. Sensory input of another modality, even if it is also weak by itself, can greatly increase the posterior probability that a target is present. Thus, the Bayes' rule model can simulate both MSE and inverse effectiveness.

The only free parameters in the model are the likelihood means and target prior probabilities, and available data leave considerable choice in their selection. Given the parameter values and input levels chosen for the example shown in Figure 16.4, %MSE ranges from 7% to 713%, but other %MSE values could be generated given alternative choices. Rather than fit any particular data set, our goal in the example is to show that there is a strong correspondence between the Bayes' rule simulation and the salient features of MSE as observed for the class of multisensory DSC neurons. This agreement provides compelling evidence in favor of the hypothesis that a DSC neuron computes the posterior probability that a target is present in its receptive fields, given its sensory input of one or more modalities. The phenomena of MSE and of inverse effectiveness are precisely what would be expected on the basis of this hypothesis.

Deriving a testable prediction from the Bayes' rule model

The correspondence between Bayes' rule simulation results and findings on MSE provides support for the hypothesis that DSC neurons use sensory input to compute target posterior probabilities (Anastasio et al., 2000). Predictions for directly testing the hypothesis can be derived by relating the parameters of the Bayes' rule model to experimentally observable quantities. Bayes' rule (Equations 2 and 5) computes target posterior probabilities on the basis of input likelihood and target prior distributions. If the input likelihood and target prior distributions for an actual DSC neuron could be accurately described, then the target posterior could be computed analytically. Comparison of the analytically determined posterior with the experimentally observed response of the DSC neuron would provide a direct test of the Bayes' rule model. The feasibility of such a test would depend on the accuracy with which the input likelihood and target prior distributions could be described. Although experimental determination of input likelihood distributions would be extremely difficult, target priors might be more accessible.

Input to a DSC neuron from a sensory system would generally arrive not over a single axon but over many axons. To determine the likelihood distribution for a specific modality using extracellular recording, it would be necessary to record from all of the axons terminating on a single DSC neuron from that sensory system. The major obstacle to this approach is in finding and recording from all of the input axons. Intracellular recording would not offer a way around that obstacle, because the membrane potential would already reflect the synaptic and dendritic processes by which the DSC neuron transforms its input. In contrast to input likelihood, the target prior distribution should depend on factors that are more readily measured.

The target prior should depend primarily on receptive field size and location, and these properties can be determined for DSC neurons. If we assume that targets are uniformly distributed in the environment, then the prior probability that a target will fall within the receptive field of a particular DSC neuron should depend on the size of the receptive field of that neuron. If receptive field size were the only factor, then individual DSC neurons with larger receptive fields should have higher target-present prior probabilities. However, receptive field location might also play an important role in the determination of the target-present prior, due to animal behavioral patterns. Animals generally will orient toward stimulus sources in the environment, bringing peripheral stimuli to more central regions of the sensory field. Thus, animals will tend to concentrate targets centrally. If receptive field location were the only factor, then individual DSC neurons with more central receptive fields should have higher target-present prior probabilities.

The Bayes' rule model predicts that the responses of DSC neurons should vary in a systematic way according to differences among DSC neurons in their target priors. Specifically, the model predicts that multisensory

DSC neurons with higher target priors should show smaller %MSE (see below). The receptive fields of DSC neurons tend to be larger peripherally than centrally (Meredith & Stein, 1990; Meredith et al., 1991; Middlebrooks & Knudsen, 1984). The topographic organization of the DSC is such that receptive field centers move from peripheral to central with movement from the back to the front of the DSC (Meredith & Stein, 1990; Meredith et al., 1991; Middlebrooks & Knudsen, 1984). The model therefore predicts that %MSE should change systematically with movement in the DSC from the back (large, peripheral receptive fields) to the front (small, central receptive fields).

If receptive field size is the predominant factor, then %MSE should increase in moving from back to front. Conversely, if orienting behavior is the predominant factor, then %MSE should decrease in moving from back to front. It is possible that the influence of orienting behavior could offset the effects of receptive field size, in which case Bayes' rule would predict no systematic change in %MSE with location in the DSC. Given some plausible assumptions, a geometric analysis reveals that orienting behavior should outweigh receptive field size in determining the target prior for individual DSC neurons.

POSSIBLE EFFECT OF ORIENTING BEHAVIOR ON TARGET-PRESENT PRIOR PROBABILITIES   The influence of orienting behavior on target prior probability is basic, and it is reasonable to suppose that it might be encoded synaptically at the level of the DSC. The multisensory responses of DSC neurons are often studied in anesthetized animals, and it is possible that the behavioral influence on target prior would remain even under anesthesia. It is also possible that target prior could be further modified by the brain in an on-line fashion, as circumstances dictate. This sort of modification of target prior could be general or more location-specific, but as it would involve conscious appraisal of current circumstances, it is not likely to operate under anesthesia.

The data on MSE were gathered primarily from the anesthetized cat, so the geometric analysis of target prior is based on DSC receptive field sizes in this animal. It focuses on vision and audition, but the principles would apply to any other modality combination. Visual receptive fields vary in diameter from 13.5 degrees to 150.5 degrees in the cat (Meredith & Stein, 1990). Cat auditory receptive field diameters vary from 20 degrees frontally to 130 degrees laterally (Middlebrooks & Knudsen, 1984). Although the auditory field extends the whole 360 degrees around the cat, the entire cat visual field has an azimuthal extent of

only about 140 degrees (Guitton, Douglas, & Volle, 1984). We model the cat's environment as a sphere. The prior probability of a target appearing anywhere in the cat's environment is $P_E(T = 1)$. The target prior for any specific receptive field is computed by comparing the surface area of the whole sphere representing the environment with the surface area of a circular region of the sphere having the same diameter as the receptive field. Using this method, the target prior for a 10-degree diameter receptive field is $1.9 \times 10^{-3} \times P_E(T = 1)$. For a 52-degree receptive field, the target prior is $5.1 \times 10^{-2} \times P_E(T = 1)$. The target prior is 27 times larger for the 52-degree than for the 10-degree receptive field. These calculations illustrate that receptive field size can have a huge influence on target prior probability for individual DSC neurons.

The possible influence of orienting behavior on the target prior for individual DSC neurons can be assessed using a simple model of saccadic undershoot. Human saccades usually undershoot their targets by 10%, and are followed by one or more corrective saccades until the target is fixated (Aitsebaomo & Bedell, 1992; Becker, 1972; Becker & Fuchs, 1969; Carpenter, 1988; Henson, 1978, 1979; Lemij & Collewjin, 1989; Lennie & Sidwell, 1978; Pelisson & Prablanc, 1988; Prablanc, Masse, & Echallier, 1978). Cats make orienting movements of their eyes and head (Evinger & Fuchs, 1978; Guitton et al., 1984; Stryker & Blakemore, 1972) and have been observed to make corrective saccades (Evinger & Fuchs, 1978). Human saccade metrics can be influenced by a variety of cognitive factors (Kowler, 1990; Viviani, 1990), but cognitive processes must play a more limited role in cat saccades.

We will assume that cat saccades also undershoot their targets by 10%, and that cats fixate with accuracy on the order of a few degrees. To assess the effect of orienting behavior on target priors, we divide the cat's environment into three concentric zones of increasing diameter: zone 0, 3.6 degrees; zone 1, 36 degrees; and zone 2, 360 degrees (Fig. 16.5). Targets appearing initially in zones 1 or 2 require one or two saccades to fixate. Targets appearing in central zone 0 are fixated. Targets that require one or more saccades to be brought to fixation are repositioned by those saccades into other zones. Such targets are counted as fresh targets in each of the sequence of zones in which they appear. Thus, every target initially appearing in zone 1 is also counted in zone 0, and every target initially appearing in zone 2 is also counted in zone 1 and zone 0.

The target prior probabilities computed separately for each zone are: zone 2, $0.975 \times P_E(T = 1)$; zone 1, $0.999 \times P_E(T = 1)$; and zone 0, $P_E(T = 1)$. Because

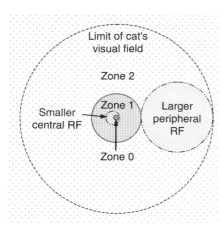

FIGURE 16.5 The sensory surroundings of a cat are divided into three circular zones. The central zone 0 represents the center of fixation of the cat's gaze. Concentric zones represent locations around the cat that require varying numbers of saccades to fixate. Stimuli presented in zone 2 require two saccades. Those in zone 1 require 1 saccade. Those in zone 0 are fixated and require no further saccades. As a very rough estimate, the three zones are assigned diameters as follows: zone 0, 3.6 degrees; zone 1, 36 degrees; zone 2, 360 degrees. The cat's visual field is roughly 140 degrees in azimuthal extent (Guitton et al., 1984). The smaller central receptive field (RF) is 10 degrees in diameter. The larger peripheral RF is 52 degrees in diameter.

orienting behavior concentrates targets centrally, it tends to equalize the target prior in each of the zones, even though zone 0 is much smaller than zone 1 and zone 1 is much smaller than zone 2. Now the effects on target prior of the receptive field size and location of a DSC neuron can both be taken into consideration. This is done by finding the amount of overlap between the receptive field of a particular DSC neuron and each of the three saccade zones, and adding up the target prior contributions from each zone to that receptive field.

A receptive field 10 degrees in diameter and containing the center of the visual field would cover zone 0 and overlap with zone 1 (Fig. 16.5). The target prior for a DSC neuron with this receptive field would be $1.3 \times P_E(T = 1)$. This value is drastically larger than that computed on the basis of receptive field size alone. This value can be compared with the target prior for a receptive field that neither contains zone 0 nor overlaps zone 1. A lateral receptive field of 52 degrees diameter that extends from the border of zone 1 to the edge of the visual field (Fig. 16.5) is the largest visual receptive field that does not overlap zone 1. This receptive field is contained entirely within zone 2. Since orienting behavior shifts targets more centrally, and never into zone 2, the target prior for this receptive field is unaffected by orienting behavior and may be computed

based on receptive field size alone as $5.1 \times 10^{-2} \times P_E(T = 1)$. The important point is that, after taking orienting behavior into consideration, the target prior for the small, central receptive field has switched from much lower to much higher than that for the larger, lateral receptive field.

The Bayes' rule model is sensitive to changes in target prior. To illustrate, we evaluate the bimodal model when inputs V and A both have the same spontaneous mean $\lambda = 4$ and driven mean $\lambda = 9$ impulses per unit time. We assume that $P_E(T = 1)$ is equal to 0.1, as in the computations of the previous sections. Then, for the central, 10-degree receptive field $P(T = 1) = 1.3 \times P_E(T = 1) = 0.13$, and for the peripheral, 52-degree receptive field $P(T = 1) = 5.1 \times 10^{-2} \times P_E(T = 1) = 0.005$. The results of using these priors in the computation of the bimodal target posterior probability and $\%MSE$ are shown in Figure 16.6A and B. The cross-modal and the modality-specific curves rise faster for the central (10 degrees, $P(T = 1) = 0.13$) than for the peripheral (52 degrees, $P(T = 1) = 0.005$) receptive field. However, the difference between the cross-modal and the modality-specific posteriors is much greater for the peripheral than for the central receptive field. This is reflected in the $\%MSE$ values, which are much higher for the peripheral than for the central receptive field. We examined $\%MSE$ as the driven means for V and A were increased together from $\lambda = 5$ to $\lambda = 14$ impulses per unit time (Fig. 16.6C). The plot shows that maximal $\%MSE$ is approximately ten times greater for the peripheral than for the central receptive field over the entire range.

Our initial assessment of the possible influence of orienting behavior on the target prior for individual DSC neurons in the cat is based on simplifying assumptions that need to be verified. Nevertheless, the Bayes' rule model is so sensitive to target prior that even our initial assessment is likely to be qualitatively correct. Our basic prediction is that maximal $\%MSE$ should be inversely correlated with target prior for individual DSC neurons. It is impossible to know a priori how target prior might be represented in the anesthetized brain, although it is likely to vary as a function of eccentricity in the DSC. If, as we assume in the illustration, the influence of orienting behavior on the target prior is coded synaptically at the level of the DSC, then we predict that maximal $\%MSE$ should be larger peripherally than centrally. On the other hand, if target prior is a function of receptive field size alone, then we predict that maximal $\%MSE$ should be larger centrally than peripherally. Showing that maximal $\%MSE$ changes in either direction with eccentricity in the DSC would provide strong support for the model.

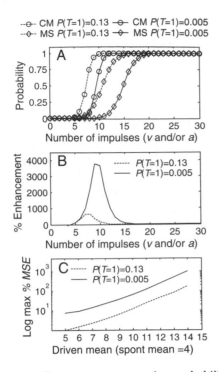

FIGURE 16.6 (A) Target-present posterior probability ($P(T = 1 | V = v, A = a)$) computed for two different prior target probability distributions using the bimodal Bayes' rule model. To simulate the results of an MSE experiment, each posterior probability is computed cross-modally (CM), in which case both modalities V and A are driven by a stimulus over the range from 0 to 30, or modality-specifically (MS), in which case one modality is driven by the stimulus while the other is held fixed at the spontaneous mean. The spontaneous and driven input likelihoods are modeled using Poisson distributions with means $\lambda = 4$ and $\lambda = 9$, respectively, for both modalities. Both the CM and MS cases are plotted for target-present prior probabilities of $P(T = 1) = 0.13$ (CM $P(T = 1) = 0.13$, dashed line with circles; MS $P(T = 1) = 0.13$, dashed line with diamonds) and $P(T = 1) = 0.005$ (CM $P(T = 1) = 0.005$, solid line with circles; MS $P(T = 1) = 0.005$, solid line with diamonds). $P(T = 1) = 0.13$ and $P(T = 1) = 0.005$ are, respectively, the estimated target-present priors for the smaller central RF and the larger peripheral RF of Figure 16.5. (B) Multisensory enhancement across a range of input levels for the peripheral ($P(T = 1) = 0.005$, solid line) and the central ($P(T = 1) = 0.13$, dashed line) receptive fields of Figure 16.5, computed using Equation 1. (C) Maximum percentage multisensory enhancement (%MSE) is compared for target-present prior probabilities of $P(T = 1) = 0.13$ (dashed line) and $P(T = 1) = 0.005$ (solid line) in the bimodal case where inputs V and A both have the same spontaneous mean $\lambda = 4$, and driven means range from $\lambda = 5$ to $\lambda = 14$. Note that the ordinate is logarithmic.

Information theoretic analysis of the Bayes' rule model

The DSC monitors the environment for targets, and its ability to do that is enhanced by the integration of multisensory input. It is natural to assume that input of another sensory modality should always increase the amount of information available to a DSC neuron concerning the environment. Under this assumption it would seem that all DSC neurons should be multisensory, but such is not the case. Only about 54% of DSC neurons in cat and 27% in monkey are multisensory (Wallace & Stein, 1996). The rest are unimodal, receiving a single, modality-specific input. Thus, the assumption that inputs of additional modalities always provide additional information may be incorrect. The use of Bayes' rule to model MSE makes it possible to evaluate this assumption quantitatively using information theory (Cover & Thomas, 1991).

Information and probability are related mathematically. The information content of an event such as the presence of a target $T = 1$ is:

$$I(T = 1) = -\log_2(P(T = 1)) \qquad (8)$$

where $\log_2$ specifies the base 2 logarithm and information is measured in units of bits. Equation 8 shows that information and probability are inversely related. Given the target priors defined as $P(T = 1) = 0.1$ and $P(T = 0) = 0.9$, the target is most often absent. The event that the target is present, therefore, is more informative. This is reflected by the information content of each event: $I(T = 1) = 3.32$ bits, whereas $I(T = 0) = 0.15$ bits. Since T is a random variable, the information content of T is also a random variable, and it is useful to find its average. The average information content of random variable T is:

$$H(T) = -[P(T = 0)\log_2(P(T = 0))$$
$$+ P(T = 1)\log_2(P(T = 1))] \qquad (9)$$

The average is computed as the expected value of the information content of binary random variable T over its two possible states: $T = 1$ and $T = 0$. The average information $H(T)$, or entropy, is a measure of our uncertainty about the target. For our target priors as defined, the unconditional target uncertainty $H(T) = 0.47$ bits.

Sensory input provides information to a DSC neuron concerning the presence of a target in its receptive field or fields. It might seem reasonable to suppose that sensory input should always reduce the uncertainty associated with a target, but such is not the case. A sensory input can reduce target uncertainty at some input levels but may actually increase target uncertainty at other input levels. We illustrate this by calculating the uncertainty of the target conditioned on specific levels of visual input $V = v$:

$$H(T | V = v)$$
$$= -[P(T = 0 | V = v)\log_2(P(T = 0 | V = v))$$
$$+ P(T = 1 | V = v)\log_2(P(T = 1 | V = v))] \qquad (10)$$

In order to calculate the conditional uncertainty $H(T \mid V = v)$ of the target we first need to compute the conditional probability that the target is present or that it is absent, given that $V = v$. The conditional probability $P(T = 1 \mid V = v)$ is computed as a posterior probability using the unimodal Bayes' rule model as described above (Equation 2). The conditional probability $P(T = 0 \mid V = v)$ is computed in the same way except that $T = 0$ is substituted for $T = 1$ in Equation 2. We model the likelihoods of V as Poisson distributions, as before (Equation 4), but we set the spontaneous mean to $\lambda = 4$ and the driven mean to $\lambda = 5$ impulses per unit time. These likelihood means are deliberately set close in value so that the spontaneous and driven likelihoods will be similar. Note that, with spontaneous and driven means of 4 and 5, these likelihoods (not shown) overlap more than those shown in Figure 16.2 that have spontaneous and driven means of 5 and 8. The modality-specific unimodal posterior probability $P(T = 1 \mid V = v)$, computed on the basis of the overlapping likelihoods, is shown in Figure 16.7A. The target-present and target-absent priors are also shown for comparison.

The modality-specific unimodal posterior probability $P(T = 1 \mid V = v)$ rises slowly with V, due to the similarity of the spontaneous and driven likelihoods. The conditional uncertainty $H(T \mid V = v)$ for these likelihoods is shown in Figure 16.7B, and the unconditional uncertainty $H(T)$ is also shown for comparison. At the extremes, for low and high values of $V = v$, the conditional uncertainty $H(T \mid V = v)$ is less than the unconditional uncertainty $H(T)$, indicating that input V has indeed reduced the uncertainty associated with the target. However, there is a broad range of values $V = v$ for which $H(T \mid V = v)$ is greater than $H(T)$. This range corresponds to the range over which $P(T = 1 \mid V = v)$ lies between the target-present and target-absent priors (Fig. 16.7A). Within this range, sensory input V has actually increased the uncertainty associated with the target.

The conditional uncertainty associated with one sensory input can be reduced by another input. We illustrate this by computing the joint conditional uncertainty of the target, given visual input $V = v$ and auditory input $A = a$:

$$H(T \mid V = v, A = a)$$
$$= -[P(T = 0 \mid V = v, A = a)$$
$$\times \log_2(P(T = 0 \mid V = v, A = a))$$
$$+ P(T = 1 \mid V = v, A = a)$$
$$\times \log_2(P(T = 1 \mid V = v, A = a))] \quad (11)$$

In order to calculate the joint conditional uncertainty of the target we first need to compute the joint conditional probability that the target is present or that it is

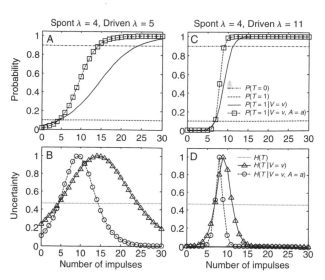

FIGURE 16.7 (A) Target-present posterior probability is plotted as the input varies from 0 to 30 in the unimodal case for modality-specific input V only (Equation 2) ($P(T = 1 \mid V = v)$, solid line with no symbols), and in the bimodal case where cross-modal inputs V and A vary together (Equation 5) ($P(T = 1 \mid V = v, A = a)$, dashed line with squares). Input likelihoods are closely spaced Poisson distributions with the indicated means. The target prior probabilities $P(T = 1) = 0.1$ (dashed line) and $P(T = 0) = 0.9$ (dot-dashed line) are shown for comparison. (B) Conditional target uncertainty is plotted in the unimodal case for modality-specific sensory input V (Equation 10) ($H(T \mid V = v)$, solid line with triangles), and in the bimodal case for cross-modal sensory inputs V and A varying together (Equation 11) ($H(T \mid V = v, A = a)$, dashed line with circles). Input likelihood means are given above panel A. The unconditional uncertainty ($H(T)$, dotted line) is plotted for comparison. (C) Target-present posterior probability is plotted in the unimodal and bimodal cases as in panel A. Input likelihoods are widely separated Poisson distributions with the indicated means. (D) Conditional target uncertainty is plotted in the unimodal and bimodal cases as in panel B. Input likelihood means are given above panel C.

absent, given that $V = v$ and $A = a$. The joint conditional probability $P(T = 1 \mid V = v, A = a)$ is computed as a posterior probability using the bimodal Bayes' rule model (Equation 5), as described above. The joint conditional probability $P(T = 0 \mid V = v, A = a)$ is computed in the same way except that $T = 0$ is substituted for $T = 1$ in Equation 5. We model the likelihoods of A using Poisson distributions and set the spontaneous mean to $\lambda = 4$ and the driven mean to $\lambda = 5$ impulses per unit time, as for V. To facilitate the comparison between the unimodal (conditional) and the bimodal (joint conditional) uncertainties, we vary v and a together over the range with $v = a$. The cross-modal bimodal posterior probability $P(T = 1 \mid V = v, A = a)$, computed on the basis of these likelihoods, is shown in Figure 16.7A. The cross-modal bimodal posterior rises faster than the modality-specific unimodal posterior probability.

The joint conditional uncertainty $H(T|V=v, A=a)$ is shown in Figure 16.7B. The range of input levels over which $H(T|V=v, A=a) > H(T)$ is only half as wide as the range over which $H(T|V=v) > H(T)$. Thus, input of a second modality has reduced the uncertainty associated with the target over a broad range of input levels. Even though the auditory input by itself is as uncertain as the visual input, the auditory input is able to reduce the uncertainty associated with the visual input when both inputs are presented together. It is also apparent in comparing $H(T|V=v)$ with $H(T|V=v, A=a)$ in Figure 16.7B that there are input levels for which $H(T|V=v, A=a) > H(T|V=v)$. Thus, at some input levels, the presence of a target is more uncertain with two inputs than with only one input. This example illustrates that multisensory interactions generally decrease target uncertainty, but can actually increase it at certain input levels.

The ability of input of one modality to reduce the uncertainty associated with the input of another modality depends on the statistical properties of the inputs. To demonstrate, we keep the spontaneous likelihood means for both V and A at $\lambda = 4$, but we increase both driven means from $\lambda = 5$ to $\lambda = 11$ impulses per unit time. Now the driven and spontaneous likelihoods are better separated. The modality-specific unimodal ($P(T=1|V=v)$) and cross-modal bimodal ($P(T=1|V=v, A=a)$) target posteriors for the better separated case are plotted in Figure 16.7C. The cross-modal bimodal target posterior rises faster than the modality-specific unimodal posterior, as before, but both curves rise faster with the better separated likelihoods (Fig. 16.7C) than with the more overlapping likelihoods (Fig. 16.7A). The conditional ($H(T|V=v)$) and the joint conditional ($H(T|V=v, A=a)$) uncertainties for the more well-separated likelihoods are plotted in Figure 16.7D. As before, the range over which $H(T|V=v, A=a) > H(T)$ is half as wide as the range over which $H(T|V=v) > H(T)$. Thus, input of a second modality can also decrease target uncertainty when the likelihoods are well-separated. However, integration of input of a second modality is of less benefit when the likelihoods are well-separated, because the range over which sensory input actually increases target uncertainty is already small with a single, modality-specific input.

The comparisons indicate that the ability of sensory inputs to reduce target uncertainty, and the effect of combining inputs of different modalities, strongly depend on the degree of separation of the spontaneous and driven likelihoods of the inputs. Inputs with better separated likelihoods reduce target uncertainty over a broader range of input levels than do inputs with more

overlapping likelihoods. By the same token, multisensory integration will provide a greater improvement in input certainty when inputs have more overlapping likelihood distributions. These effects can be explored quantitatively by defining a measure of the degree of separation between the spontaneous and driven likelihoods of a sensory input.

INPUT AMBIGUITY AND THE EFFECT OF MULTISENSORY INTEGRATION The foregoing simulations suggest that the ability of a sensory input to reduce the uncertainty associated with a target is related to the degree of separation between its spontaneous and driven likelihood distributions. This makes intuitive sense. A sensory input with well-separated spontaneous and driven likelihoods will generally show a big increase in activity in the presence of a target. Such input will indicate target presence with more certainty than a sensory input that has almost the same activity whether a target is present or absent. The simulations illustrate that inputs with similar spontaneous and driven likelihoods reduce uncertainty less that inputs with different spontaneous and driven likelihoods. It seems that inputs with similar and different spontaneous and driven likelihoods are ambiguous and unambiguous, respectively. This intuition can be grounded in quantitative terms.

The difference between the spontaneous and driven likelihoods of a sensory input can be quantified using a measure known as the Kullback-Leibler divergence D. The Kullback-Leibler divergence for a unimodal case with input V is:

$$D(P(V=v_i | T=0) \| P(V=v_i | T=1))$$

$$= \sum_{i=1}^{n} P(V=v_i | T=0) \log_2 \frac{P(V=v_i | T=0)}{P(V=v_i | T=1)} \quad (12)$$

For a bimodal case with inputs V and A the Kullback-Leibler divergence is:

$$D(P(V=v_i, A=a_j | T=0) | P(V=v_i, A=a_j | T=1))$$

$$= \sum_{i=1}^{n} \sum_{j=1}^{n} P(V=v_i | T=0) P(A=a_j | T=0)$$

$$\times \log_2 \frac{P(V=v_i | T=0) P(A=a_j | T=0)}{P(V=v_i | T=1) P(A=a_j | T=1)} \quad (13)$$

We use D to quantify the difference between the spontaneous and driven likelihoods of the input, in both the unimodal and bimodal cases, as the separation between the spontaneous and driven likelihood means is systematically increased. This is done by evaluating Equations 12 and 13 as the driven likelihood means are increased from $\lambda = 4$ to $\lambda = 30$, while the spontaneous means are fixed at $\lambda = 4$ impulses per unit time. The results are shown in Figure 16.8A. As expected, the

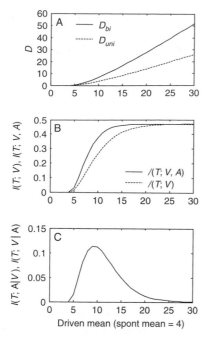

FIGURE 16.8 (*A*) Kullback-Leibler divergence (*D*) between the spontaneous and driven likelihoods is plotted versus the driven likelihood mean, which varies from $\lambda = 4$ to $\lambda = 30$. The spontaneous mean is fixed at $\lambda = 4$. All likelihoods are modeled as Poisson distributions. *D* for unimodal input *V* was computed using Equation 12 ($D_{uni} = D(P(V = v_i \mid T = 0) \parallel P(V = v_i \mid T = 1))$), dashed line). Kullback-Leibler divergence *D* for bimodal inputs *V* and *A* was computed using Equation 13 ($D_{bi} = D(P(V = v_i, A = a_j \mid T = 0) \parallel P(V = v_i, A = a_j \mid T = 1))$, solid line). For simplicity, both *V* and *A* have the same spontaneous and driven means. (*B*) The information gain due to sensory input is plotted versus the driven mean. For both modalities, the spontaneous likelihood mean is fixed at $\lambda = 4$, and the driven mean varies from $\lambda = 4$ to $\lambda = 30$. All likelihoods are Poisson distributed. Information gain for the unimodal case is computed using Equation 16 ($I(T; V)$, dashed line) and for the bimodal case using Equation 17 ($I(T; V, A)$, solid line). (*C*) The amount of information gained by the addition of a second input modality (conditional information gain, $I(T; A \mid V)$ or $I(T; V \mid A)$) is computed using Equation 18 and plotted versus the driven mean for Poisson distributed likelihoods. The spontaneous mean is held fixed at $\lambda = 4$, and the driven mean varies from $\lambda = 4$ to $\lambda = 30$.

Kullback-Leibler divergence increases as the separation between the spontaneous and driven likelihood means increases. It is interesting to note that the bimodal divergence is roughly twice as large as the unimodal divergence for driven means greater than about ten impulses per unit time. Seen from the standpoint of the Kullback-Leibler divergence, the effect of multisensory integration is to increase the apparent separation between the spontaneous and driven likelihoods of the inputs, thereby making them less ambiguous.

The Kullback-Leibler divergence measures the difference between distributions. When applied to sponta-

neous and driven likelihoods, it provides a measure of the ability of sensory inputs to indicate the presence of a target over a wide range of possible values of the input. The simulation presented above demonstrated that the ability of an input to reduce target uncertainty is related to the difference between its spontaneous and driven likelihoods, but it evaluated conditional uncertainty only at specific values of the input. In order to relate the Kullback-Leibler divergence to conditional uncertainty, it is necessary to quantify conditional uncertainty over a wide range of possible values of the input. This measure is provided by the average conditional uncertainty. For unimodal input *V*, the average conditional uncertainty $H(T \mid V)$ is:

$$
\begin{aligned}
H(T \mid V) &= -\sum_{i=1}^{n} P(v_i) H(T \mid v_i) \\
&= -\sum_{i=1}^{n} P(v_i) \left[\sum_{T=0}^{1} P(T \mid v_i) \log_2 P(T \mid v_i) \right] \\
&= -\sum_{i=1}^{n} P(v_i) \left[P(T = 0 \mid v_i) \log_2 P(T = 0 \mid v_i) \right. \\
&\quad \left. + P(T = 1 \mid v_i) \log_2 P(T = 1 \mid v_i) \right]
\end{aligned}
\tag{14}
$$

The average conditional uncertainty $H(T \mid V, A)$ for bimodal inputs *V* and *A* is:

$$
\begin{aligned}
H(T \mid V, A) &= -\sum_{i=1}^{n} \sum_{j=1}^{n} P(v_i, a_j) H(T \mid v_i, a_j) \\
&= -\sum_{i=1}^{n} \sum_{j=1}^{n} P(v_i, a_j) \left[\sum_{T=0}^{1} P(T \mid v_i, a_j) \log_2 P(T \mid v_i, a_j) \right] \\
&= -\sum_{i=1}^{n} \sum_{j=1}^{n} P(v_i, a_j) \left[P(T = 0 \mid v_i, a_j) \log_2 P(T = 0 \mid v_i, a_j) \right. \\
&\quad \left. + P(T = 1 \mid v_i, a_j) \log_2 P(T = 1 \mid v_i, a_j) \right]
\end{aligned}
\tag{15}
$$

For the unimodal case, $H(T \mid V)$ is the average of $H(T \mid V = v)$ over a wide range of values of $V = v$. Similarly, for the bimodal case, $H(T \mid V, A)$ is the average of $H(T \mid V = v, A = a)$ over a wide range of values of $V = v$ and $A = a$. As before, the needed unimodal and bimodal posterior target probabilities can be computed using Equations 2 and 5, respectively.

Reduction in uncertainty implies gain in information. When sensory input to a DSC neuron reduces target uncertainty, it has increased the information available to that neuron concerning the target. The information gained by a DSC neuron from sensory input can therefore be quantified as a decrease in target uncertainty. The average information gain $I(T; V)$ due to unimodal input *V* is the difference between the unconditional uncertainty $H(T)$ and the average uncertainty conditioned on *V*:

$$
I(T; V) = H(T) - H(T \mid V)
\tag{16}
$$

Similarly, average information gain $I(T;V,A)$ due to bimodal input V and A is:

$$I(T; V,A) = H(T) - H(T \mid V, A) \qquad (17)$$

We can now quantify the average information gain for unimodal and bimodal inputs as we increase the Kullback-Leibler divergence between the spontaneous and driven likelihoods of those inputs. This is done by evaluating Equations 16 and 17 over the same range of driven likelihood means as when computing the Kullback-Leibler divergence above. The results are shown in Figure 16.8B.

As expected, both the Kullback-Leibler divergence (Fig. 16.8A) and the average information gain (Fig. 16.8B) are zero when the spontaneous and driven likelihood means are equal. Information gain increases as the driven mean, and so the Kullback-Leibler divergence, increases. Information gain increases faster for bimodal than for unimodal inputs. Over a range of driven means (up to 15 or so) $I(T; V,A)$ exceeds $I(T; V)$, meaning that the two inputs V and A do indeed provide more information than input V does alone. It would seem the intuitive notion that two sensory inputs always provide more information than one is confirmed. However, as the driven means increase further, information gain in both the bimodal and unimodal cases reaches the same plateau. This plateau is the unconditional uncertainty $H(T)$. When the information gain equals the unconditional uncertainty, the input has completely reduced the uncertainty associated with the target. Further increases in the driven mean can further increase the Kullback-Leibler divergence but cannot further increase the amount of information that the inputs provide concerning the target.

A more direct way of assessing the amount of information gained through multisensory integration is to compute the conditional information gain $I(T; A \mid V)$. This is the gain in target information due to input of modality A after input of modality V has already been received. The average conditional information gain $I(T; A \mid V)$ is computed as the difference between the average conditional and joint conditional uncertainties:

$$I(T; A \mid V) = H(T \mid V) - H(T \mid V, A) \qquad (18)$$

We assume for simplicity that V and A have the same input likelihoods, and in that case $I(T; A \mid V) = I(T; V \mid A)$. The average conditional information gain is shown in Figure 16.8C. It clearly shows that the ability of multisensory integration to increase the amount of target information is greatest when the difference between the spontaneous and driven likelihood distributions is the least. It also clearly shows that input of a second modality does not always increase the amount of information concerning the target.

The foregoing information theoretic analysis of the Bayes' rule model offers a possible explanation for the puzzling finding that many DSC neurons are not multisensory despite the availability of cross-modal input. It hinges on the likely assumption that a sensory input indicates the presence of a target primarily in terms of its firing rate. The greater the difference in its firing rate under spontaneous as compared with driven conditions, the more certain an indication that input can give concerning the presence of the target. When the spontaneous and driven likelihoods of an input are the same, that input is completely ambiguous, and it provides no information to a DSC neuron concerning the presence of a target. Less ambiguous inputs have better separated spontaneous and driven likelihoods, and can effectively provide information to a DSC neuron concerning a target.

Inputs with very well-separated spontaneous and driven likelihoods are sufficiently unambiguous that they reduce target uncertainty to zero by themselves. Our analysis shows that it is possible for a DSC neuron to receive such unambiguous modality-specific input that it would receive little or no further information about the presence of a target by integrating input of another modality. Unimodal DSC neurons may be those that receive such unambiguous modality-specific input that integrating input of another modality is unnecessary. Conversely, a DSC neuron receiving ambiguous input of one modality could gain appreciable more information about the presence of a target by integrating inputs of one or two additional modalities. Multisensory DSC neurons may be those that combine inputs of multiple modalities and reliably detect targets despite the ambiguity of the individual inputs.

Future directions

The Bayes' rule model opens a new perspective on the function of MSE. It may also provide a new way to view the DSC within the larger context of the motor system. Future directions for modeling MSE include an exploration of the neurobiological implementation of MSE by neural networks. They also include large-scale models in which the DSC is part of a system of brain regions that work together to decide the next direction in which an orienting movement should be made.

The Bayes' rule model is consistent with findings on the multisensory responses of DSC neurons. It provides a plausible explanation for the functional role of MSE, but it does not by itself provide insight into how MSE is produced neurobiologically. In recent work we have shown that the Bayes' rule computation can be implemented using relatively simple neural models. For the case of the conditionally independent Poisson likelihoods described in this chapter, we have found that a single summing node, followed by the logistic sigmoid squashing function, can implement the needed computation (Patton & Anastasio, 2003). The Bayes' rule model is valid for any likelihood distributions, and we have found that a slightly more complicated neural model that allows inputs to be multiplied together before being summed can implement the computations needed for the more general case of conditionally dependent, Gaussian likelihoods. In this case, the multiplicative interactions are required only when the spontaneous and driven variances and covariances are unequal. In both the Poisson and Gaussian cases, MSE itself arises through weighted summation of sensory inputs, followed by the sigmoid nonlinearity. A term related to the target prior also arises as an inhibitory bias. These modeling results have interesting implications for the neurobiological mechanism of MSE.

The neural models showing how Bayes' rule might be computed by neurons suggest that MSE could arise through the simple summation of sensory influences from various sources, given a fixed inhibitory bias and the basic neuronal nonlinearities. Experimental findings regarding the role of the cortex in MSE, however, suggest a more complex arrangement. Inactivation of certain regions of parietal cortex can abolish MSE but not affect the responses of DSC neurons to modality-specific sensory inputs (Jiang, Wallace, Jiang, Vaughan, & Stein, 2001; Wallace & Stein, 1994). It seems that the cortex may be producing MSE by modulating DSC responses to ascending inputs (Anastasio & Patton, 2003). A schematic diagram illustrating some known influences on DSC is shown in Figure 16.9.

The neural models also suggest that the target prior may be represented in the brain as an inhibitory bias signal. Such a signal could arrive at the DSC from various sources, with the substantia nigra being the best-studied candidate (Appell & Behan, 1990; Ficalora & Mize, 1989; May, Sun, & Hall, 1997; Mize, 1992). Like the DSC, the substantia nigra is topographically organized (Hikosaka & Wurtz, 1983b). Neurons in the substantia nigra project to the DSC and exert an inhibitory influence on it (Anderson & Yoshida, 1977; Chevalier, Deniau, Thierry, & Feger, 1981; Chevalier, Thierry, Shibazaki, & Feger, 1981; Ficalora & Mize, 1989; Hikosaka & Wurtz, 1983a; Karabelas & Moschovakis, 1985; Niijima & Yoshida, 1982; Westby, Collinson, Redgrave, & Dean, 1994). Changes in the activity of neurons in the nigra could reflect changes in the prior expectation of targets at locations corresponding to the receptive fields of nigral neurons. These prior expectations could be derived from processing within the basal

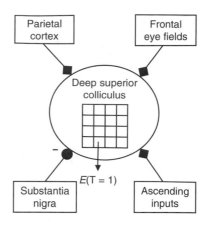

FIGURE 16.9 A schematic diagram illustrating our model of DSC function. The DSC consists of a topographic array of neurons (grid). The activity of a DSC neuron is determined by the product of the posterior probability of a target ($P(T \mid V = v, A = a)$) and the behavioral relevance of the target ($R(T = 1)$), where $E(T = 1) = P(T = 1 \mid V = v, A = a) R(T = 1)$. The posterior probability of a target (Equation 5) is essentially the prior target probability after it has been modified by sensory input. Neural signals carrying sensory input, or inputs related to target prior and behavioral relevance, may be transmitted to the DSC from various structures that may include the substantia nigra, frontal eye fields, and parietal cortex.

ganglia and relayed to the DSC through the substantia nigra. This relay might provide one way in which the basal ganglia could influence orienting behavior.

The Bayes' rule model implies that the DSC takes into account the probability that a target is present at a particular location before it initiates an orienting movement toward that location. This is behaviorally reasonable. Animals, however, do not select the targets for orienting movements on the basis of target probability alone. Higher cognitive processes, such as attention, that assess the behavioral relevance of a potential target are also involved (Kowler, Anderson, Dosher, & Blaser, 1995; Levy-Schoen, Coeffe, & Jacobs, 1989). A rewarded target stimulus, for example, produces more activity when it appears in the receptive field of a DSC neuron than does an identical stimulus when used as a distractor (Glimcher & Sparks, 1992). Attentional modulation may involve many structures that project to the DSC (Fig. 16.9), including such cortical regions as the parietal cortex and frontal eye fields (Schall, 1995; Corbetta, 1998; Schall & Bichot, 1998). It is likely that the decision to make an orienting movement toward a target is a function both of the behavioral relevance of the target and of its posterior probability.

The idea of behavioral relevance could be rigorously incorporated into the Bayes' rule model using decision theory (Berger, 1985). According to decision theory, the decision to make an orienting movement toward a particular target would involve the Bayesian expected relevance of the target, which is the behavioral relevance of the target weighted by posterior target probability. Within a decision theoretic framework, an orienting movement could be made toward a target with a low posterior probability, provided that its behavioral relevance to the organism was high.

Using Bayes' rule, the Bayesian expected relevance of the appearance of a target, as computed by a bimodal DSC neuron, could be expressed as:

$$E(T = 1) = R(T = 1)P(T = 1 \mid V = v, A = a)$$

$$= R(T = 1)\left[\frac{P(V = v, A = a \mid T = 1)}{P(V = v, A = a)}\right]P(T = 1) \quad (19)$$

where $E(T = 1)$ is the expected relevance and $R(T = 1)$ is the relevance of the target. The ratio term is related to sensory input statistics. Equation 19 illustrates how the Bayesian expected relevance of the appearance of a target could be computed from terms related to sensory input, target behavioral relevance, and prior probability. Behavioral relevance and prior target probability could be separately manipulated and explored experimentally at the level of single neurons.

A simple paradigm illustrates how this could be done (Figure 16.10). Targets appear randomly at the four corners of a square around a central fixation point. An animal that can reliably be trained to make saccades, such as a monkey, is rewarded more for saccades made to targets at the top than at the bottom of the square, so $R(T = 1)$ is higher on the top. Targets are presented more frequently on the right than on the left, so $P(T = 1)$ is higher on the right. The Bayes' rule model predicts that the sensitivity and maximal $\%MSE$ of multisensory DSC neurons should depend in opposite ways on target prior probability (see Fig. 16.6). The model predicts that DSC neuron sensitivity should be higher for targets with higher prior probabilities (Fig. 16.6A). Combined with the known attentional augmentation, the model predicts that DSC neuron sensitivity should be highest on the top right (high relevance, high prior) and lowest on the bottom left (low relevance, low prior). For multisensory DSC neurons, the Bayes' rule model predicts that $\%MSE$ should be higher for targets with lower prior probabilities (Figs. 16.6B and C). In this case, $\%MSE$ should be higher for targets on the left (low prior) at the same level of reward (top or bottom). These predictions could be tested by comparing the responses of populations of neurons with receptive fields at each of the four corners. It might also be possible to test the same neuron after retraining the monkey on different conditions of $R(T = 1)$ and $P(T = 1)$.

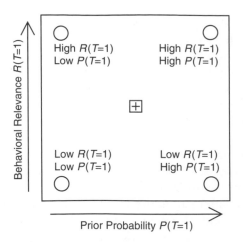

FIGURE 16.10 A proposed experiment to explore the relative effects of target prior probability $P(T = 1)$ and target behavioral relevance $R(T = 1)$ on the sensitivity and maximal $\%MSE$ of multisensory DSC neurons. A monkey is trained to saccade from the fixation point (+) to one of four targets to obtain a possible reward. Targets at the top yield a reward more frequently, and therefore have a higher behavioral relevance (high $R(T = 1)$) than those on the bottom (low $R(T = 1)$). Targets on the right appear more frequently, and therefore have a higher prior probability (high $P(T = 1)$) than those on the left (low $P(T = 1)$). The model predicts that sensitivity should be highest and lowest for DSC neurons with receptive fields on the upper right and lower left, respectively. It predicts that maximal $\%MSE$ should be higher for DSC neurons with receptive fields on the left (see text).

It is unlikely that quantities such as target prior probability, sensory input, and behavioral relevance are represented cleanly as separate signals in the brain. Even if the substantia nigra, for example, does provide an inhibitory signal to the DSC that is proportional to target prior probability, it may also provide signals related to sensory input and behavioral relevance. Substantia nigra cells are tonically active and pause in response to sensory stimulation in their receptive fields (Hikosaka & Wurtz, 1983b; Joseph & Boussaoud, 1985). Basso and Wurtz (2002) have reported evidence that changes in nigral cell activity are related to changes in target behavioral relevance. It is possible that quantities such as target prior, sensory input, and attention are combined nonuniformly and represented in a distributed fashion within brain regions such as the substantia nigra, frontal and parietal cortex, and the DSC itself. The components that make up the decision to initiate a saccade may be nonuniformly distributed, just as oculomotor commands appear to be (Anastasio & Robinson, 1989; Anastasio, 1991). Separately manipulating these components experimentally may be key to understanding how they are represented in the brain and how they combine to activate DSC neurons.

Conclusion

The Bayes' rule model offers a plausible explanation for findings on multisensory DSC neurons. It suggests that MSE arises as a consequence of the computation by DSC neurons of the probability that a target is present in their receptive fields, given cross-modal input. The Bayes' rule model is testable experimentally. It makes the robust prediction that the amount of MSE should vary systematically with the size and location of the receptive fields of DSC neurons. Analysis of the Bayes' rule model using information theory shows that, depending on the statistical properties of the inputs, multisensory integration may or may not increase the amount of information that a DSC neuron receives concerning targets. This may explain why many DSC neurons are unimodal, receiving only modality-specific input, despite the availability of cross-modal projections. By providing a rigorous interpretation of the function of MSE, the Bayes' rule model suggests how multisensory processing in the DSC may interact with other brain regions in controlling orienting behavior.

Multisensory integration certainly contributes to the power of the brain as an information processor. The Bayes' rule model opens a new perspective on multisensory integration, from which vantage point new conceptual approaches to understanding this important phenomenon can be taken.

REFERENCES

Aitsebaomo, A. P., & Bedell, H. E. (1992). Psychophysical and saccadic information about direction for briefly presented visual targets. *Vision Research, 32,* 1729–1737.

Anastasio, T. J. (1991). Distributed processing in vestibulo-ocular and other oculomotor subsystems in monkeys and cats. In M. A. Arbib & J.-P. Ewert (Eds.), *Visual structures and integrated functions* (pp. 95–109). Berlin: Springer-Verlag.

Anastasio, T. J., & Patton, P. E. (2003). A two-stage unsupervised learning algorithm reproduces multisensory enhancement in a neural network model of the corticotectal system. *Journal of Neuroscience, 23*(17), 6713–6727.

Anastasio, T. J., Patton, P. E., & Belkacem-Boussaid, K. (2000). Using Bayes' rule to model multisensory enhancement in the superior colliculus. *Neural Computation, 12,* 997–1019.

Anastasio, T. J., & Robinson, D. A. (1989). Distributed parallel processing in the vestibulo-oculomotor system. *Neural Computation, 1,* 230–241.

Anderson, M., & Yoshida, M. (1977). Electrophysiological evidence for branching nigral projections to the thalamus and the superior colliculus. *Brain Research, 137,* 361–364.

Appelbaum, D. (1996). *Probability and information: An integrated approach.* Cambridge, England: Cambridge University Press.

Appell, P. P., & Behan, M. (1990). Sources of subcortical GABAergic projections to the superior colliculus in the cat. *Journal of Comparative Neurology, 302,* 143–158.

Basso, M. A., & Wurtz, R. H. (2002). Neuronal activity in substantia nigra pars reticulata during target selection. *Journal of Neuroscience, 22,* 1883–1894.

Becker, W. (1972). The control of eye movements in the saccadic system. In J. Dichgans & E. Bizzi (Eds.), *Cerebral control of eye movements and motion perception* (pp. 233–243). Basel: Karger.

Becker, W., & Fuchs, A. F. (1969). Further properties of the human saccadic system: Eye movements and correction saccades with and without visual fixation points. *Vision Research, 9,* 1247–1258.

Berger, J. O. (1985). *Statistical decision theory and bayesian analysis* (2nd ed.). Heidelberg: Springer-Verlag.

Cadusseau, J., & Roger, M. (1985). Afferent projections to the superior colliculus in the rat, with special attention to the deep layers. *Journal für Hirnforschung, 26,* 667–681.

Carpenter, R. H. S. (1988). Saccades. In *Movements of the eyes* (2nd ed., pp. 69–101). London: Pion.

Chevalier, G., Deniau, J. M., Thierry, A. M., & Feger, J. (1981). The nigro-tectal pathway: An electrophysiological reinvestigation in the rat. *Brain Research, 213,* 253–263.

Chevalier, G., Thierry, A. M., Shibazaki T., & Feger, J. (1981). Evidence for a GABAergic inhibitory nigrotectal pathway in the rat. *Neuroscience Letters, 21,* 67–70.

Corbetta, M. (1998). Frontoparietal cortical networks for directing attention and the eye to visual locations: Identical, independent, or overlapping neural systems? *Proceedings of the National Academy of Sciences, USA, 95,* 831–838.

Cover, T. M., & Thomas, J. A. (1991). *Elements of information theory.* New York: Wiley.

Duda, R. O., Hart, P. E., & Stork, D. G. (2001). *Pattern classification* (2nd ed.). New York: Wiley.

Edwards, S. B., Ginsburgh, C. L., Henkel, C. K., & Stein, B. E. (1979). Sources of subcortical projections to the superior colliculus in the cat. *Journal of Comparative Neurology, 184,* 309–329.

Evinger, C., & Fuchs, A. F. (1978). Saccadic, smooth pursuit, and optokinetic eye movements of the trained cat. *Journal of Physiology (London), 285,* 209–229.

Ewert, J. P. (1970). Neural mechanisms of prey catching and avoidance behavior in the toad (*Bufo bufo L.*). *Brain, Behavior and Evolution, 3,* 36–56.

Ficalora, A. S., & Mize, R. R. (1989). The neurons of the substantia nigra and zona incerta which project to the cat superior colliculus are GABA immunoreactive: A double label study using GABA immunocytochemistry and lectin retrograde transport. *Neuroscience, 29,* 567–581.

Findlay, J. M., & Walker, R. (1999). A model of saccade generation based on parallel processing and competitive inhibition. *Behavioral Brain Science, 22,* 661–721.

Freedman, E. G., Stanford, T. R., & Sparks, D. L. (1996). Combined eye-head gaze shifts produced by electrical stimulation of the superior colliculus in rhesus monkeys. *Journal of Neurophysiology, 76,* 927–952.

Glimcher, P. W., & Sparks, D. L. (1992). Movement selection in advance of action in the superior colliculus. *Nature, 355,* 542–545.

Gordon, B. (1973). Receptive fields in deep layers of cat superior colliculus. *Journal of Neurophysiology, 36,* 157–178.

Guitton, D., Crommelinck, M., & Roucoux, A. (1980). Stimulation of the superior colliculus in the alert cat: I. Eye movements and neck EMG activity evoked when head is restrained. *Experimental Brain Research, 39,* 63–73.

Guitton, D., Douglas, R. M., & Volle, M. (1984). Eye-head coordination in cats. *Journal of Neurophysiology, 52,* 1030–1050.

Harris, L. R. (1980). The superior colliculus and movements of the head and eyes in cat. *Journal of Physiology (London), 300,* 367–391.

Harting, J. K., Updyke, B. V., & Van Lieshout, D. P. (1992). Corticotectal projections in the cat: Anterograde transport studies of twenty-five cortical areas. *Journal of Comparative Neurology, 324,* 379–414.

Helstrom, C. W. (1984). *Probability and stochastic processes for engineers.* New York: Macmillan.

Henson, D. B. (1978). Corrective saccades: Effects of altering visual feedback. *Vision Research, 18,* 63–67.

Henson, D. B. (1979). Investigation into corrective saccadic eye movements for refixation amplitudes of 10 degrees and below. *Vision Research, 19,* 57–61.

Hikosaka, O., & Wurtz, R. H. (1983a). Visual and oculomotor functions of monkey substantia nigra pars reticulata: IV. Relation of substantia nigra to superior colliculus. *Journal of Neurophysiology, 49,* 1285–1301.

Hikosaka, O., & Wurtz, R. H. (1983b). Visual and oculomotor functions of the monkey substantia nigra pars reticulata: I. Relation of visual and auditory responses to saccades. *Journal of Neurophysiology, 49,* 1254–1267.

Jiang, W., Wallace, M. T., Jiang, H., Vaughan, J. W., & Stein, B. E. (2001). Two cortical areas mediate multisensory integration in superior colliculus neurons. *Journal of Neurophysiology, 85,* 506–522.

Joseph, J. P., & Boussaoud, D. (1985). Role of the cat substantia nigra pars reticulata in eye and head movements: I. Neural activity. *Experimental Brain Research, 57,* 286–296.

Kadunce, D. C., Vaughan, J. W., Wallace, M. T., & Stein, B. E. (2001). The influence of visual and auditory receptive field organization on multisensory integration in the superior colliculus. *Experimental Brain Research, 139,* 303–310.

Karabelas, A. B., & Moschovakis, A. K. (1985). Nigral inhibitory termination on efferent neurons of the superior colliculus: An intracellular horseradish peroxidase study in the cat. *Journal of Comparative Neurology, 239,* 309–329.

King, A. J., & Palmer, A. R. (1985). Integration of visual and auditory information in bimodal neurones in guinea-pig superior colliculus. *Experimental Brain Research, 60,* 492–500.

Kowler, E. (1990). The role of visual and cognitive processes in the control of eye movement. In E. Kowler (Ed.), *Eye movements and their role in visual and cognitive processes* (pp. 1–70). New York: Elsevier.

Kowler, E., Anderson, E., Dosher B., & Blaser, E. (1995). The role of attention in the programming of saccades. *Vision Research, 35,* 1897–1916.

Lemij, H. G., & Collewjin, H. (1989). Differences in accuracy of human saccades between stationary and jumping targets. *Vision Research, 29,* 1737–1748.

Lennie, P., & Sidwell, A. (1978). Saccadic eye movement and visual stability. *Nature, 275,* 766–768.

Lestienne, R. (1996). Determination of the precison of spike timing in the visual cortex of anaesthetised cats. *Biology and Cybernetics, 74,* 55–61.

Levy-Schoen, A., Coeffe, C., & Jacobs, A. M. (1989). Sensory factors are insufficient to define the ocular saccade goal in complex visual fields. *Brain Behavior and Evolution, 33,* 80–84.

May, P. J., Sun, W., & Hall, W. C. (1997). Reciprocal connections between the zona incerta and the pretectum and superior colliculus of the cat. *Neuroscience, 77,* 1091–1114.

Meredith, M. A., Clemo, H. R., & Stein, B. E. (1991). Somatotopic component of the multisensory map in the deep laminae of the cat superior colliculus. *Journal of Comparative Neurology, 312,* 353–370.

Meredith, M. A., Nemitz, J. W., & Stein, B. E. (1987). Determinants of multisensory integration in superior colliculus neurons: I. Temporal factors. *Journal of Neuroscience, 7,* 3215–3229.

Meredith, M. A., & Stein, B. E. (1983). Interactions among converging sensory inputs in the superior colliculus. *Science, 221,* 389–391.

Meredith, M. A., & Stein, B. E. (1985). Descending efferents from the superior colliculus relay integrated multisensory information. *Science, 227,* 657–659.

Meredith, M. A., & Stein, B. E. (1986a). Spatial factors determine the activity of multisensory neurons in cat superior colliculus. *Brain Research, 365,* 350–354.

Meredith, M. A., & Stein, B. E. (1986b). Visual, auditory, and somatosensory convergence on cells in superior colliculus results in multisensory integration. *Journal of Neurophysiology, 56,* 640–662.

Meredith, M. A., & Stein, B. E. (1990). The visuotopic component of the multisensory map in the deep laminae of the cat superior colliculus. *Journal of Neuroscience, 10,* 3727–3742.

Meredith, M. A., &. Stein, B. E. (1996). Spatial determinants of multisensory integration in cat superior colliculus neurons. *Journal of Neurophysiology, 75,* 1843–1857.

Meredith, M. A., Wallace, M. T., & Stein, B. E. (1992). Visual, auditory and somatosensory convergence in output neurons of the cat superior colliculus: Multisensory properties of the tecto-reticulo-spinal projection. *Experimental Brain Research, 88,* 181–186.

Middlebrooks, J. C., & Knudsen, E. I. (1984). A neural code for auditory space in the cat's superior colliculus. *Journal of Neuroscience, 4,* 2621–2634.

Mize, R. R. (1992). The organization of GABAergic neurons in the mammalian superior colliculus. *Progress in Brain Research, 90,* 219–248.

Munemori, J., Hara, K., Kimura, M., & Sato, R. (1984). Statistical features of impulse trains in cat's lateral geniculate neurons. *Biology and Cybernetics, 50,* 167–172.

Munoz, D. P., & Istvan, P. J. (1998). Lateral inhibitory interactions in the intermediate layers of the monkey superior colliculus. *Journal of Neurophysiology, 79,* 1193–1209.

Niijima, K., & Yoshida, M. (1982). Electrophysiological evidence for branching nigral projections to pontine reticular formation, superior colliculus and thalamus. *Brain Research, 239,* 279–282.

Paré, M., Crommelinck, M., & Guitton, D. (1994). Gaze shifts evoked by stimulation of the superior colliculus in the head-free cat conform to the motor map but also depend on stimulus strength and fixation activity. *Experimental Brain Research, 101,* 123–139.

Patton, P., & Anastasio, T. (2003). Modeling cross-modal enhancement and modality-specific suppression in multisensory neurons. *Neural Computation, 15,* 783–810.

Patton, P., Belkacem-Boussaid, K., & Anastasio, T. (2002). Multimodality in the superior colliculus: An information theoretic analysis. *Cognitive Brain Research, 14,* 10–19.

Pelisson, D., & Prablanc, C. (1988). Kinematics of centrifugal and centripetal saccadic eye movements in man. *Vision Research, 28,* 87–94.

Prablanc, C., Masse, D., & Echallier, J. F. (1978). Error correcting mechanisms in large saccades. *Vision Research, 18,* 557–560.

Rieke, F., Warland, D., & van Stevenick, R. de Ruyter (1997). *Spikes: Exploring the neural code.* Cambrige, MA: MIT Press.

Robinson, D. A. (1972). Eye movements evoked by collicular stimulation in the alert monkey. *Vision Research, 12,* 1795–1808.

Roucoux, A., Guitton, D., & Crommelinck, M. (1980). Stimulation of the superior colliculus in the alert cat: II. Eye and head movements evoked when the head is unrestrained. *Experimental Brain Research, 39,* 75–85.

Sahibzada, N., Dean, P., & Redgrave, P. (1986). Movements resembling orientation and avoidance elicited by electrical stimulation of the superior colliculus in rats. *Journal of Neuroscience, 6,* 723–733.

Schall, J. D. (1995). Neural basis of saccade target selection. *Reviews in the Neurosciences, 6,* 63–85.

Schall, J. D., & Bichot, N. P. (1998). Neural correlates of visual and motor decision processes. *Current Opinions in Neurobiology, 8,* 211–217.

Schiller, P. H., & Stryker, M. (1972). Single-unit recording and stimulation in superior colliculus of the alert rhesus monkey. *Journal of Neurophysiology, 35,* 915–924.

Sparks, D. L., & Hartwich-Young, R. (1989). The deep layers of the superior colliculus. In R. H. Wurtz & M. Goldberg (Eds.), *The neurobiology of saccadic eye movements* (pp. 213–255). Amsterdam: Elsevier.

Stein, B. E., & Arigbede, M. O. (1972). Unimodal and multimodal response properties of neurons in the cat's superior colliculus. *Experimental Neurology, 36,* 179–196.

Stein, B. E., Huneycutt, W. S., & Meredith, M. A. (1988). Neurons and behavior: The same rules of multisensory integration apply. *Brain Research, 448,* 355–358.

Stein, B. E., Magalhaes-Castro, B., & Kruger, L. (1976). Relationship between visual and tactile representations in cat superior colliculus. *Journal of Neurophysiology, 39,* 401–419.

Stein, B. E., & Meredith, M. A. (1993). *The merging of the senses.* Cambridge, MA: MIT Press.

Stein, B. E., Meredith, M. A., Huneycutt, W. S., & McDade, L. (1989). Behavioral indicies of multisensory integration: Orientation to visual cues is affected by auditory stimuli. *Journal of Cognitive Neuroscience, 1,* 12–24.

Stryker, M., & Blakemore, C. (1972). Saccadic and disjunctive eye movements in cats. *Vision Research, 12,* 2005–2013.

Stryker, M. P., & Schiller, P. H. (1975). Eye and head movements evoked by electrical stimulation of monkey superior colliculus. *Experimental Brain Research, 23,* 103–112.

Turcott, R. G., Lowen, S. B., Li, E., Johnson, D. H., Tsuchitani, C., & Teich, M. C. (1994). A non-stationary Poisson point process describes the sequence of action potentials over long time scales in lateral-superior-olive auditory neurons. *Biology and Cybernetics, 70,* 209–217.

Viviani, P. (1990). Eye movements in visual search: Cognitive, perceptual, and motor control aspects. In E. Kowler (Ed.), *Eye movements and their role in visual and cognitive processes* (pp. 353–393). Amsterdam: Elsevier.

Wallace, M. T., Meredith, M. A., & Stein, B. E. (1998). Multisensory integration in the superior colliculus of the alert cat. *Journal of Neurophysiology, 20,* 1006–1010.

Wallace, M. T., & Stein, B. E. (1994). Cross-modal synthesis in the midbrain depends on input from cortex. *Journal of Neurophysiology, 71,* 429–432.

Wallace, M. T., & Stein, B. E. (1996). Sensory organization of the superior colliculus in cat and monkey. *Progress in Brain Research, 112,* 301–311.

Wallace, M. T., Wilkinson, L. K., & Stein, B. E. (1996). Representation and integration of multiple sensory inputs in primate superior colliculus. *Journal of Neurophysiology, 76,* 1246–1266.

Westby, G. W., Collinson, C., Redgrave, P., & Dean, P. (1994). Opposing excitatory and inhibitory influences from the cerebellum and basal ganglia converge on the superior colliculus: An electrophysiological investigation in the rat. *European Journal of Neuroscience, 6,* 1335–1342.

Wickelgren, B. G. (1971). Superior colliculus: Some receptive field properties of bimodally responsive cells. *Science, 173,* 69–72.

Wilkinson, L. K., Meredith, M. A., & Stein, B. E. (1996). The role of anterior ectosylvian cortex in cross-modality orientation and approach behavior. *Experimental Brain Research, 112,* 1–10.

Wurtz, R. L., & Goldberg, M. E. (1989). *The neurobiology of saccadic eye movements.* Amsterdam: Elsevier.

17 The Resurrection of Multisensory Cortex in Primates: Connection Patterns That Integrate Modalities

JON H. KAAS AND CHRISTINE E. COLLINS

Introduction

The classical view of cerebral cortex organization is that neocortex is subdivided into three functional types of cortex: sensory, motor, and association cortex (see Masterton & Berkley, 1974). Textbook pictures reflecting this view typically portrayed a primary area and a secondary sensory area for vision, hearing, and touch, a primary and often a secondary motor area, and association cortex (e.g., Thompson, 1967). All mammals were thought to have these sensory and motor areas but to differ in the amount of association cortex. Thus, rats, cats, monkeys, and humans were distinguished from one another by having progressively larger brains with proportionately more and more association cortex.

Over the past 30 years, this classical view has been repeatedly challenged in a number of ways. For example, this "ladder of levels" approach to describing brain differences and evolution is now seen as too simple and not reflecting the great divergences of brain organization that can be demonstrated experimentally (see Diamond & Hall, 1969; Hodos & Campbell, 1969; Preuss, 2000). Perhaps more important, regions of cortex once assigned to association cortex were rapidly being reassigned to the sensory and motor categories (see Merzenich & Kaas, 1980). In New World and Old World monkeys, as many as 35 visual areas were proposed (Felleman & Van Essen, 1991; Kaas, 1989) in regions of occipital, temporal, and parietal cortex that were formerly considered association cortex. Likewise, monkeys were found to have at least seven representations of the body (Kaas, Jain, & Qi, 2001) and approximately 12 auditory fields (Kaas & Hackett, 2000). In addition, primates appeared to have at least ten motor fields (Wu, Bichot, & Kaas, 2000). Subtracting these sensory and motor fields from the cortical sheet leaves little of the original vast expanse of association territory in these mammals. Thus, association cortex was transformed into sensory cortex (Kaas, 1999). As sensory areas of the same modality and motor areas are grouped

in the same region of cortex, they could be efficiently interconnected with short axon pathways (Young, Scannell, Burns, & Blakemore, 1994). The new view that emerged from this evidence was that processing is largely unimodal, involving an array of closely interacting, specialized cortical areas, and that little tissue is devoted to multisensory integration.

Although there is much to be said in support of this new view, it now seems that it is too extreme, for several reasons. First, a number of bimodal or multisensory areas have been identified, and they have connection patterns that are consistent with this classification. Second, more detailed studies of connection patterns, as well as more physiological data, suggest that little cortex is truly unimodal. Areas long considered to be unimodal may have inputs reflecting other modalities, and neurons in most sensory and motor areas may be under the influence of more than one modality. Thus, it may be more relevant to characterize cortical areas not by their dominant modality but by the relative weights and roles of different types of inputs.

In this chapter we describe some of the areas in the neocortex of monkeys and other primates that have connection patterns that relate them to more than one modality. These few examples serve to illustrate the importance and even the dominance of bimodal and multisensory processing in the cortex of primates. Some of the proposed subdivisions of sensory and motor cortex in macaque monkeys are shown in Figure 17.1.

Connections of unimodal auditory cortex with unimodal visual cortex

Although primary sensory areas are clearly dominated by inputs from one modality, neurons in these areas are likely to be influenced by other sensory inputs. Primary visual cortex (V1) in monkeys has widespread connections with 12 to 15 adjoining visual and more distant multisensory areas (e.g., Lyon & Kaas, 2001, 2002a, 2002b). The connections with nearby visual areas are

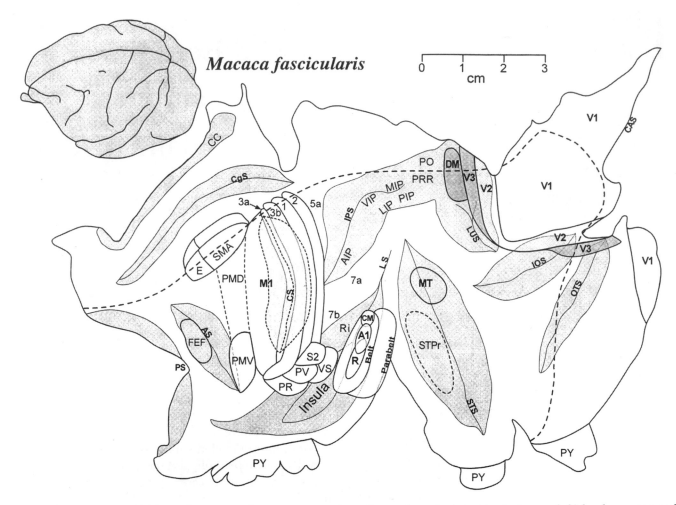

FIGURE 17.1   Some subdivisions of neocortex in macaque monkeys. Cortex from the intact brain (upper left) has been removed and flattened so that the fissures are open. The cortex normally hidden in fissures is gray. Multimodal or bimodal areas of cortex include the rostral region of the superior temporal sulcus (STPr), the anterior, lateral, ventral, and medial areas of the intraparietal sulcus (AIP, LIP, VIP, and MIP), and the parieto-occipital area (PO). Also shown are the caudomedial area (CM) of the auditory belt, the parietal ventral (PV) and ventral somatosensory (VS) areas, and the ventral premotor area (PMV). Other areas include primary visual cortex (V1, or area 17), the middle temporal visual area (MT), primary auditory cortex (A1), the rostral auditory area (R), the auditory belt of secondary areas (Belt), the auditory parabelt (Parabelt), posterior parietal areas 5a, 7a, and 7b, retroinsular cortex (Ri), anterior parietal somatosensory areas 3a, 3b, 1, and 2, primary motor cortex (M1), dorsal premotor cortex (PMD), the supplementary motor area (SMA) and its eye field (E), and the frontal eye field (FEF). Fissures include the cingulate sulcus (CgS), the principal sulcus (PS), the central sulcus (CS), the lateral sulcus (LS), the superior temporal sulcus (STS), the intraparietal sulcus (IPS), the lunate sulcus (LUS), the inferior occipital sulcus (IOS), the occipital temporal sulcus (OTS), and the calcarine sulcus (CAS). The pyriform cortex (PY) and the corpus callosum (CC) are identified.

most dense. Thus, about half of the ipsilateral cortical connections of V1 are with V2, and most of the rest are with V3, MT, and DM (see Fig. 17.1 for abbreviations). Connections with more distant regions of cortex are sparse, and in some regions there is only evidence for feedback projections to V1. Nevertheless, some sparse inputs *originate* from multisensory areas in posterior parietal cortex in the region of LIP and VIP, and in the superior temporal polysensory region (STP). Most remarkably, there is recent evidence that areas early in the auditory hierarchy of cortical processing project directly to areas early in the visual hierarchy, including V1.

Both Rockland and Ojima (2001) and Falchier, Clavagnier, Barone, and Kennedy (2002) have recently provided evidence that parabelt regions of auditory cortex in macaque monkeys project directly to primary visual cortex. Auditory cortex has been divided into a core of three primary-like areas, a surrounding belt of perhaps seven secondary areas with dense inputs from the core, and a lateral parabelt of at least two subdivisions. The core projects densely to the belt, while the parabelt represents a third level of auditory processing with dense inputs from the belt areas (see Kaas & Hackett, 2000). Visual cortex consists of a single primary area, V1, a single secondary field, V2, and an array of higher-level fields, including V3, DM (V3a), and DL (V4) (Kaas & Lyon, 2001). Rockland and Ojima (2001) placed injections in the dorsocaudal portion of the auditory parabelt and labeled terminations in the supragranular layers of V1 and V2. Falchier et al. (2002) injected tracers in V1 that were retrogradely transported to neurons in the infragranular layers of the auditory dorsocaudal parabelt. Fewer labeled cells were found in the lateral auditory parabelt and core. These connections between auditory and visual cortex are of the feedback type (see Felleman & Van Essen, 1991), and they may not be reciprocal, because projections from V1 and V2 to auditory areas have not been demonstrated. The connections are also extremely sparse, and thus they would not be expected to have a major impact on the responses of neurons in V1 and V2.

Such feedback connections are usually thought to produce weak modulatory influences on driven activity (see Salin & Bullier, 1995), although a number of functional roles have been proposed (see Falchier et al., 2002). These connections from the auditory parabelt to V1 and V2 would be difficult to detect in traditional single-unit recording experiments without an effort to reveal such weak effects, and previous studies of connections did not disclose these pathways. Rockland and Ojima (2001) suggest that the auditory inputs to V1 and V2 are related to visuospatial or attentional processes. Such a suggestion seems reasonable in that neurons in even early stations in visual pathways, such as the lateral geniculate nucleus, are modulated by information about pending visuomotor tasks (Sáry, Xu, Shostak, Schall, & Casagrande, 2001). Auditory information may also prepare neurons in visual cortex for expected visual stimuli.

Because the multisensory and auditory cortex inputs into V1 and V2 have been revealed only recently, we can expect that the more sensitive tracing methods now in use will reveal comparable inputs related to different sensory modalities in primary and secondary auditory and somatosensory fields. Toward that goal, we already know that the parietal ventral somatosensory area (PV), which also responds to auditory stimuli, projects to areas 3b (S1 proper), 3a, and 1 of anterior parietal cortex (Qi, Lyon, & Kaas, 2002).

Connections of bimodal areas of the insular cortex and the medial auditory belt

Cortex of the upper bank of the lateral sulcus and the adjoining insula of monkeys is dominated by somatosensory inputs (Augustine, 1996). Several somatosensory areas in this region have been proposed, including the parietal ventral area (PV) and the ventral somatosensory area (VS) (see Fig. 17.1). Both of these proposed areas have neurons that respond to auditory as well as somatosensory inputs (Coq et al., 1999; Cusick, Wall, Felleman, & Kaas, 1989; Krubitzer, Clarey, Tweedale, Elston, & Calford, 1995). Both areas receive inputs from a number of somatosensory areas, including areas 3b, 3a, 1, and 2 of anterior parietal cortex (Disbrow, Litinas, Recanzone, Padberg, & Krubitzer, 2003; Qi et al., 2002). The connections of VS have not been fully studied.

One of the auditory areas of the medial belt, the caudomedial auditory area (CM), contains neurons that are responsive to both auditory and somatosensory stimuli (Schroeder et al., 2001). Nearby neurons in the depths of the lateral sulcus, in a region identified as VS, also respond to both types of stimuli (Coq et al., 1999; Cusick, Seltzer, Cola, & Griggs, 1995). Because the portion of VS that is responsive to auditory stimuli is near CM, it is possible that VS and CM are parts of a larger region that is responsive to both auditory and somatosensory stimuli. The connections that mediate the somatosensory responses in CM are largely unknown. Injections placed in CM failed to identify connections with any of the established somatosensory areas; on the other hand, dense interconnections with primary auditory cortex were demonstrated (De la Mothe, Blumell, Kajikawa, & Hackett, 2002). However, the ventral intraparietal area (VIP) does appear to provide an input, and this visuosomatosensory area may provide the somatosensory activation. If so, neurons in CM may be influenced by visual stimuli as well.

In contrast to CM, both somatosensory areas PV and S2 project to the bimodal somatosensory area, VS (Krubitzer, Sesma, & Kaas, 1986; Qi et al., 2002), but the source of auditory input to VS is unknown. VS adjoins the medial auditory belt, and it seems likely that they are interconnected. However, such connections have not been established as VS connections, and those of most of the medial auditory belt have not been determined directly.

Another bimodal area of insular cortex is the gustatory region, where neurons respond to both taste substances and touch on the tongue (Scott, Plata-Salaman, & Smith-Swintosky, 1994). The somatosensory responses likely reflect the connections of anterior parietal somatosensory areas and those of S2 and PV in the region, while the taste responses likely reflect inputs from the taste nucleus of the thalamus (Ogawa, 1994). Because there are several representations of the body in cortex of the lateral sulcus, and because each of these representations should include the tongue, any or all of the areas S2, PV, and VS could also be involved in taste.

Also, the tongue representation in primary somatosensory cortex (area 3b) (Jain, Qi, Catania, & Kaas, 2001) has neurons responsive to touch and taste, with taste inputs coming directly from the taste thalamus. Finally, tactile and painful somatosensory stimuli activate an overlapping region of the human insula (Ostrowsky et al., 2002), and a thalamic nucleus specific for pain and temperature relays to insular cortex in primates (Craig, Bushnell, Zhang, & Blomquist, 1994).

Connections of the multisensory cortex of the superior temporal sulcus

In macaque monkeys, a polysensory region of cortex (STP) in the superior temporal sulcus (STS) was originally described by Desimone and Gross (1979) as responding to visual, auditory, and somatosensory stimuli. This large region has subsequently been divided by different investigators in various ways, based on differences in cortical architecture, connections, and single-neuron response properties (for an extensive review, see Cusick, 1997). Although the functionally significant subdivisions of the region remain uncertain, the existence of a mixture of unimodal and polymodal neurons responsive to visual, somatosensory, and auditory stimuli has been repeatedly demonstrated (e.g., Baylis, Rolls, & Leonard, 1987; Bruce, Desimone, & Gross, 1981; Hikosaka, Iwai, Saito, & Tanaka, 1988; Mistlin & Perrett, 1990). Only the cortex of the upper bank and fundus of the STS is polymodal. The cortex of the lower bank is visual.

The connections of the STP region include visual inputs from a number of higher-order visual areas or regions, including posterior parietal visual areas (Cusick et al., 1995; Seltzer & Pandya, 1978, 1994) and temporal lobe visual areas such as inferotemporal cortex (Saleem, Suzuki, Tanaka, & Hashikawa, 2000), the medial superior temporal area (MST), and visual cortex of the fundus of the superior temporal sulcus (FST) (Boussaoud, Ungerleider, & Desimone, 1990; Kaas & Morel, 1993). The STP region also has a sparse population of neurons with feedback connections to primary visual cortex (Falchier et al., 2002; Lyon & Kaas, 2002a, 2002b), and possibly these connections are reciprocal. Inputs from the visual pulvinar may also directly or indirectly provide some of the visual activation (Bruce, Desimone, & Gross, 1986). Auditory cortex of primates includes a core of primary or primary-like areas, a surrounding belt of auditory areas with direct inputs from the core areas, and a parabelt region of the superior temporal gyrus with inputs from the belt areas (see Kaas & Hackett, 2000, for a review). The STP region receives some auditory input from the auditory belt (Morel, Garraghty, & Kaas, 1993), but considerably more from the auditory parabelt (Seltzer & Pandya, 1978, 1994; Hackett, Stepniewska, & Kaas, 1998). Somatosensory inputs to STP appear to be less direct, with projections from the more anterior portions of posterior parietal cortex being the most prominent source (see Lewis & Van Essen, 2000b; Seltzer & Pandya, 1994). Both the predominantly somatosensory region 7b and the visuosomatosensory region 7a project to portions of the STP (Neal, Pearson, & Powell, 1988). Other inputs originate in the somatosensory cortex of the caudal insula (Seltzer & Pandya, 1994).

What is yet missing from our understanding is how inputs from different modality-related areas relate to each other in the STS region, which is functionally complex and contains several proposed areas (see Cusick et al., 1995). Visual, auditory, and somatosensory areas feeding into the STS region need to be injected with different, distinguishable tracers in the same animals so that regions of overlap, interdigitation, and segregation can be distinguished (see Sakai, Inase, & Tanji, 1996; Sakai, Stepniewska, Qi, & Kaas, 2000).

Posterior parietal cortex: Cortex of the intraparietal sulcus

The posterior parietal cortex of monkeys contains a number of functionally related areas that appear to encode the locations of objects of interest (Colby & Goldberg, 1999). In macaque monkeys, a number of different areas have been proposed, and they are generally named by location in the intraparietal sulcus (IPS). Most commonly, researchers distinguish posterior (PIP), medial (MIP), lateral (LIP), ventral (VIP), and anterior (AIP) intraparietal areas. Some of the areas have been subdivided. Thus, LIP has been divided into a dorsal, lightly myelinated zone (LIPd) and a ventral, densely myelinated zone (LIPv) (Blatt, Anderson, & Stoner, 1990). In addition, LIP has been redefined as a larger area (Ben Hamed, Duhamel, Bremmer, & Graf, 2001). Area MIP has been combined with part of a parieto-occipital area (PO) to form a parietal reach region, PRR (Snyder, Batista, & Anderson, 2000). Other ways of subdividing the intraparietal cortex have also been proposed (see Lewis & Van Essen, 2000a). All this uncertainty over how to divide the IPS region obviously complicates any discussion of connections. Collectively, the IPS areas are thought to transform sensory information into signals related to the control of hand and eye movements via projections to prefrontal, premotor, and visuomotor areas of the frontal lobe (e.g., Rizzolatti, Fogassi, & Gallese, 1997).

Visual inputs provide the predominant sensory input to the IPS areas, but auditory and somatosensory inputs access at least some of the proposed areas. Area LIP, on the posterior third of the lateral bank of the IPS, receives inputs from a number of visual areas, including V2, V3, DM (V3a), MT, MST, V4, and IT (Beck & Kaas, 1999; Blatt et al., 1990; Nakamura et al., 2001). LIP appears to have an important role in directing eye movements to visual targets, and it projects to the frontal eye field (Andersen, Asanuma, & Cowan, 1985; Huerta, Krubitzer, & Kaas, 1987; Schall, Morel, King, & Bullier, 1995). Although LIP has been implicated in multisensory functions (see Ben Hamed, Duhamel, Bremmer, & Graf, 2002), auditory and somatosensory influences appear to be very indirect, and visuomotor functions dominate, as the connection pattern suggests. Sparse somatosensory inputs to LIP appear to come from the region of 7b and insular cortex (Blatt et al., 1990). The PRR region or MIP appears to be similar to LIP, being predominantly visual and encoding the intention to reach with the hand rather than the intention to perform a saccade (Snyder et al., 2000). Yet purely somatosensory neurons and bimodal neurons responding to visual stimuli and touch are present (see Colby & Goldberg, 1999). Again, projections from LIP provide a source of visual input (Nakamura et al., 2001), although nearby visual areas also are likely sources of additional visual input (Caminiti, Ferraina, & Johnson, 1996). The sources of somatosensory inputs to PRR (MIP) are uncertain, but they could come from LIP. The functions of LIP are partially mediated through interconnections with VIP, which is more clearly multisensory. VIP has a mixture of a smaller population of unimodal visual neurons and a majority of bimodal neurons that respond to spots and bars of light as well as light touch (Duhamel, Colby, & Goldberg, 1998). The visual responses are likely mediated by the LIP inputs, although visual regions such as PO and MST provide some input (Lewis & Van Essen, 2000b). The somatosensory responses may depend on inputs from posterior parietal areas 5 and 7, and insular cortex in the region of S2 (Lewis & Van Essen, 2000b). Although it is uncertain whether neurons in VIP are responsive to auditory stimuli, auditory inputs may originate from the dorsolateral auditory belt and parabelt (Hackett et al., 1998). Other connections are with premotor and visuomotor regions of the frontal lobe, especially ventral premotor cortex, a region involved in the control of head, mouth, and hand movements. (Rizzolatti, Luppino, & Matelli, 1998). More rostrally in the IPS, AIP is another region thought to be important in visually guided reach (Colby & Goldberg, 1999). Such guidance would depend both on proprioceptive and tactile information and on visual

information. The major source of visual information appears to come from LIP (Nakamura et al., 2001). Sources of other sensory information remain to be described. However, a major output is to ventral premotor cortex (see Rizzolatti et al., 1998).

Cortex just lateral to the rostral end of IPS, area 7b, is also bimodal, responding to both visual and somatosensory stimuli (Hyvärinen & Shelepin, 1979; Krubitzer et al., 1995). Area 7b has widespread connections with multisensory cortex in STS, IPS, area 5, and the lateral sulcus, as well as with ventral premotor cortex and prefrontal cortex (Cavada & Goldman-Rakic, 1989). The region of 7a is also responsive to visual and somatosensory stimuli, and this region has connections with a number of predominantly visual higher-level visual areas and with the superior temporal polysensory area (Cavada & Goldman-Rakic, 1989; Seltzer & Pandya, 1984). There is also evidence that area 7a receives thalamic inputs related to the vestibular system (Faugier-Grimaud & Ventre, 1989).

Premotor cortex

Premotor and visuomotor areas of the frontal lobe have functions that require access to several modes of sensory information. With accumulating evidence, the precentral cortex, consisting of a primary motor area (M1), a supplementary motor area (SMA), and a premotor area (PM), has been expanded and reconfigured as dorsal and ventral premotor (PMV) areas, each with two subdivisions, a presupplementary motor area, several cingulate motor areas on the medial wall, dorsal and ventral subdivisions of SMA, and supplementary and frontal eye fields (see Wu, Bichot, & Kaas, 2000, for a review). Although it would be informative to review the connections of all of these motor regions, the ventral premotor region is of special interest because of the well-studied multisensory responses of its neurons. Neurons in PMV respond to tactile stimuli on the arm and face, as well as to visual objects near the face, (e.g., Fogassi et al., 1996; see also Graziano, Gross, Taylor, & Moore, Chap. 27, this volume). Many neurons are trimodal, responding to sounds near the head, touch, and vision (Graziano, Reiss, & Gross, 1999). Somatosensory responses could be mediated by inputs from higher-order somatosensory areas of the lateral sulcus, especially S2 and PV (Disbrow et al., 2003; Qi et al., 2001) and from areas 5, 7a, 7b, AIP, and VIP of the posterior parietal cortex (Ghosh & Gattera, 1995; Godschalk, Lemon, Kuypers, & Ronday, 1984; Kurata, 1991; Luppino, Murata, Govoni, & Matelli, 1999; Matelli, Camarda, Glickstein, & Rizzolatti, 1986). This posterior parietal region is likely to provide most of the visual activation. The sources of the auditory input are less clear. Primary auditory areas do not project to the frontal lobe, while the frontal lobe projections of belt and parabelt auditory areas are to regions rostral to premotor cortex (Hackett, Stepniewska, & Kaas, 1999; Romanski, Bates, & Goldman-Rakic, 1999). Graziano et al. (1999) suggest that the auditory responses reflect input from trimodal portions of area 7b.

Prefrontal cortex

The part of the frontal lobe anterior to premotor and visuomotor cortex is known as prefrontal cortex (see Fuster, 1997, for an extensive review). Prefrontal cortex is subdivided into a group of interconnecting cortical areas that are related to evaluative and cognitive functions. The subdivisions of prefrontal cortex are usually denoted by Brodmann's numbers, but uncertainties about how the region is functionally subdivided remain. Much of the cortex has long been considered to be multisensory (e.g., Bignall, 1970), and multisensory higher-order sensory areas provide many sources of sensory information to prefrontal regions. A few of the general regions of prefrontal cortex, each containing several subdivisions, are briefly considered here.

Medial prefrontal cortex includes several architectonically distinct areas and regions of distinct functions and sets of connections (see Barbas, Ghashghaei, Dombrowski, & Rempel-Clower, 1999, for a review). Much of the region is enriched with opiate receptors, suggesting a role in affective aspects of behavior. Major inputs to much of the cortex are from superior temporal cortex, including STP and parabelt auditory cortex (Barbas et al., 1999; Hackett et al., 1999; Romanski, Bates, et al., 1999). The dorsolateral region of prefrontal cortex is generally considered to be important for working memory. Dorsolateral prefrontal cortex has been further subdivided into a dorsal portion more related to the spatial locations of stimuli and a ventral portion related to the identity of stimulus objects (see Levy & Goldman-Rakic, 2000). Both regions receive a number of auditory, visual, and multisensory inputs, with a greater emphasis on dorsal cortex inputs related to the "where" stream of processing to dorsal prefrontal cortex and ventral cortex inputs related to the "what" stream of processing to ventral prefrontal cortex (see Cavada & Goldman-Rakic, 1989; Kaas & Hackett, 1999; Petrides & Pandya, 1988; Romanski, Tian, Mishkin, Goldman-Rakic, & Rauschecker, 1999; Selemon & Goldman-Rakic, 1988; Wilson, Scalaidhe, & Kaas, 1993). A third general region of prefrontal cortex is the orbital region, which is involved in emotive and motivational functions (see Zald & Kim, 2001, for a review). The

rostral part of the auditory parabelt and the more rostral parts of the superior temporal gyrus and sulcus provide auditory and polymodal inputs to orbitofrontal cortex (see Barbas, 1993; Carmichael & Price, 1995; Hackett et al., 1999; Romanski, Bates, et al., 1999). Visual inputs come from inferior temporal cortex and the AIP area, while somatosensory inputs come from insular cortex. Finally, part of this cortex is involved in taste, and olfactory areas may project to posterior orbitofrontal cortex. Neurons in orbitofrontal cortex are responsive to visual and auditory stimuli (Benevento, Fallon, Davis, & Rezak, 1977).

Conclusions

Over the past 30 years, major changes have occurred in the prevailing concepts of how neocortex in primates is organized. In the early years of recording from neocortex of monkeys, the anesthetics in common use depressed the responsiveness of cortical neurons, and large regions of cortex were unresponsive to sensory stimuli. Only primary and secondary sensory fields were briskly responsive, and the functional organization of most of the remaining cortex was unknown. Much of the silent cortex was assumed to be multisensory association cortex. As better anesthetics came into use, microelectrode mapping methods revealed that much of the unresponsive cortex contained orderly representations of the contralateral visual hemifield, body receptors, or auditory receptors. By the 1980s it appeared that most of the proposed association cortex was occupied by unimodal visual, somatosensory, or auditory fields (see Merzenich & Kaas, 1980). These unimodal fields were clustered together, and the clusters extended toward each other to exclude the possibility of much multisensory cortex. Connection patterns of identified areas reinforced this concept, as connections between areas tended to be concentrated between nearby and adjoining areas of the same modality (see Felleman & Van Essen, 1991; Young et al., 1994). More recently, we have begun appreciating the amount of cortex that is devoted to bimodal and multisensory processing. To a large extent, this is a consequence of the widespread use of methods that allow recordings from awake, behaving monkeys. Thus, it has become possible to study areas in posterior parietal cortex, temporal cortex, and frontal cortex that are responsive to more than one sensory modality but are connectionally distant from primary sensory areas. In addition, regions of cortex providing inputs to these strongly multisensory regions have been identified, associated with one or more of the modalities, and thus the significance of connection patterns has become more interpretable. Finally, and quite important, methods of tracing connections have become more sensitive, and previously sparse and unknown connections have been disclosed. As a dramatic and unexpected example, it now appears that even primary and secondary areas of visual cortex receive inputs from early stations of auditory cortex. Instead of having little multisensory cortex, it appears that primates have many types of multisensory and bimodal cortex with many different functional roles. The near future should further our understandings of how cortex is subdivided into functionally distinct regions and how these regions are interconnected. Most areas are unlikely to be structurally or functionally homogeneous, and the task of identifying the modular components of areas is compelling. Toward this end, we have the advantage of being able to use a number of different, distinguishable tracers to identify connections. Thus, it is now possible to see precisely how various inputs overlap or interdigitate to relate to populations of neurons to mediate unimodal or multisensory response properties and different types and magnitudes of sensory interactions.

REFERENCES

Andersen, R. A., Asanuma, C., & Cowan, W. M. (1985). Callosal and prefrontal associational projecting cell populations in area 7A of the macaque monkey: A study using retrogradely transported fluorescent dyes. *Journal of Comparative Neurology, 232*, 443–455.

Augustine, J. R. (1996). Circuitry and functional aspects of the insular lobe in primates including humans. *Brain Research Review, 3*, 229–244.

Barbas, H. (1993). Organization of cortical afferent input to orbitofrontal areas in the rhesus monkey. *Neuroscience, 56*, 841–864.

Barbas, H., Ghashghaei, H., Dombrowski, S. M., & Rempel-Clower, N. L. (1999). Medial prefrontal cortices are unified by common connections with superior temporal cortices and distinguished by input from memory-related areas in the rhesus monkey. *Journal of Comparative Neurology, 410*, 343–367.

Baylis, G. C., Rolls, E. T., & Leonard, C. M. (1987). Functional subdivisions of the temporal lobe neocortex. *Journal of Neuroscience, 2*, 330–342.

Beck, P. D., & Kaas, J. H. (1999). Cortical connections of the dorsomedial visual area in old world macaque monkeys. *Journal of Comparative Neurology, 406*, 487–502.

Ben Hamed, S., Duhamel, J. R., Bremmer, F., & Graf, W. (2001). Representation of the visual field in the lateral intraparietal area of macaque monkeys: A quantitative receptive field analysis. *Experimental Brain Research, 140*, 127–144.

Ben Hamed, S., Duhamel, J. R., Bremmer, F., & Graf, W. (2002). Visual receptive field modulation in the lateral intraparietal area during attentive fixation and free gaze. *Cerebral Cortex, 12*, 234–245.

Benevento, L. A., Fallon, J., Davis, B. J., & Rezak, M. (1977). Auditory-visual interaction in single cells in the cortex of the superior temporal sulcus and the orbital frontal cortex of the macaque monkey. *Experimental Neurology, 57*, 849–872.

Bignall, K. E. (1970). Auditory input to frontal polysensory cortex of the squirrel monkey: Possible pathways. *Brain Research, 19*, 77–86.

Blatt, G. J., Andersen, R. A., & Stoner, G. R. (1990). Visual receptive field organization and cortico-cortical connections of the lateral intraparietal area (area LIP) in the macaque. *Journal of Comparative Neurology, 299*, 421–445.

Boussaoud, D., Ungerleider, L. G., & Desimone, R. (1990). Pathways for motion analysis: Cortical connections of the medial superior temporal and fundus of the superior temporal visual areas in the macaque. *Journal of Comparative Neurology, 296*, 462–495.

Bruce, C., Desimone, R., & Gross, C. G. (1981). Visual properties of neurons in a polysensory area in superior temporal sulcus of the macaque. *Journal of Neurophysiology, 46*, 369–384.

Bruce, C. J., Desimone, R., & Gross, C. G. (1986). Both striate cortex and superior colliculus contribute to visual properties of neurons in superior temporal polysensory area of macaque monkey. *Journal of Neurophysiology, 55*, 1057–1075.

Caminiti, R., Ferraina, S., & Johnson, P. B. (1996). The sources of visual information to the primate frontal lobe: A novel role for the superior parietal lobule. *Cerebral Cortex, 6*, 319–328.

Carmichael, S. T., & Price, J. L. (1995). Sensory and premotor connections of the orbital and medial prefrontal cortex of macaque monkeys. *Journal of Comparative Neurology, 363*, 642–664.

Cavada, C., & Goldman-Rakic, P. S. (1989). Posterior parietal cortex in rhesus monkey: II. Evidence for segregated corticocortical networks linking sensory and limbic areas with the frontal lobe. *Journal of Comparative Neurology, 287*, 422–445.

Colby, C. L., & Goldberg, M. E. (1999). Space and attention in parietal cortex. *Annual Review of Neuroscience, 22*, 319–349.

Coq, J. O., Qi, H.-X., Catania, K. C., Collins, C. E., Jain, N., & Kaas, J. H. (1999). Organization of somatosensory cortex in the New World Titi monkey. *Society of Neuroscience Abstracts, 25*, 1683.

Craig, A. D., Bushnell, M. C., Zhang, E. T., & Blomquist, A. (1994). A thalamic nucleus specific for pain and temperature sensation. *Nature, 372*, 770–773.

Cusick, C. G. (1997). The superior temporal polysensory region in monkeys. In K. S. Rockland, J. H. Kaas, & A. Peters (Eds.), *Cerebral cortex: Extrastriate cortex in primates* (pp. 435–463). New York: Plenum Press.

Cusick, C. G., Seltzer, B., Cola, M., & Griggs, E. (1995). Chemoarchitectonics and corticocortical terminations within the superior temporal sulcus of the rhesus monkey: Evidence for subdivisions of superior temporal polysensory cortex. *Journal of Comparative Neurology, 360*, 513–535.

Cusick, C. G., Wall, J. T., Felleman, D. J., & Kaas, J. H. (1989). Somatotopic organization of the lateral sulcus of owl monkeys: Area 3b, S-II, and a ventral somatosensory area. *Journal of Comparative Neurology, 282*, 169–190.

De la Mothe, L., Blumell, S., Kajikawa, Y., & Hackett, T. A. (2002). Cortical connections of medial belt cortex in marmoset monkeys. *Society of Neuroscience Abstracts.*

Desimone, R., & Gross, C. G. (1979). Visual areas in the temporal cortex of the macaque. *Brain Research, 178*, 363–380.

Diamond, I. T., & Hall, W. C. (1969). Evolution of neocortex. *Science, 164*, 251–262.

Disbrow, E., Litinas, E., Recanzone, G. H., Padberg, J., & Krubitzer, L. (2003). Cortical connections of the second somatosensory area and the parietal ventral area in macaque monkeys. *Journal of Comparative Neurology, 462,* 382–399.

Duhamel, J. R., Colby, C. L., & Goldberg, M. E. (1998). Ventral intraparietal area of the macaque: Congruent visual and somatic response properties. *Journal of Neurophysiology, 79,* 126–136.

Falchier, A., Clavagnier, S., Barone, P., & Kennedy, H. (2002). Anatomical evidence of multimodal integration in primate striate cortex. *Journal of Neuroscience, 22,* 5749–5759.

Faugier-Grimaud, S., & Ventre, J. (1989). Anatomic connections of inferior parietal cortex (area 7) with subcortical structures related to vestibulo-ocular function in a monkey (*Macaca fascicularis*). *Journal of Comparative Neurology, 280,* 1–14.

Felleman, D. J., & Van Essen, D. C. (1991). Distributed hierarchical processing in the primate cerebral cortex. *Cerebral Cortex, 1,* 1–47.

Fogassi, L., Gallese, V., Fadiga, L., Luppino, G., Matelli, M., & Rizzolatti, G. (1996). Coding of peripersonal space in inferior premotor cortex (area F4). *Journal of Neurophysiology, 76,* 141–157.

Fuster, J. M. (1997). *The prefrontal cortex* (3d ed.). Philadelphia: Lippincott-Raven.

Ghosh, S., & Gattera, R. A. (1995). A comparison of the ipsilateral cortical projections to the dorsal and ventral subdivisions of the macaque premotor cortex. *Somatosensory and Motor Research, 12,* 359–378.

Godschalk, M., Lemon, R. N., Kuypers, H. G., & Ronday, H. K. (1984). Cortical afferents and efferents of monkey postarcuate area: An anatomical and electrophysiological study. *Experimental Brain Research, 56,* 410–424.

Graziano, M. S., Reiss, L. A., & Gross, C. G. (1999). A neuronal representation of the location of nearby sounds. *Nature, 397,* 428–430.

Hackett, T. A., Stepniewska, I., & Kaas, J. H. (1998). Subdivisions of auditory cortex and ipsilateral cortical connections of the parabelt auditory cortex in macaque monkeys. *Journal of Comparative Neurology, 394,* 475–495.

Hackett, T. A., Stepniewska, I., & Kaas, J. H. (1999). Prefrontal connections of the parabelt auditory cortex in macaque monkeys. *Brain Research, 817,* 45–48.

Hikosaka, K., Iwai, E., Saito, H., & Tanaka, K. (1988). Polysensory properties of neurons in the anterior bank of the caudal superior temporal sulcus of the macaque monkey. *Journal of Neurophysiology, 60,* 1615–1637.

Hodos, W., & Campbell, C. B. (1969). Scala Naturae: Why there is no theory in comparative psychology. *Psychological Review, 76,* 337–350.

Huerta, M. F., Krubitzer, L. A., & Kaas, J. H. (1987). Frontal eye field as defined by intracortical microstimulation in squirrel monkeys, owl monkeys, and macaque monkeys: II. Cortical connections. *Journal of Comparative Neurology, 265,* 332–361.

Hyvärinen, J., & Shelepin, Y. (1979). Distribution of visual and somatic functions in the parietal associative area 7 of the monkey. *Brain Research, 169,* 561–564.

Jain, N., Qi, H.-X., Catania, K. C., & Kaas, J. H. (2001). Anatomic correlates of the face and oral cavity representations in the somatosensory cortical area 3b of monkeys. *Journal of Comparative Neurology, 429,* 455–468.

Kaas, J. H. (1989). Why does the brain have so many visual areas? *Journal of Cognitive Neurosciences, 1,* 121–135.

Kaas, J. H. (1999). The transformation of association cortex into sensory cortex. *Brain Research Bulletin, 50,* 425.

Kaas, J. H., & Hackett, T. A. (1999). "What" and "where" processing in auditory cortex. *Nature Neuroscience, 2,* 1045–1047.

Kaas, J. H., & Hackett, T. A. (2000). Subdivisions of auditory cortex and processing streams in primates. *Proceedings of the National Academy of Sciences, USA, 97,* 11793–11799.

Kaas, J. H., Jain, N., & Qi, H.-X. (2001). The organization of the somatosensory system in primates. In R. J. Nelson (Ed.), *The somatosensory system: Deciphering the brain's own body image* (pp. 1–25). Boca Raton, FL: CRC Press.

Kaas, J. H., & Lyon, D. C. (2001). Visual cortex organization in primates: Theories of V3 and adjoining visual areas. *Progress in Brain Research, 134,* 285–295.

Kaas, J. H., & Morel, A. (1993). Connections of visual areas of the upper temporal lobe of owl monkeys: The MT crescent and dorsal and ventral subdivisions of FST. *Journal of Neuroscience, 13,* 534–546.

Krubitzer, L., Clarey, J., Tweedale, R., Elston, G., & Calford, M. (1995). A redefinition of somatosensory areas in the lateral sulcus of macaque monkeys. *Journal of Neuroscience, 15,* 3821–3839.

Krubitzer, L. A., Sesma, M. A., & Kaas, J. H. (1986). Microelectrode maps, myeloarchitecture, and cortical connections of three somatotopically organized representations of the body surface in the parietal cortex of squirrels. *Journal of Comparative Neurology, 250,* 403–430.

Kurata, K. (1991). Corticocortical inputs to the dorsal and ventral aspects of the premotor cortex of macaque monkeys. *Neuroscience Research, 12,* 263–280.

Levy, R., & Goldman-Rakic, P. S. (2000). Segregation of working memory functions within the dorsolateral prefrontal cortex. *Experimental Brain Research, 133,* 23–32.

Lewis, J. W., & Van Essen, D. C. (2000a). Mapping of architectonic subdivisions in the macaque monkey, with emphasis on parieto-occipital cortex. *Journal of Comparative Neurology, 428,* 79–111.

Lewis, J. W., & Van Essen, D. C. (2000b). Corticocortical connections of visual, sensorimotor, and multimodal processing areas in the parietal lobe of the macaque monkey. *Journal of Comparative Neurology, 428,* 112–137.

Luppino, G., Murata, A., Govoni, P., & Matelli, M. (1999). Largely segregated parietofrontal connections linking rostral intraparietal cortex (areas AIP and VIP) and the ventral premotor cortex (areas F5 and F4). *Experimental Brain Research, 128,* 181–187.

Lyon, D. C., & Kaas, J. H. (2001). Connectional and architectonic evidence for dorsal and ventral V3, and dorsomedial area in marmoset monkeys. *Journal of Neuroscience, 21,* 249–261.

Lyon, D. C., & Kaas, J. H. (2002a). Evidence for a modified V3 with dorsal and ventral halves in macaque monkeys. *Neuron, 33,* 453–461.

Lyon, D. C., & Kaas, J. H. (2002b). Evidence from V1 connections for both dorsal and ventral subdivisions of V3 in three species of new world monkeys. *Journal of Comparative Neurology, 449,* 281–297.

Masterton, R. B., & Berkley, M. A. (1974). Brain function: Changing ideas on the role of sensory, motor, and association cortex in behavior. *Annual Review of Psychology, 25,* 277–312.

Matelli, M., Camarda, R., Glickstein, M., & Rizzolatti, G. (1986). Afferent and efferent projections of the inferior area 6 in the macaque monkey. *Journal of Comparative Neurology, 251,* 281–298.

Merzenich, M. M., & Kaas, J. H. (1980). Principles of organization of sensory-perceptual systems in mammals. In J. M. Sprague & A. N. Epstein (Eds.), *Progress in psychobiology and physiological psychology* (pp. 1–42). New York: Academic Press.

Mistlin, A. J., & Perrett, D. I. (1990). Visual and somatosensory processing in the macaque temporal cortex: The role of "expectation." *Experimental Brain Research, 82,* 437–450.

Morel, A., Garraghty, P. E., & Kaas, J. H. (1993). Tonotopic organization, architectonic fields, and connections of auditory cortex in macaque monkeys. *Journal of Comparative Neurology, 335,* 437–459.

Nakamura, H., Kuroda, T., Wakita, M., Kusunoki, M., Kato, A., Mikami, A., et al. (2001). From three-dimensional space vision to prehensile hand movements: The lateral intraparietal area links the area V3A and the anterior intraparietal area in macaques. *Journal of Neuroscience, 21,* 8174–8187.

Neal, J. W., Pearson, R. C., & Powell, T. P. (1988). The corticocortical connections within the parieto-temporal lobe of area PG, 7a, in the monkey. *Brain Research, 438,* 343–350.

Ogawa, H. (1994). Gustatory cortex of primates: Anatomy and physiology. *Neuroscience Research, 20,* 1–13.

Ostrowsky, K., Magnin, M., Ryvlin, P., Isnard, J., Guenot, M., & Mauguiere, F. (2002). Representation of pain and somatic sensation in the human insula: A study of responses to direct electrical cortical stimulation. *Cerebral Cortex, 12,* 376–385.

Petrides, M., & Pandya, D. N. (1988). Association fiber pathways to the frontal cortex from the superior temporal region in the rhesus monkey. *Journal of Comparative Neurology, 273,* 52–66.

Preuss, T. M. (2000). Taking the measure of diversity: Comparative alternatives to the model-animal paradigm in cortical neuroscience. *Brain Behavior and Evolution, 55,* 287–299.

Qi, H.-X., Lyon, D. C., & Kaas, J. H. (2002). Cortical and thalamic connections of the parietal ventral somatosensory area in marmoset monkeys (*Callithrix jacchus*). *Journal of Comparative Neurology, 443,* 168–182.

Rizzolatti, G., Luppino, G., & Matelli, M. (1998). The organization of the cortical motor system: New concepts. *Electroencephalography and Clinical Neurophysiology, 106,* 283–296.

Rizzolatti, G., Fogassi, L., & Gallese, V. (1997). Parietal cortex: From sight to action. *Current Opinion in Neurobiology, 7,* 562–567.

Rockland, K. S., & Ojima, H. (2001). Calcarine area V1 as a multimodal convergence area. *Society for Neuroscience Abstracts, 511,* 20.

Romanski, L. M., Bates, J. F., & Goldman-Rakic, P. S. (1999). Auditory belt and parabelt projections to the prefrontal cortex in the rhesus monkey. *Journal of Comparative Neurology, 403,* 141–157.

Romanski, L. M., Tian, B., Mishkin, M., Goldman-Rakic, P. S., & Rauschecker, J. P. (1999). Dual streams of auditory afferents target multiple domains in the primate prefrontal cortex. *Nature Neuroscience, 2,* 1131–1136.

Sakai, S. T., Inase, M., & Tanji, J. (1996). Comparison of cerebellothalamic and pallidothalamic projections in the monkey (*Macaca fuscata*): A double anterograde labeling study. *Journal of Comparative Neurology, 368,* 215–228.

Sakai, S. T., Stepniewska, I., Qi, H.-X., & Kaas, J. H. (2000). Pallidal and cerebellar afferents to pre-supplementary motor area thalamocortical neurons in the owl monkey: A multiple labeling study. *Journal of Comparative Neurology, 417,* 164–180.

Saleem, K. S., Suzuki, W., Tanaka, K., & Hashikawa, T. (2000). Connections between anterior inferotemporal cortex and superior temporal sulcus regions in the macaque monkey. *Journal of Neuroscience, 20,* 5083–5101.

Salin, P. A., & Bullier, J. (1995). Corticocortical connections in the visual system: structure and function. *Physiological Review, 75,* 107–154.

Sáry, G., Xu, X., Shostak, Y., Schall, J., & Casagrande, V. (2001). Extraretinal modulation of the lateral geniculate nucleus (LGN). *Society for Neuroscience Abstracts, 723,* 15.

Schall, J. D., Morel, A., King, D. J., & Bullier, J. (1995). Topography of visual cortex connections with frontal eye field in macaque: Convergence and segregation of processing streams. *Journal of Neuroscience, 15,* 4464–4487.

Schroeder, C. E., Lindsley, R. W., Specht, C., Marcovici, A., Smiley, J. F., & Javitt, D. C. (2001). Somatosensory input to auditory association cortex in the macaque monkey. *Journal of Neurophysiology, 85,* 1322–1327.

Scott, T. R., Plata-Salaman, C. R., & Smith-Swintosky, V. L. (1994). Gustatory neural coding in the monkey cortex: The quality of saltiness. *Journal of Neurophysiology, 71,* 1692–1701.

Selemon, L. D., & Goldman-Rakic, P. S. (1988). Common cortical and subcortical targets of the dorsolateral prefrontal and posterior parietal cortices in the rhesus monkey: Evidence for a distributed neural network subserving spatially guided behavior. *Journal of Neuroscience, 8,* 4049–4068.

Seltzer, B., & Pandya, D. N. (1978). Afferent cortical connections and architectonics of the superior temporal sulcus and surrounding cortex in the rhesus monkey. *Brain Research, 149,* 1–24.

Seltzer, B., & Pandya, D. N. (1984). Further observations on parieto-temporal connections in the rhesus monkey. *Experimental Brain Research, 55,* 301–312.

Seltzer, B., & Pandya, D. N. (1994). Parietal, temporal, and occipital projections to cortex of the superior temporal sulcus in the rhesus monkey: A retrograde tracer study. *Journal of Comparative Neurology, 343,* 445–463.

Snyder, L. H., Batista, A. P., & Andersen, R. A. (2000). Intention-related activity in the posterior parietal cortex: A review. *Vision Research, 40,* 1433–1441.

Thompson, R. F. (1967). *Foundations of physiological psychology.* New York: Academic Press.

Wilson, F. A. W., Scalaidhe, S. P. Ó., & Goldman-Rakic, P. S. (1993). Dissociation of object and spatial processing domains in primate prefrontal cortex. *Science, 260,* 1955–1958.

Wu, C. W., Bichot, N. P., & Kaas, J. H. (2000). Converging evidence from microstimulation, architecture, and connections for multiple motor areas in the frontal and cingulate cortex of prosimian primates. *Journal of Comparative Neurology, 423,* 140–177.

Young, M. P., Scannell, J. W., Burns, G. A., & Blakemore, C. (1994). Analysis of connectivity: Neural systems in the cerebral cortex. *Reviews in the Neurosciences, 5,* 227–250.

Zald, D. H., & Kim, S. W. (2001). The orbitofrontal cortex. In S. P. Salloway, P. F. Malloy, & J. D. Duffy (Eds.), *The frontal lobes and neuropsychiatric illness* (pp. 33–70). Washington, DC: American Psychiatric Press.

18 Multisensory Convergence in Early Cortical Processing

CHARLES E. SCHROEDER AND JOHN J. FOXE

Introduction

Neocortical representation or "mapping" of the sensory world is a key feature of functional brain organization in most species. As exemplified by the large body of work on macaque monkeys, each sensory system is mapped onto an interconnected array of cortical areas, and within each array there appears to be a hierarchical progression from simple to complex processing (Burton & Sinclair, 1996; Felleman & Van Essen, 1991; Rauschecker, Tian, Pons, & Mishkin, 1997). The fact that the different senses sample unique aspects of physical objects should provide the brain with both a richer description of objects and converging evidence about their position, movement, and identity. Subjective experience tells us that the inputs are ultimately combined across modalities. However, our understanding of information processing in the brain is largely couched in unisensory terms. The most detailed explication of brain mechanisms of multisensory processing has come from work on the superior colliculus of cats (Stein & Meredith, 1993), although parallel work on the neocortex in humans and monkeys has progressed rapidly in recent years. In monkey studies, evidence of multisensory convergence has been obtained for numerous regions of the parietal (Duhamel, Colby, & Goldberg, 1998; Hyvarinen & Shelepin, 1979; Mazzoni, Bracewell, Barash, & Andersen, 1996; Schroeder & Foxe, 2002; Seltzer & Pandya, 1980), temporal (Benevento, Fallon, Davis, & Rezak, 1977; Bruce, Desimone, & Gross, 1981; Hikosaka, Iwai, Saito, & Tanaka, 1988; Leinonen, 1980; Leinonen, Hyvarinen, & Sovijarvi, 1980; Schroeder & Foxe, 2002; Schroeder, Lindsley, et al., 2001), and frontal lobes (Benevento et al., 1977; Graziano, Hu, & Gross, 1997; Graziano, Yap, & Gross, 1994; Rizzolatti, Scandolara, Gentilucci, & Camarda, 1981a, 1981b). Based on these findings, it is often assumed that multisensory convergence is deferred until late in processing, occurring only in high-order association cortices specialized for that purpose. However, recent findings in both monkeys and humans provide evidence of multisensory convergence at very early, putatively unisensory stages of sensory processing (Calvert, Brammer, Campbell, Iverson, & David, 1999; Foxe et al., 2000; Giard & Peronet, 1999; Levanen, Jousmaki, & Hari, 1998; Molholm et al., 2002; Schroeder & Foxe, 2002; Schroeder et al., 2001). This chapter addresses three questions about multisensory convergence during early cortical processing in humans and monkeys.

The most basic question is, how widespread is multisensory convergence early in cortical processing? If early multisensory convergence is a fundamental design feature of sensory processing architecture, we would expect it to occur across the major sensory systems. On the other hand, early multisensory convergence may be of most use in one or a few of the systems. We will examine the degree to which early sensory processing stages in the visual, auditory, and somatosensory systems receive converging afferents from one or more of the other sensory systems.

Another basic question is, what are the anatomical mechanisms of convergence? In order for interactions between different sensory inputs to occur, the neuronal projections that carry the inputs into the brain must converge at some point. Multisensory convergence can occur within a single neuron (neuronal convergence) or in adjacent neurons within a single cortical region or interconnected ensemble (areal convergence). In theory, converging sensory inputs can be mediated by feedforward, feedback, or lateral axonal projections. A firm understanding of multisensory processing requires that we define and elaborate anatomical mechanisms in terms of each of these components.

The final question concerns the temporal dimensions of multisensory processing. Multisensory convergence in the neocortex can depend on the temporal parameters of both external stimulus energy transmission and internal (neural) processing, and these parameters vary radically across different sensory modalities. As an example of the former, if we observe a man hitting a spike with a hammer at 20 meters' distance, the sound is delayed relative to the sight of the event. One reason for this perceptual incongruity is that, relative to the speed of light, the speed of sound (~1100 ft/s) is quite slow, and thus the initial sensory response in the ear begins almost 60 ms after the initial sensory response in the eye. On the other hand, at a comfortable conversational distance of about 1–2 meters, the auditory and visual stimuli generated by a speaker are perceived as synchronous, because the auditory stimulus lag due to the relatively low speed of sound is reduced to the order of 3 or 4 ms. A hidden temporal factor in multisensory convergence is the internal delay, that is, the time necessary for stimulus transduction and neural conduction up to the cortex. Interestingly, the internal processing delay for auditory stimuli is much less than that for visual stimuli, a fact which may adjust the timing offset for auditory-visual stimuli at moderate distances from the observer. Variations in stimulus energy transmission parameters, along with stimulus-related variations in the temporal parameters of processing in the central sensory pathways, contribute a rich temporal dimension to multisensory convergence. We will examine this dimension from both theoretical and empirical perspectives.

Evidence of early multisensory convergence in cortical processing

Using event-related potential (ERP) recordings, Giard and colleagues (Giard & Peronet, 1999) have demonstrated modulation of visual ERPs by concurrently presented auditory stimuli. Significantly, audiovisual interactions were detected at an extremely early time point in visual processing (40 ms) and in electrode locations overlying brain structures that lie at early stages of cortical visual processing. These findings have been replicated with higher spatial resolution by recent studies in our laboratory (Molholm et al., 2002). The location and timing of these audiovisual interactions argue for auditory input at early stages of visual processing. Both studies also showed short-latency visual-auditory interactions in electrode locations overlying auditory cortex. An additional study from our laboratory (Foxe et al., 2000) demonstrated somato-auditory interactions, with timing and topography consistent with an ERP generator in auditory cortex. Although the specific brain regions in which convergence first occurs cannot be localized with certainty by ERP methods alone, in each of these cases both the timing and the location of the interactions were consistent with the idea of multisensory convergence at early stages of the auditory pathways, in structures formerly considered to be unisensory in function. Also in each case, the conclusion was independently supported by findings from other brain imaging techniques with (arguably) better anatomical resolution. Using magnetoencephalographic (MEG)

recordings, Levanen et al. (1998) showed vibration-induced activation of auditory cortex in deaf adults, and in a functional magnetic resonance imaging (fMRI) study we subsequently confirmed localization of a somatosensory-responsive region within auditory cortex (Foxe et al., 2002). Using MEG, Sams et al. (1991) also demonstrated visual-auditory interactions in auditory cortex. Finally, with fMRI, Calvert and Bullmore (1997) demonstrated activation of auditory cortex by silent lipreading in normal adults. The same study also found auditory-visual convergence in classic "polysensory" cortex in the nearby superior temporal sulcal (STS) regions (Bruce et al., 1981). More recent fMRI studies (Calvert, Hansen, Iverson, & Brammer, 2001) suggest that audiovisual interactions are distributed across many areas that are considered to be unimodal. These areas include portions of area 19 corresponding to macaque areas V4 and V5, as well as along Heschl's gyrus, corresponding to primary auditory cortex (A1). Although it could be argued that the results reported by Levanen et al. (1998) reflect adaptive rewiring of auditory cortex during development, this argument would not apply to any of the ERP or fMRI studies conducted in normal volunteers.

Regarding auditory inputs into early visual processing, the earliest stages of visual processing, widely recognized as sites of audiovisual convergence, are the superior temporal polysensory area, or STP (Benevento et al., 1977; Bruce et al., 1981; Hikosaka et al., 1988; Seltzer & Pandya, 1978), and several regions in the intraparietal sulcus, ventral intraparietal area, or VIP (Duhamel et al., 1998), and lateral intraparietal area, or LIP (Grunewald, Linden, & Andersen, 1999). There is both anatomical and physiological evidence of multisensory convergence in STP. Similarly, there is both physiological (Grunewald et al., 1999; Linden, Grunewald, & Andersen, 1999) and anatomical (Lewis & Van Essen, 2000a, 2000b), evidence of multisensory convergence in intraparietel sulcal regions. STP is in the upper bank of the STS, while auditory cortex is on the lower bank of the adjacent lateral sulcus (LS) (Fig. 18.1; Color Plate 3). STP appears to consist of at least two divisions and occupies most of the upper bank of the STS (see, e.g., Felleman & Van Essen, 1991). The multisensory regions of the IP sulcus include both lateral and medial banks, as well as the fundus of the sulcus (Duhamel et al., 1998; Grunewald et al., 1999). Assuming audiovisual convergence by a feed-forward mechanism, the human analogues of STP and LIP are potential neural substrates for the ERP effects noted by Giard and Peronet (1999) and Molholm et al. (2002). Using more relaxed anatomical constraints, such as inclusion of feedback circuits (see below), a number of "unisensory" areas (e.g., Calvert & Bullmore, 1997;

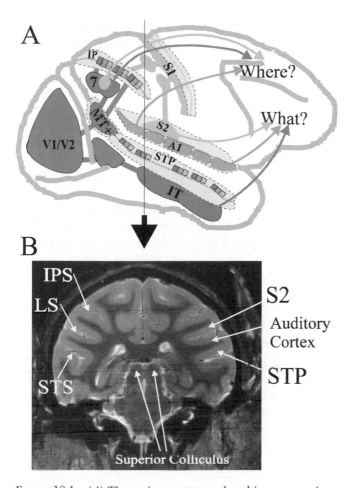

A

IP
7
SI
Where?
MT+
S2
What?
V1/V2
A1
STP
IT

B

IPS
LS
S2
Auditory
Cortex
STS
STP
Superior Colliculus

FIGURE 18.1 (*A*) The major sensory and multisensory regions of posterior sensory neocortex. The classic multisensory areas of the superior temporal polysensory (STP) and those in the intraparietal (IP) sulcus are indicated by tricolor patches and shown in relation to the proposed "where" and "what" divisions of the visual (red), auditory (blue), and somatosensory (olive) systems. Sulcal regions are depicted with dashed lines and gray shading. (*B*) Coronal MRI section through a macaque monkey brain at the level indicated by the cut line in *A*, illustrating the anatomical location of several important multisensory regions of posterior sensory neocortex. Also indicated is the position of the superior colliculus. The section is a T2-weighted image taken at 7.0 Tesla, with a section thickness of 2 mm and in-plane resolution of 0.5 × 0.5 mm. Abbreviations: IPS, intraparietal sulcus; LS, lateral sulcus; STS, superior temporal sulcus; STP, superior temporal polysensory area. (Adapted from Schroeder et al., in press.) (See Color Plate 3.)

Calvert et al., 2001) can be included as potential substrates. This is helpful, because multisensory areas of human STS and IPS are situated in ways that do not easily predict the surface ERP topography found by either Giard and Peronet (1999) or Molhom et al. (2002). However, the topography of audiovisual interactions in both of these studies is consistent with unimodal visual areas in the region of the middle occipital gyrus, such as MT+. Therefore, these data align with the possibility that some form of multisensory convergence occurs

prior to the level of STP and IP. In this regard, a few studies in cats did suggest auditory input to visual cortex in cats (e.g., Bental, Dafny, & Feldman, 1968), but because of concerns with the methodology of the studies, these reports did not gain general acceptance. Corresponding primate visual areas, such as V2, V4, and MT, that receive direct projections from V1 and thus are considered to represent "early processing stages" have not as yet been shown to be directly responsive to auditory or somatosensory stimulation. However, recent findings published by two groups (Falchier, Renaud, Barone, & Kennedy, 2001; Rockland & Ojima, 2001) indicate direct anatomical connections between auditory and visual cortices (discussed below under Anatomical Feed-forward and Feedback Circuits for Multisensory Convergence). These "cross-connections" have multilaminar termination profiles consistent with either feedback or lateral connections and extend down to the level of the primary cortices, although at this level the projections are sparse and confined to the peripheral visual field representation. An important caveat to this discussion is that although microelectrode studies in monkeys clearly can localize sites of multisensory convergence more precisely than even hemodynamic studies in humans, they have an extremely limited sampling scope and are unlikely to have detected nonvisual inputs into the early stages of the visual system unless these inputs were a target of study. Thus, the fact that prior studies in monkeys have not reported multisensory convergence in MT or MST does not rule out its occurrence in these regions.

On the other hand, findings in monkeys provide direct confirmation of multisensory convergence in auditory cortex, as indicated by the ERP, MEG, and fMRI studies in humans. Somatosensory inputs have been found in the regions immediately posterior to A1 in three macaque species to date (Fu et al., in press; Schroeder & Foxe, 2002; Schroeder, Lindsley, et al., 2001). The part of auditory cortex that we have identified as somatorecipient includes at a minimum the caudomedial (CM) belt region, and may include other belt and parabelt regions as well, but does not include primary (A1) auditory cortex (Fig. 18.2). These results merge with a complex history of findings on somatosensory representations in the region of the posterior auditory cortex (Schroeder et al., in press). About 20 years ago, Leinonen, Hyvarinen, and Sovijarvi (1980) reported extensive auditory-somatosensory corepresentation in area Tpt, the parabelt region occupying the posterior most portion of the superior temporal plane. About the same time, Robinson and Burton (1980) described a body map in a medial retroinsular (RI) region of the superior temporal plane that may correspond to the caudomedial, or CM, area in the

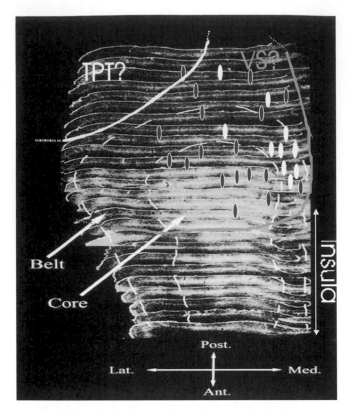

FIGURE 18.2 The distribution of somatosensory inputs in auditory cortex. Histological (80 μm) sections were stained for parvalbumin to help localize the borders between the core, belt, and parabelt regions of auditory cortex. To make this figure, the pattern of penetrations in each of the six brain hemispheres we sampled was reconstructed with respect to the caudal border of A1, and these were collapsed across hemispheres and subjects and registered onto the histological reconstruction of the caudal superior temporal plane in one subject. Also illustrated are the proposed regions of overlap between the multisensory region identified by Schroeder, Lindsley, et al. (2001) and the ventral somatosensory (VS) area, as identified by Krubitzer et al. (1995), and area Tpt, as identified by Leinonen et al. (1980). (Adapted from Schroeder, Lindsley, et al., 2001.)

terminology adopted by Kaas and colleagues. Subsequently, Krubitzer, Clarey, Tweedale, Elston, and Calford (1995) suggested that one or more body surface maps, referred to as ventral somatosensory (VS) area, adjoin the medial edge (foot representation) of parietal operculum areas S2 and PV and extend out over the surface of the posterior superior temporal plane. Some portion of VS may correspond to the RI of Robinson and Burton (1980). In any case, the somatosensory region extending over the caudal superior temporal plane probably corresponds to belt area CM, and possibly also to belt area caudolateral (CL) and the posterior parabelt (Tpt), but neither Burton et al. nor Krubitzer et al. investigated overlap with the auditory representations in the region. Our recent studies confirm somatosen-

sory input into CM, as well as its corepresentation with the local auditory fields (Fu et al., in press; Schroeder, Lindsley, et al., 2001), and, in combination with the results of Leinonen et al. (1980), suggest multiple somato-auditory fields in the superior temporal plane. Likewise, examination of the partial maps (e.g., Fig. 6 in Krubitzer et al., 1995) suggest the possibility of two or more body maps in the superior temporal plane. The proposed overlap of the fields mapped by Leinonen et al. and by Krubitzer et al., with the somato-auditory convergence region identified by Schroeder et al., is outlined in Figure 18.2. At this point, the number of body maps, as well as the content of the maps in the posterior superior temporal plane, is unclear. In the following section we consider anatomical sources of multisensory convergence in auditory association cortex and other locations in which convergence occurs.

Mechanisms of multisensory convergence at early processing stages

What circuits make multisensory interactions possible at early, putatively unisensory, processing stages, in normal individuals? Current models of visual (Felleman & Van Essen, 1991), auditory (Rauschecker et al., 1997), and somatosensory (Burton & Sinclair, 1996) organization clearly illustrate the point that, using feed-forward, feedback, or lateral projection circuits, input from any sensory source can be routed to nearly any cortical region, and even to most subcortical regions. At this time, there is a growing understanding of the brain circuits that promote multisensory convergence, from both structural and functional perspectives. Structurally, feed-forward and feedback inputs into a cortical area can be distinguished by the laminar pattern of axon terminations (Felleman & Van Essen, 1991; Rockland & Pandya, 1979) (Fig. 18.3). Feed-forward input terminations are concentrated in and near lamina 4, whereas feedback projections largely exclude lamina 4, terminating either in the supragranular laminae or in a "bilaminar" pattern above and below lamina 4. Lateral projections have a "columnar" pattern, terminating without any particular laminar focus (Felleman & Van Essen, 1991). These laminar termination patterns make predictions about laminar patterns of sensory responses, which can be addressed physiologically.

FUNCTIONAL MANIFESTATIONS OF FEED-FORWARD CONVERGENCE Recording of laminar response profiles with linear array multielectrodes is an established means of defining the functional correlates of feed-forward inputs in visual (Givre, Arezzo, & Schroeder, 1995; Givre, Schroeder, & Arezzo, 1994; Mehta, Ulbert, & Schroeder,

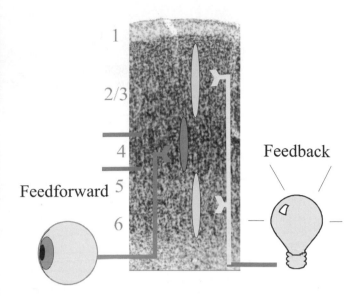

FIGURE 18.3 A depiction of the laminar patterns of feed-forward (red eyeball) and feedback (yellow light bulb) inputs in neocortex. The predominant targeting of lamina 4 and lower lamina 3 by feed-forward afferents, and the contrasting avoidance of this zone by feedback afferents, are based on the original findings of Rockland and Pandya (1979) and their extension by Felleman and Van Essen (1991). (From Schroeder et al., in press.)

2000a, 2000b; Schroeder, Tenke, Arezzo, et al., 1990; Schroeder, Lindsley, et al., 1997; Schroeder, Mehta, & Givre, 1998; Schroeder, Tenke, & Givre, 1992; Schroeder, Tenke, Givre, Arezzo, & Vaughan, 1991), somatosensory (Peterson, Schroeder, & Arezzo, 1995; Schroeder, Seto, et al., 1995; Schroeder, Seto, et al., 1997), and auditory (Schroeder & Foxe, 2002; Steinschneider, Reser, Fishman, Schroeder, & Arezzo, 1998; Steinschneider, Schroeder, Arezzo, & Vaughan, 1994, 1995) cortices. Such recordings in areas of multisensory convergence with linear array multielectrodes (Schroeder, Lindsley, et al., 2001) provide an opportunity to investigate the functional correlates of these input patterns. The laminar profile of auditory response in auditory association cortex, for example (Fig. 18.4), has the pattern predicted by the anatomy of feed-forward input: an initial response centered on lamina 4, followed by responses in the extragranular laminae. Feed-forward auditory input to the region in question, CM auditory cortex, is well established (Hackett, Stepniewska, & Kaas, 1998; Kosaki, Hashikawa, He, & Jones, 1997). In the same location, the overall timing and the laminar activation sequence for a convergent somatosensory input are nearly indentical to the timing and sequence of the auditory input. This suggests that the somatosensory input, like the auditory input, is conveyed by a feed-forward projection. The source of the somatosensory input is unclear at this time, because the anatomical interface between the auditory and somatosensory areas of the lateral sulcus region is not clearly delineated. This issue is considered further in a following section.

FUNCTIONAL MANIFESTATIONS OF FEEDBACK CONVERGENCE Our laminar activity analysis findings also point to a "feedback-mediated" visual input into auditory cortex (Fig. 18.5). This form of visual-auditory convergence has been observed to date in three monkeys, in all cases in posterior auditory association cortices (Schroeder & Foxe, 2002). Thus far, visual-auditory and somato-auditory convergence regions appear to be in nonoverlapping zones, although we have observed one example of trimodal (visual-auditory-somatosensory) convergence in posterior auditory cortex. As shown in Figure 18.4, auditory inputs have the characteristics of a feed-forward anatomical projection, that is, with initial activation centered on lamina 4. This is typical throughout the core and belt regions of auditory cortex (Schroeder, Lindsley, et al., 2001). The visual input profile, in contrast, has a bilaminar pattern, with initial responses beginning simultaneously in the supra- and infragranular laminae. This is the physiological pattern predicted by the anatomy of feedback projections (Felleman & Van Essen, 1991; Rockland & Pandya, 1979). Another point of contrast between the colocated auditory and visual response profiles concerns response timing. Visual response latency (~50 ms) is considerably longer than the auditory response latency (~11 ms). The large timing difference between convergent visual and auditory inputs to a single location contrasts with the lack of any corresponding timing difference between convergent somatosensory and auditory inputs to single auditory cortical locations (Fig. 18.5). With proper analysis and interpretation, these latency data can help to identify input sources and possibly also to predict the characteristics of multisensory interactions. This issue is treated in a subsequent section.

ANATOMICAL FEED-FORWARD AND FEEDBACK CIRCUITS FOR MULTISENSORY CONVERGENCE The known connectivity patterns of the primate brain provide a number of routes by which sensory inputs can converge in a given cortical area. A number of these cases are illustrated in Figure 18.6 (see also Color Plate 4). In identifying potential sources of somatosensory input to auditory association area CM (Fig. 18.6A), it is important to consider how the position and boundaries of CM relate to known somatosensory fields. It is possible, and even likely, that this somatosensory representation in CM corresponds to one defined by earlier unit mapping studies that did not test for auditory responsiveness. For example, somatorecipient CM may correspond to the VS area as

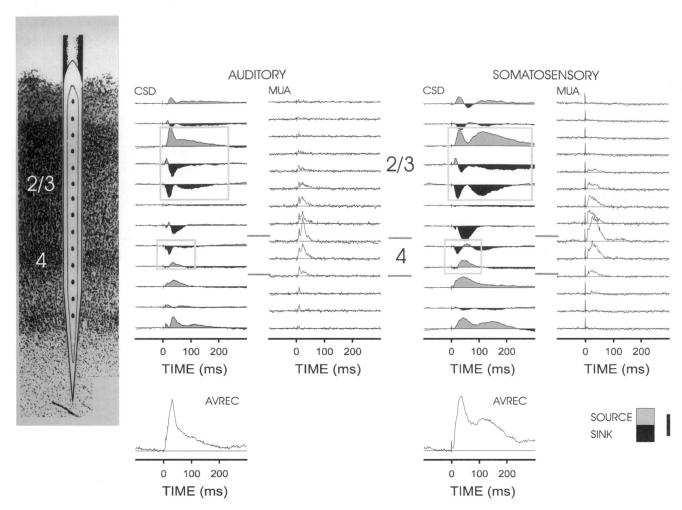

FIGURE 18.4 Laminar activity profiles consisting of current source density (CSD) and concomitant multiunit activity (MUA) patterns. (At left is a schematic illustration of the recording multielectrode positioned and scaled with respect to the laminae of auditory cortex.) Intercontact spacing is 150 μm. The CSD (one-dimensional) and MUA patterns were sampled simultaneously using a multielectrode array straddling auditory association cortex in the superior temporal plane, posteromedial to A1, in an awake macaque. Each tracing represents an average of 100 stimulus-evoked responses. Those on the left represent the averaged responses to binaural 65 dB clicks. Those on the right were elicited by electrical stimulation (2–3 mA, 100 ns square pulse) of the contralateral median nerve at the wrist. The CSD reflects local postsynaptic potential (PSP) patterns, and the MUA reflects the concomitant action potential patterns. In the CSD profile, downward deflections (dark-shaded) signify net extracellular current sinks (representing inward transmembrane currents), and upward deflections (stippled) indicate net extracellular current sources (representing outward currents); sinks and sources are associated with local depolarization and hyperpolarization in local neuronal ensembles, respectively. At the bottom of each CSD profile is the average rectified current flow (AVREC) pattern obtained by averaging together the absolute value of the CSD across all sites in the laminar profile. The AVREC waveform is a simplification of the CSD used for quantification and comparison. MUA patterns are obtained by full-wave rectification and averaging of the high-frequency activity at each electrode contact (upward deflection represents excitation). Each MUA trace is in effect a multiunit histogram. The boxes circumscribe CSD configurations that reflect the initial excitatory response at the depth of lamina 4 (lower boxes) and the subsequent excitation of the pyramidal cell ensembles in laminae 2/3 (upper boxes). Scale bar (lower right) = 1.4 mV/mm^2 for CSD, 0.1 mV/mm^2 for AVREC, and 1.6 μV for MUA. (Adapted from Schroeder, Lindsley, et al., 2001.)

defined by Krubitzer et al. (1995). (The approximate location of VS relative to auditory cortex is illustrated in Figure 18.2.) This being the case, the input could be provided by nearby areas S2 or PV. If CM/VS corresponds to the RI region (Robinson & Burton, 1980), possible additional sources of feed-forward input include areas 3b, 1, 2, and 5 (Burton & Sinclair, 1996). Finally,

the input could originate in the somatorecipient zones of a number of multisensory regions, including those in the intraparietal sulcus, STP and PfC. These areas, as well as anterior cingulate (AS) cortex, are emerging as possible sources in our ongoing tracer studies.

As suggested above, early audiovisual interaction effects in the occipital ERP (Giard & Peronet, 1999;

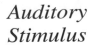

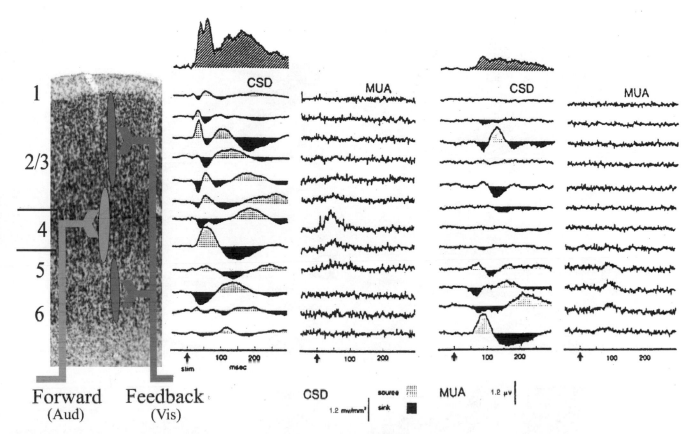

FIGURE 18.5   Laminar activity profiles elicited by auditory stimulation (65 dB binaural clicks) and visual stimulation (binocular light flash), sampled from posterior auditory association cortex in an awake macaque monkey. Conventions are like those in Figure 18.1, except that the AVREC waveforms are shown at the top of the associated CSD profiles. At left is a schematic illustration of the feed-forward and feedback anatomical input patterns that are proposed to account for the differences between the laminar profiles of auditory and visual responses in this region. (Adapted from Schroeder & Foxe, 2002.)

Molholm et al., 2002) could be a physiological manifestation of the feed-forward convergence of auditory and visual inputs in STP. The connections supporting this convergence are well described (Bruce et al., 1981; Pandya, Hallett, & Kmukherjee, 1969; Pandya & Sanides, 1973). However, another possibility is that early visual-auditory interactions in posterior brain regions are mediated by feedback of auditory input into classical visual regions such as MST or even MT. It should be noted that the contribution of the lower-order ventral stream areas, such as V4, to the early audiovisual interaction in the scalp ERP is considered unlikely. Although auditory input could reach these areas at a very short latency, the first visual response in these areas, as extrapolated from macaque data (Schroeder, Mehta, et al., 1998), would be at a minimum latency of about 60 ms. This is much too late to account for the effects

noted by Molhom et al. (2001). On the other hand, extrapolated visual latencies in MT/MST are on the order of 40–45 ms, and thus reciprocal connections between MT/MST and the frankly multisensory regions of the dorsal STS, intraparietal sulcus, and prefrontal cortex (reviewed by Felleman & Van Essen, 1991) all provide potential substrates for feedback-mediated auditory input to MT+ (Fig. 18.6B). Although the MT+ complex represents an early visual processing stage, especially in terms of response timing (Schroeder, Mehta, et al., 1998), recent findings from two laboratories (Falchier, et al., 2001) indicate projections from auditory regions including A1 and posterior auditory association areas, to areas V1 and V2 (Fig. 18.6C). According to Rockland (Rockland & Ojima, 2001, in press), the projections to V1 are sparse and focused in the uppermost layers, but those to V2 are much more dense and extend

SCHROEDER AND FOXE: MULTISENSORY CONVERGENCE IN EARLY CORTICAL PROCESSING   301

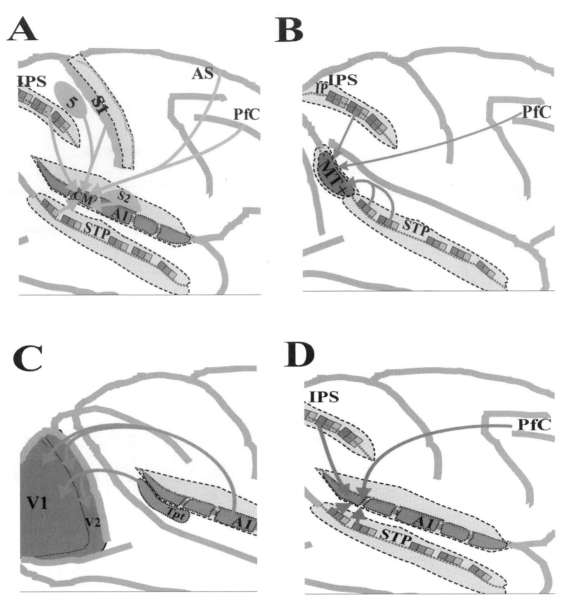

FIGURE 18.6   Schematic diagrams of known projections that are potential substrates for multisensory convergence at early stages of auditory and visual processing. (*A*) Potential sources of somatosensory input to auditory area CM. Abbreviations: IPS, intraparietal sulcus; 5, area 5; S1, somatosensory areas 3a, 3b, 1, and 2; AS, anterior cingulate cortex; PfC, prefrontal cortex; S2, areas "S2" and posteroventral somatosensory cortex; A1, primary auditory cortex; CM, caudomedial auditory cortex; STP, superior temporal polysensory area. (*B*) Potential sources of auditory feedback input into MT+ (MT plus MST). (*C*) Sources of auditory input to V1 (primary visual cortex) and V2 (secondary visual cortex), as identified by Falchier et al. (2001) and Rockland and Ojima (2001). (*D*) Potential sources of visual feedback input into posterior auditory association cortex. (Adapted from Schroeder et al., in press.) (See Color Plate 4.)

through both the upper and lower layers of the cortex. The basic laminar profiles of these projections fit into the feedback/lateral categories of projections (K. S. Rockland, personal communication). Although it is too early to conclude that all the auditory afferents into visual cortex are feedback-mediated, the mere presence of these connections indicates a substrate for multisensory convergence at the earliest stages of the cortical visual hierarchy.

Just as feedback circuits have been invoked in the case of auditory input into early visual processing, one could account for early visual-auditory interactions in auditory processing (Calvert & Bullmore, 1997; Giard & Peronet, 1999; Molholm et al., 2002) by positing that auditory inputs progress up their processing hierarchy until they converge with visual input (e.g., in STP or PfC), and then are conveyed by feedback projections to the putative "unisensory" auditory areas. A set of connections that could support feedback-mediated visual input to auditory cortex from STP (Hackett et al., 1998; Pandya et al., 1969), intraparietal sulcal regions (Lewis & Van Essen, 2000a, 2000b), and prefrontal regions (Romanski, Bates, & Goldman-Rakic, 1999; Romanski et al., 2000) is illustrated in Figure 18.6D. Our findings on visual-auditory convergence in auditory cortex (Fig. 18.5) outline a physiological response pattern that conforms to the expected (bilaminar) profile of a feedback input (Schroeder & Foxe, 2002).

Suborning of activity in unisensory cortex by feedback-mediated input from another sensory modality is an intriguing phenomenon. Both visual and auditory cortices appear to contain the substrates for very early multisensory integration. In view of the multiple possible feedback routes for multisensory convergence in auditory cortex (or, for that matter, in any sensory area), it is in some respects remarkable that there is enough sensory segregation to promote unimodal sensory representation at early cortical processing stages. Obviously, under normal circumstances, there is a strong bias in favor of specific patterns of unimodal representation and processing in lower-order cortical areas. However, the striking findings in the congenitally deaf human (Levanen et al., 1998), along with the earlier work on developmental sensory rewiring in ferrets (Pallas, Roe, & Sur, 1990; Sur, Pallas, & Roe, 1990), indicate that there is great potential for altering this bias during development.

KONIOCELLULAR INPUT: AN ADDITIONAL MECHANISM OF CONVERGENCE   Koniocellular projections from the thalamus (see review by Jones, 1998) provide an additional potential mechanism for multisensory convergence. These projections parallel the main or "core" thalamic projections into the neocortex, and although they generally target cortex appropriate for the sense modality from which they originate, there are exceptions. For example, the ventral posterior complex, which mainly carries somatosensory inputs, contains koniocellular neurons that project sparsely to posterior auditory cortex. These neurons could provide a means for somatosensory inputs to cross over into the auditory system. However, koniocellular mediation of the somatosensory input into auditory cortex does not appear to account completely for the results of Schroeder, Lindsley, et al. (2001), because these projections terminate heavily in the superficial laminae (Jones, 1998; Rausell, Bae, Vinuela, Huntley, & Jones, 1992; Rausell & Jones, 1991) and thus would not produce the feedforward (layer 4-centered) activation profile observed in Schroeder, Lindsley, et al. (2001). Although koniocellular projections thus do not seem to produce the initial somatosensory response in auditory cortex, they may yet contribute to a later portion of the response. In any case, because of their tendency to violate the rather rigid connectional order of the "core" sensory projection systems, koniocellular projections pose an interesting potential substrate for multisensory convergence at many levels of sensory processing.

Temporal parameters of multisensory convergence

In the context of early sensory processing, it is extremely interesting to note that through its access to the M-system, the dorsal or parietal visual pathway as a whole (which includes the STP area) responds very quickly to visual stimulation. In fact, the average latency of response in the region of STP cortex (Schroeder, Mehta, et al., 1998) is only slightly longer than the average latency in V1, and is actually shorter than the average response latency in V2 and V4 (see also Nowak & Bullier, 1997; Schmolesky et al., 1998) (Fig. 18.7). To underscore the rapid response characteristics in STP, we have placed time lines at the onset and mean of the STP onset latency distribution in Figure 18.7. Thus, by the standard of timing, all of the areas in the dorsal visual pathway, including those already shown to be sites of multisensory convergence, participate in early visual processing.

Because of their relatively longer activation latencies, ventral stream visual areas are unlikely to contribute to the very early audiovisual interactions observed in ERP studies (Giard & Peronet, 1999; Molholm et al., 2002). Average latency in V4, for example, is 33 ms in the Schroeder, Mehta, et al. (1998) study. Using a 3/5 rule for extrapolating from monkey to human sensory response latencies (Schroeder, Steinschneider, et al., 1995), monkey V4 latency corresponds to a human V4 latency of 55 ms. The corresponding extrapolations for MT and STP are 37 ms and 48 ms, respectively. Obviously, these extrapolations are not quite that straightforward, because the range of latency values in each structure should also be considered. However, based on mean response latency, MT is a likely candidate site for very early audiovisual interactions. The human ERP findings converge on this point, in that the early audiovisual interactions occur at sites overlying the anatomical location of human MT+ (Giard & Peronet, 1999; Molholm et al., 2002). Interestingly, although there appear to be auditory inputs into very early stages of the visual hierarchy in monkeys (i.e., V1 and V2; see earlier discussion), any early audiovisual interactions in V1 and V2 that may result from this anatomical convergence do not have an obvious impact on the scalp ERP distribution.

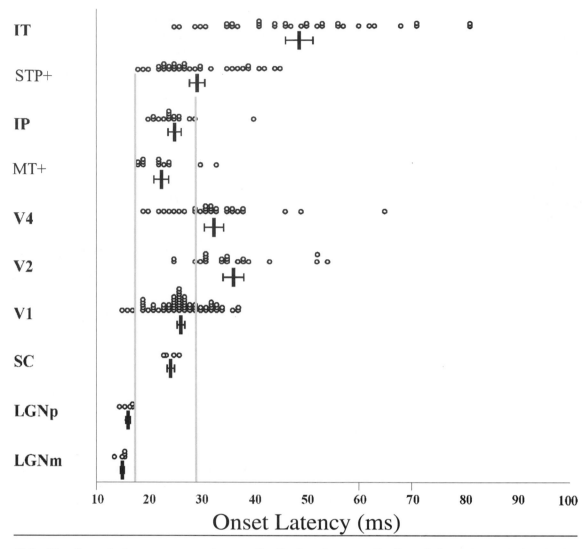

FIGURE 18.7 Visually evoked response onset latency distributions for areas distributed along the cortical and subcortical visual pathways in awake monkeys. Data were taken from nine subjects under identical stimulation conditions. Each entry indicates one onset latency, scored for one electrode penetration. Mean and SED for each area are also shown. Drop lines are placed at the shortest and mean latency points in the STP distribution, as explained in the text. (Adapted from Schroeder, Mehta, et al., 1998.)

Beyond constraining the set of areas that could contribute to multisensory interactions, there are a number of ways in which the precise temporal pattern of convergent inputs could have an impact on neuronal responding. For example, the first input to arrive in a location could gain preferential access to local excitability and thus might be able to "dominate" or otherwise modulate the processing of later-arriving inputs. On the other hand, a weak input may not evoke a significant response unless it arrives within the time frame of excitation caused by a convergent input. This latter case is illustrated with data from a visual-somatosensory convergence site in the macaque lateral intraparietal sulcus (Fig. 18.8). In this case, we can see that that somatosensory stimulation by itself has no discernible impact on action potentials and only a small effect on transmembrane current flow; this pattern of effects indicates a weak (subthreshold) input. However, somatosensory stimulation clearly enhances the amplitude of a concurrently presented visual stimulus. This example of multisensory response enhancement, consistent with earlier findings in this region of macaque neocortex (Duhamel et al., 1998), illustrates the point that at least within broad limits, neuronal integration of inputs requires some degree of temporal as well as spatial coincidence. Although the specific temporal integration requirements of neurons are likely to vary as a function of stimulus type and brain location (for a review, see Stein &

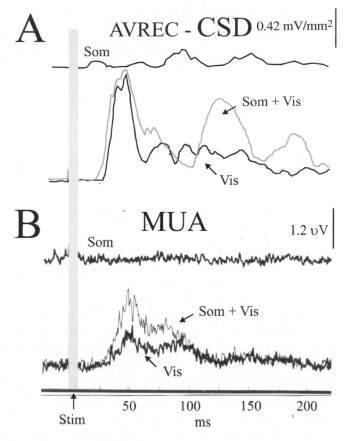

A AVREC - CSD 0.42 mV/mm²

Som

Som + Vis

Vis

B MUA 1.2 υV

Som

Som + Vis

Vis

Stim   50   100   150   200

ms

FIGURE 18.8   Illustration of multisensory interaction in intraparietal sulcal area VIP. (*A*) AVREC representations of CSD responses to somatosensory stimulation alone (top), visual stimulation alone (bottom, black), and combined visual-somatosensory stimulation (bottom, gray). (*B*) MUA responses in the same three stimulation conditions, recorded from a midcortical depth at which the maximal unisensory MUA response was observed. (From Schroeder & Foxe, 2002.)

post-stimulus and exhibits synchrony dependence. Although our observations on the onset latency of actual multisensory interactions are quite limited at this point, we have a much wider sample of unisensory response latencies across brain regions, including those regions in which convergence occurs. As reviewed next, these data make certain predictions about temporal parameters of multisensory interactions.

TIMING OF CONVERGING SENSORY INPUTS   As mentioned earlier, when auditory and somatosensory stimuli are presented less than 1 meter from the head (i.e., within arm's reach), the response in classic multisensory area STP is rapid and approximately simultaneous for both input modalities. Visual-auditory convergence in auditory cortex, however, contrasts greatly with this pattern of effects. That is, for stimuli presented within arm's reach, there is a large delay for visual relative to auditory responses. In order to gain an overall impression of the temporal patterns of visual-auditory, visual-somatosensory, and somato-auditory convergence across different neocortical areas, we assembled a set of grand mean activation patterns for separate sensory inputs that converge in three of the brain regions we have studied (Fig. 18.9). The waveforms shown in Figure 18.9 are based on a condensed average rectified current flow (AVREC) representation of the laminar current source density (CSD) profile, obtained by taking the absolute value of the CSD at each point in the laminar profile and averaging across the points in the profile, for each point in time (Schroeder & Foxe, 2002). The single-penetration AVREC waveforms are then averaged across penetrations and subjects for a given area.

Two aspects of the temporal pattern of multisensory convergence for "peripersonal space"—visual, auditory, and somatosensory—are evident in the summary figure. First, somatosensory input, when present in any structure, is as early as or earlier than either auditory or visual input to the same region. However, these somatosensory responses, were elicited by electrical stimulation of median nerve, and these latencies slightly underestimate the latency of a response to stimulation of the volar hand surface (Schroeder, Steinschneider, et al., 1995). Also, the relative timing of the somatosensory, visual, and auditory components of a multisensory stimulus (e.g., an object held in the hand, looked at, and listened to) would vary considerably depending on whether the object is active or inert, that is whether it moves actively or must be turned with the hand. Thus, whereas the neural processing of somatosensory inputs might be faster than the processing of other, particularly visual, inputs, the significance of this factor relative

Meredith, 1993), at some level, in every brain location, the temporal pattern of multisensory convergence that exists in a given situation should have an impact on processing. It is therefore of interest to characterize temporal as well as anatomical patterns of multisensory convergence. We have only recently begun to characterize the timing of multisensory interactions in monkey neocortex, and at this point, we can make only anecdotal comments. For example, based on experiments in one monkey, it seems that audiovisual interaction can have an onset latency of as early as 25 ms in STP, and furthermore it adheres to the temporal principle of multisensory integration (Stein & Meredith, 1993), that is, it depends on a modicum of input synchrony. However, the timing of audiovisual interaction in auditory association cortex has not yet been studied. Again, based on a sample in one monkey, we note that somatovisual interaction in the IP sulcus region can begin as early as 25 ms

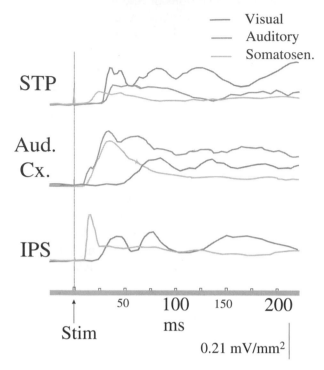

Grand Mean AVREC

— Visual
— Auditory
— Somatosen.

STP

Aud. Cx.

IPS

Stim   50   **100**   150   **200**
                        ms
                              0.21 mV/mm²

FIGURE 18.9   Grand mean AVREC waveforms illustrating the onset timing and temporal pattern of CSD responses to standard forms of unisensory visual, auditory, and somatosensory stimulation in three regions receiving multisensory convergence of inputs. These waveforms were obtained by averaging together single-penetration waveforms (e.g., see Figs. 18.4 and 18.5) across penetrations and subjects. (From Schroeder & Foxe, 2002.)

to the complex temporal dynamics of the physical stimuli is open to speculation.

MULTISENSORY PERCEPTUAL CONTOURS?   A second point of temporal patterning that is evident in Figure 18.9 may be more interpretable. That is, for an audiovisual stimulus presented at 1 meter, the degree of synchrony between convergent visual and auditory inputs varies markedly across different structures. For example, our preliminary findings in posterior auditory cortex (Figs. 18.6 and 18.9) suggest that auditory input is very fast (~10 ms), while visual input is relatively slow (~50 ms). Thus, given an audiovisual stimulus at a typical conversational distance, auditory and visual inputs would be asynchronous and unable to support the precise temporal ordering necessary for audiovisual speech perception. However, with the relatively slow speed of sound (~1100 ft/s) relative to the speed of light, the relative timing of inputs in such a location would be appropriate for synchronization of inputs generated by audiovisual stimuli at a distance of approximately

40 feet from the observer. In STP, on the other hand, the response latency for auditory input from a sound source at 1 meter (~25 ms latency; see Fig. 18.9) is comparable to that of a visual input from the same source, so that the inputs are in synchrony. Note that for audiovisual sources located at greater distances (e.g., ~40 feet) from the observer, inputs into STP would become asynchronous when auditory and visual inputs into posterior auditory cortex began to synchronize. Based on the timing relationship between auditory and visual inputs, posterior auditory cortex and STP, respectively, may contain complementary representations of near "peripersonal" and far "extrapersonal" space. There are two caveats to this suggestion. The first is that although these simple unisensory response latency estimates set a lower boundary on the timing of auditory-visual interactions in each brain region for audiovisual stimuli located at different distances from the observer, they do not specify the time point at which a significant interaction occurs. This issue will require additional experimentation. Second, the findings in macaque monkeys have implications for understanding the temporal pattern of brain activation in humans, but multisensory interaction latencies, like unisensory response-onset latencies, differ between monkeys and humans. Additional experiments will be required to firm up the comparison of monkey and human findings.

Concluding note: Early multisensory convergence and the "sensory hierarchy"

In current models of brain organization, there appears to be a hierarchical progression from the processing of simple to more complex aspects of unimodal stimuli within each sensory system (Burton & Sinclair, 1996; Felleman & Van Essen, 1991; Rauschecker et al., 1997). How does early multisensory convergence fit into the hierarchical model of brain organization? The view that multisensory convergence and integration are deferred until relatively late in processing is directly challenged by the convergence between separate sensory systems at early, putatively "unisensory" processing stages and at extremely short poststimulus latencies. The fact that early multisensory convergence can occur through feedback as well as feed-forward circuits highlights the potential higher-order functions of low-level sensory cortices. On a very basic level, our understanding of "low-level (uni)sensory processing" needs to incorporate the fact that multisensory interaction is already possible at or near the onset of response, in the earliest cortical processing stages. On a larger scale, it appears that in multisensory processing, as in sensory contextual processing (Lamme, 1995; Zipzer, Lamme, & Schiller,

1996) and attentional modulation of processing (Bullier, 2001; Mehta et al., 2000a, 2000b; Schroeder, Mehta, et al., 2001), recruitment of low-level sensory areas into the cognitive-perceptual process is partially attributable to feedback-dependent processes that occur relatively late in poststimulus time. Thus, the evolving concept of the sensory processing hierarchy must encompass temporal as well as anatomical dimensions (Schroeder, Mehta, et al., 2001).

ACKNOWLEDGMENTS Work was supported by grants MH61989 and TW05674 from the National Institute of Mental Health.

REFERENCES

Benevento, L. A., Fallon, J., Davis, B. J., & Rezak, M. (1977). Auditory–visual interaction in single cells in the cortex of the superior temporal sulcus and the orbital frontal cortex of the macaque monkey. *Experimental Neurology, 57*(3), 849–872.

Bental, E., Dafny, N., & Feldman, S. (1968). Convergence of auditory and visual stimuli on single cells in the primary visual cortex of unanesthetized and unrestrained cats. *Experimental Neurology, 20,* 341–351.

Bruce, C., Desimone, R., & Gross, C. G. (1981). Visual properties of neurons in a polysensory area in superior temporal sulcus of the macaque. *Journal of Neurophysiology, 46*(2), 369–384.

Bullier, J. (2001). Feedback connections and conscious vision. *Trends in Cognitive Sciences, 5*(9), 369–370.

Burton, H., & Sinclair, R. (1996). Somatosensory cortex and tactile perceptions. In *Pain and touch* (chap. 3). San Diego, CA: Academic Press.

Calvert, G., Brammer, M., Campbell, R., Iverson, L., & David, A. (1999). Response amplification in sensory-specific cortices during crossmodal binding. *NeuroReport, 10,* 2619–2623.

Calvert, G. A., & Bullmore, E. T. (1997). Activation of auditory cortex during silent lipreading. *Science, 276*(5312), 593–596.

Calvert, G., Hansen, P. C., Iverson, L., & Brammer, M. J. (2001). Detection of audio-visual integration sites in humans by application of electrophysiological criteria to the bold effect. *Neuroimage, 14,* 428–438.

Duhamel, J. R., Colby, C. L., & Goldberg, M. E. (1998). Ventral intraparietal area of the macaque: Convergent visual and somatic response properties. *Journal of Neurophysiology, 79,* 126–136.

Falchier, A., Renaud, L., Barone, H., & Kennedy, H. (2001). Extensive projections from primary auditory cortex and area STP to peripheral V1 in the macaque. *Society of Neuroscience Abstracts, 27,* 511.21.

Felleman, D. J., & Van Essen, D. C. (1991). Distributed hierarchical processing in the primate cerebral cortex. *Cerebral Cortex, 1,* 1–47.

Foxe, J. J., Morocz, I. A., Murray, M. M., Higgins, B. A., Javitt, D. C., & Schroeder, C. E. (2000). Multisensory auditory-somatosensory interactions in early cortical processing revealed by high-density electrical mapping. *Brain Research: Cognitive Brain Research, 10*(1–2), 77–83.

Foxe, J. J., Wylie, G. R., Martinez, A., Schroeder, C. E., Javitt, D. C., Guilfoyle, D., et al. (2002). Auditory-somatosensory multisensory processing in auditory association cortex: An fMRI study. *Journal of Neurophysiology, 88*(1), 540–543.

Fu, K. G., Johnston, T. A., Shah, A. S., Arnold, L., Smiley, J., Hackett, T. A., et al. (in press). Auditory cortical neurons respond to somatosensory input. *Journal of Neuroscience.*

Giard, M., & Peronet, F. (1999). Auditory-visual integration during multimodal object recognition in humans: A behavioral and electrophysiological study. *Journal of Cognitive Neuroscience, 11,* 473–490.

Givre, S. J., Arezzo, J. C., & Schroeder, C. E. (1995). Effects of wavelength on the timing and laminar distribution of illuminance-evoked activity in macaque V1. *Visual Neuroscience, 12,* 229–239.

Givre, S. J., Schroeder, C. E., & Arezzo, J. C. (1994). Contribution of extrastriate area V4 to the surface-recorded flash VEP in the awake macaque. *Vision Research, 34,* 415–438.

Graziano, M. S., Hu, X. T., & Gross, C. G. (1997). Visuospatial properties of ventral premotor cortex. *Journal of Neurophysiology, 77*(5), 2268–2292.

Graziano, M. S., Yap, G. S., & Gross, C. G. (1994). Coding of visual space by premotor neurons. *Science, 266*(5187), 1054–1057.

Grunewald, A., Linden, J. F., & Andersen, R. A. (1999). Responses to auditory stimuli in macaque lateral intraparietal area: I. Effects of training. *Journal of Neurophysiology, 82*(1), 330–342.

Hackett, T. A., Stepniewska, I., & Kaas, J. H. (1998). Subdivisions of auditory cortex and ipsilateral cortical connections of the parabelt auditory cortex in macaque monkeys. *Journal of Comparative Neurology, 394*(4), 475–495.

Hikosaka, K., Iwai, E., Saito, H., & Tanaka, K. (1988). Polysensory properties of neurons in the anterior bank of the caudal superior temporal sulcus of the macaque monkey. *Journal of Neurophysiology, 60*(5), 1615–1637.

Hyvarinen, J., & Shelepin, Y. (1979). Distribution of visual and somatic functions in the parietal associative area 7 of the monkey. *Brain Research, 169*(3), 561–564.

Jones, E. (1998). Viewpoint: The core and matrix of thalamic organization. *Neuroscience, 85*(2), 331–345.

Kosaki, H., Hashikawa, T., He, J., & Jones, E. G. (1997). Tonotopic organization of auditory cortical fields delineated by parvalbumin immunoreactivity in macaque monkeys. *Journal of Comparative Neurology, 386,* 304–316.

Krubitzer, L., Clarey, J., Tweedale, R., Elston, G., & Calford, M. (1995). A re-definition of somatosensory areas in the lateral sulcus of macaque monkeys. *Journal of Neuroscience, 15,* 3821–3839.

Lamme, V. (1995). The neurophysiology of figure-ground segregation in primary visual cortex. *Journal of Neuroscience, 15,* 1605–1615.

Leinonen, L. (1980). Functional properties of neurones in the parietal retroinsular cortex in awake monkey. *Acta Physiologica Scandinavica, 108*(4), 381–384.

Leinonen, L., Hyvarinen, J., & Sovijarvi, A. R. (1980). Functional properties of neurons in the temporo-parietal association cortex of awake monkey. *Experimental Brain Research, 39*(2), 203–215.

Levanen, S., Jousmaki, V., & Hari, R. (1998). Vibration-induced auditory cortex activation in a congenitally deaf adult. *Current Biology, 8,* 869–872.

Lewis, J. W., & Van Essen, D. C. (2000a). Mapping of architectonic subdivisions in the macaque monkey, with emphasis on parieto-occipital cortex. *Journal of Comparative Neurology, 428*(1), 79–111.

Lewis, J. W., & Van Essen, D. C. (2000b). Corticocortical connections of visual, sensorimotor, and multimodal processing areas in the parietal lobe of the macaque monkey. *Journal of Comparative Neurology, 428*(1), 112–137.

Linden, J. F., Grunewald, A., & Andersen, R. A. (1999). Responses to auditory stimuli in macaque lateral intraparietal area: II. Behavioral modulation. *Journal of Neurophysiology, 82*(1), 343–458.

Mazzoni, P., Bracewell, R. M., Barash, S., & Andersen, R. A. (1996). Spatially tuned auditory responses in area LIP of macaques performing delayed memory saccades to acoustic targets. *Journal of Neurophysiology, 75*(3), 1233–1241.

Mehta, A. D., Ulbert, I., & Schroeder, C. E. (2000a). Intermodal selective attention in monkeys: I. Distribution and timing of effects across visual areas. *Cerebral Cortex, 10*, 343–358.

Mehta, A. D., Ulbert, I., & Schroeder, C. E. (2000b). Intermodal selective attention in monkeys: II. Physiologic mechanisms of modulation. *Cerebral Cortex, 10*, 359–370.

Molholm, S., Ritter, W., Murray, M. M., Javitt, D. C., Schroeder, C. E., & Foxe, J. J. (2002). Multisensory auditory-visual interactions during early sensory processing in humans: A high-density electrical mapping study. *Brain Research: Cognitive Brain Research, 14*(1), 115–128.

Nowak, L. G., & Bullier, J. (1997). The timing of information transfer in the visual system. *Cerebral Cortex, Extrastriate Cortex, 12*, 205–241.

Pallas, S. L., Roe, A. W., & Sur, M. (1990). Visual projections induced into the auditory pathway of ferrets: I. Novel inputs to primary auditory cortex (AI) from the LP/pulvinar complex and the topography of the MGN-AI projection. *Journal of Comparative Neurology, 298*(1), 50–68.

Pandya, D. N., Hallett, M., & Kmukherjee, S. K. (1969). Intra- and interhemispheric connections of the neocortical auditory system in the rhesus monkey. *Brain Research, 14*(1), 49–65.

Pandya, D. N., & Sanides, F. (1973). Architectonic parcellation of the temporal operculum in rhesus monkey and its projection pattern. *Zeitschrift für Anatomische Entwicklungsgeschichte, 139*(2), 127–161.

Peterson, N. N., Schroeder, C. E., & Arezzo, J. C. (1995). Neural generators of early cortical somatosensory evoked potentials in the awake monkey. *Electroencephalography and Clinical Neurophysiology, 96*(3), 248–260.

Rauschecker, J. P., Tian, B., Pons, T., & Mishkin, M. (1997). Serial and parallel processing in rhesus monkey auditory cortex. *Journal of Comparative Neurology, 382*, 89–103.

Rausell, E., Bae, C. S., Vinuela, A., Huntley, G. W., & Jones, E. G. (1992). Calbindin and parvalbumin cells in monkey VPL thalamic nucleus: distribution, laminar cortical projections, and relations to spinothalamic terminations. *Journal of Neuroscience, 12*(10), 4088–4111.

Rausell, E., & Jones, E. G. (1991). Chemically distinct compartments of the thalamic VPM nucleus in monkeys relay principal and spinal trigeminal pathways to different layers of the somatosensory cortex. *Journal of Neuroscience, 11*(1), 226–237.

Rizzolatti, G., Scandolara, C., Gentilucci, M., & Camarda, R. (1981a). Response properties and behavioral modulation of "mouth" neurons of the postarcuate cortex (area 6) in macaque monkeys. *Brain Research, 225*(2), 421–424.

Rizzolatti, G., Scandolara, C., Gentilucci, M., & Camarda, R. (1981b). Afferent properties of periarcuate neurons in macaque monkeys: I. Somatosensory responses. *Behavioural Brain Research, 2*(2), 125–146.

Robinson, C. J., & Burton, H. (1980). Organization of somatosensory fields in areas 7b, retroinsula, postauditoru, and granular insula of *M. fascicularis. Journal of Comparative Neurology, 192*, 69–92.

Rockland, K. S., & Pandya, D. N. (1979). Laminar origins and terminations of cortical connections in the occipital lobe in the rhesus monkey. *Brain Research, 179*, 3–20.

Rockland, K. S., & Ojima, K. (2001). Calcarine area V1 as a multimodal convergence area. *Society of Neuroscience Abstracts, 27*, 511.20.

Rockland, K. S., & Ojima, K. (2001). V1 as a multimodal area. *International Journal of Psychophysiology.*

Roe, A. W., Pallas, S. L., Hahm, J. O., & Sur, M. (1990). A map of visual space induced in primary auditory cortex. *Science, 250*(4982), 818–820.

Romanski, L. M., Bates, J. F., & Goldman-Rakic, P. S. (1999). Auditory belt and parabelt projections to the prefrontal cortex in the rhesus monkeys. *Journal of Comparative Neurology, 403*, 141–157.

Romanski, L. M., Tian, B., Fritz, J., Mishkin, M., Goldman-Rakic, P. S., & Rauschecker, J. P. (2000). Dual streams of auditory afferents target multiple domains in the primate prefrontal cortex. *Nature Neuroscience, 2*, 1131–1136.

Sams, M., Aulanko, R., Hamalainen, M., Hari, R., Lounasmaa, O. V., Lu, S. T., et al. (1991). Seeing speech: Visual information from lip movements modifies activity in the human auditory cortex. *Neuroscience Letters, 127*, 141–145.

Schmolesky, M., Wang, Y., Hanes, D. P., Thompson, K. G., Leutgeb, S., Schall, J. D., et al. (1998). Signal timing across the macaque visual system. *Journal of Neurophysiology, 79*, 3272–3278.

Schroeder, C. E., & Foxe, J. J. (2002). The timing and laminar profile of converging inputs to multisensory areas of the macaque neocortex. *Brain Research: Cognitive Brain Research, 14*(1), 187–198.

Schroeder, C. E., Javitt, D. C., Steinschneider, M., Mehta, A. D., Givre, S. J., Vaughan, H. G., Jr., et al. (1997). *N*-methyl-D-aspartate enhancement of phasic responses in primate neocortex. *Experimental Brain Research, 114*, 271–278.

Schroeder, C. E., Lindsley, R. W., Specht, C., Marcovici, A., Smiley, J. F., & Javitt, D. C. (2001). Somatosensory input to auditory association cortex in the macaque monkey. *Journal of Neurophysiology, 85*(3), 1322–1327.

Schroeder, C. E., Mehta, A. D., & Foxe, J. J. (2001). Determinants and mechanisms of attentional modulation of neural processing. *Frontiers in Bioscience, 6*, D672–D684.

Schroeder, C. E., Mehta, A. D., & Givre, S. J. (1998). A spatiotemporal profile of visual system activation revealed by current source density analysis in the awake macaque. *Cerebral Cortex, 8*, 575–592.

Schroeder, C. E., Seto, S., Arezzo, J. C., & Garraghty, P. E. (1995). Electrophysiologic evidence for overlapping dominant and latent inputs to somatosensory cortex in squirrel monkeys. *Journal of Neurophysiology, 74*(2), 722–732.

Schroeder, C. E., Seto, S., & Garraghty, P. E. (1997). Emergence of radial nerve dominance in median nerve cortex after median nerve transection in an adult squirrel monkey. *Journal of Neurophysiology, 77*, 522–526.

Schroeder, C. E., Smiley, J., Fu, K. G., McGinnis, T., O'Connell, M. N., & Hackett, T. A. (in press). Mechanisms and implications of multisensory convergence in early cortical processing. *International Journal of Psychophysiology.*

Schroeder, C. E., Steinschneider, M., Javitt, D. C., Tenke, C. E., Givre, S. J., Mehta, A. D., et al. (1995). Localization of ERP generators and identification of underlying neural processes. *Electroencephalography and Clinical Neurophysiology, 44*(Suppl.), 55–75.

Schroeder, C. E., Tenke, C. E., Arezzo, J. C., & Vaughan, H. G., Jr. (1990). Binocularity in the lateral geniculate nucleus of the alert macaque. *Brain Research, 521*, 303–310.

Schroeder, C. E., Tenke, C. E., & Givre, S. J. (1992). Subcortical contributions to the surface-recorded flash-VEP in the awake macaque. *Electroencephalography and Clinical Neurophysiology, 84*, 219–231.

Schroeder, C. E., Tenke, C. E., Givre, S. J., Arezzo, J. C., & Vaughan, H. G., Jr. (1990). Laminar analysis of bicuculline-induced epileptiform activity in area 17 of the awake macaque. *Brain Research, 515*, 326–330.

Schroeder, C. E., Tenke, C. E., Givre, S. J., Arezzo, J. C., & Vaughan, H. G., Jr. (1991). Striate cortical contribution to the surface-recorded pattern-reversal VEP in the alert monkey. *Vision Research, 31*(11), 1143–1157.

Seltzer, B., & Pandya, D. N. (1980). Converging visual and somatic sensory cortical input to the intraparietal sulcus of the rhesus monkey. *Brain Research, 192*(2), 339–351.

Seltzer, B., & Pandya, D. (1978). Afferent cortical connections and architechtonics of the superior temporal sulcus and surrounding cortex in the rhesus monkey. *Brain Research, 149*, 1–24.

Stein, B. E., & Meredith, M. A. (1993). *The merging of the senses.* Cambridge, MA: MIT Press.

Steinschneider, M., Reser, D. H., Fishman, Y. I., Schroeder, C. E., & Arezzo, J. C. (1998). Click train encoding in primary auditory cortex of the awake monkey: Evidence for two mechanisms subserving pitch perception. *Journal of the Acoustical Society of America, 104*(5), 2935–2955.

Steinschneider, M., Schroeder, C. E., Arezzo, J. C., & Vaughan, H. G., Jr. (1994). Speech-evoked activity in primary auditory cortex: Effects of voice onset time. *Electroencephalography and Clinical Neurophysiology, 92*, 30–43.

Steinschneider, M., Schroeder, C. E., Arezzo, J. C., & Vaughan, H. G., Jr. (1995). Physiologic correlates of the voice onset time (VOT) boundary in primary auditory cortex (A1) of the awake monkey: Temporal response patterns. *Brain and Language, 48*, 326–340.

Sur, M., Pallas, S. L., & Roe, A. W. (1990). Cross-modal plasticity in cortical development: Differentiation and specification of sensory neocortex. *Trends in Neuroscience, 13*(6), 227–233.

Zipzer, K., Lamme, P., & Schiller, P. (1996). Contextual modulation in primary visual cortex. *Journal of Neuroscience, 16*, 7376–7389.

19 Multisensory Neuronal Convergence of Taste, Somatosensory, Visual, Olfactory, and Auditory Inputs

EDMUND T. ROLLS

Introduction

Many single neurons in the primate orbitofrontal cortex respond to different combinations of taste, somatosensory, visual, olfactory, and auditory inputs. Multisensory convergence is achieved by these neurons in that many of the neurons in the preceding cortical areas (such as the primary taste cortex and the inferior temporal visual cortex) are unimodal. (For example, there are no or few visual and olfactory neurons in the primary taste cortex, and no taste, olfactory, or somatosensory neurons in the inferior temporal visual cortex.) The visual-to-taste convergence is organized by associative learning with synaptic modification of the visual inputs onto taste-responsive neurons. This associative learning can reverse (in a visual discrimination reversal task) in as little as one trial, and is an important function performed by the orbitofrontal cortex. Olfactory-to-taste associations are learned in a similar way but reverse less rapidly, providing some stability in the representation of flavor. The taste (and somatosensory) neuronal representation is of the reward value of the sensory input, in that feeding to satiety decreases the responses of the neurons and the reward value of the food. The multisensory convergence in the orbitofrontal cortex at the ends of the "what" processing systems (for vision, taste, and smell) thus enables a rich, multisensory representation of the reward (and punishment) value of stimuli that allows rapid relearning of which visual stimuli are currently associated with primary reinforcers. The roles of this convergence at the single-neuron level are to build representations that reflect the whole combination of sensory inputs needed to define a stimulus so that behavior to just that stimulus and not to others can be produced (as in sensory-specific satiety), and to enable behavior to, for example, visual stimuli to be made to depend on the taste, or more generally the reinforcer, with which the visual stimulus is

currently associated. These functions provide a basis for understanding the role of the orbitofrontal cortex in emotions, which can be construed as states elicited by reinforcers. Neurons in the amygdala also respond to similar sensory inputs from two or more sensory modalities, but the learning of associations between stimuli in different sensory modalities is less flexible than that of neurons in the orbitofrontal cortex. Neurons in the cortex in the macaque superior temporal sulcus frequently respond to moving objects, including the lips of a speaker, and other neurons respond to auditory stimuli, including vocalization. This is therefore likely to be an important multisensory convergence zone for dynamically changing stimuli that correspond to a particular type of biological motion, and that can give rise to phenomena such as the McGurk effect. A formal model of coupled networks is described that can account for phenomena, including illusions, that can arise due to multisensory convergence, including the McGurk effect. Neurons in the primate hippocampus have very different representations of visual space in an allocentric coordinate frame, and combine these representations with idiothetic (self-motion) inputs from the vestibular and proprioceptive systems. The integration in the hippocampus requires path integration of the idiothetic inputs so that they can be combined with allocentric visual spatial representations, and a model of how this path integration can be performed is described. An analogous model can also account for how single neurons in the primate presubiculum respond to both visual cues anchored to head direction and to signals of vestibular origin related to changes of head direction that require path integration before they are combined with the visual inputs. These investigations provide a basis for understanding the functions of and the underlying mechanisms for the multisensory convergence found at the ends of the unimodal cortical sensory processing streams.

This chapter describes some of the rules of the cortical processing at the ends of the ventral stream cortical processing areas that build multisensory representations of "what" object is present. These ventral stream systems include the visual pathways to the inferior temporal visual cortex, where what object is being seen is represented (E. T. Rolls & Deco, 2002), and the taste and olfactory systems, which define what smell or taste is being presented (E. T. Rolls, 1999a). To understand the general architecture of these processing streams, we need evidence from neuroanatomy. To understand whether inputs from different sensory systems show convergence within a cortical area, evidence about whether single neurons respond to both types of sensory input is the direct and best measure, and using a single-neuron recording approach also allows the rules of sensory convergence (such as whether the convergence reflects a learned association between the sensory inputs) to be discovered. Finally, because each single neuron has different tuning to each sensory stimulus, the nature of the representations built by multisensory convergence can be best understood by considering populations of different single neurons at the network level, and indeed this neuronal network level enables precise models to be constructed of how whole populations of neurons interact with each other to produce interesting phenomena, including attention. Because all these approaches are necessary to define the nature and mechanisms of multisensory convergence, all are included and combined in this chapter. An introduction to this computational approach to understanding brain function that builds on single-neuron neurophysiology but leads to models that make predictions at the more global level of what is being measured in, for example, a neuroimaging experiment is provided by E. T. Rolls and Deco (2002).

One of the cortical areas that builds multisensory representations from the outputs of mainly unimodal processing streams is the orbitofrontal cortex. Because the sensory modalities that project into this region include the taste and somatosensory systems, the orbitofrontal cortex plays an important role in representing primary reinforcers, that is, stimuli that can produce reward or punishment innately, without learning (E. T. Rolls, 1999a). (A reward is a stimulus that an animal will work to obtain. A punisher is a stimulus that an animal will work to escape from or avoid. Taste is a primary reinforcer in that the first time that an animal is salt-deprived, it shows a preference for salt taste [see E. T. Rolls, 1999a]. Similarly, a painful stimulus is innately a punisher.) We will see that the orbitofrontal cortex builds multisensory representations by association learning, learning, for example, that a particular visual stimulus is associated with a particular taste.

Some of the anatomical pathways that provide the basis of the multisensory representations to be described are shown in Figure 19.1. Most of the areas that precede the orbitofrontal cortex, and the amygdala, which has similar connectivity, are mainly unimodal. This is part of the evidence that multisensory representations are formed in the orbitofrontal cortex and amygdala. An interesting aspect of the architecture shown in Figure 19.1 is that the representation of objects and faces in the inferior temporal visual cortex is in an ideal form for the pattern association learning that enables visual-to-taste associations to be formed, as will be described.

Much of the fundamental evidence for multisensory convergence comes from single-neuron recording studies, because such studies are the direct and unequivocal method by which it can be shown whether real convergence from different modalities actually occurs in a brain region, in contrast to a neuroimaging study, in which nearby (within millimeters) or even intermingled neuronal populations may not be connected to each other. Single-neuron recording also allows direct study of the nature of what is being represented from each sensory modality in the convergent neurons to be analyzed, and the rules that underlie the formation of the multisensory convergence to be directly studied.

To enable the neurophysiological studies to provide a fundamental basis for understanding multisensory convergence in these systems in humans, and thus to advance our understanding of disorders of these brain areas in humans, the studies described were performed in nonhuman primates, macaques, in which both the temporal lobe cortical visual areas and the orbitofrontal cortex are well developed, as in humans. Because visual and olfactory processing in the primate orbitofrontal cortex is closely linked to that for taste, a summary of the cortical representation of taste in the primate orbitofrontal cortex is provided first.

Taste processing in the primate brain

PATHWAYS The diagram of the taste and related visual, olfactory, and somatosensory pathways in primates (Fig. 19.1) shows a direct projection from the rostral part of the nucleus of the solitary tract (NTS) to the taste thalamus and thus to the primary taste cortex in the frontal operculum and adjoining insula, with no pontine taste area and associated subcortical projections as in rodents (Norgren, 1984; Pritchard, Hamilton, Morse, & Norgren, 1986). This emphasis on cortical processing of taste in primates may be related to the great development of the cerebral cortex in primates and the advantage of using extensive and similar

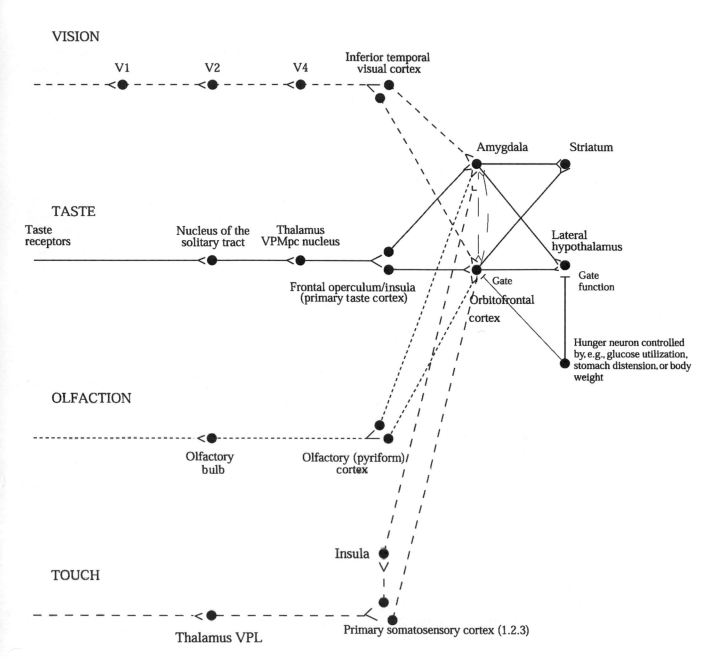

VISION

V1   V2   V4   Inferior temporal
                  visual cortex

Amygdala   Striatum

TASTE

Taste   Nucleus of the   Thalamus
receptors   solitary tract   VPMpc nucleus

Lateral
hypothalamus

Frontal operculum/insula
(primary taste cortex)

Gate   Gate
        function

Orbitofrontal
cortex

Hunger neuron controlled
by, e.g., glucose utilization,
stomach distension, or body
weight

OLFACTION

Olfactory   Olfactory (pyriform)/
bulb   cortex

Insula

TOUCH

Thalamus VPL   Primary somatosensory cortex (1.2.3)

FIGURE 19.1   Schematic diagram of the taste and olfactory pathways in primates showing how they converge with each other and with visual pathways. The gate functions shown refer to the finding that the responses of taste neurons in the orbitofrontal cortex and the lateral hypothalamus are modulated by hunger. VPMpc, ventral-posteromedial thalamic nucleus; V1, V2, V4, visual cortical areas; VL, ventral-posterolateral group of thalamic nuclei.

cortical analysis of inputs from every sensory modality before the analyzed representations from each modality are brought together in multisensory regions.

THE SECONDARY TASTE CORTEX, PART OF THE ORBITOFRONTAL CORTEX   A secondary cortical taste area in primates was discovered by E. T. Rolls, Yaxley, and Sienkiewicz (1990) in the caudolateral orbitofrontal cortex, extending several millimeters in front of the primary taste cortex and receiving from it (Baylis, Rolls, &

Baylis, 1994). One principle of taste processing is that by the secondary taste cortex, the tuning of neurons can become quite specific compared with earlier stages in the taste pathways, with some neurons responding, for example, only to sweet taste (E. T. Rolls, 1995; E. T. Rolls & Scott, 2003; cf. Scott, Yaxley, Sienkiewicz, & Rolls, 1986b; Yaxley, Rolls, & Sienkiewicz, 1990). This specific tuning (especially when combined with olfactory inputs) helps to provide a basis for changes in appetite for some but not other foods eaten during a meal.

FIVE PROTOTYPICAL TASTES, INCLUDING UMAMI   In the primary and secondary taste cortex, there are many neurons that respond best to each of the four classical prototypical tastes sweet, salt, bitter and sour (E. T. Rolls, 1997), but there are also many neurons that respond best to umami tastants, such as glutamate (which is present in many natural foods such as tomatoes, mushrooms, and milk; Baylis & Rolls, 1991) and inosine monophosphate (which is present in many green vegetables; E. T. Rolls, Critchley, Wakeman, & Mason, 1996). This evidence, together with the identification of the glutamate taste receptor (Chaudhari, Landin, & Roper, 2000), leads to the view that there are five prototypical types of taste information channels, with umami contributing, often in combination with corresponding olfactory inputs (E. T. Rolls, Critchley, Browning, & Hernadi, 1998), to the flavor of protein.

THE PLEASANTNESS OF THE TASTE OF FOOD   The modulation of the reward value of a sensory stimulus such as the taste of food by motivational state, for example hunger, is one important way in which motivational behavior is controlled (E. T. Rolls, 1999a). The subjective correlate of this modulation is that food tastes pleasant when one is hungry but tastes hedonically neutral when it has been eaten to satiety (see E. T. Rolls, 1999a). We have found that the modulation of taste-evoked signals by motivation is not a property found in early stages of the primate gustatory system. The responsiveness of taste neurons in the nucleus of the solitary tract (Yaxley, Rolls, Sienkiewicz, & Scott, 1985) and in the primary taste cortex (frontal opercular: E. T. Rolls, Scott, Sienkiewicz, & Yaxley, 1988; insular: Yaxley, Rolls, & Sienkiewicz, 1988) is not attenuated by feeding to satiety. In contrast, in the secondary taste cortex, in the caudolateral part of the orbitofrontal cortex, the responses of the neurons to the taste of the glucose decreased to zero while the monkey ate it to satiety, during the course of which the animal's behavior turned from avid acceptance to active rejection (E. T. Rolls, Sienkiewicz, & Yaxley, 1989). This modulation of responsiveness of the gustatory responses of the orbitofrontal cortex neurons by satiety could not have been due to peripheral adaptation in the gustatory system or to altered efficacy of gustatory stimulation after satiety was reached, because modulation of neuronal responsiveness by satiety was not seen at earlier stages of the gustatory system, including the nucleus of the solitary tract, the frontal opercular taste cortex, and the insular taste cortex (E. T. Rolls et al., 1988; Yaxley et al., 1985, 1988). (The changes in human subjective ratings of the pleasantness of food that occur during a meal [B. J. Rolls, Rowe, Rolls, Kingston, & Megson, 1981; E. T. Rolls, 1999a; E. T. Rolls & Rolls, 1997] are highly correlated with changes in the reward value of food, measured by whether the food is worked for and accepted. Further, human subjective ratings of the pleasantness of food are highly correlated with activation of the same part of the orbitofrontal cortex in which neurons in macaques respond in relation to the reward value of food [Critchley & Rolls, 1996b; O'Doherty et al., 2000; E. T. Rolls, 1999a; E. T. Rolls, Sienkiewicz, et al., 1989].)

SENSORY-SPECIFIC SATIETY   In the secondary taste cortex, it was also found that decreases in the responsiveness of the neurons were relatively specific to the food with which the monkey had been fed to satiety. For example, in seven experiments in which the monkey was fed glucose solution, neuronal responsiveness to the taste of the glucose decreased, but neuronal responsiveness to the taste of black currant juice did not (see examples in Fig. 19.2). Conversely, in two experiments in which the monkey was fed to satiety with fruit juice, the responses of the neurons decreased to fruit juice but not to glucose (E. T. Rolls, Sienkiewicz, et al., 1989).

This evidence shows that the reduced acceptance of food that occurs when food is eaten to satiety, and the reduction in the pleasantness of its taste (Cabanac, 1971; B. J. Rolls, Rolls, & Rowe, 1983; B. J. Rolls, Rolls, Rowe, & Sweeney, 1981; B. J. Rolls, Rowe, et al., 1981; B. J. Rolls, Rowe, & Rolls, 1982; E. T. Rolls & Rolls, 1977, 1982), are not produced by a reduction in the responses of neurons in the nucleus of the solitary tract or frontal opercular or insular (both parts of the primary) gustatory cortices to gustatory stimuli. Indeed, after feeding to satiety, humans reported that the taste of the food on which they had been satiated tasted almost as intense as when they were hungry, though much less pleasant (E. T. Rolls, Rolls, & Rowe, 1983). This comparison is consistent with the possibility that activity in the frontal opercular and insular taste cortices, as well as in the nucleus of the solitary tract, does not reflect the pleasantness of the taste of a food but rather its sensory qualities, and independently of motivational state. On the other hand, the responses of the neurons in the caudolateral orbitofrontal cortex taste area and in the lateral hypothalamus (E. T. Rolls, Murzi, Yaxley, Thorpe, & Simpson, 1986) are modulated by satiety, and it is presumably in areas such as these that neuronal activity may be related to whether a food tastes pleasant and to whether the food should be eaten (see further Critchley & Rolls, 1996b; E. T. Rolls, 1996a, 1999a, 2000d, 2000g; Scott, Yan, & Rolls, 1995).

It is an important principle that the identity of a taste and its intensity are represented separately from its pleasantness. Thus it is possible to represent what a taste is, and to learn about it, even when we are not hungry (E. T. Rolls, 1999a).

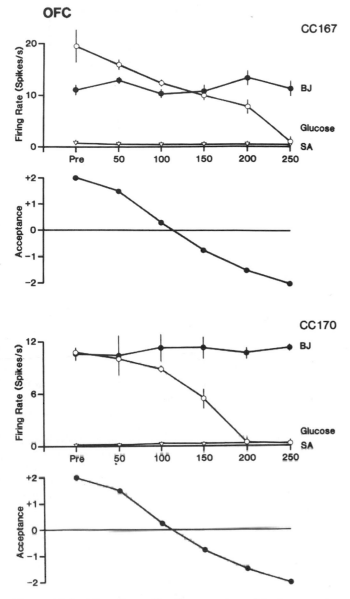

OFC

CC167

BJ

Glucose

SA

FIGURE 19.2 The effect of feeding to satiety with glucose solution on the responses of two neurons in the secondary taste cortex to the taste of glucose and of black currant juice (BJ). The spontaneous firing rate (SA) is also indicated. Below the neuronal response data, the behavioral measure of the acceptance or rejection of the solution on a scale from +2 to −2 (see text) is shown. The solution used to feed to satiety was 20% glucose. The monkey was fed 50 mL of the solution at each stage of the experiment, as indicated along the abscissa, until he was satiated, as shown by whether he accepted or rejected the solution. Pre, the firing rate of the neuron before the satiety experiment started. Values shown are the mean firing rate and SE. (After E. T. Rolls, Sienkiewicz, & Yaxley, 1989.)

The representation of flavor: Convergence of olfactory and taste inputs in the orbitofrontal cortex

At some stage in taste processing, it is likely that taste representations are brought together with inputs from different modalities, for example with olfactory inputs, to form a representation of flavor (see Fig. 19.1). We found (E. T. Rolls & Baylis, 1994) that in the orbitofrontal cortex taste areas, of 112 single neurons that responded to any of these modalities, many were unimodal (taste 34%, olfactory 13%, visual 21%), but they were found in close proximity to each other. Some single neurons showed convergence, responding, for example, to taste and visual inputs (13%), taste and olfactory inputs (13%), and olfactory and visual inputs (5%). Some of these multisensory single neurons had corresponding sensitivities in the two modalities, in that they responded best to sweet tastes (e.g., 1M glucose) and responded more on a visual discrimination task to the visual stimulus that signified sweet fruit juice than to that which signified saline; or they responded to sweet taste and on an olfactory discrimination task to fruit odor. The different types of neurons (unimodal in different modalities, and multisensory) were frequently found intermingled in tracks made into this region (E. T. Rolls & Baylis, 1994), consistent with the hypothesis that the multisensory representations are actually being formed from unimodal inputs to this region.

It thus appears to be in these orbitofrontal cortex areas that flavor representations are built, where flavor is taken to mean a representation that is evoked best by a combination of gustatory and olfactory input. This orbitofrontal region does appear to be an important region for convergence, for there is only a low proportion of bimodal taste and olfactory neurons in the primary taste cortex (E. T. Rolls & Baylis, 1994; E. T. Rolls & Scott, 2003).

The rules underlying the formation of olfactory representations in the primate cortex

Critchley and Rolls (1996a) showed that 35% of orbitofrontal cortex olfactory neurons categorized odors based on their taste association in an olfactory-to-taste discrimination task. This categorization was evident in the fact that 35% of the neurons either responded to all the odors associated with the taste of glucose and to none of the odors associated with the taste of aversive saline (0.1M NaCl), or vice versa. E. T. Rolls, Critchley, Mason, and Wakeman (1996) found that 68% of orbitofrontal cortex odor-responsive neurons modified their responses in some way following changes in the taste reward associations of the odorants during olfactory-taste discrimination learning and its reversal. (In an olfactory discrimination experiment, if a lick response to one odor, the S+, is made, a drop of glucose, the taste reward, is obtained; if incorrectly a lick response is made to another odor, the S−, a drop of aversive saline is obtained.

At some time in the experiment, the contingency between the odor and the taste is reversed, and when the "meaning" of the two odors alters, so does the behavior. It is of interest to investigate in which parts of the olfactory system the neurons show reversal, for where they do, it can be concluded that the neuronal response to the odor depends on the taste with which it is associated, and does not depend primarily on the physicochemical structure of the odor.) Full reversal of the neuronal responses was seen in 25% of the neurons analyzed. (In full reversal, the odor to which the neuron responded reversed when the taste with which it was associated reversed.) Extinction of the differential neuronal responses after task reversal was seen in 43% of these neurons. (These neurons simply stopped discriminating between the two odors after the reversal. This is termed conditional reversal.) These findings demonstrate directly a coding principle in primate olfaction whereby the responses of some orbitofrontal cortex olfactory neurons are modified by, and depend upon, the taste with which the odor is associated.

It was of interest, however, that this modification was less complete, and much slower, often requiring more than 30 trials, than the modifications found for orbitofrontal visual neurons during visual—taste reversal, which take one or two trials (E. T. Rolls, Critchley, Mason, et al., 1996; Thorpe, Rolls, & Maddison, 1983). This relative inflexibility of olfactory responses is consistent with the need for some stability in odor-taste associations to facilitate the formation and perception of flavors. In addition, some orbitofrontal cortex olfactory neurons did not code in relation to the taste with which the odor was associated (Critchley & Rolls, 1996a), indicating that there is also a taste-independent representation of odor in this region.

Visual inputs to the orbitofrontal cortex and the rules of their multisensory convergence

Many of the neurons with visual responses in the primate orbitofrontal cortex also show olfactory or taste responses (E. T. Rolls & Baylis, 1994), reverse rapidly in visual discrimination reversal (Rolls, Critchley, Mason, et al., 1996; see example in Fig. 19.3), often in as little as one trial (Thorpe et al., 1983), and only respond to the sight of food if hunger is present (Critchley & Rolls, 1996b). The orbitofrontal cortex thus seems to implement a mechanism that can flexibly alter the responses to visual stimuli depending on the reinforcement (e.g., the taste) associated with the visual stimulus (see E. T. Rolls, 1996a; Thorpe et al., 1983). This enables prediction of the taste associated with ingestion of what is

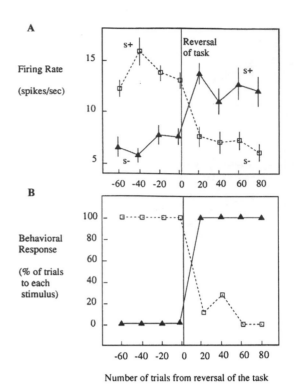

FIGURE 19.3 Orbitofrontal cortex: visual discrimination reversal. The activity of an orbitofrontal visual neuron during performance of a visual discrimination task and its reversal. The stimuli were a triangle and a square presented on a video monitor. (A) Each point represents the mean poststimulus activity of the neuron in a 500 ms period on approximately 10 trials of the different visual stimuli. The standard errors (SE) of these responses are shown. After 60 trials of the task, the reward associations of the visual stimuli were reversed. (A + indicates that a lick response to that visual stimulus produced a fruit juice reward; a − indicates that a lick response to that visual stimulus resulted in a small drop of aversive tasting saline.) This neuron reversed its responses to the visual stimuli following the task reversal. (B) The behavioral response of the monkey to the task. The monkey performed well, in that he rapidly learned to lick only in response to the visual stimulus associated with the fruit juice reward. (After E. T. Rolls, Critchley, Mason, & Wakeman, 1996.)

seen, and thus is important in the visual selection of foods (see E. T. Rolls, 1993, 1994, 1999a, 2000g). It also provides a mechanism for the sight of a food to influence its flavor.

The general underlying mechanism that provides the basis for this learning is likely to be a pattern associator, with associatively modifiable synapses from visual projection neurons from the inferior temporal visual cortex onto orbitofrontal cortex taste neurons, as shown in Figure 19.4. (The inferior temporal visual cortex is the last unimodal cortical area in the visual ventral stream that builds a representation of "what" object is being seen [E. T. Rolls & Deco, 2002]. Neurons in the inferior

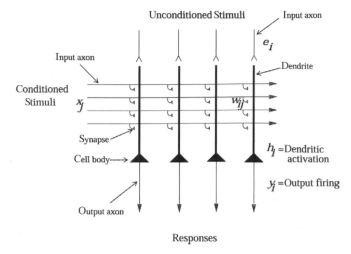

Unconditioned Stimuli

Input axon

e_i

Input axon

Dendrite

Conditioned Stimuli

x_j

w_{ij}

Synapse

h_i = Dendritic activation

Cell body

y_i = Output firing

Output axon

Responses

FIGURE 19.4 A Pattern association network that could underlie the learning and reversal of stimulus-reinforcement association learning in the orbitofrontal cortex (see text). The unconditioned stimulus might be a taste, and the conditioned stimulus a visual astimulus. The synapses w_{ij} are modifiable by an associative (Hebb-like) learning rule. (After E. T. Rolls & Deco, 2002.)

temporal visual cortex do not reflect whether an object is associated with the taste of food, and do not reflect the reward value of the object when this is devalued by feeding to satiety [E. T. Rolls & Rolls, 1977].) The way in which these pattern associators operate in a biologically plausible way has been described by E. T. Rolls and Treves (1998), E. T. Rolls (1999a), and E. T. Rolls and Deco (2002). Long-term potentiation allows the correct associations to be formed, and a process such as long-term depression when the pre- and postsynaptic terms are no longer correlated contributes to allowing the associations to be reversed. A key feature of what is implemented is that the representation of objects (and faces) in the primate inferior temporal visual cortex shows translation, size, and view invariance (Booth & Rolls, 1998; see E. T. Rolls, 2000a; E. T. Rolls & Deco, 2002). This enables correct generalization, after an association has been learned to one view of an object, to another view of the same object, a property of fundamentally important adaptive value conferred by this systems-level design of the brain. The representation provided by the inferior temporal visual cortex is also in a form in which the information conveyed by different neurons about objects is largely independent, so that the number of stimuli that can be represented is very large (increasing exponentially with the number of neurons in the population) (E. T. Rolls, Treves, & Tovee, 1997). Moreover, the representation is in a form that can be read quite efficiently by a dot product operation in which one vector is the set of firing rates of the inferior temporal visual

cortex neurons and the "decoding" vector is the set of synaptic weights set up by associative learning onto single orbitofrontal cortex neurons (see Fig. 19.4) (see E. T. Rolls, 1999a; E. T. Rolls & Deco, 2002; E. T. Rolls & Treves, 1998). Moreover, the inferior temporal cortex representation is in a sufficiently distributed form (for the multisensory integration performed using it in the orbitofrontal cortex) that is allows correct generalization and graceful degradation of performance when the visual stimulus is similar to but not identical to one learned about previously, or is partially obscured, or the system is partially damaged (see E. T. Rolls, 1999a; E. T. Rolls & Deco, 2002; E. T. Rolls & Treves, 1998).

It is also the case that the multisensory integration is performed in the orbitofrontal cortex and not before it in the inferior temporal visual cortex itself, in that inferior temporal cortex neurons do not respond to taste stimuli and do not reverse their responses in the reversal of a visual discrimination reversal task (E. T. Rolls, Judge, & Sanghera, 1977). (Multisensory convergence in the orbitofrontal cortex is present in that some single neurons in it respond to different combinations of visual, olfactory, taste, and/or texture inputs, and that the visual and olfactory representations provided by some of the neurons depend on the taste with which the visual or olfactory representation is associated.) Indeed, it is an important part of brain design that the representation of objects provided in the inferior temporal visual cortex is not influenced by properties such as the (taste) reward association or reward value, so that other brain areas can use the visual object representations for other functions, such as episodic memory, including spatial context memory (involving projections that reach the hippocampus), long-term familiarity memory (via projections to the perirhinal cortex), and short-term or working memory (by projections to the prefrontal cortex) (see E. T. Rolls & Deco, 2002). The point here is that if inferior temporal cortex representations of objects did represent their reward value, and the neurons did not respond when an object was not rewarding (as is the case in the orbitofrontal cortex), then we would not be able to learn about the locations of objects, or even see the objects, if they were not rewarding.

In a visual discrimination reversal task, there is an interesting subpopulation of orbitofrontal cortex neurons (3.5% in the study by Thorpe et al., 1983) that respond for several seconds only when a visual stimulus is not followed by the expected taste reward. These neurons are likely to be an important part of the mechanism by which visual-to-taste and similar multisensory representations can be rapidly reversed. In the context of multisensory processing, these neurons have interesting responses, which occur when an expected correspondence between the sensory inputs in different sensory modalities is not present and there is a mismatch or error.

These classes of neurons appear to be important in rapidly adjusting behavior in line with reinforcers received and thus in emotion, for patients with damage to the orbitofrontal cortex who have some emotional problems may be impaired at visual discrimination reversal or extinction (E. T. Rolls, 1999b; E. T. Rolls, Hornak, Wade, & McGrath, 1994).

In addition to these visual neurons, there are further populations of orbitofrontal cortex neurons that are tuned to respond to the sight of faces (E. T. Rolls, Critchley, Browning, & Inoue, 2004), and others with auditory responses that respond in some cases to vocalization. These neurons are likely in some cases to be multisensory and may be involved, for example, in face expression and voice expression identification, both potential reinforcers and thus important in emotion, and both impaired in some patients with damage to the orbitofrontal cortex (Hornak, Rolls, & Wade, 1996; E. T. Rolls, 1999b).

The representation of the pleasantness of olfactory and visual stimuli in the brain: Olfactory and visual sensory-specific satiety, and their representation in the primate orbitofrontal cortex

It has also been possible to investigate whether the olfactory representation in the orbitofrontal cortex is affected by hunger, and thus whether the pleasantness of odor is represented in the orbitofrontal cortex. In satiety experiments, Critchley and Rolls (1996b) showed that the responses of some olfactory neurons to a food odor decrease during feeding to satiety with a food (e.g., fruit juice) containing that odor. In particular, seven of nine olfactory neurons that were responsive to the odors of foods, such as black currant juice, were found to decrease their responses to the odor of the satiating food. The decrease was typically at least partly specific to the odor of the food that had been eaten to satiety, potentially providing part of the basis for sensory-specific satiety. It was also found that eight of nine neurons that had selective responses to the sight of food demonstrated a sensory-specific reduction in their visual responses to foods following satiation. These findings show that the olfactory and visual representations of food, as well as the taste representation of food, in the primate orbitofrontal cortex are modulated by hunger. Usually a component related to sensory-specific satiety can be demonstrated.

These findings link at least part of the processing of olfactory and visual information in this brain region to the control of feeding-related behavior. This is further evidence that part of the olfactory representation in this region is related to the hedonic value of the olfactory stimulus, and in particular that at this level of the olfactory system in primates, the pleasure elicited by the food odor is at least part of what is represented.

As a result of the neurophysiological and behavioral observations showing the specificity of satiety in the monkey (see E. T. Rolls, 1999a), experiments were performed to determine whether satiety is specific to foods eaten in humans. It was found that the pleasantness of the taste of food eaten to satiety decreased more than the pleasantness of foods that had not been eaten (B. J. Rolls, Rolls, et al., 1981). One consequence of this is that if one food is eaten to satiety, appetite reduction for other foods is often incomplete, and this situation will lead to enhanced eating when a variety of foods is offered (relative to the amount eaten if one food is offered) (B. J. Rolls, Rolls, et al., 1981; B. J. Rolls, Rowe, et al., 1981; B. J. Rolls, Van Duijenvoorde, & Rolls, 1984). Because sensory factors such as similarity of color, shape, flavor, and texture are usually more important than metabolic equivalence in terms of protein, carbohydrate, and fat content in influencing how foods interact in this type of satiety, it has been termed "sensory-specific satiety" (B. J. Rolls, 1990; B. J. Rolls, Rolls, et al., 1981; B. J. Rolls, Rowe, et al., 1981, 1982; E. T. Rolls & Rolls, 1977, 1982). It should be noted that this effect is distinct from alliesthesia, in that alliesthesia is a change in the pleasantness of sensory inputs produced by internal signals (such as glucose in the gut) (see Cabanac, 1971; Cabanac & Duclaux, 1970; Cabanac & Fantino, 1977), whereas sensory-specific satiety is a change in the pleasantness of sensory inputs that is accounted for at least partly by the external sensory stimulation received (such as the taste of a particular food), in that as shown above it is at least partly specific to the external sensory stimulation received.

To investigate whether the sensory-specific reduction in the responsiveness of the orbitofrontal olfactory neurons might be related to a sensory-specific reduction in the pleasure produced by the odor of a food when it is eaten to satiety, E. T. Rolls and Rolls (1997) measured humans' responses to the smell of a food that was eaten to satiety. It was found that the pleasantness of the odor of a food, but much less significantly its intensity, was decreased when subjects ate it to satiety. It was also found that the pleasantness of the smell of other foods (i.e., foods not eaten in the meal) showed much less decrease. This finding has clear implications for the control of food intake, for ways to keep foods presented in a meal appetitive, and for effects on odor pleasantness ratings that could occur following meals. In an investigation of the mechanisms of this odor-specific, sensory-specific satiety, E. T. Rolls and Rolls (1997) allowed humans to chew a food without swallowing, for approximately as long as the food is normally in the mouth during eating. They demonstrated some sensory-specific satiety with this procedure, showing that the sensory-specific satiety does not depend on food reaching the stomach. They were also able to demonstrate some sensory-specific satiety produced by smelling the food for approximately as long as the food is normally in the mouth during eating. Thus at least part of the mechanism is likely to be produced by a change in processing in the olfactory pathways. The earliest stage of olfactory processing at which this modulation occurs is not yet known. It is unlikely to be in the receptors, because the change in pleasantness found was much more significant than the change in intensity (E. T. Rolls & Rolls, 1997).

This sensory-specific satiety is found for all four sensory modalities, taste, olfaction, vision, and texture, in neurons in the orbitofrontal cortex, and individual neurons that respond to up to three of four of these types of sensory input show the effect in all the sensory modalities (Fig. 19.5) (Critchley & Rolls, 1996b; E. T. Rolls, Critchley, Browning, Hernadi, & Lenard, 1999). Sensory-specific satiety is also shown in all these sensory modalities in humans (E. T. Rolls & Rolls, 1997; see E. T. Rolls, 1999a).

The enhanced eating when a variety of foods is available, as a result of the operation of sensory-specific satiety, may have been advantageous in evolution in ensuring that different foods with important different nutrients were consumed, but today in humans, when a wide variety of foods is readily available, it may be a factor that can lead to overeating and obesity. In a test of this in the rat, it has been found that variety itself can lead to obesity (B. J. Rolls, Van Duijenvoorde, & Rowe, 1983; see further B. J. Rolls & Hetherington, 1989).

The responses of orbitofrontal cortex taste and olfactory neurons to the texture of food

The orbitofrontal cortex of primates is also important as an area of convergence for somatosensory inputs, related for example to the texture of food, including fat in the mouth. We have shown in recent recordings that the responses of single neurons influenced by taste in this region can in some cases be modulated by the texture of the food. This was shown in experiments in which the texture of food was manipulated by the addition of methylcellulose or gelatine, or by puréeing a semisolid food (E. T. Rolls, 1997, 1999a; E. T. Rolls & Critchley, in prep.).

THE MOUTH FEEL OF FAT Texture in the mouth is an important indicator of whether *fat* is present in a food, which is important not only as a high-value energy source, but also as a potential source of essential fatty acids. In the orbitofrontal cortex, E. T. Rolls, Critchley, et al. (1999) have found a population of neurons that responds when fat is in the mouth. An example of the responses of such a neuron is shown in Figure 19.6. It is evident that information about fat as well as about taste can converge onto the same neuron in this region. The neuron responded to taste in that its firing rate was significantly different within the group of tastants sweet, salt, bitter, sour, and umami (i.e., MSG, to which it did respond). However, its response to fat in the mouth was larger. The fat-related responses of these neurons are produced at least in part by the texture of the food rather than by chemical receptors, in that such neurons typically respond not only to foods such as cream and milk containing fat, but also to nonfat chemicals with a similar texture to fat, such as paraffin oil (which is a pure hydrocarbon) and silicone oil $(Si(CH_3)_2O)_n)$. Some of the fat-related neurons do, though, have convergent inputs from the chemical senses, in that in addition to taste inputs, some of these neurons respond to the odor associated with a fat, such as the odor of cream (E. T. Rolls, Critchley, et al., 1999). Feeding to satiety with fat (e.g., cream) decreases the responses of these neurons to zero on the food eaten to satiety, but if the neuron receives a taste input from, for example, glucose taste, that is not decreased by feeding to satiety with cream. Thus there is a representation of the macronutrient fat in this brain area, and the activation produced by fat is reduced by eating fat to satiety.

We have now shown that the (slick) texture of fat is represented separately from a texture information processing channel that enables some orbitofrontal cortex neurons to respond to the viscosity of a stimulus (such as methylcellulose in the viscosity range 1–10,000 centipoise), and that each of these texture channels is combined with other sensory modalities in the primate orbitofrontal cortex to enable different single neurons to respond to different sensory combinations of taste, texture, and also temperature (Verhagen, Rolls, & Kadohisa, 2002).

The neuronal representation in the primate orbitofrontal cortex is thus extremely rich in providing an encoding system in which populations of different neurons, each responding to different combinations of sensory inputs, provide as a population a system that encodes very efficiently the very rich set of different sensory inputs provided by the sensory receptor systems, and that enables very simple read-out of the information by neurons that receive from these neuronal

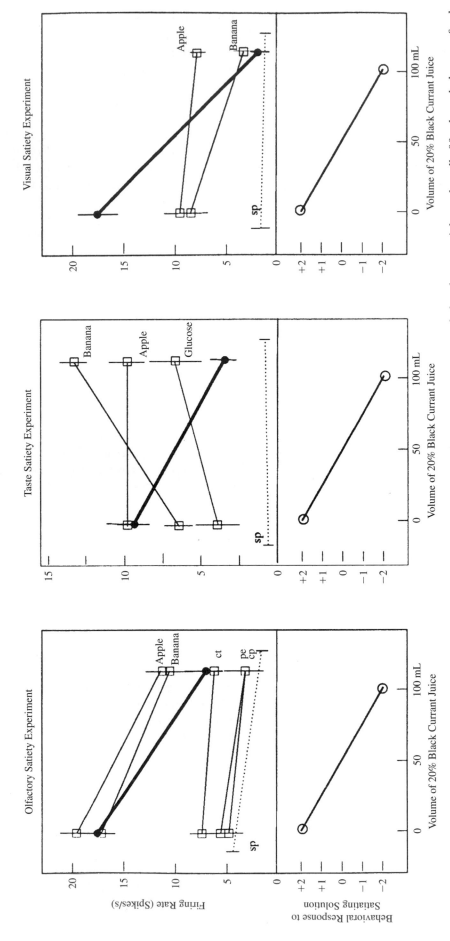

FIGURE 19.5   Taste, olfactory, and visual sensory-specific satiety in a multisensory neuron. The same neuron responded to the taste, sight, and smell of foods; and when one food (black currant juice, thick line, solid black circles) was eaten to satiety, the responses of the neuron to that food produced through each sensory modality decreased relative to the responses to other foods, which included apple (ap) and banana (ba). The abscissa shows the amount of black currant juice consumed. On the behavioral rating scale, +2 is strongly accepted and −2 is strongly rejected. Abbreviations: sp, spontaneous firing rate; cp, caprylic acid; ct, citral; pe, phenyl ethanol. (After Critchley & Rolls, 1996b.)

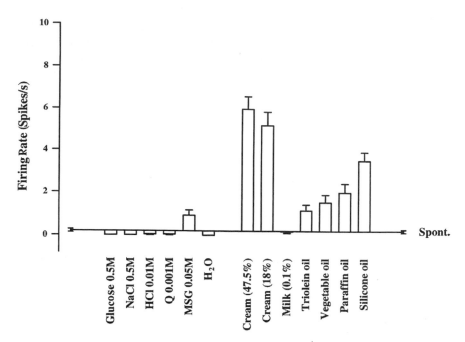

FIGURE 19.6   A neuron in the primate orbitofrontal cortex responding to the texture of fat in the mouth. The cell (Be047) increased its firing rate to cream (double and single cream), and responded to texture rather than the chemical structure of the fat in that it also responded to 0.5 mL of silicone oil (SiO$_2$) or paraffin oil (hydrocarbon). The cell has a taste input, too, in that it had a consistent but small response to umami taste (monosodium glutamate, MSG). Abbreviations: Gluc, glucose; NaCl, salt; HCl, sour; Q-HCl, quinine, bitter. The spontaneous firing rate of the cell is also shown. (From E. T. Rolls, Critchley, et al., 1999.)

populations (see E. T. Rolls, 1999a; E. T. Rolls & Deco, 2002; E. T. Rolls & Treves, 1998).

THE AMYGDALA   The amygdala has many similar connections to the orbitofrontal cortex (see Fig. 19.1), and also shows many similar types of multisensory convergence (E. T. Rolls, 2000c). One apparent difference is that in primates, the amygdala does not show such rapid visual-to-taste reversal learning (E. T. Rolls, 2000c; Sanghera, Rolls, & Roper-Hall, 1979) as the orbitofrontal cortex. It may be that as a noncortical structure that has been present throughout vertebrate evolutionary history, is has less well-developed synaptic mechanisms for learning, and in particular for rapid relearning. The relearning process is likely to involve long-term synaptic depression (LTD) to weaken synapses from presynaptic (e.g., visual) inputs that are no longer coactive with postsynaptic (e.g., taste-produced) activation (see Fig. 19.4), and it may be that LTD in particular operates less rapidly in the amygdala. LTD is an important feature of neocortical plasticity (Fregnac, 1996) that is likely to be important not just in the reversal of previous learning but also in ensuring a close match between each input firing rate vector and the postsynaptic activation associated with it. To optimize this matching when multiple associations are learned, and when the neurons show positive-only firing rates (heterosynaptic), LTD becomes very important (E. T. Rolls & Treves, 1998).

Temporal cortex multisensory convergence areas

There are a number of areas in the temporal lobe neocortex where multisensory sensory convergence occurs. Many of these are in and closely related to cortex in the superior temporal sulcus, where within individually defined cytoarchitectonic areas different single neurons can respond to visual, auditory, or somatosensory inputs (Baylis, Rolls, & Leonard, 1987). In recent experiments we have shown that some of these neurons show convergence from more than one input. For example, some neurons in the cortex in the superior temporal sulcus respond to the sight of lip movements; other neurons in the same region respond to vocalization. It seems very likely that these areas are important in multisensory convergence to produce representations in which the inputs from different modalities all combine to describe the object or event in the world, and in which mutual support (in, e.g., noisy signal conditions) is implemented. (The mutual support refers to the situation in which different modules have inputs that correspond to the same object or event in the world, and in which cross-connections between the modules then are consistent.) Once the multisensory representations have been formed, backprojections to earlier cortical areas may enable top-down influences, which are important in perception, to operate (see E. T. Rolls & Deco, 2002).

Formal analyses of how such cortical systems, which are characterized by recurrent collateral feedback connections within modules and by forward and backward connections between modules, could operate have been performed by Renart, Parga, and Rolls (1999a, 1999b). The operation of these systems is described using the architecture shown in Figure 19.7, and in the context of coupled attractor networks that capture important aspects of the operation of networks of single neurons with the architecture just described (see Rolls & Deco, 2002, pp. 224–228). In the trimodular attractor architecture shown in Figure 19.7 (which has recurrent collateral connections within each module), interesting interactions occur that account for effects such as the McGurk effect, in which what is seen affects what is heard (Renart et al., 1999a, 1999b). The effect was originally demonstrated with the perception of auditory syllables, which were influenced by what was seen (McGurk & MacDonald, 1976). An important parameter in the

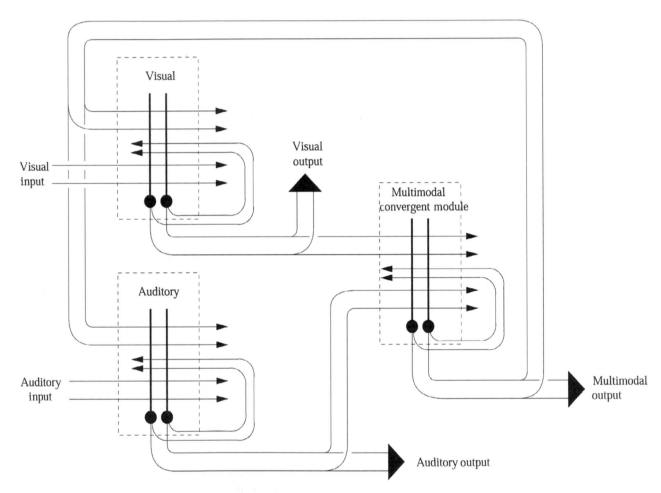

FIGURE 19.7   A two-layer set of attractor (or autoassociation) nets in which feedback from layer 2 (labeled the multimodal convergent module) can influence the states reached in the modules (labeled visual and auditory) in layer 1. Layer 2 could be a higher cortical visual area with convergence from earlier cortical visual areas. Layer 2 could also be a multisensory area receiving inputs from unimodal visual and auditory cortical areas, as labeled. Each of the three modules has recurrent collateral synapses that are trained by an associative synaptic learning rule, and also intermodular synaptic connections in the forward and backward direction that are also associatively trained. Attractors are formed within modules, the different modules interact, and attractors are also formed by the forward and backward intermodular connections. The higher area not only may affect the states reached during attractor settling in the input layers but also, as a result of this, may influence the representations that are learned in earlier cortical areas. A similar principle may operate in any multilayer hierarchical cortical processing system, such as the ventral visual system, in that the categories that can be formed only at later stages of processing may help earlier stages to form categories relevant to what can be diagnosed at later stages. (For further description, see E. T. Rolls & Deco, 2002.)

architecture is g, the relative average strength of the backprojection synapses from one module to the preceding module, relative to the average strength of the recurrent collateral connections within a module. The trimodular architecture (studied using scenarios in which first a stimulus was presented to a module, then removed during a memory delay period in which stimuli were applied to other modules) showed a phase with $g < 0.005$ in which the modules operated in an isolated way. With g in the range of 0.005–0.012, an "independent" regime existed in which each module could be in a separate state to the others, but in which interactions between the modules occurred that could assist or hinder retrieval in a module, depending on whether the states in the other modules were consistent or inconsistent. It is in this "independent" regime that a module can be in a continuing attractor that can provide other modules with a persistent external modulatory input that is helpful for tasks such as making comparisons between stimuli processed sequentially (as in delayed match-to-sample tasks and visual search tasks) (see E. T. Rolls & Deco, 2002). In this regime, if the modules are initially quiescent, then a stimulus applied to one input module propagates to the central module, and from it to the nonstimulated input module as well (see Fig. 19.7). When g grows beyond 0.012, the picture changes, and the independence between the modules is lost. The delay activity states found in this region (of the phase space) always involve the three modules in attractors correlated with consistent features associated in the synaptic connections. Also, because g is now larger, changes in the properties of the external stimuli have more impact on the delay activity states. The general trend seen in this phase under the change of stimulus after a previous consistent attractor has been reached is that, first, if the second stimulus is not effective enough (if it is weak or brief), it is unable to move any of the modules from their current delay activity states. If the stimulus is made more effective, then as soon as it is able to change the state of the stimulated input module, the internal and nonstimulated input modules follow, and the whole network moves into the new consistent attractor selected by the second stimulus. In this case, the interaction between the modules is so large that it does not allow contradictory local delay activity states to coexist, and the network is described as being in a "locked" state.

The conclusion is that the most interesting scenario for coupled attractor networks is when they are weakly coupled (in the trimodular architecture, $0.005 < g < 0.012$), for then interactions occur whereby how well one module responds to its own inputs can be influenced by

the states of the other modules, but it can retain partly independent representations. This emphasizes the importance of weak interactions between coupled modules in the brain (see E. T. Rolls & Deco, 2002).

These generally useful interactions between coupled attractor networks can be useful in implementing top-down constraint satisfaction and short-term memory. One type of constraint satisfaction in which they are also probably important is cross-modal constraint satisfaction, which occurs, for example, when the sight of the lips moving assists the hearing of syllables. If the experimenter mismatches the visual and auditory inputs, then auditory misperception can occur, as in the McGurk effect. In such experiments (McGurk & MacDonald, 1976) the subject receives one stimulus through the auditory pathway (e.g., the syllables *ga-ga*) and a different stimulus through the visual pathway (e.g., the lips of a person performing the movements corresponding to the syllables *ba-ba* on a video monitor). These stimuli are such that their acoustic waveforms as well as the lip motions needed to pronounce them are rather different. One can then assume that although they share the same vowel *a*, the internal representation of the syllables is dominated by the consonant, so that the representations of the syllables *ga-ga* and *ba-ba* are not correlated either in the primary visual cortical areas or in the primary auditory ones. At the end of the experiment, the subject is asked to repeat what he heard. When this procedure is repeated with many subjects, roughly 50% of them claim to have heard either the auditory stimulus (*ga-ga*) or the visual one (*ba-ba*). The rest of the subjects report having heard neither the auditory nor the visual stimulus but some combination of the two (e.g., *gabga*), or even something else, including phonemes not presented auditorally or visually (e.g., *gagla*).

Renart et al. (1999b) were able to show that the McGurk effect can be accounted for by the operation of coupled attractor networks of the form shown in Figure 19.7. One input module is for the auditory input, the second is for the visual input, and both converge on a higher area that represents the syllable formed on the evidence of combination of the two inputs. There are backprojections from the convergent module back to the input modules. Persistent (continuing) inputs were applied to both the inputs, and during associative training of all the weights, the visual and auditory inputs corresponded to the same syllable. When tested with inconsistent visual and auditory inputs, it was found that for g between approximately 0.10 and 0.11, the convergent module can either remain in a symmetric state, in which it represents a mixture of the two inputs, or it can choose between the inputs, with either situation being stable. For lower g the convergent module always settles into a state corresponding to the input in one of the input modules. It is the random fluctuations produced during the convergence to the attractor that determine the pattern selected by the convergent module. When the convergent module becomes correlated with one of its stored patterns, the signal backprojected to the input module stimulated with the feature associated to that pattern becomes stronger, and the overlap in this module is increased. Thus, with low values of the intermodule coupling parameter g, situations are found in which sometimes the input to one module dominates, and sometimes the input to the other module dominates what is represented in the convergent module, and sometimes mixture states are stable in the convergent module. This model can thus account for the influences that visual inputs can have on what is heard, for example in the McGurk effect.

The interactions between coupled attractor networks can lead to the following effects. Facilitation can occur in a module if its external input is matched (in terms of the vector of firing rates on the axons, which constitutes the input to the module) by an input from another module, whereas suppression in a module of its response to an external input can occur if the two inputs mismatch. This type of interaction can be used in imaging studies to identify brain regions where different signals interact with each other. One example is to locate brain regions where multisensory inputs converge. If the inputs in two sensory modalities are consistent based on previous experience, then facilitation will occur, whereas if they are inconsistent, suppression of the activity in a module can occur. This is one of the effects described in the bimodular and trimodular architectures investigated by Renart et al. (1999a, 1999b) and E. T. Rolls and Stringer (2001), and found in architectures such as that illustrated in Figure 19.7.

An interesting issue that arises is how rapidly a system of interacting attractor networks such as that illustrated in Figure 19.7 settles into a stable state. Is it sufficiently rapid for the interacting attractor effects described to contribute to cortical information processing? It is likely that the settling of the whole system is quite rapid, if it is implemented (as it is in the brain) with synapses and neurons that operate with continuous dynamics, where the time constant of the synapses dominates the retrieval speed, and is on the order of 15 ms for each module, as described by E. T. Rolls and Deco (2002) and Panzeri, Rolls, Battaglia, and Treves (2001). These investigators showed that a multimodular attractor network architecture can process information in approximately 17 ms per module (assuming an inactivation time constant for the synapses of 10 ms), and similarly fast settling may be expected of a system of the type shown in Figure 19.7.

The hippocampus

Another brain region in which multisensory integration is somewhat understood at the neuronal level is the primate hippocampus. The anatomical basis for this convergence in regions such as the CA3 and CA1 neurons of the hippocampus is shown in Figure 19.8. The anatomical evidence indicates that the hippocampus receives from the end of every sensory processing stream (including visual from the inferior temporal visual cortex, auditory from the superior temporal auditory cortex, and somatosensory, olfactory, and spatial information from the parietal cortex) and is thus in a position to combine these inputs. The neurophysiology to be described shows that different single hippocampal neurons do respond to each of these inputs and others to their combinations. This provides a basis for a multisensory memory of events, as exemplified by episodic and object-place memory.

Indeed, it has been found that the primate hippocampus contains populations of neurons that reflect not only the location in allocentric space "out there" at which a monkey is looking (see E. T. Rolls, 1999c; E. T. Rolls, Robertson, & Georges-François, 1997; E. T. Rolls, Treves, Robertson, Georges-François, & Panzeri, 1998) but also the object being seen (E. T. Rolls, Critchley, et al., 1989). In a task in which monkeys had to make a behavioral choice that depended not only on the object shown on a video monitor but also on where the monitor was located in the room (a conditional object-place response task), some hippocampal neurons responded in relation to which object had been shown (6%), some responded in relation to where the monitor was located in allocentric space (9%), and some responded to a combination of which object was shown and where it was shown (15%) (E. T. Rolls, Xiang, & Franco, in prep.). These latter neurons thus reflected multisensory convergence of an allocentric spatial representation and an object representation, and, in representing this arbitrary (unique and not predefined) association, provided an important basis for the hippocampus to contribute to solving such a task. Indeed, once such combination neurons have been formed, only a simple pattern association is required to associate each particular object-place combination with reward versus punishment.

Episodic memories typically involve spatial and nonspatial information. An example might be where a particular object has been left. A quantitative model

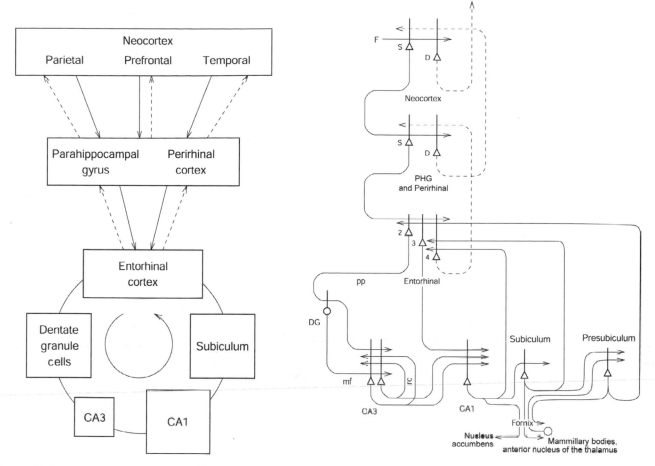

FIGURE 19.8   Forward connections (solid lines) from areas of cerebral association neocortex via the parahippocampal gyrus and perirhinal cortex, and entorhinal cortex, to the hippocampus, and backprojections (dashed lines) via the hippocampal CA1 pyramidal cells, subiculum, and parahippocampal gyrus to the neocortex. There is great convergence in the forward connections down to the single network implemented in the CA3 pyramidal cells, and great divergence again in the backprojections. On the left is a block diagram. On the right is a more detailed representation of some of the principal excitatory neurons in the pathways. Abbreviations: D, deep pyramidal cells; DG, dentate granule cells; F, forward inputs to areas of the association cortex from preceding cortical areas in the hierarchy; mf, mossy fibers; PHG, parahippocampal gyrus and perirhinal cortex; pp, perforant path; rc, recurrent collaterals of the CA3 hippocampal pyramidal cells; S, superficial pyramidal cells; 2, pyramidal cells in layer 2 of the entorhinal cortex; 3, pyramidal cells in layer 3 of the entorhinal cortex; 5, 6, pyramidal cells in the deep layers of the entorhinal cortex. The thick lines above the cell bodies represent the dendrites.

has been developed that shows how the CA3 recurrent collateral system could operate as an autoassociation (attractor) network crucial in forming such episodic memories by allowing multisensory information occurring at one particular time to be associated together, and later the whole memory to be retrieved from any of its parts (E. T. Rolls, 1996b; E. T. Rolls & Treves, 1998; Treves & Rolls, 1992, 1994). The theory also shows how corticocortical backprojections could be used to implement recall of, for example, visual neurons firing in high-order, primarily unimodal visual cortical areas in response to a retrieval cue in another sensory modality (Treves & Rolls, 1994). In a development of this model to deal with the inherently continuous nature of spatial representations, it has been shown

that associating together discrete representations of objects with continuous spatial representations can occur in a single network that combines the properties of discrete and continuous attractor dynamics (E. T. Rolls, Trappenberg, & Stringer, 2002). Such a network, implemented in the hippocampus, could enable episodic memories involving object and spatial information to be stored, and for a memory to be retrieved from either its spatial or its object component (E. T. Rolls & Deco, 2002).

The hippocampus also contains single neurons that combine information about allocentric "spatial view" with idiothetic (self-motion) information. In particular, hippocampal spatial view cells, which respond to allocentrically encoded locations in space "out there"

(Georges-François, Rolls, & Robertson, 1999), continue to respond when the view details are obscured and in the dark, responding when the eyes move to look toward a particular location in space (Robertson, Rolls, & Georges-François, 1998). This neuronal response is triggered by internal eye movement–related signals, in that the view fields tend to drift in the dark, and are reset by the spatial view when it is shown again (Robertson et al., 1998). The process by which idiothetic signals update the representation of where one is in space or where one is looking in space is known as path integration, and is reflected in the responses of these hippocampal neurons. Path integration involves updating by idiothetic signals a spatial representation that is reflected in the ongoing activity of neurons, with the set of active neurons being shifted by the idiothetic signals. Given that space is inherently continuous, the most likely network to implement this representation is a continuous attractor network. This is a network with associatively modifiable recurrent connections (implemented by, for example, recurrent collateral connections between neurons), where the patterns stored are continuous (e.g., Gaussian) because they are spatial, rather than discrete as in point attractor networks (see E. T. Rolls & Deco, 2002). To learn the direction and magnitude of the shift in the activity packet of neuronal activity that represents the current remembered spatial view by the idiothetic eye velocity and head direction signals requires true integration and not just association (which is adequate for many forms of multisensory integration, such as that in the orbitofrontal cortex and amygdala), because the shift must be correct for every starting location in the state space. A network that can self-organize (teach itself) using the visual inputs from the scene and the idiothetic signals has been described by Stringer, Rolls, and Trappenberg (2002) and Stringer, Trappenberg, Rolls, and Araujo (2002). It uses a short-term-memory-traced synaptic input term from other neurons in the continuous attractor in order to detect the recent change in the location being represented, and learns combinations of these shifts with the associated idiothetic signals.

A related type of sensory integration is found in the primate presubiculum, where cells are found that respond to head direction. These cells can be updated in the dark by path integration using idiothetic inputs, and any drift is reset by visual cues when these cues become available again (Robertson, Rolls, Georges-François, & Panzeri, 1999). A self-organizing continuous attractor network performing path integration and activated by both visual and idiothetic inputs could implement the multisensory integration performed by

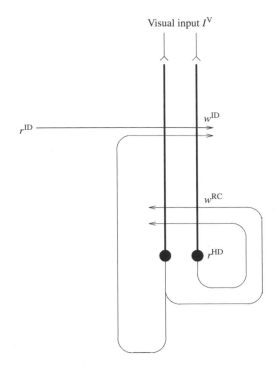

FIGURE 19.9 General network architecture for a one-dimensional continuous attractor model of head direction cells that can be updated by idiothetic inputs produced by head rotation cell firing r^{ID}. The head direction cell firing is r^{HD}, the continuous attractor synaptic weights are w^{RC}, the idiothetic synaptic weights are w^{ID}, and the external visual input is I^V.

these neurons (Stringer, Rolls, Trappenberg, & Araujo, 2004) (Fig. 19.9).

Attention

Another fascinating type of interaction between functionally partly separate sensory processing streams is exemplified by the attention-related interactions between the ventral and dorsal visual cortical processing streams in primates, including humans. In a visual search task, attention can be object-based, and the location of the specified target in the scene must be found. Alternatively, attention can be based on spatial location, and the object at that location must be identified. A model of these interactions between sensory processing streams that can account for single-neuron, fMRI, and neuropsychological findings on these attentional processes has been described by E. T. Rolls and Deco (2002), who also review the literature on attention and its brain mechanisms. This biased competition model utilizes the architecture shown in Figure 19.10 and is implemented with mean field theory–based dynamics. Although the model analyzed in detail is for

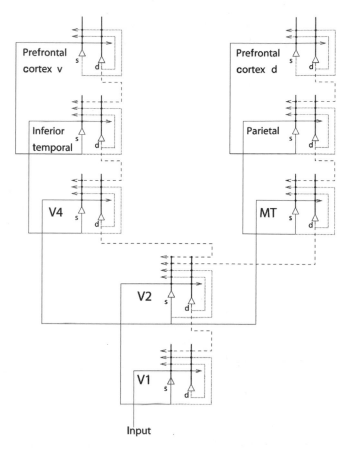

FIGURE 19.10   The overall architecture of the model of object and spatial processing and attention, including the prefrontal cortical areas that provide the short-term memory required to hold the object or spatial target of attention active. Forward projections between areas are shown as solid lines and backprojections are shown as dashed lines. The triangles represent pyramidal cell bodies, with the thick vertical line above them the dendritic trees. The cortical layers in which the cells are concentrated are indicated by s (superficial, layers 2 and 3) and d (deep, layers 5 and 6). The prefrontal cortical areas most strongly reciprocally connected to the inferior temporal cortex "what" processing stream are labeled v to indicate that they are in the more ventral part of the lateral prefrontal cortex, area 46, close to the inferior convexity in macaques. The prefrontal cortical areas most strongly reciprocally connected to the parietal visual cortical "where" processing stream are labeled d to indicate that they are in the more dorsal part of the lateral prefrontal cortex, area 46, in and close to the banks of the principal sulcus in macaques (see text).

the interaction between two visual processing streams, the model is generic and applies in principle to interactions between different sensory modalities, as described by E. T. Rolls and Deco (2002).

In an object-based visual search task, the object that is to be the target of the search is loaded into the short-term memory attractor network in the ventral (v) part of the prefrontal cortex. Via backprojections to the inferior temporal visual cortex (which does not have any visual field-related topological organization) and V4, the representations of features that are part of the object are facilitated in early topologically mapped visual areas such as V2 and V1. Wherever those features are present in the visual scene (presented to V1 via the input pathway from the lateral geniculate nucleus), there is somewhat increased activity in that part of V1 and V2 (because of the summation of the forward and corresponding backprojected inputs). That enhanced activity in V1 and V2 is fed up through the topologically mapped dorsal stream areas MT and parietal cortex, leading to the spotlight of covert attention developing in the parietal cortex in just the location where the object is present. In this way, the network finds the location of the target object and represents the location in the parietal cortex.

In a spatial cue–based visual search task, the location in which the object is to be identified is loaded into the dorsal stream short-term memory attractor network (labeled Prefrontal cortex d in Fig. 19.10). Via the backprojections to parietal cortical visual areas and MT, neurons in early topologically organized visual areas such as V2 and V1 become facilitated. This facilitation sums with the forward inputs from the visual scene, resulting in enhanced activity for features in just those parts of the visual scene where the spotlight of spatial attention (held in the prefrontal cortex d short-term memory) is located. The effects of just those features being facilitated are fed up through the ventral visual stream via V4 to the inferior temporal cortex, producing preferential activation of neurons representing objects containing the facilitated features. In this way, the correct object neurons in the inferior temporal cortex respond for the object at the specified attentional location, even though the inferior temporal cortex itself has no spatial topological organization.

This model can account not only for object and spatial search but also, because it is a full dynamical model, for temporal aspects of covert visual search. For example, covert (that is, without eye movements) so-called "serial search," which seems to occur as the number of distracter objects in the visual scene increases, is accounted for instead by the dynamics of a fully parallel processing system in which the constraints are more difficult to satisfy with multiple distractors, so that the network takes longer to settle into an energy minimum, resulting in a longer "search" (E. T. Rolls & Deco, 2002).

This model of attention thus shows a very interesting way in which different sensory processing streams, in this case the dorsal visual stream for spatial location and motion and the ventral visual stream for object identification, can interact, and by doing so in the way specified, lead to a model of attention that models neuronal, neuroimaging, neuropsychological, and psychophysical phenomena (see further E. T. Rolls & Deco, 2002).

Conclusions

The primate orbitofrontal cortex is an important site for the convergence of representations of the taste, smell, sight, and mouth feel of food, and this convergence allows the sensory properties of each food to be represented and defined in detail. The primate orbitofrontal cortex is also the region where short-term, sensory-specific control of appetite and eating is implemented. Moreover, it is likely that visceral and other satiety-related signals reach the orbitofrontal cortex and there modulate the representation of food, resulting in an output that reflects the reward (or appetitive) value of each food (see E. T. Rolls, 1999a). The learning and reversal of associations between olfactory and taste stimuli that occur in the orbitofrontal cortex could be implemented by Hebbian modification of synapses conveying visual input onto taste-responsive neurons, implementing a pattern association network (E. T. Rolls & Treves, 1998; E. T. Rolls, 1999a, 2000b). The orbitofrontal cortex (and amygdala) thus provide for the multisensory integration of signals from the "what" sensory systems, with an emphasis on associations with primary reinforcers such as taste and touch because the reward value of these is represented in the orbitofrontal cortex. This is part of the basis for the important role of the orbitofrontal cortex (and amygdala) in emotion (E. T. Rolls, 1999a).

The hippocampus combines information from all sensory modalities, including spatial information, in order to form multisensory memories of particular events. The hippocampus again receives inputs from the end of the "what" processing streams, where objects are represented, but combines these inputs with spatial information, including internal vestibular and other idiothetic information, which must undergo path integration before it can be combined with visual and auditory information.

The rule underlying much multisensory integration involving object representations is that once objects have become represented in mainly unimodal information processing streams, then associative learning can be performed in convergence areas. When these associations are with a primary reinforcer, then a pattern association network is appropriate so that the reinforcer associated with a particular object can be determined. If the convergence provides for a multisensory representation of an object or event, then convergence of the different inputs into an autoassociation network enables a representation to be formed in which the full representation can be retrieved from any part. Feedforward convergence of different inputs can also be used to form categories that define particular combinations of the inputs. These processes are described by E. T. Rolls and Deco (2002). In the case of path integration, the rules of the integration are more complex, because the correct location must be selected based on the current location and the idiothetically signaled shift that is required, and this could be implemented by a special form of continuous attractor network.

Finally, it may be useful to clarify the distinction between "sensory integration" and "sensory convergence." The distinction that is suggested by the editors of this handbook is that integration involves nonlinear processing, whereas convergence does not. One reason for making the distinction may be that with neuroimaging, convergence between modalities can only be detected if there is nonlinear enhancement or a reduced signal when corresponding versus noncorresponding sensory inputs are applied. This is not, of course, a limitation of single-neuron recording, in which the convergence can be detected directly, by whether single neurons respond to inputs in more than one sensory modality. Moreover, the single-neuron recording approach allows the rules of the convergence to be examined, in the ways described in this chapter. Of course, nonlinear processing is necessary for useful computation by the brain, as described by E. T. Rolls and Deco (2002) and E. T. Rolls and Treves (1998). But frequently different sensory modalities may converge in a way that does not involve supra-additive overall effects of inputs, or subadditive overall effects of inputs. Many examples have been provided in this chapter, one of which is visual-to-taste association learning. Moreover, the types of interaction between modules are better captured by, for example, the coupled attractor models described here, which show how the signals interact, without necessarily producing a gross change in overall activation of an area that can be measured using, for example, neuroimaging. Indeed, whether nonlinearity and interaction between modules are captured by nonadditivity of two sensory inputs is a matter that is largely determined by the feedback regulation by inhibitory neurons in an area. Many of the important interactions between modules may be produced without nonadditivity of inputs expressed in the gross level of activity in an area, and indeed the interactions and convergence that do occur between processing streams can perhaps be usefully captured by the single-neuron recording and neuronal network models described in this chapter, which allow much richness in these interactions to be demonstrated.

ACKNOWLEDGMENTS Research from the author's laboratory was supported by Medical Research Council grants PG8513790 and PG9826105, by the Human Frontier Science Program, and by the Oxford McDonnell Centre for Cognitive Neuroscience.

REFERENCES

Baylis, L. L., & Rolls, E. T. (1991). Responses of neurons in the primate taste cortex to glutamate. *Physiology and Behavior, 49*, 973–979.

Baylis, L. L., Rolls, E. T., & Baylis, G. C. (1994). Afferent connections of the orbitofrontal cortex taste area of the primate. *Neuroscience, 64*, 801–812.

Baylis, G. C., Rolls, E. T., & Leonard, C. M. (1987). Functional subdivisions of temporal lobe neocortex. *Journal of Neuroscience, 7*, 330–342.

Booth, M. C. A., & Rolls, E. T. (1998). View-invariant representations of familiar objects by neurons in the inferior temporal visual cortex. *Cerebral Cortex, 8*, 510–523.

Cabanac, M. (1971). Physiological role of pleasure. *Science, 173*, 103–1107.

Cabanac, M., & Duclaux, R. (1970). Specificity of internal signals in producing satiety for taste stimuli. *Nature, 227*, 966–967.

Cabanac, M., & Fantino, M. (1977). Origin of olfacto-gustatory alliesthesia: Intestinal sensitivity to carbohydrate concentration? *Physiology and Behavior, 10*, 1039–1045.

Chaudhari, N., Landin, A. M., & Roper, S. D. (2000). A metabotropic glutamate receptor variant functions as a taste receptor. *Nature Neuroscience, 3*, 113–119.

Critchley, H. D., & Rolls, E. T. (1996a). Olfactory neuronal responses in the primate orbitofrontal cortex: Analysis in an olfactory discrimination task. *Journal of Neurophysiology, 75*, 1659–1672.

Critchley, H. D., & Rolls, E. T. (1996b). Hunger and satiety modify the responses of olfactory and visual neurons in the primate orbitofrontal cortex. *Journal of Neurophysiology, 75*, 1673–1686.

Fregnac, Y. (1996). Dynamics of cortical connectivity in visual cortical networks: An overview. *Journal of Physiology, Paris, 90*, 113–139.

Georges-François, P., Rolls, E. T., & Robertson, R. G. (1999). Spatial view cells in the primate hippocampus: Allocentric view not head direction or eye position or place. *Cerebral Cortex, 9*, 197–212.

Hornak, J., Rolls, E. T., & Wade, D. (1996). Face and voice expression identification in patients with emotional and behavioural changes following ventral frontal lobe damage. *Neuropsychologia, 34*, 247–261.

McGurk, H., & MacDonald, J. (1976). Hearing lips and seeing voices. *Nature, 264*, 746–748.

Norgren, R. (1984). Central neural mechanisms of taste. In I. Darien-Smith (Ed.), *Handbook of physiology: The nervous system. Section III. Sensory processes* (J. Brookhart & V. B. Mountcastle, Section Eds.). Bethesda, MD: American Physiological Society.

Panzeri, S., Rolls, E. T., Battaglia, F., & Lavis, R. (2001). Speed of information retrieval in multilayer networks of integrate-and-fire neurons. *Network: Computation in Neural Systems, 12*, 423–440.

Pritchard, T. C., Hamilton, R. B., Morse, J. R., & Norgren, R. (1986). Projections of thalamic gustatory and lingual areas in the monkey, *Macaca fascicularis. Journal of Comparative Neurology, 244*, 213–228.

Renart, A., Parga, N., & Rolls, E. T. (1999a). Backprojections in the cerebral cortex: Implications for memory storage. *Neural Computation, 11*, 1349–1388.

Renart, A., Parga, N., & Rolls, E. T. (1999b). Associative memory properties of multiple cortical modules. *Network, 10*, 237–255.

Robertson, R. G., Rolls, E. T., & Georges-François, P. (1998). Spatial view cells in the primate hippocampus: Effects of removal of view details. *Journal of Neurophysiology, 79*, 1145–1156.

Robertson, R. G., Rolls, E. T., Georges-François, P., & Panzeri, S. (1999). Head direction cells in the primate pre-subiculum. *Hippocampus, 9*, 206–219.

Rolls, B. J. (1990). The role of sensory-specific satiety in food intake and food selection. In E. D. Capaldi & T. L. Powley (Eds.), *Taste, experience, and feeding* (pp. 197–209). Washington, DC: American Psychological Association.

Rolls, B. J., & Hetherington, M. (1989). The role of variety in eating and body weight regulation. In R. Shepherd (Ed.), *Handbook of the psychophysiology of human eating* (pp. 57–84). Chichester, England: Wiley.

Rolls, B. J., Rolls, E. T., & Rowe, E. A. (1983). Body fat control and obesity. *Behavioural Brain Science, 4*, 744–745.

Rolls, B. J., Rolls, E. T., Rowe, E. A., & Sweeney, K. (1981). Sensory-specific satiety in man. *Physiology and Behavior, 27*, 137–142.

Rolls, B. J., Rowe, E. A., & Rolls, E. T. (1982). How sensory properties of foods affect human feeding behavior. *Physiology and Behavior, 29*, 409–417.

Rolls, B. J., Rowe, E. A., Rolls, E. T., Kingston, B., & Megson, A. (1981). Variety in a meal enhances food intake in man. *Physiology and Behavior, 26*, 215–221.

Rolls, B. J., Van Duijenvoorde, P. M., & Rolls, E. T. (1984). Pleasantness changes and food intake in a varied four course meal. *Appetite, 5*, 337–348.

Rolls, B. J., Van Duijenvoorde, P. M., & Rowe, E. A. (1983). Variety in the diet enhances intake in a meal and contributes to the development of obesity in the rat. *Physiology and Behavior, 31*, 21–27.

Rolls, E. T. (1993). The neural control of feeding in primates. In D. A. Booth (Ed.), *Neurophysiology of ingestion* (pp. 137–169). Oxford, England: Pergamon Press.

Rolls, E. T. (1994). Neural processing related to feeding in primates. In C. R. Legg & D. A. Booth (Eds.), *Appetite: Neural and behavioural bases* (pp. 11–53). Oxford, England: Oxford University Press.

Rolls, E. T. (1995). Central taste anatomy and neurophysiology. In R. L. Doty (Ed.), *Handbook of olfaction and gustation* (pp. 549–573). New York: Dekker.

Rolls, E. T. (1996a). The orbitofrontal cortex. *Philosophical Transactions of the Royal Society of London. Series B: Biological Sciences, 351*, 1433–1444.

Rolls, E. T. (1996b). A theory of hippocampal function in memory. *Hippocampus, 6*, 601–620.

Rolls, E. T. (1997). Taste and olfactory processing in the brain and its relation to the control of eating. *Critical Reviews in Neurobiology, 11*, 263–287.

Rolls, E. T. (1999a). *The brain and emotion*. Oxford, England: Oxford University Press.

Rolls, E. T. (1999b). The functions of the orbitofrontal cortex. *Neurocase, 5*, 301–312.

Rolls, E. T. (1999c). Spatial view cells and the representation of place in the primate hippocampus. *Hippocampus, 9*, 467–480.

Rolls, E. T. (2000a). Functions of the primate temporal lobe cortical visual areas in invariant visual object and face recognition. *Neuron, 27*, 205–218.

Rolls, E. T. (2000b). Memory systems in the brain. *Annual Review of Psychology, 51*, 599–630.

Rolls, E. T. (2000c). Neurophysiology and functions of the primate amygdala, and the neural basis of emotion. In J. P. Aggleton (Ed.), *The amygdala: A functional analysis* (pp. 447–478). Oxford, England: Oxford University Press.

Rolls, E. T. (2000d). The orbitofrontal cortex and reward. *Cerebral Cortex, 10*, 284–294.

Rolls, E. T. (2000e). Précis of *The brain and emotion*. *Behavioural Brain Sciences, 23*, 177–233.

Rolls, E. T. (2000f). The representation of umami taste in the taste cortex. *Journal of Nutrition, 130*, S960–S965.

Rolls, E. T. (2000g). Taste, olfactory, visual and somatosensory representations of the sensory properties of foods in the brain, and their relation to the control of food intake. In H.-R. Berthoud & R. J. Seeley (Eds.), *Neural and metabolic control of macronutrient intake* (pp. 247–262). Boca Raton, FL: CRC Press.

Rolls, E. T., & Baylis, L. L. (1994). Gustatory, olfactory and visual convergence within the primate orbitofrontal cortex. *Journal of Neuroscience, 14*, 5437–5452.

Rolls, E. T., Critchley, H. D., Browning, A., & Hernadi, I. (1998). The neurophysiology of taste and olfaction in primates, and umami flavor. *Annals of the New York Academy of Sciences, 855*, 426–437.

Rolls, E. T., Critchley, H. D., Browning, A. S., Hernadi, A., & Lenard, L. (1999). Responses to the sensory properties of fat of neurons in the primate orbitofrontal cortex. *Journal of Neuroscience, 19*, 1532–1540.

Rolls, E. T., Critchley, H. D., Browning, A. S., & Inoue, K. (2004). *Face-selective and auditory neurons in the primate orbitofrontal cortex*. Manuscript submitted for publication.

Rolls, E. T., Critchley, H., Mason, R., & Wakeman, E. A. (1996). Orbitofrontal cortex neurons: Role in olfactory and visual association learning. *Journal of Neurophysiology, 75*, 1970–1981.

Rolls, E. T., Critchley, H., Wakeman, E. A., & Mason, R. (1996). Responses of neurons in the primate taste cortex to the glutamate ion and to inosine 5'-monophosphate. *Physiology and Behavior, 59*, 991–1000.

Rolls, E. T., & Deco, G. (2002). *Computational neuroscience of vision*. Oxford, England: Oxford University Press.

Rolls, E. T., Hornak, J., Wade, D., & McGrath, J. (1994). Emotion-related learning in patients with social and emotional changes associated with frontal lobe damage. *Journal of Neurology, Neurosurgery and Psychiatry, 57*, 1518–1524.

Rolls, E. T., Judge, S. J., & Sanghera, M. (1977). Activity of neurones in the inferotemporal cortex of the alert monkey. *Brain Research, 130*, 229–238.

Rolls, E. T., Murzi, E., Yaxley, S., Thorpe, S. J., & Simpson, S. J. (1986). Sensory-specific satiety: Food-specific reduction in responsiveness of ventral forebrain neurons after feeding in the monkey. *Brain Research, 368*, 79–86.

Rolls, E. T., Robertson, R. G., & Georges-François, P. (1997). Spatial view cells in the primate hippocampus. *European Journal of Neuroscience, 9*, 1789–1794.

Rolls, E. T., & Rolls, B. J. (1977). Activity of neurons in sensory, hypothalamic and motor areas during feeding in the monkey. In Y. Katsuki, M. Sato, S. Takagi, & Y. Oomura (Eds.), *Food intake and chemical senses* (pp. 525–549). Tokyo: University of Tokyo Press.

Rolls, E. T., & Rolls, B. J. (1982). Brain mechanisms involved in feeding. In L. M. Barker (Ed.), *Psychobiology of human food selection* (pp. 33–62). Westport, CT: AVI.

Rolls, E. T., Rolls, B. J., & Rowe, E. A. (1983). Sensory-specific and motivation-specific satiety for the sight and taste of food and water in man. *Physiology and Behavior, 30*, 185–192.

Rolls, E. T., & Rolls, J. H. (1997). Olfactory sensory-specific satiety in humans. *Physiology and Behavior, 61*, 461–473.

Rolls, E. T., & Scott, T. R. (2003). Central taste anatomy and neurophysiology. In R. L. Doty (Ed.), *Handbook of olfaction and gustation* (2nd ed., ch. 33, pp. 679–705). New York: Dekker.

Rolls, E. T., Scott, T. R., Sienkiewicz, Z. J., & Yaxley, S. (1988). The responsiveness of neurones in the frontal opercular gustatory cortex of the macaque monkey is independent of hunger. *Journal of Physiology, 397*, 1–12.

Rolls, E. T., Sienkiewicz, Z. J., & Yaxley, S. (1989). Hunger modulates the responses to gustatory stimuli of single neurons in the orbitofrontal cortex. *European Journal of Neuroscience, 1*, 53–60.

Rolls, E. T., & Stringer, S. M. (2001). A model of the interaction between mood and memory. *Network: Computation in Neural Systems, 12*, 89–109.

Rolls, E. T., Trappenberg, T. P., & Stringer, S. M. (2002). A unified model of spatial and episodic memory. *Proceedings of the Royal Society of London, Series B: Biological Sciences, 269*, 1087–1093.

Rolls, E. T., & Treves, A. (1998). *Neural networks and brain function*. Oxford, England: Oxford University Press.

Rolls, E. T., Treves, A., & Tovee, M. J. (1997). The representational capacity of the distributed encoding of information provided by populations of neurons in the primate temporal visual cortex. *Experimental Brain Research, 114*, 149–162.

Rolls, E. T., Treves, A., Robertson, R. G., Georges-François, P., & Panzeri, S. (1998). Information about spatial view in an ensemble of primate hippocampal cells. *Journal of Neurophysiology, 79*, 1797–1813.

Rolls, E. T., Yaxley, S., & Sienkiewicz, Z. J. (1990). Gustatory responses of single neurons in the orbitofrontal cortex of the macaque monkey. *Journal of Neurophysiology, 64*, 1055–1066.

Sanghera, M. K., Rolls, E. T., & Roper-Hall, A. (1979). Visual responses of neurons in the dorsolateral amygdala of the alert monkey. *Experimental Neurology, 63*, 610–626.

Scott, T. R., Yan, J., & Rolls, E. T. (1995). Brain mechanisms of satiety and taste in macaques. *Neurobiology, 3*, 281–292.

Scott, T. R., Yaxley, S., Sienkiewicz, Z. J., & Rolls, E. T. (1986a). Taste responses in the nucleus tractus solitarius of the behaving monkey. *Journal of Neurophysiology, 55*, 182–200.

Scott, T. R., Yaxley, S., Sienkiewicz, Z. J., & Rolls, E. T. (1986b). Gustatory responses in the frontal opercular cortex of the alert cynomolgus monkey. *Journal of Neurophysiology, 56*, 876–890.

Stringer, S. M., Rolls, E. T., & Trappenberg, T. P. (2004). *Self-organising continuous attractor network models of hippocampal spatial view cells*. Manuscript submitted for publication.

Stringer, S. M., Rolls, E. T., Trappenberg, T. P., & Araujo, I. E. T. (2002). Self-organising continuous attractor networks and path integration: Two-dimensional models of place cells. *Network, 13,* 1–18.

Stringer, S. M., Trappenberg, T. P., Rolls, E. T., & Araujo, I. E. T. (2002). Self-organising continuous attractor networks and path integration: One-dimensional models of head direction cells. *Network, 13,* 217–242.

Thorpe, S. J., Rolls, E. T., & Maddison, S. (1983). Neuronal activity in the orbitofrontal cortex of the behaving monkey. *Experimental Brain Research, 49,* 93–115.

Treves, A., & Rolls, E. T. (1992). Computational constraints suggest the need for two distinct input systems to the hippocampal CA3 network. *Hippocampus, 2,* 189–199.

Treves, A., & Rolls, E. T. (1994). A computational analysis of the role of the hippocampus in memory. *Hippocampus, 4,* 374–391.

Verhagen, J. V., Rolls, E. T., & Kadohisa, M. (2002). Taste, texture, and fat representations in the primate orbitofrontal cortex. *Chemical Senses* (in press).

Yaxley, S., Rolls, E. T., Sienkiewicz, Z. J., & Scott, T. R. (1985). Satiety does not affect gustatory activity in the nucleus of the solitary tract of the alert monkey. *Brain Research, 347,* 85–93.

Yaxley, S., Rolls, E. T., & Sienkiewicz, Z. J. (1988). The responsiveness of neurones in the insular gustatory cortex of the macaque monkey is independent of hunger. *Physiology and Behavior, 42,* 223–229.

Yaxley, S., Rolls, E. T., & Sienkiewicz, Z. J. (1990). Gustatory responses of single neurons in the insula of the macaque monkey. *Journal of Neurophysiology, 63,* 689–700.

20 Cross-Modal Memory in Primates: The Neural Basis of Learning About the Multisensory Properties of Objects and Events

AMANDA PARKER AND ALEXANDER EASTON

Introduction

Much is now understood about the neural mechanisms that underlie the learning of visual object representations in the primate. We propose that within this context, it is possible to reevaluate previous work on the mechanisms of multisensory processes in primates. We also consider the importance of cross-modal memory in episodic and semantic memory, which necessarily comprise components from different sensory modalities.

Early work in the area of cross-modal memory in nonhuman primates implicated the amygdala as crucial for forming cross-modal associations, but more recent evidence indicates that the rhinal cortex (the entorhinal and perirhinal cortices), in particular the perirhinal cortex, is critically involved in the formation of a multimodal representation of an object as a whole. In this chapter we review recent advances in the area of cross-modal memory formation in primates, then propose a likely mechanism for the encoding of cross-modal memories.

Functions of cross-modal memory in primates

Cross-modal learning is an important part of primate life. A monkey or ape that can associate, for example, a pleasant taste with a red fruit and an unpleasant taste with a green fruit of the same type will be able to modify its foraging behavior in a highly efficient way. However, early laboratory studies of such cross-modal learning in monkeys proved disappointing (Ettlinger, 1960; Ettlinger & Blakemore, 1967). Later studies in apes (Davenport & Rogers, 1970; Davenport, Rogers, & Steele Russell, 1973) showed that cross-modal learning

could occur, leading to the view that such learning was possible in apes but not in monkeys.

Cross-modal learning was first shown in monkeys when animals were taught to discriminate, in darkness, palatable food of one shape, for example star-shaped, from nonpalatable food of another shape. Later, both shapes of food were presented in the light for visual discrimination, in which case the palatable food was chosen in roughly 80% of the cross-modal trials (Cowey & Weiskrantz, 1975; Weiskrantz & Cowey, 1975). Subsequent studies expanded on these early observations. Jarvis and Ettlinger (1977) used a similar experimental paradigm but with several discrimination problems presented within a single test session. A similar (though slightly lower) level of performance was seen relative to that observed in the experiments of Weiskrantz and Cowey. Cross-modal learning has also been seen in monkeys on a tactual-to-visual, delayed non-matching-to-sample (DNMS) task (Goulet & Murray, 1996; Malkova & Murray, 1996; Murray & Mishkin, 1985) with a set of highly familiar objects.

Studies of cross-modal learning in lesioned monkeys

Much work on the neural basis of cross-modal learning entails studies in lesioned animals. To demonstrate a lack of learning that is specific to cross-modal learning, however, researchers must show that the same lesion does not impair intramodal learning, and therefore that the impairment is not simply a generalized learning impairment. For example, early lesion studies using the cross-modal recognition method implicated various regions of the frontal lobe, the arcuate cortex (Petrides &

Iversen, 1976), the anterior cingulate cortex (Aitken, 1980), and combined lesions of the frontal and parieto-occipital polysensory areas (Streicher & Ettlinger, 1987). However, a later study using the technique of cooling the dorsolateral region of the prefrontal cortex found that although cross-modal (tactual-to-visual and visual-to-tactual) learning was impaired, intramodal learning (tactual to tactual) was also impaired (Shindy, Posley, & Fuster, 1994). This implies that prefrontal cooling was having a generalized effect on learning rather than solely on cross-modal learning. The results of earlier studies in animals with permanent frontal ablations should therefore be viewed with caution.

The first study to show convincing evidence of intact intramodal learning and impaired cross-modal learning (Murray & Mishkin, 1985) used a tactual-to-visual DNMS task, on which animals with aspiration lesions of the amygdala and subjacent cortex showed impaired performance. The cross-modal impairment observed was very severe, with results barely better than chance, whereas the same monkeys showed normal performance on intramodal DNMS tasks. From this striking impairment it was proposed that the amygdala was a crucial structure for the formation of cross-modal stimulus-stimulus associations.

In addition to the finding that aspiration lesions (created by removal of neural tissue by suction) of the amygdala impaired performance on cross-modal NMS tasks (Murray & Mishkin, 1985), other studies showed that such lesions also impaired learning of tasks requiring intermodal secondary reinforcer association learning. In tasks of this type, correct trials are not rewarded. Instead, the monkey must learn to pay attention to a cue in another modality (the secondary reinforcer), which signals whether the problem was correctly solved. After several such trials, in which the monkey learns about the reward properties of the choice stimuli on the basis of the secondary reinforcer, a reward is dispatched when a certain number of correct choices have been made.

For example, in the experiment of D. Gaffan and Harrison (1987), the only information concerning correct or incorrect choices in each problem was the presentation of one of two auditory stimuli that had previously been associated with either food reward (the auditory reinforcer) or no food reward (the nonreinforcer). The monkey had to choose, based only on the auditory feedback, the correct stimulus four times in a row to obtain a food reward. Aspiration lesions of the amygdala impaired this learning more severely than they impaired learning a similar discrimination when the visual object was directly associated with a reward (e.g., E. A. Gaffan, D. Gaffan, & Harrison, 1988). However, more recently experiments using more selec-

tive lesions of the amygdala have shed new light on the role of the amygdala itself in a variety of forms of learning. In aspiration lesions of the amygdala, the cell bodies of the amygdala are not the only cells damaged by the lesion. The overlying cortex that must be removed to expose the amygdala is damaged as well. There is also damage to the white matter running near the amygdala, and damage to fibers that course through the amygdala on their way to and from other structures. To study the effects of damage to the amygdala alone it is important to minimize this collateral damage, and for this purpose neurotoxins injected into the amygdala can be used. These toxins will selectively lesion the cells within a region while sparing those fibers passing through the structure, and because the lesions are stereotaxically placed, cortical and white matter damage is minimal.

Studies that have used neurotoxic lesions of the amygdala have shown that the cell bodies of the amygdala themselves are not important for the cross-modal NMS task (Goulet & Murray, 1996, 2001; Malkova & Murray, 1996). Similarly, large excitotoxic lesions of the amygdala do not impair performance on the secondary auditory reinforcer task of Gaffan and Harrison (Malkova, Gaffan, & Murray, 1997). This lack of effect of neurotoxic lesions of the amygdala on tasks that had been impaired by aspiration lesions implied that theoretical assumptions about the amygdala's role in cross-modal memory had to be reevaluated. Current research is focusing on alternative explanations for the effects of aspiration lesions of the amygdala, the likely candidates being first, damage to the anterior portion of the rhinal cortex during exposure of the amygdala, and second, damage to the white matter surrounding the amygdala. As discussed in the next section, the rhinal cortex appears to play a critical role in cross-modal learning, and damage to it may be sufficient to explain the effects of aspiration amygdalectomy. The second possible explanation, white matter damage, should also be examined, and we return to what the nature of this damage might be later in the chapter.

Role of the rhinal cortex in cross-modal learning

The rhinal cortex appears to be crucial for learning about visual stimuli. Figure 20.1 indicates the position of the perirhinal cortex on the ventral surface of the macaque brain. Lesions of the rhinal cortex, or of the perirhinal cortex alone, impair recognition memory (Eacott, Gaffan, & Murray, 1994; D. Gaffan & Murray, 1992; Meunier, Bachevalier, Mishkin, & Murray, 1993; Zola-Morgan, Squire, Amaral, & Suzuki, 1989) and visual object-reward association learning (Buckley & Gaffan, 1997, 1998a, 1998b; Easton & Gaffan, 2000b).

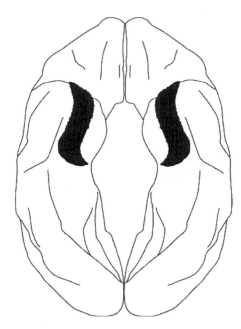

FIGURE 20.1   Ventral view of the macaque brain. Perirhinal cortex (in black) extends laterally from the rhinal sulcus.

Indeed, lesions of the perirhinal cortex alone result in an impairment that is large enough to account for all of the impairment seen following rhinal cortex lesions (Meunier et al., 1993). Very similar effects of suction ablations and neurotoxic ablations of the rhinal cortex suggest that the cortex in this area itself, rather than fibers passing near it, is important in learning about visual stimuli (Baxter & Murray, 2001).

The effect of rhinal or perirhinal cortex ablations, however, appears to depend on the perceptual difficulty of the task. Although it is hard to precisely define perceptual difficulty in terms of currently published experiments, manipulations have concentrated on increasing the number of items to be discriminated, making the discrimination finer-grained, or manipulating the amount of preoperative experience that monkeys acquire with objects of the same type. For example, in recognition memory monkeys with lesions of the rhinal cortex were impaired when a large set of stimuli was used but not when a small stimulus set was used (Eacott et al., 1994). Similarly, Buckley and Gaffan (1997) showed that visual object-reward association learning was unimpaired when 20 problems were learned concurrently and only one foil object (the unrewarded member of the discrimination pair) was presented with the correct object. However, when the number of foils was increased or the number of problems learned concurrently was increased, performance in animals with lesions of the perirhinal cortex was significantly impaired. Similarly, monkeys with lesions of the perirhinal cortex showed significant impairment on discriminat-

ing objects presented in different views on each trial (Buckley & Gaffan, 1998a) or within a visual scene (Buckley & Gaffan, 1998b).

That these differences depend on the perceptual difficulty of a task is supported by a study that used a small number of concurrent visual object-reward associations with only one foil (the task not impaired in the monkeys with perirhinal lesions in the study of Buckley & Gaffan, 1997) and showed monkeys with perirhinal cortex lesions to be very severely impaired (Easton & Gaffan, 2000b). The difference between this study and the study of Buckley and Gaffan is that the earlier study used very little preoperative training, whereas Easton and Gaffan trained the animals preoperatively with hundreds of similar visual objects. This manipulation increases the similarity between objects and so increases the perceptual difficulty of the task, because objects in memory must be discriminated among using much more subtle differences than when an animal has seen very few of these similar objects.

That the perirhinal cortex appears to be involved in learning, but in a way that depends on the perceptual demands of the task, has led to the proposal that it serves both a mnemonic and a perceptual role (Buckley & Gaffan, 1998b; Murray & Bussey, 1999). As part of these mnemonic and perceptual roles, the perirhinal cortex would store representations of visual objects. The nature of this object representation might hold the key to why the rhinal cortex is important for cross-modal learning. The study by Buckley and Gaffan (1998a) showed that monkeys with lesions of the perirhinal cortex were impaired at discriminating objects that were presented in different views on each trial. One explanation for this result is that the perirhinal cortex stores a representation of the complete object, rather than simply visual features that can combine to form one view of an object, as might be seen in other areas of the visual temporal cortex (Tanaka, 1996). This proposal for an integrative role for perirhinal cortex is supported by the observation that cells within the inferior temporal cortex of the monkey (including perirhinal cortex) show view-invariant responses to objects (Booth & Rolls, 1998). That is, some of the cells in this region will respond when shown a visual object, irrespective of the view of that object. It seems unlikely, then, that these cells are responding to specific visual features of the object and more likely that they are responding to some higher-order object property.

The proposal that perirhinal cortical cells store a view-invariant representation of an object is supported by a recent study in which monkeys with perirhinal cortex lesions were specifically impaired in an odd-one-out task when alternative photographic views of the same object were used (Buckley, Booth, Rolls, & Gaffan, 2001). In this experiment, six items were presented on a computer touch screen to a monkey. In all cases, five of the items were the same and one was different, and the monkey was required to respond to the different object. In some instances, the five "same" incorrect choice items were an identical view of an object. In the other instances the five incorrect choice items were alternative views of an object, showing the object from a variety of angles. Monkeys with perirhinal lesions were impaired only if the incorrect object was presented in alternative views. For example, a monkey with a perirhinal cortex lesion might be able to select an image of a ball from five identical images of a rattle. However, it would have great difficulty selecting a ball displayed with five different views of a rattle. This effect seems to hold true even when the perceptual difficulty of the tasks using the same view of the distracter object is high, suggesting that at least one perceptual role of the perirhinal cortex is to represent a higher-order property of the object rather than simply the differentiation of similar items.

If the perirhinal cortex is storing a representation of an object rather than individual features of that object, this might also explain why cross-modal learning is impaired following rhinal cortex lesions. In representing an object, one would want to characterize an object not only on the basis of its visual features but also on the basis of all salient features in all modalities. For example, if the perirhinal cortex stored a representation of an apple as an object, as well as storing its visual features, one would also wish to link the taste and texture properties of that apple into the representation. In this way the perirhinal cortex would store a representation of a complete object, not just a visual object. This hypothesis is supported by anatomical evidence showing that the perirhinal cortex is the first region in the ventromedial temporal lobe to receive a wide variety of sensory inputs: somatosensory from the insula, auditory from the superior temporal sulcus, olfactory and gustatory from the orbital prefrontal cortex (Friedman, Murray, O'Neill, & Mishkin, 1986; Suzuki & Amaral, 1994; Van Hoesen, Pandya, & Butters, 1975). Some of these sensory inputs into the perirhinal cortex are from modality-specific sensory areas and others are from polymodal regions (Suzuki & Amaral, 1994).

Evidence for this proposed representational role of rhinal cortex in cross-modal flavor-visual association memory comes from a study of macaque monkeys, in which the flavor of a cue item predicted which of two visually presented junk objects covered another food item of the same type (Parker & Gaffan, 1998a). We trained the monkeys in stages using a conditional task in which the flavor of a food item presented at the beginning of each trial, either a peanut or a raisin, signaled which of two objects would be rewarded with a further reward of the same type. The task was learned first in conditions of illumination, then in darkness. Although the first stage of training took many weeks, the monkeys learned the task in darkness in 100 trials or less. After a rest period of three weeks, all three animals were performing at close to perfect levels. After surgery to remove the rhinal cortex and a further rest period of three weeks, however, the performance of all three of the monkeys failed to rise above chance. The animals were also very impaired on a food preference test, being willing to eat foodstuffs like meat and olives that normal monkeys assiduously avoid.

The conclusion that can be drawn from this experiment is that the rhinal cortex is of fundamental importance in flavor-visual associative memory. This is most likely due to the large input the entorhinal cortex receives from piriform olfactory cortex and a substantial direct projection from the olfactory bulb. Insofar as human psychophysical experiments have indicated that 70%–80% of flavor is produced by the olfactory properties of foods as they are eaten (Murphy & Cain, 1980; Murphy, Cain, & Bartoshuk, 1977), this input will provide the majority of the flavor input needed to perform the task on the basis of food flavor. Because the entorhinal cortex then projects to perirhinal cortex, which receives visual object information from the ventral visual stream, the rhinal cortex is in an optimal position to integrate cross-modal flavor-visual memories.

For progress to be made in understanding cross-modal memory, it is important to consider the effects of both excitotoxic amygdala lesions and removal of the rhinal cortex in monkeys within the same experiment. A direct comparison of amygdala and rhinal cortex lesion effects on cross-modal memory can be found in a recent study by Goulet and Murray (2001). They trained three groups of macaques on visual, tactual, and cross-modal (tactual to visual) DNMS tasks. One group underwent bilateral amygdalectomies, one group underwent aspiration lesions of the rhinal cortex, and a third group served as nonoperate controls. Postoperatively, all three groups of monkeys were first tested on cross-modal DNMS tasks, with both rhinal and amygdalectomized animals showing a deficit relative to controls. They were then tested on tactual DNMS tasks, on which only the group with rhinal cortex lesions showed impairment. This overall tactual impairment in the rhinal group was further broken down into the three problems learned, with only one of the three, the first postoperative problem, showing a significant impairment.

Postoperative performance on relearning the visual version of the task for the DNMS task was not impaired in any of the three experimental groups. Finally, the cross-modal version of the task was re-tested, with the rhinal group showing a persisting deficit, whereas the amygdalectomized group performed at a level similar to controls. The authors concluded that this persistent and robust deficit in cross-modal memory after rhinal lesion was due to a combination of two functions of the rhinal cortex. First, rhinal cortex is a critical component of the "what" pathway in the ventral visual stream, serving as a site of visual representations. Second, rhinal cortex is essential for the association of stimuli within and across sensory modalities. As the authors note, "Thus, the rhinal cortex may be the anatomical site through which information from visual, tactual, gustatory, and perhaps other sensory properties of objects, as appropriate, are linked and through which environmental stimuli are invested with meaning" (Goulet & Murray, 2001, p. 283).

Mechanisms of memory encoding and storage in the inferior temporal lobe: Issues relevant to cross-modal memory formation

Although the rhinal cortex appears to be an essential component in the system responsible for the formation of cross-modal memories, it is important to understand how these memories are encoded and which other cortical regions are involved. Although much of the research on memory encoding has focused on the hippocampal complex, recently it has been proposed that the cholinergic cells of the basal forebrain reinforce representations of objects or events. This would imply that the cholinergic cells of the basal forebrain reinforce the representation of the whole multimodal object in rhinal cortex. To understand how this object representation might be encoded by the cholinergic afferents to rhinal cortex, it is important to know something of the background to the debate on where and how memories are encoded in the brain.

The early focus on the hippocampus as the site of memory storage was due to the dramatic amnesia shown by patients after medial temporal lobe surgery (Scoville & Milner, 1957). One group of patients, however, that may be of importance in studying the effects of hippocampal damage alone in humans may be those patients who suffer bilateral anoxic damage to the hippocampus early in life (Vargha-Khadem et al., 1997). Anoxia is damage caused by lack of oxygen, and the pyramidal cells of the hippocampus, being large, are particularly susceptible to anoxic damage. Bilateral damage to the fornix, which is the major output pathway of the hippocampus, causes a similar impairment (D. Gaffan & E. A. Gaffan, 1991). Observations in these patient groups suggest that the role of the hippocampus in memory encoding is specifically an inability to remember events, that is, episodic memory. Of relevance to the topic of semantic memory, it is also critical to note that children with early hippocampal damage can develop a nearly normal level of knowledge about the world, indicating that object memories continue to be encoded normally in the inferior temporal lobe. Similarly, monkeys with bilateral transection of the fornix are impaired on a scene memory task that may be considered a primate model of episodic memory (D. Gaffan, 1994), but are unimpaired on tasks of recognition memory (D. Gaffan, Shields, & Harrison, 1984; for a review, see D. Gaffan, 1992). These observations have led to the hypothesis that the hippocampus is part of a system that is specifically adapted for episodic memory and that includes the mammillary bodies and anterior thalamus (Aggleton & Brown, 1999; Delay & Brion, 1969; Parker & Gaffan, 1997a, 1997b).

Densely amnesic patients, however, are severely impaired not only on tests of visual recognition memory, as seen in nonhuman primates with lesions of medial temporal lobe structures, but also on object discrimination learning (Aggleton, Nicol, Huston, & Fairburn, 1988; Hood, Postle, & Corkin, 1996; Oscar-Berman & Zola-Morgan, 1980). An alternative explanation of the dense amnesia seen following medial temporal lobe surgery, namely, damage to the white matter of the anterior temporal stem, was put forward by Horel (1978). The temporal stem is the band of white matter within the temporal lobe, dorsolateral to the amygdala and hippocampus. Many important fibers that may be involved in learning pass through the temporal stem, running close to the amygdala, and therefore are unlikely to be spared by complete ablation of the gray matter of the amygdala. This, then, may be part of the explanation of the effects of aspiration amygdalectomy on both object discrimination learning and cross-modal associative memory. The fibers projecting through the temporal stem white matter to the temporal lobe are those from the cholinergic basal forebrain (consisting of substantia innominata, nucleus basalis of Meynert, nucleus of the diagonal band, the septal nuclei, and the hypothalamus), and recent work in the monkey has indicated that this projection may be vital to new memory formation in both episodic and semantic learning (Easton & Gaffan, 2000a, 2000b, 2001; Easton, Parker, & Gaffan, 2001; D. Gaffan, Parker, & Easton, 2001; Parker, Easton, & Gaffan, 2002). It therefore seems very likely that cross-modal memories would be affected in the same way. Figure 20.2 illustrates the location and extent

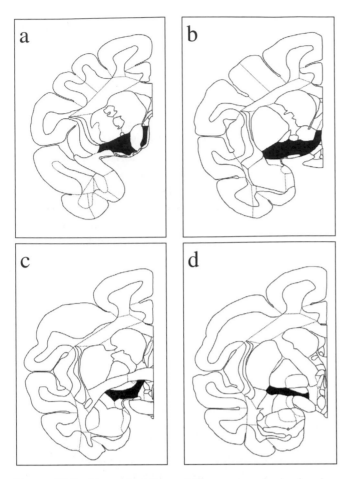

FIGURE 20.2   Coronal sections of the macaque brain showing the region of the basal forebrain (in black; substantia innominata, nucleus basalis of Meynert, and nucleus of the diagonal band). Sections are located 4 mm anterior to the anterior commisure (A), 2 mm anterior (B), at the level of the anterior commisure (C), and 2 mm posterior to the anterior commisure (D). Sections are reproduced and adapted from the maps of Martin and Bowden (1996).

of the basal forebrain in the macaque brain. Projections from the basal forebrain reach structures of the temporal and medial temporal lobe and travel through three main routes, which can be described as the ventral and lateral pathways and the fornix (Kitt, Mitchell, DeLong, Wainer, & Price, 1987; Mesulam, Mufson, Levey, & Wainer, 1983). With David Gaffan, we proposed (D. Gaffan et al., 2001) that some of the variability in the results of Horel and colleagues could be due to only partial transection of these basal forebrain fibers. Transection of the anterior temporal stem alone would leave fibers in the fornix and those in the ventral pathway running through, or near to, the amygdala intact. D. Gaffan et al. (2001) more completely isolated the temporal lobe from these basal forebrain inputs by making a combined section of the white matter tracts of the fornix, amygdala, and anterior temporal stem.

These animals were tested on a variety of new learning tasks with various combinations of lesions. In agreement with the variable effects seen after temporal stem sections alone (Cirillo, Horel, & George, 1989), it was noted that animals with lesions of the temporal stem alone were only partially impaired on visual discriminations, improving significantly over three sets of ten concurrent discriminations postoperatively. A combined lesion of all three white matter tracts resulted in substantial and persistent impairment in the learning of concurrent visual discrimination problems (D. Gaffan et al., 2001). We also showed that sections of the temporal stem and amygdala, even with the fornix intact, produced a very severe impairment of postoperative performance on a DMS task (D. Gaffan et al., 2001).

Dense amnesia is characterized by a deficit in encoding memories of a variety of types, so we also measured performance on a scene-based object-in-place task that can be considered a useful model of episodic memory in the monkey (D. Gaffan, 1994, 1998). After the anterior temporal stem and amygdala were sectioned bilaterally, animals showed significant impairment on this task, similar in severity to that seen after fornix section alone (D. Gaffan, 1994; D. Gaffan et al., 2001). Addition of a fornix section to this lesion, however, resulted in very severe impairment in performance, with animals showing no improvement from chance within a session where preoperatively they were performing at nearly 90% correct after one presentation of each scene. This effect of adding the fornix section to the amygdala and anterior temporal stem section was very much greater than the additive effects of fornix section and amygdala and anterior temporal stem section separately. This finding led us to propose that the complete isolation of the temporal lobe from its basal forebrain afferents resulted in a severe anterograde amnesia in the monkey.

We were interested to see if, like human amnesics, our monkeys had preserved memories of well-learned objects from before the operations. In contrast to previous results obtained with rhinal cortex ablations, their postoperative retention of preoperatively learned material was well-preserved. One animal was taught 100 visual discrimination problems preoperatively and tested on postoperative retention. Although this animal did not perform at preoperative levels on the first presentation of the problems postoperatively, its performance was significantly above chance. Also, it rapidly relearned these 100 problems postoperatively (within four presentations it was performing at over 90% correct). This rapid relearning, then, is an effect of retention of preoperatively learned material, which resembles the situation of relative sparing of retrograde memory in densely amnesic patients despite their severe impairment on new learning tasks (Dusoir, Kapur, Byrnes, McKinstry, & Hoare, 1990; Kapur, Thompson, Cook, Lang, & Brice, 1996; Milner, Corkin, & Teuber, 1968; Scoville & Milner, 1957; Teuber, Milner, & Vaughan, 1968).

On the basis of our findings, we proposed the basal forebrain to be a site of corticocortical communication between frontal and inferior temporal cortex, and further that this is the basis of the role it plays in learning (D. Gaffan et al., 2001). Both frontal and inferior temporal cortex are required for new learning in tasks such as recognition memory or visual discrimination. In tasks such as visual discrimination, it is known that lesions of the frontal cortex in one hemisphere and of the inferior temporal cortex in the opposite hemisphere have no effect on learning (Parker & Gaffan, 1998b), so this communication must be interhemispheric and subcortical. The basal forebrain is ideally suited for such communication. The entire basal forebrain receives projections from the frontal cortex and in turn projects to the inferior temporal cortex (Mesulam et al., 1983; Ongur, An, & Price, 1998). The cells of the basal forebrain are responsive to reward, and also to predictors of reward (Fukuda, Masuda, Ono, & Tabuchi, 1993; Fukuda, Ono, Nishino, & Nakamura, 1986; Rolls, Sanghera, & Roper-Hall, 1979; Wilson & Rolls, 1990). A major way in which the basal forebrain may contribute to the communication between frontal and inferior temporal cortex is likely to be the signaling of reinforcement.

Recent work in the monkey has shown that interruption of the communication between midbrain reward centers and the basal forebrain, by lesions of the medial forebrain bundle in one hemisphere and of the inferior temporal cortex in the opposite hemisphere, impairs learning of object discriminations (Easton & Gaffan, 2000b, 2001), scenes (Easton & Gaffan, 2000b), and recognition memory (Easton et al., 2001) to a similar extent as lesions of the temporal stem, amygdala, and fornix (D. Gaffan et al., 2001) or the cholinergic basal forebrain (Easton, Ridley, Baker, & Gaffan, 2002). We have proposed a model of frontotemporal interactions via the basal forebrain based on these results (Easton et al., 2001). In this model the frontal cortex determines the current goal of the animal. This goal is then signaled to the midbrain reward centers, where peripheral signals of reward are integrated with the goal signal. In this way the animal can determine whether it has succeeded in achieving its goal. This integrated signal of reward and goal is then sent to the cholinergic basal forebrain via the medial forebrain bundle. The cholinergic basal forebrain then signals the information to the structures involved in encoding the memory (such as the hippocampal-anterior thalamic circuit for episodic memories, or perirhinal cortex for visual memories), where the event or object is then reinforced if it coincides with the animal's goals.

Implications for cross-modal memory encoding

We propose that, as the cholinergic basal forebrain has been shown to be essential for new memory encoding in structures, including the rhinal cortex, it is likely to be essential for the encoding of cross-modal memories in this region. One potentially interesting modification to the hypothesis that rhinal cortex stores a cross-modal representation of an object can be adduced from the work on the basal forebrain. In our presentation of the basal forebrain as essential for new learning, we discussed how crossed unilateral lesions of the basal forebrain and inferior temporal cortex impaired new learning but spared recall of preoperatively learned material (Easton & Gaffan, 2000b). This study also included a group of animals with bilateral lesions of the perirhinal cortex. The interesting difference between these animals and animals in earlier studies of discrimination learning (e.g., Buckley & Gaffan, 1997) is that the animals in Easton and Gaffan's study were massively overtrained preoperatively on the type of objects seen on the discrimination task, as discussed earlier. Another unexpected result of overtraining these animals prior to lesion creation was that their recall of preoperatively taught discriminations was better than would have been expected on the basis of previous studies examining recall in animals with lesions of the rhinal cortex (Buckley & Gaffan, 1997; Thornton, Rothblat, & Murray, 1997). It is somewhat difficult to account for this increased reliance on the perirhinal cortex for new learning but decreased reliance on perirhinal cortex for recall by overtraining of the animals preoperatively. However, Easton and Gaffan (2000b) argued that potentially, the perirhinal cortex and other areas in the inferior temporal cortex (such as area TE) might act as a distributed network, and that the preoperative training changed the way the perirhinal cortex behaved on a discrimination task. Where previously (in line with the argument presented at the beginning of this chapter) we would have considered that representation of the image (or the multimodal object) as residing in the rhinal cortex, Easton and Gaffan proposed that increased demand placed on the perirhinal cortex by new learning (due to the perceptual difficulty of the task) reduces the capability of perirhinal cortex to store representations of the images (or multimodal objects). Instead, this representation is more reliant on other areas in the inferior temporal cortex (such as area TE).

If this hypothesis is correct, then it opens up the possibility that cross-modal representations of objects are not confined to the region of the rhinal cortex alone but might spread out within the inferior temporal cortex as a whole. However, the findings of Easton and Gaffan were restricted to two-dimensional visual objects, and so may not generalize to multimodal object representations. Nonetheless, the result is potentially of great interest in an explanation of the structures critical for cross-modal object learning, and should be investigated further.

Conclusions

Although early work on the neuroanatomy of memory formation focused on the hippocampus, it now appears that this structure is essential only for episodic memories. In this type of learning, the hippocampus is part of a unified system that includes the mamillary bodies and anterior thalamus. In contrast, the rhinal cortex appears to be required for the type of learning that can be classed as semantic and object representation learning, a major component of which is multisensory. Despite the existence of a variety of memory structures in the brain, each with a different function, recent work strongly suggests that the cholinergic basal forebrain acts to modulate these different systems. In modulating these systems the basal forebrain provokes memory formation, but it does not affect memories once they are encoded in these temporal lobe structures.

The implications of this work on memory encoding for the study of multisensory integration are clear. In early studies of cross-modal memory in which the amygdala was removed by aspiration, such procedures would have damaged the white matter of the temporal lobe surrounding the amygdala (referred to as the anterior temporal stem). Although anatomical studies show that many of the fibers in the anterior temporal stem connect the rhinal cortex to regions such as the mediodorsal nucleus of the thalamus (Goulet, Dore, & Murray, 1998) and the frontal cortex (Baxter, Hadfield, & Murray, 1999), there are many other fibers in the temporal stem, including those that arise from the cholinergic cells of the basal forebrain and project to the inferior temporal cortex (including rhinal cortex). The studies discussed in this account that have investigated the function of these cells in monkeys have shown them to be essential for new learning of many types. Specifically, the inferior temporal cortex and the medial temporal lobe can be isolated from these cholinergic projections by sectioning the three main pathways that these fibers take, the anterior temporal stem, the amygdala, and the fornix. Sectioning these pathways bilaterally results in a severe anterograde amnesia (D. Gaffan et al., 2001; MacLean, Gaffan, Baker, & Ridley, 2001) while sparing retrograde memory (D. Gaffan et al., 2001). Without the modulating influence of basal forebrain afferents to inferior temporal cortex, new memories, whether unimodal or cross-modal, cannot be encoded.

REFERENCES

Aggleton, J. P., & Brown, M. W. (1999). Episodic memory, amnesia and the hippocampal-anterior thalamic axis. *Behavioral and Brain Sciences, 22*, 425–444.

Aggleton, J. P., Nicol, R. M., Huston, A. E., & Fairburn, A. F. (1988). The performance of amnesic subjects on tests of experimental amnesia in animals: Delayed matching-to-sample and concurrent learning. *Neuropsychologia, 26*, 265–272.

Aitken, P. G. (1980). Lesion effects on tactual to visual cross-modal matching in the monkey. *Neuropsychologia, 18*, 575–578.

Baxter, M. G., Hadfield, W. S., & Murray, E. A. (1999). Rhinal cortex lesions produce mild deficits in visual discrimination learning for an auditory secondary reinforcer in rhesus monkeys. *Behavioral Neuroscience, 113*, 243–252.

Baxter, M. G., & Murray, E. A. (2001). Impairments in visual discrimination learning and recognition memory produced by neurotoxic lesions of rhinal cortex in rhesus monkeys. *European Journal of Neuroscience, 13*, 1228–1238.

Booth, M. C. A., & Rolls, E. T. (1998). View-invariant representations of familiar objects by neurons in the inferior temporal visual cortex. *Cerebral Cortex, 8*, 510–523.

Buckley, M. J., Booth, M. C., Rolls, E. T., & Gaffan, D. (2001). Selective perceptual impairments after perirhinal cortex ablation. *Journal of Neuroscience, 21*, 9824–9836.

Buckley, M. J., & Gaffan, D. (1997). Impairment of visual object-discrimination learning after perirhinal cortex ablation. *Behavioral Neuroscience, 111*, 467–475.

Buckley, M. J., & Gaffan, D. (1998a). Learning and transfer of object-reward associations and the role of the perirhinal cortex. *Behavioral Neuroscience, 112*, 15–23.

Buckley, M. J., & Gaffan, D. (1998b). Perirhinal cortex ablation impairs visual object identification. *Journal of Neuroscience, 18*, 2268–2275.

Cirillo, R. A., Horel, J. A., & George, P. J. (1989). Lesions of the anterior temporal stem and the performance of delayed match-to-sample and visual discriminations in monkeys. *Behavioral Brain Research, 34*, 55–69.

Cowey, A., & Weiskrantz, L. (1975). Demonstration of cross-modal matching in rhesus monkeys, *Macaca mulatta. Neuropsychologia, 13*, 117–120.

Davenport, R. K., & Rogers, C. M. (1970). Intermodal equivalence of stimuli in apes. *Science, 168*, 279–280.

Davenport, R. K., Rogers, C. M., & Steele Russell, I. (1973). Cross-modal perception in apes. *Neuropsychologia, 11*, 21–28.

Delay, J., & Brion, S. (1969). *Le syndrome de Korsakoff* (*Korsakoff's syndrome*). Paris: Masson.

Dusoir, H., Kapur, N., Byrnes, D. P., McKinstry, S., & Hoare, R. D. (1990). The role of diencephalic pathology in human memory disorder: Evidence from a penetrating paranasal brain injury. *Brain, 113*, 1695–1706.

Eacott, M. J., Gaffan, D., & Murray, E. A. (1994). Preserved recognition memory for small sets, and impaired stimulus identification for large sets, following rhinal cortex ablation in monkeys. *European Journal of Neuroscience, 6*, 1466–1478.

Easton, A., & Gaffan, D. (2000a). Amygdala and the memory of reward: The importance of fibers of passage from the basal forebrain. In J. P. Aggleton (Ed.), *The amygdala: A functional analysis* (pp. 569–586). Oxford, England: Oxford University Press.

Easton, A., & Gaffan, D. (2000b). Comparison of perirhinal cortex ablation and crossed unilateral lesions of medial forebrain bundle from inferior temporal cortex in the Rhesus monkey: Effects on learning and retrieval. *Behavioral Neuroscience, 114,* 1041–1057.

Easton, A., & Gaffan, D. (2001). Crossed unilateral lesions of the medial forebrain bundle and either inferior temporal or frontal cortex impair object-reward association learning in Rhesus monkeys. *Neuropsychologia, 39,* 71–82.

Easton, A., Parker, A., & Gaffan, D. (2001). Crossed unilateral lesions of medial forebrain bundle and either inferior temporal or frontal cortex impair object recognition memory in Rhesus monkeys. *Behavioural Brain Research, 121,* 1–10.

Easton, A., Ridley, R. M., Baker, H. F., & Gaffan, D. (2002). Lesions of the cholinergic basal forebrain and fornix in one hemisphere and inferior temporal cortex in the opposite hemisphere produce severe learning impairments in rhesus monkeys. *Cerebral Cortex, 12,* 729–736.

Ettlinger, G. (1960). Cross-modal transfer of training in monkeys. *Behaviour, 16,* 56–65.

Ettlinger, G., & Blakemore, C. B. (1967). Cross-modal matching in the monkey. *Neuropsychologia, 5,* 147–154.

Friedman, D. P., Murray, E. A., O'Neill, J. B., & Mishkin, M. (1986). Cortical connections of the somatosensory fields of the lateral sulcus of macaques: Evidence for a cortico-limbic pathway for touch. *Journal of Comparative Neurology, 252,* 323–347.

Fukuda, M., Masuda, R., Ono, T., & Tabuchi, E. (1993). Responses of monkey basal forebrain neurons during a visual discrimination task. *Progress in Brain Research, 95,* 359–369.

Fukuda, M., Ono, T., Nishino, H., & Nakamura, K. (1986). Neuronal responses in monkey lateral hypothalamus during operant feeding behaviour. *Brain Research Bulletin, 17,* 879–884.

Gaffan, D. (1992). The role of the hippocampus-fornix-mammillary system in episodic memory. In L. R. Squire & N. Butters (Eds.), *Neuropsychology of memory* (pp. 336–346). New York: Guilford Press.

Gaffan, D. (1994). Scene-specific memory for objects: A model of episodic memory impairment in monkeys with fornix transection. *Journal of Cognitive Neuroscience, 6,* 305–320.

Gaffan, D. (1996). Memory, action and the corpus striatum: Current developments in the memory-habit distinction. *Seminars in the Neurosciences, 8,* 33–38.

Gaffan, D. (1998). Idiothetic input into object-place configuration as the contribution to memory of the monkey and human hippocampus: A review. *Experimental Brain Research, 123,* 201–209.

Gaffan, D., & Eacott, M. J. (1995). Uncinate fascicle section leaves delayed matching-to-sample intact, both with large and small stimulus sets. *Experimental Brain Research, 105,* 175–180.

Gaffan, D., & Gaffan, E. A. (1991). Amnesia in man following transection of the fornix: A review. *Brain, 114,* 2611–2618.

Gaffan, D., & Harrison, S. (1987). Amygdalectomy and disconnection in visual learning for auditory secondary reinforcement by monkeys. *Journal of Neuroscience, 7,* 2285–2292.

Gaffan, D., & Murray, E. A. (1992). Monkeys (*Macaca fascicularis*) with rhinal cortex ablations succeed in object discrim-

ination learning despite 24-hr intertial intervals and fail at matching to sample despite double sample presentations. *Behavioral Neuroscience, 106,* 30–38.

Gaffan, D., Parker, A., & Easton, A. (2001). Dense amnesia in the monkey after transection of fornix, amygdala and anterior temporal stem. *Neuropsychologia, 39,* 51–70.

Gaffan, D., Shields, S., & Harrison, S. (1984). Delayed matching by fornix-transected monkeys: The sample, the push and the bait. *Quarterly Journal of Experimental Psychology. B, Comparative and Physiological Psychology, 36,* 305–317.

Gaffan, E. A., Gaffan, D., & Harrison, S. (1988). Disconnection of the amygdala from visual association cortex impairs visual reward-association learning in monkeys. *Journal of Neuroscience, 8,* 3144–3150.

Goulet, S., Dore, F. Y., & Murray, E. A. (1998). Aspiration lesions of the amygdala disrupt the rhinal corticothalamic projection system in rhesus monkeys. *Experimental Brain Research, 119,* 131–140.

Goulet, S., & Murray, E. A. (1996). Neural substrate of intramodal and cross-modal memory in rhesus monkeys. *International Journal of Psychology, 31,* 307.

Goulet, S., & Murray, E. A. (2001). Neural substrates of cross-modal association memory in monkeys: The amygdala versus the anterior rhinal cortex. *Behavioral Neuroscience, 115,* 271–284.

Hood, K. L., Postle, B. R., & Corkin, S. (1996). Habit learning in H.M.: Results from a concurrent discrimination task. *Society for Neuroscience Abstracts, 22,* 732.18.

Horel, J. A. (1978). The neuroanatomy of amnesia: A critique of the hippocampal memory hypothesis. *Brain, 101,* 403–445.

Jarvis, M. J., & Ettlinger, G. (1977). Cross-modal recognition in chimpanzees and monkeys. *Neuropsychologia, 15,* 499–506.

Kapur, N., Thompson, S., Cook, P., Lang, D., & Brice, J. (1996). Anterograde but not retrograde memory loss following combined mamillary body and medial thalamic lesions. *Neuropsychologia, 34,* 1–8.

Kitt, C. A., Mitchell, S. J., DeLong, M. R., Wainer, B. H., & Price, D. L. (1987). Fiber pathways of basal forebrain cholinergic neurons in monkeys. *Brain Research, 406,* 192–206.

Malkova, L., Gaffan, D., & Murray, E. A. (1997). Excitotoxic lesions of the amygdala fail to produce impairment in visual learning for auditory secondary reinforcement but interfere with reinforcer devaluation effects in rhesus monkeys. *Journal of Neuroscience, 17,* 6011–6020.

Malkova, L., & Murray, E. A. (1996). Effects of partial versus complete lesions of the amygdala on cross-modal associations in rhesus monkeys. *Psychobiology, 24,* 255–264.

MacLean, C. J., Gaffan, D., Baker, H. F., Ridley, R. M. (2001). Visual discrimination learning impairments produced by combined transections of the anterior temporal stem, amygdala and fornix in marmoset monkeys. *Brain Research, 888,* 34–50.

Martin, R. F., & Bowden, D. M. (1996). A stereotaxic template atlas of the macaque brain for digital imaging and quantitative neuroanatomy. *Neuroimage, 4,* 119–150.

McMackin, D., Cockburn, J., Anslow, P., & Gaffan, D. (1995). Correlation of fornix damage with memory impairment in six cases of colloid cyst removal. *Acta Neurochirurgica, 135,* 12–18.

Mesulam, M.-M., & Mufson, E. J. (1984). Neural inputs into the nucleus basalis of the substantia innominata (Ch4) in the rhesus monkey. *Brain, 107,* 253–274.

Mesulam, M.-M., Mufson, E. J., Levey, A. I., & Wainer, B. H. (1983). Cholinergic innervation of cortex by the basal forebrain: Cytochemistry and cortical connections of the septal area, diagonal band nuclei, nucleus basalis (substantia innominata), and hypothalamus in the rhesus monkey. *Journal of Comparative Neurology, 214,* 170–197.

Meunier, M., Bachevalier, J., Mishkin, M., & Murray, E. A. (1993). Effects on visual recognition of combined and separate ablations of the entorhinal and perirhinal cortex in rhesus monkeys. *Journal of Neuroscience, 13,* 5418–5432.

Milner, B., Corkin, S., & Teuber, H.-L. (1968). Further analysis of the hippocampal amnesic syndrome: 14-year follow-up study of H.M. *Neuropsychologia, 6,* 215–234.

Murphy, C., & Cain, W. S. (1980). Taste and olfaction: Independence *vs* interaction. *Physiology and Behavior, 24,* 601–605.

Murphy, C., Cain, W. S., & Bartoshuk, L. M. (1977). Mutual action of taste and olfaction. *Sensory Processes, 1,* 204–211.

Murray, E. A., & Bussey, T. J. (1999). Perceptual-mnemonic function of the perirhinal cortex. *Trends in Cognitive Sciences, 3,* 142–151.

Murray, E. A., & Mishkin, M. (1985). Amygdalectomy impairs crossmodal association in monkeys. *Science, 228,* 604–606.

Ongur, D., An, X., & Price, J. L. (1998). Prefrontal cortical projections to the hypothalamus in macaque monkeys. *Journal of Comparative Neurology, 401,* 480–505.

Oscar-Berman, M., & Zola-Morgan, S. (1980). Comparative neuropsychology and Korsakoff's syndrome: II—two-choice visual discrimination learning. *Neuropsychologia, 18,* 513–525.

Parker, A., Easton, A., & Gaffan, D. (2002). Memory encoding in the primate brain: The role of the basal forebrain. In A. Parker, E. Wilding, & T. J. Bussey (Eds.), *The cognitive neuroscience of memory: Encoding and retrieval.* Hove, England: Psychology Press.

Parker, A., & Gaffan, D. (1997a). The effect of anterior thalamic and cingulate cortex lesions on object-in-place memory in monkeys. *Neuropsychologia, 35,* 1093–1102.

Parker, A., & Gaffan, D. (1997b). Mamillary body lesions in monkeys impair object-in-place memory: Functional unity of the fornix-mamillary system. *Journal of Cognitive Neuroscience, 9,* 512–521.

Parker, A., & Gaffan, D. (1998a). Lesions of the primate rhinal cortex cause deficits in flavour-visual associative memory. *Behavioral Brain Research, 93,* 99–105.

Parker, A., & Gaffan, D. (1998b). Memory after frontal-temporal disconnection in monkeys: Conditional and nonconditional tasks, unilateral and bilateral frontal lesions. *Neuropsychologia, 36,* 259–271.

Petrides, M., & Iversen, S. D. (1976). Cross-modal matching and the primate frontal cortex. *Science, 192,* 1023–1024.

Rolls, E. T., Sanghera, M. K., & Roper-Hall, A. (1979). The latency of activation of neurones in the lateral hypothalamus and substantia innominata during feeding in the monkey. *Brain Research, 164,* 121–135.

Scoville, W. B., & Milner, B. (1957). Loss of recent memory after bilateral hippocampal lesions. *Journal of Neurology, Neurosurgery and Psychiatry, 20,* 11–21.

Shindy, W. W., Posley, K. A., & Fuster, J. M. (1994). Reversible deficit in haptic delay tasks from cooling prefrontal cortex. *Cerebral Cortex, 4,* 443–450.

Streicher, M., & Ettlinger, G. (1987). Cross-modal recognition of familiar and unfamiliar objects by the monkey: The effects of ablation of polysensory neocortex of the amygdaloid complex. *Behavioural Brain Research, 23,* 95–107.

Suzuki, W. A., & Amaral, D. G. (1994). Perirhinal and parahippocampal cortices of the macaque monkey: Cortical afferents. *Journal of Comparative Neurology, 350,* 497–533.

Tanaka, K. (1996). Inferotemporal cortex and object vision. *Annual Review of Neuroscience, 19,* 109–139.

Teuber, H.-L., Milner, B., & Vaughan, H. G. J. (1968). Persistent anterograde amnesia after stab wound of the basal brain. *Neuropsychologia, 6,* 267–282.

Thornton, J. A., Rothblat, L. A., & Murray, E. A. (1997). Rhinal cortex removal produces amnesia for preoperatively learned problems but fails to disrupt postoperative acquisition and retention in monkeys. *Journal of Neurosciences, 17,* 8536–8549.

Van Hoesen, G. W., Pandya, D. N., & Butters, N. (1975). Some connections of the entorhinal (area 28) and perirhinal (area 35) cortices of the rhesus monkey: II. Frontal lobe afferents. *Brain Research, 95,* 25–38.

Vargha-Khadem, F., Gadian, D. G., Watkins, K. E., Connelly, A., Paesschen, W. V., & Mishkin, M. (1997). Differential effects of early hippocampal pathology on episodic and semantic memory. *Science, 277,* 376–380.

Weiskrantz, L., & Cowey, A. (1975). Cross-modal matching in the rhesus monkey using a single pair of stimuli. *Neuropsychologia, 13,* 257–261.

Wilson, F. A., & Rolls, E. T. (1990). Learning and memory is reflected in the responses of reinforcement-related neurons in the primate basal forebrain. *Journal of Neuroscience, 10,* 1254–1267.

Zola-Morgan, S., Squire, L. R., Amaral, D. G., & Suzuki, W. A. (1989). Lesions of perirhinal and parahippocampal cortex that spare the amygdala and hippocampal formation produce severe memory impairment. *Journal of Neuroscience, 9,* 4355–4370.

21 Corticocortical Connectivity of Cross-Modal Circuits

M. ALEX MEREDITH

Introduction

The activity of a multisensory neuron, like that of any other neuron, is the result of the physical properties of its membrane and the collective effect of its inputs. Although little is known about the membrane properties of multisensory neurons *per se* and how they might differ from the properties of unimodal neurons, multisensory neurons are *defined* by their multiple sensory inputs. Beyond this essential feature, however, little detailed information is known about the organization of inputs to identified multisensory neurons. From what has been reported to date, it has been generalized that multisensory neurons are generated by the convergence of basically excitatory inputs from different sensory modalities (see, e.g., Stein & Meredith, 1993). Inhibition, when it occurs, has been observed as an accompaniment to complex receptive field properties such as spatial inhibition and postexcitatory inhibition. Thus, the well-known designations of bimodal and trimodal aptly apply to neurons responsive to two or three different sensory modalities, respectively. How these properties arise and are distributed within a given area (e.g., areal convergence) has been the subject of a number of investigations not only of the well-known multisensory layers of the superior colliculus but also of "polymodal" or multisensory regions of cortex (see, e.g., Jones & Powell, 1970; Seltzer & Pandya, 1994). Although the documentation of multiple sensory inputs to lower-level, "unimodal" cortical areas has received a great deal of recent attention (Falchier, Clavagnier, Barone, & Kennedy, 2002; Schroeder & Foxe, 2002; Schroeder et al., 2001), the patterns of convergence that generate multisensory neuronal properties in any region largely remain unexplored. This chapter examines the areal and circuit-level relationships of cortical association areas representing different sensory modalities with the intention of revealing organizational patterns that expand our current appreciation of the structure of multisensory convergence at the neuronal level.

Higher-order, modality-specific cortical representations

A particularly fertile region for the study of relationships among the representations of different sensory modalities is the cortex surrounding the cat anterior ectosylvian sulcus (AES), where representations of three different sensory modalities share borders with one another. The AES is found at the juncture of the frontal, parietal, and temporal regions of the cat cortex (Fig. 21.1) and is composed of an anterior (horizontal) limb and a posterior (vertical) limb. Within the dorsal bank of the anterior limb, there is a representation of the body surface, identified as SIV (Clemo & Stein, 1982, 1983). Medially and deep within the dorsal bank of the AES, SIV transitions into an area of the fundus termed the para-SIV. Para-SIV lacks a somatotopic organization and contains neurons with large, sometimes bilateral receptive fields that often also respond to inputs from other sensory modalities (Clemo & Stein, 1983). Posterior to SIV, within the banks of the posterior limb of the AES, lies the anterior ectosylvian sulcus auditory field (FAES; also termed FAES by Clarey & Irvine, 1990a, 1990b; Meredith & Clemo, 1989; Wallace, Meredith, & Stein, 1992, 1993; but see Korte & Rauschecker, 1993; Rauschecker & Korte, 1993). Auditory FAES lacks a tonotopic organization and contains neurons that are tuned not for sound frequency but for the spatial features of auditory cues (Clarey & Irvine, 1990a; Middlebrooks, Clock, Xu, & Green, 1994; Rauschecker, 1996; Korte & Rauschecker, 1993). In fact, the FAES is thought to represent a cortical locus subserving sound localization (Korte & Rauschecker, 1993; Middlebrooks et al., 1994; Nelken, BarYosef, & Rotman, 1997; Rauschecker & Korte, 1993), although no map of auditory space has as yet been revealed in this region. Vision is the third modality represented in AES cortex. The anterior ectosylvian visual area (AEV) is found on the inferior (ventral) bank from the base of the vertical limb of the sulcus to its posterior end (Benedek et al., 1988; Mucke et al., 1982; Olson & Graybiel, 1983, 1987;

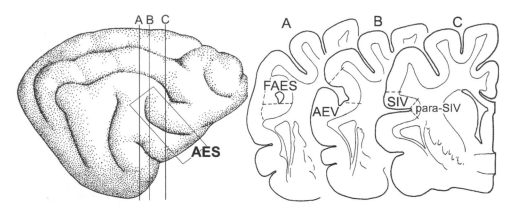

FIGURE 21.1 Lateral view of cat cortex showing the location of the anterior ectosylvian sulcus (AES) and its associated cortex (rectangle). The vertical lines labeled A, B, and C indicate the levels from which the coronal sections on the right are taken. In A, the most posterior section, the AES is not evident on the surface of the cortex but lies beneath the middle ectosylvian gyrus. The auditory FAES is located in the dorsal portions of this region of the sulcal cortex. Section B is taken just anterior to the point where the dorsal and ventral lips of the AES become apparent on the lateral surface of the cortex. The ventral bank of the AES here contains the visual representation of the anterior ectosylvian visual area (AEV). Section C is taken at the midpoint of the anteroposterior extent of the AES, where the somatosensory area SIV is found in its dorsal bank. Dashed lines represent the approximate borders between the different sensory representations. These conventions are used throughout the remaining figures in this chapter.

Rauschecker & Korte, 1993; Scannell et al., 1996). This area is unique among feline visual areas because of its sensitivity to pattern motion (Scannell et al., 1996). Visually responsive neurons in this area exhibit local rather than global retinotopies and generally have large receptive fields that include the fovea (Benedek et al., 1988; Mucke et al., 1982; Olson & Graybiel, 1987). In addition, some authors report visually responsive neurons further anteriorly along the ventral bank of the AES (Benedek et al., 1988; Mucke et al., 1982) in a region adjacent to and continuous with the agranular insular area.

Multisensory neurons in unimodal cortex: Correspondence with organization of external inputs?

Thus, the cortex surrounding the AES hosts contiguous, higher-order representations of three different sensory modalities. As described in the previous section, these regions are regarded as unimodal, not multisensory, cortices. In addition, a modest proportion of neurons responsive to more than one sensory modality have been consistently identified within some of these areas (Clemo & Stein, 1983; Jiang et al., 1994a, 1994b; Kimura et al., 1996; Minciacchi, Tassinari, & Antonini, 1987; Wallace et al., 1992). However, the pattern of distribution of multisensory neurons here has been enigmatic. A few investigators have argued for a dispersed distribution of multisensory neurons within the different unimodal representations of the AES cortex (Jiang et al., 1994a, 1994b; Kimura et al., 1996; Minciacchi et al.,

1987); others have reported that multisensory neurons preferentially reside along the shared borders of, or the transition regions between, the different subregions (Wallace et al., 1992, 1993). Because the issue of multisensory dispersion versus restriction to transitional zones probably applies to many other areas of cortex, an examination of this problem should provide insight into the general principles of multisensory convergence.

EXTERNAL AFFERENTS TO AES CORTEX Tracer experiments were conducted to examine whether external inputs to the functionally different areas of the AES cortex are coextensive, as schematically depicted in Figure 21.2A (consistent with a dispersed arrangement of multisensory neurons), or are largely discrete from one another except at border zones, as illustrated in Figure 21.2B (consistent with multisensory neuronal segregation within transition zones). Using standard neuroanatomical techniques (see Meredith, Miller, Ramoa, Clemo, & Behan, 2001, for details), we injected the highly sensitive orthograde tracer, biotinylated dextran amine (BDA), into modality-specific cortices known to project to AES cortex. These injection sites, shown in Figure 21.3, include the auditory posterior ectosylvian gyral cortex, PEG (Fig. 21.3A), the somatosensory area, SV (Fig. 21.3B), and the visual posterior medial lateral suprasylvian cortex, PMLS (Fig. 21.3C). BDA injections were placed in one of these areas per animal, and the terminal labeling in AES cortex was examined. As the micrographs in Figure 21.3 show, in each case, labeled axons and terminal boutons were observed within AES cortex. Bouton profiles included both terminal and

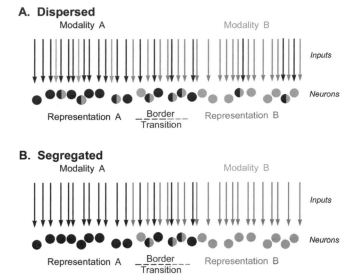

A. Dispersed

B. Segregated

FIGURE 21.2 Hypothetical arrangements for external inputs to adjoining sensory representations and their relationship with the distribution of multisensory neurons. Inputs from modality A (black arrows) target neurons (black circles) primarily within representation A, while those from modality B (gray arrows) target neurons (gray circles) in representation B. Where black and gray arrows intermingle, multisensory neurons (half-black, half-gray circles) result from the convergence of the different external inputs. (*A*) If external inputs from one modality are intermingled among those from the other modality throughout each representation, multisensory neurons are likely to be found dispersed throughout both areas. (*B*) Alternatively, if external inputs are largely segregated from one another, such that intermingling occurs only at the borders between the different representations, multisensory neurons are most likely to be segregated within the border/ transition region between the different representations.

en passant varieties, although the latter appeared to predominate. However, in each case terminal label was not distributed throughout the AES cortex. Instead, as shown in Figure 21.4*A*, auditory projections originating in PEG were extremely dense in the posterior quarter but were virtually absent from the anterior aspects of the AES cortex. The terminal label occupied essentially the same area of the AES cortex as that obtained with BDA injections placed in and around the thalamic medial geniculate nucleus (MGB; not shown). Therefore, those projections from PEG (or MGB) found most posteriorly in the AES cortex undoubtedly contribute to and delineate the auditory FAES. The distribution of somatosensory projections from area SV to AES cortex was regionally restricted (Fig. 21.4*B*) to the dorsal bank of the anterior limb of the sulcal cortex. Moreover, the projections from SV terminated in an area that corresponds closely with SIV, as physiologically described by several investigators (Burton & Kopf, 1984; Clemo & Stein, 1983; Rauschecker & Korte, 1993). Projections from

SV to AES cortex essentially avoided the ventral bank (where AEV is found), the fundus (where para-SIV is located), and the posterior region (where FAES is positioned). The visual projection to AES cortex was even more restricted in its distribution, as illustrated in Figure 21.4*C*. Terminal boutons from visual PMLS cortex were observed almost exclusively on the ventral bank at the point where the AES begins to submerge under the middle ectosylvian gyrus (MEG). This is precisely where Olson and Graybiel (1987) functionally and anatomically identified the AEV. Except for the projections to AEV (Olson & Graybiel, 1987), none of these terminal distributions within AES cortex has been reported before. The spatial distribution of these distinct auditory, somatosensory, and visual inputs within AES cortex is summarized in Figure 21.5. Collectively, these data indicate, for at least the afferent sources examined, that modality-specific inputs to AES cortex largely target exclusive zones of termination, with overlap or mixture of the different external inputs occurring predominantly at borders or transition zones. These results are consistent with the alternative illustrated in Figure 21.2*B*.

CORRESPONDENCE OF EXTERNAL INPUTS TO FUNCTIONAL REPRESENTATIONS Electrophysiological recordings showed that the anatomical extent and distribution of each modality-specific representation in AES cortex were largely coextensive with the corresponding modality-specific external inputs as detailed here, as well as in previous reports (Clemo & Stein, 1983; Meredith & Clemo, 1989; Olson & Graybiel, 1987; Rauschecker & Korte, 1993; Wallace et al., 1992, 1993). In the present experiments, four animals chronically prepared for repeated recording sessions (for detailed methodology, see Wallace et al., 1992) yielded a total of 489 identified neurons, each tested with stimuli from three modalities (auditory, visual, somatosensory), within the AES cortex. The sensory responsiveness of this sample is detailed in Table 21.1. The histological location of these identified neurons is summarized for three of the cases in Figure 21.6. Figures 21.6*A* and *B* show recordings made throughout the anterior-posterior extent of the AES cortex, while the recording shown in Figure 21.6*C* concentrates specifically on the posterior aspect of the region. From these data, it is evident that neurons with auditory responsiveness predominate in the posterior end of the AES cortex and are quite infrequent at more anterior locations of either the dorsal or ventral banks. This region in which auditory responsiveness predominates corresponds to the region that receives external auditory inputs described above and in previous reports (Meredith & Clemo, 1989; Rauschecker & Korte, 1993). These data also

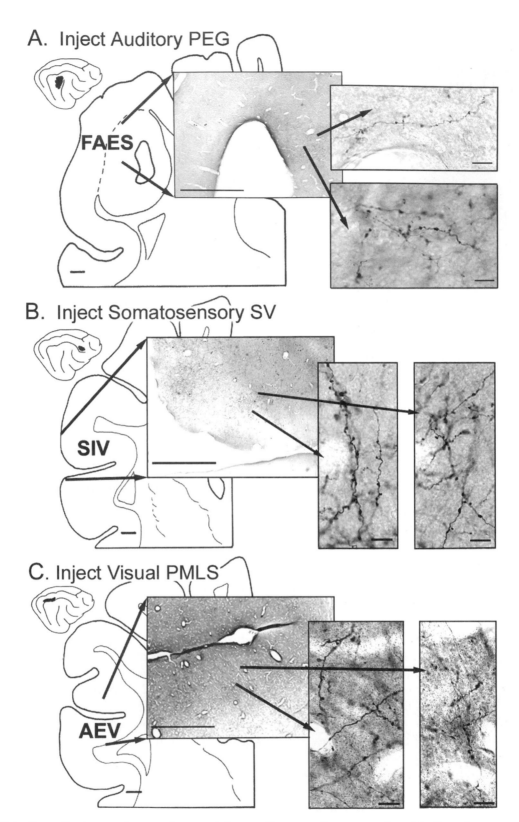

FIGURE 21.3 Injections of anterograde tracer into modality-specific areas of cortex produce labeling of axons and terminal boutons within AES cortex. (*A*) Injection of the tracer biotinylated dextran amine (BDA) into the PEG (dark spot on lateral view of cat cortex) produced labeling in the posterior AES cortex. The coronal section (scale bar = 1 mm) shows where the midmagnification view was taken (inset, scale bar = 1 mm). At highest magnification (right insets, magnification 1000×, scale bar = 10 μm), labeled axons as well as swellings characteristic of terminal boutons are visible. (*B*) Similar treatment, with injection sites in the somatosensory (SV) area. (*C*) Similar treatment, with injection sites in the visual (PMLS) area.

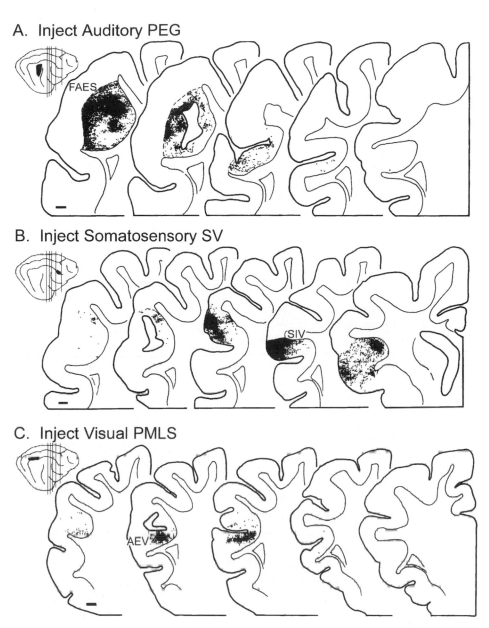

A. Inject Auditory PEG

FAES

B. Inject Somatosensory SV

SIV

C. Inject Visual PMLS

AEV

FIGURE 21.4   The pattern of terminal label for each of the cases presented in Figure 21.3 reveals modality-specific distribution patterns within the AES cortex. (*A*) BDA injection into auditory PEG produced the heaviest terminal label (each dot = 1 labeled bouton) within the FAES. (*B*) A different pattern of terminal label within AES cortex was observed following BDA injections into somatosensory area SV, which primarily filled the dorsal bank in its middle and anterior regions. Note that the ventral bank and fundus were almost completely unlabeled. (*C*) In contrast, BDA injections into visual area PMLS yielded terminal label within the ventral bank of the AES cortex, almost to its posterior limit. Vertical lines on the schematics indicate the levels of cortex from which the coronal sections, displayed on the right, were taken. The blackened area of the schematic represents the BDA injection site for each case. Scale bar = 1 mm.

reveal that the region of AES cortex in which visual activity predominates is found on the ventral bank near the point where the AES disappears from view on the lateral surface of the cortex. This concentration of visual activity corresponds well with the location of external visual inputs (described above) and the location of the AEV as defined by Olson and Graybiel (1987). Somatosensory responses predominated anteriorly on

the dorsal bank, corresponding with the location of external inputs from SV (described above) as well as with that of SIV as defined by Clemo and Stein (1983).

In addition to unimodal neurons, a small proportion (19.2%; 94/489; see Table 21.1) of multisensory neurons were also identified within the AES cortex. These values correspond closely to those identified in earlier reports (Wallace et al., 1992). Multisensory neurons

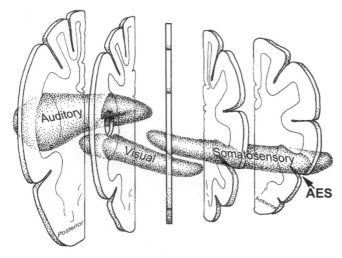

FIGURE 21.5 A summary of the distribution of the different modality-specific representations within AES cortex. In this figure, five coronal sections are displayed in fanlike perspective in order to demonstrate the three-dimensional distribution of the different modality-specific areas (stippled forms) in relation to cortical landmarks. Auditory inputs to FAES terminate in the most posterior aspects of the AES (left) but become progressively more dorsal as the AES reaches the lateral surface of the brain (center, shown edge-on). Anteriorly, somatosensory inputs to SIV primarily terminate in the dorsal bank of the AES. Visual inputs to AEV end in a relatively restricted region of the ventral bank near the point where the AES is no longer apparent on the lateral surface of the cortex.

were generally encountered posteriorly, with the largest number of bimodal auditory-somatosensory neurons (93%; 28/30) or visual-auditory/visual-somatosensory neurons (82%; 52/63) found in this region. In contrast, few multisensory neurons (6%; 6/94) of any type were found in the anterior dorsal bank where SIV was located. The distribution of these multisensory neurons

TABLE 21.1
Sensory response patterns of neurons in AES cortex

Modality	Number	% of Sample
Unimodal		
Visual	155	31.7
Auditory	84	17.2
Somatosensory	126	25.8
Total	**365**	**74.7**
Multisensory		
Visual-auditory	39	8.0
Visual-somatosensory	24	4.9
Auditory-somatosensory	30	6.1
Visual-auditory-somatosensory	1	0.4
Total	**94**	**19.2**
Unresponsive	30	6.1
Total	**489**	**100**

was examined further to determine whether they were colocated with unimodal neurons or were generally segregated from them.

Within a given representation, the position of each unimodal and multisensory neuron (unresponsive neurons were not included) was established according to anatomical landmarks using the reconstructed recording tracks like those shown in Figure 21.6. Neurons were assigned to categories of "within designated representation" or "transition zones between representations." These values were then normalized to accommodate the different sampling rates in the different representations. The results, shown in Figure 21.7, indicate that for areas within a given representation, the proportion of unimodal neurons was substantially higher than that found at the borders. Conversely, the proportion of multisensory neurons increased in the transition areas between representations, and the differences in values were statistically significant (χ^2 test; $P < 0.01$). Although it is not possible with these methods to establish with absolute certainty the exact location of the borders between the different representations, the overall trend is apparent even in the recording track reconstructions provided in Figure 21.6. Therefore, these observations are also consistent with the hypothesis that the incidence of multisensory neurons increases in zones of transition between representations of different sensory modalities.

Multisensory neurons in unimodal cortex: Contribution of local inputs

The preponderance of multisensory neurons at the border or transition region between representations of different sensory modalities is also consistent with the anatomical overlap of projections from the different external sources, especially posterior in the AES cortex, where the three representations closely appose one another. These same anatomical data show that there is very little cross-modal connectivity to the central regions of any of the modality-specific representations (see Fig. 21.4). Yet electrophysiological data indicate that multisensory neurons can also be found within as well as between representations, and the distribution of external inputs does not appear to account for these. Because proximity is a strong factor in corticocortical connectivity (Young, Scannell, & Burns, 1995), it seemed possible that local cross-modal projections could occur among the different representations within the AES cortex that might contribute to the generation of multisensory properties. Such a local arrangement could account for the distribution of multisensory neurons where convergence of external

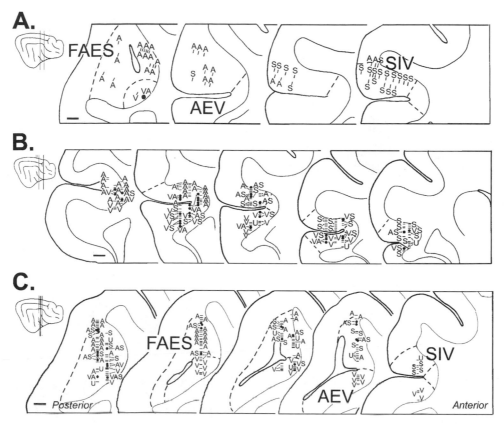

FIGURE 21.6 Electrophysiological mapping of modality distribution within the AES cortex in three cases. (A, B) Recordings along the anterior-posterior length of AES in two cases, (C) Recording concentrated on the responses found in the posterior aspect of AES. In each case, responses to auditory stimuli predominated in FAES. The examples of auditory responses found farther anteriorly along the AES cortex were found in association with transition zones between regions or within fundic cortex where para-SIV is located. Visual responses were found almost exclusively on the ventral bank, although some examples were identified within the anterior fundic region. In contrast, somatosensory responses were encountered throughout the AES cortex, although unimodal somatosensory responses predominated on the anterior dorsal bank, corresponding to the location of SIV. Multisensory neurons (solid circles) also appear to be distributed throughout the AES cortex. However, they are most concentrated in fundic and transitional regions. In addition, as expected from the distribution of somatosensory responses, multisensory neurons that responded to somatosensory cues were often found paired with auditory responses in FAES and coupled with visual responses in AEV. Abbreviations: A, auditory; V, visual; S, somatosensory; U, unresponsive; dashed line, unimodal; solid circle, multisensory. Scale bar = 1 mm.

inputs is apparently lacking, as depicted schematically in Figure 21.8.

INTRINSIC CROSS-MODAL CONNECTIVITY OF AES CORTEX
To test the hypothesis that adjacent modality-specific representations may be cross-modally linked by local projections, the intrinsic connectivity of the AES cortex was examined using the same neuroanatomical techniques used to identify the external inputs, as described earlier. Of particular interest was whether such intrinsic connectivity would cross modality-specific borders, and if so, whether the pattern of connectivity would reflect the distribution of multisensory neurons identified electrophysiologically. Representative examples of terminal labeling in the AES following anterograde injec-

tion of tracer into either SIV, AEV, or FAES are shown in Figure 21.9. Injection of BDA tracer into somatosensory SIV consistently revealed a projection to the posterior AES cortex, including the FAES (Fig. 21.9A). Other experiments (not shown) in which the SIV injection did not spread into the fundic, para-SIV region also preferentially targeted the FAES. Injection of tracer within the auditory FAES labeled boutons almost exclusively within the anterior, dorsal bank corresponding to SIV (Fig. 21.9B). Tracer injection into the region of the visual AEV on the ventral bank (Fig. 21.9C) produced terminal label rostrally on the anterior ventral bank as well as in the fundic, para-SIV region of the AES. In these cases, however, terminal label was conspicuously absent in SIV and FAES.

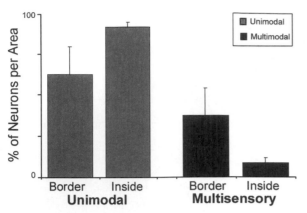

FIGURE 21.7 Multisensory neurons tend to occur at borders or transition zones between modality-specific representations. From the histological reconstructions of recording penetrations through the AES cortex, the location of each identified neuron was categorized as being either "inside" or "between (bordering)" the three different modality-specific representations. These data show that average percentage of unimodal neurons per subregion was highest within the representations, while the proportion of multisensory neurons was largest between representations, and these differences were statistically significant (χ^2, $P < 0.01$). Values exceed 100% because designations for "inside" and for "bordering" were calculated separately. Error bars = standard deviation.

In each of these experiments, local projections from discrete modality-specific regions (e.g., SIV) generally terminated within at least one of the other modality-specific areas of the AES (as summarized in Fig. 21.10). These local cross-modal projections form synaptic terminals within a representation of another modality, and it seems logical to assume that such connectivity could

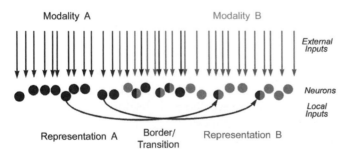

FIGURE 21.8 A small proportion of multisensory neurons are present within modality-specific representations, and it is possible that they might arise by means of local, cross-modal projections. In this hypothetical schematic, external inputs A and B largely target modality-specific representations A and B, respectively, with multisensory neurons (half-black, half-gray circles) occurring primarily at their zone of overlap (see also Fig. 21.2B). Multisensory neurons occurring outside the border zone, or within the representation, may arise from the convergence of external inputs for modality B with local, cross-modal inputs from representation A.

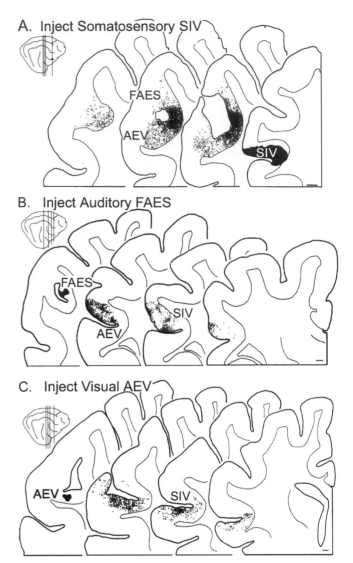

FIGURE 21.9 Intrinsic connections of subregions of the AES cortex. (A) Tracer placed using electrophysiological guidance into SIV (solid black = injection site) shows a projection posteriorly to FAES. (B) Tracer placed within the posterior region corresponding to FAES produced terminal label throughout the anterior dorsal bank in the area corresponding to SIV. (C) Tracer placed in the ventral bank where AEV is located yielded terminal label in zones exclusive of those identified by the more dorsal injections described in A and B, but projected to the anterior aspects of the ventral bank as well as to the fundus. Scale bar = 1 mm.

render the target neurons multisensory. Because AEV projects into adjoining regions of para-SIV, this may help facilitate the generation of visual-somatosensory properties described in neurons there (Clemo & Stein, 1982, 1983). Similarly, SIV projects posteriorly to the FAES and may thereby convey somatosensory properties to auditory neurons in that region; such bimodal neurons have been observed, if infrequently, in the current study as well as in published studies (Jiang et al., 1994a).

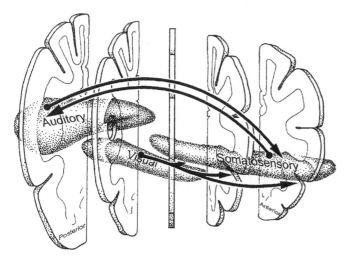

FIGURE 21.10 Summary of the intrinsic connectivity of the AES cortex. Regions found dorsally (FAES, SIV) are reciprocally innervated and avoid connecting to the ventral bank and fundus. The ventrally located AEV projects primarily to the anterior ventral bank and to the fundus. The paths of the arrows do not reflect the anatomical course of the projection, only connectivity between specified areas.

However, while cross-modal convergence between external inputs and local connections may generate the multisensory neurons in the posterior AES cortex, the same mechanisms do not appear to apply to its anterior sector. Although both the present experiments and those by Dehner, Clemo, and Meredith (2000) and by Burton and Kopf (1984) show that auditory FAES projects to somatosensory SIV, the expected bimodal auditory-somatosensory neurons within SIV have rarely been encountered. None were reported by Clemo and Stein (1983), who made an exhaustive analysis of SIV and the adjoining regions. The present experiments observed only a single bimodal auditory-somatosensory neuron in SIV, with the remaining 29 such neurons in the sample located within the transition zone between FAES and SIV or more posteriorly. Thus, although there is anatomical evidence for local auditory projections into somatosensory SIV, the bimodal result of such convergence has not been observed (see Clemo & Stein, 1983; Jiang et al., 1994a, 1994b; Kimura et al., 1996; Minciacchi et al., 1987; Rauschecker & Korte, 1993). These conflicting data suggest that whereas some local cross-modal projections could support the generation of multisensory neurons as they are presently known, other projections might not. This possibility has been explored further, as follows.

A NEW FORM OF MULTISENSORY CONVERGENCE: EXCITATORY-INHIBITORY MULTISENSORY NEURONS Despite the presence of a consistent cross-modal projection from FAES, SIV neurons have not and were not shown to be excited by free-field auditory stimulation. Thus, the FAES-SIV projection does not appear to elicit an excitatory response. Alternatively, the cross-modal projection from FAES to SIV may result in inhibition, not excitation, which would not be observed using extracellular recording methods unless SIV neurons exhibited regular spontaneous activity or auditory stimulation was combined with effective (e.g., somatosensory) stimulation. To examine this possibility, a series of preliminary experiments was conducted (Clemo, Dehner, & Meredith, 2000) in which cats were chronically implanted for recording from neurons in SIV, with rows of stimulating electrodes positioned within auditory FAES. Of the more than 100 somatosensory neurons identified in SIV in four animals, none was excited by free-field auditory stimuli presented alone, nor was any excited by electrical stimulation of FAES through the implanted electrodes. In addition, although auditory free-field stimulation seemed to reduce the activity of some SIV neurons, it did not significantly inhibit their spontaneous activity or tactile responses.

On the other hand, as shown in the peristimulus time histograms in Figure 21.11, SIV somatosensory responsiveness was significantly suppressed by the concurrent activation of the auditory FAES. This form of FAES stimulation-induced somatosensory suppression occurred in nearly 70% of the neurons tested. That FAES stimulation was effective was not surprising, because these procedures synchronously activated a nearby segment of the auditory pathway rather than rely on the faithful transmission of activity along the entire auditory projection in an anesthetized animal. Controls for current spread and site specificity revealed that the projection corresponded well with the anatomically identified FAES-SIV pathway. In addition, this stimulation-induced suppression was blocked by the application of the competitive antagonist of the inhibitory neurotransmitter γ-aminobutyric acid (GABA) (see Fig. 21.11), bicuculline methiodide. Stimulation-induced suppression reappeared after the drug was discontinued (after a waiting period). Therefore, it is apparent that this form of multisensory convergence involves a cross-modal inhibitory signal. Because the FAES-SIV projection originates from pyramidal neurons that are presumably glutamatergic, it seems most likely that the signal from FAES is converted to inhibition by GABAergic interneurons within SIV. Although such a circuit is novel to multisensory studies, there is a great deal of evidence in the neocortical literature showing that inhibition is mediated successfully by local circuits involving interneurons (e.g., Ebner & Armstrong-James, 1990; Gilbert, 1993, 1998; Richter, Hess, &

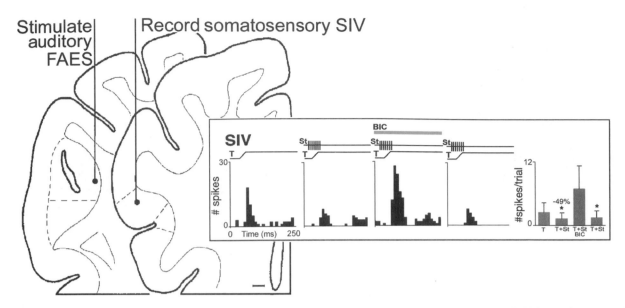

FIGURE 21.11 The cross-modal suppression of SIV responses by the FAES is based on GABA-ergic inhibition. The coronal sections show the position of stimulating (auditory FAES) and recording (somatosensory SIV) electrodes. The rectangle outlines the responses of an SIV neuron to somatosensory stimulation (left, ramp labeled T), the reduction in response to the same stimulus when combined with FAES stimulation (waveforms labeled St), the blockade of the stimulation-induced inhibition by the application of the GABA$_A$ antagonist bicuculline methiodide (bar labeled BIC; 50 μM continuously applied), and the recovery of FAES-induced suppression following 15-minute washout of the bicuculline. Data in each peristimulus-time histogram are derived from 10 stimulus presentations; bin width = 10 ms. The bar graph at the far right summarizes these responses and shows that the significant levels ($^*P < 0.05$, paired t-test) of FAES-induced suppression was reversed by concurrent application of the inhibitory antagonist.

Scheich, 1999; Wang, Caspary, & Salvi, 2000), and there is an abundance of GABAergic neurons within SIV through which this cross-modal effect could occur (e.g., Clemo, Keniston, & Meredith, 2003).

That cross-modal inhibition occurs is not a new finding in multisensory studies. Numerous investigations have shown that combined-modality stimulation can lead to a significant reduction in response, termed response depression (see, e.g., Meredith & Stein, 1986). However, in these published cases, inhibition was an accompanying property of one or more excitatory inputs, manifested as inhibitory receptive field surrounds (Kadunce et al., 1997; Meredith & Stein, 1996) or postexcitatory inhibition (Meredith, Nemitz, & Stein, 1987). In this fashion, the excitatory effects of combined-modality stimuli that occurred out of spatial or temporal register, respectively, could be nullified by inhibition. In contrast, in this study free-field auditory or FAES stimulation completely failed to excite SIV neurons, and only inhibition was manifest in the comprehensive series of tests that was presented. Furthermore, when free-field auditory stimuli were used, they were always presented within spatial and temporal alignment with the effective somatosensory stimulus, thereby avoiding the effects of spatiotemporal misalignments. Thus, it is apparent that this form of multisensory inhibitory convergence is

quite distinct from that which accompanies converging excitatory inputs from different modalities.

Conclusions

These results confirm that AES cortex is, indeed, a fertile region for examination of multisensory circuitry, in this case permitting the examination of several features of multisensory convergence. First, these data show that external inputs to the different modality-specific representations within the AES cortex are largely segregated. When multisensory neurons occur in this area, they tend to occur in the transition regions between the different representations, where inputs from the different modality-specific sources have the highest likelihood of overlapping one another. Whether is this a feature peculiar to the organization of AES cortex or broadly applies to other cortical regions with multiple sensory representations has yet to be determined. However, bimodal auditory-visual neurons have been observed in PEG between the posterior auditory fields and the visual areas of 20/21 in the posterior suprasylvian sulcal cortex (Bowman & Olson, 1988). Similarly, multisensory neurons have been reported within the rostral suprasylvian area, where somatosensory areas SII and SV abut the auditory fringe and the anterior medial/

anterior lateral suprasylvian visual areas (Palmer, Rosenquist, & Tusa, 1978). Thus, it seems possible, absent an abrupt transition or a physical barrier between areas, that the transition between adjoining representations of different sensory modalities is gradual. Under these conditions, an intermingling of external, modality-specific inputs can occur that generates multisensory properties in some neurons within the zone of transition.

An interesting question arises as a consequence of multisensory convergence in transition zones between different sensory representations: Is the resulting multisensory output signal incorporated into the overall efferent product of either (or both) area, or are the projections from multisensory neurons distinct from those of the modality-specific representations that they separate? If the answer is the former, then it should be expected that the output signal of unimodal areas might be "tainted" by cross-modal signals. If the latter, then unimodal signals would largely be preserved as such, with the segregated multisensory information redirected toward a processing stream that has yet to be examined. In either case, carefully crafted experimentation to address this fundamental issue would seem appropriate.

Second, although multisensory neurons tended to cluster in transition zones between the different sensory representations, some multisensory neurons were also encountered within areas that appeared to be innervated by external inputs from only one modality. Although it is possible that, like their transition-zone counterparts, these centrally located multisensory neurons could also result from the convergence of different external inputs, such a scenario seems improbable. Anatomical evidence shows that external inputs to AES cortex are largely segregated according to their related, modality-specific representation (of course, not every afferent source for every representation was investigated). Given the cross-modal connectivity of local projections among the AES representations, it seems possible that a convergence of external inputs from one modality with local cross-modal projections could provide a viable substrate for these multisensory neurons. However, local cross-modal projections were observed only between selected representations within the AES cortex. Auditory FAES and somatosensory SIV were reciprocally connected, but neither projected to nor received inputs from visual AEV. In contrast, AEV projected to the fundic regions of the AES, where para-SIV resides. Thus, local projections might account for only a portion of the multisensory convergence seen in AES cortex.

Third, while neurons excited by more than one sensory modality predominantly occur in the posterior, transitional portions of the AES cortex, few if any have been reported anteriorly within the SIV representation despite receiving a consistent, local projection from auditory FAES. Furthermore, electrical activation of FAES or natural auditory stimuli also failed to excite SIV neurons. However, in nearly 70% of the SIV neurons tested, activation of FAES suppressed their responses to somatosensory stimulation, and this suppression appears to be GABAergically mediated. Therefore, a likely explanation for these effects is that the FAES projection to SIV conveys an inhibitory signal. Thus, it appears that many SIV neurons represent a novel form of excitatory (from somatosensory inputs)-inhibitory (from auditory FAES) multisensory convergence.

It is generally accepted that multisensory neurons are those whose activity is significantly *influenced* by stimuli from more than one sensory modality (e.g., Meredith & Stein, 1986). To date, the multisensory neurons that have been most readily identified have been those that were excited by independent, sequential stimuli from different modalities. Using extracellular recording techniques, it is simply much easier to employ a series of different, manually presented search stimuli than to search with their electronically generated combinations. However, such search parameters would miss those neurons that were excited by one modality but inhibited by another, as in the case of SIV neurons. Therefore, while the excitatory-excitatory form of multisensory neuron depicted in Figure 21.12A is familiar and well established, it is possible that the number of multisensory neurons resulting from excitatory-inhibitory convergence, as schematically illustrated in Figure 21.12B, is vastly underestimated. Although the precise anatomical architecture that underlies this excitatory-inhibitory pattern has yet to be deciphered, that this modulatory role is mediated through short, or local, connections is consistent with a wealth of literature on the role of local circuits in cortex (Ebner & Armstrong-James, 1990; Gilbert, 1993, 1998; Richter et al., 1999; Wang et al., 2000), as well as the inhibitory immunocytochemistry of the AES region (Clemo et al., 2003). In fact, modulation of excitatory activity by local inhibitory circuits is well documented throughout the different primary sensory cortices (Ebner & Armstrong-James, 1990; Gilbert, 1993, 1998; Richter et al., 1999; Wang et al., 2000). In summary, then, excitatory-inhibitory convergence among cross-modal projections produces a form of neuron whose *multisensory* properties are virtually silent during conventional multisensory search techniques and which therefore represents a substantially undersampled form of multisensory neuron. Therefore, future examinations of the incidence or distribution of multiple sensory convergence

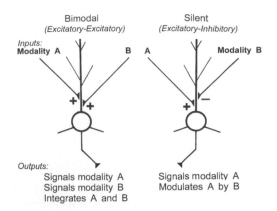

Bimodal
(Excitatory-Excitatory)

Silent
(Excitatory-Inhibitory)

Inputs:
Modality A   B   A   **Modality B**

Outputs:

Signals modality A
Signals modality B
Integrates A and B

Signals modality A
Modulates A by B

FIGURE 21.12   Idealized convergence patterns for different types of multisensory neurons. For the well-known "bimodal" multisensory neuron, principally excitatory inputs from at least two different sensory modalities converge to produce three basic forms of response: (1) response to the presence of one modality (e.g., A) alone, (2) response to the presence of a second modality (e.g., B) alone, and (3) when A and B are active together, an integrated response that is significantly different from either of the modalities active alone. However, it should be noted that some forms of bimodal, excitatory-excitatory neurons have been shown not to integrate combined responses (see Wallace et al., 1996). A second form a multisensory convergence results from the merging of excitatory inputs from one modality with inhibitory effects directed by another. The *multisensory* properties of these neurons are silent unless stimulation of the inhibitory modality is paired with spontaneous activity or simultaneous excitation from the other modality. This convergence architecture yields two forms of response: response to the presence of the excitatory modality (e.g., A) alone, and modulation of excitatory activity by inhibition and disinhibition mediated by inputs from the inhibitory modality (e.g., B).

at the neuronal level should use a search strategy that can reveal combinations of excitatory as well as inhibitory inputs.

REFERENCES

Benedek, G., Mucke, L., Norita, M., Albowitz, M., & Creutzfeldt, O. (1988). Anterior ectosylvian visual area (AEV) of the cat: Physiological properties. *Progress in Brain Research, 75,* 245–255.

Bowman, E. M., & Olson, C. R. (1988). Visual and auditory association areas of the cat's posterior ectosylvian gyrus: Cortical afferents. *Journal of Comparative Neurology, 272,* 30–42.

Burton, H., & Kopf, E. (1984). Ipsilateral cortical connections from the second and fourth somatic sensory areas in the cat. *Journal of Comparative Neurology, 225,* 527–553.

Clarey, J. C., & Irvine, D. R. F. (1990a). The anterior ectosylvian sulcal auditory field in the cat: I. An electrophysiological study of its relationship to surrounding auditory cortical fields. *Journal of Comparative Neurology, 301,* 289–303.

Clarey, J. C., & Irvine, D. R. F. (1990b). The anterior ectosylvian sulcal auditory field in the cat: II. A horseradish perox-

idase study of its thalamic and cortical connections. *Journal of Comparative Neurology, 301,* 304–324.

Clemo, H. R., Dehner, L. R., & Meredith, M. A. (2000). Cross-modal circuitry of anterior ectosylvian sulcal (AES) cortex: II. Functional connections from auditory field AES to somatosensory SIV. *Society of Neuroscience Abstracts, 26,* 1221.

Clemo, H. R. H., Keniston, L. P., & Meredith, M. A. (2003). GABAergic neurons show similar distribution patterns within cortical areas representing different sensory modalities. *Journal of Chemical Neuroanatomy, 26,* 51–63.

Clemo, H. R., & Stein, B. E. (1982). Somatosensory cortex: A "new" somatotopic representation. *Brain Research, 235,* 162–168.

Clemo, H. R., & Stein, B. E. (1983). Organization of a fourth somatosensory area of cortex in cat. *Journal of Neurophysiology, 50,* 910–925.

Dehner, L. R., Clemo, H. R. H., & Meredith, M. A. (2000). Cross-modal circuitry of anterior ectosylvian sulcal (AES) cortex: I. Anatomical connections from auditory Field AES to somatosensory SIV. *Society of Neuroscience Abstracts, 26,* 1221.

Ebner, F. F., & Armstrong-James, M. A. (1990). Intracortical processes regulating the integration of sensory information. *Progress in Brain Research, 86,* 129–141.

Falchier, A., Clavagnier, C., Barone, P., & Kennedy, H. (2002). Anatomical evidence of multimodal integration in primate striate cortex. *Journal of Neuroscience, 22,* 5749–5759.

Gilbert, C. D. (1993). Circuitry, architecture, and functional dynamics of visual cortex. *Cerebral Cortex, 3,* 373–386.

Gilbert, C. D. (1998). Adult cortical dynamics. *Physiological Review, 78,* 467–485.

Jiang, H., Lepore, F., Ptito, M., & Guillemont, J. P. (1994a). Sensory modality distribution in the anterior ectosylvian cortex of cats. *Experimental Brain Research, 97,* 404–414.

Jiang, H., Lepore, F., Ptito, M., & Guillemont, J. P. (1994b). Sensory interactions in the anterior ectosylvian cortex of cats. *Experimental Brain Research, 101,* 385–396.

Jones, E. G., & Powell, T. P. S. (1970). An anatomical study of converging sensory pathways within the cerebral cortex of the monkey. *Brain, 93,* 793–820.

Kadunce, D. C., Vaughan, J. W., Wallace, M. T., Benedek, G., & Stein, B. E. (1997). Mechanisms of within- and cross-modality suppression in the superior colliculus. *Journal of Neurophysiology, 78,* 2834–2847.

Kimura, A., Hamada, Y., Kawai, Y., & Tamai, Y. (1996). Sensory response properties of cortical neurons in the anterior ectosylvian sulcus of cats: Intracellular recording and labeling. *Neuroscience Research, 26,* 357–367.

Korte, M., & Rauschecker, J. P. (1993). Auditory spatial tuning of cortical neurons is sharpened in cats with early blindness. *Journal of Neurophysiology, 70,* 1717–1721.

Meredith, M. A., & Clemo, H. R. (1989). Auditory cortical projection from the anterior ectosylvian sulcus (AES) to the superior colliculus in the cat: An anatomical and electrophysiological study. *Journal of Comparative Neurology, 289,* 687–707.

Meredith, M. A., Miller, L. F., Ramoa, A. S., Clemo, H. R. H., & Behan, M. (2001). Organization of neurons of origin of the descending output pathways from the ferret superior colliculus. *Neuroscience Research, 40,* 301–313.

Meredith, M. A., Nemitz, J. W., & Stein, B. E. (1987). Determinants of multisensory integration in superior colliculus neurons: I. Temporal factors. *Journal of Neuroscience, 7,* 3215–3229.

Meredith, M. A., & Stein, B. E. (1986). Visual, auditory, and somatosensory convergence on cells in the superior colliculus results in multisensory integration. *Journal of Neurophysiology, 56,* 640–662.

Meredith, M. A., & Stein, B. E. (1996). Spatial determinants of multisensory integration in cat superior colliculus neurons. *Journal of Neurophysiology, 75,* 1843–1857.

Minciacchi, D., Tassinari, G., & Antonini, A. (1987). Visual and somatosensory integration in the anterior ectosylvian sulcus. *Brain Research, 410,* 21–31.

Middlebrooks, J. C., Clock, A. E., Xu, L., & Green, D. M. (1994). A panoramic code for sound location by cortical neurons. *Science, 264,* 842–844.

Mucke, L., Norita, M., Benedek, G., & Creutzfeldt, O. (1982). Physiologic and anatomic investigation of a visual cortical area situated in the ventral bank of the anterior ectosylvian sulcus of the cat. *Experimental Brain Research, 46,* 1–11.

Nelken, I., BarYosef, O., & Rotman, Y. (1997). Responses of field AES neurons to virtual space stimuli. *Society of Neuroscience Abstracts, 23,* 2071.

Olson, C. R., & Graybiel, A. M. (1983). An outlying visual area in the cerebral cortex of the cat. *Progress in Brain Research, 58,* 239–245.

Olson, C. R., & Graybiel, A. M. (1987). Ectosylvian visual area of the cat: Location, retinotopic organization and connections. *Journal of Comparative Neurology, 261,* 277–294.

Palmer, L. A., Rosenquist, A. C., & Tusa, R. J. (1978). The retinotopic organization of lateral suprasylvian visual areas in the cat. *Journal of Comparative Neurology, 177,* 237–256.

Rauschecker, J. P. (1996), Substitution of visual by auditory inputs in the cat's anterior ectosylvian cortex. *Progress in Brain Research, 112,* 313–323.

Raushchecker, J. P., & Korte, M. (1993). Auditory compensation for early blindness in cat cerebral cortex. *Journal of Neuroscience, 13,* 4538–4548.

Richter, K., Hess, A., & Scheich, H. (1999). Functional mapping of transsynaptic effects of local manipulation of inhibition in gerbil auditory cortex. *Brain Research, 831,* 184–199.

Scannell, J. W., Sengpiel, F., Tovee, M., Benson, P. J., Blakemore, C., & Young, M. P. (1996). Visual motion processing in the anterior ectosylvian sulcus of the cat. *Journal of Neurophysiology, 76,* 895–907.

Schroeder, C. E., & Foxe, J. J. (2002). The timing and laminar profile of converging inputs to multisensory areas of the macaque neocortex. *Brain Research: Cognitive Brain Research, 14,* 187–198.

Schroeder, C. E., Lindsley, R. W., Specht, C., Marcovici, A., Smiley, J. F., & Javitt, D. C. (2001). Somatosensory input to auditory association cortex in the macaque monkey. *Journal of Neurophysiology, 85,* 1322–1327.

Seltzer, B., & Pandya, D. N. (1994). Parietal, temporal, and occipital projections to cortex of the superior temporal sulcus in the rhesus monkey: A retrograde tracer study. *Journal of Comparative Neurology, 343,* 445–463.

Stein, B. E., & Meredith, M. A. (1993). *The merging of the senses.* Cambridge, MA: MIT Press.

Wallace, M. T., Meredith, M. A., & Stein, B. E. (1992). Integration of multiple sensory modalities in cat cortex. *Experimental Brain Research, 91,* 484–488.

Wallace, M. T., Meredith, M. A., & Stein, B. E. (1993). Converging influences from visual, auditory, and somatosensory cortices onto output neurons of the superior colliculus. *Journal of Neurophysiology, 69,* 1797–1809.

Wallace, M. T., Wilkinson, L. K., & Stein, B. E. (1996). Representation and integration of multiple sensory inputs in primate superior colliculus, *Journal of Neurophysiology, 76,* 1246–1266.

Wang, J., Caspary, D., & Salvi, R. J. (2000). GABA-A antagonist causes dramatic expansion of tuning in primary auditory cortex. *NeuroReport, 11,* 1137–1140.

Young, M. P., Scannell, J. W., & Burns, G. (1995). *The analysis of cortical connectivity.* New York: Springer.

22 Multisensory-Evoked Potentials in Rat Cortex

DANIEL S. BARTH AND BARBARA BRETT-GREEN

Introduction

Although the experience of our different sensory modalities is unique, the brain integrates information across modalities to form a coherent picture of the environment, enhancing our existence and survival. Numerous perceptual studies in humans have demonstrated that stimulation in one sensory modality can alter the response to stimulation in another sensory modality (Welch & Warren, 1986). However, noninvasive evoked potential recording is one of the few means available to study the neurophysiology of human multisensory integration.

Original evoked potential work by Walter demonstrated that large regions of the human cortex are responsive to multiple types of sensory stimulation (Walter, 1965). In addition, it was shown that the simultaneous presentation of stimuli in two different sensory modalities produces significantly larger evoked responses than unimodal stimulation, concurrent with a reduced reaction time on behavioral tests (Andreassi & Greco, 1975; Cigánek, 1966; Hershenson, 1962; Morrell, 1968; Nickerson, 1973). Currently, event-related potentials are being used to study features of multisensory integration, confirming and extending the earlier results (Aunon & Keirn, 1990; Costin, Neville, et al., 1991; Fort, Delpuech, et al., 2002a, 2002b; Foxe, Morocz, et al., 2000; Foxe, Wylie, et al., 2002; Giard & Peronnet, 1999; Hansen & Hillyard, 1983; Kenemans, Kok, et al., 1993; Molholm, Ritter, et al., 2002; Naatanen, Paavilainen, et al., 1993). Yet the interpretation of human multisensory-evoked potential studies is limited by a lack of basic understanding about the neurogenesis of these responses. Thus, there is a need to conduct invasive multisensory-evoked potential studies in animals to provide an essential bridge to understanding the physiological basis of similar phenomena recorded noninvasively in the extracranial human response.

Early evoked potential mapping studies in animals began this task by systematically mapping evoked responses from numerous cortical locations and defining putative multisensory cortex, typically corresponding to regions where unimodal responses converged or overlapped (Berman, 1961a, 1961b; Bignall & Imbert, 1969; Bignall & Singer, 1967; Thompson, Johnson, et al., 1963; Thompson, Smith, et al., 1963; Woolsey, 1967; Woolsey & Fairman, 1946). With the introduction of the microelectrode, multisensory electrophysiology became increasingly focused on information obtainable through single-cell and unit recording. Although this research has led to the discovery of individual multisensory neurons in the cortex and other structures, as well as to the establishment of many basic principles governing multisensory integration (for a review, see Stein & Meredith, 1993), the reliance on recording from single cells or small groups of cells has biased our understanding of these phenomena toward single-cell response properties and away from how larger populations of cells may participate in multisensory integration. Thus, multisensory-evoked potential studies in animals not only provide a method for establishing the neurogenesis of similar population responses in humans, they also provide another essential link, that between the multisensory responses of single cells and those of larger cellular aggregates. In this way, evoked potentials permit exploration of the spatiotemporal properties of multisensory integration in wide areas of multisensory cortex and functional delineation of the location and borders of both multisensory and unimodal cortex for more detailed electrophysiological and anatomical investigation.

Although the closest animal model in which to study the electrophysiology of human multisensory integration is the monkey (Schroeder & Foxe, 2002; Schroeder, Lindsley, et al., 2001), there is growing interest in evoked potential analysis of multisensory integration in rat (Barth, Goldberg, et al., 1995; Brett-Green, Walsh, et al., 2000; Di, Brett, et al., 1994; Mirmiran, Brenner, et al., 1986; Ramachandran, Wallace, et al., 1993; Toldi, Fehér, et al., 1986) and cat (Toldi, Fehér, et al., 1984; Toldi, Rojik, et al., 1981) cortex, where the functional anatomy of multisensory-evoked responses may be studied in a more thoroughly understood nervous system and tentatively extrapolated to higher mammals.

357

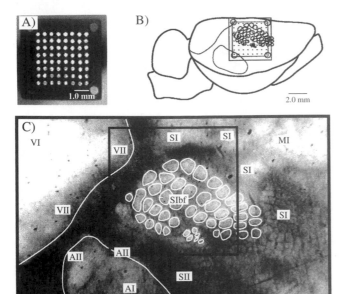

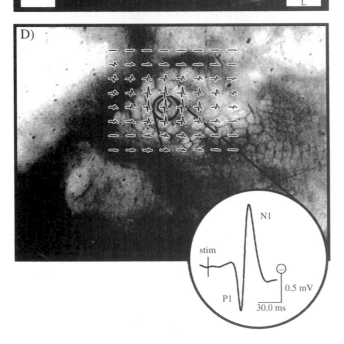

In this chapter we describe new methods for high spatial resolution mapping of unimodal and multisensory-evoked potentials in rat cortex. We demonstrate how these new methods can be used to identify cortical regions that are uniquely responsive to multisensory stimulation, and how the locus of putative multisensory-zones may be defined relative to the cortical anatomy revealed with cytochrome oxidase staining. Finally, we discuss preliminary results obtained with multisensory-evoked-potential-guided intracellular recording and anatomical tracing, which has implications for discriminating the functional anatomy of thalamocortical multisensory integration in the rat and perhaps in higher species, including man.

High-resolution cortical mapping of unimodal evoked potentials

Electrophysiological identification of the locus and limits of multisensory cortex, particularly in smaller species such as the rodent, has been constrained by the presumably small size of these zones and the difficulty of searching for multisensory-evoked responses with single electrodes. We have therefore developed methods for high spatial resolution mapping of unimodal and multisensory-evoked potentials with multielectrode arrays placed directly on the cortical surface. In fact, epicortical mapping of sensory evoked potentials is particularly useful in lissencephalic cortex such as that of the rat, where a spatially continuous electrophysiological map of evoked responses may be obtained and correlated directly with the underlying anatomy in tangential cortical sections. To introduce these methods, Figure 22.1A depicts a typical recording array, which consists of an 8 × 8 grid of electrodes with 100-μm tip diameters and 0.5-mm spacing, covering a 3.5 × 3.5 mm

on the contralateral mystacial pad (highlighted with white outlines). Rostral and medial to SIbf are areas of primary somatosensory cortex (SI) representing other regions of the body and face. Other CO-rich areas are associated with primary auditory (AI) and visual (VI) cortex. Surrounding these primary areas and extending into the more lightly staining dysgranular cortex are secondary somatosensory (SII), auditory (AII), and visual (VII) cortex. Primary motor cortex (MI) may also be seen in the rostromedial region of this section. (D) The somatosensory-evoked potential (SEP) evoked by displacement of a single contralateral vibrissa is of largest amplitude over the cortical column representing that vibrissa in SIbf (highlighted with a black outline). An enlargement of the primary SEP (insert) consists of a biphasic positive/negative slow wave with amplitude peaks referred to as P1 and N1, to reflect their surface polarity and sequence of occurrence.

FIGURE 22.1 High resolution mapping of sensory-evoked potentials from the cortical surface. (A) A typical 8 × 8 grid of electrodes with 100-μm tips and 0.5-mm center spacing covers 3.5 × 3.5 mm. Holes machined into the perimeter of the array permit placement of fiducial marks in the cortex after a recording session for subsequent correlation of electrode positions with underlying anatomy. (B) A single placement of the array is sufficient to record from primary and secondary regions of a given sensory modality. In this example, the array is positioned above the vibrissal representation of primary somatosensory cortex (SIbf). (C) A similar recording area (square box) is superimposed on a flattened hemisphere that has been stained with cytochrome oxidase (CO) and tangentially sectioned through layer IV to reveal the somatotopic organization of SIbf, corresponding to the pattern of vibrissae

area of the cortical surface in a single placement (Fig. 22.1*B*). Holes machined into the perimeter of some arrays permit placement of fiducial marks in the cortex for subsequent alignment of electrodes with the cortical anatomy.

In this example, the array has been placed over the vibrissa representation of primary somatosensory cortex (SI). This area is unique in that there is a somatotopic organization of cortical columns in spatial register with afferent input from individual vibrissae on the contralateral mystacial pad (Tracey, 1985). Furthermore, this area may be visualized in flattened tangential sections of cortical layer IV stained with cytochrome oxidase (CO) (Land & Simons, 1985; Wong-Riley & Welt, 1980) (Fig. 22.1*C*). Areas of layer IV granular cortex (white) that receive dense thalamocortical input exhibit high CO reactivity, whereas intervening regions of dysgranular cortex (black) that receive more sparse thalamocortical input exhibit low CO reactivity. The barrel-like pattern of CO staining apparent in the vibrissa region of SI is labeled SIbf (primary somatosensory cortex, barrel field). SIbf is flanked on its rostral and medial borders by other body representations of primary somatosensory cortex (Fig. 22.1*C*; SI) and laterally by secondary somatosensory cortex (Fig. 22.1*C*; SII). Lateral to SII is primary auditory cortex (Fig. 22.1*C*; AI), which is surrounded by secondary auditory or belt cortex (Fig. 22.1*C*; AII). In the most caudal and medial locations of the hemisphere, primary visual cortex (VI) is surrounded by secondary visual cortex (VII). High CO reactivity has also been shown to colocalize with the primary auditory and visual cortices (Wallace, 1987). Finally, primary motor cortex (MI) is located in the most rostral and medial region of the template. Although far more detailed and precise delineations of the organization of rat cortex have been published (see Chapin & Lin, 1990, for a review), the anatomical template and nomenclature shown in Figure 22.1*C* will be used in this chapter for simplicity.

When the surface array is placed above SIbf, transient stimulation of a single vibrissa evokes a highly stereotyped cortical response that is of greatest amplitude over the appropriate barrel (Fig. 22.1*D*). Yet the somatosensory evoked potential (SEP) is distributed over a wider region than just the principal barrel. Volume-conducted currents are unlikely to contribute significantly to this spatial distribution, insofar as recent studies in SIbf with optical imaging, a technique that is not affected by volume currents, reveal similar spatial distributions of responsive cortex (Brett, Chen-Bee, et al., 1997, 2001). The SEP consists of a positive/negative slow wave sequence whose amplitude peaks are referred to as P1 and N1, reflecting their polarity and

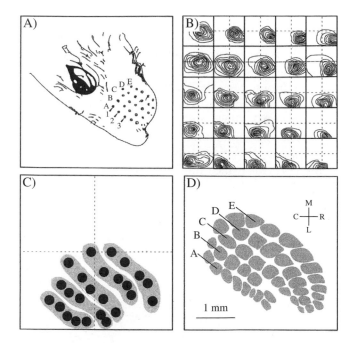

FIGURE 22.2   Topographic mapping of the P1 evoked by individually stimulating each of the 25 major vibrissae provides a rapid functional verification of the location, extent, and orientation of SIbf that is useful for consistent alignment of the electrode array across animals and experiments. (*A*) The rows of vibrissae are labeled with letters and the columns with numbers. (*B*) Isopotential maps of the initial P1 of the SEP systematically shift position according to the vibrissa stimulated. (*C*) A composite plot of the maximum amplitude of each single vibrissa SEP reveals the underlying locations of corresponding cortical columns in SIbf. (*D*) A template of these columns has been labeled according to the somatotopic representation of the contralateral vibrissae for comparison with the electrophysiological map.

order of occurrence (Fig. 22.1*D*, insert). The evoked potential is highly localized at the onset of the SEP, providing a spatial resolution capable of discriminating activity within individual cortical columns. Thus, isopotential maps of the initial P1 wave generated by single vibrissa stimulation may provide a complete functional map of SIbf (Fig. 22.2) that is useful for consistently aligning the array across animals and experiments, eliminating the need for reliance on stereotaxic coordinates or anatomical landmarks.

Neurogenesis of the P1/N1 slow wave

Before exploring unique evoked responses to multisensory stimulation, it is instructive to briefly examine the morphology and neurogenesis of unimodal responses, because these responses have been more thoroughly investigated. The P1/N1 wave of the SEP is quite similar to the auditory-evoked potential (AEP) and the visual-evoked potential (VEP) recorded over the auditory and visual cortices, respectively. The P1/N1 wave is considered an archetypal response sequence (Steriade, 1984) that reflects the systematic vertical cascade of excitation of lamina-specific cell populations upon the arrival of afferent input, regardless of the sensory modality in which it is elicited (Barth & Di, 1990; Di, Baumgartner, et al., 1990; Mitzdorf, 1985). This cascade of excitation is best visualized in laminar recordings obtained using a linear array of electrodes that is inserted perpendicular to the cortical surface until the top electrode is flush. To spatially resolve the laminar locations of extracellular current sinks and sources (transmembrane currents) along the axis of the linear electrode array, spatially smoothed current source density (CSD; Mitzdorf, 1985; Nicholson & Freeman, 1975; Rappelsberger, Pockberger, et al., 1981; Vaknin, DiScenna, et al., 1988) is typically computed according to the method of Vaknin et al. (1988), using the following equation (Rappelsberger et al., 1981):

with only two independent components (Fig. 22.3C), reflecting a vertically oriented current dipole in the supragranular (Fig. 22.3E) and infragranular (Fig. 22.3G) layers, and with component scores reflecting the P1 (Fig. 22.3D) and N1 (Fig. 22.3F), respectively. P1 therefore appears to reflect depolarization of the proximal apical dendrites of supragranular pyramidal cells, either by direct or indirect (via layer IV stellate cells) thalamocortical projections, whereas N1 reflects depolarization of the distal apical dendrites of predominantly infragranular pyramidal cells, probably by way of intracortical projections. This sequence closely resembles the classic type A and C activation patterns noted in cat primary visual cortex (Mitzdorf, 1985). Analogous sequential and hierarchical models for the processing of thalamic input to the cortex have also emerged from single-unit studies of sensory receptive field properties (Hubel & Wiesel, 1968; Simons, 1978). P1 is attenuated or absent during intracortical activation from the direct

$$\frac{\mathrm{d}^2\phi}{\mathrm{d}z^2} = \frac{0.23\ \phi\ (z-2h) + 0.08\ \phi\ (z-h) - 0.62\ \phi\ (z) + 0.08\ \phi\ (z+h) + 0.23\ \phi\ (z+2h)}{h^2}$$

This equation expresses CSD as the second spatial derivative of the smoothed values of potential (Ø) measured in 150-μm increments (h) along an axis (z) perpendicular to the cortical surface. In addition, principal components analysis (PCA) may used to separate independent sources of covariance in the CSD across the laminar electrodes (Ruchkin, Villegas, et al., 1964; Barth, Di, et al., 1988). A physiological interpretation of PCA in this application is that the principal components represent separate cellular populations that project distinct spatial patterns of CSD onto the laminar electrode array. The principal component loadings reflect these spatial patterns, or how each identified cellular population makes a weighted contribution to the CSD recorded at each electrode. The principal component scores reflect the time course and polarity of CSD in each cellular population as it contributes to the recorded signal. Typically the first two principal components account for more than 90% of the variance of laminar CSD profile.

Both P1 and N1 recorded at the cortical surface reverse polarity in the depth (Fig. 22.3A), indicating that they are generated by vertically oriented current dipoles formed by synchronized postsynaptic activation of the parallel apical dendrites of pyramidal cells (Nicholson, 1979). Yet the laminar spatiotemporal pattern is more complex than a single polarity reversal, suggesting that multiple pyramidal cell populations are activated. PCA models the data (Fig. 22.3B) well

cortical response (Barth & Sutherling, 1988), by transcallosal activation from the contralateral hemisphere (Barth, Kithas, et al., 1994), or by cortical activation through nonspecific projections from the intralaminar nuclei of the thalamus that terminate in the uppermost as opposed to the middle layers (Barth & MacDonald, 1996). Although more complex intralaminar evoked potential patterns have been reported in other species, particularly in unanesthetized preparations (Givre, Schroeder, et al., 1994; Peterson, Schroeder, et al., 1995; Schroeder, 1995; Schroeder, Mehta, et al., 1998; Schroeder, Tenke, et al., 1991; Steinschneider, Tenke, et al., 1992), in the ketamine/xylazine anesthetized rat, the existence of P1 appears to be a distinct indicator of the cortical response to afferent input from the thalamus, a factor that will figure importantly in our interpretation of the functional anatomy of multisensory-evoked potentials in this preparation.

Evoked potential mapping of auditory and somatosensory cortex

Four placements of the 64-channel array in adjacent quadrants permits mapping of both unimodal and multisensory-evoked potentials from nearly an entire hemisphere (Figs. 22.4 to 22.7). Unimodal evoked potentials mapped from all 256 locations provide a detailed picture of the locus and limits of both primary and secondary sensory cortex, and also permit the

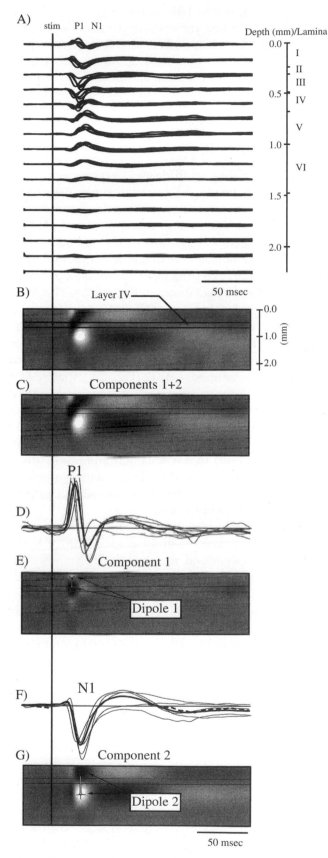

identification of small multisensory zones and their spatial relationship to, and partial overlap with, these larger unimodal cortical regions. For example, when a click stimulus is presented, the resulting AEP covers AI (Fig. 22.4A), but also spreads substantially into the belt of dysgranular cortex, including much of AII (Fig. 22.4A). At first glance, Figure 22.4A may give the impression that it would be impossible to distinguish AI from AII based on the AEP alone. However, because the AEP in AII is systematically delayed by approximately 4.0 ms compared with that of AI (Fig. 22.4B), spatiotemporal analysis may be used to separate their distinct spatial distributions (Di & Barth, 1993). A similar separation between SIbf and SII may be discriminated in the SEP evoked by silent transient simultaneous displacement of the 25 contralateral vibrissae (Fig. 22.4C). Again, the earliest and largest-amplitude response is in SIbf, but it extends well beyond these borders, into surrounding cortex, with an approximately 4.0 ms latency shift from the primary response. The delayed secondary response forms a spatially distinct pattern in the lateral region of the array over SII that is separated from the SIbf response region. Close examination of the AEP and SEP mapped in this way reveals substantial spatial overlap between the unimodal responses in

sequential activation of supra- and infragranular pyramidal cells. (A) Superimposed laminar recordings of the evoked potentials from five animals. CSD of P1 and N1 reverse polarity at depth, indicating that they are generated by vertically oriented current dipoles in the gray matter. This dipole pattern is typical for synchronous postsynaptic potentials imposed on the apical dendrites of both supra- and infragranular pyramidal cells. (B) Gray-scale maps of the laminar CSD averaged across animals indicate that the surface positivity (current source, white) of P1 is associated with a layer IV negativity (current sink, black), whereas the surface negativity (current sink, black) of the later N1 is associated with a layer V + VI negativity (current sink, black). (C) PCA accounts for more than 90% of the system variance with only two components. (D) Scores for the first component reflect the timing of P1. (E) Reconstruction of the first component indicates a vertically oriented dipole confined to the supragranular layers, reflecting depolarization of the proximal apical dendrites of supragranular pyramidal cells either directly or indirectly (via excitatory stellate cells) by thalamocortical afferent fibers preferentially terminating in the middle cortical laminae. (F) The subsequent surface negativity of N1 is reflected in the scores of the second component. (G) The N1 component indicates a vertically oriented dipole spanning both the infra- and supragranular layers, probably resulting from depolarization of the distal ends of apical dendrites of predominantly infragranular pyramidal cells via intralaminar axonal projections. This intralaminar cascade of excitation is typical for evoked potentials in any area of sensory cortex, with P1 distinctly representing initial thalamocortical as opposed to intracortical or interhemispheric activation.

FIGURE 22.3 Laminar current source density (CSD) recording of the P1/N1 complex indicates that it is produced by

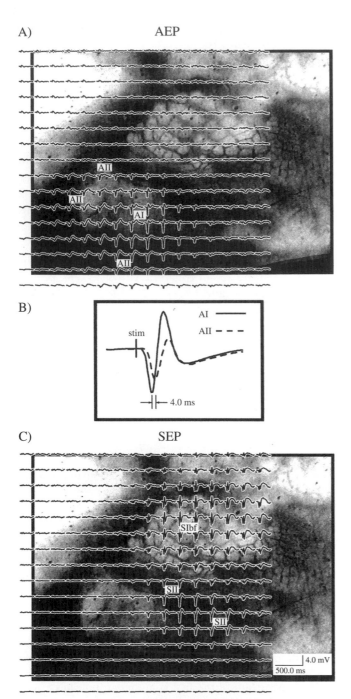

A) AEP

AII

AII

AI

AII

B)

stim

AI ———
AII - - - -

|— 4.0 ms

C) SEP

SIbf

SII

SII

4.0 mV
500.0 ms

FIGURE 22.4 Unimodal auditory- and somatosensory-evoked potentials (AEP and SEP, respectively) mapped from 256 sites in the right hemisphere correspond to the location and extent of both primary and secondary sensory cortex. (*A*) The AEP produced by click stimuli is of largest amplitude over AI, but may also be seen in surrounding areas of auditory belt cortex or AII. (*B*) Contributions from AI and AII to the AEP may be easily separated by spatiotemporal analysis because of a systematic delay of the AII response by approximately 4.0 ms. (*C*) A similar map of the SEP evoked by simultaneous silent stimulation of all 25 major vibrissae is of largest amplitude and earliest poststimulus latency above SIbf. A spatially separate and longer latency response may also be seen over SII.

each condition, particularly in the regions of SII and AII that extend along the dysgranular zone separating AI and SIbf. A large number of cells in this region may therefore be expected to respond to either auditory or somatosensory stimuli, and perhaps to respond uniquely to a combination of both.

*Evoked potential mapping
of multisensory cortex*

To test for unique multisensory responsiveness, we compared the results of simultaneously presenting both auditory and somatosensory stimuli, producing an auditory/somatosensory-evoked potential (ASEP), with the summed distributions of the unimodal AEP and SEP. Whole hemisphere mapping of the ASEP (Fig. 22.5*A*) appears as expected from the simple sum of the AEP and SEP responses shown in Figure 22.4. The ASEP covers all of SIbf, SII, AI, and AII and is of particularly large amplitude in the region of overlap between the unimodal AII and SII responses. Indeed, a linear model of the ASEP (Fig. 22.5*B*, ASEPmod), computed by adding the unimodal AEP (Fig. 22.4*A*) and SEP (Fig. 22.4*C*), appears identical to the actual ASEP complex. However, subtraction of each waveform of the ASEPmod from corresponding waveforms of the actual ASEP complex reveals a difference waveform (Fig. 22.6, ASEPdif) that is of largest amplitude where AII and SII responses overlap. Thus, there is a unique and spatially localized response to multisensory stimulation that is nonlinear and cannot be anticipated from the unimodal responses alone. We label the area of nonlinear response the multisensory zone, or MZas, to reflect its specialized multisensory response characteristics to combined auditory and somatosensory stimulation.

Similar results may be obtained for combined auditory and visual stimulation (Fig. 22.7). Here, auditory stimulation is again limited to simple clicks, and visual stimulation is provided by a strobe light located in a separate room with fiber-optic cable used to transmit the light flash to the animal. This effort is mandated by the need to provide absolutely silent visual stimulation. The combined auditory-visual-evoked response (Fig. 22.7*A*; AVEP) consists of an AEP with similar spatiotemporal distribution to that of Figure 22.4*A*, combined with the flash-evoked VEP covering all of VI and VII. Again, the AVEP complex is not the same as a linear sum of the unimodal AEP and VEP, and yields a difference waveform (Fig. 22.7*B*) that indicates two additional multisensory zones (Fig. 22.7*B*; MZav), one in the medial region of VII and a more lateral zone overlapping caudal AII.

A) ASEP

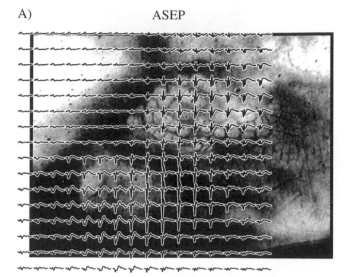

B) ASEP_{mod}

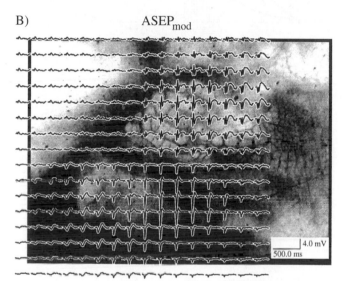

FIGURE 22.5 Multisensory responses evoked by combined auditory and somatosensory stimulation (ASEP) approximate that expected from the linear sum of the AEP and SEP evoked separately. (*A*) The ASEP covers all areas of SIbf, SII, AI, and AII. (*B*) The ASEP is similar to a model computed as the sum of the unimodal AEP and SEP (ASEPmod) depicted in Figure 22.4. However, the spatiotemporal distribution of the ASEP differs from the model, particularly in the region of dysgranular cortex separating auditory and somatosensory cortex, where the spatial distributions of the unimodal AEP and SEP overlap the most.

Intracellular correlates
of multisensory-evoked potentials

Although surface-recorded evoked potentials are quite useful for identifying and localizing multisensory zones, they tell us little about the cellular generation of nonlinear multisensory responses. To achieve this, we have recently developed a method for mapping extracellular

ASEP_{dif}

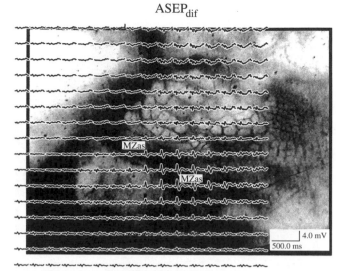

FIGURE 22.6 Subtraction of the ASEP from the ASEPmod produces a difference waveform (ASEPdif), reflecting a region of nonlinear response to multisensory stimulation that defines a multisensory zone for these modalities (MZas). MZas extends along the diagonal band of dysgranular cortex separating AI from SIbf and is approximately concentric with the area where unimodal responses from AII and SII maximally overlap.

field potentials at the surface concurrently with intracellular responses in vivo. This is achieved using a specially designed surface array with split leads and a centralized access hole through which microelectrodes can be lowered into the cortex (Fig. 22.8*A*). With this apparatus, preliminary surface mapping is used to functionally identify the precise locus for intracellular recording. Micropipettes can be similarly used with this apparatus to inject small quantities of anatomical tracers, thus revealing the morphology of cells participating in multisensory responses as well as the intracortical and thalamocortical circuits giving rise to these responses.

In the example of Figure 22.8, extracellular field potentials and intracellular potentials were recorded within MZas (see Fig. 22.6). Examining first the surface potentials recorded from an electrode immediately adjacent to the central access hole in the array, the classic P1/N1 wave of the unimodal AEP (Fig. 22.8*B*, thin trace) and SEP (Fig. 22.8*B*, thin trace) is apparent. It should be noted that even though these potentials were recorded from MZas and not directly from primary sensory cortex, they maintain a P1/N1 morphology suggestive of strong thalamocortical as opposed to intracortical activation. As seen in previous illustrations, the ASEP in this zone, evoked by simultaneous auditory and somatosensory stimulation (Fig. 22.8*D*, thin solid trace), is both larger in amplitude and of earlier

A)
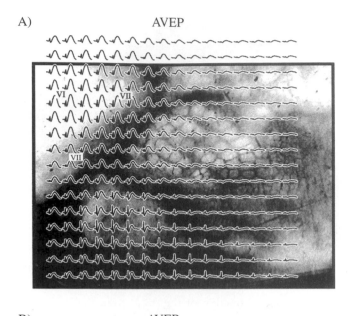
AVEP

B)
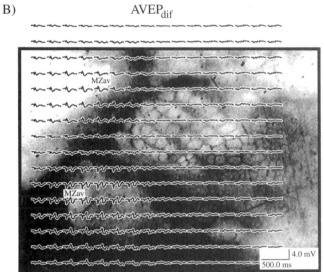
AVEP$_{dif}$

4.0 mV
500.0 ms

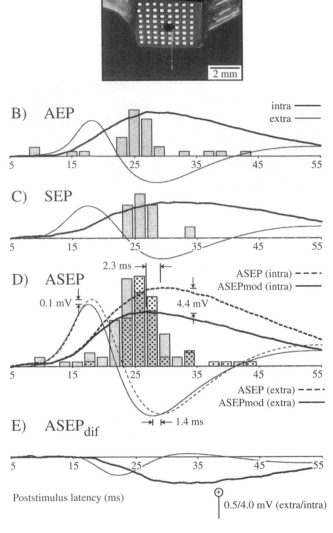

A)
2 mm

B) AEP
intra ——
extra ——

5   15   25   35   45   55

C) SEP

5   15   25   35   45   55

D) ASEP
2.3 ms →
↑
0.1 mV
4.4 mV
ASEP (intra) - - - -
ASEPmod (intra) ——

5   15   25   35   45   55

ASEP (extra) - - - -
ASEPmod (extra) ——
→ ← 1.4 ms

E) ASEP$_{dif}$

5   15   25   35   45   55

Poststimulus latency (ms)

⊕
0.5/4.0 mV (extra/intra)

FIGURE 22.7 Multisensory responses evoked by combined auditory and visual stimulation reveal two additional multisensory zones. (*A*) The auditory-visual response (AVEP) covers primary and secondary regions of both auditory and visual cortex in the caudal regions of the array. (*B*) Difference waveforms (AVEPdif), computed in the same way as for the ASEP, show two regions of nonlinear interaction during multisensory stimulation. These auditory-visual multisensory zones (MZav) are located in the medial region of VII and at the caudal border of AII, where AII and VII spatially overlap.

poststimulus latency than either unimodal stimulus. Again, a linear model waveform computed from the sum of the unimodal AEP and SEP (Fig. 22.8*D*, thin dashed trace) is of larger amplitude and longer poststimulus latency than the actual ASEP. It is this nonlinearity that yields the distinct difference waveform, or ASEPdif (Fig. 22.8*E*, thin trace), used to identify MZas from surface mapping alone.

FIGURE 22.8 Extracellular and intracellular multisensory response from MZas. (*A*) A 64-electrode surface array is modified with a central access hole through which intracellular microelectrodes can be lowered into the cortex. (*B*) The averaged extracellular unimodal AEP (thin trace) recorded from a surface electrode adjacent to the access hole shows a typical P1/N1 morphology. Simultaneously recorded postsynaptic potentials (PSPs, thick trace) in MZas are averaged by injecting QX-314, which blocks action potentials and permits averaging the intracellular PSP alone without contamination. The averaged PSP has a similar poststimulus onset latency and duration as the extracellular AEP and a peak amplitude corresponding to the peak of N1. In cells where QX-314 was not administered, poststimulus time histograms (PSTH; gray bars denote evoked multisensory responses; dotted bars denote sum of unimodal auditory and somatosensory responses) indicate a maximum firing probability at the rising crest of the PSP. (*C*) Same as *B*, but recorded in the same cells during somatosensory stimulation. (*D*) The extracellular ASEP (thin solid trace) is of earlier latency and larger amplitude than either of the unimodal responses in these cells. However, the

Intracellular recording reveals that nearly all cells we recorded within MZas are multisensory, that is, they respond with both postsynaptic potentials (PSPs) and action potentials (APs) to auditory, somatosensory, and combined auditory-somatosensory stimulation. Furthermore, as suggested by surface-evoked potential recording, their response to multisensory stimuli is enhanced and nonlinear. Both the AEP and SEP are associated with slow intracellular depolarization (Figs. 22.8B–E, thick traces) beginning at the onset of the surface response, peaking at the maximum of the surface NI, and returning to baseline at the same time as the termination of the surface N1. These intracellular traces represent an average of many responses across a number of animals. To obtain averages of PSPs alone that are uncontaminated by APs, the sodium channel blocker QX-314 is administered iontophoretically. QX-314 blocks APs but leaves PSPs unaffected (Connors & Prince, 1982), permitting direct comparison of intracellular PSPs to extracellular PSPs, which are the main contributors to potentials recorded at the cortical surface. However, if QX-314 is not applied, poststimulus time histograms (PSTH) revealing the temporal distribution of evoked action potentials (AP; Figs. 22.8B–D, bars) indicate maximum suprathreshold responses during the rising phase and crest of the averaged evoked PSPs. Similar to the extracellular record, the intracellular PSP produced by auditory-somatosensory stimulation (Fig. 22.8D, thick solid trace) is of larger amplitude and shorter poststimulus latency than either unimodal response, but is again nonlinear, in that it is of lower amplitude and shorter poststimulus latency (Fig. 22.8D, thick dashed trace) than that anticipated from the sum of the unimodal PSPs, resulting in an intracellular difference waveform (Fig. 22.8E, thick trace) that corresponds in latency and duration to that of the surface response. These differences are also reflected in the PSTH of the ASEP (Fig. 22.8D, gray bars). Combined stimulation elicited more numerous APs than either stimulus alone. The maximum number of APs elicited during combined stimulation did not differ noticeably from that predicted from the sum of the unimodal PSTHs (Fig. 22.8D, dotted bars); however, similar to the averaged EPSPs, the latency of the maximum was earlier.

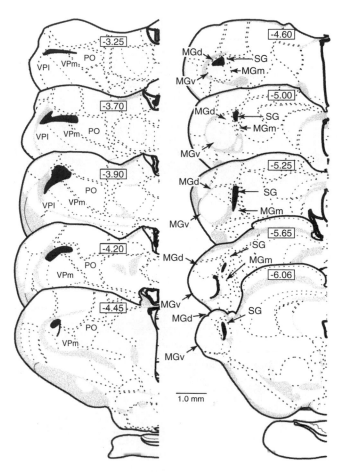

FIGURE 22.9 Retrograde labeling in coronal sections of the thalamus from WGA-HRP injections made into the caudal portion of MZas summarized across animals (n = 9). Cell bodies are labeled in both the somatosensory and auditory thalamocortical projection nuclei, including the ventral posterior medial nucleus (VPm), the ventral posterior lateral nucleus (VPl), and the ventral division of the medial geniculate nucleus (MGv). Cell bodies are also labeled in putative multisensory nuclei of the thalamus, including the posterior nucleus (PO), the suprageniculate nucleus (SG), and the dorsal and medial divisions of the medial geniculate (MGd, MGm).

Histological tracing of multisensory pathways

To obtain evidence concerning the anatomical circuitry underlying multisensory responses, we inject small quantities of tracers, again targeted by surface mapping of the evoked potential. Figures 22.9 and 22.10 show labeling in thalamus and cortex, respectively, when injections of WGA-HRP are made into portions of the MZas. Similar studies have not yet been performed in MZav. From initial results it is clear that the MZas represents a principal site of multisensory convergence of both thalamocortical and intracortical fiber paths. Subcortical labeling density (Fig. 22.9) is heavy in the somatosensory thalamus, including the posterior

---

ASEP is also of shorter latency and lower amplitude than the sum of the unimodal responses (thin dashed trace), showing nonlinear integration of the multisensory inputs. Similar results are seen for averaged multisensory PSPs (thick solid and dashed traces). (*E*) Nonlinear interactions in MZas produce difference waveforms for the extracellular (thin trace) and intracellular (thick trace) with similar onset latency and duration.

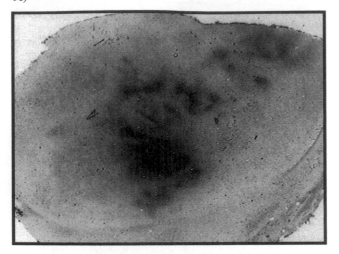

A)

B)

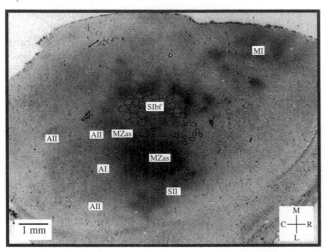

FIGURE 22.10 WGA-HRP labeling from an injection made into the MZas close to the posterior portion of SII (see Fig. 22.6). Part *A* depicts labeling alone, and part *B* includes a template of SIbf derived from a tangential cytochrome oxidase (CO)-stained section in the same animals. In this example, cell bodies and fibers are heavily labeled in the dysgranular region surrounding SIbf and in the septa between barrels, such that a barrel-like pattern may be discerned without examining sequential tangential section stained for CO. Portions of the dysgranular zone between SIbf and AI are also labeled in the region where SII and AII overlap (see Fig. 22.4). Additional staining is apparent in the motor cortex and in an additional lateral area, possibly the posterior lateral cortex.

nucleus (PO) and segments of the medial and lateral ventral posterior nucleus (VPm and VPl, respectively). Staining of cells is also observed in areas of acoustic thalamus, including the suprageniculate nucleus (SG) and limited sections of the dorsal, medial, and ventral divisions of the medial geniculate nucleus (MGd, MGm, and MGv, respectively).

We have found that intracortical connections to MZas are best viewed in tangential sections (Fig. 22.10). In this example, a large injection made in the MZas near the posterior portion of SII demonstrates that the MZas receives clear ipsilateral input from dysgranular regions of SIbf and from areas of AII and SII that extend beyond the borders of MZas defined by surface mapping (see Fig. 22.6) (However, it is apparent from unimodal maps of the AEP and SEP [see Fig. 22.4] that MZas also represents an area of overlap between AII and SII.) Additional staining is apparent in the motor cortex and in a lateral region, possibly the posterior lateral region (PL). Intracortical projections to MZas through the corpus callosum from a small (<1.0 mm) corresponding region of the contralateral hemisphere are also typically observed. Finally, although projections to MZas from distant areas of AI are not clear, MZas appears to overlap the most medial border of AI, and therefore may have direct access to auditory information from this region as well. We are continuing to explore the anatomy of MZas to further define its connectivity at both the cortical and subcortical levels.

Summary and conclusions

We have provided examples in this chapter that demonstrate the efficiency and accuracy of multichannel evoked potential mapping not only for determining the location and extent of unimodal cortex in the lissencephalic animal, but also for identifying smaller regions of putative multisensory cortex, based on their unique response to multisensory stimulation. We have also introduced preliminary data obtained from newly developed techniques using surface-evoked potentials to functionally target both intracellular recording and the injection of anatomical tracers to further examine the cellular generators and circuitry responsible for multisensory responses. Some features of rat MZas recall properties of the cat anterior ectosylvian sulcus (Wallace, Meredith, et al., 1992) and possibly portions of the superior temporal plane in both monkeys and humans (Foxe et al., 2000; Krubitzer, Clarey, et al., 1995; Pandya & Yeterian, 1985; Schroeder et al., 2001), regions that also exhibit auditory and somatosensory convergence. Although our results remain preliminary, several conclusions can be drawn concerning the neurogenesis of multisensory-evoked potentials in rat cortex.

The identification of multisensory zones from surface-recorded evoked potentials alone relies on determining spatially localized areas where the multisensory responses are unique and nonlinear. The nonlinearity of the multisensory responses has two important implications. First, the overlapping ASEP or AVEP complex is not simply an addition of volume-conducted currents of the otherwise unimodal responses at the cortical surface; volume-conducted currents sum linearly. Second, nonlinear difference waveforms suggest an active interaction between multisensory-responsive cells in the region of overlap during combined stimulation that is not recorded in other primary or secondary areas of sensory cortex. Multisensory cells in MZas and MZav must generate both subthreshold and suprathreshold responses to multisensory input that are quite different from the simple sum of their responses to unimodal stimulation. Nonlinear interactions during multisensory stimulation like those described here have been reported in other studies (Foxe et al., 2000; Giard & Peronnet, 1999; Molholm et al., 2002; Toldi & Fehér, 1984; Toldi et al., 1981, 1984, 1986) suggesting that this feature of the evoked potential may be useful for identifying and localizing multisensory cortex in recordings performed in other species, including man.

With simultaneous intra- and extracellular recording, we have begun to obtain insights into cellular mechanisms producing multisensory-evoked potentials. Nearly all cells we have recorded in MZas (other multisensory zones have not yet been similarly studied) respond to both auditory and somatosensory stimuli, and yet respond uniquely when the stimuli are presented simultaneously—evidence of true multisensory integration. This intracellular pattern is not seen from cells within the primary sensory regions, which show preference for a given sensory modality. Whether cells in multisensory cortex can be identified as a distinct type that differs from cells in either primary or secondary unimodal cortex or are distinguishable only by their unique connectivity remains to be determined.

Multisensory cells show enhanced and shorter latency responses during the ASEP. They therefore appear to integrate PSPs from the separate auditory and somatosensory pathways. The fact that this multisensory response is also nonlinear indicates that the difference waveform of the surface ASEP is produced by nonlinear addition of PSPs evoked by the separate modalities. There are several possible explanations for nonlinearities recorded intracellularly. Amplitude attenuation of combined PSPs may be due to lower effective membrane resistance from multiple active synapses (Koch, Poggio, et al., 1983; Kogo & Ariel, 1999; Lev-Tov, Miller, et al., 1983; Shepherd & Koch, 1990). Additionally, PSPs produced by each unimodal input may temporarily drive the membrane potential toward the reversal potential. Ionic driving forces of multisensory PSPs may therefore be less than the linear sum of forces underlying those evoked separately by unimodal

stimuli (Kuno & Miyahara, 1969; Lev-Tov et al., 1983), resulting in nonlinear or "sublinear" (Shepherd & Koch, 1990) summation observed here. Additionally, there may be a contribution of N-methyl-D-aspartate (NMDA) receptors to nonlinear multisensory responsiveness in these cells. NMDA receptors have been strongly implicated in nonlinear amplification of event-related potential components (Javitt, Steinschneider, et al., 1996) and in nonlinear components of multisensory integration in other studies (Binns & Salt, 1996). Finally, occlusion and facilitation of multisensory responses have also been attributed to changes in the relative balances between excitatory and inhibitory influences on multisensory cells by combined stimulation (Toldi et al., 1984), a balance that may be sensitive to the spatial register between auditory and somatosensory stimuli (Stein & Wallace, 1996; Wallace et al., 1992). Although auditory and somatosensory stimuli were in approximate spatial register in the study described here, systematic manipulation of this parameter and its effect on both intracellular responses as well as on multisensory-evoked potentials will be essential for further elucidating the topographic organization of multisensory cortex.

Intracellular injections of anatomical tracers targeted by surface-evoked potential mapping have begun to provide insights into the connectivity of multisensory cortex that make these areas unique. Yet these results have also raised several fundamental questions. It is not yet clear whether multisensory cortex is distinct from secondary sensory cortex or is simply a region where the secondary cortical areas from multiple sensory modalities spatially overlap. Our evidence from histological analysis of MZas would seem to favor the latter conclusion. Like classic secondary sensory cortex, MZas is reciprocally connected to primary sensory cortex. It is also densely interconnected to homologous regions in the contralateral hemisphere, a characteristic that is in accordance with established preferential commissural connections between dysgranular as opposed to granular cortex (Akers & Killackey, 1978; Olavarria, Van Sluyters, et al., 1984; Wise & Jones, 1978; Záborszky & Wolff, 1982). Patterns of thalamocortical connectivity to MZas are not unlike what would be expected from projections typically attributed to SII (VPM, VPL, and PO) or AII (MGv, MGm, and SG). However, it is clear from the spatial distributions of unimodal and multisensory-evoked potential maps that, whereas MZas may share patterns of connectivity that are typically associated with secondary sensory cortex, it appears to be only a subset of these secondary regions; unimodal evoked responses in AII and SII extend well beyond the borders of MZas. Furthermore, although interhemispheric connections are thought to characterize secondary cortex in general, previous studies of commissurally evoked potentials in the rat (Barth et al., 1994) have shown the strongest responses to be within a subregion of dysgranular cortex corresponding approximately to caudal region of MZas. The caudal MZas therefore appears to be one of the least lateralized areas of parietotemporal cortex in the rat, possibly establishing a bilateral spatial representation of multisensory receptive fields.

The combination of anatomical and electrophysiological results described here for MZas raises questions about the relative influence of intracortical as opposed to thalamocortical pathways on multisensory integration. Although MZas must integrate unimodal auditory and somatosensory information arriving through intracortical pathways, the thalamus is a direct source of input as well. Thalamocortical projections suggest a convergence in MZas of unimodal projections from VPM, VPL, and MGv. However, the distinct multisensory evoked potentials in MZas may also reflect influences of a multisensory pathway arising from PO, MGm, and SG, thalamic nuclei that are known to have multisensory response characteristics. Interestingly, the morphology of the multisensory ASEP is quite similar to the AEP or SEP, with a clear P1/N1 slow wave complex. This morphology suggests that, like the unimodal response, multisensory responses are dominated by thalamocortical as opposed to intracortical projections, at least in the anesthetized animal. The possibility that multisensory responses are strongly influenced by parallel projections from the thalamus should not be that surprising in light of previous work in auditory cortex indicating that AEP in AI and AII can be evoked independently by stimulating subnuclei of the medial geniculate, with little apparent influence of established intracortical projections between these cortical regions (Di & Barth, 1992). Again, these results were obtained in anesthetized animals. In the unanesthetized preaparation, intracortical responses may have a much stronger influence on the evoked potential complex. Perhaps multisensory cortex should not be viewed as a place of hierarchical convergence, where unimodal afferent flow passes first from thalamus to unimodal cortex and is then secondarily integrated in multisensory cortex by way of intracortical pathways. Instead, multisensory cortex appears to be a place of dense parallel convergence between intracortical, interhemispheric, and, significantly, unimodal and multisensory thalamocortical input. In all cases, connections are reciprocal, suggesting that multisensory cortex actively collaborates with both subcortical and cortical areas but is by no means an end-point where multisensory convergence is realized.

REFERENCES

Akers, R. M., & Killackey, H. P. (1978). Organization of corticocortical connections in the parietal cortex of the rat. *Journal of Comparative Neurology, 181,* 513–538.

Andreassi, J. L., & Greco, J. R. (1975). Effects of bisensory stimulation on reaction time and the evoked cortical potential. *Physiological Psychology, 3,* 189–194.

Aunon, J. I., & Keirn, Z. A. (1990). On intersensory evoked potentials. *Biomedical Sciences Instrumentation, 26,* 33–39.

Barth, D. S., & Di, S. (1990). Three dimensional analysis of auditory evoked potentials in rat neocortex. *Journal of Neurophysiology, 64,* 1527–1536.

Barth, D. S., Di, S., et al. (1988). Principal component analysis of laminar currents produced by penicillin spikes in rat cortex. *Society for Neuroscience Abstracts, 14,* 6.

Barth, D. S., Goldberg, N., et al. (1995). The spatiotemporal organization of auditory, visual, and polysensory evoked potentials in rat cortex. *Brain Research, 678,* 177–180.

Barth, D. S., Kithas, J., et al. (1994). Anatomic organization of evoked potentials in rat parietotemporal cortex: Electrically evoked commissural responses. *Journal of Neurophysiology, 72,* 139–149.

Barth, D. S., & MacDonald, K. D. (1996). Thalamic modulation of high-frequency oscillating potentials in auditory cortex. *Nature, 383,* 78–81.

Barth, D. S., & Sutherling, W. W. (1988). Current source-density and neuromagnetic analysis of the direct cortical response in rat cortex. *Brain Research, 450,* 280–294.

Berman, A. L. (1961a). Overlap of somatic and auditory cortical response fields in anterior ectosylvian gyrus of cat. *Journal of Neurophysiology, 24,* 595–607.

Berman, A. L. (1961b). Interaction of cortical responses to somatic and auditory stimuli in anterior ectosylvian gyrus of cat. *Journal of Neurophysiology, 24,* 608–620.

Bignall, K. E., & Imbert, M. (1969). Polysensory and corticocortical projections to frontal lobe of squirrel and rhesus monkeys. *Electroencephalography and Clinical Neurophysiology, 26,* 206–215.

Bignall, K. E., & Singer, P. (1967). Auditory, somatic and visual input to association and motor cortex of the squirrel monkey. *Experimental Neurology, 18,* 300–312.

Binns, K. E., & Salt, T. E. (1996). Importance of NMDA receptors for multimodal integration in the deep layers of the cat superior colliculus. *Journal of Neurophysiology, 75,* 920–930.

Brett, B., Chen-Bee, C., et al. (1997). Intrinsic signal optical imaging of sensory evoked activity in rat parietal-temporal cortex. *Society of Neuroscience Abstracts, 23,* 2343.

Brett-Green, B., Chen-Bee, C., et al. (2000). Comparing the functional representations of central and border whiskers in rat primary somatosensory cortex. *Journal of Neuroscience, 21,* 9944–9954.

Brett-Green, B., Walsh, K., et al. (2000). Polysensory cortex in the rat: Field potential mapping and intracellular recording. *Society of Neuroscience Abstracts, 26,* 1976.

Chapin, J. K., & Lin, C. S. (1990). The somatic sensory cortex of the rat. In B. Kolb & R. C. Tees (Eds.), *The cerebral cortex of the rat* (pp. 341–380). Cambridge, MA: MIT Press.

Cigánek, L. (1966). Evoked potentials in man: Interaction of sound and light. *Electroencephalography and Clinical Neurophysiology, 21,* 28–33.

Connors, B. W., & Prince, D. A. (1982). Effects of local anesthetic QX-314 on the membrane properties of hippocampal pyramidal neurons. *Journal of Pharmacology and Experimental Therapeutics, 220,* 476–481.

Costin, D., Neville, H. J., et al. (1991). Rules of multisensory integration and attention: ERP and behavioral evidence in humans. *Society of Neuroscience Abstracts, 00,* 656.

Di, S., & Barth, D. S. (1992). The functional anatomy of middle latency auditory evoked potentials: Thalamocortical connections. *Journal of Neurophysiology, 68,* 425–431.

Di, S., & Barth, D. S. (1993). Binaural vs. monaural auditory evoked potentials in rat neocortex. *Brain Research, 630,* 303–314.

Di, S., Baumgartner, C., et al. (1990). Laminar analysis of extracellular field potentials in rat vibrissa/barrel cortex. *Journal of Neurophysiology, 63,* 832–840.

Di, S., Brett, B., et al. (1994). Polysensory evoked potentials in rat parietotemporal cortex: Auditory and somatosensory responses. *Brain Research, 64,* 267–280.

Fort, A., Delpuech, C., et al. (2002a). Dynamics of cortico-subcortical cross-modal operations involved in audio-visual object detection in humans. *Cerebral Cortex, 12,* 1031–1039.

Fort, A., Delpuech, C., et al. (2002b). Early auditory-visual interactions in human cortex during nonredundant target identification. *Brain Research: Cognitive Brain Research, 14,* 20–30.

Foxe, J., Morocz, I., et al. (2000). Multisensory auditory-somatosensory interactions in early cortical processing revealed by high density electrical mapping. *Cognitive Brain Research, 10,* 77–83.

Foxe, J. J., Wylie, G. R., et al. (2002). Auditory-somatosensory multisensory processing in auditory association cortex: An fMRI study. *Journal of Neurophysiology, 88,* 540–543.

Giard, M., & Peronnet, F., (1999). Auditory-visual integration during multimodal object recognition in humans: A behavioral and electrophysiological study. *Journal of Cognitive Neuroscience, 11,* 473–490.

Givre, S. J., Schroeder, C. E., et al. (1994). Contribution of extrastriate area V4 to the surface-recorded flash VEP in the awake macaque. *Vision Research, 34,* 415–428.

Hansen, J. C., & Hillyard, S. A. (1983). Selective attention to multidimensional auditory stimuli. *Journal of Experimental Psychology: Human Perception and Performance, 9,* 1–19.

Hershenson, M. (1962). Reaction time as a measure of intersensory facilitation. *Journal of Experimental Psychology, 63,* 289–293.

Hubel, D. H., & Wiesel, T. N. (1968). Receptive fields and functional architecture of monkey striate cortex. *Journal of Physiology (London), 195,* 215–243.

Javitt, D. C., Steinschneider, M., et al. (1996). Role of cortical N-methyl-D-aspartate receptors in auditory sensory memory and mismatch negativity generation: Implications for schizophrenia. *Proceedings of the National Academy of Sciences, USA, 93,* 11962–11967.

Kenemans, J. L., Kok, A., et al. (1993). Event related potentials to conjunction of spatial frequency and orientation as a function of stimulus parameters and response requirements. *Electroencephalography and Clinical Neurophysiology, 88,* 51–63.

Koch, C., Poggio, T., et al. (1983). Nonlinear interactions in a dendritic tree: Localization, timing, and role in information processing. *Proceedings of the National Academy of Sciences, USA, 80,* 2799–2802.

Kogo, N., & Ariel, M. (1999). Response attenuation during coincident afferent excitatory inputs. *Journal of Neurophysiology, 81,* 2945–2955.

Krubitzer, L., Clarey, J., et al. (1995). A redefinition of somatosensory areas in the lateral sulcus of macaque monkeys. *Journal of Neuroscience, 15,* 3821–3839.

Kuno, M., & Miyahara, J. (1969). Non-linear summation of unit synaptic potentials in spinal motoneurones of the cat. *Journal of Physiology (London), 201,* 465–477.

Land, P. W., & Simons, D. J. (1985). Cytochrome oxidase staining in the rat SmI barrel cortex. *Journal of Comparative Neurology, 238,* 225–235.

Lev-Tov, A., Miller, J., et al. (1983). Factors that control amplitude of EPSPs in dendritic neurons. *Journal of Neurophysiology, 50,* 399–412.

Mirmiran, M., Brenner, E., et al. (1986). Visual and auditory evoked potentials in different areas of rat cerebral cortex. *Neuroscience Letters, 72,* 272–276.

Mitzdorf, U. (1985). Current source-density method and application in cat cerebral cortex: Investigation of evoked potentials and EEG phenomena. *Physiological Review, 65,* 37–100.

Molholm, S., Ritter, W., et al. (2002). Multisensory auditory-visual interactions during early sensory processing in humans: A high-density electrical mapping study. *Brain Research: Cognitive Brain Research, 14,* 115–128.

Morrell, L. K. (1968). Sensory interaction: Evoked potential interaction in man. *Experimental Brain Research, 6,* 146–155.

Naatanen, R., Paavilainen, P., et al. (1993). Attention and mismatch negativity. *Psychophysiology, 30,* 436–450.

Nicholson, C. (1979). Generation and analysis of extracellular field potentials. *In Electrophysiological techniques: Society for Neuroscience short course* (pp. 93–149).

Nicholson, C., & Freeman, J. A. (1975). Theory of current source-density analysis and determination of conductivity tensor for anuran cerebellum. *Journal of Neurophysiology, 38,* 356–368.

Nickerson, R. S. (1973). Intersensory facilitation of reaction time. *Psychology Review, 80,* 489–509.

Olavarria, J., Van Sluyters, R. C., et al. (1984). Evidence for the complementary organization of callosal and thalamic connections within rat somatosensory cortex. *Brain Research, 291,* 364–368.

Pandya, D. N., & Yeterian, E. H. (1985). Architecture and connections of cortical association areas. In A. Peters & E. G. Jones (Eds.), *Association and auditory cortices* (pp. 3–61). New York: Plenum Press.

Peterson, N. N., Schroeder, C. E., et al. (1995). Neural generators of early cortical somatosensory evoked potentials in the awake monkey. *Electroencephalography and Clinical Neurophysiology, 96,* 248–260.

Ramachandran, R., Wallace, M. T., et al. (1993). Multisensory convergence and integration in rat cortex. *Society of Neuroscience Abstracts, 19,* 1447.

Rappelsberger, P., Pockberger, H., et al. (1981). Current source density analysis: Methods and application to simultaneously recorded field potentials of the rabbit's visual cortex. *Pflügers Archiv, 389,* 159–170.

Ruchkin, D. S., Villegas, J., et al. (1964). An analysis of average evoked potentials making use of least mean square techniques. *Annals of the New York Academy of Sciences, 115,* 799–821.

Schroeder, C. E. (1995). Defining the neural bases of visual selective attention: Conceptual and empirical issues. *International Journal of Neuroscience, 80,* 65–78.

Schroeder, C. E., & Foxe, J. J. (2002). The timing and laminar profile of converging inputs to multisensory areas of the macaque neocortex. *Brain Research: Cognitive Brain Research, 14,* 187–198.

Schroeder, C. E., Lindsley, R. W., et al. (2001). Somatosensory input to auditory association cortex in the macaque monkey. *Journal of Neurophysiology, 85,* 1322–1327.

Schroeder, C. E., Mehta, A. D., et al. (1998). A spatiotemporal profile of visual system activation revealed by current source density analysis in the awake macaque. *Cerebral Cortex, 8,* 575–592.

Schroeder, C. E., Tenke, C. E., et al. (1991). Striate cortical contribution to the surface-recorded pattern-reversal VEP in the alert monkey. *Vision Research, 31,* 1143–1157.

Shepherd, G. M., Koch, C. (1990). Dendritic electrotonus and synaptic integration. In G. M. Shepherd (Ed.), *The synaptic organization of the brain* (pp. 439–473). Oxford, England: Oxford University Press.

Simons, D. J. (1978). Response properties of vibrissa units in the rat SI somatosensory neocortex. *Journal of Neurophysiology, 41,* 798–820.

Stein, B., & Wallace, M. (1996). Comparisons of cross-modality integration in midbrain and cortex. *Progress in Brain Research, 112,* 289–299.

Stein, B. E., & Meredith, M. A. (1993). *The merging of the senses.* Cambridge, MA: MIT Press.

Steinschneider, M., Tenke, C. E., et al. (1992). Cellular generators of the cortical auditory evoked potential initial component. *Electroencephalography and Clinical Neurophysiology, 84,* 196–200.

Steriade, M. (1984). The excitatory-inhibitory response sequence in thalamic and neocortical cells: State-related changes and regulatory systems. In G. M. Edelman, W. E. Gall, & W. M. Cowan (Eds.), *Dynamic aspects of neocortical function* (pp. 107–157). New York: Wiley.

Thompson, R. F., Johnson, R. H., et al. (1963). Organization of auditory, somatic sensory, and visual projection to associational fields of cerebral cortex in the cat. *Journal of Neurophysiology, 33,* 343–364.

Thompson, R. F., Smith, H. E., et al. (1963). Auditory, somatosensory, and visual response interactions and interrelations in association and primary cortical fields of the cat. *Journal of Neurophysiology, 00,* 365–378.

Toldi, J., & Fehér, O. (1984). Acoustic sensitivity and bimodal properties of cells in the anterior suprasylvian gyrus of the cat. *Experimental Brain Research, 55,* 180–183.

Toldi, J., Fehér, O., et al. (1984). Dynamic interactions of evoked potentials in a polysensory cortex of the cat. *Neuroscience, 13,* 645–652.

Toldi, J., Fehér, O., et al. (1986). Sensory interactive zones in the rat cerebral cortex, *Neuroscience, 18,* 461–465.

Toldi, J., Rojik, I., et al. (1981). Two different polysensory systems in the suprasylvian gyrus of the cat: An electrophysiological and autoradiographic study, *Neuroscience, 6,* 2539–2545.

Tracey, D. J. (1985). Somatosensory system. In G. Paxinos (Ed.), *The rat nervous system: Hindbrain and spinal cord* (pp. 129–152). Sydney: Academic Press.

Vaknin, G., DiScenna, P. G., et al. (1988). A method for calculating current source-density (CSD) analysis without resorting to recording sites outside the sampling volume. *Journal of Neuroscience Methods, 24,* 131–135.

Wallace, M. N. (1987). Histochemical demonstration of sensory maps in the rat and mouse cerebral cortex. *Brain Research, 418,* 178–182.

Wallace, M. T., Meredith, M. A., et al. (1992). Integration of multiple sensory modalities in cat cortex. *Experimental Brain Research, 91,* 484–488.

Walter, W. G. (1965). The convergence and interaction of visual, auditory, and tactile responses in human nonspecific cortex. *Annals of the New York Academy of Sciences, 112,* 320–361.

Welch, R. B., & Warren, D. H. (1986). Intersensory interactions. In K. R. Boff, L. Kaufman, & J. P. Thomas (Eds.), *Handbook of perception and human performance* (pp. 1–36). New York: Wiley.

Wise, S. P., & Jones, E. G. (1978). Developmental studies of thalamocortical and commissural connections in the rat somatic sensory cortex. *Journal of Comparative Neurology, 178,* 187–208.

Wong-Riley, M. T. T., & Welt, C. (1980). Histochemical changes in cytochrome oxidase of cortical barrels after vibrissal removal in neonatal and adult mice. *Proceedings of the National Academy of Sciences, 77,* 2333–2337.

Woolsey, C. N., & Fairman, D. (1946). Contralateral, ipsilateral and bilateral representation of cutaneous receptors in somatic areas I and II of the cerebral cortex of pig, sheep and other mammals. *Surgery, 19,* 684–702.

Woolsey, T. A. (1967). Somatosensory, auditory and visual cortical areas of the mouse. *Johns Hopkins Medical Journal, 121,* 91–112.

Záborszky, L., & Wolff, J. R. (1982). Distribution patterns and individual variations of callosal connections in the albino rat. *Anatomy and Embryology, 165,* 213–232.

IV MULTISENSORY MECHANISMS IN ORIENTATION

23 Auditory-Visual Interactions Subserving Primate Gaze Orienting

A. J. VAN OPSTAL AND D. P. MUNOZ

Introduction

The visual and auditory systems are the *exteroceptive* senses that provide information about objects and events in the outside world. Both are involved in identifying and localizing stimuli in space. Often, an object may simultaneously emit both visual and acoustic signals, in which case the brain should decide that the stimuli indeed emanated from the same object. However, for that to happen, the sensory signals need to be integrated. Multisensory integration is of paramount importance for any nervous system coping with a multitude of potential stimuli that simultaneously compete for attention in the natural world. To process this information successfully, the brain must weed out irrelevant stimuli, resolve potential ambiguities in the sensory inputs arising from blurred, partially occluded, or noisy signals, and select a unique target from all the potential possibilities. The result of this process may be the generation of a rapid orienting response, allowing further detailed analysis with foveal vision. While programming or executing the movement, however, objects may change their position or their multimodal attributes, or new stimuli may appear elsewhere in the environment. The need for continuous updating of the multisensory world poses a major challenge to the brain. A crucial neural structure involved in multisensory-evoked orienting behavior is the midbrain superior colliculus (SC).

In this chapter, we focus on the integration of auditory and visual stimuli when evoking a rapid goal-directed orienting response of the eyes and head (a so-called gaze saccade, i.e., eye in space). We first describe the relevant sensorimotor response properties of SC cells in awake, behaving rhesus monkeys, and some of the multisensory characteristics of these neurons. We then describe the problems underlying auditory-visual orienting behavior, and present and discuss recent experimental results obtained in human subjects.

Role of the SC in multisensory processing

The intermediate layers of the mammalian SC offer a rich diversity of multisensory neurons. Pioneering work by Stein and Meredith (reviewed in Stein & Meredith, 1993) revealed that neurons in the intermediate and deep layers of the SC in anesthetized cats respond to visual, auditory, and somatosensory stimuli. Many neurons respond to more than one modality, giving these multisensory neurons visual, auditory, and/or somatosensory receptive fields. The organizational structure and distribution of these receptive fields across sensory space are not haphazard but highly organized, so that there is spatial congruence of receptive fields for many multisensory neurons. For example, a visual-auditory neuron that responds to a visual stimulus in the right visual hemifield at 20 degrees of eccentricity will also respond to an auditory stimulus positioned at the same location. When multimodal stimuli are combined, a significant interaction may occur, with the result that the response is either enhanced or depressed (Meredith & Stein, 1986a). These interactions depend critically on the spatial and temporal alignment of the stimuli. In general, greatest enhancement occurs when the visual and auditory stimuli coincide in space and time. As the stimuli move out of spatial-temporal alignment, the magnitude of the enhancement diminishes and often reverses into depression (Meredith, Nemitz, & Stein, 1987; Meredith & Stein, 1986b).

Wallace, Wilkinson, and Stein (1996) have demonstrated similar multisensory integration properties in single neurons of the superficial and deeper layers of the anesthetized monkey SC. Figure 23.1 illustrates the overlap in the visual and auditory response fields for a representative auditory-visual cell from their study.

More recently, Wallace, Meredith, and Stein (1998), Frens and Van Opstal (1998), and Bell and colleagues (Bell, Corneil, Meredith, & Munoz, 2001; Bell,

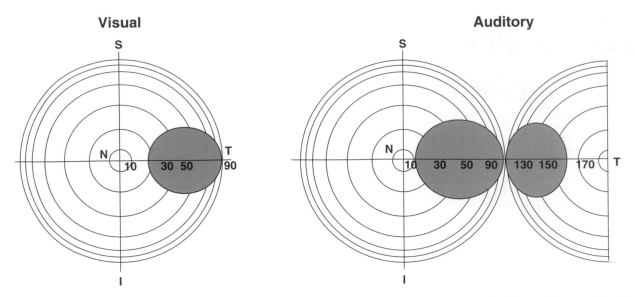

FIGURE 23.1   Visual (left) and auditory (right) receptive fields of bimodal neurons in the monkey SC overlap considerably, as shown here for a representative example. (Modified from Wallace et al., 1996.)

Everling, & Munoz, 2000; Bell et al., in press) have begun to investigate multisensory processing in the SC of awake preparations. Figure 23.2 shows the distribution of visual and auditory responses among neurons in the intermediate layers of the SC collected in the awake monkey (Bell et al., 2001). The intermediate layers were identified based on the depth of saccade-related neurons (Munoz & Wurtz, 1995a). Many of the neurons with sensory responses recorded in the awake animal also have motor responses linked to saccade generation. Qualitatively, the distribution of multisen-

sory neurons is similar to that described by Wallace et al. (1996). Neurons in the SC of the awake monkey could also be classified as visual, auditory, or bimodal (i.e., responsive to individual presentation of visual and auditory stimuli).

The SC plays a critical role in the control of both visual fixation and the generation of saccadic eye-head gaze shifts (see Corneil, Olivier, & Munoz, 2002; Freedman & Sparks, 1997; Munoz, Dorris, Paré, & Everling, 2000, for review). Cortical and subcortical inputs converge on the SC, which then projects to the brainstem premotor circuitry (Fig. 23.3A). The superficial layers of the SC contain neurons that receive direct retinal inputs as well as inputs from other visual areas, and are organized in a map representing the contralateral visual hemifield. The intermediate layers of the SC contain neurons whose discharges are modulated by saccadic eye movements and visual fixation (e.g., Sparks, & Mays, 1980; Munoz & Wurtz, 1993a, 1995a; Schiller & Koerner, 1971; Wurtz & Goldberg, 1972). These neurons are organized into a motor map that encodes saccades in the contralateral visual field (Robinson, 1972; Fig. 23.3B). Neurons that increase their discharge before and during saccades, referred to as *saccade neurons* (SN, Fig. 23.3C), are distributed throughout the intermediate layers of the SC. Neurons that are tonically active during visual fixation and pause during saccades, referred to as *fixation neurons* (FN, Fig. 23.3C), are located in the rostrolateral pole of the SC where the fovea is represented. It is believed that a local inhibitory network shapes this reciprocal pattern (Lee, Helms, Augustine, & Hall, 1997; Meredith &

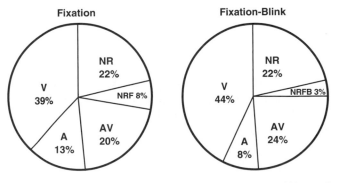

FIGURE 23.2   Proportions of visual (V), auditory (A), and auditory-visual (AV) neurons in SC of awake monkeys. The sensory responses of 84 cells in two monkeys were tested in two conditions. In the fixation condition (left), a visual fixation light was continuously present. In the fixation-blink condition (right), the fixation light disappeared. In both conditions, the monkey maintained active fixation. Note that the sensory response properties of the cells are similar for the two conditions. NR, not responsive in none of the conditions; NRF(B), not responsive in fixation-blink condition.

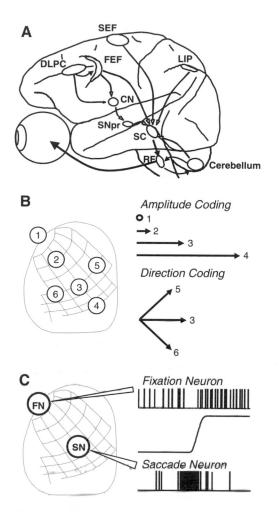

A

SEF

DLPC   FEF   LIP

CN

SNpr

SC

RF

Cerebellum

B

Amplitude Coding

1
2
3
4

Direction Coding

5
3
6

C

Fixation Neuron

FN

SN

Saccade Neuron

FIGURE 23.3   (*A*) Schematic of lateral view of the hemisphere of a nonhuman primate (rhesus monkey) brain highlighting the cortical and subcortical structures involved in controlling saccadic eye movements. (*B*) Dorsal view of the saccadic motor map in the intermediate layers of the SC. Vectors on the right side correspond to the collicular locations highlighted on the left. (*C*) Discharge recorded from a fixation neuron (FN) in the rostrolateral pole of the left SC and a saccade neuron (SN) in the caudal SC during the execution of a large rightward visually guided saccade. Note that FN and SN have reciprocal discharge during this behavior. (*B* adapted from Robinson, 1972.)

Ramoa, 1998; Munoz & Istvan, 1998). Most SNs and FNs are inhibited at very short latency (often monosynaptically) after microstimulation of other regions of the ipsilateral and contralateral SC (Munoz & Istvan, 1998). These strong inhibitory connections include interactions between remote populations of SNs. The role of this local inhibitory network in multisensory integration has been largely ignored so far. Inputs from many sources, including sensory inputs of different modalities, converge on the intermediate layers of the SC and provide critical inputs to selectively activate either FNs or SNs. The signals are then passed to the brainstem

burst generator to direct the appropriate behavior: saccade or fixate.

Collicular SNs can be subdivided into two classes based on (1) the presence or absence of long-lead prelude activity prior to saccade initiation, (2) the shape of their movement fields, and (3) their depth below the dorsal surface of the SC (Munoz & Wurtz, 1995a, 1995b). *Superior colliculus burst neurons* (SCBNs) lack any significant long-lead preparatory activity before saccades, discharge a vigorous burst of action potentials for a restricted range of saccade vectors that defines a closed movement field, and tend to be located in the dorsal part of the intermediate layers. *Superior colliculus buildup neurons* (SCBUNs) have long-lead anticipatory discharges before saccades, discharge for all saccades whose amplitudes are equal to or greater than optimal (i.e., open-ended movement fields), and tend to reside in the ventral part of the intermediate layers.

The discharges of a representative SCBN, SCBUN, and SCFN are illustrated in Figure 23.4. These neurons were recorded in the gap saccade paradigm in which the visual fixation point (FP) disappears prior to appearance of the saccade target (T). The FN is tonically active during fixation; during the gap period, the FN has a modest reduction in discharge, followed by an abrupt pause for the visually triggered saccade. The SCBUN has a reciprocal discharge: it is silent during visual fixation but presents a low-frequency buildup of activity that coincides with the modest reduction in FN activity (Dorris, Paré, & Munoz, 1997). The SCBN remains silent during visual fixation and during the gap period. Both the SCBN and the SCBUN discharge a high-frequency burst of action potentials following the appearance of the saccade target in their response fields.

Recent models describing saccade initiation have used a rise-to-threshold concept in which there is a fixed threshold for a saccade (e.g., Carpenter & Williams, 1995). Reaction time is influenced by both the baseline (pretarget) activity and the rate of rise of activity toward the threshold after the target has appeared (posttarget). Pretarget processes such as anticipation or early preparation influence the baseline, while posttarget processes such as target selection influence the subsequent rate of rise to the threshold. The gap saccade task illustrated in Figure 23.4 offers the opportunity to separate pretarget from posttarget processes. The low-frequency, long-lead buildup activity of SCBUNs that occurs during the gap period represents an early motor preparation signal. The intensity of this pretarget activity correlates well with saccadic reaction time (Dorris & Munoz, 1998): the greater the activation of SCBUNs prior to target appearance, the shorter the subsequent reaction time. Many saccade-related neurons in the

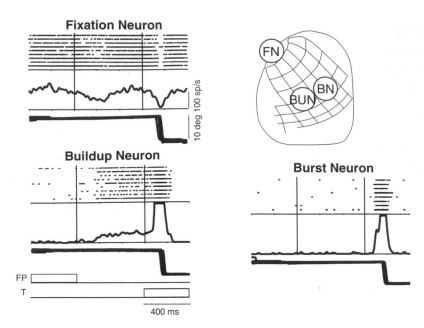

Fixation Neuron

Buildup Neuron

FP

T

Burst Neuron

10 deg 100 sp/s

400 ms

FIGURE 23.4   Activity of SCFN, SCBUN, and SCBN during the gap paradigm. Rasters, spike density, and eye position traces are aligned on fixation point disappearance (left vertical line) and target appearance (right vertical line). The gap duration was fixed at 600 ms. The SCFN has a slight drop in activity early in the gap period that coincides with the increase in low-frequency buildup activity of the SCBUN. The SCBN remains silent during the gap period. Both the SCBN and SCBUN discharge a high-frequency burst of action potentials for the generation of the visually guided saccade, while the SCFN has a pause in its tonic discharge.

SC also respond phasically following the onset of visual and/or auditory stimuli (Fig. 23.4). How these posttarget sensory responses interact with pretarget processes to influence reaction time remains unanswered.

FNs and SNs in the intermediate layers of the SC project to the reticular formation (Gandhi & Keller, 1997), where the premotor saccade burst generator is located (e.g., Fuchs, Kaneko, & Scudder, 1985; Moschovakis, Scudder & Highstein, 1996; see also Corneil, Olivier, et al., 2002). Reticular burst neurons are silent during fixation and discharge a vigorous burst of action potentials for saccades into the ipsilateral hemifield. These burst neurons receive excitatory input from the SC and in turn innervate the extraocular motor neurons to provide the appropriate motor commands (Raybourn & Keller, 1977). The burst neurons are subject to potent inhibition from so-called omnipause neurons (OPNs), which discharge tonically during all fixations and pause for saccades in all directions (Everling, Paré, Dorris, & Munoz, 1998; Luschei & Fuchs, 1972). To drive a saccade, the OPNs must first be silenced to disinhibit the burst neurons. It is thought that FNs and SCBUNs project monosynaptically onto OPNs, while SCBUNs and SCBNs project to the brainstem burst neurons (Everling et al., 1998). Thus, during early motor preparation in the gap saccade paradigm, when activity of the FNs decreases while the buildup activity in SCBUNs increases, the OPN discharge remains constant, as their net excitatory input does not change during the gap.

Fundamental problems for orienting to multimodal stimuli

Combining a visual and an auditory stimulus as a target for a saccade is far from a trivial problem, for reasons that are illustrated in Figures 23.5 and 23.6. First, visual and auditory signals are represented in very different neural encoding formats at the level of the retina and cochlea, respectively (Fig. 23.5). As light enters the eye, it is projected onto the retina in a point-to-point fashion (i.e., retinotopically coded). The retina is organized in a circular-symmetric fashion, where the density of receptor cells decreases as a function of distance from the fovea (Fig. 23.5A), with no preferred direction. In contrast, because of mechanical interactions within the cochlea, acoustic input causes a traveling wave along the basilar membrane (BM) that peaks at a frequency-dependent location. High-frequency sounds yield maximum excitation of the BM at its base, low sound frequencies peak at the apex. In this way, sounds are represented *tonotopically*. As a result, the auditory system must derive the location of a sound on the basis of acoustic cues that arise as a consequence of the geometry of head and ears.

Differences in path length to either ear induce interaural differences in arrival time (ITDs), while the

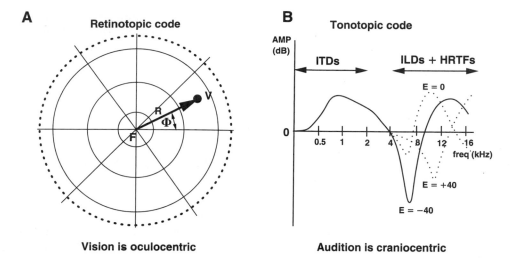

A Retinotopic code

B Tonotopic code

Vision is oculocentric

Audition is craniocentric

FIGURE 23.5   The visual and auditory systems encode and represent the sensory input in very different ways. (*A*) The visual input is organized retinotopically in oculocentric polar coordinates, referencing the location of the target (V) by its eccentricity (R) and direction (Φ) relative to the fovea (F). (*B*) Acoustic input is encoded tonotopically (frequency code). Interaural difference cues in timing (ITDs < 1.5 kHz) and level (ILDs > 2kHz) determine sound location in the horizontal plane (azimuth). The overall spectral shape of the input (the so-called head-related transfer function, or HRTF) differs for changes in target elevation for frequencies above 4 kHz (here schematized for E = −40, 0, and +40 degrees). As the cues are ear- (or head-) fixed, they refer to the sound in ear or craniocentric coordinates.

acoustic shadow of the head causes an interaural difference in sound level (ILDs). Both cues are monotonically related to sound location in the horizontal plane (azimuth), but they dominate at different frequency bands (see Fig. 23.5*B*). To localize a sound in the medial plane (elevation) and to resolve front-back confusions, the auditory system relies on the detailed

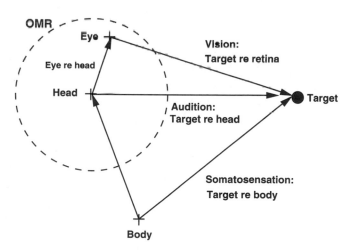

FIGURE 23.6   The relationship between the different sensory systems is determined by the orientation of the eye in the head and by the orientation of the head in space (or on the body). For example, to determine the location of the auditory target in oculocentric coordinates, eye position in the head should be subtracted from the head-centered target representation. Likewise, a somatosensory stimulus can be expressed in oculocentric coordinates by subtracting both eye and head orientation from the somatotopic representation.

geometry of the pinnae, causing acoustic waves to diffract and to undergo direction-dependent reflections. This results in a sound interference pattern containing attenuations and magnifications at specific frequencies (Fig. 23.5*B*), known as the *head-related transfer function* (HRTF; see Blauert, 1997, for a review). Different elevations give rise to different HRTFs (Fig. 23.5*B*). Because the HRTFs change in a complex way during growth, it is generally assumed that the auditory system obtains knowledge about these functions through learning (e.g., Hofman, Van Riswick, & Van Opstal, 1998). Presumably, this learning process necessitates a visual teaching signal (Zwiers, Van Opstal, & Cruysberg, 2001; Zwiers, Van Opstal, & Paige, 2003).

Apart from fundamental differences in spatial encoding, the visual and auditory systems also employ different frames of reference. Because the retina is fixed to the eye, visual input is expressed in an eye-centered (oculocentric) frame of reference. On the other hand, the acoustic cues are encoded in ear-centered or, for immobile ears such as in humans, craniocentric coordinates. These different coordinate systems introduce additional problems for gaze orienting to multimodal stimuli, because in normal behavior the different reference frames usually are not aligned. Thus, neural updating mechanisms are needed to ensure that the spatial coordinates of different sensory events are maintained within a common frame of reference.

The coordinate transformations that relate the reference frames of the different sensory systems are schematically illustrated in Figure 23.6. For example, to transform the craniocentric coordinates of an auditory target into the oculocentric reference frame of the visuomotor system, a signal about eye position in the head should be subtracted from the head-centered auditory coordinates: $T_E = T_H - E_H$. In this way, a saccadic eye movement can be programmed toward an auditory target despite changes in eye position. Conversely, if a head movement is made toward a visual target, the oculocentric visual coordinates should be transformed into the craniocentric coordinates of the head motor system. This is achieved by adding eye position to the retinal target coordinates: $T_H = T_E + E_H$. In the same fashion, somatosensory signals in body-centered coordinates are transformed into oculocentric or head-centered coordinates by incorporating signals about eye and head position, respectively.

How would these neural transformations become manifest in the brain? To appreciate this problem at the level of the SC, we can consider the following simple examples of auditory-visual stimulation (Fig. 23.7). In Figure 23.7A the eyes and head are both looking straight ahead, while an auditory stimulus (A) is presented 20 degrees to the right (in head-centered coordinates). If the visual stimulus is also presented 20 degrees to the right (in eye-centered coordinates), the two stimuli emanate from the same location in space. Note that the receptive fields for a putative bimodal cell in the SC overlap (Fig. 23.7A, bottom left; see also Fig. 23.1).

However, when the eyes look 20 degrees to the left (Fig. 23.7B), a light spot again presented 20 degrees to the right of fixation (V) is now located straight ahead. This situation represents the case in which the putative SC neuron has a craniocentric auditory and an oculocentric visual receptive field. In such a case, both receptive fields would still overlap, although the stimuli would emanate from quite different locations in space (dotted AV areas at bottom right). Only when the visual stimulus was 40 degrees to the right of fixation would the stimuli again be at the same spatial location. However, for this hypothetical SC neuron, the response would be quite different, as the two receptive fields (A and V′) would no longer overlap in this condition. Interestingly, however, sound localization recording

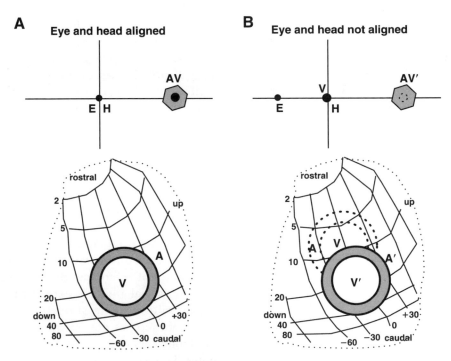

FIGURE 23.7   Auditory (A) and visual (V) receptive fields of bimodal cells overlap (see also Fig. 23.1). This figure shows two cases. (A) In this case, the eyes (E) and head (H) are aligned. The craniocentric and oculocentric reference frames are identical, and the auditory and visual stimuli both excite the receptive fields of the cell (bottom left). The neural excitations are shown superimposed on Robinson's (1972) sensorimotor map of the SC. (B) In this case, the eyes look to the left. The point images of the visual and auditory targets (dotted lines, bottom right) would still overlap for a cell encoding sound in craniocentric coordinates and light in oculocentric coordinates. However, the spatial locations are different. When the visual target moves to the right (V′), it again overlaps in space with the sound (A). The point images for the putative cell, however, V′ and dotted A, will not overlap, and hence may not invoke integration. Jay and Sparks (1984, 1987) have shown, however, that in monkey SC, the point image of the sound moves to A′, i.e., the oculocentric representation of the sound. In that case, both the spatial locations and the neural representations overlap.

studies in awake monkeys (Jay & Sparks, 1984, 1987) have shown that in the latter fixation condition, the auditory receptive field of many SC neurons actually shifts to the eye-centered representation (A'). Although these experiments have so far not been conducted with bimodal stimuli, one would expect that since the visual and auditory receptive fields again overlap (A'V'), neural integration would take place.

The fundamental differences in neural encoding and reference frames of auditory and visual inputs extends to the somatosensory system, too. Although the somatosensory system has a somatotopic representation in a body-centered reference frame, Groh and Sparks (1996) have shown that somatosensory receptive fields in the (head-fixed) monkey SC are again represented in oculocentric coordinates.

To summarize, orienting to a multimodal object requires the different sensory signals to be expressed in a similar representational format, as well as in the same frame of reference. At the level of the deep layers of the primate SC, the common frame of reference appears to be oculocentric, specifying a gaze motor-error signal. In this way, stimuli presented at the same location in space will always yield overlapping response fields, despite changes in the alignment of the different sensory systems.

Multisensory integration could serve several functions related to goal-directed orienting behavior. First, it might speed up the response, as neural activity levels in the SC increase for spatially and temporally coincident stimuli. A second important function is the need to calibrate and align the different sensory systems, especially in the light of their different encoding formats, differences in receptive range and spatial resolution, and different reference frames. A third consideration relates to the behavioral task: spatial attention, target versus nontarget, the act of fixation, and so on, may all strongly influence the effects of multisensory integration.

The rest of this chapter addresses these issues by discussing recent experimental evidence obtained in humans and trained rhesus monkeys. It will become apparent that many of the behavioral effects seen in multisensory integration can be understood from known neural mechanisms at the level of the SC.

Experimental results

INFLUENCE OF MULTISENSORY INTEGRATION ON SACCADE REACTION TIMES   It is well known that bimodal stimuli affect the reaction times of goal-directed saccadic eye movements (Arndt & Colonius, 2001; Corneil, Van Wanrooij, Munoz, & Van Opstal, 2002; Engelken & Stevens, 1989; Frens, Van Opstal, & Van der Willigen,

1995; Harrington & Peck, 1998; Hughes, Reuter-Lorenz, Nozawa, & Fendrich, 1994; Nozawa, Reuter-Lorenz, & Hughes, 1994). In particular, when the two stimuli are aligned in space and time, a considerable reduction of the saccade reaction time (SRT) is typically observed. This is also true for combined eye and head movements (Corneil & Munoz, 1996; Goldring, Dorris, Corneil, Ballantyne, & Munoz, 1996), or for auditory-visually evoked hand movements (Simon & Craft, 1970; Gielen, Schmidt, & Van den Heuvel, 1983; Hughes et al., 1994). It was already argued by Raab (1962) that it is not straightforward to assign this reduction to multisensory integration, because several other factors may induce shorter reaction times (see also Diederich & Colonius, Chap. 24, this volume).

The most obvious one is that in general, SRTs to auditory stimuli are shorter than SRTs to visual targets (e.g., Frens et al., 1995). Thus, it could be that subjects were merely responding to the onset of the auditory stimulus rather than to the appearance of the visual stimulus. This factor will be denominated here as the *warning effect* (Ross & Ross, 1981). Note that this effect is nonspecific to the orienting task, because the spatial location of the auditory stimulus is irrelevant and does not influence the programming of the saccade coordinates.

A second factor to be considered in auditory-visual orienting is that the spatial range of the auditory system is much larger than that of vision. Thus, the spatially cruder sound localization system could aid the visuomotor system in getting the fovea quickly near the target location (Perrott, Saberi, Brown, & Strybel, 1990; Perrott, Sadralodabai, Saberi, & Strybel, 1991). According to this idea, the first phase of the response is entirely auditorily guided, after which the visual system takes over as soon as the target is within the parafoveal range. Experimental evidence suggests that this strategy is operational not only for peripheral and rear target locations (Perrott et al., 1990), but also in the central frontal hemifield (Perrott et al., 1991).

A subtler factor leading to a reduction of SRTs is *statistical facilitation* (Raab, 1962; Gielen et al., 1983), a concept formalized by the so-called race model (Fig. 23.8*A*). According to this idea, the brain processes visual and auditory stimuli independently, and the saccade is triggered by whichever process finishes first. The SRTs produced by this model are therefore distributed as the minima of the auditory ($A(\tau)$) and visual ($V(\tau)$) SRT distributions (τ is a given SRT). Formally, this bimodal race distribution, $AV_R(\tau)$, can be computed by (Gielen et al., 1983):

$$AV_R(\tau) = A(\tau)\int_\tau^\infty V(s)\,ds + V(\tau)\int_\tau^\infty A(s)\,ds \qquad (1)$$

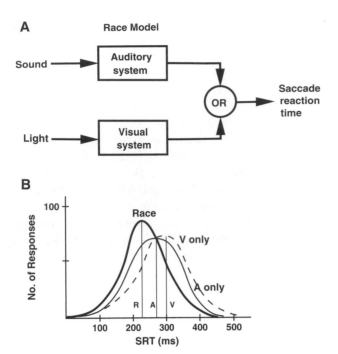

FIGURE 23.8   The race model assumes entirely independent channels for auditory and visual signals. (*A*) A saccade is triggered by whichever process arrives first at the saccade generator. (*B*) The unimodal SRT distributions are shown, as well as the race model prediction, based on Equation 1. The race prediction is shifted toward shorter reaction times, a phenomenon known as statistical facilitation.

As Figure 23.8*B* shows, the race distribution of bimodal SRTs is shifted toward shorter values whenever the two unimodal distributions overlap sufficiently. This shortening of SRTs is, however, a purely statistical effect, one that does not require any neural integration of signals. In fact, the race model operates as a simple logical OR gate.

This important concept is often taken as a benchmark for experiments to test whether or not neural integration explains observed SRTs. Often, in experimental studies an upper bound is determined by simply summing the $A(\tau)$ and $V(\tau)$ reaction time distributions, yielding the non-normalized summed distribution: $AV_S(\tau) \leq A(\tau) + V(\tau)$. Whenever SRTs are shorter than predicted by the race model, a facilitating neural integration process has to be assumed. Unfortunately, the model does not allow firm statements for saccades that fail the race prediction with longer reaction times, although bimodal neural inhibitory processes could also be involved in preventing the generation of saccades (see earlier discussion on the neural mechanisms underlying fixation and saccade generation). The reason for this failure of the race model is that subjects could in principle adopt many different strategies to withhold a saccade, and these strategies might not

require neural integration. For example, subjects could simply decide not to make a saccade at all, leading to infinitely long reaction times.

Despite its importance as a conceptual model, it is now generally agreed that SRTs elicited by bimodal stimuli can be explained neither by the race model nor by a warning effect. Rather, their explanation requires some form of neural integration. One crucial aspect is that the spatial and temporal arrangement of the two stimuli influences SRT, a factor not accounted for by the race model (Arndt & Colonius, 2001; Frens et al., 1995; Harrington & Peck, 1998; Hughes, Nelson, & Aronchik, 1998). This feature is illustrated in Figure 23.9, which shows data from Frens et al. (1995; Fig. 23.9*A*) and Arndt and Colonius (2001; Fig. 23.9*B*). Both sets of data show a qualitatively similar gradual decrease in the change in SRT as the auditory and visual stimuli are separated from each other. A simple linear regression line, $\Delta SRT = a.\Delta R + b$, was used to describe the observed change in SRT, where ΔR is the spatial separation (in degrees) of the two stimuli, a is the sensitivity of the effect (in ms/degree), and b is the offset (in ms). Note that b contains the summed effect of MI, auditory warning, auditory-assisted search, or statistical facilitation, and is estimated in both studies to be about -30 ms. The spatial sensitivity was found to be non-zero in both studies, although different values were obtained (about 0.7 ms/degree by Frens et al., 1995, and about 0.2 ms/degree by Arndt & Colonius, 2001). This quantitative difference may be due to differences in experimental procedures.

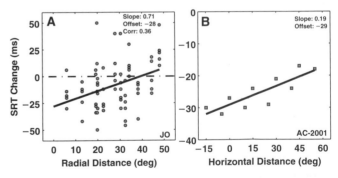

FIGURE 23.9   The change in saccade reaction time (relative to visually evoked saccades to the same location) depends weakly but systematically on the spatial separation between the visual target and auditory distractor. (*A*) Data on one subject (from Frens et al., 1995) for saccades evoked in two dimensions, with the free-field acoustic stimulus at many different locations in relation to the visual target. (*B*) Averaged data (from Arndt & Colonius, 2001) for saccades to visual targets in the horizontal plane, with the acoustic distracter simulated over head phones. Both data sets are qualitatively similar.

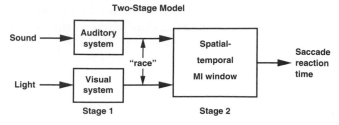

Two-Stage Model

FIGURE 23.10   The two-stage model of Arndt and Colonius (2001) accounts for the effects of both statistical facilitation and neural integration. In the first stage, the auditory and visual signals race against each other. Integration in the second stage occurs only when the auditory signal wins the race, and both stimuli are presented within a restricted spatial-temporal window.

Recently, Arndt and Colonius (2001) have proposed a two-stage model to account for these behavioral findings (Fig. 23.10). In this model, the change in SRT is explained by two mechanisms: a race between auditory and visual signals in the first stage of signal processing, followed by a neural integration stage. In the model, neural integration is task dependent (e.g., when the task is to orient to the visual stimulus, integration is effective only when the auditory process wins the race). Neural integration also depends on the spatial-temporal separation of the stimuli. It does not depend on modality-specific factors such as stimulus intensity, because these factors determine the speed of the processes in the first stage. The neural integration stage therefore shares features that have also been observed in single-cell recordings of the SC.

Recent experiments involving recordings from neurons in the intermediate layers of the SC in awake, behaving monkeys (Bell, Meredith, et al., 2001) illustrate how pretarget anticipatory responses combine with posttarget visual and auditory responses to accumulate toward a saccade threshold. Figure 23.11 illustrates the discharges of an SCBN and an SCBUN that were recorded in the gap condition with either a visual (V; dotted spike density waveform) or a combined visual-auditory (VA; solid spike density waveform) target. Only the SCBUN had a sensory response. There was no difference in the magnitude or latency of the initial sensory response, a feature that was consistent in the sensory responses of SCBNs and SCBUNs (Bell et al., in press). What was different was the time to threshold to trigger the orienting saccade following target appearance. The

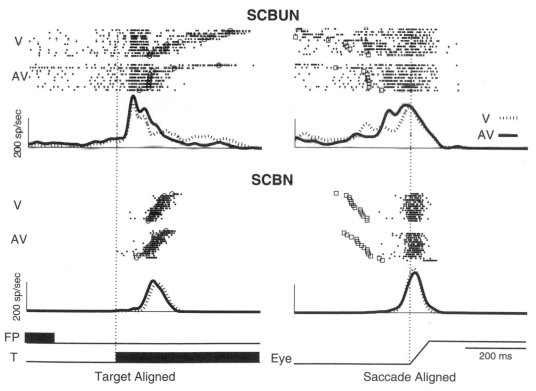

FIGURE 23.11   Discharge of an SCBUN and an SCBN in the gap saccade condition when the target appeared in the cell's response field and was either visual (V) or a combined visual-auditory (VA) target. The SCBUN had a visual response (left panels aligned on target appearance). There was no difference in the timing of the visual response in the two conditions. Rather, the time required for the cell activity to accumulate to a threshold level was reduced in the VA condition, leading to a reduced SRT. From the saccade-aligned activity (right panels), it is evident that there was no difference in peak burst magnitude for V and VA saccades, consistent with the fact that the peak velocity of the saccades was identical in V and VA conditions.

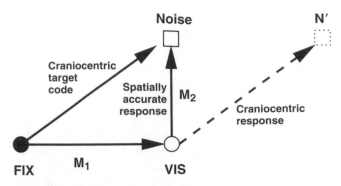

FIGURE 23.12   The eye-head double-step paradigm. The subject starts with eyes and head pointing toward FIX. Then two targets briefly appear at V (visual) and N (acoustic noise burst), respectively. The subject first makes an eye-head gaze shift toward V (M_1). To program a spatially correct second gaze shift to N (M_2), M_1 should be accounted for. If the sound is maintained in craniocentric coordinates, the second gaze shift will be directed toward N' (M_2').

saccade-related burst occurred earlier for both the SCBN and the SCBUN and was highly correlated with a reduction in SRT; the time to threshold for both the SCBN and SCBUN was reduced. Thus, in an awake animal, multisensory integration facilitates the rise to threshold and leads to a reduction in SRT. The neural correlate for this phenomenon is found in the increased pretarget activity of SCBUNs (Bell, Meredith, Van Opstal, & Munoz, 2003).

HUMAN EYE-HEAD COORDINATION TO AUDITORY-VISUAL STIMULI   We recently tested whether the required updating mechanisms outlined in Figure 23.6 are indeed operational in human gaze orienting, by performing the following double-step experiment (Fig. 23.12; Goossens & Van Opstal, 1999). At the start of a trial the subject looked straight ahead at a fixation point, with eyes and head aligned. Then the fixation point vanished and, after a brief gap of darkness (50 ms), two targets were presented briefly at different locations—a visual flash (V, 50 ms duration), followed 100 ms later by a white noise sound burst (N, duration 50 ms). The subject had to reorient eyes and head as quickly and as accurately as possible, first to the visual and then to the auditory target location. Both stimuli were extinguished well before the subject initiated the first gaze shift. Therefore, both gaze shifts were executed in total darkness and silence, and were therefore open loop (no visual or auditory feedback). At the start of the trial, the stimuli provide oculocentric information about the visual target and craniocentric information about the sound. If the auditory system keeps the target in head-centered coordinates, the second gaze shift, M_2', should be directed to the location determined by the craniocentric displacement vector alone (Fig. 23.7A, gaze shift

M_2', to N'). For the task to be performed correctly, the gaze control system must update the coordinates of the auditory target on the basis of the intervening gaze shift (gaze shift M_2 to N). Moreover, it has to account for the fact that the eyes and head are no longer aligned after the first gaze shift, M_1, by an amount that varies considerably from trial to trial. Thus, only if the eyes and head were driven by signals expressed in their own reference frame would both motor systems move toward the spatial target location. Alternatively, if the eyes and head were driven by the same (say, oculocentric) signal, the eyes would foveate the target, but the head would not.

The left-hand side of Figure 23.13 shows the result of two typical trials in this experiment. Note that in both cases, eyes and head were directed toward the spatially accurate location (N) instead of toward the craniocentric location (N'). To determine whether the movements of eyes and head are indeed guided by their oculocentric and craniocentric error signals, respectively, Figures 23.13C and D show the data acquired over a large number of trials in one subject. Figure 23.13C shows the (horizontal) displacements of the eye in space as a function of the remaining motor error after the first gaze shift (open symbols). The data are indistinguishable from the control condition, in which only a single visual or auditory target was presented (closed symbols). The same is true for the head movements in this experiment, which correlate well with the craniocentric motor error (Fig. 23.13D).

Further quantitative analysis of the data was performed to reveal which signals are incorporated in the generation of the second gaze shift. To that end, multiple linear regression related all potentially relevant signals to the second gaze displacement:

$$M_2 = aT_H + bE_H + c\Delta H + d \qquad (2)$$

where T_H is the initial head-centered location of the auditory target, E_H is the eye-in-head position after the first gaze shift (note that the eye is no longer aligned with the head), and ΔH is the head displacement of the first gaze shift (not necessarily equal to the total gaze shift). Parameters a, b, and c are dimensionless gains, and d is an offset (in degrees). If the first gaze shift, $M_1 = \Delta H + E_H$, is not accounted for, coefficients b and c are close to zero. This corresponds to the hypothetical case of a gaze shift toward N' (Figs. 23.12 and 23.13). On the other hand, if the gaze control system incorporated only changes in eye position and ignored the change in head position (as illustrated in Fig. 23.7, and extrapolating from the electrophysiological findings of Jay & Sparks, 1984, 1987), c would be near zero, but a would equal $+1$ and b would equal -1.

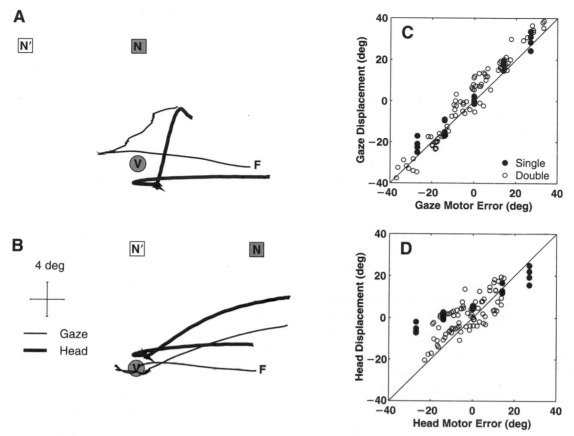

FIGURE 23.13 Spatially correct behavior in the double-step paradigm (after Goossens & Van Opstal, 1999). On the left are shown two representative eye (thin trace) and head (thick trace) movement responses (*A*, *B*). Eye-in-space (gaze) and head-in-space are both directed toward the acoustic target. (*C*) Gaze displacement is highly correlated with gaze motor error. The gaze shift of the second step (open symbols) is as accurate as the single-step control responses to the same locations (closed symbols). (*D*) Head displacement has a strong linear relation with the head motor error after the first gaze shift. Thus, eyes and head are both driven toward the sound.

In fact, the regression coefficients were close to $a = +1$, $b = -1$, $c = -1$, and $d = 0$ for all subjects tested. These are the values required for a system that takes the first gaze shift fully into account in programming the second one. In other words, the most succinct description of the data is given by the following simple equation:

$$M_2 = T_H - M_1 \qquad (3)$$

Results such as these provide good evidence that the gaze orienting system is capable of rapid and accurate updating of the required movement signals for eyes and head in demanding visual-auditory localization tasks. The experiment also shows that eyes and head are eventually driven by signals expressed in different reference frames (oculocentric and craniocentric, respectively), allowing both to capture the target.

INFLUENCE OF TASK CONSTRAINTS ON MULTISENSORY INTEGRATION Multisensory integration also depends on task requirements. In most behavioral studies, the visual stimulus is usually taken as the target, while the auditory costimulus is a distracter that may or may not coincide in space and time with the visual stimulus. In either case, the task for the subject is to ignore the auditory distracter altogether. Even so, spatiotemporal effects on SRT are observed in such a paradigm (Arndt & Colonius, 2001; Frens et al., 1995; Harrington & Peck, 1998; Hughes et al., 1998).

But what if the task is different? For example, are similar effects observed when the auditory stimulus serves as the target and the visual stimulus acts as a distracter, or when the distracter could occur in either modality? This question has recently been investigated in human subjects engaged in an eye-head orienting task (Corneil & Munoz, 1996). In the experiments, subjects generated a rapid eye-head gaze shift toward a stimulus that could be presented at either of two locations on the horizontal meridian 200 ms after the fixation light disappeared (gap trials). On each trial, an additional costimulus was presented that could either coincide with the target location (enhancer trials) or be on the opposite side (distracter trials). Depending on the task, the subject had to orient toward a visual or an auditory target, and the costimulus, which had to be ignored, could occur in the same or in the other modality. Eight different trial types were thus studied, four enhancer conditions and four distracter conditions. For each of these trial types, the temporal asynchrony between the stimuli was systematically varied between −200 and +200 ms (minus sign: costimulus first). In the distracter condition, subjects would often make a mistake by first responding to the distracter. The probability of such an error was larger, the earlier the distracter was presented, but it also depended on the modality of the task. The averaged data are shown in Figure 23.14A. Errors were most likely when the target was visual (VA and VV trials) and were least likely in the auditory orienting task (AV and AA trials). Errors approached zero when the distracter was presented after the target (about 60–100 ms) for all conditions. A similar pattern was observed for the SRT difference between the distracter and enhancer conditions (typically, enhancer trials yielded shorter latencies when the costimulus preceded or was synchronous with the target). As is shown in Figure 23.14B, there was a strong correlation between these two quantities (slope about 0.6%/ms; correlation = 0.94). The observed fraction of error responses in the distracter condition, however, was less than expected from the (upper limit) race model prediction for all distracter stimulus combinations (Fig. 23.14C).

Finally, when the SRT data of enhancer and distracter trials were compared, only the VA condition (visual target, auditory costimulus) surpassed the race model (Fig. 23.14D); the AV, AA, and VV conditions clearly did not. This occurred only for temporal asynchronies around zero. Thus, a task constraint that requires target selection (and hence suppression of movement initiation toward the distracter) appears to affect the processes underlying multisensory integration.

An intriguing aspect of orienting gaze shifts made in a gap paradigm in which there are only two possible target locations is that the head sometimes begins to move in advance of the gaze shift. In the distracter condition, when the distracter preceded the target, the head sometimes began to move toward the distracter before turning around in midflight to move in the same direction as the correct gaze shift (Corneil & Munoz, 1999). The presence of these early incorrect head movements accompanying correct gaze shifts suggests that in the distracter condition, an orienting signal can influence the head premotor system independently of the eye premotor system. There is also evidence that the premotor signal sent to the head premotor circuitry is augmented by the saccadic burst signal in the SC (Corneil, Olivier, et al., 2002).

Relatively little is known about how multisensory integration at the neuronal level is influenced by task-related factors seen only in awake, behaving animals. One such factor that has been shown previously to influence visual responses and motor activity in the SC is the state of fixation. During active fixation on a visible fixation point, sensory responses and motor activity are suppressed compared to what is observed when the fixation point disappears (Dorris & Munoz, 1995; Dorris et al., 1997). Multisensory integration may also be suppressed when fixation is actively engaged. To address this question, Bell et al. (2000) varied the state of fixation while recording sensory activity from neurons in the SC of behaving monkeys. Monkeys were trained to fixate a central visual fixation point (FP) while visual and/or auditory stimuli were presented in the periphery. Two fixation conditions were employed: a fixation (FIX) condition in which the FP remained

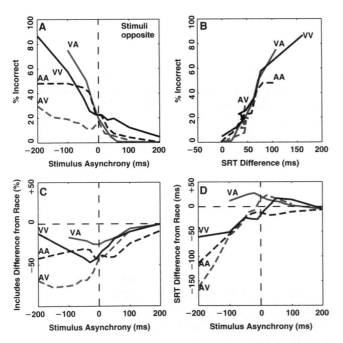

FIGURE 23.14 Task dependence of auditory-visual integration in an eye-head orienting task (after Corneil & Munoz, 1996). (A) The probability of an error response is largest when the distracter (presented on the opposite side) is presented first (negative asynchronies). This effect depends on target modality and is largest when the visual stimulus is the target (VA or VV trials). The error rate, however, is less than predicted by the race model for all conditions (C). The larger the difference in SRT between distracter and enhancer conditions, the larger the error rate (B). Note that all stimulus conditions follow the same relationship. (D) Only the VA enhancer condition (visual target, auditory irrelevant) produces SRTs that surpass the race model.

visible for the duration of the trial, and a fixation-blink (FIX-BLINK) condition in which the FP was extinguished prior to the presentation of the peripheral stimuli. Although both conditions required the monkey to maintain central fixation and the same eye position, the FIX condition included a visible FP and required exogenous visual fixation during stimulus presentation, whereas in the FIX-BLINK condition, the animal was required to fixate in the absence of a visible fixation spot. Bell et al. (2000) found that both the unimodal and multimodal sensory responses (Fig. 23.15) and multisensory interaction (Fig. 23.16) of

many of the neurons in the intermediate layers of the monkey SC were influenced by the state of fixation. Several neurons showed significantly stronger unimodal and combined responses in the FIX-BLINK condition than in the FIX condition (e.g., Fig. 23.15). This trend was significant across the population for visual and combined visual-auditory responses. When the visual and auditory stimuli were presented simultaneously, a larger proportion of neurons showed multisensory enhancement in the FIX-BLINK condition compared to the FIX condition (e.g., Fig. 23.16). These data demonstrate that multisensory processing

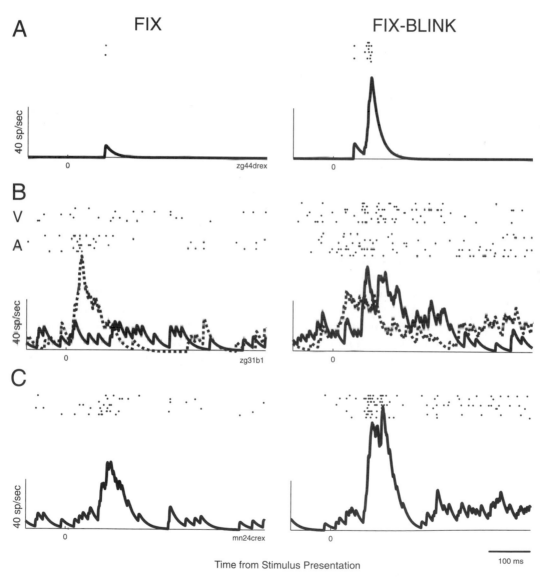

FIGURE 23.15   Sensory responses of SC neurons are modulated by the state of visual fixation. (A) SC neuron whose visual response was revealed only in the FIX-BLINK condition. During the FIX condition, the response was inhibited. (B) Example of an SC neuron that had only an auditory response in the FIX condition but both an auditory and a visual response in the FIX-BLINK condition. (C) Responses from an SC neuron with a visual response that was significantly augmented in the FIX-BLINK condition compared to the FIX condition.

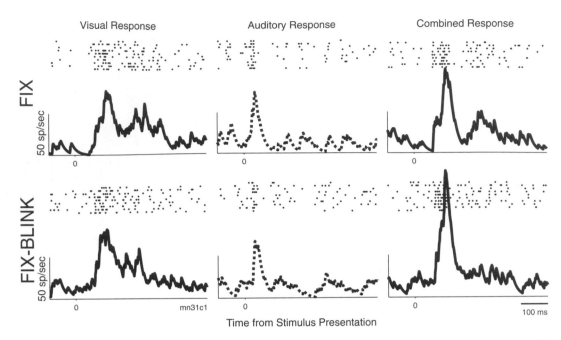

FIGURE 23.16 Multisensory integration of an SC neuron was enhanced in the FIX-BLINK condition. The cell had both visual (left panel) and auditory (middle panel) responses. The combined auditory-visual response was significantly enhanced during the FIX-BLINK condition when compared to the AV FIX condition and the unimodal responses for both fixation conditions.

can be influenced by the state of fixation of the animal.

AUDITORY-VISUAL INTEGRATION IN COMPLEX ENVIRONMENTS The experiments described so far involved orienting to auditory-visual stimuli presented well above the detection threshold and in the absence of a structured environment. Under more natural conditions, however, the saccadic system is typically challenged by a myriad of possible unimodal and multimodal targets to which gaze could be directed, and stimuli may be partially occluded or masked by complex backgrounds. Under such conditions, the gaze control system has to detect and select the relevant targets and ignore the irrelevant ones. This requires substantial additional processing time, and likely involves neural pathways (presumably cortical) that have not been discussed so far.

In the midbrain SC, neuronal multisensory interactions have been reported to be particularly strong when stimulus intensities are presented near response threshold (*inverse effectiveness;* Meredith & Stein 1986a). This situation might approach natural conditions in that the unimodal stimuli by themselves would hardly be sufficient to evoke a rapid and accurate orienting response. However, these neurophysiological results were obtained for sensory responses in an anesthetized preparation that is incapable of eliciting an orienting response. If similar mechanisms also influenced the saccade-generating mechanisms of awake and behaving subjects, the behavioral benefits afforded by multisensory integration (e.g., speed and accuracy) should also be largest for low-intensity stimuli.

Indeed, improved orienting (or approaching) to low-intensity stimuli was demonstrated in cats (Stein, Hunneycutt, & Meredith, 1988), although in that study saccadic eye movements were not measured and response time was not constrained. Until recently, human studies using low-intensity stimuli had not demonstrated the dramatic behavioral benefits expected from inverse effectiveness: the SRT reductions afforded by pairing low-intensity stimuli typically approximated similar magnitudes than for high-intensity stimuli (Frens et al., 1995; Hughes et al., 1994). Although this finding is in line with the assumptions underlying the two-stage model discussed earlier, perhaps the stimuli employed in those studies were not weak enough to invoke inverse effectiveness.

To approach this issue experimentally, we studied auditory-visual integration in human saccades (head fixed) evoked by low-intensity auditory and visual stimuli hidden in a complex auditory-visual background. Both stimuli served as potential targets (Corneil, Van Wanrooij, et al., 2002). Unimodal or bimodal targets could be presented at any of 24 possible target locations within the two-dimensional oculomotor range (Fig. 23.17A). Both the signal-to-noise ratio (S/N) of the auditory target relative to the acoustic background and the temporal asynchrony of the auditory and visual

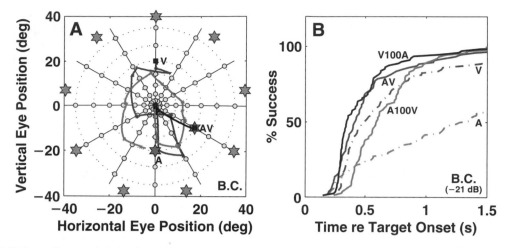

FIGURE 23.17   (*A*) Saccadic search behavior of human subject, B.C., in the presence of an auditory-visual background when the target was visual (V, dim red LED), auditory (A, broad-band buzzer at −21 dB in relation to background), or bimodal. Green LEDs (n = 85; light gray circles) served as a visual background. Nine speakers (solid stars) produced a broad-band white noise backgroud at 60 dB. The background was on for 4500 ms; targets were on for 3300 ms. The response to the visual target (black square at 20 degrees up; dark gray trace) took ten saccades to reach the target. The auditory trial (gray star at 20 degrees down; light gray trace) was initially goal-directed but followed by a sequence of saccades quite similar to the visual search. The AV target (synchronous presentation at (*R*, Φ = 20, 330 degrees; black trace) acquired the target with one saccadic eye movement. (*B*) Cumulative success rate as a function of time for the V, A, and three types of AV trials (A100V, AV, and V100A) for subject B.C. (about 100 trials per condition). The most successful conditions were the AV and V100A trials, showing the behavioral benefit of AV integration. See text for further explanation.

targets in bimodal trials were systematically varied. All trial types were randomly interleaved across trials. In this demanding task, subjects generated saccade scan patterns that consisted of anywhere from one to more than ten saccades before localizing the target.

An example of this behavior (occurring in about 15% of the trials) is illustrated in Figure 23.17*A*. It shows the scanning patterns for three different trial types superimposed on the AV background scene: a visual-only scan path (dark gray trace), an auditory-only response (S/N −21 dB; light gray trace), and an auditory-visual response (synchronous presentation; black trace). The initial A-only response appeared to be directed toward the target. Yet the subject was quite uncertain about this response, as subsequent saccades did not revisit that first location. The V-only response consisted of a series of ten saccades, in which only the last saccade led to target foveation. A similarity in scan patterns for both A-only and V-only saccades under these low-intensity stimulation conditions is evident.

In contrast, the bimodal condition necessitated only one saccadic eye movement to identify the target. This behavior was quite typical of AV trials, for which multiple-saccade scan patterns were quite rare. The benefit of AV integration is further illustrated in Figure 23.17*B*, which shows how the cumulative success rate evolved over time within the first 1.5 s. A trial was considered a success as soon as the end-point of a saccade landed within a small window around the target.

The A-only trials (−21 dB condition) were the least successful in acquiring the target (light gray dash-dotted line; Fig. 23.17*A* shows a successful example), because only 50% of the trials met this criterion within 1.5 s. The V-only trials were considerably more successful: on roughly 85% of the trials the target was foveated within 1.5 s (dark gray dash-dotted line). As is evident from the graphs, the different AV conditions (i.e., three temporal asynchronies) are clearly different from the unimodal trials. The AV (synchronous) and V100A (V leads auditory by 100 ms) trials were obviously the most beneficial stimulus combinations, with subjects exceeding a 90% success score within 500 ms (i.e., within two saccades). Interestingly, the A100V saccades were much worse (only 50% success after 500 ms), even though for this stimulus the first stimulus-evoked neural responses would have been by far the earliest of all the trial types. Thus, under complex stimulus conditions such as these, a race mechanism does not appear to be operational.

Sound localization behavior was strongly affected by the S/N: as the sound intensity in relation to background decreased, reaction times of the first localization response became progressively longer and the first-saccade response became more and more inaccurate (Corneil, Van Wanrooij, et al., 2002). Interestingly, the latter was predominantly observed in the elevation response component, as azimuth response accuracy was quite robust, even down to a −18 dB S/N. Bimodal stimuli led to a marked improvement in response behavior

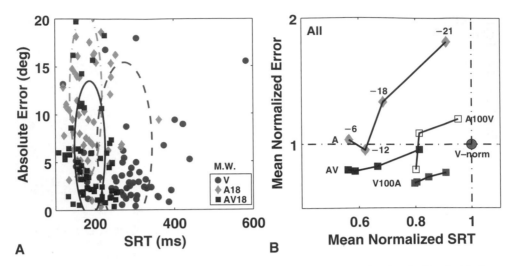

A

B

FIGURE 23.18 (*A*) First-saccade reaction time versus absolute error of the saccade end-point for V-only (dark gray circles), A-only (−18 dB S/N; light gray diamonds) and synchronous AV saccades (black squares). The latter capture the best of both modalities: AV saccades are as fast as A-only saccades and as accurate as V-only saccades, and have less end-point scatter (ellipses). (*B*) Summary of the results averaged and normalized in relation to V-only across subjects. All AV conditions show signs of integration, because none of the AV results coincide with the unimodal conditions. See text for explanation. (Modified from Corneil, Van Wanrooij, et al., 2002.) (See Color Plate 5.)

that was already noticeable in the first saccadic eye movement. A summary of the results of a typical experimental session of one subject is shown in Figure 23.18*A* (Color Plate 5). Here, the first saccade in each trial is represented by plotting the SRT against the absolute localization error for V-only saccades (light gray circles), A-only responses (evoked at −18 dB; light gray diamonds), and AV-saccades (synchronous condition; dark gray squares). The ellipses circumscribing the data are drawn around the mean with 1 SD. The V-only saccades have long SRTs but are accurate on average. The scatter, however, is large. A-only saccades, on the other hand, have shorter reaction times but are much more inaccurate. Moreover, the scatter is larger than for the V-only responses. The AV saccades have the lowest errors and yield the shortest reaction times. In addition, the scatter of the responses is lowest in both dimensions. Quantitative analysis showed that the reaction time data followed the prediction of the race model (Corneil, Van Wanrooij, et al., 2002). This was a consistent finding across subjects. Apparently, in more complex stimulus environments, the reaction times to synchronous AV stimuli do not surpass the race prediction, as reported for simpler stimulus conditions (Arndt & Colonius, 2001; Harrington & Peck, 1998; see also Fig. 23.9).

A quantitative comparison of the SRTs with the race model for the different stimulus conditions (i.e., S/N and temporal order) revealed the following pattern: (1) The differences of the SRTs with the race model predictions were invariant for the different S/N ratios (this is in line with the two-stage model). (2) The differences

depended strongly on the temporal asynchrony. (3) Fast SRTs for AV saccades required spatial alignment of the stimuli. The A100V stimuli yielded SRTs that were much longer than predicted by the race model, while for the AV condition the SRT data were indistinguishable from the race model. The V100A trials yielded SRTs that were shorter than predicted.

As shown in Figure 23.18*B* (Color Plate 5) for the averaged and pooled data, the effects of AV integration depended strongly on both the S/N and the relative timing of the two stimuli. The largest differences with the unimodal results were obtained at the lowest S/N, which shows that inverse effectiveness is observed for saccadic eye movements also. Moreover, the temporal order of the stimuli was important, too. In line with the results in Figure 23.17, the least beneficial configuration was the one in which the auditory stimulus preceded the visual target by 100 ms (A100V conditions; open squares in Fig. 23.18*B*). For those stimuli, the mean accuracy was worse than for V-only trials, although better than for the A-only stimuli. Interestingly, the SRTs for this stimulus configuration were shorter than for V-only saccades but longer than for A-only responses. This finding hints at an inhibitory interaction between the two modalities. The highest accuracy was obtained for the V100A saccades, whereas the SRTs for this condition surpassed the prediction of the race model. The latter suggests an excitatory AV interaction (Corneil, Van Wanrooij, et al., 2002). The results for the synchronous AV stimuli fall between the two asynchronous conditions. Thus, it appears that auditory-visual integration evolves from inhibitory to excitatory within a 100–150 ms time window and its strength is largest for spatially aligned, low-intensity stimuli. Because the AV data almost never lined up with the unimodal responses, it could be argued that nearly all bimodal stimulus conditions gave rise to neural integration. The only exception was the synchronous AV condition at −6 dB S/N.

Summary and conclusions

The experiments described in this chapter provide ample evidence for neural integration of multisensory stimuli evoking an orienting response of the eyes and head. Many of the results suggest similar neural mechanisms as have been described for sensory responses and multisensory integration in anesthetized preparations. In addition, behavioral experiments with human subjects suggest further neurophysiological studies in awake and trained animals that should provide important insight into the functional role of multisensory integration in the programming and generation of rapid orienting gaze shifts.

SACCADE REACTION TIMES The experimental data show that neural integration rather than auditory-assisted search, an acoustic warning effect, or statistical facilitation underlies the reduction in SRT. The neural correlate for this effect is found in an enhancement of SCBUN prelude activity rather than in an increase of the peak firing rate of the saccade-related burst of SCBNs or SCBUNs. We believe that these neural responses cannot be explained by a warning mechanism, as in that case the SCBUN activity for AV saccades would have to be the same as auditory-evoked responses. Although auditory saccades were not measured in the animal experiments described here, Van Opstal and Frens (1996) have shown that auditory-related movement activity is lower rather than higher for the majority of SC cells when compared with visually evoked responses. Despite these lower firing rates, however, auditory-evoked saccades typically have shorter reaction times than visually evoked saccades (in the non-gap condition). One reason for this effect lies in the shorter conduction delays of acoustic input (between 15 and 20 ms in the SC) compared with visual signals (about 60–70 ms). In addition, the recruited population of SCBUNs may be larger for auditory saccades than for visual saccades. Although the latter factor has not been studied so far, auditory receptive fields are typically much larger than visual receptive fields (see, e.g., Fig. 23.1). This property might extend to the preparatory activity of SCBUNs. Both factors would lead to an earlier crossing of the threshold for initiating an auditory saccade.

The neural responses observed in the SC do not provide a basis for statistical facilitation, as the early sensory responses do not change their timing for bimodal stimuli at all. This finding is consistent with the assumption of the two-stage model that the race between the sensory channels takes place upstream from the SC, and that the SC itself is part of the second stage (Arndt & Colonius, 2001; Fig. 23.10).

Finally, the experiments of Bell and colleagues have also been performed with the A-stimuli and V-stimuli out of spatial-temporal alignment (data not shown). As shown by Frens and Van Opstal (1998), the reduction in monkey SRT then decreases systematically as the auditory and visual stimuli are moved out of alignment, just as it does for human saccades (Fig. 23.9). In line with this observation, the prelude buildup activity in SCBUNs is no longer enhanced when the stimuli are misaligned. Instead, they are often depressed (Bell et al., in preparation).

Taken together, multisensory integration is observable in the preparatory phase of saccade programming rather than in the sensory-evoked responses or in the movement-related saccadic burst. Some caution is warranted, however, because stimuli were always presented well above threshold. It is therefore conceivable that both the timing and the intensity of the sensory and motor bursts could change substantially under near-threshold conditions, and that AV integration may affect these parameters too.

COORDINATE TRANSFORMATIONS The visual-auditory double-step experiments show that eye-head gaze shifts fully compensate for the intervening eye and head movements in planning the coordinates of the subsequent gaze shift. The neural mapping stages involved encode the desired displacement of eyes and head in different reference frames (Figs. 23.13C and D): whereas the eye is guided by oculocentric motor error, the head is driven by a head-centered error signal. The neural transformations involved are also quite different for the different sensory modalities (Fig. 23.6), yet the gaze control system is able to achieve this task on a time scale of several tens of milliseconds. It is unlikely that the eye and head movement vectors of the second gaze shift in the double-step trials are already programmed before the start of the first gaze shift. Because the contributions of eyes and head to the first gaze shift vary considerably from trial to trial (e.g., Corneil, Hing, Bautista, & Munoz, 1999; Goossens & Van Opstal, 1997), the motor errors after the first response will also vary. An updating mechanism that is based on feedback of the actual gaze shift is more flexible and robust against perturbations, and has been proposed in the literature to account for gaze control behavior (e.g., Goossens & Van Opstal, 1997; Munoz & Guitton, 1989; Munoz, Pélisson, & Guitton, 1991).

There is good evidence that in nonhuman primates, the oculocentric code for the eye in space is represented by a localized population of cells in the deeper layers of the SC (e.g., Fig. 23.7A; Freedman & Sparks, 1997; Munoz & Guitton, 1989). So far, it is not clear how and where the craniocentric head motor-error signal is determined, but it has been proposed that the decomposition of eye and head motor-error signals occurs downstream from the collicular gaze displacement command (Goossens & Van Opstal, 1997).

Although auditory-receptive fields of many SC cells shift with eye position so as to align with an oculocentric target representation (Fig. 23.7B), it is not known whether under conditions of eye-head misalignment AV integration still takes place at the level of SCBUNs and SCBNs.

Interestingly, for a substantial subset of auditory-responsive neurons in the SC, the head-centered to eye-centered transformation was incomplete: the responses of these cells aligned neither with the oculocentric motor error nor with the craniocentric target coordinates (Jay & Sparks, 1984, 1987). For these cells, the responses could be best described by an intermediate coordinate system. It would be interesting to know the auditory-visual response properties of such "hybrid" cells. For example, does auditory-visual integration for such neurons occur when the stimuli are (not) aligned in space?

EFFECT OF TASK CONSTRAINTS ON MULTISENSORY INTEGRATION The neurophysiological data show that the state of visual fixation (presence or absence of a visual target on the fovea) exerts a prominent influence on both the unimodal sensory responses to peripheral targets and the neural integration of AV stimuli. This factor has so far been largely ignored in the literature. The neural basis for this phenomenon is likely to be found in the intracollicular inhibitory network between rostral FNs and the more caudal SCBUNs and SCBNs (Munoz & Istvan, 1998). Introducing a gap between the disappearance of the visual fixation point and the onset of the peripheral targets, the masking effects of this potent inhibition are circumvented, allowing multisensory integration to be revealed also in the alert animal.

EFFECT OF A COMPLEX ENVIRONMENT ON MULTISENSORY INTEGRATION Multisensory integration is clearly beneficial when the saccadic system is confronted with a complex environment. In such environments neither

the visual system nor the auditory system alone is capable of generating a rapid and accurate saccadic eye movement (e.g., Corneil, Van Wanrooij, et al., 2002). The experiments, so far performed only in human subjects, show clearly that both saccade accuracy and saccade timing improve for AV stimulation. Neural integration thus brings about the optimal performance of both systems: visual accuracy paired with auditory speed. The improvement in saccadic performance is largest for the weakest stimuli. These data therefore show that inverse effectiveness is also manifest in the human saccadic system. A control experiment with a nonlocalizable auditory stimulus showed that then the effect disappears completely, which shows that spatial alignment of the stimuli is crucial (Corneil, Van Wanrooij, et al., 2002). It should be noted that the SRTs surpassed the race model prediction only when the auditory target followed the visual target. Thus, the relative timing of the stimuli also influences the amount of multisensory integration on saccades. As predicted by the two-stage model, these effects did not depend on the S/N. Taken together, these behavioral results are nicely in line with earlier neurophysiological recordings of low-intensity sensory responses in SC cells of anesthetized cats. The next step would be to study these phenomena in the awake, behaving preparation.

CONCEPTUAL MODEL OF MULTISENSORY INTEGRATION As described in the previous sections, the two-stage model can accommodate the behavioral data (Fig. 23.10; Arndt & Colonius, 2001). In our closing discussion we incorporate the neurophysiological findings from awake monkey SC into the neural integration stage of the model. Our conceptual model is presented in Figure 23.19. In the first stage of the model, the visual and auditory channels provide input to the deeper layers of the SC. It is assumed that the processing speed within these channels is influenced by the S/N. In the SC motor map, both modalities superimpose at the same location for spatially aligned targets. Updating mechanisms that transform the acoustic input into oculocentric coordinates encoding the desired gaze shift are also assumed to be implemented upstream from the motor SC (e.g., Sparks & Mays, 1990). Visual and auditory noise broadens the population activity patterns in the motor map (Fig. 23.19B) and lowers the firing rates (Fig. 23.19C). The population activity for auditory saccades is also broader and less vigorous than for visual saccades. Thus, SRT is prolonged in the presence of noise, as the rise to threshold takes more time (indicated by $\tau(v)$, etc.). Broader activity profiles cause more scatter in the saccade end-points. The saccade is triggered as soon as the population activity reaches a fixed

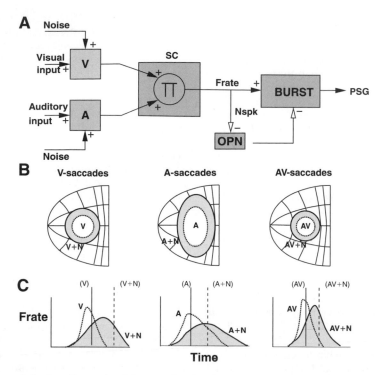

FIGURE 23.19   Conceptual model of auditory-visual integration in the primate saccadic system. See text for explanation.

threshold (here indicated by the number of spikes, Nspk, emitted by the population), leading to full inhibition of the OPNs. The firing rate (Frate) modulates the reticular burst neurons, so that lower firing rates generate saccades with lower peak velocities. A nonlinearity in the SC neurons accounts for the inverse effectiveness for low-intensity stimuli (Π). An alternative for such a nonlinearity has recently been provided by Anastasio, Patton, and Belkacem-Boussaid (2000), who proposed that Bayesian computations at the single-neuron level can in principle account for this phenomenon. Auditory-visual stimuli would pass the threshold earlier than unimodal stimuli, provided they are properly timed and spatially aligned. When stimuli are not in spatial and temporal register, lateral inhibition within the motor map prevents the full development of simultaneously active sites (e.g., Munoz & Istvan, 1998; Meredith & Romoa, 1998). This in turn leads to lower firing rates and hence longer SRTs. An asymmetry in temporal behavior of MI has to be assumed: multisensory interactions are supposed to develop from inhibitory (when auditory leads) to excitatory (when visual leads).

REFERENCES

Anastasio, T. J., Patton, P. E., & Belkacem-Boussaid, K. (2000). Using Bayes' rule to model multisensory enhancement in the superior colliculus. *Neural Computation, 12,* 1165–1187.

Arndt, P. A., & Colonius, H. (2001). A two-stage model for visual-auditory interaction in saccadic latencies. *Perception & Psychophysics, 63,* 126–147.

Bell, A. H., Corneil, B. D., Meredith, M. A., & Munoz, D. P. (2001). The influence of stimulus properties on multisensory processing in the awake primate superior colliculus. *Canadian Journal of Experimental Psychology, 55,* 123–132.

Bell, A. H., Everling, D., & Munoz, D. P. (2000). Influence of stimulus eccentricity and direction on characteristics of pro- and antisaccades in non-human primates. *Journal of Neurophysiology, 84,* 2595–2604.

Bell, A. H., Meredith, M. A., Van Opstal, A. J., & Munoz, D. P. (2003). *Audio-visual integration in monkey superior colliculus underlying the preparation and initiation of saccadic eye movements.* Manuscript submitted for publication.

Bell, A. H., Meredith, M. A., Van Opstal, A. J., Van Wanrooij, M., Corneil, B. D., & Munoz, D. P. (2001). Multisensory integration in the primate superior colliculus: Saccades to visual and audio-visual stimuli. *Society of Neuroscience Abstracts, 27,* 681.2.

Blauert, J. (1997). *Spatial hearing: The psychophysics of human sound localization* (2nd ed.). Cambridge, MA: MIT Press.

Carpenter, R. H., & Williams, M. L. (1995). Neural computation of log-likelihood in control of saccadic eye movements. *Nature, 377,* 59–62.

Corneil, B. D., Hing, C. A., Bautista, D. V., & Munoz, D. P. (1999). Human eye-head gaze shifts in a distractor task: I. Truncated gaze shifts. *Journal of Neurophysiology, 82,* 1390–1405.

Corneil, B. D., & Munoz, D. P. (1996). The influence of auditory and visual distractors on human orienting gaze shifts. *Journal of Neuroscience, 16,* 8193–8207.

Corneil, B. D., & Munoz, D. P. (1999). Human eye-head gaze shifts in a distractor task: II. Reduced threshold for initiation of early head movements. *Journal of Neurophysiology, 82,* 1406–1421.

Corneil, B. D., Olivier, E., & Munoz, D. P. (2002). *Neck muscle activity evoked by stimulation of the monkey superior colliculus: II. Relationships with gaze shift initiation.* Manuscript submitted for publication.

Corneil, B. D., Van Wanrooij, M., Munoz, D. P., & Van Opstal, A. J. (2002). Auditory-visual interactions subserving goal-directed saccades in a complex scene. *Journal of Neurophysiology, 88,* 438–454.

Dorris, M. C., & Munoz, D. P. (1995). A neural correlate for the gap effect on saccadic reaction times in monkey. *Journal of Neurophysiology, 73,* 2558–2562.

Dorris, M. C., & Munoz, D. P. (1998). Saccadic probability influences motor preparation signals and time to saccadic initiation. *Journal of Neuroscience, 18,* 7015–7026.

Dorris, M. C., Paré, M., & Munoz, D. P. (1997). Neural activity in monkey superior colliculus related to the initiation of saccadic eye movements. *Journal of Neuroscience, 17,* 8566–8579.

Engelken, E. J., & Stevens, K. W. (1989). Saccadic eye movements in response to visual, auditory and bisensory stimuli. *Aviation, Space, and Environmental Medicine, 60,* 762–768.

Everling, S., Paré, M., Dorris, M. C., & Munoz, D. P. (1998). Comparison of the discharge characteristics of brain stem omnipause neurons and superior colliculus fixation neurons in monkey: Implications for control of fixation and saccade behavior. *Journal of Neurophysiology, 79,* 511–528.

Freedman, E. G., & Sparks, D. L. (1997). Activity of cells in the deeper layers of the superior colliculus of the rhesus monkey: Evidence for a gaze displacement command. *Journal of Neurophysiology, 78,* 1669–1690.

Frens, M. A., & Van Opstal, A. J. (1995). A quantitative study of auditory-evoked saccadic eye movements in two dimensions. *Experimental Brain Research, 107,* 103–117.

Frens, M. A., & Van Opstal, A. J. (1998). Visual-auditory interactions in the superior colliculus of the behaving monkey. *Brain Research Bulletin, 46,* 211–224.

Frens, M. A., Van Opstal, A. J., & Van der Willigen, R. F. (1995). Spatial and temporal factors determine audio-visual interactions in human saccadic eye movements. *Perception & Psychophysics, 57,* 802–816.

Fuchs, A. F., Kaneko, C. R., & Scudder, C. A. (1985). Brainstem control of saccadic eye movements. *Annual Review of Neuroscience, 8,* 307–337.

Gandhi, N. J., & Keller, E. L. (1997). Spatial distribution and discharge characteristics of superior colliculus neurons antidromically activated from the omnipause region in monkey. *Journal of Neurophysiology, 78,* 2221–2225.

Gielen, C. C. A. M., Schmidt, R. A., & Van den Heuvel, P. J. M. (1983). On the nature of intersensory facilitation of reaction time. *Perception & Psychophysics, 34,* 161–168.

Goldring, J. E., Dorris, M. C., Corneil, B. D., Ballantyne, P. A., & Munoz, D. P. (1996). Combined eye-head gaze shifts to visual and auditory targets in humans. *Experimental Brain Research, 111,* 68–78.

Goossens, H. H. L. M., & Van Opstal, A. J. (1997). Human eye-head coordination in two dimensions under different sensorimotor conditions. *Experimental Brain Research, 114,* 542–560.

Goossens, H. H. L. M., & Van Opstal, A. J. (1999). Influence of head position on the spatial representation of acoustic targets. *Journal of Neurophysiology, 81,* 2720–2736.

Groh, J. M., & Sparks, D. L. (1996). Saccades to somatosensory targets: III. Eye-position-dependent somatosensory activity in primate superior colliculus. *Journal of Neurophysiology, 75,* 439–453.

Harrington, L. K., & Peck, C. K. (1998). Spatial disparity affects visual-auditory interactions in human sensorimotor processing. *Experimental Brain Research, 122,* 247–252.

Hofman, P. M., Van Riswick, J. G., & Van Opstal, A. J. (1998). Relearning sound localization with new ears. *Nature Neuroscience, 1,* 417–421.

Hughes, H. C., Nelson, M. D., & Aronchick, D. M. (1998). Spatial characteristics of visual-auditory summation in human saccades. *Vision Research, 38,* 3955–3963.

Hughes, H. C., Reuter-Lorenz, P. A., Nozawa, G., & Fendrich, R. (1994). Visual-auditory interactions in sensorimotor processing: Saccades versus manual responses. *Journal of Experimental Psychology: Human Perception and Performance, 20,* 131–153.

Jay, M. F., & Sparks, D. L. (1984). Auditory receptive fields in primate superior colliculus shift with eye position. *Nature, 309,* 345–347.

Jay, M. F., & Sparks, D. L. (1987). Sensorimotor integration in the primate superior colliculus: II. Coordinates of auditory signals. *Journal of Neurophysiology, 57,* 35–55.

Lee, P. H., Helms, M. C., Augustine, G. J., & Hall, W. C. (1997). Role of intrinsic synaptic circuitry in collicular sensorimotor integration. *Proceedings of the National Academy of Sciences, USA, 94,* 13299–13304.

Luschei, E. S., & Fuchs, A. F. (1972). Activity of brainstem neurons during eye movements of alert monkeys. *Journal of Neurophysiology, 35,* 445–461.

Meredith, M. A., Nemitz, J. W., & Stein, B. E. (1987). Determinants of multisensory integration in superior colliculus neurons: I. Temporal factors. *Journal of Neuroscience, 10,* 3215–3229.

Meredith, M. A., & Ramoa, A. S. (1998). Intrinsic circuitry of the superior colliculus: Pharmacophysiological identification of horizontally oriented inhibitory interneurons. *Journal of Neurophysiology, 79,* 1597–1602.

Meredith, M. A., & Stein, B. E. (1986a). Visual, auditory and somatosensory convergence on cells in superior colliculus results in multisensory integration. *Journal of Neurophysiology, 56,* 640–662.

Meredith, M. A., & Stein, B. E. (1986b). Spatial factors determine the activity of multisensory neurons in cat superior colliculus. *Brain Research, 365,* 350–354.

Moschovakis, A. K., Scudder, C. A., & Highstein, S. M. (1996). The microscopic anatomy and physiology of the mammalian saccadic system. *Progress in Neurobiology, 50,* 133–254.

Munoz, D. P., Dorris, M. C., Paré, M., & Everling, S. (2000). On your mark, get set: Brainstem circuitry underlying saccadic initiation. *Canadian Journal of Physiology and Pharmacology, 78,* 934–944.

Munoz, D. P., & Guitton, D. (1989). Fixation and orientation control by the tecto-reticulo-spinal system in the cat whose head is unrestrained. *Review of Neurology (Paris), 145,* 567–579.

Munoz, D. P., & Istvan, P. J. (1998). Lateral inhibitory interactions in the intermediate layers of the monkey superior colliculus. *Journal of Neurophysiology, 79*, 1193–1209.

Munoz, D. P., Pélisson, D., & Guitton, D. (1991). Movement of neural activity on the superior colliculus motor map during gaze shifts. *Science, 251*, 1358–1360.

Munoz, D. P., & Wurtz, R. H. (1993a). Fixation cells in monkey superior colliculus: I. Characteristics of cell discharge. *Journal of Neurophysiology, 70*, 559–575.

Munoz, D. P., & Wurtz, R. H. (1993b). Fixation cells in monkey superior colliculus: II. Reversible activation and deactivation. *Journal of Neurophysiology, 70*, 576–589.

Munoz, D. P., & Wurtz, R. H. (1995a). Saccade-related activity in monkey superior colliculus: I. Characteristics of burst and buildup cells. *Journal of Neurophysiology, 73*, 2313–2333.

Munoz, D. P., & Wurtz, R. H. (1995b). Saccade-related activity in monkey superior colliculus. II. Spread of activity during saccades. *Journal of Neurophysiology, 73*, 2334–2348.

Nozawa, G., Reuter-Lorenz, P. A., & Hughes, H. C. (1994). Parallel and serial processes in the human oculomotor system: Bimodal integration and express saccades. *Biology and Cybernetics, 72*, 19–34.

Perrott, D. R., Saberi, K., Brown, K., & Strybel, T. Z. (1990). Auditory psychomotor coordination and visual search performance. *Perception & Psychophysics, 48*, 214–226.

Perrott, D. R., Sadralodabai, T., Saberi, K., & Strybel, T. Z. (1991). Aurally aided visual search in the central visual field: Effects of visual load and visual enhancement of the target. *Human Factors, 33*, 389–400.

Raab, D. H. (1962). Statistical facilitation of simple reaction times. *Transactions of the New York Academy of Sciences, 24*, 574–590.

Raybourn, M. S., & Keller, E. L. (1977). Colliculoreticular organization in primate oculomotor system. *Journal of Neurophysiology, 40*, 861–878.

Robinson, D. A. (1972). Eye movements evoked by collicular stimulation in the alert monkey. *Vision Research, 12*, 1795–1808.

Ross, S. M., & Ross, L. E. (1981). Saccade latency and warning signals: Effect of auditory and visual stimuls onset and offset. *Perception & Psychophysics, 29*, 429–437.

Schiller, P. H., & Koerner, F. (1971). Discharge characteristics of single units in superior colliculus of the alert rhesus monkey. *Journal of Neurophysiology, 34*, 920–936.

Simon, J. R., & Craft, J. L. (1970). Effects of an irrelevant auditory stimulus on visual choice reaction time. *Journal of Experimental Psychology, 86*, 272–274.

Sparks, D. L., & Mays, L. E. (1980). Movement fields of saccade-related burst neurons in the monkey superior colliculus. *Brain Research, 190*, 39–50.

Sparks, D. L., & Mays, L. E. (1990). Signal transformations required for the generation of saccadic eye movements. *Annual Review of Neuroscience, 13*, 309–336.

Stein, B. E., & Meredith, M. A. (1993). *The merging of the senses.* Cambridge, MA: MIT Press.

Stein, B. E., Hunneycutt, W. S., & Meredith, M. A. (1988). Neurons and behavior: The same rules of multisensory integration apply. *Brain Research, 448*, 355–358.

Van Opstal, A. J., & Frens, M. A. (1996). Task-dependence of saccade-related activity in monkey superior colliculus: Implications for models of the saccadic system. *Progress in Brain Research, 112*, 179–194.

Wallace, M. T., Wilkinson, L. K., & Stein, B. E. (1996). Representation and integration of multiple sensory inputs in primate superior colliculus. *Journal of Neurophysiology, 76*, 1246–1266.

Wallace, M. T., Meredith, M. A., & Stein, B. E. (1998). Multisensory integration in the superior colliculus of the alert cat. *Journal of Neurophysiology, 80*, 1006–1010.

Wurtz, R. H., & Goldberg, M. E. (1972). Activity of superior colliculus in behaving monkey: 3. Cells discharging before eye movements. *Journal of Neurophysiology, 35*, 575–586.

Zwiers, M. P., Van Opstal, A. J., & Cruysberg, J. R. M. (2001). A spatial hearing deficit in early-blind humans. *Journal of Neuroscience, 21*, RC142, 1–5.

Zwiers, M. P., Van Opstal, A. J., & Paige, G. D. (2003). Plasticity in human sound localization induced by compressed spatial vision. *Nature Neuroscience, 6*, 175–181.

24 Modeling the Time Course of Multisensory Interaction in Manual and Saccadic Responses

ADELE DIEDERICH AND HANS COLONIUS

Introduction

Numerous effects of multisensory stimulation on perception and action have been described in the psychological literature for more than a century (see Welch & Warren, 1986). Although many phenomena, such as synesthetic experiences, can only be described at a qualitative level, other cross-modal effects are amenable to standard psychophysical measurement techniques. A prominent example is the ventriloquism effect, in which the presentation of a visual stimulus can shift the apparent location of a sound in the direction of the visual stimulus (see Vroomen & de Gelder, Chap. 9, this volume). However, as long as researchers must rely on participants' subjective estimates (e.g., about sound localization), it is difficult to determine whether the observed cross-modal effect is a genuine perceptual effect or due to some kind of response bias. Similar qualifications apply to numerous studies that try to determine, for example, the influence of a nonspecific accessory stimulus from one modality on detection thresholds of a second modality. Such effects are generally small and unreliable, but the role of bias in threshold measurements can be assessed by using techniques from the theory of signal detection (e.g., Lovelace, Stein, & Wallace, 2002).

RESPONSE SPEED AS A MEASURE OF MULTISENSORY INTERACTION   Another measure of perceptual sensitivity is the speed with which an observer is able to respond to the presence of a stimulus above threshold. Response time (RT) is a measure that has been used in experimental psychology for more than 150 years to investigate hypotheses about the mental and motor processes leading to the generation of a response. Thus, it is not surprising that some of the first psychological studies of intersensory interaction employed RTs to assess the effect of combining stimuli from different modalities and of varying their intensities (Todd, 1912). Although RT is measured on a physical (ratio) scale and seems not to be contaminated by judgment or response

bias effects, the interpretation of RT data in the context of a specific experimental paradigm is subtle and requires a high level of technical skill. Fortunately, this skill has been developed within experimental psychology (e.g., Van Zandt, 2002).

RT analysis is most powerful in uncovering underlying processes when it is based on explicit quantitative hypotheses (Luce, 1986). Thus, this chapter emphasizes mathematical models of RT that have been developed to explain and predict cross-modal stimulus effects resulting from a manipulation of their spatial-temporal configuration and of physical stimulus dimensions such as intensity. One feature of the models discussed is that they are based on a few relatively simple principles—if not mathematically, then at least conceptually—and thus they do not reflect the full complexity of the underlying multisensory processes. This should be considered a virtue rather than a defect at this stage: these models can be tested rigorously and, hopefully, shown to converge on those principles that constitute a valid framework for a more detailed account to be developed as more evidence is collected.

One simple reason to use RT as a measure of multimodal effects is that, whatever happens as an organism processes stimulus information from several sensory modalities, it must unfold over time. One of the main experimental findings in behavioral studies is that the occurrence of cross-modal effects critically depends on the temporal arrangement of the stimulus sets. For example, the speeding up of the RT to a visual stimulus resulting from the presentation of say, an accessory auditory stimulus typically is greatest when the visual stimulus precedes the auditory stimulus by an interval that equals the difference in RT between response to the visual stimulus alone and response to the auditory stimulus alone (Hershenson, 1962). Interestingly, temporal integration rules similar to this one have been discerned for responses at the level of individual multisensory neurons. Specifically, bimodal cells in cat superior colliculus (SC) show maximal levels of response enhancement when the peak discharge periods evoked by each modality overlap in time (Meredith, Nemitz, & Stein, 1987). This overlap often is not correlated with simultaneous stimulus presentation or with differences in stimulus presentation that match their latency differences. Because multisensory SC neurons project to premotor areas of the brainstem that control orientation of the eyes, pinnae, and head, the temporal relationships of stimulus complexes that control the activity of these neurons should ultimately contribute to orientation behavior as well. Of course, individual neurons differ in their temporal response properties, and behavior is the result of a large number of neurons at different sites of the brain. Nonetheless, it is a distinct possibility that the temporal integration rules observed in behavioral experiments can ultimately be deduced from certain principles holding at the level of the individual neuron or an assembly of neurons (see Colonius & Diederich, 2002a).

CROSS-MODAL PARADIGMS Experimental paradigms to elicit a response to a cross-modal stimulus set differ with respect to the instructions given to the participant, and these differences must be taken into account in models of response speed. In the *redundant target* paradigm, stimuli from different modalities are presented simultaneously or at certain interstimulus intervals, and the subject is instructed to respond to whatever stimulus is detected first. The participant is not asked to identify the modality that elicited his or her response and often is not able to. In the *focused attention* paradigm, cross-modal stimulus sets are presented in the same manner, but participants are instructed to respond only to the onset of a stimulus from a specific target modality. If in some of the trials no stimulus from the target modality is presented, these trials are called *catch* trials.

In all paradigms, participants are prone to make certain types of errors. *Anticipation errors* are responses made before any stimulus appears, and *misses* occur if no response is made at all. These two types of errors can often be attributed to slips of attention, are minimized by training, and are typically not part of the modeling effort. Another type of error consists of responses made in catch trials. Their frequency depends on whether the participant is explicitly instructed to respond as fast as possible and not to worry about avoiding erroneous catch trial responses or, alternatively, to respond at a speed that minimizes these errors. In the models discussed in this chapter, no mechanism to explain catch trial responses is adopted, because catch trial error frequency is typically kept at a negligible level (less than 1% or 2%).

MANUAL VERSUS SACCADIC RESPONSES The most common mode of assessing speed of response has been to measure the time it takes to press a button, or to release it, by a finger or foot movement (see Donders, 1868/1969). With the advent of modern eye movement registration techniques, the measurement of *saccadic reaction time*, i.e., the time from the presentation of the target stimulus to the beginning of the eye movement, is gaining in popularity. Because SC is an important site of oculomotor control (e.g., Munoz & Würtz, 1995), measuring saccadic RT is an obvious choice to study the behavioral consequences of multisensory integration.

An important distinction in measuring response speed is whether a correct response requires the participant to make a choice. For example, a participant may be asked to respond to a visual stimulus with the left hand and to an auditory stimulus with the right hand, or to respond to a stimulus on the right, irrespective of modality, with the right hand and to a stimulus on the left with the left hand (or vice versa). In any event, the possible number of stimulus-response mappings is somewhat restricted (even if responding with different fingers is employed, a procedure that adds possibly unwanted compatibility effects) as long as manual responses are employed.

For saccadic eye movements, however, this restriction does not apply, given that the possible number of target positions in space is limited only by the spatial resolution of the oculomotor system. Thus, saccadic responses are ideally suited for studying the spatial rules of cross-modal interaction in parallel with the determination of the temporal rules. Eye movement registration is possible under both the redundant target paradigm and the focused attention paradigm, and participants can be asked to move their eyes in response to visual, auditory, or somatosensory targets. Nevertheless, the model builder should be aware of certain idiosyncrasies that arise from the simple fact that the ocular system is dominated by the visual system. For example, it is well known that saccades to visual targets have a higher level of accuracy than those to auditory or somatosensory stimuli (see Van Opstal & Munoz, Chap. 23, this volume).

PREVIEW Current models of response time can roughly be divided into two classes, *separate activation models* and *coactivation models* (a terminology suggested in Miller, 1982). Some models of either type will be described in subsequent sections, along with their empirical merits, but for a complete coverage of experimental results we must refer to the literature. Finally, we present the recently developed *time-window-of-integration model*, which combines features of both model types (see Colonius & Diederich, 2002b).

Separate activation models

Separate activation models, also known as *race models*, assume (1) that presenting a multisensory stimulus produces parallel, separate activation in different sensory channels that build to the level at which they can produce a response, and (2) that the response is triggered by the signal that reaches that level first. Assuming statistical variability in the channel processing times, separate activation models predict faster average reaction time to multisensory stimuli than to unimodal stimuli because the average of the winner's processing time is smaller than the average processing time in each single channel ("statistical facilitation"; see Raab, 1962).

For example, let T, V, and A denote the random processing time for a tactile, visual, and auditory stimulus, respectively. Then

$$E[\min(T, V, A)] \leq \min(E[T], E[V], E[A]) \quad (1)$$

where $E[\ ]$ indicates the expected value of the random variables (*Jensen's inequality*; see. Billingsley, 1979). Thus, statistical facilitation predicts faster mean responses to multisensory stimuli as a statistical phenomenon without assuming an additional neural mechanism.

To illustrate, we can consider a visual and an auditory stimulus, say, with processing time distributions f_V, f_A, and f_{VA} for the visual, auditory, and the bimodal (visual-auditory) condition, respectively. Now let us suppose the subject consistently responds faster to the unimodal auditory stimulus than to the unimodal visual stimulus. In that case, distribution f_A would lie completely to the left of distribution f_V (no overlap) (Fig. 24.1). Thus, in the bimodal condition the subject's reaction time would be determined by the time needed to process the auditory stimulus only. More realistically, however, f_V and f_A do overlap, and thus some of the long reactions to the

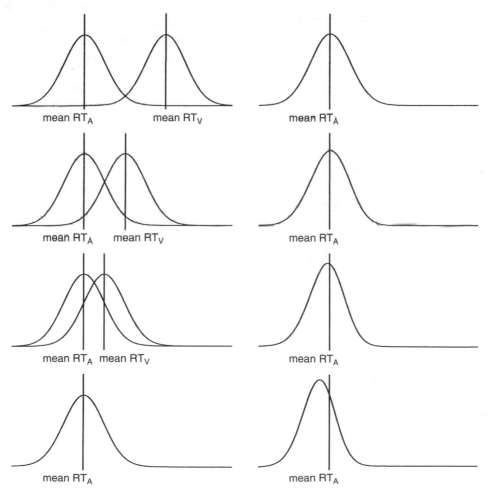

FIGURE 24.1   Graphs on the left depict processing time distributions f_A and f_V for the visual and auditory condition, respectively, graphs on the right depict the distributions of minima, f_{VA}, for the bimodal (visual-auditory) condition. In the top graph, f_A and f_V are fairly well separated—they barely overlap. Thus, the mean for f_{VA} (on the right) is about the same as for f_A. As the overlap between f_A and f_V increases, the distribution of minima shifts left and becomes most pronounced in the bottom graphs, where f_A and f_V overlap completely.

auditory stimulus will be replaced by shorter reactions to the visual stimulus in the bimodal condition. Therefore, mean bimodal RT will tend to be smaller than mean RT to the auditory stimulus. The more the distributions overlap, the more often long reactions to the auditory stimulus will be replaced by shorter reactions to the visual stimulus, resulting in a smaller bimodal mean RT. Figure 24.1 illustrates this effect. Maximal overlap and thus maximal statistical facilitation are expected if presentation of the faster processed stimulus (e.g., the auditory stimulus) is delayed by an amount of time equal to the difference in mean RT in the unimodal stimulus conditions, that is, when *physiological synchrony,* rather than stimulus presentation synchrony, is achieved.

TESTING SEPARATE ACTIVATION MODELS Assuming independent Gaussian distributions for the processing times, Raab's model (1962) fell slightly short of predicting the facilitation observed in Hershenson (1962). Gielen, Schmidt, and van den Heuvel (1983) generalized Raab's model by employing the observed unimodal distributions to estimate the minimum distribution in the bimodal conditions. Nevertheless, statistical facilitation alone could not account for the facilitation observed in their data.

It should be noted that separate activation models need not assume processing times in the multimodal conditions to be statistically independent. Specifically, the amount of statistical facilitation increases with negatively dependent processing times because longer processing times of one modality then tend to occur more often with shorter processing times of the other modality (see Colonius, 1990).

The prevailing test of separate activation models was proposed by Miller (1982). It is based on a simple inequality (Boole's inequality; see Billingsley, 1979) holding for arbitrary events E_1 and E_2 in a probability space,

$$P(E_1 \cup E_2) \le P(E_1) + P(E_2) \qquad (2)$$

Identifying E_1 with the event $\{V \le t\}$, E_2 with $\{A \le t\}$ yields $E_1 \cup E_2 = \{\min(V, A) \le t\}$, so that Equation 2 becomes, for all t,

$$P(\min(V, A) \le t) \le P(V \le t) + P(A \le t) \qquad (3)$$

Assuming that the observable reaction times in the unimodal and bimodal conditions, RT_V, RT_A, and RT_{VA}, follow the same distribution as V, A, and $\min(V, A)$, respectively, puts an upper bound on the facilitation produced by bimodal stimuli (see Miller, 1982):

$$P(RT_{VA} \le t) \le P(RT_V \le t) + P(RT_A \le t) \qquad \text{for all } t \qquad (4)$$

If this inequality is violated for some value of time t, all separate activation models, whether statistical independence among the channel processing times is assumed or not, can be rejected.

Miller's test has become the standard tool to assess whether statistical facilitation suffices to explain the response speed-up of bimodal stimulus presentations (Townsend & Nozawa, 1995). Nevertheless, there are a number of caveats to be aware of when employing this test. First, the inequality is not yet amenable to sound statistical testing. The problem is that its right-hand side is not a probability distribution (it converges toward 2 for large t values). For the same reason, violations can only be expected for small enough values of t. Second, the inequality is based on the assumption of *context independence* (Colonius, 1990; Townsend & Ashby, 1983). Although different from statistical independence, context independence means that the distribution of V (or A) should be the same whether the stimulus is presented in the unimodal or in the bimodal condition, and it is not clear how to test this empirically. Third, it should be noted that nonviolation of the inequality does not provide evidence in favor of separate activation models (Colonius, 1986, 1990; Diederich & Colonius, 1987; Miller, 1982; Ulrich & Giray, 1986).

The amount of violation of the inequality can also be utilized as an indicator of the amount of statistical facilitation that is present in the data. Subtracting the right-hand side of Equation 4 from the left-hand side and plotting the difference as a function of t yields a curve that takes on positive values wherever the inequality is violated. Thus, the area under the (positive part of the) difference function is a measure of the degree of violation.

As an example, Figure 24.2 presents saccadic RT data from a visual-auditory focused attention study in which both the spatial disparity between the visual target and the auditory accessory and the intensity of the auditory stimulus were orthogonally combined at 3×3 levels (Arndt & Colonius, 2003). The area indicating violation is about constant within each row, with obvious violations for coincident stimuli (0 degree), whereas for disparate stimuli very little (25 degrees) or no violation at all (50 degrees) is exhibited. It is noteworthy that the intensity level of the auditory accessory has no discernible influence on the amount of violation (for an explanation, see below).

Following the same rationale as before, Inequality 4 can be extended to test separate activation models with trimodal (e.g., tactile-visual-auditory) stimulus sets:

$$P(RT_{TVA} \le t) \le P(RT_T \le t) + P(RT_V \le t) + P(RT_A \le t) \qquad (5)$$

where RT_{TVA} refers to the observable reaction time to the tactile-visual-auditory stimulus. This inequality places an

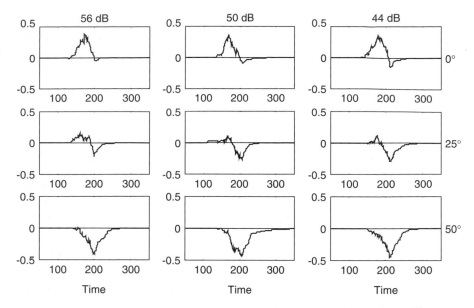

FIGURE 24.2   Test of separate activation model in a visual-auditory focused attention task; the area above the line indicates the degree of violation of Inequality 4. Auditory intensity decreases from left to right, visual-auditory distance increases from top to bottom.

upper bound on the facilitation produced by trimodal stimuli. However, because it is the sum of three probabilities approaching 3 for increasing values of t, this bound is often not of much use in testing separate activation. Interestingly, the upper bound can be sharpened in various ways. Let $E_1, \ldots, E_m$ be m arbitrary events in some probability space. Worsley (1982) proved that

$$P\left(\bigcup_{i=1}^{m} E_i\right) \le \sum_{i=1}^{m} P(E_i) - \sum_{i=1}^{m-1} P(E_i \cap E_{i+1}) \qquad (6)$$

holds. Taking $m = 3$ and identifying $E_1, E_2,$ and E_3 with the events $\{T \le t\}, \{V \le t\},$ and $\{A \le t\}$ for processing a tactile, visual, and auditory stimulus before time t, respectively, yields $P(E_1 \cup E_2 \cup E_3) = P(\min(T, V, A) \le t)$. As shown in Diederich (1992), this leads to three different inequalities relating the observable reaction time distributions in uni-, bi-, and trimodal conditions. One of them is

$$P(RT_{TVA} \le t) = P(\min(T, V, A) \le t)$$
$$\le P(\min(T, V) \le t) + P(\min(V, A) \le t)$$
$$\quad - P(RT_V \le t)$$
$$= P(RT_{TV} \le t) + P(RT_{VA} \le t)$$
$$\quad - P(RT_V \le t)$$

and the other two follow by combining other pairs of modalities analogously. The upper bound should be sharper now, because it approaches 1 for large enough t values. Moreover, taking at each t the minimum of all three upper bounds may lead to an even sharper upper bound.

This extension of the inequality test to three modalities is illustrated here with data from an experiment in which a tactile stimulus was presented first, followed by a visual stimulus after τ_1 ms, followed by an auditory stimulus $\tau_2 - \tau_1$ ms later (Diederich, 1995). Writing $RT_{T\tau_1 V(\tau_2 - \tau_1)A}$ for the RT of this trimodal stimulus, $RT_{T\tau_1 V}$ for the RT to a tactile stimulus followed by a visual stimulus τ_1 ms later, and so on, the following inequality test obtains:

$$P(RT_{T\tau_1 V(\tau_2 - \tau_1)A} \le t) \le P(RT_{T\tau_1 V} \le t)$$
$$\quad + P(RT_{V(\tau_2 - \tau_1)A} \le t) - P(RT_V + \tau_1 \le t) \qquad (7)$$

Figure 24.3 shows the trimodal RT data (stars) together with (1) the upper bound of Inequality 7, obtained from the sum of two bimodal RT data minus the unimodal RT data (diamonds) and (2) the upper bound of Inequality 5, obtained from the sum of three unimodal RT data (circles). A separate activation model would predict an ordering of the curves opposite to what is seen (up to about 160 ms), so these data constitute further evidence against this class of models.

Coactivation models

Because of the frequent empirical failure of separate activation models, an alternative model type has been considered to explain intersensory facilitation. *Coactivation models* assume that activation raised in different sensory channels by presenting multimodal stimuli is combined to satisfy a single criterion for response initiation. Coactivation models predict a faster average RT to

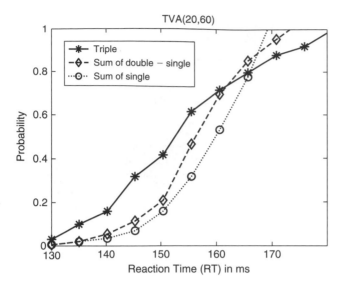

TVA(20,60)

FIGURE 24.3 Graph showing the trimodal RT data (stars) together with (1) the upper bound of Inequality 7, obtained from the sum of two bimodal RT data minus the unimodal RT data (diamonds), and (2) the upper bound of Inequality 5, obtained from the sum of three unimodal RT data (circles). A separate activation model would predict an ordering of the curves opposite to what is seen (up to about 160 ms).

multiple stimuli than to single stimuli because the combined activation reaches that criterion faster.

An early version of this concept is the *energy summation* hypothesis, according to which the energy from the different sensory modalities, determined by stimulus intensities, is assumed to be added during some peripheral stage of processing. Bernstein, Rose, and Ashe (1970) presented an energy integration model according to which the intensities of visual and auditory stimuli integrate at some common point in the nervous system. Presenting two different stimuli amounts to the same thing as increasing the intensity of either stimulus. Empirical evidence with respect to the energy summation hypothesis proved to be mixed. For example, decreasing auditory intensity often only slightly affected facilitation. Moreover, the fact that the spatial configuration of the stimuli has a clear effect on facilitation is not easily reconcilable with the hypothesis (for a review, see Nickerson, 1973). As an alternative to energy summation, Nickerson proposed the *preparation enhancement model*. In this model one stimulus plays an alerting role at many of the processing stages, so that the affected stages are terminated more quickly and the response comes earlier. These models are formulated mainly at a descriptive level, however, which makes testing them rigorously a difficult task. The two coactivation models considered next have a clear mathematical basis.

SUPERPOSITION MODELS Assume that the presentation of a stimulus triggers a sequence of "events" occurring randomly over time. In a neurophysiological context, these events are typically interpreted as the spikings of a neuron, say, but the model can be formulated at a more abstract level (see Tuckwell, 1995). The only relevant property of the events is their time of occurrence, and all information about the stimulus is contained in the time course of the events. For example, the rate of the event sequence—that is, the mean number of events per unit time interval—is typically thought to be related to signal intensity. Let $N(t)$ denote the number of events that have occurred by time t after stimulus presentation. *Counter models* assume that $N(t)$ has some internal representation registering the number of events over the course of time.

Let us assume a counter model in which separate counters exist for each modality, $N_V(t)$, $N_A(t)$, $N_T(t)$, for a visual, auditory, and tactile stimulus, respectively. The presentation of a multimodal stimulus triggers all counters to start registering their sequence of modality-specific events, and the counter that reaches a preset criterion first initiates the response. Obviously, under this assumption we are back to the class of separate activation (race) models, in which a race between counters takes place and the winner determines the response.

Alternatively, in *superposition models* the counters activated by a cross-modal stimulus will be summed. For example, a visual-auditory stimulus would trigger a composite counter, $N_2(t) \equiv N_V(t) + N_A(t)$, and a trimodal stimulus would trigger a composite counter corresponding to $N_3(t) \equiv N_V(t) + N_A(t) + N_T(t)$, analogously. Intuitively, the more counters that are combined in the composite counter, the faster a fixed criterion number of counts, c, say, will be reached on average. Figure 24.4 illustrates this intuition.

To compute the distribution of the (random) *waiting time* S_c for the cth count to occur, note that

$$P(S_c \le t) = P(N(t) \ge c)$$

The most tractable case from which to derive exact quantitative predictions is the *Poisson (counting) process,* where it is assumed that for each counter the times between successive events (*interarrival times*) are independent exponentially distributed random variables. Each Poisson process is characterized by a single constant, the *intensity parameter* λ. The expected waiting time for the cth count then simply is c/λ.

Superposition models represent RT by the waiting time S_c for the cth count. The criterion c is a (bias) parameter describing the subject's strategic behavior. Specifically, requiring high accuracy from the subject,

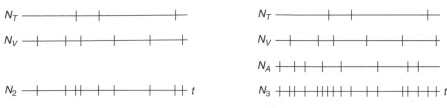

FIGURE 24.4   Superposition of visual, auditory, and tactile counters.

e.g., avoiding anticipation responses, may raise the criterion, whereas requiring a high response speed may lower it. It is assumed to be a constant, however, over a given experimental condition (see Luce, 1986, for a comprehensive discussion).

A superposition model for RT in redundant target experiments with two modalities was proposed by Schwarz (1989). Diederich (1992, 1995) extended the model to deal with trimodal stimulus data. In the Poisson superposition model with λ_T, λ_V, and λ_A denoting the intensity parameters of the tactile, visual, and auditory stimulus, respectively, the expected waiting time for the cth count to occur when all three stimuli are presented is:

$$E[S_c \mid trimodal] = \frac{c}{\lambda_T + \lambda_V + \lambda_A} \qquad (8)$$

At the level of mean RTs, the following model predictions are obvious:

1. The smaller the intensity parameter λ, the fewer counts are registered within a given time interval, and the longer it takes to reach the criterion to initiate a response. Thus, if λ is assumed to be an increasing function of stimulus intensity, mean RT to weak stimuli should be longer than to strong stimuli. For example, using a 50-dB and a 70-dB tone with $\lambda_{50} < \lambda_{70}$,

$$E[S_c \mid 50\ \mathrm{dB}] = \frac{c}{\lambda_{50}} > E[S_c \mid 70\ \mathrm{dB}] = \frac{c}{\lambda_{70}}$$

2. Mean RT to multimodal stimuli should be shorter than mean RT to unimodal stimuli, and should decrease with the number of modalities involved.

Figure 24.5 presents the fit of the model to data from a redundant target experiment with trimodal and bimodal stimuli, including various stimulus onset asynchrony (SOA) conditions (Diederich, 1992). In particular, the tactile stimulus and the visual stimulus were presented with SOA τ_1 indicated at the abscissa. For the trimodal stimulus condition the auditory stimulus was presented τ_2 ms after the tactile stimulus (upper graph in Fig. 24.5: $\tau_2 = 40$ ms; lower graph: $\tau_2 = 60$ ms). As predicted, mean RT to trimodal stimuli was shorter than to bimodal stimuli. Overall, at the level of the

means the model gave a very satisfactory fit for this rather large set of data. In particular, it was possible to predict mean RT values in the bimodal condition by using parameter values estimated in the trimodal condition (for details, see Diederich, 1992, 1995). On the negative side, the variability in the response speed, as

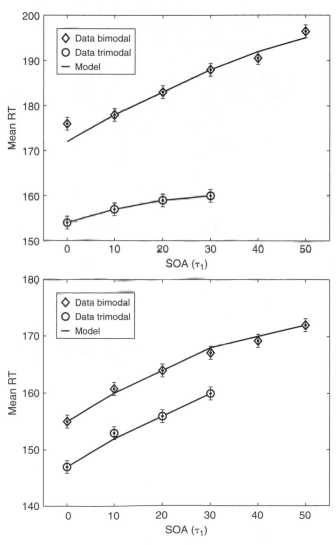

FIGURE 24.5   Fit of the superposition model to data from a redundant target experiment with trimodal and bimodal stimuli, including various stimulus onset asynchrony (SOA) conditions (Diederich, 1992).

measured by RT variance (derived in Diederich & Colonius, 1991), was not adequately captured by the model. This may be due to the fact that for the exponential distribution of the interarrival times (in the Poisson process), mean and variance are strictly coupled. It is not evidence against the superposition model in general.

On the other hand, the direct representation of stimulus intensity by the intensity parameter falls short of two common empirical observations. First, the model predicts that increasing the stimulus intensity should lead to ever faster responses, without being able to account for any saturation effects. Second, it is not clear how the observation of "inverse effectiveness," according to which cross-modal facilitation is strongest when stimulus strengths are weak, can be predicted by the superposition model. These shortcomings of superposition models have led to consideration of still another version of the coactivation idea.

THE MULTICHANNEL DIFFUSION MODEL This model resembles the superposition model in many ways. Its mathematical foundation is again a class of stochastic processes, but whereas superposition models are based on counting processes, the multichannel diffusion model is based on *Brownian motion,* or *diffusion* processes (see Billingsley, 1979). Generalizing the counter concept, response initiation depends on a stimulus-triggered activation accumulation process to cross a criterion level of activation. The level of activation varies continuously rather than in discrete counts. The main determinant of the process is its *drift (rate)* μ, a parameter that can intuitively be considered as the instantaneous propensity for the activation to go up or down by an infinitely small amount. Each presentation of a stimulus triggers the realization of a function describing the course of activation over time, called a *trajectory* (Fig. 24.6). The drift parameter is constant over time, but in a particular type of diffusion process, the *Ornstein-Uhlenbeck process* (OUP), it is a function of the activation level:

$$\mu(x) = \delta - \gamma \cdot x \qquad (9)$$

where δ refers to the constant part of the drift driving the process to the criterion (absorbing boundary). Diffusion models of RT assume that δ is a monotonic function of stimulus intensity: strong stimuli have large δ values, implying that the trajectories first have a tendency to be steep and to quickly approach the criterion level to initiate a response. Note, however, that for positive values of γ (the *decay parameter*), the drift $\mu(x)$ decreases the faster the larger the activation level x becomes, that is, the closer activation gets to the criterion level. This is responsible for the trajectories leveling off rather than increasing linearly over time (Fig. 24.6, upper graphs). Moreover, when the stimulus signal is

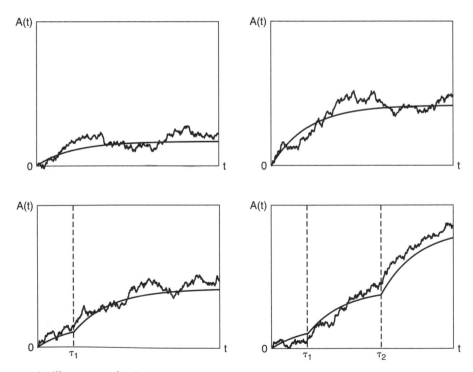

FIGURE 24.6   Upper graphs illustrate activation processes for different rates (drifts): the left-hand side, the one with the smaller drift, representing a stimulus with weaker intensity. The lower graphs demonstrate the processes for multimodal stimuli with different onset times.

switched off, the drift becomes negative and activation is assumed to decay to its starting level, since δ takes on a value of zero. It is assumed that activation never drops below its initial level. This decay process, which cannot be represented in a superposition or a counter model has been discussed in studies of neuronal activity dynamics (Ricciardi, 1977; Tuckwell, 1995).

For multimodal stimuli, the δ values corresponding to the unimodal stimuli are added:

$$\mu(x) = (\delta_T + \delta_V + \delta_A) - \gamma \cdot x \qquad (10)$$

Figure 24.6 (lower graphs) illustrates the effect of the drift change when modalities are added after certain SOAs. It is not difficult to see that the multichannel diffusion model affords the same predictions as the superposition model with respect to the effect of stimulus intensity and the number of modalities involved. Moreover, a parametric fit of the diffusion model to the bi- and trimodal data of the redundant target experiment with different SOAs was very close to the fit using the superposition model (for details, see Diederich, 1992, 1995).

SUPERPOSITION VERSUS DIFFUSION MODELS Although the database for evaluating the relative merits of both types of coactivation models is not large enough to yield a definite answer, the diffusion model seems to be more flexible in dealing with the problems that arise with certain intensity variations mentioned previously. First, the OUP diffusion model does not predict that RT will to go to zero with a high enough stimulus intensity; an increase in δ can, in principle, be compensated for by a corresponding increase in the decay parameter γ. Second, inverse effectiveness could be introduced by an appropriate elaboration of the drift function. For example, replacing the term $\delta_T + \delta_V + \delta_A$ in Equation 10 by

$$(\delta_T + \delta_V + \delta_A)[1 + (\delta_T^{\max} - \delta_T)(\delta_V^{\max} - \delta_V)(\delta_A^{\max} - \delta_A)] \qquad (11)$$

or something similar would yield an additive effect of intensity if at least one modality was close to maximum level, but an overadditive effect if all stimuli were far away from the their maximum levels. In principle, superposition models could be developed along this line, but deriving the ensuing multimodal mean RT predictions seems much more difficult.

The time-window-of-integration (TWIN) modeling scheme

One feature of all models considered so far, whether of separate activation or of coactivation type, is their complete functional symmetry with respect to the stimulus modalities involved. In other words, these models have no mechanism to account for possible effects caused by distinguishing a target signal modality from an accessory or distracter signal modality in experimental paradigms like the focused attention paradigm. The modeling scheme proposed in this section incorporates explicit assumptions about possible target/nontarget modality distinctions.

Although there is increasing evidence for a complex network of largely parallel neural subprocesses underlying performance even in simple cross-modal tasks (Driver & Spence, 2000), the initial separation of the afferent pathways for the different sensory modalities suggests that one can distinguish at least two serial stages of the entire saccadic reaction time: an early, afferent stage of peripheral processing (first stage), followed by a compound stage of converging subprocesses (second stage). As discussed below, in conjunction with a number of additional weak assumptions, some interesting and empirically testable predictions can be derived from this simple setup.

First-Stage Assumption: The first stage consists of a race among the peripheral neural excitations in the visual, auditory, and/or somatosensory pathways triggered by a multimodal stimulus complex.

Because the first stage refers to very early sensory processing, in general, random processing times for visual, auditory, and somatosensory stimuli are assumed to be statistically independent.

Second-Stage Assumption: The second stage comprises neural integration of the input and preparation of an ocular motor response. Multisensory integration manifests in an increase or decrease in second-stage processing time.

Distinguishing only between two stages is clearly an oversimplification. But the second stage is defined by default: it includes all subsequent, possibly overlapping, processes that are not part of the peripheral processes in the first stage.

Time-Window-of-Integration Assumption: Multisensory interaction occurs only if the peripheral processes of the first stage all terminate within a given time interval, the "window of integration."

This window of integration acts like a filter, determining whether the afferent information delivered from different sensory organs is registered close enough in time to allow for multisensory integration. Passing the filter is a necessary but not a sufficient condition for multisensory integration to occur. The reason is that multisensory integration also depends on the spatial configuration of the stimuli. However, rather than assuming the existence of a joint spatial-temporal window of integration permitting interaction to occur only for both spatially and temporally neighbored stimuli, the TWIN model allows multisensory integration to occur even for rather distant stimuli (of different modality), as long as they fall within the time window. The interaction will typically be an inhibition or only a small facilitation. It should be noted that this arrangement affords the organism more flexibility in a complex environment. For example, response depression may occur with nearly simultaneous but distant stimuli, making it easier for the organism to focus attention on the more important event.

QUANTIFYING MULTISENSORY INTEGRATION IN THE TWIN MODEL   According to the two-stage assumption, total reaction time in the multimodal condition can be written as a sum of two random variables:

$$RT_{\text{multimodal}} = W_1 + W_2 \qquad (12)$$

where W_1 and W_2 refer to the first- and second-stage processing time, respectively. Let I denote the event that multisensory integration occurs, having probability $Pr(I)$. For the expected saccadic RT in the multimodal condition then follows:

$$
\begin{aligned}
E[RT_{\text{multimodal}}] &= E[W_1] + E[W_2] \\
&= E[W_1] + Pr[I]E[W_2 \mid I] \\
&\quad + (1 - Pr[I])E[W_2 \mid \text{not-}I] \\
&= E[W_1] + E[W_2 \mid \text{not-}I] \\
&\quad - Pr[I](E[W_2 \mid \text{not-}I] - E[W_2 \mid I])
\end{aligned}
$$

where $E[W_2 \mid I]$ and $E[W_2 \mid \text{not-}I]$ denote the expected second-stage processing time conditioned on the interaction occurring (I) or not occurring (not-I), respectively. Putting $\Delta \equiv E[W_2 \mid \text{not-}I] - E[W_2 \mid I]$, this becomes

$$E[RT_{\text{multimodal}}] = E[W_1] + E[W_2 \mid \text{not-}I] - Pr[I] * \Delta \qquad (13)$$

The term $Pr[I] * \Delta$ can be interpreted as a measure of the expected saccadic RT speed-up in the second stage, with positive Δ values corresponding to facilitation and negative ones to inhibition. In the unimodal condition, no interaction is possible. Thus,

$$E[RT_{\text{unimodal}}] = E[W_1] + E[W_2 \mid \text{not-}I] \qquad (14)$$

and

$$E[RT_{\text{unimodal}}] - E[RT_{\text{multimodal}}] = Pr[I] * \Delta \qquad (15)$$

PREDICTIONS   The TWIN model makes a number of empirical predictions. First, the amount of multisensory integration should depend on the SOA between the stimuli. Indeed, the effect of multisensory integration tends to be most prominent when there is some characteristic temporal asynchrony between the stimuli (Frens, Van Opstal, & van der Willigen, 1995). In the model, this simply means that a stimulus with faster peripheral processing has to be delayed in such a way that the arrival times of both stimuli have a higher probability of falling into the window of integration.

Second, the probability of interaction, $Pr[I]$, should depend on unimodal features that affect the speed of processing in the first stage, such as stimulus intensity or eccentricity. For example, if a stimulus from one modality is very strong compared with the other stimulus's intensity, the chances that both peripheral processes terminate within the time window are small (assuming simultaneous stimulus presentations). The resulting low value of $Pr(I)$ is in line with the empirical observation that a very strong target signal will effectively suppress any interaction with other modalities.

On the other hand, the principle of inverse effectiveness, according to which multisensory integration is strongest when stimulus strengths are weak or close to threshold level (Meredith & Stein, 1986), can be accommodated in the model by adjusting the width of the time window: for low-level stimuli the window should become larger to increase the likelihood of cross-modal integration.

Finally, the amount of multisensory integration (Δ) and its direction (facilitation or inhibition) occurring in the second stage depend on cross-modal features of the stimulus set, in particular on spatial disparity and laterality (laterality here refers to whether or not all stimuli appear in the same hemisphere). Cross-modal features cannot have an influence on first-stage processing time because the modalities are still being processed in separate pathways. More specific predictions require an explication of the rules governing the window-of-integration mechanism in specific task requirements, to be discussed next.

INTEGRATION RULE ASSUMPTIONS

Focused Attention Task: When the task is to orient toward the target stimulus and ignore stimuli from other modalities, the duration of the first stage is determined by the target peripheral process, but multisensory integration is effective only if the nontarget stimulus wins the race in the first stage.

In other words, in the focused attention situation, the window of integration is "opened" only by activity triggered by the nontarget stimulus.

Redundant Target Task: When the task is to orient toward the first stimulus detected, no matter which modality, the duration of the first stage is determined by the winner's peripheral processing time, and the window of integration is opened by whichever stimulus wins the race.

From these assumptions, further predictions concerning the effects of varying stimulus intensity follow. Let us consider, for example, a focused attention task with a visual target and an auditory nontarget stimulus. Increasing the intensity of the visual stimulus will increase the chances for the visual target to win the race. Thus, the probability that the window of integration opens decreases, predicting less cross-modal interaction. This result is again in line with the observation that a very strong target signal will tend to suppress interaction with any other modality. Increasing the intensity of the nontarget auditory stimulus, however, leads to the opposite prediction: the auditory stimulus will have a better chance to win the race and to open the window of integration, hence predicting more multisensory integration to occur on average.

SEPARATING SPATIAL AND TEMPORAL FACTORS OF INTEGRATION Expected multisensory integration is defined as the difference between mean RT in the unimodal and the cross-modal condition. An important property of the TWIN model is the factoring of expected cross-modal interaction. In other words, expected multisensory integration is simply the product of the probability of interaction $Pr(I)$ and the amount and sign of interaction (Δ) (see Equation 15). According to the assumptions, the first factor depends on the temporal configuration of the stimuli (SOA), whereas the second factor depends on their spatial configuration. This separation of temporal and spatial factors is in accordance with the definition of the window of integration: the incidence of multisensory interaction hinges on the stimuli occurring close in time, whereas the amount and sign of the interaction (Δ) are modulated by spatial proximity, ranging from enhancement for close stimuli to possible inhibition for distant stimuli.

TWIN MODEL FOR VISUAL-TACTILE INTERACTION IN FOCUSED ATTENTION To illustrate the modeling scheme, we sketch here a TWIN model application to a visual-tactile interaction experiment under focused attention (see Colonius & Diederich, 2002b, in press, for details). Subjects were asked to make a saccade as quickly and as accurately as possible toward a visual stimulus appearing randomly left or right of the fixation point. They were instructed to ignore a tactile accessory stimulus that, in bimodal trials, was applied at different hand positions ipsilateral or contralateral to the visual target. The SOA between visual and tactile stimulus was -100, -50, 0, and 50 ms.

With V denoting visual peripheral processing time, T tactile peripheral processing time, τ stimulus onset asynchrony, and ω the width of the integration window, cross-modal interaction depends on the event I that the tactile stimulus wins the race in the first stage and that visual peripheral processing terminates within the window of integration:

$$I = \{T + \tau < V < T + \tau + \omega\}$$

For a quantitative prediction, the peripheral processes in the first stage are assumed to have stochastically independent exponentially distributed durations. The exponential assumption is motivated by mathematical simplicity and, together with a Gaussian distribution assumption for second-stage processing time, results in an ex-Gaussian distribution that has been demonstrated to be a reasonably adequate description for many empirically observed RT data (see Van Zandt, 2002). The duration of the first stage is determined by the target peripheral process of random duration V, say, yielding $E[W_1] = E[V] = 1/\lambda_V$ (λ_V denotes the intensity parameter of the exponential distribution of V). From the assumptions stated in the last section, straightforward calculation yields

$$\Pr[I] = \frac{\lambda_T}{\lambda_T + \lambda_V} \{\exp[-\lambda_V \tau] - \exp[-\lambda_V (\tau + \omega)]\} \tag{16}$$

where λ_T refers to the tactile intensity parameter. It is obvious from Equation 16 that the probability of interaction increases both with λ_T and the window width ω, as it should. Expected saccadic reaction time then is (see Colonius & Diederich, 2002b):

$$E[RT_{\text{multimodal}}] = 1/\lambda_V + \mu - \frac{\Delta \lambda_T}{\lambda_T + \lambda_V} \{\exp[-\lambda_V \tau]$$
$$- \exp[-\lambda_V (\tau + \omega)]\}$$

where $\mu = E[W_2 \mid \text{not-}I]$, the mean duration of the second stage when no interaction occurs.

The choice of the second-stage distribution is irrelevant as long as only mean latencies are considered. For predictions of the entire saccade latency distribution, however, it should be noted that owing to conditioning on the event of interaction I, the two-stage durations W_1 and W_2 are not stochastically independent. For the model version considered in this section, it can be shown that they are negatively dependent if Δ is positive: in any given trial, whenever the visual peripheral process ($V \equiv W_1$) is relatively slow, the tactile peripheral process has a better chance of winning the race and opening the integration window, thus increasing the likelihood of facilitation in the second stage, and

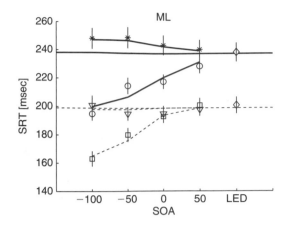

FIGURE 24.7 Saccadic RT to a visual target presented randomly left or right of fixation was reduced by up to 22% when accompanied by a spatially nonpredictive tactile stimulus. This facilitation effect was larger for spatially aligned visual-tactile stimulus configurations than for contralateral presentation, and it increased with stimulus eccentricity (20 degrees vs 70 degrees). Data are from one participant.

vice versa. Data from one of the subjects (Fig. 24.7) show that saccadic RT to a visual target presented randomly left or right from fixation was reduced by up to 22% when accompanied by a spatially nonpredictive tactile stimulus. This facilitation effect was larger for spatially aligned visual-tactile stimulus configurations than for contralateral presentations, and it increased with stimulus eccentricity (20 degrees vs 70 degrees). Moreover, responses were the faster the earlier the tactile stimulus was presented (in a range of the tactile stimulus preceding the visual stimulus by 100 ms to following it by 50 ms). These results extend previous findings to nonsimultaneous visual-tactile stimulus presentations (Diederich, Colonius, Bockhorst, & Tabeling, 2003). Obviously, the model captures the main features of the data at the level of the means. Mean saccadic RT is increasing with SOA for all stimulus configurations, except for the 70-degree contralateral condition, where monotonicity is reversed, owing to inhibition, consistent with the model. The estimate for the window width was 200 ms.

Conclusions

In evaluating the TWIN model, it is important to realize that it is not meant to mirror the processes at the level of an individual neuron. There are many different types of multisensory convergence occurring in individual neurons (for a recent review, see Meredith, 2002), and some of their activities are consistent with the TWIN assumptions, while others are not. For example, for certain neurons in cat SC, given a visual stimulus that is always presented in the visual receptive field of the

bimodal (visual-auditory) neuron, an auditory stimulus presented outside its receptive field will generate only response depression (or no interaction), regardless of the SOA between the stimuli (Stein & Meredith, 1993, p. 140). This observation accords nicely with the separation of temporal and spatial factors postulated by the TWIN model. However, in other visual-auditory neurons, changing the temporal order and interval between the stimuli can change enhancement to depression, even if their spatial arrangement is left unchanged (Meredith et al., 1987). This latter type of behavior could only be accounted for in the TWIN model if two stimuli, after having passed the filter of the temporal window of integration, could still carry over information about their temporal distance to the subsequent convergence stage. Moreover, besides the common excitatory-excitatory type of multisensory convergence, there is evidence for an excitatory-inhibitory type of neural circuit by which inputs from one modality inhibit those from the other (see Meredith, 2002). These circuits could play a specific role in focused attention situations (Meredith, 2002, p. 37). In any event, at this stage of development, the TWIN model operates at the level of behavioral data resulting from the combined activity of a possibly large number of neurons and from the specific task instructions, so that the existence of different types of multisensory convergence in individual neurons does not provide a strong modeling constraint.

Insofar as stimulation from different modalities like vision and touch cannot interact (e.g., on the retina), the main assumption of the two-stage model, the existence of a first stage of parallel independent modality-specific activations in the afferent pathways, seems noncontroversial. It refers to a very early stage of processing in which detection of the stimuli, but possibly no "higher" processes such as localization and identification, takes place. It should be noted that the two-stage assumption does not preclude the possibility of interaction between modality-specific pathways, or between modality-specific and cross-modal areas, at a later stage. In fact, there is increasing evidence that cross-modal processing does not take place entirely in feed-forward convergent pathways but that it can also modulate early cortical unisensory processing, as suggested by recent functional magnetic resonance imaging (fMRI) and event-related potential (ERP) studies (fMRI: Laurienti et al., 2002; Macaluso, Frith, & Driver, 2000; ERP: Molholm et al., 2002).

Even if certain assumptions of the TWIN model eventually turn out to be inconsistent with experimental results, an advantage of this modeling framework is that it facilitates the statement of clear-cut hypotheses about the rules of multisensory integration. A case in point is the hypothesis of "restricted influence," which holds that unimodal stimulus properties, such as stimulus intensity, do not have a direct effect on processing in the second stage. Of course, unimodal properties may influence the resulting multisensory integration indirectly by modulating the opening of the integration window. We may note here that the restricted influence hypothesis is a strengthening of the (obvious) TWIN model assumption that unimodal properties affect the race among the modalities in the first stage of processing. This is consistent with the focused attention study mentioned before (Arndt & Colonius, 2003). In a similar vein, in a redundant target experiment, Corneil, Wanrooij, Munoz, and Van Opstal (2002) did not find an effect of auditory signal-to-noise ratio on the amount of multisensory integration.

Further work on the TWIN model should include specification of the second-stage mechanisms, in particular with respect to the spatial stimulus configuration effects. A large database on the receptive field properties of multisensory neurons is now available (see Kadunce et al., 2001), and connecting these data with behavioral data via an appropriate elaboration of the TWIN model should be a rewarding task.

REFERENCES

Arndt, A., & Colonius, H. (2003). Two separate stages in crossmodal saccadic integration: Evidence from varying intensity of an auditory accessory stimulus. *Experimental Brain Research, 150,* 417–426.

Billingsley, P. (1979). *Probability and measure.* New York: Wiley.

Bernstein, I. H., Rose, R., & Ashe, V. M. (1970). Energy integration in intersensory facilitation. *Journal of Experimental Psychology, 86,* 196–203.

Colonius, H. (1986). Measuring channel dependence in separate activation models. *Perception & Psychophysics, 40,* 251–255.

Colonius, H. (1990). Possibly dependent probability summation of reaction time. *Journal of Mathematical Psychology, 34,* 253–275.

Colonius, H., & Arndt, P. (2001). A two-stage model for visual-auditory interaction in saccadic latencies. *Perception & Psychophysics, 63,* 126–147.

Colonius, H., & Diederich, A. (2002a). A maximum-likelihood approach to modeling multisensory enhancement. In T. G. Dietterich, S. Becker, & Z. Ghahramani (Eds.), *Advances in neural information processing systems 14* (pp. 181–187). Cambridge, MA: MIT Press.

Colonius, H., & Diederich, A. (2002b). A stochastic model of multimodal integration in saccadic responses. In R. P. Würtz & M. Lappe (Eds.), *Dynamic perception* (pp. 321–326). Berlin: Akademische Verlagsgesellschaft.

Colonius, H., & Diederich, A. (in press). The time-window-of-integration model: Visual-tactile interaction in saccade generation. *Journal of Cognitive Neuroscience.*

Corneil, B. D., Van Wanrooij, M., Munoz, D. P., & Van Opstal, A. J. (2002). Auditory-visual interactions subserving goal-directed saccades in a complex scene. *Journal of Neurophysiology, 88,* 438–454.

Diederich, A. (1992). Probability inequalities for testing separate activation models of divided attention. *Perception & Psychophysics, 52,* 714–716.

Diederich, A. (1995). Intersensory facilitation of reactin time: Evaluation of counter and diffusion coactivation models. *Journal of Mathematical Psychology, 39,* 197–215.

Diederich, A., & Colonius, H. (1987). Intersensory facilitation in the motor component? *Psychological Research, 49,* 23–29.

Diederich, A., & Colonius, H. (1991). A further test of the superposition model for the redundant-signals effect in bimodal detection. *Perception & Psychophysics, 50,* 83–86.

Diederich, A., Colonius, H., Bockhorst, D., & Tabeling, S. (2003). Visual-tactile spatial interaction in saccade generation. *Experimental Brain Research, 148,* 328–337.

Donders, F. C. (1868/1969). On the speed of mental processes (W. G. Koster, Trans.). *Acta Psychologia, 30,* 412–431.

Driver, J., & Spence, C. (2000). Beyond modularity and convergence. *Current Biology, 10,* 731–735.

Frens, M. A., Van Opstal, A. J., & van der Willigen, R. F. (1995). Spatial and temporal factors determine auditory-visual interactions in human saccadic eye movements. *Perception & Psychophysics, 57,* 802–816.

Gielen, S. C. A. M., Schmidt, R. A., & Van den Heuvel, P. Y. M. (1983). On the nature of intersensory facilitation of reaction time. *Perception & Psychophysics, 34,* 161–168.

Hershenson, M. (1962). Reaction time as a measure of intersensory facilitation. *Journal of Experimental Psychology, 63,* 289–293.

Kadunce, D. C., Vaughan, J. W., Wallace, M. T., & Stein, B. E. (2001). The influence of visual and auditory receptive field organization on multisensory integration in the superior colliculus. *Experimental Brain Research, 139,* 303–310.

Laurienti, P. J., Burdette, J. H., Wallace, M. T., Yen, Y., Field, A. S., & Stein, B. E. (2002). Deactivation of sensory-specific cortex by cross-modal stimuli. *Journal of Cognitive Neuroscience, 14,* 420–429.

Lovelace, C. T., Stein, B. E., & Wallace, M. T. (2002). *Now you hear it, now you don't: A light improves detection of a sound.* Poster presented at the Neural Control of Movement conference, Naples, FL.

Luce, R. D. (1986). *Response times: Their role in inferring elementary mental organization.* New York: Oxford University Press.

Macaluso, E., Frith, C. D., & Driver, J. (2000). Modulation of human visual cortex by crossmodal spatial attention. *Science, 289,* 1206–1208.

Meredith, M. A. (2002). On the neural basis for multisensory convergence: A brief overview. *Cognitive Brain Research, 14,* 31–40.

Meredith, M. A., Nemitz, J. W., & Stein, B. E. (1987). Determinants of multisensory integration in superior colliculus neurons: I. Temporal factors. *Journal of Neuroscience, 10,* 3215–3229.

Meredith, M. A., & Stein, B. E. (1986). Visual, auditory, and somatosensory convergence on cells in superior colliculus results in multisensory integration. *Journal of Neurophysiology, 56,* 640–662.

Miller, J. O. (1982). Divided attention: Evidence for coactivation with redundant signals. *Cognitive Psychology, 14,* 247–279.

Molholm, S., Ritter, W., Murray, M. M., Javitt, D. C., Schroeder, C. E., & Foxe, J. J. (2002). Multisensory auditory-visual interactions during early sensory processing in humans: A high-density electrical mapping study. *Cognitive Brain Research, 14,* 115–128.

Munoz, D. P., & Würtz, R. H. (1995). Saccade-related activity in monkey superior colliculus: I. Characteristics of burst and buildup cells. *Journal of Neurophysiology, 73,* 2313–2333.

Nickerson, R. S. (1973). Intersensory facilitation of reaction time: Energy summation or preparation enhancement. *Psychological Review, 80,* 489–509.

Raab, D. H. (1962). Statistical facilitation of simple reaction times. *Transactions of the New York Academy of Sciences, 24,* 574–590.

Ricciardi, L. M. (1977). *Diffusion processes and related topics in biology.* Berlin: Springer-Verlag.

Schwarz, W. (1989). A new model to explain the redundant-signal effect. *Perception & Psychophysics, 46,* 498–500.

Stein, B. E., & Meredith, M. A. (1993). *The merging of the senses.* Cambridge, MA: MIT Press.

Todd, J. W. (1912). Reaction to multiple stimuli. In R. S. Woodworth (Ed.), *Archives of psychology,* 25 (Columbia Contributions to Philosophy and Psychology, Vol. XXI, No. 8). New York: Science Press.

Townsend, J. T., & Ashby, F. G. (1983). *Stochastic modeling of elementary psychological processes.* Cambridge, England: Cambridge University Press.

Townsend, J. T., & Nozawa, G. (1995). Spatio-temporal properties of elementary perception: An investigation of parallel, serial, and coactive theories. *Journal of Mathematical Psychology, 39,* 321–359.

Tuckwell, H. C. (1995). *Elementary applications of probability theory.* (2nd ed.), London: Chapman and Hall.

Ulrich, R., & Giray, M. (1986). Separate-activation models with variable base times: Testability and checking of cross-channel dependency. *Perception & Psychophysics, 34,* 248–254.

Van Zandt, T. (2002). Analysis of response time distributions. In H. Pashler (Series Ed.), *Stevens' handbook of experimental psychology* (3rd ed.), Vol. 4. *Methodology in experimental psychology* (J. T. Wixted, Vol. Ed., pp. 461–516). New York: Wiley.

Welch, R. B., & Warren, D. H. (1986). Intersensory interactions. In *Handbook of perception and human performance:* Vol. 1. *Sensory processes and perception* (K. R. Boff, L. Kaufmann, & J. P. Thomas, Eds., pp. 25-1–25-36). New York: Wiley.

Worsley, K. J. (1982). An improved Bonferroni inequality and applications. *Biometrika, 69,* 297–302.

25 Multisensory Influences on Orientation and Movement Control

JAMES R. LACKNER AND PAUL DIZIO

Introduction

The perception of body orientation is influenced by multiple sensory and motor systems. Vision provides information about body orientation relative to the external environment. The semicircular canals of the inner ear are responsive to angular acceleration of the head and the otolith organs are sensitive to linear acceleration, including gravity. Somatosensory receptors provide information about body contact and orientation in relation to the ground or support surface. Proprioceptive receptors, Golgi tendon organs, and muscle spindles and joint receptors provide signals that, when interrelated with motor signals, provide information about body configuration. Audition can also provide spatially relevant signals about body orientation. Normally the information provided by these systems is congruent and redundant.

It is well known that unusual patterns of sensory stimulation can elicit errors in the representation of ongoing orientation. Visually induced illusions of self-motion are perhaps the most familiar. A person viewing a wide-field display of objects or stripes moving at constant velocity will soon experience the display to be stationary and her- or himself to be moving in the direction opposite the display motion (cf. Dichgans & Brandt, 1972). Rotary visual motion can evoke illusions of body tilt (Held, Dichgans, & Bauer, 1975). In the absence of vision, constant motion transduced by nearly any sensory modality can elicit illusory self-motion. A rotating auditory field can elicit illusory self-displacement and a pattern of compensatory motion of the eyes like that which occurs during actual body motion (Lackner, 1977). Moving tactile stimulation of the body surface can elicit apparent body motion (Lackner & DiZio, 1984). Vibrating skeletal muscles of the body to activate muscle spindle receptors can elicit various proprioceptive illusions in which the apparent configuration of the body is modified or illusory motion

of the whole body relative to the environment is experienced (Lackner, 1988). Motor-based illusions of apparent body motion can also be generated when a seated, stationary, blindfolded individual pedals a platform under his or her feet. If it has the same inertia as the individual, compelling illusory self-motion will be evoked (Lackner & DiZio, 1984).

The situations described represent perceptual "good fits" with the available patterns of sensory and motor stimulation. For example, illusions of constant-velocity self-motion evoked by moving visual, auditory, or somatosensory stimulation patterns are consistent with a nonchanging vestibular input from the semicircular canals and otolith organs. Voluntary tilting movements of the head can often suppress the elicitation of sensory-induced illusions of body rotation, because the patterns of vestibular and proprioceptive feedback elicited by the head movements are inconsistent with those that would be generated during actual body rotation. The mechanisms and processes underlying the perception of self-motion and orientation are complex and not fully understood (cf. Lackner, 1978).

Exposure to unusual force conditions also affects the normal patterning of sensory stimulation and has profound influences on spatial orientation and the control of body movements. The otolith organs of the inner ear respond to linear acceleration. Consequently, their effective stimulus is gravitoinertial force, which is the result of gravity and imposed inertial forces arising from self-motion or from transport in a vehicle of some sort. Figure 25.1 illustrates how gravitoinertial force (gif) affects the otolith organs. Exposure to altered levels and directions of gravitoinertial force can elicit postural illusions, orientation illusions, and errors in sensory localization. In addition, it affects the control of body movements, because the effective weight of the body changes in altered force environments. Vestibulospinal reflexes are also modulated and alter the effective tonus of the antigravity musculature of the body (Lackner, Dizio, &

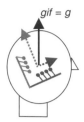 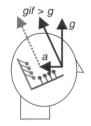

Upright, stationary   Upright, backward
translatory acceleration

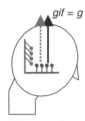 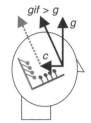

Tilt re gravity,   Upright, centrifugation
stationary   with back toward center

FIGURE 25.1 A side view of simplified otolith organs stimulated by head tilt relative to gravitational acceleration, by acceleration relative to an inertial reference frame, and by centripetal force. The black arrows represent the contact force of support opposing gravity (*g*), the force that must be applied in order to accelerate the body relative to inertial space (*a*), centripetal force (*c*), and the vector resulting from contact forces (*gif*). These forces are applied to the body surface and are transmitted through the skeleton to the saccular (red) and utricular (blue) surfaces, which are represented as idealized orthogonal planes pitched up about 30 degrees relative to the naso-occipital axis of the head. When the head is in a natural upright posture (upper left), the saccular and utricular otoconial masses are displaced from their viscoelastic equilibria and deflect their hair cells in proportion to the components (dotted lines) of gif parallel to their respective planes. Static 30-degree pitch forward of the head (lower left) relative to gravity alters the ratio of saccular to utricular deflection relative to that in upright stationary conditions (upper left). Backward acceleration relative to space (upper right) and centrifugation while facing away from the rotation axis (lower right) can rotate the gif 30 degrees backward relative to the head and produce the same ratio of saccular to utricular deflection as a 30-degree forward tilt.

Fisk, 1992; Watt, Money, & Tomi, 1986; Wilson & Peterson, 1978). This overall pattern of changes means that to bring about any posture or body movement relative to the immediate surroundings requires different patterns of muscle innervation than those employed prior to the change in gravitoinertial force.

Centrifuges and slow-rotation rooms have been a valuable way of studying alterations in spatial orientation and sensory localization associated with unusual force conditions. In these devices, alterations in gravitoinertial force result from the centripetal force generated by rotation. The object on the rotating vehicle moves in a circular path because the centripetal force applied by the vehicle deflects it accordingly; otherwise the object would move in a straight path. Centripetal force is proprotional to the square of the velocity of rotation (in radians) times the radius of rotation. Consequently, the farther the object or person from the center of rotation and the faster the rate of rotation, the greater will be the increase in the resulting gravitoinertial force (gravity and centripetal force combined).

Rotating vehicles are of special interest because of the possibility of using them to generate artificial gravity in long-duration space flight. Humans in weightless conditions undergo progressive loss of bone and muscle strength. Approximately 1% of bone mineral content is lost per month of weightlessness in space flight (Holick, 1992, 1997). This degree of bone mineral loss is acceptable for brief missions but is a severe problem for very long-duration missions because of the possibility of bone fractures and severe skeletal-muscular control problems on return to Earth. The centripetal force or artificial gravity associated with rotation could in principle be substituted for Earth's gravity in space flight. One complication of rotating artificial gravity vehicles is the generation of Coriolis forces by body movements in relation to the vehicle. For example, if an object translates in the plane of rotation, as shown in Figure 25.2, a transient Coriolis force will be generated on it. This force is proportional to the velocity of rotation of the vehicle (ω) and the velocity of linear motion of the object (v): $F_{\mathrm{Cor}} = -2m(\omega \times v)$, where m is the mass of the object.

Coriolis forces are generated by any linear body movement and by tilting movements of the head as well. The latter movements can evoke motion sickness because of the unusual pattern of vestibular stimulation generated. Early studies of rotating environments suggested that 3–4 rpm would be the highest feasible rotation velocity for an artificial gravity vehicle in space flight because it was thought that astronauts would become severely motion sick and disoriented at higher velocities (Graybiel, Clark, & Zarriello, 1960; Graybiel et al., 1965; Guedry, Kennedy, Harris, & Graybiel, 1964; Kennedy & Graybiel, 1962). In fact, as will be discussed later, quite high Coriolis forces are generated during our natural everyday movements when simultaneous torso and limb motions occur, so it is not unusual for humans to experience Coriolis forces.

The emphasis in this chapter will be on human orientation and movement control in unusual force environments, on adaptive changes in motor control that can occur in such environments, and on how static and dynamic patterns of somatosensory and haptic stimulation can affect apparent orientation and postural control.

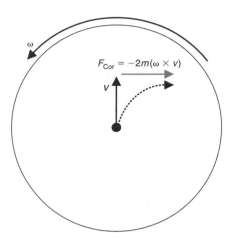

FIGURE 25.2 Illustration of Coriolis force (F_{Cor}) on a projectile (black circle) whose mass is m and whose instantaneous linear velocity is v relative to an environment rotating with angular velocity equal to ω. The dashed arrow indicates the object's trajectory.

Throughout we will highlight the constant interplay and interaction of multiple sensory and motor influences in determining orientation, sensory localization, and movement control.

Somatogravic illusions and errors in visual and auditory localization

Typically, when we move and change position in our natural environment, we maintain accurate perception of our body orientation and of external objects in relation to our surroundings. However, when we are exposed to inertial accelerations, in a centrifuge or in an aircraft, the net linear acceleration acting on our body (the gravitoinertial acceleration) is greater than the $1g$ ($9.8 \, \mathrm{m/s^2}$) acceleration of Earth's gravity. In this circumstance, sensory and orientation illusions will be experienced. Exposure to rotary acceleration also gives rise to errors in sensory localization and body orientation. Such illusions have been attributed to stimulation of the vestibular system because of the sensitivity of the otolith receptors to linear acceleration and the semicircular canals to angular acceleration and their conjoint influences on oculomotor and postural control. However, acceleration also affects the sensorimotor control of the eyes, head, and entire body as inertial masses. As a result, the control patterns that are normally used to coordinate body movements and to maintain posture are no longer fully adequate in non-$1g$ acceleration fields. Many illusory effects traditionally attributed solely to vestibular function actually reflect sensory and orientation remappings elicited by altered sensorimotor control of the body, as will be discussed later. These remappings can be quite complex.

Individuals exposed to a resultant linear force vector increased in magnitude and rotated relative to gravity experience illusory tilt of themselves and of their vehicle relative to external space. The body tilt component is typically referred to as the *somatogravic illusion* and the visual change as the *oculogravic illusion* (cf. Graybiel, 1952). Figure 25.3 illustrates the illusions as experienced in rooms that rotate to generate centripetal forces on the body. The illusions take much longer to develop fully (minutes rather than seconds) and do not reach as great a magnitude in people who lack labyrinthine function (Clark & Graybiel, 1966; Graybiel & Clark, 1962). If a person stands rather than sits during exposure, the illusory postural and visual changes that are experienced are attenuated (Clark & Graybiel, 1968).

The traditional explanation of the somatogravic and oculogravic illusions is that the gravitoinertial resultant force is interpreted by the central nervous system (CNS) as the direction of down, just as under normal static conditions the direction of gravity represents the direction

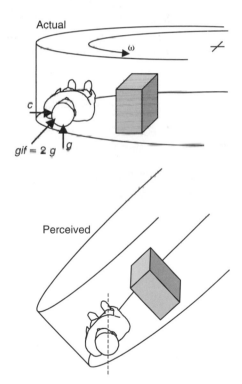

FIGURE 25.3 Illustrations of the illusions experienced in a rotating (ω) centrifuge where the resultant (*gif*) of gravity (*g*) and centripetal force (*c*) has a magnitude of 2*g* and is tilted 60 degrees toward the subject's right ear. The somatogravic illusion is apparent self-tilt relative to the subjective vertical (dashed line) and the oculogravic is apparent visual tilt of the surroundings relative to the subjective vertical. The shaded box represents the actual and perceived orientation of environmental objects.

of down. Consequently, as long as the body and the vehicle are not aligned with the gravitoinertial force, self-tilt and vehicle tilt will be experienced as illustrated in Figure 25.3. An auditory analogue of the oculogravic illusion, referred to as the *audiogravic illusion,* also occurs (Graybiel & Niven, 1951). Typically, these sensory effects are measured by having individuals set a visual or an auditory target to the apparent horizon. The settings to the horizon usually undershoot by about 20%–30% what would be predicted if the resultant direction were accurately represented as the vertical.

Recent studies of body-relative sensory localization during exposure to increased force levels indicate that when a somatogravic illusion is induced, changes in body-relative sensory localization are evoked as well (DiZio, Lackner, Held, Shinn-Cunningham, & Durlach, 2001). This is illustrated in Figure 25.4, which shows a test subject in the periphery of a slow-rotation room. The physically horizontal subject is being exposed to a $2g$ force that is rotated 60 degrees rightward with respect to his midsagittal plane. In this circumstance, the subject will experience leftward body tilt and simultaneously will mislocalize sounds and visual targets presented in the otherwise dark experimental chamber. A sound or visual target that is physically in the head median plane will be heard or seen leftward of the body. The targets have to be moved rightward to be localized in the body midline. The magnitude of change in sensory localization is a joint function of the rotation and magnitude of the gravitoinerital force vector. For a $2g$ force level, the localization change is approximately 15% of the shift in the force direction relative to the body. The shifts in visual and auditory localization are in the same direction and of comparable magnitude. When the subject manipulates a joystick to align it with the apparent median plane of his or her head, it will be displaced in the direction opposite the shifts in sensory localization by a comparable amount. This means that the apparent median plane of the head is displaced in the direction opposite the physical rotation of the resultant vector. Conjoint changes in auditory and visual localization and in the head apparent median plane strongly suggest that a common central reference frame has been shifted, rather than that multiple independent remappings of each sensory modality and of the head midline have occurred.

Figure 25.5 shows the time course of shifts in auditory and visual localization in subjects exposed to rotation in a slow-rotation room. At constant velocity, the gravitoinertial force level has increased to $2g$ and rotated 60 degrees rightward with respect to the subject. Separate runs were made for the auditory and visual settings. The nearly identical magnitudes and time course of the changes suggest a shift of a common reference coordinate system.

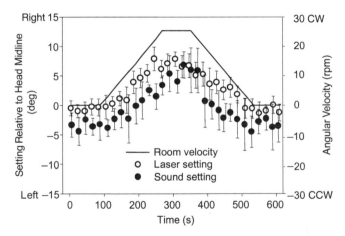

FIGURE 25.5 Plots illustrating the changes in visual and auditory localization of targets relative to the head during exposure to altered gravitoinertial force. Subjects are presented either with a binaural acoustic stimulus simulating a lateralized external sound or with an eccentric laser spot, in darkness, and are asked to make adjustments until they perceive the target on their head midline. When the gif increases to $2g$ and rotates 60 degrees right relative to midline (see Fig. 25.4), subjects set both types of stimuli about 8 degrees to their right to hear them as centered, consistent with a leftward perceptual shift of fixed stimuli. The time courses and magnitudes of shift are similar in both sensory modalities.

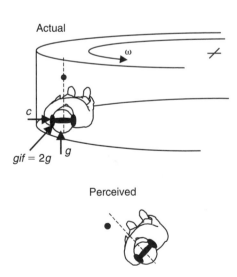

FIGURE 25.4 *Top:* Illustration of a subject exposed to a resultant force (gif) that is greater than $1g$ and is tilted right with respect to the midline, and simultaneously being presented through earphones with a binaural sound (black dot) that is physically consistent with a location on the head's midline (dashed line). *Bottom:* The sound is perceived to be to the left of midline and the subject experiences leftward body tilt.

Head movement control in rotating environments

Head movements made in unusual force environments have long been recognized to be disorienting and to evoke motion sickness. For example, head movements made in non-1*g* environments, such as the weightless conditions of space flight or in high-force conditions in an aircraft, can produce visual illusions and nausea. Head movements made during passive rotation are especially disruptive and have been the focus of much experimentation and theorizing because of the possible use of rotating artificial gravity vehicles in space flight (Graybiel & Knepton, 1978).

To understand why head movements during rotation are disorienting, it is useful to consider their influence on the semicircular canals of the inner ear, which respond to angular acceleration. Figure 25.6 illustrates what happens to the semicircular canals if the head is tilted forward during constant-velocity, counterclockwise rotation. For simplicity, we will refer to the three orthogonally oriented semicircular canals on each side of the head as "yaw," "roll," and "pitch" canals.

As the head pitches forward during constant-velocity rotation, the yaw canals are moved out of the plane of rotation and thus lose angular momentum. This generates a signal specifying clockwise yaw rotation of the head. Simultaneously, the roll canals are moved into the plane of rotation and thus gain angular momentum,

thereby producing a signal specifying leftward roll of the head relative to the trunk. The remaining pitch canals accurately indicate pitch of the head because they are moved perpendicular to the plane of rotation and are not affected abnormally. These unusual patterns of canal stimulation produce the sensation of simultaneous rotation about multiple axes, which is highly confusing and disorienting. Such vestibular stimulation is often referred to as Coriolis cross-coupling and is highly *g* force-dependent in terms of its disorienting and nauseogenic effects. One of the early space flight experiments on vestibular function, the *Skylab* M-131 experiment, evaluated the influence of being weightless on responses to Coriolis cross-coupling stimulation. The experiment required astronauts to make head movements during constant-velocity body rotation preflight, in-flight, and postflight (Graybiel, Miller, & Homick, 1977). All astronauts experienced disorientation and motion sickness symptoms preflight, but they were totally insusceptible when tested in-flight in the weightless conditions of orbital flight. Moreover, they did not find the head movements at all disorienting. After a day or two postflight, they returned to preflight sensitivity. In the M-131 experiment, the first in-flight head movements made during rotation did not take place until the sixth day in orbit. To determine whether the decreased provocativeness of in-flight head movements was related to exposure to weightlessness per se or to some adaptive process occurring over time, later experiments were conducted in an aircraft flying a parabolic path to create alternating periods of high force and weightlessness (DiZio, Lackner, & Evanoff, 1987; Lackner & Graybiel, 1984). Figure 25.7 illustrates the

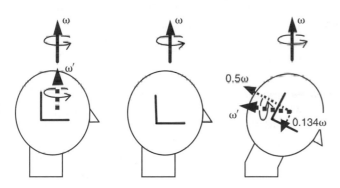

FIGURE 25.6   Schematic of vestibular cross-coupled stimulation of idealized roll and yaw plane semicircular canals elicited by a pitch head movement during clockwise rotation. Solid arrows indicate body rotation velocity (ω). The thin dashed arrows represent the encoding of body rotation velocity by individual semicircular canals, and the heavy dashed arrows represent the resultant encoded body velocity (ω'). The left figure shows the yaw canal accurately encoding body angular velocity after a brief acceleration. The center illustrates the canals equilibrated to resting discharge levels after constant velocity rotation has been maintained for about a minute. At this point, the subject will feel stationary if denied vision as well as auditory and wind cues. Pitching the head 30° forward (right) elicits cross-coupled stimulation of the roll and yaw canals which jointly encode rotation about a nearly horizontal axis.

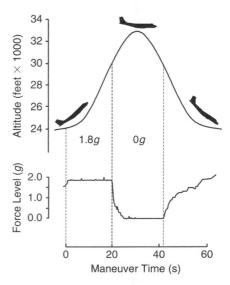

FIGURE 25.7   Flight profile of the KC-135 aircraft and a recording of gravitoinertial force during parabolic flight maneuvers.

associated gravitoinertial force profile: approximately 25–30 s periods of 0g and 1.8g alternate, separated by rapid force transitions. It was found that head movements made during constant-velocity rotation immediately became much less provocative and disorienting on transition into weightlessness than in 1g. Importantly, on transition to 1.8g, head movements became much more disorienting and evocative of motion sickness than in 1g conditions. This pattern means the M-131 results are related to exposure to weightlessness per se and not to adaptive changes occurring in weightlessness.

This g dependence of Coriolis cross-coupling stimulation cannot be accounted for solely by the unusual patterns of semicircular canal stimulation associated with head movements made during rotation. In the parabolic flight experiments, the semicircular canal stimulation was the same across background force levels, yet the disorientation and motion sickness evoked were drastically different. Factors related to the sensorimotor control of the head as an inertial mass are also involved. In fact, when a head movement is made during rotation, it turns out that the head does not go through its intended trajectory. Figure 25.8 shows what the head

does during an attempted pitch-forward head movement under nonrotating and rotating conditions when the eyes are closed. In the nonrotating condition, the head achieves its goal quite accurately; however, during passive counterclockwise body rotation, the path is quite different from that intended. As the head pitches forward, it deviates laterally rightward (Fig. 25.8). In addition, it also yaws and rolls in relation to the trunk (Lackner & DiZio, 1998).

The angular motions of the head in yaw and roll are the result of vestibulocollic reflexes induced by the activation of the yaw and roll canals, whereas the lateral deviation component of the head movement is related to the action of a Coriolis force acting on the head as an inertial mass. As mentioned earlier, Coriolis forces are inertial forces that arise in a rotating reference frame when an object moves linearly in the plane of rotation, and are dependent on the velocity (v) of the object, its mass (m), and the angular velocity in radians of rotation (ω): $F_{Cor} = -2m(v \times \omega)$. As the head is tilted forward in pitch during counterclockwise rotation, its center of mass moves forward in the plane of rotation, generating a Coriolis force that displaces the head laterally rightward.

When test subjects make many head movements during rotation, they gradually become less disoriented, and their head trajectory more closely approaches that intended. Adaptation to the lateral Coriolis force generated by head movements occurs with relatively few movements. Usually within 20–40 movements, subjects regain the desired head path. It takes much longer to adapt to the unusual vestibular stimulation and eliminate the undesired yaw and roll components of the head movement.

Arm movement control in rotating environments

The Coriolis forces generated during reaching movements in a rotating environment have great practical and theoretical significance because they can affect movement path and end-point. From a practical standpoint, the disruptive effects of Coriolis forces and the ability to adapt to them will influence the feasibility of using rotating vehicles to generate artificial gravity in space missions. If movements are greatly disturbed and adaptive accommodations cannot be made with relative ease, then rotating vehicles will have little operational value. From a theoretical standpoint, rotating environments, and the Coriolis forces generated on objects moving within them, provide a means to evaluate theories of movement control. Equilibrium-point theories of movement control, for example, posit that limb movements result from an evolving series of movement commands that specify the ongoing activity of motor

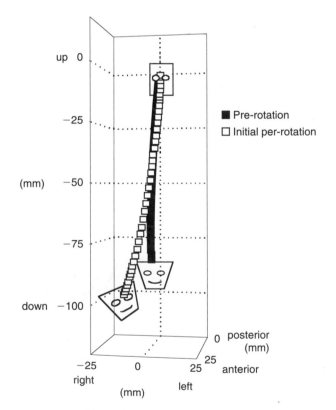

FIGURE 25.8 Plots of the paths of the initial voluntary pitch head movement (a point between the eyes) attempted during 10 rpm counterclockwise rotation, compared to a prerotation baseline movement. During rotation, the end-point is deviated in the direction of the Coriolis force. Data from four subjects are averaged.

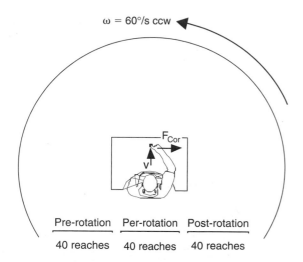

ω = 60°/s ccw

F_{Cor}

V

Pre-rotation   Per-rotation   Post-rotation

40 reaches   40 reaches   40 reaches

FIGURE 25.9   Illustration of Coriolis force (F_{Cor}) generated by reaching movements during 10 rpm counterclockwise rotation. The figure also illustrates the experimental paradigm for assessing the initial effects of and the adaptation to Coriolis forces generated during rotation, as well the aftereffects on returning to stationary conditions, in relation to the prerotation baseline conditions.

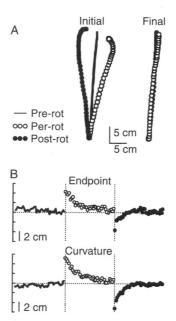

A

Initial   Final

— Pre-rot
ooo Per-rot
••• Post-rot

5 cm
5 cm

B

Endpoint

2 cm

Curvature

2 cm

FIGURE 25.10   (A) Top view of the finger paths of the initial reaches made before, during, and after rotation (n = 11). (B) Lateral end-point errors and curvatures of 40 reaching movements made before, during, and after rotation (n = 11 per reaching movement).

neurons innervating the muscles involved in producing the desired movement. The end-point of a movement is thought to be determined by the relative final balance of prespecified innervations of agonist and antagonist muscles. Equilibrium-point theories predict that movement paths but not movement end-points will be disturbed by the Coriolis forces associated with movements made in rotating environments. Such predictions are a cornerstone of these theories.

A simple test situation for evaluating the influence of Coriolis forces on reaching movements made to a visual target in a rotating environment is illustrated in Figure 25.9. A subject is seated at the center of a large, fully enclosed room that is very slowly brought up to a constant velocity of 10 rpm so that the subject never experiences any sense of rotation. The rate of acceleration is below the threshold of the angular acceleration-sensitive semicircular canals. The subject is at the center of rotation and during rotation is not exposed to a significant centrifugal force such as would be present if he or she were seated in the periphery. The subject, although being rotated at constant velocity, feels completely stationary as long as head movements are not made. This is because the subject's semicircular canals, if stimulated above threshold during acceleration to constant velocity, will have returned to resting discharge levels, and there are no visual motion cues to signal rotation in the fully enclosed room. Reaching movements made to the target prerotation will be straight and accurate. However, during constant-velocity rota-

tion, reaching movements will be laterally deviated in the direction opposite rotation and miss the target (Lackner & DiZio, 1994). This deviation is due to the Coriolis force generated by the forward velocity of the arm relative to the rotating room.

Importantly, as additional reaching movements are made, even in the absence of visual feedback, movement control will soon improve, with reaches becoming straighter and more accurate. Figure 25.10 shows the adaptation of movement trajectories and end-points that subjects exhibit with repeated movements. The lateral deviation of the arm by Coriolis forces is analogous to the lateral deviation of the head caused by pitch-forward head movements during body rotation, as discussed earlier. In both cases, the Coriolis forces are influencing the controlled appendage, causing deviations from the intended path. And, in both cases, adaptation to the Coriolis forces generated is achieved rapidly with additional movements.

These findings are of special significance because they show that if the cardinal predictions of equilibrium-point theories of movement control are wrong, movement end-point errors are initially huge. They show also that movement errors will initially be made in rotating environments, but that with additional movements, accurate trajectories and end-points will be regained. This adaptability supports the feasibility of artificial gravity environments from a human-factor standpoint.

During everyday activities, we commonly turn and reach for objects or turn and move our head out of the axis of body rotation. The question arises whether such movements create significant Coriolis forces on the head and arm or whether the peak velocities of head, trunk, and arm are staggered so as to minimize the generation of Coriolis forces. Alternatively, the nervous system could program anticipatory compensations to counteract the influence of self-generated Coriolis forces on movement paths. Figure 25.11A illustrates a test paradigm that was designed to answer this question

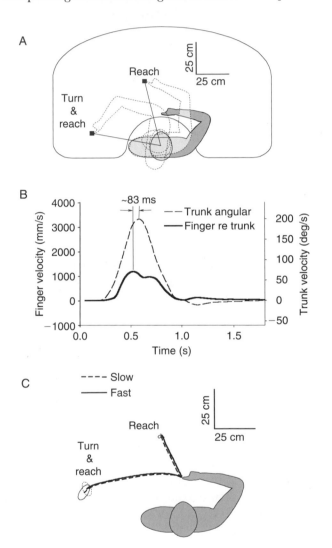

FIGURE 25.11 (A) Top view of the location of targets for studying self-generated Coriolis forces during natural turn-and-reach movements. The shaded silhouette shows the starting posture and the outlined figures show the terminal postures. (B) Traces of trunk angular velocity relative to space and finger linear velocity relative to the trunk during a typical turn-and-reach movement. (C) Top view of finger paths during turn-and-reach movements and simple reaching movements, executed at fast and slow speeds, in the dark. Coriolis forces scale with movement speed (not illustrated), but the movement paths are constant.

(Pigeon, Bortolami, DiZio, & Lackner, 2003). A subject makes natural pointing movements to each of three targets. Reaching to one of the targets requires only motion of the arm, reaching to the second one requires only motion of the torso, and reaching to the final one requires rotation of the torso and extension of the arm. It turns out that when subjects make natural, unconstrained movements involving both arm extension and trunk rotation, the extension of the arm falls completely within the period of trunk rotation (Fig. 25.11B). As a consequence, large Coriolis forces are generated on the arm during its forward projection. Nevertheless, as Figure 25.11C illustrates, such pointing movements are accurate. The magnitude of the Coriolis forces on the arm during natural turn and reach movements is actually much greater than in the slow-rotation room experiments described earlier, in which control of arm movements is initially severely disrupted. In voluntary turn-and-reach movements, therefore, the CNS must anticipate and precisely compensate for the Coriolis forces generated by arm extension during voluntary trunk rotation. These self-generated Coriolis forces are not sensed or perceived. By contrast, the smaller Coriolis forces generated by arm movements during passive body rotation are perceptually experienced as large, magnetlike forces deviating the arm from its intended path and goal.

Signals related to impending and/or ongoing self-rotation must be critical for the CNS in determining how to anticipate and compensate for the Coriolis forces that will be generated by voluntary limb movements. It is clear from the slow-rotation room studies that without such anticipatory compensations, movement paths and end-points are distorted. Figure 25.12 illustrates a technique that has been used to demonstrate compensation for Coriolis forces when subjects experience self-rotation while they are physically stationary (Cohn, DiZio, & Lackner, 2000). Subjects wear a wide-field head-mounted display that receives input from video cameras viewing a laboratory room. The cameras are mounted on a servo-controlled turntable that can be rotated and view a work surface that is also mounted on the turntable. The surface seen in the head-mounted display corresponds spatially and in all dimensions to the one at which the physically stationary subject is seated. When the remotely viewed turntable is rotated, the subject receives a moving visual input of the room in which it is located. Within a few seconds, the subject experiences compelling illusory self-rotation and displacement in relation to a visually stationary environment.

When the subject makes reaching movements to a target presented on the workspace surface, large errors result. During experienced counterclockwise rotation,

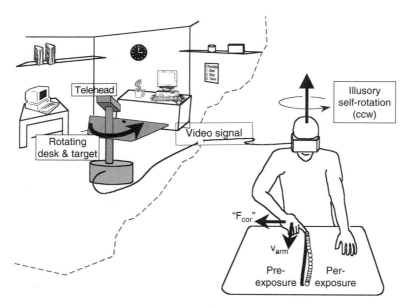

FIGURE 25.12   Illustration of an experiment assessing whether subjects automatically generate motor compensations for Coriolis forces during their reaches if they are experiencing self-motion. Powerful illusory self-rotation is elicited in a stationary subject (right), who remotely views the world from the perspective of a "Telehead" on a chair rotating in a complex natural environment (left). If the subject were really rotating in this fashion, rightward Coriolis forces ("F_{Cor}") would be generated during forward reaching movements and leftward compensation would be necessary to maintain a straight, accurate movement. No Coriolis force is present during illusory self-rotation, and the subject's reaching movements (open symbols) deviate to the left of reaches made while the subject views a stationary scene (closed symbols). The subject's arm is not present in the visual display.

the reaching movements will deviate leftward and end far to the left of the target location. The path of the reach viewed from above is a mirror image of what happens during counterclockwise rotation in the slow-rotation room. Subjects also report that their hand is deviated from its intended path by an intangible force, that their arm did not do what they intended. What is being experienced is a centrally generated compensation for an anticipated Coriolis force, a Coriolis force that would be present if the subjects were actually rotating. The leftward deviation of the arm results from a "correction" that is inappropriate in the actual context and that is perceived as an external force deviating the arm. These results mean that the experience of self-rotation—the sensing of self-rotation and displacement through space—is taken into account by the CNS in planning movement coordination. The CNS thus models and plans appropriate compensations for movement-dependent Coriolis forces contingent on sensed and anticipated body rotation.

A key issue is whether compensation during normal voluntary movements is entirely feed-forward in character (that is, not dependent on sensory feedback, e.g., semicircular canal activity) but preplanned so as to compensate precisely for the action of Coriolis forces as they are generated. Inherent feedback delays associated with using feedback control, and the time constants associated with neuromuscular force genera-

tion, make it likely that under normal conditions, feed-forward control is employed. For example, the generation of virtually straight-line reaches in relation to external space during voluntary turn-and-reach movements indicates central anticipation and feed-forward control consistent with the CNS establishing internal models of the body and its neuromuscular dynamics, and the ongoing and anticipated force environment. However, feedback must be used to update the calibration of internal models for movement control because adaptive changes occur after a few additional perturbed movements.

Vertical linear oscillation and visual stimulation

Vertical linear oscillation has been used as a means of determining thresholds of the linear acceleration-sensitive otolith organs of the inner ear. In threshold measurements, test subjects are usually exposed to brief periods of acceleration and report up-down motion. Interestingly, during periods of suprathreshold linear oscillation lasting more than about a minute, more complex movement paths with fore-aft and lateral body motion will be reported as well. Figure 25.13 illustrates some of the paths reported. The otolith organs are not flat structures and have receptors polarized for different directions of stimulation; as a consequence, vertical linear oscillation may activate receptors related to multiple

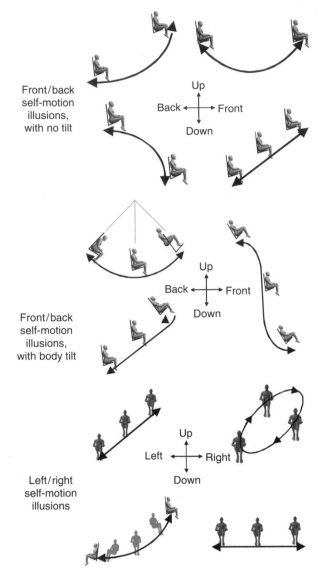

Front/back
self-motion
illusions,
with no tilt

Up
Back ← → Front
Down

Front/back
self-motion
illusions,
with body tilt

Up
Back ← → Front
Down

Left/right
self-motion
illusions

Up
Left ← → Right
Down

FIGURE 25.13 Paths of body translation and rotation perceived during exposure to vertical linear oscillation at 0.2 Hz, 1.7 m peak to peak. Fourteen subjects, seated upright, were tested in the dark.

directions of motion, thus resulting in complex patterns of stimulation, giving rise to additional directions of experienced motion.

Studies of multisensory influences on orientation and movement control often emphasize how illusions of self-motion can be induced in stationary subjects by patterns of visual, auditory, or somatosensory stimulation. Vertical linear oscillation coupled with visual stimulation allows the creation of the converse, that is, situations in which subjects undergoing physical motion can experience very different patterns of motion and even feel stationary. These studies also reveal the influence of "top-down" cognitive effects. If test subjects on a vertical oscillator wear a wide-field-of-view, head-mounted

video display, it is possible to provide them with visual stimulation that is either concordant or discordant with their actual physical motion. This can be achieved by making recordings using a video camera mounted at the position the subject's head occupies when he or she is in the apparatus. These recordings can be made with the oscillator moving or stationary, and then later played back in the head-mounted display. For example, it is possible to display a stationary view of the test chamber while the subject is oscillating up and down, or to present a view of the room displacing up and down while the subject is stationary. Horizontal oscillatory camera motion can also be used to generate a visual scene moving horizontally.

When a stationary visual recording of the test chamber is presented to the subject as he or she is oscillating vertically, the subject will feel completely stationary viewing a stable room. The sense of motion is totally suppressed despite the continuously changing inputs from the otolith organs and from tactile and pressure receptors stimulated by body contact with the apparatus and from displacements of the viscera and other movable tissues of the body. If a horizontally oscillating visual scene of the test chamber is presented while the subject is undergoing vertical oscillation, he or she will initially experience vertical and then diagonal oscillation (cf. Fig. 25.14). After about 10–60 s, the vertically oscillating subject will come to experience purely horizontal self-oscillation in a visually stationary environment.

If a visual array of stationary or moving horizontal or vertical stripes is presented to the subject, then the dominance of vision that occurs with views of the actual

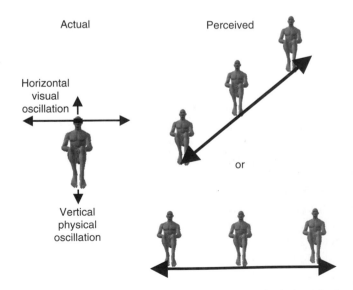

Actual   Perceived

Horizontal
visual
oscillation

or

Vertical
physical
oscillation

FIGURE 25.14 Perceived paths of self-motion during vertical, linear, 0.2 Hz oscillation while subjects view a visual scene oscillating horizontally at the same rate.

test chamber does not occur. Vertical linear oscillation of the subject coupled with horizontal stationary stripes leads to the perception of vertical self-motion in which the visual array moves with the body. Exposure to linearly vertical oscillation and horizontally oscillating vertical stripes produces some apparent side-to-side motion superimposed on up-down motion. This means that cognitive factors are influencing the effects of visual stimulation. When the visual scene depicted represents the actual visual scene that would be visible from the subject's real-world position, then that visual array dominates the subject's perception of orientation. It is possible that a visual scene depicting any possible real environment would show stronger influences on orientation than patterns of stripes.

Somatosensory influences on orientation and movement control

Multisensory influences on body orientation and their dependence on frequency are especially prominent during "barbecue spit rotation." Rotation about an Earth-horizontal body axis generates continuously changing stimulation of the otolith organs and of the body surface because of the continued reorientation of the body with respect to gravity. After a minute has elapsed at constant velocity, the activity of the semicircular canals elicited during the period of angular acceleration will have decayed to baseline, so that these receptors will no longer be indicating body rotation. In this circumstance, with vision permitted, subjects will accurately perceive self-rotation about their long-body axis, or z-axis, when rotation speeds are below about 6 rpm. Above this speed, subjects will perceive rotation about a displaced axis (Fig. 25.15).

When vision is denied during barbecue spit rotation, very different patterns are experienced (Lackner & Graybiel, 1978b). At velocities of rotation less than about 6 rpm, subjects veridically experience their body rotation. However, at progressively higher velocities, subjects begin to feel displaced from the axis of rotation and cease to experience 360-degree body rotation. Instead, they experience orbital motion, in which they feel either face-up or face-down as they go through their apparent orbital path. Each time they "complete" one revolution of their orbit they actually rotate 360 degrees in the test apparatus. The relationship between physical position in relation to the apparatus and the experienced face-up or face-down orbit is illustrated in Figure 25.16. As can be seen, there is a 180-degree phase shift in actual body position between the experienced face-up and face-down patterns. With vision allowed, subjects experience full 360-degree rotation but feel themselves to be displaced from the center of rotation.

From Figure 25.16 it can be seen that the directions of experienced orbital motion and of actual body rotation are opposite. A subject undergoing clockwise rotation experiences counterclockwise orbital motion even though the otolith organs, which are sensitive to the

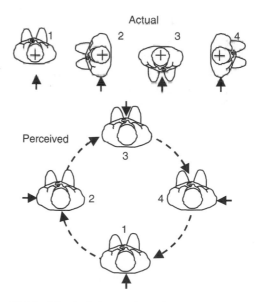

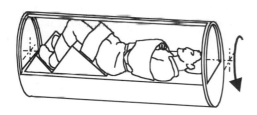

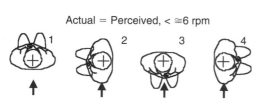

Actual = Perceived, < ≅6 rpm

FIGURE 25.15 The top part of the figure illustrates a subject in the z-axis recumbent rotation device. At constant-velocity rotation, subjects allowed vision perceive rotation about their horizontal z-body axis (sequence of lower figures). The arrows indicate the locus on the body of the contact forces of support against gravity.

FIGURE 25.16 Physical (upper) and perceived (lower) sequence of body orientations during z-axis recumbent rotation in darkness at speeds greater than 6 rpm. If the body were really undergoing the perceived pattern of orbital motion, a centripetal contact force on the body (arrow) would be present, which matches the actual contact forces. Different subjects experience face-up or face-down orbital motion, but face-up is illustrated.

direction of gravity, must be providing signals that are only consistent with the actual direction of rotation. Subjects without labyrinthine function also experience orbital motion during off-axis vertical rotation, and their experienced orbital diameter can be greater than that of normal subjects (Graybiel & Johnson, 1963). This means that nonvestibular factors must account both for the experienced orbital motion and for the fact that a constant direction of facing is experienced. Experiments in parabolic flight have made it possible to identify the key role of somatosensation in giving rise to these illusions experienced during horizontal axis rotation.

In an aircraft flying parabolic maneuvers, the resultant force of gravity and other linear accelerations varies from $0g$ to about $1.8g$. Figure 25.7 illustrates a typical flight profile. In the "$0g$" or weightless period, the otolith organs of a subject undergoing barbecue spit rotation are not differentially activated because they are unloaded, nor are touch and pressure receptors differentially activated by contact with the apparatus because the subject and the apparatus are in a state of free fall. By contrast in $1.8g$, the subject's otoliths are stimulated by a much greater than normal acceleration vector and touch and pressure receptors of the body surface and viscera are activated much more than on Earth, because body weight has nearly doubled. A blindfolded subject spinning at 30 rpm constant velocity during straight and level flight will experience the pattern illustrated in Figure 25.16; however when exposed to the weightless period of flight, the subject will experience the orbit to shrink in diameter and will soon feel no motion whatsoever, even though spinning at 30 rpm (Lackner & Graybiel, 1979). As soon as the weightless period is over the subject will begin to experience a progressively larger and larger orbit. At "steady state" $1.8g$, the apparent orbital diameter will be much greater than in $1g$. The subject always "completes" one orbital revolution each time the apparatus rotates 360 degrees; consequently, the subject's apparent orbital velocity is much greater in $1.8g$ because the orbital circumference is so much larger.

Other experiments have shown that by manipulating the pattern of somatosensory stimulation of the body surface, subjects can dramatically influence their experienced orientation (Lackner & Graybiel, 1978a, 1979). This is illustrated in Figure 25.17, which shows the patterns experienced when a subject pushes the top of his or her head or feet against the end of the apparatus. With such added pressure cues, the subject feels progressively less compellingly in the current experienced pattern and then progressively experiences a new pattern until it is totally vivid. The subject's experienced orientation can

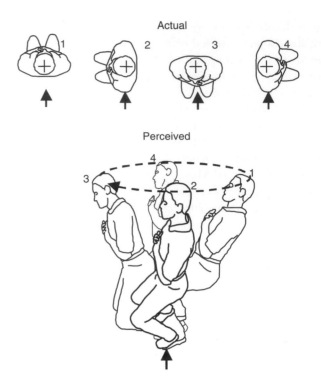

FIGURE 25.17 Illustration of the perceived conical pattern of body motion and orientation experienced when a subject pushes against the foot restraints of the apparatus during z-axis recumbent rotation in darkness. Compare with Figure 25.16.

thus be predictably changed by manipulating the touch and pressure cues on the body surface.

Figure 25.17 also shows the relationship between experienced orbital position and actual body position. As can be seen, when there is physically pressure on the chest, the subject is at the top of the apparent orbit for face-up experienced motion and at the bottom for face-down motion. The pattern of touch and pressure stimulation of the body is determining the subject's experienced motion. Consequently, there is a 180-degree phase shift between experienced face-up and face-down orbital motion. The dominance of somatosensory stimulation during body recumbent rotation could be in part because the otolith organs may serve as low-pass filters and saturate at higher velocities of rotation (e.g., >6 rpm). The key point, however, is that the orientation experienced is multimodally determined and that the relative contribution of different receptor systems depends on rotation velocity.

Haptic influences on postural control and locomotion

Somatosensory stimulation can also have a stabilizing effect on orientation. Contact of the hand with a surface or object, for example, has surprisingly large influences on balance control. Freely standing subjects always exhibit body sway and the magnitude of this sway increases if the eyes are closed. However, if a subject is allowed to touch a stationary surface with the finger of one hand, the postural sway will be attenuated (Holden, Ventura, & Lackner, 1994). Such light touch contact (subjects spontaneously adopt about $40g$ of applied force, which is mechanically nonsupportive) is even more effective than vision in stabilizing the body. Contact with the index fingers of each hand on laterally placed surfaces attenuates sway even more. The stabilizing effect of light touch is quite profound. Labyrinthine-defective subjects can only stand for seconds in the dark before losing balance, yet when allowed light touch at nonsupportive force levels, they can stand as stably as normal subjects (Lackner et al., 1999).

Finger contact at virtually any force level, even a few grams, is stabilizing (Lackner, Rabin, & DiZio, 2001). If the object contacted is a filament that can bend, body sway will be attenuated as long as the subject maintains finger contact, but less so than with contact on a rigid surface. If unbeknownst to subjects the surface they are touching is oscillated at low frequency and amplitude, then, over a considerable range of frequencies, body sway will be entrained to the frequency of the moving contact surface. Subjects will perceive the touched surface as stationary and will be unaware that they are swaying at the frequency of the surface (Jeka, Schoner, Dijkstra, Ribeiro, & Lackner, 1997).

The stabilizing effect of hand contact is partly related to "top-down" effects. If a subject is aware that the contacted surface can oscillate, then sway will still be entrained, although to a somewhat lesser extent than when the subject is unaware of potential surface motion. But the contacted surface will also no longer be perceived as stationary. Even in trials in which the contacted surface is physically stationary the subject may feel it to be oscillating. Thus, the perception of spatial stability of the contacted surface is critically dependent on cognitive assumptions and knowledge about the surface (Rabin et al., 2004).

Touch can enhance posture even under conditions of extreme destabilization. For example, the body sway of subjects standing in a room rotating at constant velocity generates Coriolis forces that are further destabilizing (Soeda, DiZio, & Lackner, 2003). (These are the same Coriolis forces that also affect arm and head movement control, as described earlier.) If such subjects are allowed light, mechanically unsupportive finger contact, they will be as stable during rotation as when the room is stationary. The touch allows them to maintain body sway velocity below levels that would generate significant Coriolis forces.

Touch stabilizes posture even when balance is perturbed by aberrant inputs. When the Achilles tendons of a standing subject are vibrated, reflexive contraction of the muscles will result and displace the subject backward about the ankles (Lackner, Rabin, & DiZio, 2000). However, the lightest touch of a finger with a stationary surface will completely suppress the destabilizing effects of vibration. Still other observations have shown that locomotion is stabilized by touch contact cues. Subjects walking on a treadmill show greater synchronization of their step cycle with touch. With eyes closed and finger touch, they also do not drift off the treadmill, as they do without the touch cue (Rabin et al., 2004).

Haptic cues from hand contact with a surface have great importance as a means for preventing falling in elderly individuals with reduced vestibular and proprioceptive function and for balance rehabilitation after sensory loss. Experiments in parabolic flight also point to the importance of haptic cues for maintaining an accurate sense of orientation and for suppressing the debilitating postural aftereffects that occur transiently after space flight (Lackner & Graybiel, 1983). Eventually it may be possible for astronauts to use such cues to suppress the reentry disturbances of posture, locomotion, and movement control that are commonplace after return from prolonged space flight.

Conclusions

Exposure to unusual force environments has widespread influences on sensory localization, spatial orientation, and movement control. Remappings of body-relative auditory and visual localization occur in non-1g force fields and are paralleled by a deviation of the apparent body midline of comparable magnitude. Such conjoint remappings imply that coordinates of a common underlying reference frame have been transformed.

Head and body movements initially made in a rotating environment generate Coriolis forces that disrupt movement path and end-point. However, with additional exposure, movements soon become accurate again as the CNS institutes adaptive motor compensations that precisely cancel the Coriolis forces generated by voluntary movements. During everyday life, it is commonplace to simultaneously turn and reach for objects. Such reaching movements are straight and accurate even though Coriolis forces much larger than those studied in passively rotating environments are generated. This means that the CNS automatically anticipates and compensates for the influence of self-generated Coriolis forces on movement path. Stationary subjects experiencing illusory self-rotation and displacement initially make errors in movement paths and end-points, errors that reflect compensations being made for Coriolis forces that are being anticipated but are actually absent.

Vertical linear oscillation and z-axis recumbent (barbecue spit) rotation are two experimental situations in which multisensory influences on perceived orientation are especially striking, with visual and somatosensory cues largely dominating perceived orientation. In the case of vertical linear oscillation, a stationary subject can be made to feel that he or she is oscillating up and down by the scene of the test chamber moving up and down in a head-mounted display. Analogously, a stationary scene of the test chamber will make an oscillating subject feel stationary. During z-axis recumbent rotation at velocities above 6 rpm, perceived orientation is driven by somatosensory, and possibly visceral, afferent signals, and blindfolded subjects no longer experience rotary motion but an orbital motion, the diameter of which is determined by background gravitoinertial force level.

Somatosensory cues can also serve to stabilize posture and locomotion. Contact of the hand with a stationary surface allows even subjects without functioning labyrinths to stand as stably in the dark as normal subjects. Even a few grams of applied force is stabilizing, and such light touch of the hand is more effective than vision in enhancing balance. If the contacted surface is oscillated without the subject's awareness, the subject will become entrained to its motion and perceive the surface as stationary. By contrast, when subjects are aware that the touched surface can move, they will no longer perceive it to be stationary even when it is.

The situations that have been described underscore the critical role of multisensory and motor factors as well as cognitive knowledge in the control and appreciation of body orientation and movement.

ACKNOWLEDGMENTS   Work was supported by AFOSR grant F49620-01-1-0171 and NASA grant NAG9-1263.

REFERENCES

Clark, B., & Graybiel, A. (1966). Factors contributing to the delay in the perception of the oculogravic illusion. *American Journal of Psychology, 79*(3), 377–388.

Clark, B., & Graybiel, A. (1968). Influence of contact cues on the perception of the oculogravic illusion. *Acta Otolaryngology, 65*, 373–380.

Cohn, J., DiZio, P., & Lackner, J. R. (2000). Reaching during virtual rotation: Context-specific compensation for expected Coriolis forces. *Journal of Neurophysiology, 83*(6), 3230–3240.

Dichgans, J., & Brandt, T. (1972). Visual-vestibular interaction and motion perception. In J. Dichgans & E. Bizzi (Eds.), *Cerebral control of eye movements and motion perception* (pp. 327–338). Basel: Karger.

DiZio, P., Lackner, J. R., & Evanoff, J. N. (1987). The influence of gravitointertial force level on oculomotor and perceptual responses to Coriolis, cross-coupling stimulation. *Aviation, Space and Environmental Medicine, 58*, A218–A223.

DiZio, P., Lackner, J. R., Held, R. M., Shinn-Cunningham, B., & Durlach, N. I. (2001). Gravitoinertial force magnitude and direction influence head-centric auditory localization. *Journal of Neurophysiology, 85*, 2455–2460.

Graybiel, A. (1952). The oculogravic illusion. *AMA Archives of Ophthalmology, 48*, 605–615.

Graybiel, A., & Clark, B. (1962). The validity of the oculogravic illusion as a specific indicator of otolith function (BuMed Project MR005.13-6001 Subtask 1, Report No. 67 and NASA Order No. R-37). Pensacola, FL: Naval School of Aviation Medicine.

Graybiel, A., Clark, B., & Zarriello, J. J. (1960). Observations on human subjects living in a "slow rotation room" for periods of two days. *Archives of Neurology, 3*, 55–73.

Graybiel, A., & Johnson, W. H. (1963). A comparison of the symptomatology experienced by healthy persons and subjects with loss of labyrinthine function when exposed to unusual patterns of centripetal force in a counter-rotating room. *Annals of Otology, 72*, 357–373.

Graybiel, A., Kennedy, R. S., Knoblock, E. C., Guedry, F. E., Jr., Mertz, W., McLeod, M. W., et al. (1965). The effects of exposure to a rotating environment (10 rpm) on four aviators for a period of twelve days. *Aerospace Medicine, 36*, 733–754.

Graybiel, A., & Knepton, J. (1978). Bidirectional overadaptation achieved by executing leftward or rightward head movements during unidirectional rotation. *Aviation, Space and Environmental Medicine, 49*, 1–4.

Graybiel, A., Miller, E. F. II, & Homick, J. L. (1977). Experiment M131: Human vestibular function. In R. S. Johnston & L. F. Dietlein (Eds.), *Biomedical results from Skylab* (pp. 74–103). Washington, DC: NASA.

Graybiel, A., & Niven, J. I. (1951). The effect of a change in direction of resultant force on sound localization: The audiogravic illusion. *Journal of Experimental Psychology, 42*, 227–230.

Guedry, F. E., Kennedy, R. S., Harris, C. S., & Graybiel, A. (1964). Human performance during two weeks in a room rotating at three RPM. *Aerospace Medicine, 35*, 1071–1082.

Held, R., Dichgans, J., & Bauer, J. (1975). Characteristics of moving visual scenes influencing spatial orientation. *Vision Research, 15*, 357–365.

Holden, M., Ventura, J., & Lackner, J. R. (1994). Stabilization of posture by precision contact of the index finger. *Journal of Vestibular Research, 4*(4), 285–301.

Holick, M. F. (1992). Microgravity, calcium and bone metabolism: A new perspective. *Acta Astronautica, 27*, 75–81.

Holick, M. F. (1997). *Connective tissue/biomineralization*. Presented at an NIA-NASA forum.

Jeka, J. J., Schoner, G., Dijkstra, T., Ribeiro, P., & Lackner, J. R. (1997). Coupling of fingertip somatosensory information to head and body sway. *Experimental Brain Research, 113*, 475–483.

Kennedy, R. S., & Graybiel, A. (1962). Symptomatology during prolonged exposure in a constantly rotating environment at a velocity of one revolution per minute. *Aerospace Medicine, 33*, 817–825.

Lackner, J. R. (1977). Induction of illusory self-rotation and nystagmus by a rotating sound-field. *Aviation, Space and Environmental Medicine, 48*, 129–131.

Lackner, J. R. (1978). Some mechanisms underlying sensory and postural stability in man. In R. Held, H. Leibowitz, &

H. L. Teuber (Eds.), *Handbook of sensory physiology* (Vol. VIII, pp. 805–845). New York: Springer-Verlag.

Lackner, J. R. (1988). Some proprioceptive influences on the perceptual representation of body shape and orientation. *Brain, 111,* 281–297.

Lackner, J. R., & DiZio, P. (1984). Some efferent and somatosensory influences on body orientation and oculomotor control. In L. Spillman & B. R. Wooten (Eds.), *Sensory experience, adaptation, and perception* (pp. 281–301). Clifton, NJ: Erlbaum.

Lackner, J. R., & DiZio, P. (1994). Rapid adaptation to Coriolis force perturbations of arm trajectory. *Journal of Neurophysiology, 72*(1), 299–313.

Lackner, J. R., & DiZio, P. (1998). Adaptation in a rotating artificial gravity environment. *Brain Research Review, 28,* 194–202.

Lackner, J. R., DiZio, P., & Fisk, J. D. (1992). Tonic vibration reflexes and background force level. *Acta Astronautica, 26*(2), 133–136.

Lackner, J. R., DiZio, P., Jeka, J. J., Horak, F., Krebs, D., & Rabin, E. (1999). Precision contact of the fingertip reduces postural sway of individuals with bilateral vestibular loss. *Experimental Brain Research, 126,* 459–466.

Lackner, J. R., & Graybiel, A. (1978a). Postural illusions experienced during Z-axis recumbent rotation and their dependence on somatosensory stimulation of the body surface. *Aviation, Space and Environmental Medicine, 49,* 484–488.

Lackner, J. R., & Graybiel, A. (1978b). Some influences of touch and pressure cues on human spatial orientation. *Aviation, Space and Environmental Medicine, 49,* 798–804.

Lackner, J. R., & Graybiel, A. (1979). Parabolic flight: Loss of sense of orientation. *Science, 206,* 1105–1108.

Lackner, J. R., & Graybiel, A. (1983). Perceived orientation in free fall depends on visual, postural, and architectural factors. *Aviation, Space and Environmental Medicine, 54,* 47–51.

Lackner, J. R., & Graybiel, A. (1984). Influence of gravitoinertial force level on apparent magnitude of Coriolis cross-coupled angular accelerations and motion sickness. In *NATO-AGARD Aerospace Medical Panel Symposium on Motion Sickness: Mechanisms, prediction, prevention and treatment* (pp. 1–7). AGARD-CP-372, 22.

Lackner, J. R., Rabin, E., & DiZio, P. (2000). Fingertip contact suppresses the destabilizing influence of leg muscle vibration. *Journal of Neurophysiology, 84*(5), 2217–2224.

Lackner, J. R., Rabin, E., & DiZio, P. (2001). Stabilization of posture by precision touch of the index finger with rigid and flexible filaments. *Experimental Brain Research, 139,* 454–464.

Pigeon, P., Bortolami, S. B., DiZio, P., & Lackner, J. R. (2003). Coordinated turn and reach movements: I. Anticipatory compensation for self-generated Coriolis and interaction torques. *Journal of Neurophysiology, 89,* 276–289.

Rabin, E., DiZio, P., & Lackner, J. R. (2004). The control of the fingertip as a spatial sensor: Entrainment of posture to dynamic haptic stimuli. *Experimental Brain Research,* submitted.

Soeda, K., DiZio, P., & Lackner, J. R. (2003). Balance in a rotating artificial gravity environment. *Experimental Brain Research, 148,* 266–271.

Watt, D. G. D., Money, K. E., & Tomi, L. M. (1986). MIT/Canadian vestibular experiments on the Spacelab-1 mission. 3. Effects of prolonged weightlessness on a human otolith-spinal reflex. *Experimental Brain Research, 64,* 308–315.

Wilson, V. J., & Peterson, B. W. (1978). Peripheral and central substrates of vestibulospinal reflexes. *Physiological Review, 50,* 80–105.

26 Action as a Binding Key to Multisensory Integration

LEONARDO FOGASSI AND VITTORIO GALLESE

Introduction

One of the classic roles attributed to multisensory integration is that of producing a unitary percept of objects. We can recognize a spoon not only by looking at it but also by touching it when it is out of view. We can recognize a species of bird by seeing it, by using visual information about its size, shape, and colors, and also by hearing its song. We can guess that a bee is approaching one side of our face by seeing it enter one side of our visual field or by hearing its buzzing near one of our ears.

Another fundamental role of multisensory integration is to help us recognize and understand what other individuals are doing. Even without seeing a person pouring water into a glass, we can recognize this action from the sound made by the flowing liquid.

In addition, action execution depends on multisensory integration. Indeed, in our daily life most of the actions we perform rely on sensory information, and in order to act appropriately, we often have to process in parallel information arriving via more than one sensory modality. The act of kicking a ball, for example, requires the integration of visual, proprioceptive, and tactile modalities. Writing is another example of an action that, to be accomplished accurately, requires the integration of visual, proprioceptive, and tactile information.

Thus, the retrieval in our brain of the representation of a given object, individual, or action greatly benefits from information arriving through different and multiple sensory modalities. Where and how are the different sensory modalities integrated?

According to the classic view, the cerebral cortex consists of sensory, motor, and associative areas that are functionally separate from one another. In particular, it has been assumed that perception constitutes the highest level in the elaboration of sensory inputs through several serial steps. According to this view, the task of associative areas is to integrate several modalities, producing a final percept, such as that of space or that of objects. The content of perception is then provided to motor areas to drive movement execution. The basis of this view is a serial model of the processes that occur in the cerebral cortex, in which the role of the motor cortices is to deal with already elaborated sensory information, thus playing little or no role in its elaboration.

A more recent conceptualization of the relationship between action and perception limns a dichotomy between a perceptuocognitive brain, which basically relies on visual information elaborated in the ventral stream, and an executive brain, which exploits the visual information elaborated in the dorsal stream for the on-line control of action (see, e.g., Goodale, 2000; for a somewhat different view, see Martin, Ungerleider, & Haxby, 2000).

Recent empirical evidence has contributed to a change in these views by emphasizing the role of the motor system not only in the control of action but also in the perceptuocognitive domain. Neuroanatomical data show that a basic architectural feature of the cerebral cortex is the presence of multiple parallel cortico-cortical circuits, each involving areas tightly linked with one another. Many of these circuits consist of specific parietal and frontal areas linked by reciprocal connections (for a review, see Rizzolatti & Luppino, 2001; Rizzolatti, Luppino, & Matelli, 1998). In these circuits, sensory inputs are transformed in order to accomplish not only motor but also cognitive tasks, such as space perception and action understanding.

Neurophysiological data show that the neurons of motor areas not only discharge during a monkey's active movements but can also be driven by different types of sensory stimuli, such as tactile, visual, or auditory stimuli, previously considered the typical inputs for driving neurons in the posterior part of the cerebral cortex. Particularly interesting is the demonstration of polymodal neurons in the premotor cortex. Other functional data provide evidence that the parietal cortex contains not only neurons activated by several sensory inputs but also neurons that discharge during active movements performed with different effectors. Therefore, it is possible to conclude that parietal areas are endowed with motor properties and motor areas are endowed with uni- or polymodal sensory properties (Andersen, Snyder, Bradley, & Xing, 1997; Colby & Goldberg, 1999; Hyvärinen, 1982; Mountcastle, 1995; Mountcastle, Lynch, Georgopoulos, Sakata, & Acuna, 1975; Rizzolatti, Fogassi, & Gallese, 1997, 2002; Sakata & Taira, 1994).

In this chapter we will show that multisensory integration is a pervasive feature of parietofrontal centers involved in sensorimotor planning and control. We will present and discuss three parallel parietofrontal circuits: those involved in sensorimotor transformations for action, those involved in space perception, and those involved in action understanding. We propose that motor representations play a major role by providing a binding key to multisensory integration.

F4-VIP: A circuit for action in space and space perception

Area F4 of the ventral premotor cortex and the ventral intraparietal (VIP) area of the inferior parietal lobule constitute a frontoparietal circuit. The microinjection of neural tracers into both F4 and VIP demonstrates their reciprocal connections (Lewis & Van Essen, 2000; Luppino, Murata, Govoni, & Matelli, 1999). The properties of these two areas will be presented separately. Special emphasis will be placed on premotor area F4.

ANATOMICAL LOCATION AND FUNCTIONAL PROPERTIES OF AREA F4   Area F4 is one of the areas in which agranular frontal cortex is subdivided, as shown by cytoarchitectonic and histochemical studies (Matelli, Luppino, & Rizzolatti, 1985, 1991). As shown in Figure 26.1, area F4 is located in front of area F1 (primary motor cortex) and is bordered rostrally by area F5. The two areas together form the ventral premotor cortex. Area F4 is connected with other areas of the agranular frontal cortex (F1, F2, F5) and with posterior parietal area VIP (Luppino et al., 1999; Matelli, Camarda, Glickstein, & Rizzolatti, 1986; Matelli, Marconi, Caminiti, & Luppino, 1999). F4 projects subcortically to both the spinal cord and the brainstem (Keizer & Kuypers, 1989).

Electric stimulation of area F4 evokes axial, proximal, and facial movements with relatively low-intensity currents (Fogassi, Gallese, Fadiga, & Rizzolatti, 1996; Gentilucci et al., 1988). Arm and neck movements are represented more medially while orofacial movements are represented more laterally, although there is a large overlap among these representations.

Most F4 neurons are activated by sensory stimuli. According to the effective stimulus, F4 neurons can be subdivided into three main categories: (1) somatosensory neurons, (2) visual neurons, and (3) bimodal, somatosensory and visual neurons (Fogassi, Gallese,

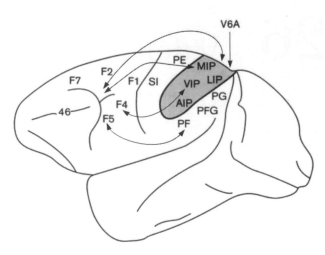

FIGURE 26.1   Lateral view of the macaque monkey cerebral cortex, showing the main subdivisions of frontal agranular and parietal cortex and some frontoparietal circuits. Frontal agranular cortical areas are classified according to Matelli et al. (1985, 1991). Parietal areas are classified according to Pandya and Seltzer (1982). The intraparietal sulcus is opened (shaded gray) to show areas located in its medial and lateral banks. The location of area V6A, in the anterior bank (not visible) of the parieto-occipital sulcus, is shown by an arrow. AIP, anterior intraparietal area; LIP, lateral intraparietal area; MIP, medial intraparietal area; SI, primary somatosensory cortex; VIP, ventral intraparietal area.

Fadiga, Luppino, et al., 1996; Fogassi, Gallese, Fadiga, & Rizzolatti, 1996; Fogassi et al., 1992; Gentilucci, Scandolara, Pigarev, & Rizzolatti, 1983; Gentilucci et al., 1988; Graziano & Gross, 1995; Graziano, Hu, & Gross, 1997a; Graziano, Yap, & Gross, 1994; Rizzolatti, Scandolara, Matelli, & Gentilucci, 1981a, 1981b). Recently, trimodal neurons were also described. These neurons respond to auditory stimuli in addition to somatosensory and visual stimuli (Graziano, Reiss, & Gross, 1999).

Somatosensory F4 neurons typically (82%) respond to superficial tactile stimuli. A small percentage (8%) are also activated by deep pressure on the skin or joint manipulation. About 10% are activated by both light touch and joint rotation or deep pressure. The receptive fields (RFs) of neurons responding to superficial tactile stimuli are generally large and located on the face, chest, arm, and hand, whereas proprioceptive and deep responses are mostly evoked by trunk and arm stimulation. Most somatosensory neurons have contralateral (66%) or bilateral (22%) RFs (Fogassi, Gallese, Fadiga, & Rizzolatti, 1996).

F4 visual neurons are activated by different types of static and moving visual stimuli. Visual responses are evoked by the abrupt presentation of objects in space, by object motion along a tangential plane, or by object rotation. Neurons responding to motion often prefer a particular direction or sense of rotation.

The most interesting category of F4 neurons is represented by bimodal, somatosensory and visual neurons, which account for 80% of all visually responding neurons. Their somatosensory properties are the same as those of purely somatosensory neurons. The visual stimuli most effective in evoking the neurons' discharge are three-dimensional (3D) static or moving objects. Some neurons (2%) discharge phasically to object presentation, others (4%) discharge tonically to objects kept still in their RF (Fogassi, Gallese, Fadiga, & Rizzolatti, 1996). Graziano, Hu, and Gross (1997b) described a particularly interesting subcategory of F4 bimodal neurons that, in addition to their tonic response to object presentation, also fire when the light is turned off, but the monkey "imagines" that the stimulus is still there. When the stimulus is withdrawn without the monkey noticing it, the neuron discharge is still present, but it stops as soon as the monkey is aware that the stimulus is not there anymore.

The vast majority (89%) of bimodal neurons prefer moving to stationary stimuli. The preferred motion direction is along a sagittal trajectory pointing toward the monkey. These neurons typically prefer stimuli approaching the tactile RF. Neurons activated by stimuli withdrawn from the monkey are much less common.

The visual RFs of F4 bimodal neurons are 3D, that is, they extend to a given depth from the monkey's body (Fig. 26.2). Their extension in depth ranges from a few centimeters to 40 cm, calculated starting from the tactile RF. Visual stimuli presented outside this 3D visual field do not evoke any response. As shown in Figure 26.2, in the great majority of these neurons the visual RF is large and generally in register with the tactile RF.

For example, a neuron with a tactile RF on the upper face will also respond to an object approaching the forehead and the eyes. Similarly, a neuron with a tactile RF on the shoulder and neck will be activated by stimuli directed to these areas of the skin. On the basis of this direct matching between tactile and visual RFs, the 3D visual RFs can be considered to originate from the skin, forming a "projection" in space of the tactile RF. They have been called peripersonal RFs. Like tactile RFs, visual peripersonal RFs are mostly contralateral (60%) to the recorded side or bilateral (32%).

Quantitative studies of the visual properties of F4 bimodal neurons have shown that most neurons of this area (90%) have visual RFs coded in somatocentered coordinates. Only 10% of the studied neurons could be defined as retinocentric. This was demonstrated by verifying whether, in monkeys trained to fixate a spot of light located in different spatial locations, the position of the visual RF shifted with the eyes or not (Fig. 26.3). In most F4 neurons, the position in space of the visual RF did not change when the eyes shifted. Thus, F4 visual responses do not depend on the retinal position of the stimulus (Fogassi, Gallese, Fadiga, Luppino, et al., 1996; Fogassi et al., 1992; see also Gentilucci et al., 1983, Graziano et al., 1994, 1997a).

The response of bimodal F4 neurons is also independent of visual cues present in the environment. In an experiment in which the position of the monkey was changed with respect to the walls of the recording room, it was observed that in none of the tested bimodal F4 neurons did the location in space of their visual RF depend on allocentric cues (Fogassi, Gallese, Fadiga, Luppino, et al., 1996).

The spatial coordinates of the visual RF of F4 bimodal neurons are not centered on a single frame of reference but are referred to a multiplicity of spatial reference points, that is, to different body parts, as originally proposed by Rizzolatti and Gentilucci (1988). Graziano et al. (1994; see also Graziano et al., 1997a), in an experiment in which presumably F4 bimodal neurons were studied, moved the body part (e.g., arm) around which the previously defined visual peripersonal RF was located. They found that the visual RF moved together with the involved body part.

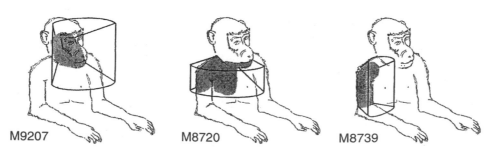

FIGURE 26.2 Examples of different types of bimodal (tactile and visual) receptive fields (RFs) of F4 neurons. Shaded areas indicate tactile RFs. Solids drawn around different body parts indicate visual RFs. (Modified from Fogassi, Gallese, Fadiga, Luppino, et al., 1996).

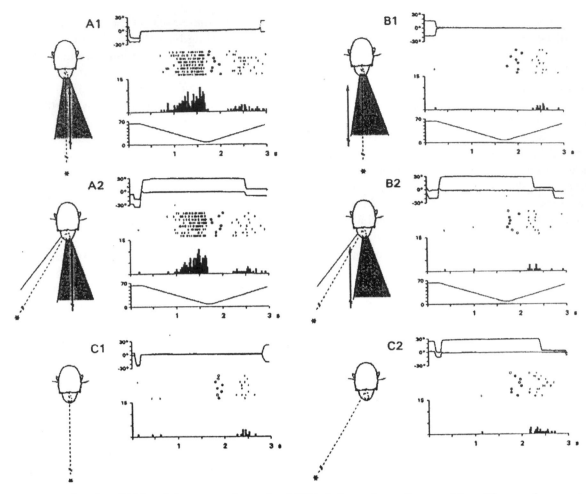

FIGURE 26.3 Example of an F4 bimodal neuron whose visual RF is independent of eye position. The monkey was trained to fixate an LED for a variable time and to release a bar when it dimmed. During fixation, a 3D stimulus was moved toward the monkey at constant velocity (40 cm/s), inside and outside the visual RF. Each panel shows horizontal and vertical eye movements, rasters and histograms representing the neuronal response, and a plot indicating the variation over time of the distance between the stimulus and the monkey. The large dots in the rasters indicate the dimming of the fixation point. After foveation to the LED, the monkey's eyes remained in the fixation position (indicated by the asterisk at the end of each dotted line) until after the LED was dimmed. The neuron tactile RF was bilateral, located on the central part of the face. In *A1* and *A2*, the stimulus was moved inside the visual RF. The stimulus direction reversed when the stimulus was 8 cm from the orbital plane. In *B1* and *B2*, the stimulus was moved outside the visual RF. *C1* and *C2* are control trials in which the monkey fixated the same two points as in *A* and *B*, but no stimulus other than the LED was introduced. The discharge was present when the visual stimulus was moved into the somatocentric RF and was independent of eye position; consequently, it is not related to a specific point on the retina. Time is charted on the abscissa and spikes per bin are charted on the ordinate. The bin width was 20 ms. (Modified from Fogassi, Gallese, Fadiga, Luppino, et al., 1996).

The extension in depth of F4 neurons' visual RFs is not fixed but can be modulated by the velocity of the approaching stimulus. In most F4 bimodal neurons tested with stimuli of different velocities, the visual RF expands with an increase in stimulus velocity (Fig. 26.4). The neuron discharge begins earlier in time and farther away in space with increasing stimulus velocity.

Recently, Graziano et al. (1999) showed that some F4 bimodal neurons can also be activated by acoustic stimuli. These neurons respond when an auditory stimulus is introduced in the space around the monkey's head. The auditory RFs of these neurons are in register with the tactile and the visual peripersonal RFs. Some of these neurons are also sensitive to the intensity of the auditory stimulus.

Taken together, the properties of F4 bimodal and trimodal neurons indicate that information about object position in somatocentered space can be provided by different sensory inputs. In all multisensory neurons, the location of the tactile RF constrains the location of the visual and auditory RFs.

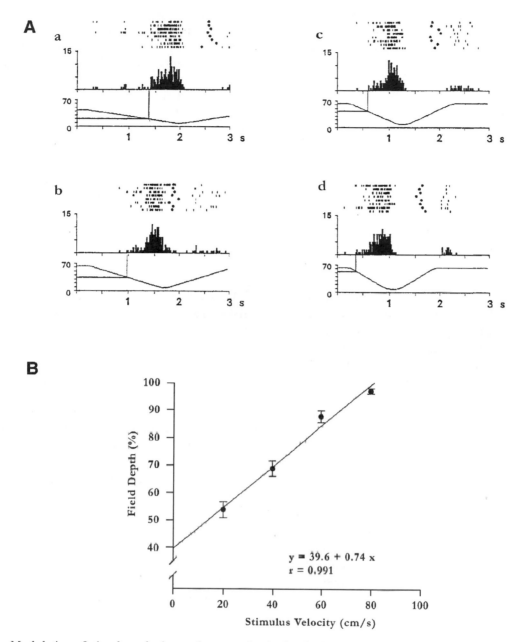

FIGURE 26.4   Modulation of stimulus velocity on the extension in depth of visual RFs in F4. (*A*) Example of a somatocentered F4 neuron whose visual RF expands in depth with increasing stimulus velocity. The behavioral paradigm was the same as that described in Figure 26.3, except that four different stimulus velocities in separate blocks were employed: 20 cm/s (*a*), 40 cm/s (*b*), 60 cm/s (*c*), and 80 cm/s (*d*). The value of the ordinate at the intersection between the vertical line indicating the beginning of the neural discharge and the curve representing the stimulus movement corresponds to the outer border of the visual RF at different velocities. There is a clear shift in time and space of the beginning of the discharge, when stimulus velocity increases. (*B*) Correlation between field depth change as function of stimulus velocity in 25 F4 neurons modulated by the velocity of the approaching stimulus. (Modified from Fogassi, Gallese, Fadiga, Luppino, et al., 1996).

The characterization of the motor properties of all F4 neurons demonstrated that more than 50% of them have motor properties, as would be expected from a cortical sector endowed with projections to the spinal cord and the brainstem. These F4 motor neurons discharge during movements of the upper or lower face (10%), such as blinking or lifting the eyebrows, grimacing or retracting the lips for food grasping, movements of the neck and lower trunk (28%) such as orienting or avoiding, and movements of the arm (25%) such as reaching or bringing to the mouth (Fogassi, Gallese, Fadiga, & Rizzolatti, 1996; see also Gentilucci et al., 1988; Godschalk, Lemon, Nijs, & Kuypers, 1981; Graziano et al., 1997a). A more detailed study of F4 "arm-reaching" neurons revealed that they discharge when the arm is moved toward a given spatial location, although their directional specificity is broad (Gentilucci et al., 1988). Many motor neurons (33%) discharge during active movements that associate different effectors, such as bringing food to the mouth plus mouth opening, or arm reaching plus trunk orienting. It is interesting to note that microstimulation frequently evokes the combined movements of different effectors, such as arm and mouth (Gentilucci et al., 1988). Thus, the movement representation based on active movements is in agreement with that revealed by intracortical microstimulation.

Of all the motor neurons, 36% are activated by both somatosensory and visual stimuli. Systematic quantitative studies in which the sensory and motor properties of F4 neurons were investigated in the same neurons are lacking. However, in those cells in which this relation was examined, a good congruence was found between the visual RF location of the neuron and the spatial position toward which the effector (arm or head) had to be moved in order to excite it (Gentilucci et al., 1988; Graziano et al., 1997a).

ANATOMICAL LOCATION AND FUNCTIONAL PROPERTIES OF AREA VIP   Area VIP (see Fig. 26.1) occupies the fundus of the intraparietal sulcus, approximately along its middle third, and extends from the sulcus onto both its lateral and medial banks (Colby, Duhamel, & Goldberg, 1993). Area VIP receives visual inputs from the middle temporal visual area, the medial superior temporal area, the fundus of the superior temporal sulcus, area MIP in the intraparietal sulcus, and the parieto-occipital area (Boussaoud, Ungerleider, & Desimone, 1990; Lewis & Van Essen, 2000; Maunsell & Van Essen, 1983; Ungerleider & Desimone, 1986). Somatosensory information is fed to area VIP by several parietal areas (Lewis & Van Essen, 2000; Seltzer & Pandya, 1986).

The functional properties of area VIP have been investigated by Colby and co-workers (Colby & Duhamel, 1991; Colby et al., 1993; Duhamel, Colby, & Golderg, 1998). Area VIP contains both purely visual and bimodal—visual and tactile—neurons. Purely visual VIP neurons are strongly selective for the direction and speed of the stimuli. Their RFs are typically large. Some respond preferentially to expanding and contracting stimuli (Colby et al., 1993; Schaafsma, Duysens, & Gielen, 1997).

Bimodal neurons of area VIP share many features with F4 bimodal neurons. As for the latter, VIP bimodal neurons also respond independently to both visual and tactile stimulation. Tactile RFs are located predominantly on the face. The preferred visual stimuli are those moving with a specific direction and speed. Tactile and visual RFs are usually "in register": neurons with visual RFs coding central vision have tactile fields on the nose and mouth region, while neurons with peripheral visual RFs have tactile fields on the side of the head or of the body. Directional selectivity is also the same in both modalities. In contrast to F4, however, only a small percentage of bimodal VIP neurons respond to 3D objects presented in the peripersonal space and moved toward or away from the monkey. Again in contrast to F4, the vast majority of the visual RFs of VIP visual neurons are organized in retinotopic coordinates. In only 30% is the position of the RF independent of gaze direction (Colby et al., 1993), remaining anchored to the tactile field. It is interesting to note that all VIP neurons that responded to stimuli moved into the monkey's peripersonal space have somatocentered visual RFs. These data suggest that in area VIP, an initial transformation from retinal to egocentric coordinates occurs (Colby, Gattass, Olson, & Gross, 1998; Duhamel et al., 1998).

Neurophysiological studies of the motor properties of area VIP are lacking. However, Thier and Andersen (1998), in an intracortical microstimulation study of several areas of the intraparietal sulcus, were able to evoke, with high current intensity, head, face, and arm movements from a region of the floor of the intraparietal sulcus that could partially overlap with area VIP, as defined by Colby et al. (1993). These findings corroborate the suggestion that VIP neurons play a role in coding visual targets for head movements (see Colby, 1998).

ROLE OF MULTISENSORY INTEGRATION IN THE F4-VIP CIRCUIT   The visual and auditory responses of F4 polymodal neurons are peculiar because their RFs are limited to a portion of space located around a particular body part, that is, a specific, although large, tactile RF. This organization seems to reflect a mechanism through which the presence of a body carves a limited (peripersonal) space sector out of space, which in principle is infinite. The location of the peripersonal spatial RF is prespecified by the tactile RF.

A striking feature of these peripersonal visual RFs is that, in contrast to the typical RFs of striate and extrastriate visual cortices, they extend in depth. What defines the depth of these RF? The visual RFs of area F4 neurons may span a very short distance or a longer distance from the animal skin, but they always remain inside reaching distance. This limitation in depth strongly suggests that these RFs are related to the various types of movements that are normally made inside this space, such as mouth grasping (pericutaneous RFs) or arm reaching or trunk orienting (distant peripersonal RFs). Thus, the obvious conclusion would be that the visual and auditory inputs are instrumental for providing spatial *sensory* information for the different types of actions represented in area F4.

This type of sensory interpretation is very much related to the classic concept of serial processing of sensory information, with the motor output constituting the final outcome of a process in which perception has occurred upstream.

We suggest here a different account of the role of multisensory neurons of the F4-VIP circuit, namely, that what the different sensory modalities evokes is always a motor representation of the perceived object, whether it is seen or heard. This *motor representation* interpretation fits the conceptualization that has been proposed to explain the visuomotor properties of area F4 (Fogassi, Gallese, Fadiga, Luppino, et al., 1996; Fogassi, Gallese, Fadiga, & Rizzolatti, 1996; Rizzolatti, Fogassi, & Gallese, 1997). As summarized earlier, area F4 is endowed with visuomotor neurons that discharge when the monkey executes orienting and reaching actions and when visual stimuli approach the same body parts motorically controlled by the same neurons (Fogassi, Gallese, Fadiga, Luppino, et al., 1996; Fogassi, Gallese, Fadiga, & Rizzolatti, 1996; Gentilucci et al., 1988; Graziano et al., 1994, 1997a). It must be emphasized that the "visual" responses evoked by objects moving inside the peripersonal somatocentered RF are present in the absence of any impending movement of the monkey directed toward those objects. These "visual" responses can be interpreted as a motor representation of the working space of a given effector. In other words, every time an object is introduced into the monkey's peripersonal space, a pragmatic representation of the associated action is immediately retrieved. This representation, depending on the context, can be turned into overt action.

The motor representation interpretation of the multisensory responses within the F4-VIP circuits posits that the function of the different sensory inputs is to retrieve different types of motor representations according to the body part on or near which the tactile, visual, or auditory stimuli are applied. A visual stimulus near the monkey could evoke an avoiding action, a mouth approaching action, or a reaching action directed toward the body. Similarly, a far peripersonal stimulus could elicit an orienting action or a reaching action away from the body. If the context is suitable, these actions will be executed; if not, they remain as *potential actions,* enabling space perception (discussed in the next section). Thus, the motor representations of F4 neurons can accomplish two tasks. First, they can play a major role in

the sensorimotor transformation for facial, axial, and proximal actions. Second, they can code space directly, in motor terms, using the same coordinate system of the effector acting in that portion of peripersonal space.

The strict relation between the sensory responses of F4 bimodal neurons and their motor valence is corroborated by the expansion in depth of their visual RFs determined by the increase in stimulus velocity (see Fig. 26.4). The behavior of these neurons reflects what has been demonstrated in human subjects. Typically, if an individual wants to reach an approaching object, his or her nervous system must compute the object velocity in order to lift the arm at the right time. If the velocity of the approaching target increases, the reaching action must start earlier in time. Chieffi, Fogassi, Gallese, and Gentilucci (1992), in an experiment in which human subjects were required to reach and grasp an object approaching at different velocities, demonstrated that, when the velocity of the approaching object increased, a subject's arm began to move earlier in time when the object was farther from the subject's starting hand position. This change in time and depth is exactly what happens in F4 bimodal neurons whose RF depth is modulated by the stimulus velocity. These data are compatible with a motor, and therefore dynamic, coding of space.

NEUROLOGICAL DEFICITS RELATED TO PERIPERSONAL SPACE
In the previous section we emphasized that within the F4-VIP circuit, sensory stimuli can evoke the motor representation of a given action without leading to its overt execution. We have proposed that such a mechanism may generate space perception. Lesion studies in monkeys and humans seem to confirm the involvement of the F4-VIP circuit in space perception.

Unilateral lesions of ventral premotor cortex that include area F4 produce two types of deficits, motor deficits and perceptual deficits (Rizzolatti, Matelli, & Pavesi, 1983; see also Fogassi et al., 2001; Schieber, 2000). Motor deficits consist in a reluctance to use the contralesional arm, spontaneously or in response to tactile and visual stimuli, and in impaired grasping with the mouth of food presented contralesionally near the mouth. Movements of the contralateral arm are slower, and in some cases misreaching is also observed.

Perceptual deficits consist in the neglect of stimuli introduced in the peripersonal space, especially around the mouth, the face, and the contralateral arm. Stimulation of the lips produces either no response or the opening of the mouth not accompanied by any attempt to bite. Licking movements cannot be elicited by wetting the contralateral lip with water or juice; the same stimulation promptly evokes the response on the ipsilateral side. Blinking in response to threatening stimuli moved toward the contralateral hemiface is absent. In contrast, facial movements are easily elicited by emotional stimuli presented far from the animal. When two stimuli are simultaneously moved in the peribuccal space, the monkey always tries to reach for the one ipsilateral to the lesion. Similarly, when the animal is fixating a central stimulus, it ignores another stimulus introduced into the peripersonal space contralateral to the lesion but responds normally to stimuli introduced into the ipsilateral visual field. Conversely, stimuli presented in the far space, outside the animal's reach, are immediately detected, and the presentation of two simultaneous stimuli, one ipsilateral, the other contralateral to the lesion, does not produce any clear side preference. Eye movements are difficult to elicit with tactile or visual peribuccal stimuli but are easily evoked with visual stimuli presented far from the monkey.

Selective lesions of area VIP were performed by J.-R. Duhamel (personal communication) in an experiment aimed at evaluating the role of area VIP in eye movements directed at moving objects. After lesion, no effects were observed in eye movements. Instead, there was a consistent, although mild, unilateral neglect for near space. The deficit consisted in a tendency to ignore or orient away from visual stimuli presented near the face contralaterally to the lesion. However, the monkey oriented normally to stimuli presented at distant locations. The monkey also failed to orient toward tactile stimuli applied to the contralateral hemiface, even when a piece of food was moved toward the mouth in full vision, whereas tactile stimuli applied to or moved toward the ipsilateral hemiface elicited normal orienting and mouth grasping.

In humans, spatial neglect normally occurs after lesions of the right inferior parietal lobule and, less frequently, after lesions of the posterior part of the frontal lobe. Patients with unilateral neglect typically fail to respond to visual stimuli presented in the contralesional half field and to tactile stimuli delivered to the contralesional limbs (see Bisiach & Vallar, 2000; Rizzolatti, Berti, & Gallese, 2000). As in monkeys, neglect in humans may also selectively affect the peripersonal space. It has been reported that in a line bisection task, when the bisection was made in near space, patients with neglect displaced the midpoint mark to the right. Bisection was normal in far space (Halligan & Marshall, 1991; see also Berti & Frassinetti, 2000). Other authors described the opposite dissociation (Cowey, Small, & Ellis, 1994, 1999; Shelton, Bowers, & Heilman, 1990). All these data indicate that space perception can be selectively impaired in relation to space sectors that can be uniquely defined in motor terms.

The relevance of action for space perception is further corroborated by evidence showing that in humans, as in monkeys, spatial maps are not fixed but are dynamically modulated by action requirements. Berti and Frassinetti (2000) showed that when the cerebral representation of body space is extended to include tools that the subject uses, space previously mapped as far is treated as near. In a patient with neglect who exhibited a clear dissociation between near and far space on the line bisection task, they tested line bisection in far space, asking him to use a stick by means of which he could *reach* the line. Neglect reappeared and was as severe as neglect in near space. Therefore, as in monkeys (see Iriki, Tanaka, & Iwamura, 1996), the use of a tool extended the patient's peripersonal space. Through action, the far space was remapped as near space. As a consequence, neglect reappeared.

Thus, both in humans and in monkeys it is possible to demonstrate separate systems for peripersonal and extrapersonal space. Furthermore, peripersonal space can be dynamically modulated by action. Because of the large lesions that cause neglect in humans, however, it is difficult to establish a homology between areas whose damage causes neglect in these two species. It is interesting to note, however, that in a recent fMRI study, Bremmer et al. (2001) reported activation in a region in the depth of the intraparietal sulcus and one in the ventral premotor cortex at the border between ventral area 6 and area 44 following application of tactile stimuli to the forehead and the presentation of moving visual stimuli and auditory stimuli near the face. These activated parietal and frontal regions could correspond to areas VIP and F4 of the monkey, respectively (see Rizzolatti et al., 2002).

F2 ventrorostral-V6A/MIP: A circuit for the control of reaching in space

Area F2 of the dorsal premotor cortex and parietal areas V6A and MIP constitute a frontoparietal circuit. The microinjection of neural tracers into these three areas demonstrates their connections (Marconi et al., 2001; Matelli, Govoni, Galletti, Kutz, & Luppino, 1998). The properties of these three areas will be separately presented.

ANATOMICAL LOCATION AND FUNCTIONAL PROPERTIES OF AREA F2   Area F2 of the monkey occupies the caudal two-thirds of dorsal premotor cortex. Microstimulation and neuronal recording show that this area contains a representation of the whole body, except the face (Fogassi et al., 1999; Raos, Franchi, Gallese, & Fogassi, 2003). The hind limb is represented in its medial half, the forelimb in its lateral half, and the trunk in between the hind limb and the forelimb representations. The sensory input to area F2 is mostly somatosensory, proprioception being the most represented submodality (Fogassi et al., 1999; see also Matelli et al., 1998). Recently, however, visual neurons were described in the ventrorostral part of area F2 (Fogassi et al., 1999). Neurons of this sector discharge during arm and hand movements (Raos, Umiltà, Gallese, & Fogassi, 1999) and are driven mainly by proprioceptive stimulation. Visual neurons can be subdivided into four classes. Neurons included in three of these categories generally are not activated by somatosensory stimulation. They are (1) object presentation neurons, discharging in response to the presentation of a specific object; (2) extrapersonal neurons, activated by stimuli moved or rotated along a tangential plane, showing also directional or rotational preference; and (3) peripersonal neurons, activated by 3D visual stimuli moved toward the forelimb or the upper trunk of the monkey or rotated within its peripersonal space. The responses of neurons of the first two classes are independent of the distance from the monkey at which the visual stimulation is performed. The fourth class of visual neurons consists of bimodal neurons that are activated by both tactile and visual stimuli. These neurons have large tactile RFs on the forelimb and upper trunk. As in F4, visual RFs are 3D, limited to the peripersonal space, and in register with the somatosensory RFs. The best stimuli are 3D stimuli moved toward or away from the tactile RFs.

Bimodal neurons of F2 have some similarities with and differences from those of F4. Neurons of both areas have large, 3D peripersonal RFs, and in both areas the best visual stimulus is that directed toward the tactile RF. In contrast to F4, however, the RFs of F2 neurons are more related to the forelimb; face-related neurons, which are prominent in F4, are virtually absent in F2. Because F4 is located lateral to the spur of the arcuate sulcus and the lateral part of F2 is located medial to the spur, the bimodal representation of area F2 could be considered an extension of the F4 properties, except that the somatotopy of the RFs is different in the two areas. Although the two areas share many properties, some considerations seem to suggest that they play different functional roles. For example, they have different cytoarchitectonic properties (Matelli et al., 1985, 1991), different subcortical projections (see He, Dum, & Strick, 1993; Keizer & Kuypers, 1989), and different corticocortical connections. In particular, although area F4 is connected to the inferior parietal lobule, lateral F2 is linked to areas of the superior parietal lobule. Its sector endowed with visual properties receives projections from area MIP and area V6A (Marconi et al., 2001; Matelli et al., 1998).

ANATOMICAL LOCATION AND FUNCTIONAL PROPERTIES OF AREAS MIP AND V6A   Area MIP is located in the dorsal bank of the intraparietal sulcus. This area was originally defined on the basis of its connections with the parieto-occipital area (PO)/V6 (Colby et al., 1988). Area V6A is located in the anterior bank of the parieto-occipital sulcus (Galletti, Fattori, Battaglini, Shipp, & Zeki, 1996). It receives its input from extrastriate, lateral, and medial parietal areas (Shipp, Blanton, & Zeki, 1998). In particular, V6A is connected to MIP (Marconi et al., 2001; Shipp et al., 1998). In both V6A and MIP there are neurons responding to visual stimuli. In V6A, among visually responding neurons, there are neurons selective for stimulus direction (Galletti et al., 1996). In most neurons the visual stimulus is coded in retinocentric coordinates, but there is a small group of neurons whose response is independent of the retinal position of the stimulus (Galletti, Battaglini, & Fattori, 1993). In addition to visual neurons, there are also neurons responding to somatosensory stimuli applied to the forelimb (Galletti, Fattori, Kutz, & Gamberini, 1997) and during the execution of arm movements (Galletti et al., 1997). In MIP there are purely visual neurons, purely somatosensory neurons, and neurons with bimodal properties (see Colby, 1998). Bimodal neurons respond to passive touch on the contralateral forelimb and to the presentation of a visual stimulus. Their activity is very high when the monkey executes a reaching movement toward a visual target. It is interesting to note that deep in the sulcus, below these bimodal neurons, there are purely visual neurons whose response increases when the target is moved within reaching distance. Finally, there are motor neurons that discharge during reaching movements (Colby & Duhamel, 1991; see also Johnson, Ferraina, Bianchi, & Caminiti, 1996).

The somatosensory properties of V6A and MIP and some of their visual properties (directional selectivity, responses in near space) resemble those of F2 bimodal neurons. Because the connections from both V6A and MIP terminate in the same F2 ventrorostral region, it is not possible at present to disentangle the specific contribution of each of these two superior parietal areas. Furthermore, in only a few neurons of V6A does the location of visual stimuli seem to be coded in nonretinotopic coordinates. What can create a functional link between these areas of superior parietal and dorsal premotor cortex is their common involvement in forelimb movements in space. What is the function of these forelimb movements? Because most visual RFs in V6A and MIP are large and encompass the periphery of the visual field (Colby et al., 1991; Galletti, Fattori, Kutz, & Gamberini, 1999), it is likely that, although a transformation from a retinotopic to a somatocentered frame of reference takes place, as suggested by the properties of bimodal neurons, the coding of space in this circuit could subserve a monitoring function of the transport phase of the hand toward a static or a moving target.

There is rich evidence from clinical studies in human patients that lesions centered on the superior parietal lobule produce reaching disorders (optic ataxia). Unilateral lesions often determine the deficit in the contralesional half field in the absence of hemianopia (Ratcliff & Davies-Jones, 1972). Perenin and Vighetto (1988) carefully studied lesions causing optic ataxia and those producing hemispatial neglect. Their results showed that the two syndromes result as a consequence of lesions of different posterior parietal sectors. Damage to the inferior parietal lobule produces unilateral neglect, while damage to the superior parietal lobule produces optic ataxia. Similar findings were also reported by Vallar and Perani (1987). These clinical data could be explained by an impairment of a circuit homologue to the F2 ventrorostral-V6A/MIP circuit in monkeys.

F5-PF: A circuit for action understanding

Ventral premotor area F5 and area PF of the inferior parietal lobule constitute a frontoparietal circuit. The microinjection of neural tracers into both F5 and PF demonstrates their reciprocal connections (Cavada & Goldman-Rakic, 1989; Matelli et al., 1986; Rizzolatti & Luppino, 2001). The properties of these two areas will be presented separately.

Anatomical Location and Functional Properties of Area F5 Area F5 forms the rostral part of ventral premotor cortex. It is bordered caudally by area F4 and rostrally by the inferior limb of the arcuate sulcus (see Fig. 26.1). It is subdivided into two parts, F5 bank and F5 convexity. In the F5 convexity there is a peculiar class of visuomotor neurons, called mirror neurons. *Mirror neurons* discharge both when the monkey executes a goal-directed hand action (grasping, tearing, manipulating) and when it observes a similar hand action performed by another individual (Gallese, Fadiga, Fogassi, & Rizzolatti, 1996; Rizzolatti, Fadiga, Gallese, & Fogassi, 1996).

Their main functional properties can be briefly described. The effective visual stimulus evoking mirror neurons' discharge is the interaction between the hand of an agent (human being or monkey) and a target object. The pure visual presentation of objects such as pieces of food or other interesting objects does not evoke any response. When the observed action effective in driving the neuron response is mimed without the object, the mirror neurons' responses are weak or absent. Similarly ineffective in driving mirror neurons' responses are observed actions that, although achieving the same goal and looking similar to those performed by the experimenter's hand, are performed with tools such as pliers or pincers. Thus, mirror neurons respond only to hand-object interactions.

The observed actions coded by mirror neurons are grasping, manipulating, tearing, holding, and releasing objects. These neurons can respond to only one observed action or to two or three actions. The observed and the executed action effective in triggering mirror neurons' discharge often correspond both in terms of the general action (e.g., grasping) and in terms of the way in which that action is executed (e.g., precision grip). It has been proposed that mirror neurons are part of a system that matches action observation with action execution. The resonance between the observed action made by another individual and the neural circuit of the observer coding the same action could be the basis of action understanding. Actions, however, can also be understood on the basis of sensory modalities other than vision.

In everyday life, many actions produce sounds, and these sounds are a cue to recognizing these actions when the actions are not visible. Sound-producing actions are also present in the behavioral repertoire of the monkey. Recently, our laboratory discovered a subset of mirror neurons that can also be activated by auditory stimuli (Kohler et al., 2001, 2002). The experiment consisted of three main sensory conditions. In the first condition, the monkey observed a hand action accompanied by its sound; in the second condition, the monkey could see the action but not hear its sound; and in the third condition the monkey could hear the sound but not see the action. Figure 26.5 shows an example of one of these "audiovisual mirror neurons."

The sounds that most effectively evoke the discharge of these mirror neurons are those produced by tearing actions (breaking a peanut, ripping paper), by manipulating objects such as plastic, or by dropping objects to the floor. Typically, audiovisual mirror neurons do not respond to unspecific, arousing sounds such as loud noises, animal calls, and so on. Both the auditory and the visual responses are specific to a particular type of action. Neurons responding to peanut breaking do not respond to plastic manipulation or paper ripping. The same neurons also respond when the monkey performs a specific hand action similar to that observed and heard (Fig. 26.5).

Audiovisual mirror neurons are different from the previously described premotor neurons, which respond to somatosensory, visual, and acoustic stimuli. The latter

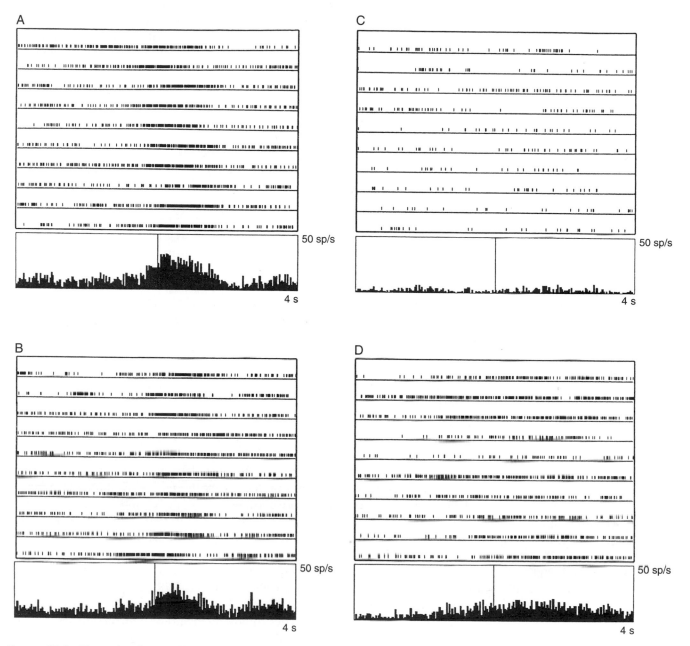

FIGURE 26.5   Example of an audiovisual mirror neuron. In each panel the raster representing the neuronal discharge during each trial and the histogram representing the average neural frequency are shown. (*A*) The experimenter ripped a piece of paper in full vision (vision and sound). (*B*) The experimenter ripped a piece of paper out of the monkey's vision. The animal could only hear the sound of the action (sound only). (*C*) White noise was delivered through loudspeakers. (*D*) The monkey ripped a piece of paper. Histograms are aligned (vertical line) with the beginning of the ripping action (*A*, *B*, *D*) or with the onset of the control sound (*C*). The discharge in the vision and sound condition and in the sound-only condition have similar intensity. Time is graphed on the abscissa; number of spikes/s is graphed on the ordinate.

are related to actions in space and to space representation. Instead, audiovisual mirror neurons allow retrieval of the meaning of a hand action on the basis of its sound alone, and, if the context is suitable, also allow execution of the same action. The importance of these neurons is also related to the fact that they are present in an area of monkey premotor cortex that has been considered a homologue of Broca's area in humans.

ANATOMICAL LOCATION AND FUNCTIONAL PROPERTIES OF AREA PF   According to the classification of Pandya and Seltzer (1982), the convexity of the inferior parietal lobule is formed by three different cytoarchitectonic areas: PF (7b), in its rostral part; PG (7a), in its caudal part; and PFG, located between PF and PG (see Fig. 26.1). Area PF is reciprocally connected to the ventral premotor cortex (Cavada & Goldman-Rakic, 1989; Matelli et al., 1986; Matsumura & Kubota, 1979; Muakkassa & Strick, 1979; Petrides & Pandya, 1984; see also Rizzolatti et al., 1998). Several authors have reported the presence in this area of many bimodal neurons with tactile RFs on the face, arm, and upper trunk (Graziano & Gross, 1995; Hyvärinen, 1981; Leinonen & Nyman, 1979; Leinonen et al., 1979). The visual RFs are large and often very close to the tactile RFs.

Area PF could play an important role in the action observation-execution matching system. In fact, area PF is connected, on one side, to superior temporal sulcus (STS; Cavada & Goldman-Rakic, 1989; Seltzer & Pandya, 1994), in the anterior part of which (STSa) Perrett and co-workers described neurons that respond to the observation of hand-object interactions and apparently do not discharge during the monkey's actions (Perrett et al., 1989, 1990). On the other side, area PF is reciprocally connected to area F5 (Luppino et al., 1999). Therefore, area PF appears to be an ideal candidate as a relay center between a visual description of actions provided by STSa neurons and their motor description occurring in area F5.

Following this hypothesis, we reinvestigated the neuronal properties of the rostral part of PF, confirming previous findings. Our investigation showed that most somatosensory neurons have RFs on the face (64%), while the remaining have RFs on the hand (18%) or the arm (5%). Among bimodal (somatosensory and visual) neurons, visual peripersonal RFs are located around the tactile RFs (face, 73%; hand, 8%; arm, 6%). The best stimuli are rotating stimuli or stimuli that are moved in a horizontal, vertical, or sagittal direction (Fogassi, Gallese, Fadiga, & Rizzolatti, 1998; Gallese, Fogassi, Fadiga, & Rizzolatti, 2002).

In addition, in the same PF region we discovered neurons responding while the monkey observed hand actions performed by the experimenter (Fogassi et al., 1998; Gallese et al., 2002). Neurons that discharge during action observation constituted about 25% of the total number of recorded neurons and 40% of all visually responsive recorded neurons. Of these, 70% also have motor properties, becoming active when the monkey performs mouth or hand actions, or both. We designated these latter neurons "PF mirror neurons." Similar to F5 mirror neurons, PF mirror neurons respond to the observation of several types of single or combined actions. A grasping action, alone or in combination with other hand actions, is the most represented one. As for F5 mirror neurons, simple object observation or the observation of a mimed action is not effective.

In contrast to area F5, about 30% of PF mirror neurons are also activated by superficial tactile stimuli applied to the monkey's face and by peripersonal visual stimuli (Fig. 26.6). The visual peripersonal and the "action observation" responses of each mirror neuron of this subcategory are evoked independently and cannot be interpreted as the same visual response, because the neuron discharge during action observation is evoked by hand actions made by the experimenter far from the monkey (at least three times the reaching distance), whereas the peripersonal response is evoked by *any* type of 3D stimulus introduced near the monkey's face, and disappears as soon as the stimulus is moved out of the reaching space.

The presence in area PF of this peculiar class of mirror neurons is quite surprising, because these neurons seem to associate a sensitivity to biological actions with bimodal properties related to space. Moreover, when motor activity is present, the controlled effector (the mouth) is not congruent with the effector (the hand) performing the action that, when observed, evokes a visual response.

How can such multiple sensory responses with apparently different meaning can be framed together? The *motor valence* of these neurons could be a key to understanding their role.

The starting point is to consider both the bimodal and the motor properties of all neurons we recorded in area PF. With regard to the bimodal properties, a visual peripersonal RF located around a mouth tactile RF can be interpreted, as proposed for F4 bimodal neurons (see previous sections), as a motor space. If this is accepted, the visual stimuli that cross this RF are translated into suitable motor plans (e.g., a mouth grasping action), enabling the organism endowed with such RFs to successfully interact with the same stimuli (see Fogassi, Gallese, Fadiga, & Rizzolatti, 1996; Rizzolatti, Fogassi, & Gallese, 1997). Concerning their motor properties, almost all PF motor neurons are activated by hand actions, mouth actions, or both hand and mouth actions. Motor neurons in this latter class are likely to be endowed with anatomical connections with both the circuits controlling hand movements and those controlling mouth movements.

The most likely explanation for the apparently incongruent matching between observed hand actions and executed mouth actions seems to be in terms of a more abstract action coding. That is, both hand and mouth, although independent effectors, code the same goal of grasping. How might such a putative abstract level coding of action have evolved in area PF?

Two possible, although not mutually exclusive, ontogenetic hypotheses can be proposed. First, during development, the matching between observed and executed action occurs not only in neurons endowed

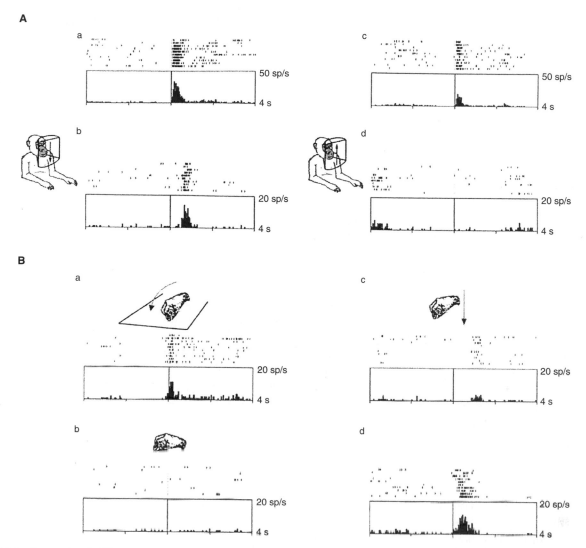

A

a
c
50 sp/s
4 s
50 sp/s
4 s

b
d
20 sp/s
4 s
20 sp/s
4 s

B

a
c
20 sp/s
4 s
20 sp/s
4 s

b
d
20 sp/s
4 s
20 sp/s
4 s

FIGURE 26.6 Example of a PF mirror neuron with bimodal (visual and somatosensory) properties. (*A*) Bimodal responses. A tactile 3D stimulus was moved on the face along a top-down (*a*) or a bottom-up (*c*) trajectory; a visual 3D stimulus was moved near the tactile RF along a top-down (*b*) or a bottom-up trajectory (*d*). The tactile and the visual 3D RFs and the direction of the stimulation are shown in the drawings to the left of the corresponding panels. The tactile RF (shaded area) covered the entire hemiface; the peripersonal visual RF (solid) extended about 15 cm from the monkey's face. Note that this neuron is selective for the top-down direction of stimulation in both modalities. Rasters and histograms are aligned with the moment in which the tactile stimulus touched the monkey's skin (*a, c*) and the visual stimulus entered the monkey's visual field (*b, d*). (*B*) Responses to action observation of the same neuron. (*a*) The experimenter grasped an object placed on a tray, moving the hand along a top-down trajectory. (*b*) The experimenter showed the same object to the monkey with a steady hand. (*c*) The experimenter moved the object along the same trajectory as in *a*. (*d*) The monkeys grasped a piece of food. Rasters and histograms are aligned with the moment in which the experimenter's (*a*) or the monkey's (*d*) hand touched the object, with the moment in which the experimenter started object presentation (*b*), or with the moment in which the experimenter began moving the object (*c*). Note that observation of a grasping action (*a*), but not of a particular motion direction (*c*), is effective in evoking the neuron discharge. Time is graphed on the abscissa: number of spikes/s is graphed on the ordinate. (Modified from Gallese et al., 2002.)

with hand motor properties (as in classic mirror neurons), but also in those controlling both hand and mouth actions. Once neurons of this latter type acquire mirror properties, some of them may lose the anatomical connections with the circuit controlling the hand (it should be noted that a feature of motor development is indeed the progressive disappearance of hand

and mouth synergism). In the adult individual, these neurons may therefore appear as "mouth" grasping neurons that are also endowed with the property to respond during the observation of hand actions.

Second, the visual stimulus that most frequently crosses the peripersonal visual RFs of these PF mirror neurons is likely to be the monkey's own hand as it brings food to the mouth. A hand approaching the mouth can therefore preset the motor programs controlling grasping with the mouth. During development, through a process of generalization between the monkey's own moving hand—treated as a signal to grasp with the mouth—and the object-directed moving hands of others, any time the monkey observes another individual's hand interacting with food, the same mouth action representation will be evoked. The peripersonal visual RF around the mouth would enable a primitive form of matching to occur between the vision of the monkey's own hand and the motor program controlling mouth grasping. Once this equivalence is put in place, a mirror system matching hand action (observation) with mouth action (execution) can be established.

Whatever hypothesis is accepted, the "primitive" matching system would also be beneficial during adulthood, when a more sophisticated hand-hand matching system has developed, in order to provide an abstract categorization of the observed actions: what is recognized is a particular action goal, regardless of the effector enabling its achievement.

It is not clear how PF bimodal mirror neurons might achieve this peculiar type of multisensory integration. The answer to this question can be found in the cortico-cortical circuits in which PF is involved. As far as the convergence of somatosensory and visual peripersonal responses is concerned, this can be explained by a mechanism similar to that proposed for F4 bimodal neurons. The motor information on mouth grasping action could be provided by the mouth representation of ventral premotor cortex. Visual information about the hand could be provided by STSa neurons: the pictorial representation of the hand would be directly matched with PF motor properties. An alternative source could be represented by an efferent copy of the hand motor representation fed by area F5. In that latter case, it might be that PF bimodal mirror neurons match the *motor representations* of effectors—the hand and the mouth—that are different but are endowed with the same *goal* (grasp).

The properties of bimodal PF mirror neurons, although partially different from those of other F5 and PF mirror neurons, seem to reflect the same general concept as is valid for the neurons of the F5-PF circuit: the sensory input, whether visual, acoustic, or bimodal, is used to retrieve the representation of an action. In this circuit, however, different from F4-VIP and from the F2vr-MIP/V6A circuit, the action representation is used for understanding the actions made by others. Moreover, bimodal PF mirror neurons show another property: they can generalize the action meaning in an effector-independent way.

Conclusions

In this chapter, we have addressed the issue of multisensory integration by illustrating and discussing the functional properties of three parallel frontoparietal circuits. We have shown that multisensory integration is a pervasive feature of cortical areas involved in motor planning and control. The neuroscientific evidence that has accumulated over the past two decades has contributed to changing our views of sensorimotor integration, and more generally to redefining the relationship between action and perception. As discussed in this chapter, cortical premotor areas are endowed with sensory properties, and posterior parietal areas, traditionally considered association areas, are endowed with motor properties. Parietal areas, together with the frontal areas to which they are connected, constitute cortical networks that process and integrate multisensory information for the purpose of action execution, but also for the purpose of representing the environment in which action takes place.

This functional architecture can be interpreted in two different ways. According to the sensory hypothesis, sensory information is integrated within posterior parietal areas and fed to the motor centers of the frontal lobe as a prespecified perceptual database.

According to the motor representation hypothesis, which we have proposed throughout this chapter, action constitutes the binding key to multisensory integration: premotor areas, through their connections with the posterior parietal areas, play a major role in binding together different sensory attributes of stimuli. Following this perspective, multisensory integration is instrumental for attaining three different goals:

1. To provide a coherent action environment. As we have seen, perceptual information is specified in formats that are not only compatible with but determined by the type of effector and action control centers that will be using this information for action planning and control purposes.

2. To enable a coherent perceptual environment. The same sensory information integrated for action is also available to provide the agent with a perceptual account of the environment, of which the agent is aware and that the agent can understand. Thus, motor cortical centers play a major role not only in action but also in perception. Space, actions, and objects are perceived by exploiting the same neural resources used to act.

3. To enable the possibility of generalizing across different sensory instances of the same perceptual object, thus paving the road to semantic categorization. This categorization greatly enhances the possibility of

exploiting the implicit action-related knowledge of the perceiving subject. The multimodal coding of actions provided by auditory mirror neurons, for example, can be interpreted as the dawning of a distinctive feature of the human mind, the capacity to categorize objects and events in an abstract and context-independent way.

REFERENCES

Andersen, R. A., Asanuma, C., Essick, G. K., & Siegel, R. M. (1990). Cortico-cortical connections of anatomically and physiologically defined subdivisions within the inferior parietal lobule. *Journal of Comparative Neurology, 296,* 65–113.

Andersen, R. A., Snyder, L. H., Bradley, D. C., & Xing, J. (1997). Multimodal representation of space in the posterior parietal cortex and its use in planning movements. *Annual Review of Neuroscience, 20,* 303–330.

Berti, A., & Frassinetti, F. (2000). When far becomes near: Re-mapping of space by tool use. *Journal of Cognitive Neuroscience, 12,* 415–420.

Bisiach, E., & Vallar, G. (2000). Unilateral neglect in humans. In F. Boller & J. Grafman (Eds.), *Handbook of neuropsychology* (2nd ed., pp. 459–502). Amsterdam: Elsevier.

Boussaoud, D., Ungerleider, L., & Desimone, R. (1990). Pathways for motion analysis: Cortical connections of the medial superior temporal and fundus of the superior temporal visual areas in the macaque. *Journal of Comparative Neurology, 296,* 462–495.

Bremmer, F., Schlack, A., Jon Shah, N., Zafiris, O., Kubischik, M., Hoffmann, K. P., et al. (2001). Polymodal motion processing in posterior parietal and premotor cortex: A human fMRI study strongly implies equivalences between humans and monkeys. *Neuron, 29,* 287–296.

Cavada, C., & Goldman-Rakic, P. (1989). Posterior parietal cortex in rhesus monkey: II. Evidence for segregated cortico-cortical networks linking sensory and limbic areas with the frontal lobe. *Journal of Comparative Neurology, 287,* 422–445.

Chieffi, S., Fogassi, L., Gallese, V., & Gentilucci, M. (1992). Prehension movements directed to approaching objects: Influence of stimulus velocity on the transport and the grasp components. *Neuropsychologia, 30,* 877–897.

Colby, C. (1998). Action-oriented spatial reference frames in cortex. *Neuron, 20,* 15–24.

Colby, C., & Duhamel, J.-R. (1991). Heterogeneity of extrastriate visual areas and multiple parietal areas in the macaque monkey. *Neuropsychologia, 29,* 517–537.

Colby, C. L., Duhamel, J.-R., & Goldberg, M. E. (1993). Ventral intraparietal area of the macaque: Anatomic location and visual response properties. *Journal of Neurophysiology, 69,* 902–914.

Colby, C. L., Gattass, R., Olson, C. R., & Gross, C. G. (1988). Topographic organization of cortical afferents to extrastriate visual area PO in the macaque: A dual tracer study. *Journal of Comparative Neurology, 269,* 392–413.

Colby, C. L., & Goldberg, M. E. (1999). Space and attention in parietal cortex. *Annual Review of Neuroscience, 22,* 319–349.

Cowey, A., Small, M., & Ellis, S. (1994). Left visuo-spatial neglect can be worse in far than near space. *Neuropsychologia, 32,* 1059–1066.

Cowey, A., Small, M., & Ellis, S. (1999). No abrupt change in visual hemineglect from near to far space. *Neuropsychologia, 37,* 1–6.

Duhamel, J.-R., Colby, C. L., & Goldberg, M. E. (1998). Ventral intraparietal area of the macaque: Congruent visual and somatic response properties. *Journal of Neurophysiology, 79,* 126–136.

Fogassi, L., Gallese, V., Buccino, G., Craighero, L., Fadiga, L., & Rizzolatti, G. (2001). Cortical mechanism for the visual guidance of hand grasping movements in the monkey: A reversible inactivation study. *Brain, 124,* 571–586.

Fogassi, L., Gallese, V., di Pellegrino, G., Fadiga, L., Gentilucci, M., Luppino, G., et al. (1992). Space coding by premotor cortex. *Experimental Brain Research, 89,* 686–690.

Fogassi, L., Gallese, V., Fadiga, L., Luppino, G., Matelli, M., & Rizzolatti, G. (1996). Coding of peripersonal space in inferior premotor cortex (area F4). *Journal of Neurophysiology, 76,* 141–157.

Fogassi, L., Gallese, V., Fadiga, L., & Rizzolatti, G. (1996). Space coding in inferior premotor cortex (area F4): Facts and speculations. In F. Laquaniti & P. Viviani (Eds.), *Neural basis of motor behavior* (pp. 99–120). NATO ASI Series. Dordrecht: Kluwer.

Fogassi, L., Gallese, V., Fadiga, L., & Rizzolatti, G. (1998). Neurons responding to the sight of goal-directed hand/arm actions in the parietal area PF (7b) of the macaque monkey. *Society of Neuroscience Abstracts, 24,* 257.5.

Fogassi, L., Raos, V., Franchi, G., Gallese, V., Luppino, G., & Matelli, M. (1999). Visual responses in the dorsal premotor area F2 of the macaque monkey. *Experimental Brain Research, 128,* 194–199.

Gallese, V., Fadiga, L., Fogassi, L., & Rizzolatti, G. (1996). Action recognition in the premotor cortex. *Brain, 119,* 593–609.

Gallese, V., Fogassi, L., Fadiga, L., & Rizzolatti, G. (2002). Action representation and the inferior parietal lobule. In W. Prinz & B. Hommel (Eds.), *Attention and performance XIX* (pp. 334–355). Oxford, England: Oxford University Press.

Galletti, C., Battaglini, P. P., & Fattori, P. (1993). Parietal neurons encoding spatial locations in craniotopic coordinates. *Experimental Brain Research, 96,* 221–229.

Galletti, C., Fattori, P., Battaglini, P. P., Shipp, S., & Zeki, S. (1996). Functional demarcation of a border between areas V6 and V6A in the superior parietal gyrus of the macaque monkey. *European Journal of Neuroscience, 8,* 30–52.

Galletti, C., Fattori, P., Kutz, D. F., & Battaglini, P. P. (1997). Arm movement-related neurons in visual area V6A of the macaque superior parietal lobule. *European Journal of Neuroscience, 9,* 410–413.

Galletti, C., Fattori, P., Kutz, D. F., & Gamberini, M. (1999). Brain location and visual topography of cortical area V6A in the macaque monkey. *European Journal of Neuroscience, 11,* 575–582.

Gentilucci, M., Fogassi, L., Luppino, G., Matelli, M., Camarda, R., & Rizzolatti, G. (1988). Functional organization of inferior area 6 in the macaque monkey: I. Somatotopy and the control of proximal movements. *Experimental Brain Research, 71,* 475–490.

Gentilucci, M., Scandolara, C., Pigarev, I. N., & Rizzolatti, G. (1983). Visual responses in the postarcuate cortex (area 6) of the monkey that are independent of eye position. *Experimental Brain Research, 50,* 464–468.

Godschalk, M., Lemon, R. N., Nijs, H. G. T., & Kuypers, H. G. J. M. (1981). Behaviour of neurons in monkey periarcuate and precentral cortex before and during visually guided arm and hand movements. *Experimental Brain Research, 44,* 113–116.

Goodale, M. A. (2000). Perception and action in the human visual system. In M. S. Gazzaniga (Ed.), *The new cognitive neurosciences* (2nd ed., pp. 365–378). Cambridge, MA: MIT Press/Bradford Books.

Graziano, M. S. A., & Gross, C. G. (1995). The representation of extrapersonal space: A possible role for bimodal visual-tactile neurons. In M. S. Gazzaniga (Ed.), *The cognitive neurosciences* (pp. 1021–1034). Cambridge, MA: MIT Press.

Graziano, M. S. A., Hu, X., & Gross, C. G. (1997a). Visuospatial properties of ventral premotor cortex. *Journal of Neurophysiology, 77,* 2268–2292.

Graziano, M. S. A., Hu, X., & Gross, C. G. (1997b). Coding the locations of objects in the dark. *Science, 277,* 239–241.

Graziano, M. S. A., Reiss, L. A. J., & Gross, C. G. (1999). A neuronal representation of the location of nearby sounds. *Nature, 397,* 428–430.

Graziano, M. S. A., Yap, G. S., & Gross, C. G. (1994). Coding of visual space by premotor neurons. *Science, 266,* 1054–1057.

Halligan, P. W., & Marshall, J. C. (1991). Left neglect for near but not far space in man. *Nature, 350,* 498–500.

He, S.-Q., Dum, R. P., & Strick, P. L. (1993). Topographic organization of corticospinal projections from the frontal lobe: Motor areas on the lateral surface of the hemisphere. *Journal of Neuroscience, 13,* 952–980.

Hyvärinen, J. (1981). Regional distribution of functions in parietal association area 7 of the monkey. *Brain Research, 206,* 287–303.

Hyvärinen, J. (1982). Posterior parietal lobe of the primate brain. *Physiological Review, 62,* 1060–1129.

Iriki, A., Tanaka, M., & Iwamura, Y. (1996). Coding of modified body schema during tool use by macaque postcentral neurones. *NeuroReport, 7,* 2325–2330.

Johnson, P. B., Ferraina, S., Bianchi, L., & Caminiti, R. (1996). Cortical networks for visual reaching: Physiological and anatomical organization of frontal and parietal lobe arm regions. *Cerebral Cortex, 6,* 102–119.

Keizer, K., & Kuypers, H. G. J. M. (1989). Distribution of corticospinal neurons with collaterals to the lower brain stem reticular formation in monkey (*Macaca fascicularis*). *Experimental Brain Research, 74,* 311–318.

Kohler, E., Umiltà, M. A., Keysers, C., Gallese, V., Fogassi, L., & Rizzolatti, G. (2001). Auditory mirror neurons in ventral premotor cortex. *Society for Neuroscience Abstracts, 27,* 129.9.

Kohler, E., Keysers, C., Umiltà, M. A., Fogassi, L., Gallese, V., & Rizzolatti, G. (2002). Hearing sounds, understanding actions: Action representation in mirror neurons. *Science, 297,* 846–848.

Leinonen, L., Hyvärinen, J., Nyman, G., & Linnankoski, I. (1979). I. Function properties of neurons in lateral part of associative area 7 in awake monkeys. *Experimental Brain Research, 34,* 299–320.

Leinonen, L., & Nyman, G. (1979). II. Functional properties of cells in anterolateral part of area 7 associative face area of awake monkeys. *Experimental Brain Research, 34,* 321–333.

Lewis, J. W., & Van Essen, D. C. (2000). Corticocortical connections of visual, sensorimotor, and multimodal processing areas in the parietal lobe of the macaque monkey. *Journal of Comparative Neurology, 428,* 112–137.

Luppino, G., Murata, A., Govoni, P., & Matelli, M. (1999). Largely segregated parietofrontal connections linking rostral intraparietal cortex (areas AIP and VIP) and the ventral premotor cortex (areas F5 and F4). *Experimental Brain Research, 128,* 181–187.

Marconi, B., Genovesio, A., Battaglia-Mayer, A., Ferraina, S., Squatrito, S., Molinari, M., et al. (2001). Eye-hand coordination during reaching: I. Anatomical relationships between parietal and frontal cortex. *Cerebral Cortex, 11,* 513–527.

Martin, A., Ungerleider, L. G., & Haxby, J. V. (2000). Category specificity and the brain: The sensory/motor model of semantic representations of objects. In M. S. Gazzaniga (Ed.), *The new cognitive neurosciences* (2nd ed., pp. 1023–1036). Cambridge, MA: MIT Press/Bradford Books.

Matelli, M., Camarda, R., Glickstein, M., & Rizzolatti, G. (1986). Afferent and efferent projections of the inferior area 6 in the macaque monkey. *Journal of Comparative Neurology, 251,* 281–298.

Matelli, M., Govoni, P., Galletti, C., Kutz, D. F., & Luppino, G. (1998). Superior area 6 afferents from the superior parietal lobule in the macaque monkey. *Journal of Comparative Neurology, 402,* 327–352.

Matelli, M., Luppino, G., & Rizzolatti, G. (1985). Patterns of cytochrome oxidase activity in the frontal agranular cortex of the macaque monkey. *Behavioural Brain Research, 18,* 125–137.

Matelli, M., Luppino, G., & Rizzolatti, G. (1991). Architecture of superior and mesial area 6 and of the adjacent cingulate cortex. *Journal of Comparative Neurology, 311,* 445–462.

Matelli, M., Marconi, B., Caminiti, R., & Luppino, G. (1999). Arm representations of dorsal and ventral premotor cortices are reciprocally connected. *Society for Neuroscience Abstracts, 25*(Pt. 1), 382.

Matsumura, M., & Kubota, K. (1979). Cortical projection of hand-arm motor area from post-arcuate area in macaque monkeys: A histological study of retrograde transport of horse-radish peroxidase. *Neuroscience Letters, 11,* 241–246.

Maunsell, J. H. R., & Van Essen, D. C. (1983). The connections of the middle temporal visual area (MT) and their relationship to a cortical hierarchy in the macaque monkey. *Journal of Neuroscience, 3,* 2563–2586.

Mountcastle, V. B. (1995). The parietal system and some higher brain functions. *Cerebral Cortex, 5,* 377–390.

Mountcastle, V. B., Lynch, J. C., Georgopoulos, A., Sakata, H., & Acuna, C. (1975). Posterior parietal association cortex of the monkey: Command functions for operations within extrapersonal space. *Journal of Neurophysiology, 38,* 871–908.

Muakkassa, K. F., & Strick, P. L. (1979). Frontal lobe inputs to primate motor cortex: Evidence for four somatotopically organized "premotor" areas. *Brain Research, 177,* 176–182.

Pandya, D. N., & Seltzer, B. (1982). Intrinsic connections and architectonics of posterior parietal cortex in the rhesus monkey. *Journal of Comparative Neurology, 204,* 196–210.

Perenin, M.-T., & Vighetto, A. (1988). Optic ataxia: A specific disruption in visuomotor mechanisms. I. Different aspects of the deficit in reaching for objects. *Brain, 111,* 643–674.

Perrett, D. I., Harries, M. H., Bevan, R., Thomas, S., Benson, P. J., Mistlin, A. J., et al. (1989). Frameworks of analysis for the neural representation of animate objects and actions. *Journal of Experimental Biology, 146,* 87–113.

Perrett, D. I., Mistlin, A. J., Harries, M. H., & Chitty, A. K. (1990). Understanding the visual appearance and consequence of hand actions. In M. A. Goodale (Ed.), *vision and action: The control of grasping* (pp. 163–180). Norwood, NJ: Ablex.

Petrides, M., & Pandya, D. N. (1984). Projections to the frontal cortex from the posterior parietal region in the rhesus monkey. *Journal of Comparative Neurology, 228,* 105–116.

Raos, V., Franchi, G., Gallese, V., & Fogassi, L. (2003). Somatotopic organization of the lateral part of area F2 (dorsal premotor cortex) of the macaque monkey. *Journal of Neurophysiology, 89,* 1503–1518.

Raos, V., Umiltà, M. A., Gallese, V., & Fogassi, L. (1999). Hand representation in the dorsal premotor area F2 of the macaque monkey. *Society for Neuroscience Abstracts, 25,* 381.

Ratcliff, G., & Davies-Jones, G. A. B. (1972). Defective visual localization in focal brain wounds. *Brain, 95,* 49–60.

Rizzolatti, G., Berti, A., & Gallese, V. (2000). Spatial neglect: Neurophysiological bases, cortical circuits and theories. In F. Boller & J. Grafman (Eds.), *Handbook of neuropsychology* (2nd ed., pp. 503–537). Amsterdam: Elsevier.

Rizzolatti, G., Fadiga, L., Fogassi, L., & Gallese, V. (1996). The space around us. *Science, 277,* 190–191.

Rizzolatti, G., Fadiga, L., Gallese, V., & Fogassi, L. (1996). Premotor cortex and the recognition of motor actions. *Brain Research: Cognitive Brain Research, 3,* 131–141.

Rizzolatti, G., Fogassi, L., & Gallese, V. (1997). Parietal cortex: From sight to action. *Current Opinion in Neurobiology, 7,* 562–567.

Rizzolatti, G., Fogassi, L., & Gallese, V. (2002). Motor and cognitive functions of the ventral premotor cortex. *Current Opinion in Neurobiology, 12,* 149–154.

Rizzolatti, G., & Gentilucci, M. (1988). Motor and visuomotor functions of the premotor cortex. In P. Rakic & W. Singer (Eds.), *Neurobiology of neocortex* (pp. 269–284). Chichester, England: Wiley.

Rizzolatti, G., & Luppino, G. (2001). The cortical motor system. *Neuron, 31,* 889–901.

Rizzolatti, G., Luppino, G., & Matelli, M. (1998). The organization of the cortical motor system: New concepts. *Electroencephalography and Clinical Neurophysiology, 106,* 283–296.

Rizzolatti, G., Matelli, M., & Pavesi, G. (1983). Deficits in attention and movement following the removal of postarcuate (area 6) and prearcuate (area 8) cortex in macaque monkeys. *Brain, 106,* 655–673.

Rizzolatti, G., Scandolara, C., Matelli, M., & Gentilucci, M. (1981a). Afferent properties of periarcuate neurons in macaque monkeys: I. Somatosensory responses. *Behavioural Brain Research, 2,* 125–146.

Rizzolatti, G., Scandolara, C., Matelli, M., & Gentilucci, M. (1981b). Afferent properties of periarcuate neurons in macaque monkeys: II. Visual responses. *Behavioural Brain Research, 2,* 147–163.

Sakata, H., & Taira, M. (1994). Parietal control of hand action. *Current Opinion in Neurobiology, 4,* 847–856.

Schaafsma, S. J., Duysens, J., & Gielen, C. C. (1997). Responses in ventral intraparietal area of awake macaque monkey to optic flow patterns corresponding to rotation of planes in depth can be explained by translation and expansion effects. *Visual Neuroscience, 14,* 633–646.

Schieber, M. (2000). Inactivation of the ventral premotor cortex biases the laterality of motoric choices. *Experimental Brain Research, 130,* 497–507.

Seltzer, B., & Pandya, D. N. (1984). Further observations on parieto-temporal connections in the rhesus monkey. *Experimental Brain Research, 55,* 301–312.

Seltzer, B., & Pandya, D. N. (1986). Posterior parietal projections to the intraparietal sulcus of the rhesus monkey. *Experimental Brain Research, 62,* 459–469.

Shelton, P. A., Bowers, D., & Heilman, K. M. (1990). Peripersonal and vertical neglect. *Brain, 113,* 191–205.

Shipp, S., Blanton, M., & Zeki, S. (1998). A visuo-somatomotor pathway through superior parietal cortex in the macaque monkey: Cortical connections of areas V6 and V6A. *European Journal of Neuroscience, 10,* 3171–3193.

Thier, P., & Andersen, R. A. (1998). Electrical microstimulation distinguishes distinct saccade-related areas in the posterior parietal cortex. *Journal of Neurophysiology, 80,* 1713–1735.

Ungerleider, L., & Desimone, R. (1986). Cortical projections of visual area MT in the macaque. *Journal of Comparative Neurology, 248,* 190–222.

Vallar, G., & Perani, D. (1987). The anatomy of spatial neglect in humans. In M. Jeannerod (Ed.), *Neurophysiological and neuropsychological aspects of spatial neglect* (pp. 235–258). Amsterdam: North-Holland/Elsevier.

27 Multisensory Neurons for the Control of Defensive Movements

MICHAEL S. A. GRAZIANO, CHARLES G. GROSS, CHARLOTTE S. R. TAYLOR, AND TIRIN MOORE

Introduction

If a hornet flies toward your face, you might duck, squint, and lift your hand to block it. If the insect touches your hand, you might withdraw your hand, even pulling it behind your back. These defensive movements have a reflexive quality. They are fast and can occur without conscious planning or thought. They are similar in all people (Fig. 27.1; Color Plate 6). Although they seem reflexive, however, defensive movements are also highly sophisticated. They can be elicited by touch, sight, or sound. They involve coordination between different body parts, such as the arm and head. They are spatially specific: the body parts that move and the direction of movement are appropriate for the location of the threat. The movements can be stronger or weaker, depending on external context or the internal state of the person. For example, someone whose "nerves are on edge" may give an exaggerated alerting response to an unexpected stimulus.

What sensorimotor pathways in the brain coordinate this rich and complex behavior? We suggest that a special set of interconnected areas in the monkey brain monitors the location and movement of objects near the body and controls flinch and other defensive responses. This hypothesized "defensive" system, shown in Figure 27.2, includes the ventral intraparietal area (VIP), parietal area 7b, the polysensory zone (PZ) in the precentral gyrus, and the putamen. These brain areas are monosynaptically interconnected (Cavada & Goldman-Rakic, 1989a, 1989b, 1991; Kunzle, 1978; Luppino, Murata, Govoni, & Matelli, 1999; Matelli, Camarda, Glickstein, & Rizzolatti, 1986; Mesulam, Van Hoesen, Pandya, & Geschwind, 1977; Parthasarathy, Schall, & Graybiel, 1992; Weber & Yin, 1984). Of the four areas, PZ is closest to the motor output, sending direct projections to the spinal cord (Dum & Strick, 1991). Electrical stimulation of PZ evokes defensive movements, such as withdrawal of the hand, squinting, turning of the head, ducking, or lifting the hand as if

to defend the side of the head (Graziano, Taylor, & Moore, 2002).

In the following sections we review experimental results on this system of areas and discuss the evidence that they are involved in representing the space near the body and in controlling defensive movements. We concentrate mainly on areas VIP and PZ in the monkey brain, because they are the most thoroughly studied of these multisensory areas. We then discuss the general question of coordinate transformations from sensory input to motor output. Finally, we discuss the evidence that the human brain contains a similar set of multisensory areas processing the space near the body.

The brain contains many multisensory areas in addition to the set of areas described in this chapter. These other areas are thought to have a variety of specific functions. For example, the superior colliculus contains neurons that respond to tactile, visual, and auditory stimuli. This structure is thought to be involved in orienting of the eyes, ears, or body toward salient stimuli (see Stein, Jiang, & Stanford, Chap. 15, this volume; Meredith, Chap. 21, this volume; Van Opstal & Munoz, Chap. 23, this volume). Regions of the parietal and premotor cortex appear to be involved in the multisensory task of coordinating hand actions for grasping objects (see Fogassi & Gallese, Chap. 26, this volume; Ishibashi, Obayashi, & Iriki, Chap. 28, this volume). Work in human stroke patients and normal human subjects suggests that multisensory processing is crucial for directing spatial attention around the body (see Spence & McDonald, Chap. 1, this volume). A common view a century ago was that the brain contained association areas, regions that served the general purpose of combining the senses. These association areas did not have specific functions; they provided a general understanding of the environment and helped in choosing a path of action. Work over the past 20 years on multisensory integration paints a different picture, one in which the brain contains many distinct multisensory areas, each with its specific set of functions.

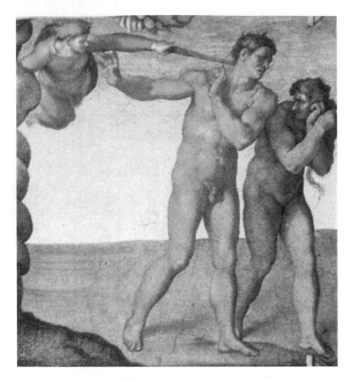

FIGURE 27.1 Detail from Michelangelo's *Fall and Expulsion from Eden*. Both Adam and Eve are in classic defensive poses, with the head turned and the hands raised to defend the face. Compare with Figure 27.5*B*. (See Color Plate 6).

The polysensory zone

The precentral gyrus of monkeys contains a restricted zone in which the neurons respond with short latency to tactile, visual, and sometimes auditory stimuli. This zone is variously termed ventral premotor (PMv) or inferior area 6. Recent mapping experiments (Graziano &

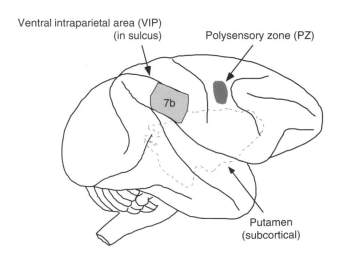

FIGURE 27.2 Side view of a macaque monkey brain showing the location of four interconnected multisensory areas.

Gandhi, 2000) show that the region of multisensory responses does not encompass the entire ventral premotor cortex. Its location varies slightly from monkey to monkey, and whether it lies entirely within premotor cortex is not yet clear. We have therefore adopted a new, more descriptive term, polysensory zone (PZ), to describe this restricted and functionally distinct region (see Fig. 27.2).

Neurons in other parts of motor and premotor cortex also respond to sensory stimuli, especially in animals trained to use those stimuli to perform a task (e.g., Boussaoud, Barth, & Wise, 1993; Kwan, MacKay, Murphy, & Wong, 1985; Mauritz & Wise, 1986). The sensory responses found in PZ, however, do not depend on training the animal. Instead, the neurons respond to passively presented stimuli. The responses can even be found in anesthetized animals (Graziano, Hu, & Gross, 1997a). These sensory responses may derive from the direct projections to PZ from the parietal lobe, especially from areas VIP and 7b (Cavada & Goldman-Rakic, 1989b; Luppino et al., 1999; Matelli et al., 1986). PZ in turn can influence movement through its projections to the rest of the motor cortex and to the spinal cord (Dum & Strick, 1991). PZ therefore is not strictly a sensory or a motor area but, like much of the brain, lies on the pathway from sensory input to motor output.

Most neurons in PZ respond to tactile and visual stimuli (Fogassi et al., 1996; Graziano, Yap, & Gross, 1994; Graziano et al., 1997a; Rizzolatti, Scandolara, Matelli, & Gentilucci, 1981). For these bimodal cells, the tactile receptive field is located on the face, shoulder, arm, or upper torso, and the visual receptive field extends from the approximate region of the tactile receptive field into the immediately adjacent space. For almost all cells (93%), the visual receptive field is confined in depth (Graziano et al., 1997a). The visual receptive fields usually extend out from the body less than 30 cm. Most of the bimodal cells are directionally selective (Graziano et al., 1997a). All directions of motion are represented; different cells prefer movement to the left, right, up, down, and even movement of objects toward or away from the monkey. The directional preference is usually the same for both the tactile and the visual modality. For example, a cell that responds best to the sight of a nearby object moving to the right may also respond best to the felt movement of an object in the same direction, across the tactile receptive field. Figure 27.3 shows the tactile receptive fields and the associated visual receptive fields for two typical bimodal neurons related to the face and arm.

For almost all bimodal cells with a tactile receptive field on the arm, when the arm is placed in different

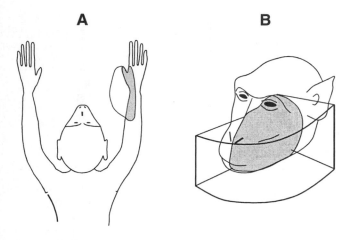

FIGURE 27.3 Two examples of bimodal, visual-tactile neurons from the polysensory zone in the precentral gyrus. In both cases the tactile receptive field (stippled) matched the location of the visual receptive field (outlined). (*A*) Arm; (*B*) face.

positions, the visual receptive field moves with the arm (Graziano, 1999; Graziano, Yap, et al., 1994; Graziano et al., 1997a). In contrast, when the eyes move, the visual receptive field does not move but remains anchored to the arm (Fogassi et al., 1992, 1996; Gentilucci, Scandolara, Pigarev, & Rizzolatti, 1983; Graziano & Gross, 1998; Graziano, Yap, et al., 1994; Graziano et al., 1997a). Thus these cells encode the locations of nearby visual stimuli with respect to the arm. Such information could be used to guide the arm away from nearby objects.

Similarly, for most bimodal cells with a tactile receptive field on the face, when the head is rotated, the visual receptive field moves with the head (Graziano et al., 1997a, 1997b). When the eyes move the visual receptive field does not move but remains anchored to the head (Fogassi et al., 1992, 1996; Gentilucci et al., 1983; Graziano, Yap, et al., 1994; Graziano & Gross, 1998; Graziano et al., 1997a). Such visual receptive fields encode the locations of nearby stimuli relative to the head and would be useful for guiding the head away from an impending threat.

The buzzing of an insect near the ear can sometimes elicit a flinch reaction. Therefore, we might expect neurons in PZ to be responsive to auditory stimuli. Indeed, neurons with a tactile response on the side and back of the head often respond to auditory stimuli near the head, within about 30 cm (Graziano, Reiss, & Gross, 1999). Regardless of the intensity of the sound, if the source is more than about 30 cm from the head, these neurons respond weakly or not at all. Figure 27.4 shows an example of a cell tested with bursts of white noise presented over a speaker at different distances from the head in the dark. At 10 cm from the head, the white noise evoked a response at all loudness levels. At 25 cm from the head, the sound bursts evoked a smaller response. At 50 cm from the head, the sound bursts evoked little or no response. The auditory parameter that is used by these neurons to encode the distance to the stimulus is not known, but it is thought that primates use the amount of reverberation of sound to estimate the distance to the source (Blauert, 1997). Auditory responses were never found in association with tactile responses on the arm. It may be that auditory localization in nearby space is most precise near the head and is not adequate to determine whether a stimulus is approaching the arm. Thus, a defensive or flinch mechanism might use auditory information mainly to protect the head.

About 20% of the multisensory neurons in PZ continue to respond to objects in the visual receptive field even after the lights are turned out and the object is no longer visible (Graziano et al., 1997b). Such neurons apparently "remember" the locations of nearby objects. When the lights are turned on, revealing the presence of an object in the visual receptive field, the neuron will begin to respond. When the lights are turned off, the neuron will continue to respond. When the lights are turned on again, revealing the absence of the object in the receptive field, the response stops. The firing of these neurons therefore reflects the most recent visual information about the presence or absence of the object near the face. Such mnemonic information could be useful in maintaining a margin of safety around the body even when the eyes are closed, in the dark, or for objects out of view behind the head. The neuronal signal, essentially "alerting" the motor system to the presence of a stimulus immediately adjacent to the head, could be used for collision avoidance. The effectiveness of this remembered spatial information can be demonstrated by walking toward a wall or other known obstacle in a dark room. One experiences a strong, uneasy compulsion to cringe when the face approaches the remembered location of the object.

In summary, the multisensory neurons in PZ represent the space immediately surrounding the body through touch, audition, vision, and even visual memory. These neurons monitor the location and movement of nearby objects. In the following section we describe the results of electrical stimulation in PZ. These studies suggest that neurons in PZ control a specific type of motor output, namely, movements that protect the body against an impending threat.

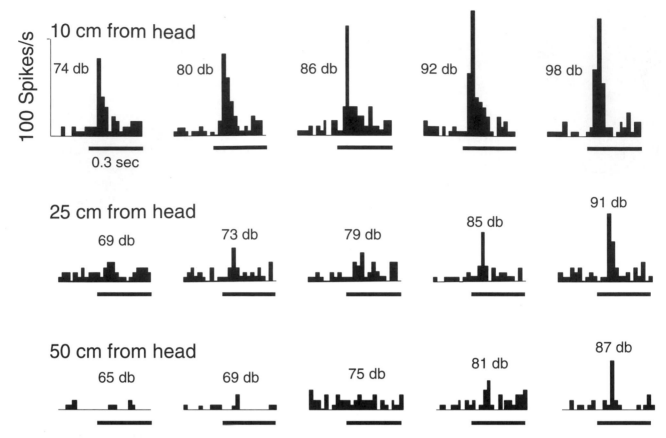

FIGURE 27.4 Auditory responses of a trimodal, visual-tactile-auditory neuron in PZ. This neuron had a tactile receptive field on the right side of the head and a visual receptive field near the right side of the face. It also responded to sounds presented near the right side of the face. Each histogram shows the response of the neuron to white noise presented over a loudspeaker in the dark (average of 10 trials). The intensity of the sound was measured in decibels by a small microphone at the monkey's ear. When the speaker was 10 cm away from the head, the neuron responded to all sound intensities presented. When the speaker was 25 cm from the head, the neuron responded less well. When the speaker was 50 cm from the head, the neuron responded weakly or not at all, regardless of the intensity of the sound.

Electrical stimulation of the polysensory zone

The function of the multisensory neurons in the precentral gyrus has been the subject of speculation for two decades. Rizzolatti and colleagues (1981) first suggested that the multisensory neurons help guide movement on the basis of sensory input. We elaborated on Rizzolatti's suggestion, hypothesizing that the neurons guide individual body parts toward or away from nearby objects, such as for flinching, kissing, reaching, or ducking (Graziano & Gross, 1995; Graziano et al., 1997a). Recent results from mapping the precentral gyrus, however, suggest that the multisensory neurons are unlikely to have such a general role in the control of movement (Graziano & Gandhi, 2000). The multisensory cells are clustered in a small zone in the center of the precentral gyrus, covering relatively little of the motor representation. What function could be served by this restricted zone? We set out to test the motor output of PZ by elec-

trically stimulating sites within it (Graziano et al., 2002). For each cortical site tested, we advanced a microelectrode into the cortex and first studied single neuron and multineuron activity. We then passed current through the same electrode. We used a train of biphasic pulses, typically at 200 Hz, 25–150 μA, and 0.5 s train duration. Such electrical stimulation directly activates a cluster of neurons around the tip of the electrode. The neuronal activity then spreads to other neurons through transsynaptic signals. Thus, the effect of electrical stimulation is thought to depend on the recruitment of physiologically relevant brain circuits.

The results from one example site are shown in Figure 27.5A. Neurons at this site had a tactile receptive field on the left arm and a visual receptive field in space near the left arm. The visual response was strongest to objects approaching the tactile receptive field from any direction, but there was a response to stationary stimuli as well. We electrically stimulated this cortical site at

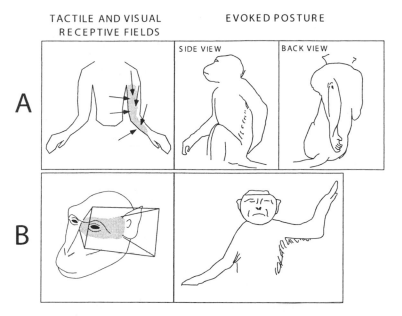

TACTILE AND VISUAL
RECEPTIVE FIELDS

EVOKED POSTURE

SIDE VIEW

BACK VIEW

FIGURE 27.5 Electrical stimulation of PZ evokes defensive movements. (*A*) Neurons at this site responded to a touch on the arm (within the shaded area) and to nearby visual stimuli moving toward the arm (indicated by arrows). Microstimulation caused the arm to move to a posture behind the back. (*B*) Multineuron activity at this site responded to a touch on the contralateral upper part of the face and to visual stimuli in the space near this tactile receptive field. Microstimulation evoked a complex defensive posture involving a facial squint, a head turn, and the arm and hand moving to a guarding position. Compare with Figure 27.1.

200 Hz and 100 μA for 0.5 s. During each stimulation train, the arm moved rapidly to a posture behind the monkey's back. This linking of a response to nearby objects approaching the arm with a motor output that withdraws the arm suggests that these neurons help to guard the arm from an impending threat. Regardless of the initial position of the arm, stimulation always evoked this final "guarding" posture.

Another example is shown in Figure 27.5*B*. When the eyes were covered, the neurons at this site responded to touching the left temple. When the eyes were open, the neurons responded to the sight of objects in the space near the temple. Electrical stimulation of this site caused the left eye to close entirely, the right eye to close partially, the face to contract into a grimace, the head to turn toward the right, the left arm to extend rapidly into the upper left space, and the left hand to turn such that the palm faced outward. That is, stimulation caused the monkey to mimic the actions of flinching from an object near the side of the head and thrusting out a hand to fend off the object (compare Fig. 27.5*B* with Fig. 27.1.) Stimulation using lower currents evoked a weaker defensive reaction. At the lowest current that was above threshold, only a closure of the eye occurred. This finding suggests that the strength of the flinch response is determined by the amount of neuronal activation in PZ. One possibility is that the salience of a nearby sensory stimulus will determine the magnitude of the

neuronal response, which in turn will determine the strength of the flinching movement.

At another site, the neurons responded to a touch on the forehead and to the sight of objects approaching the forehead. Stimulation of that site caused the eyes to close and the head to pull downward. At yet another site, the neurons responded to touching the back of the arm near the elbow and to the sight of objects moving in the periphery. Stimulation caused the elbow to pull rapidly forward and inward toward the midline.

For all 50 sites that we tested within PZ, in two monkeys, the evoked postures were consistent with flinching, avoiding, or defending against an object located in the multisensory receptive field. These defensive movements usually involved a retraction of body parts from the region of the multisensory receptive field, but in some cases also involved a palm-out thrusting of the hand toward the region of the multisensory receptive field. Thus these evoked movements appeared to include a complex mixture of withdrawal and blocking. Stimulation of sites outside PZ did not evoke defensive postures but instead evoked a different class of movements, such as reaching movements, shaping of the hand into grip postures, or movements of the tongue and jaw (Graziano et al., 2002).

Does the electrical stimulation cause a sensory percept such as pain on a part of the body, causing the monkey to flinch in reaction to that sensation? We believe that this is not the case. Instead, the stimulation appears to evoke a specific motor plan devoid of any sensory component or emotional valence. Two observations support this view. First, after each stimulation, as soon as the stimulation train ended, the monkey returned to a normal resting posture or to feeding itself pieces of fruit. Second, we found that the same defensive movements could be elicited from an anesthetized monkey. For several stimulation sites, we tested the effect of stimulation in the awake preparation, then injected the monkey with an anesthetic (pentobarbital sodium [Nembutal] and/or ketamine) and waited until the animal was unresponsive. To ensure that the monkey could not flinch from externally applied stimuli, we touched the monkey, manipulated the limbs, blew on the face, and finally pricked the eyelid. None of these stimuli elicited a response from the anesthetized monkey, suggesting that the monkey was not reacting to normally startling or painful stimuli. Electrical stimulation of the bimodal site, however, elicited a flinching movement that included a facial grimace and a clenching shut of the eyelids. This finding suggests that the stimulation does not operate indirectly by way of a sensory percept but instead directly stimulates a motor output.

Is the control of defensive movements the main or only function of area PZ, or does it have other functions, such as the control of reaching and grasping in the space near the body? Thus far, for all multimodal sites that we have tested within PZ, stimulation evoked an apparent defensive movement, not a reach or a grasp. One possibility is that this defensive function is somehow more electrically excitable than other functions, and thus, on stimulation, it dominates. Another possibility is that the defensive function is the main or only function of the brain area. This question remains unanswered, but we hope that studies using reversible deactivation will be able to address the issue in the future. On the basis of the data thus far, we tentatively suggest that PZ is primarily involved in the control of defensive movements.

In the next two sections we discuss areas VIP and 7b in the parietal lobe. Vision, touch, and audition converge in VIP and 7b. These two areas project directly to PZ and may be a source of the multisensory input to PZ. Neurons in VIP and 7b have response properties that are similar to but less complex than the properties in PZ, suggesting that there is a hierarchy of areas that process the space near the body.

The ventral intraparietal area

The ventral intraparietal area (VIP) was first defined as the projection zone of the middle temporal visual area (MT) onto the floor of the intraparietal sulcus (Maunsell & Van Essen, 1983a). The neuronal response properties in VIP may be related to this input from area MT. Area MT is thought to be specialized for the processing of visual motion; most of its neurons respond to moving visual stimuli and are tuned to the direction of movement (e.g., Albright, 1984; Allman & Kass, 1971; Dubner & Zeki, 1971; Maunsell & Van Essen, 1983b). Most neurons in VIP also respond to visual stimuli and are tuned to the direction of motion of the stimulus (Colby, Duhamel, & Goldberg, 1993; Duhamel, Colby, & Goldberg, 1998). Some neurons in VIP are even tuned to motion toward the animal, that is, to an expanding visual stimulus; other neurons prefer a contracting visual stimulus (Schaafsma & Duysens, 1996). These responses to complex motion patterns have been found in other visual areas that receive a projection from MT, such as MST and caudal STP (Graziano, Andersen, & Snowden, 1994; Hikosaka, Iwai, Saito, & Tanaka, 1988; Tanaka et al., 1986).

VIP, however, is strikingly different from the other visual motion areas in two respects. First, about half of VIP cells respond best to nearby visual stimuli, usually within 30 cm, sometimes only within a few centimeters (Colby et al., 1993). This preference for nearby stimuli is independent of the size of the stimulus. The depth cues that are used by VIP neurons are not yet known but probably include binocular disparity.

A second property of VIP that sets it apart from other visual motion areas is that almost all of its neurons have a tactile receptive field in addition to a visual receptive field (Duhamel et al., 1998). The tactile receptive field is typically on the face and roughly matches the location of the visual receptive field. Cells with a tactile receptive field on the forehead, for example, tend to have a visual receptive field in upper space, near the forehead. Cells with a tactile receptive field on the chin tend to have a visual receptive field in lower space near the chin. The visual and tactile modalities match not only in location but also in directional preference. For example, cells that prefer a leftward-moving visual stimulus usually also prefer a tactile stimulus that moves leftward across the skin.

At least some VIP neurons are trimodal, responding to visual, tactile, and auditory stimuli; for these neurons, the three receptive fields are spatially aligned (Schlack, Sterbing, Hartung, Hoffmann, & Bremmer, 2000).

In summary, neurons in area VIP receive convergent visual, somesthetic, and auditory input. They encode the location and motion of objects near the body, whether those objects are felt, seen, or heard. These response properties are strikingly similar to the properties found in PZ, to which area VIP projects. VIP and PZ do not, however, have identical response properties, as described in the next section. The differences suggest that the two areas are arranged in a hierarchy in which spatial information is more fully processed in PZ.

From sensory input to motor output

Protecting the body requires locating the threat with respect to the body surface, that is, in somatotopic coordinates. Is the object threatening the right forearm, the left side of the face, the forehead? The tactile modality, organized somatotopically, can provide this information for objects that are already touching the body. The auditory modality, anchored to the head, can be used to locate nearby stimuli at least with respect to the head. Visual stimuli, however, are not easily referenced to the body surface. A visual stimulus is first encoded as a location on the retina, but the retina is constantly in motion with respect to the body. In this section we discuss how visual information might be transformed from a spatial coordinate frame centered on the retina to a coordinate frame centered on the body surface that can guide movement.

How do neurons encode the location of visual stimuli? In the retina, a ganglion cell will respond only when light falls on a particular part of the retina, the cell's receptive field. Similar receptive fields, anchored to a location on the retina, are found in cortical areas that are near the retinal input, such as areas V1, V2, MT, V4, and others.

In contrast, in area PZ, many synapses from the retina and only one or two synapses from the motor output, almost none of the visual receptive fields are anchored to the retina. When the eyes move, these visual receptive fields remain stationary. Instead, they are anchored to the body surface. Some visual receptive fields are anchored to the arm, moving as the arm moves; others are anchored to the head, moving as the head moves. These body-part-centered visual receptive fields must require a massive amount of computation to construct. In effect, a neuron in PZ receives input from every part of the retina. Somehow, inputs from different parts of the retina can be turned on and off depending on the position of the eyes, the head, and the arms. How is visual information transformed from the simple retinal receptive fields at the input end to the complex body-part-centered receptive fields found near the motor output?

Area VIP in the parietal lobe may be a crucial intermediate step. As described above, it receives input from retinocentric visual areas such as MT and projects to PZ. Many neurons in VIP have visual receptive fields that are anchored to the retina, moving as the eyes move

(Duhamel, Bremmer, BenHamed, & Gref, 1997). About a third of the neurons have visual receptive fields that do not move as the eyes move. These visual receptive fields remain at the same location on a projection screen in front of the monkey even when the monkey is fixating different locations. Many neurons have intermediate properties; they have visual receptive fields that move in the same direction that the eyes move, but not to the same extent. This mixture of properties suggests that VIP is an intermediate step in the transformation from retinocentric receptive fields to body-part-centered receptive fields.

Several groups have created neural network models that transform retinal receptive fields into head or arm centered receptive fields (Pouget, Fisher, & Sejnowski, 1993; Salinas & Abbott, 1995; Zipser & Andersen, 1988). These neural network models have somewhat different properties, but they all demonstrate certain underlying constraints. (1) In order to construct a head-centered visual receptive field, it is necessary to combine visual information with information about eye position. In order to construct a limb-centered visual receptive field, it is necessary to use additional information about the position of the head on the trunk and the limb with respect to the trunk. (2) When these different types of visual and proprioceptive information converge on a single simulated neuron, the neuron often has complex and intermediate response properties such as a visual receptive field that is modulated by eye position, or that shifts partially with the eye, similar to the properties actually found in area VIP.

In summary, we suggest that there is a cortical pathway for locating nearby objects and organizing defensive reactions. This pathway begins in the visual system, where stimuli are located on the retina. This visual information converges with tactile and auditory information in area VIP. In addition to the multisensory convergence in VIP, the visual information also begins to be transformed such that visual stimuli can be located with respect to the body surface rather than on the retina. Finally, in area PZ, this transformation is completed; the neurons respond on the basis of the proximity of objects to specific body parts. The output of area PZ then triggers the appropriate defensive movement.

Area 7b

Multisensory responses similar to those found in PZ and VIP have been reported in other brain areas, including parietal area 7b (Graziano & Gross, 1995; Hyvarinen, 1981; Hyvarinen & Poranen, 1974; Leinonen, Hyvarinen, Nyman, & Linnankoski, 1979; Leinonen & Nyman, 1979; Robinson & Burton, 1980a,

1980b). This area, shown in Figure 27.2, is monosynaptically connected to VIP and PZ and may be part of the same brain system.

We studied single neurons in area 7b in anesthestized monkeys by plotting tactile and visual receptive fields (Graziano, Fernandez, & Gross, 1996; Graziano & Gross, 1995). Tactile stimuli included light touch with a cotton swab, manual palpation, and joint rotation. Visual stimuli included bars and spots of light projected onto a tangent screen, and also objects on the end of a wand, moved by hand in the space near the monkey's body. The objects on a wand were used because most neurons appeared to respond best to real objects rather than to two-dimensional stimuli on a screen. We found a high proportion of bimodal neurons in area 7b, in agreement with previous reports. In at least one part of area 7b, in the upper bank of the lateral sulcus, we found trimodal neurons responding to visual, tactile, and auditory stimuli. Bimodal and trimodal cells had somatosensory receptive fields on the face (13%), the arm (48%), both face and arm (33%), the chest (2%), and the whole upper body (4%). We obtained visual receptive field plots for 50 bimodal cells. Of these, 42% preferred stimuli within 20 cm of the animal, 42% preferred stimuli within 1 meter, and 16% responded well to stimuli at greater distances. When the arm was moved to different locations in front of the monkey, the visual receptive fields did not move with the arm. In no case did we observe an apparent shift of the visual receptive field. These results suggest that the visual receptive fields in 7b, like those in VIP, are not entirely in a coordinate system fixed to the body surface.

The putamen

The putamen is a large subcortical structure that is part of the basal ganglia and appears to play a role in the control of movement. Neurons in the putamen respond to tactile stimuli and also during voluntary movements; these tactile and motor fields are arranged to form a map of the body, with the legs represented at the top of the putamen and the inside of the mouth represented at the bottom (Alexander, 1987; Crutcher & DeLong, 1984a, 1984b; Kimura, Aosaki, Hu, Ishida, & Watanabe, 1992; Liles, 1985; Schultz & Romo, 1988). We studied the putamen in anesthetized monkeys, testing single neurons for tactile and visual responses (Graziano & Gross, 1993). Tactile stimuli included light touch with a cotton swab, manual palpation, and joint rotation. Visual stimuli included bars and spots of light projected onto a tangent screen, and also objects on the end of a wand, moved by hand in the space near the monkey's body. In the arm and face part of the map, about 25% of the neurons responded to both visual and tactile stimuli. For these bimodal neurons, the visual receptive field was confined to the space near the body, within about 30 cm, and matched the location of the tactile receptive field on the face or arm. For bimodal cells with a tactile receptive field on the arm, when the arm was moved to different locations, the visual receptive field also moved, remaining in register with the arm. Because these studies of visual responses in the putamen were done in anesthetized monkeys with a fixed eye position, it is not known how eye position affects the visual receptive fields. Auditory responses have not yet been studied in the putamen.

Multisensory areas in the human brain

Recent evidence suggests that the human brain contains a set of multisensory areas much like the ones described in this chapter for the monkey brain. In one experiment (Bremmer et al., 2001), subjects in a magnetic resonance imaging (MRI) scanner were exposed to tactile, visual, and auditory stimuli in separate trials. A small set of cortical areas appeared to be multisensory; that is, they could be activated above baseline by any of the three sensory modalities. One of the multisensory areas was located in the parietal lobe, on the floor of the intraparietal sulcus, closely matching the location of area VIP in the monkey brain. A second multisensory area was located in the frontal lobe, just in front of the central sulcus, closely matching the location of PZ in the monkey brain. A third multisensory area was located in the upper bank of the lateral sulcus. The correspondence to the monkey brain is less clear in this case, but this region of the human brain might correspond to part of area 7b in the monkey brain. Alternatively, it might represent a new multisensory area not yet found in the monkey brain. Deep structures, such as the putamen, were not investigated in this human study.

In another study (Vallar et al., 1999), human subjects in an MRI scanner made judgments about the location of a visual stimulus with respect to the head, or, in control trials, about the movement of the stimulus. The task that required referencing spatial locations to the body activated an area in the frontal lobe closely matching PZ in the monkey brain.

These brain imaging studies suggest that the human brain contains a set of multisensory cortical areas, many of which match the location of the multisensory areas in the monkey brain. It will be important to ascertain whether these areas in the human brain are engaged during tasks that tap into a defensive or flinch mechanism.

Summary

In this chapter we described a specific system of brain areas that are multisensory; they combine vision, audition, and touch. Neurons in these multisensory areas encode the location and movement of objects that are in the space near the body, within about 30 cm. Electrical stimulation experiments suggest that this particular set of multisensory areas serves the purpose of defending the body against nearby, threatening objects. In this view, objects that enter the space near the body will activate neurons in this system of areas, and these neurons will in turn induce the appropriate flinch or defensive movement. This system might serve as a model for understanding how sensory information is transformed by the brain into motor output.

REFERENCES

Albright, T. D. (1984). Direction and orientation selectivity of neurons in visual area MT of the macaque. *Journal of Neurophysiology, 52,* 1106–1130.

Alexander, G. E. (1987). Selective neuronal discharge in monkey putamen reflects intended direction of planned limb movements. *Experimental Brain Research, 67,* 623–634.

Allman, J. M., & Kass, J. H. (1971). A representation of the visual field in the caudal third of the middle temporal gyrus of the owl monkey (*Aotus trivirgatus*). *Brain Research, 31,* 85–105.

Blauert, J. (1997). *Spatial hearing: The psychophysics of human sound localization* (J. S. Allen, Trans.). Cambridge, MA: MIT Press.

Bremmer, F., Schlack, A., Shah, N. J., Zafiris, O., Kubischik, M., Hoffmann, K., et al. (2001). Polymodal motion processing in posterior parietal and premotor cortex: A human fMRI study strongly implies equivalencies between humans and monkeys. *Neuron, 29,* 287–296.

Boussaoud, D., Barth, T. M., & Wise, S. P. (1993). Effects of gaze on apparent visual responses of frontal cortex neurons. *Experimental Brain Research, 93,* 423–434.

Cavada, C., & Goldman-Rakic, P. S. (1989a). Posterior parietal cortex in rhesus monkey: I. Parcellation of areas based on distinctive limbic and sensory corticocortical connections. *Journal of Comparative Neurology, 287,* 393–421.

Cavada, C., & Goldman-Rakic, P. S. (1989b). Posterior parietal cortex in rhesus monkey: II. Evidence for segregated corticocortical networks linking sensory and limbic areas with the frontal lobe. *Journal of Comparative Neurology, 287,* 422–444.

Cavada, C., & Goldman-Rakic, P. S. (1991). Topographic segregation of corticostriatal projections from posterior parietal subdivisions in the macaque monkey. *Neuroscience, 42,* 683–696.

Colby, C. L., Duhamel, J.-R., & Goldberg, M. E. (1993). Ventral intraparietal area of the macaque: Anatomic location and visual response properties. *Journal of Neurophysiology, 69,* 902–914.

Crutcher, M. D., & DeLong, M. R. (1984a). Single cell studies of the primate putamen: I. Functional organization. *Experimental Brain Research, 53,* 233–243.

Crutcher, M. D., & DeLong, M. R. (1984b). Single cell studies of the primate putamen: I. Relations to direction of movement and pattern of muscular activity. *Experimental Brain Research, 53,* 244–258.

Dubner, R., & Zeki, S. M. (1971). Response properties and receptive fields of cells in an anatomically defined region of the superior temporal sulcus in the monkey. *Brain Research, 35,* 528–532.

Duhamel, J., Bremmer, F., BenHamed, S., & Gref, W. (1997). Spatial invariance of visual receptive fields in parietal cortex neurons. *Nature, 389,* 845–848.

Duhamel, J. R., Colby, C. L., & Goldberg, M. E. (1998). Ventral intraparietal area of the macaque: Congruent visual and somatic response properties. *Journal of Neurophysiology, 79,* 126–136.

Dum, R. P., & Strick, P. L. (1991). The origin of corticospinal projections from the premotor areas in the frontal lobe. *Journal of Neuroscience, 11,* 667–689.

Fogassi, L., Gallese, V., di Pellegrino, G., Fadiga, L., Gentilucci, M., Luppino, M., et al. (1992). Space coding by premotor cortex. *Experimental Brain Research, 89,* 686–690.

Fogassi, L., Gallese, V., Fadiga, L., Luppino, G., Matelli, M., & Rizzolatti, G. (1996). Coding of peripersonal space in inferior premotor cortex (area F4). *Journal of Neurophysics, 76,* 141–157.

Gentilucci, M., Scandolara, C., Pigarev, I. N., & Rizzolatti, G. (1983). Visual responses in the postarcuate cortex (area 6) of the monkey that are independent of eye position. *Experimental Brain Research, 50,* 464–468.

Graziano, M. S. A. (1999). Where is my arm? The relative role of vision and proprioception in the neuronal representation of limb position. *Proceedings of the National Academy of Sciences, USA, 96,* 10418–10421.

Graziano, M. S. A., Andersen, R. A., & Snowden, R. J. (1994). Tuning of MST neurons to spiral motions. *Journal of Neuroscience, 14,* 54–67.

Graziano, M. S. A., Fernandez, T., & Gross, C. G. (1996). Bimodal, visual-tactile neurons in parietal area 7b are not influenced by arm position. *Society of Neuroscience Abstracts, 22,* 398.

Graziano, M. S. A., & Gandhi, S. (2000). Location of the polysensory zone in the precentral gyrus of anesthetized monkeys. *Experimental Brain Research, 135,* 259–266.

Graziano, M. S. A., & Gross, C. G. (1993). A bimodal map of space: Somatosensory receptive fields in the macaque putamen with corresponding visual receptive fields. *Experimental Brain Research, 97,* 96–109.

Graziano, M. S. A., & Gross, C. G. (1995). The representation of extrapersonal space: A possible role for bimodal, visual-tactile neurons. In M. S. Gazzaniga (Ed.), *The cognitive neurosciences* (pp. 1021–1034). Cambridge, MA: MIT Press.

Graziano, M. S. A., & Gross, C. G. (1998). Visual responses with and without fixation: Neurons in premotor cortex encode spatial locations independently of eye position. *Experimental Brain Research, 118,* 373–380.

Graziano, M. S. A., Hu, X., & Gross, C. G. (1997a). Visuospatial properties of ventral premotor cortex. *Journal of Neurophysics, 77,* 2268–2292.

Graziano, M. S. A., Hu, X., & Gross, C. G. (1997b). Coding the locations of objects in the dark. *Science, 277,* 239–241.

Graziano, M. S. A., Reiss, L. A. J., & Gross, C. G. (1999). A neuronal representation of the location of nearby sounds. *Nature, 397,* 428–430.

Graziano, M. S. A., Taylor, C. S. R., & Moore, T. (2002). Complex movements evoked by microstimulation of precentral cortex. *Neuron, 34,* 841–851.

Graziano, M. S. A., Yap, G. S., & Gross, C. G. (1994). Coding of visual space by premotor neurons. *Science, 266,* 1054–1057.

Hikosaka, K., Iwai, E., Saito, H., & Tanaka, K. (1988). Polysensory properties of neurons in the anterior bank of the caudal superior temporal sulcus of the macaque monkey. *Journal of Neurophysiology, 60,* 1615–1637.

Hyvarinen, J. (1981). Regional distribution of functions in parietal association area 7 of the monkey. *Brain Research, 206,* 287–303.

Hyvarinen, J., & Poranen, A. (1974). Function of the parietal associative area 7 as revealed from cellular discharges in alert monkeys. *Brain, 97,* 673–692.

Kimura, M., Aosaki, T., Hu, Y., Ishida, A., & Watanabe, K. (1992). Activity of primate putamen neurons is selective to the mode of voluntary movement: Visually guided, self-initiated or memory-guided. *Experimental Brain Research, 89,* 473–477.

Kunzle, H. (1978). An autoradiographic analysis of the efferent connections from premotor and adjacent prefrontal regions (areas 6 and 8) in *Macaca fascicularis. Brain, Behavior and Evolution, 15,* 185–236.

Kwan, H. C., MacKay, W. A., Murphy, J. T., & Wong, Y. C. (1985). Properties of visual cue responses in primate precentral cortex. *Brain Research, 343,* 24–35.

Leinonen, L., Hyvarinen, J., Nyman, G., & Linnankoski, I. (1979). I. Functional properties of neurons in the lateral part of associative area 7 in awake monkeys. *Experimental Brain Research, 34,* 299–320.

Leinonen, L., & Nyman, G. (1979). II. Functional properties of cells in anterolateral part of area 7 associative face area of awake monkeys. *Experimental Brain Research, 34,* 321–333.

Liles, S. L. (1985). Activity of neurons in putamen during active and passive movement of wrist. *Journal of Neurophysiology, 53,* 217–236.

Luppino, G., Murata, A., Govoni, P., & Matelli, M. (1999). Largely segregated parietofrontal connections linking rostral intraparietal cortex (areas AIP and VIP) and the premotor cortex (areas F5 and F4). *Experimental Brain Research, 128,* 181–187.

Matelli, M., Camarda, R., Glickstein, M., & Rizzolatti, G. (1986). Afferent and efferent projections of the inferior area 6 in the macaque monkey. *Journal of Comparative Neurology, 255,* 281–298.

Maunsell, J. H. R., & Van Essen, D. C. (1983a). The connections of the middle temporal visual area (MT) and their relationship to a cortical hierarchy in the macaque monkey. *Journal of Neuroscience, 3,* 2563–2580.

Maunsell, J. H. R., & Van Essen, D. C. (1983b). Functional properties of neurons in middle temporal visual area of the macaque monkey: I. Selectivity for stimulus direction, speed, and orientation. *Journal of Neurophysiology, 49,* 1127–1147.

Mauritz, K.-H., & Wise, S. P. (1986). Premotor cortex of the rhesus monkey: Neuronal activity in anticipation of predictable environmental events. *Experimental Brain Research, 61,* 229–244.

Mesulam, M.-M., Van Hoesen, G. W., Pandya, D. N., & Geschwind, N. (1977). Limbic and sensory connection of the inferior parietal lobule (area PG) in the rhesus monkey: A study with a new method for horseradish peroxidase histochemistry. *Brain Research, 136,* 393–414.

Parthasarathy, H. B., Schall, J. D., & Graybiel, A. M. (1992). Distributed but convergent ordering of corticostriatal projections: Analysis of the frontal eye field and the supplementary eye field in the macaque monkey. *Journal of Neuroscience, 12,* 4468–4488.

Pouget, A., Fisher, S. A., & Sejnowski, T. J. (1993). Egocentric spatial representation in early vision. *Journal of Cognitive Neuroscience, 5,* 150–161.

Rizzolatti, G., Scandolara, C., Matelli, M., & Gentilucci, M. (1981). Afferent properties of periarcuate neurons in macaque monkeys: II. Visual responses. *Behavioural Brain Research, 2,* 147–163.

Robinson, C. J., & Burton, H. (1980a). Organization of somatosensory receptive fields in cortical areas 7b, retroinsula, postauditory and granular insula of *M. fascicularis. Journal of Comparative Neurology, 192,* 69–92.

Robinson, C. J., & Burton, H. (1980b). Somatic submodality distribution within the second somatosensory (SII), 7b, retroinsular, postauditory, and granular insular cortical areas of *M. fascicularis. Journal of Comparative Neurology, 192,* 93–108.

Salinas, E., & Abbott, L. F. (1995). Transfer of coded information from sensory to motor networks. *Journal of Neuroscience, 15,* 6461–6474.

Schaafsma, S. J., & Duysens, J. (1996). Neurons in the ventral intraparietal area of awake macaque monkey closely resemble neurons in the dorsal part of the medial superior temporal area in their responses to optic flow patterns. *Journal of Neurophysiology, 76,* 4056–4068.

Schlack, A., Sterbing, S., Hartung, K., Hoffmann, K.-P., & Bremmer, F. (2000). Auditory responsiveness in the macaque ventral intraparietal area (VIP). *Society of Neuroscience Abstracts, 26.*

Schultz, W., & Romo, R. (1988). Neuronal activity in the monkey striatum during the initiation of movements. *Experimental Brain Research, 71,* 431–436.

Tanaka, K., Hikosaka, K., Saito, H., Yukie, M., Fukada, Y., & Iwai, E. (1986). Analysis of local and wide-field movements in the superior temporal visual areas of the macaque monkey. *Journal of Neuroscience, 6,* 134–144.

Vallar, G., Lobel, E., Galati, G., Berthoz, A., Pizzamiglio, L., & Le Bihan, D. (1999). A fronto-parietal system for computing the egocentric spatial frame of reference in humans. *Experimental Brain Research, 124,* 281–286.

Weber, J. T., & Yin, T. C. T. (1984). Subcortical projections of the inferior parietal cortex (area 7) in the stump-tailed monkey. *Journal of Comparative Neurology, 224,* 206–230.

Zipser, D., & Andersen, R. A. (1988). A back-propagation programmed network that simulates response properties of a subset of posterior parietal neurons. *Nature, 311,* 679–684.

28 Cortical Mechanisms of Tool Use Subserved by Multisensory Integration

HIDETOSHI ISHIBASHI, SHIGERU OBAYASHI, AND ATSUSHI IRIKI

Introduction

From the viewpoint of developmental psychology, human cognitive growth proceeds in a hierarchically organized manner during sensorimotor maturation. According to Piaget, an infant is initially able to conceive of himself and others only in terms of the direct effects of and on his body; for example, the infant is only able to conceive of graspable objects that are within reach (Piaget, 1953). The initially random and spontaneous actions, or motor bubblings, of the infant come to be internally associated with the visual, kinesthetic, and somatosensory information that is contingent upon and highly correlated with them, leading to the emergence of an unconscious "enactive" body schema that is action dependent. As they become familiar with the surrounding space, thus resulting in overlearning with regard to object manipulation, by the age of 9 to 10 months children gain the abilities needed to handle action-free visual images, or "ikonic" representations of their own body; these abilities enable a child to dissociate a spatially organized internal schema from supporting actions, thus becoming free from the actions (Bruner, Oliver, & Greenfield, 1966). The ikonic representation would admit the dissociation of self from others, thus permitting self-awareness.

What are the neural bases for a body schema or body image? The idea that the construction of an internal representation of the body is based on the synthesis of visual and somatosensory sensations is almost a century old (Head & Holmes, 1911). This chapter considers how the body schema, a representation of the spatial relations among the parts of the body, is represented in the monkey and human brain, and how it is modified by experience. We also discuss how research on the body schema can be used to understand the neural mechanisms related to body image (i.e., the conscious and manipulable body schema) and self-awareness.

Body schema of one's own body

Human patients with a lesion in the parietal cortex often show unilateral neglect syndrome, which is characterized by a lack of awareness of sensory information, usually on the side contralateral to the lesion. In some cases there is dissociation between neglect for the human body and neglect for objects in the external environment. Case studies have shown that visual-spatial neglect for extrapersonal space can occur without personal neglect (Halligan & Marshall, 1991), and that severe unilateral personal neglect can exist in the absence of an extrapersonal space deficit (Guariglia & Antonucci, 1992). These findings suggest the existence of a body-specific attentional system that is separate from other attentional systems (for reviews, see Denes, 1989; Fredriks, 1985).

The parietal cortex is the primary site for creating the body schema. This brain area receives inputs conveying intrinsic information about the current posture. It is also fed (via a dorsal stream of visual information processing) with extrinsic information about the spatial locations and movements of objects and our own body parts (Colby, Gattass, Olson, & Gross, 1988; Ungerleider & Mishkin, 1982) (Fig. 28.1). Thus, the monkey intraparietal cortex possesses multimodal representations of the body-centered space and some planning of movements (Andersen, Snyder, Bradley, & Xing, 1997; Cohen & Andersen, 2002; but see Graziano, 2001). Neurons in this area project onto the higher motor cortices, including the premotor areas (Jones & Powell, 1970), where motor planning for purposeful actions—such as to reach, catch, or manipulate objects—is refined.

Neural representation of another's body

For most animal species, the visual perception of motion is a particularly crucial source of sensory input.

453

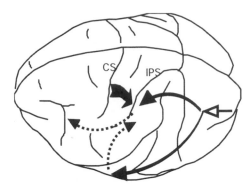

FIGURE 28.1 An anteroposteriorly running somatosensory pathway with increasing complexity of somatosensory information and the dorsal visual pathway ("where" pathway) converge in the intraparietal sulcus (IPS) area. CS, the central sulcus.

The ability to pick out the motion of biological forms from other types of motion in the natural environment is essential to predicting the actions of other individuals. An animal's survival depends on its ability to identify the movements of prey, predators, and mates, and to predict their future actions, the consequences of which differ radically and could in some cases be fatal. As social animals, humans behave largely on the basis of their interpretations of and predictions about the actions of others.

Humans' superior perception of biological motion without interference from shape was first reported by Johansson (1973), who attached light sources to an actor's joints and recorded the actor's movements in a dark environment. Naive participants rapidly and effortlessly recognized the moving dots as a person walking. Proprioceptive information concerning one's own body position facilitates, but does not interfere with, the visual perception of others' body positions (Reed & Farah, 1995), suggesting that body schema for one's own body and that for another individual's body share some representation or interact in some way.

Brain imaging studies have investigated whether a specific neural network subserves the perception of biological motion. One such study used functional magnetic resonance imaging (fMRI) to compare brain regions activated by dot displays showing biological motion and regions activated by dot displays showing coherent motion, within which all the dots moved at equal velocity in the same direction (Grossman et al., 2000). The authors found a specific area that was responsive to biological motion, located within the ventral bank of the occipital extent of the superior temporal sulcus (STS).

In the macaque monkey, the cerebral cortex in the anterior section of the STS has been implicated as a focus for the perceptual processing of the visual appearance of the face and body (reviewed by Emery & Perrett, 2000). Several types of neurons are relevant to understanding actions. One type of cell encodes the visual appearance of the face and body while the face and are static or in motion. A second type encodes particular face and body movements but is unresponsive to static images or still frames of the face and body. A third type of cell in the STS, especially in TEa, encodes face and body movements as goal-directed actions. This type of cell responds only to particular body movements made in relation to particular objects or positions in space (e.g., a hand reaching for an object, but not hand movements alone). The STS neurons respond when the subject sees another individual's actions (Jellema, Baker, Wicker, & Perrett, 2000), but no STS neurons were found to respond to the subject's own actions. Thus, based on the neurophysiological studies and functional imaging studies done so far, the inferior temporal cortex of both humans and monkeys is considered to be responsible for the processing of information about another individual's body.

Mirror neurons and body schema

Of special relevance to our model is a subset of such action-coding neurons identified in the ventral premotor cortex (area F5) in monkeys (Gallese, Fadiga, Fogassi, & Rizzolatti, 1996; Rizzolatti, & Arbib, 1998). Such neurons will fire when the monkey performs a specific action, such as a precision grip, but also when an equivalent action (a precision grip, in this example) is performed by another individual (either an experimenter or another monkey) that the monkey is watching. These neurons, called mirror neurons, appear to form a cortical system that matches the observation and execution of motor actions, which might be the basis of an understanding of motor events.

There are at least two hypotheses, not necessarily mutually exclusive, that might explain how the brain implements action understanding (Rizzolatti, Fogassi, & Gallese, 2001; see also Fogassi & Gallese, Chap. 26, this volume). The visual hypothesis states that action understanding is based on a visual analysis of the different elements that form an action, with no motor involvement. The direct-matching hypothesis holds that we understand actions when we map the visual representation of the observed action onto our motor representation of the same action. The visual properties of some monkey STS neurons (as described earlier) support the visual hypothesis. On the other hand, properties of the mirror neurons support the direct-matching hypothesis (Gallese & Goldman, 1998).

Although mirror neurons cannot be directly studied in the same way in humans, the belief that a system with the properties of mirror neurons exists is supported by several functional imaging studies. The sight of hand actions produces activity in frontal regions (the premotor cortex and Broca's area) (Grafton, Arbib, Fadiga, & Rizzolatti, 1996; Rizzolatti, Fadiga, Gallese, Fogassi, 1996), which may be homologous to F5 in the monkey (Rizzolatti & Arbib, 1998). Motor-evoked potentials from the hand muscles induced by transcranial magnetic stimulation over the motor cortex increase when the participant observes an actor grasping an object (Fadiga, Fogassi, Pavesi, & Rizzolatti, 1995). The activation of the left Broca's area during observation of finger movements became more intense when the same action was simultaneously executed (Iacoboni et al., 1999). These imaging studies have also revealed activity in the parietal cortex, which also provides some evidence of mirror neuron activity (Fogassi, Gallese, Fadiga, & Rizzolatti, 1998). The STS region is connected with the anterior part of the inferior parietal lobule (area PF or 7b), which in turn is reciprocally connected with area F5 (Matelli, Camarda, Glickstein, Rizzolatti, 1986). Thus, these three brain regions are likely to work together in the understanding of actions made by other individuals.

Body image developed through tool use

A body schema is not static but changes plastically, depending on one's experience. For example, it can be altered through tool use, which was defined by Beck (1980) as the alteration of the place, shape, or size of a target object with another inanimate object. When humans repeatedly use a tool, our body image alters until we feel introspectively that the tool has become a part or extension of the body. We trained macaque monkeys to use rake-shaped tools to extend their reaching distance (Iriki, Tanaka, & Iwamura, 1996). The training was usually completed in two or three weeks (Ishibashi, Hihara, & Iriki, 2000) and typically consisted of three stages. Stage 1: All the monkeys we examined started using the tool in the first few days. However, they used the tool in a typical manner and could retrieve food only when the tool was placed close to the food. Stage 2: In the first week, the monkeys became able to manipulate the tool in various ways and able to retrieve the food regardless of its position relative to the tool. Stage 3: They developed the level of skill required for efficient retrieval. Further experiments revealed that the monkeys attempted to use unfamiliar objects that were similar to the original tool in shape but different in size, color, and weight to rake in the food. However,

they did not use spherical or ring-shaped objects to retrieve food. These results suggest that the monkeys "conceptualized" the stick-shaped object as a tool to rake in the food. After the training, response properties of the neurons in the anterior (medial) bank of the intraparietal sulcus (IPS, the posterior extension of the primary somatosensory area) markedly changed. In naive animals, neurons in this area had essentially somatosensory responses, and thus they exhibited scant to no visual responses (Iwamura, Tanaka, Sakamoto, & Hikosaka, 1993). After the training was completed, a group of bimodal neurons appeared that exhibited clear visual responses in addition to the somatosensory responses. Around the somatosensory receptive field was formed the visual receptive field, defined as a territory in the space where a neuron responded to the moving visual stimuli. Tool use induced an expansion of the visual receptive field only when monkeys used tools to retrieve distant objects, but the modification was never induced when the monkeys simply held a tool as an external object (Fig. 28.2; Iriki et al. 1996). Thus, two maps exist in the brains of well-trained monkeys. One map, which corresponds to the ordinary body schema, is made of body-part-centered neural response properties. The other map, which corresponds to the expanded body schema, is made of tool-centered neural response properties. Switching between the two maps, or changes in the neuronal response properties, is subjective or context dependent and occurs within no more than five minutes. Bottom-up information alone is unlikely to explain this switch. Rather, we suppose that there is some mechanism that drives this switching, which is similar to the body image we humans have, although we do not claim that monkeys are aware of the switching.

We further examined whether the internal representation of the body was restricted to the real body or could be enhanced to include the image of the body parts projected onto a video monitor (Fig. 28.3). We trained monkeys to use the image of their hands shown on a video monitor to guide their hands, and examined the visual receptive field of the bimodal neurons. Bimodal neurons, having somatosensory receptive fields on the hand and visual receptive fields near the hand, were newly formed around the image of the hand projected onto the video screen; these neurons responded when the moving visual stimulus was present near the image of the hand in the video monitor. Moreover, the visual receptive field of the bimodal neurons that had been restricted to the space near the hand on the video monitor expanded to include the image of the tool in the monitor. These results indicate that monkeys can have an extended body image not only of their real body and

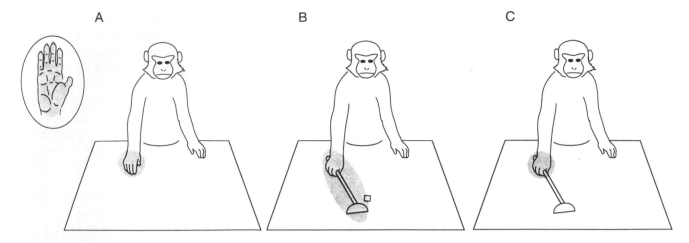

A   B   C

FIGURE 28.2 Example of modification of body image through experience. (A) Visual receptive field of bimodal neurons, somatosensory receptive field on the hand (inset) and visual receptive field near the hand in the anterior bank of the intraparietal sulcus. (B) Immediately after the cessation of tool use there is extended visual receptive field that includes the tool head. (C) Five minutes after the monkey stopped using the tool, the visual receptive field had shrunk back.

the real tool, but also of images shown on a video monitor (Iriki, Tanaka, Obayashi, & Iwamura, 2001).

If the coded image is truly a subjective one, those neurons should also respond to an image that is not actually visible but exists only as an internal representation. We examined whether those newly formed neuronal response properties in trained monkeys are also responsible for the perceptual image of an occluded hand by using the same method to detect visual receptive fields as in an earlier study (Iriki et al., 1996) for

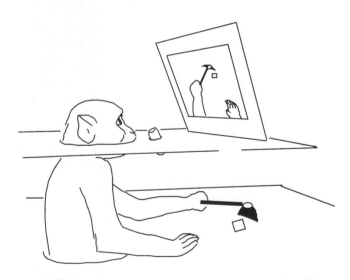

FIGURE 28.3 Monkey using an image of its hidden hand on a monitor to retrieve food with a tool in its hand. Initially, the monkeys were trained to use a rake-shaped tool. After this training an opaque panel was installed under the monkeys' eyes to mask their view, and instead of viewing the table directly, monkeys were trained to retrieve food relying entirely on the video monitor screen on which a real-time video image of their retrieval as captured by the camera was projected.

comparison. We examined whether IPS neurons encoding a body image also respond to an image that is not actually visible but exists only as an internal representation (Obayashi, Tanaka, & Iriki, 1998, 2000). After the monkey's hand was occluded from view by an opaque plate, the location of the visual receptive field coincided exactly with the area where the hand was located beneath the plate. Furthermore, when the hand was moved under the plate, the visual receptive field moved over the plate to follow the nonvisible hand. These findings suggest that the visual response properties of monkey intraparietal neurons may represent internal processes to create and sustain the body image as a higher-order representation that is linked to the internal state and arises from a complex integration of multisensory modalities, such as vision, proprioception, touch, and feedback of motor output, and not simply from proprioceptive signals (Graziano, Cooke, & Taylor, 2000; Obayashi et al., 2000). This may be similar to ikonic body image.

Dynamic properties of the body image in humans have also been reported (see also Làdavas & Farnè, Chap. 50, this volume; Maravita & Driver, Chap. 51, this volume). A subject with right hemisphere damage showed rightward error on a line bisection test on which the subject was asked to mark the approximate midpoint of a straight line with a laser pointer within the near, but not far, visual space. However, when the subject was asked to bisect far lines with a long stick, the visual neglect returned, which suggests that wielding the tool extended the subject's body schema (Berti & Frassinetti, 2000). A similar remapping of space through tool use is also seen in cross-modal extinction. Patients with right hemisphere damage are often unaware of stimulation on the side opposite the lesion if presented concurrently with stimulation on the same side as the lesion, even though they typically detect isolated stimuli on either side; the latter is said to extinguish awareness of the former. The cross-modal extinction of patients who had right hemisphere damage was reduced when the right visual stimulus was placed far from the patient's hands, but was restored when the patient manipulated the sticks and the visual stimulus came close to the tool head (Farnè & Làdavas, 2000; Maravita, Husain, Clarke, & Driver, 2001). These three human studies did not require intensive training (although patients in the study by Farnè and Làdavas engaged in some tool use), in contrast to our monkey study, where the monkeys required massive training. This may well be in accordance with the increased visual responsiveness in the anterior bank of the IPS: few neurons in this area, unlike those in the VIP and MIP, show a visual response in naive monkeys, whereas it is rather common to find neurons showing a visual response in monkeys trained for tool use. There is a possibility, at this point highly speculative, that acquiring visual properties in this area contributes to developing a body image so that the animal becomes more vision dependent and less somatosensory dependent, and forms an ikonic body image more easily. In the next section we discuss our attempts to investigate how tool use increases the visual projection into the IPS region.

Molecular processes subserving tool use learning

One possible mechanism for altering the body image through tool use is that projections from the vision-related cortex form new synapses with neurons processing somatosensory signals in the IPS region. Such newly formed synapses may be silent synapses—that is, silent at the resting membrane potential but active at the depolarized membrane potential (Isaac et al., 1995)—that are active only during the use of the tool.

Our interest in the development of new synapses between visual projections and the somatosensory cortex led us to consider the role of neurotrophins. Neurotrophins, such as nerve growth factor (NGF), brain-derived neurotrophic factor (BDNF), and neurotrophin 3 (NT-3), regulate not only long-term neuronal survival and differentiation but also neurite arborization and synaptic formation, synaptic transmission and plasticity, and learning and memory (for a review, see Poo, 2001). For example, neurotrophins are involved in activity-dependent modulation of dendritic and axonal growth in the cortex (McAllister, Katz, & Lo, 1996, 1997; McAllister, Lo, & Katz, 1995), the formation of the ocular dominance column in the visual cortex

(Cabelli, Hohn, & Shatz, 1995; Cabelli, Shelton, Segal, & Shatz, 1997; Domenici, Berardi, Carmignoto, Vantini, & Maffei, 1991; Maffei, Berardi, Domenici, Parisi, & Pizzorusso, 1992), and acute modification of the functional representation of a stimulated whisker in the barrel subdivision of the rat somatosensory cortex (Prakash, Cohen-Cory, & Frostig, 1996). Neurotrophins acutely enhance synaptic transmission at neuromuscular synapses (Lohof, Ip, & Poo, 1993; Stoop & Poo, 1996; Wang & Poo, 1997; Xie, Wang, Olafsson, Mizuno, & Lu, 1997). The impairment of CA1 hippocampal long-term potentiation in BDNF knockout mice is reversed by introducing the exogenous BDNF gene (Korte, Staiger, Griesbeck, Thoenen, & Bonhoeffer, 1996). The expression of BDNF is enhanced in the rat hippocampus by contextual learning (Hall, Thomas, & Everitt, 2000) and in the monkey inferior temporal cortex by a paired association task (Tokuyama, Okuno, Hashimoto, Xin, & Miyashita, 2000). Thus, we investigated whether the expression of neurotrophins is altered when monkeys are learning to use a tool.

To examine the expression of neurotrophins, we first introduced a method of tissue sampling suitable for examining the expression of messenger RNA (mRNA) in the monkey brain, since the conventional method—cutting out the brain tissue after removing the skull—was laborious and time-consuming. The brain tissue was collected by the biopsy method just after the training and following anesthesia induction. The tissue from the IPS region contralateral to the tool-using hand contained more mRNA for BDNF, its receptor trkB, and NT-3 than the tissue from the corresponding ipsilateral region (Ishibashi et al., 2002b). We evaluated the gene expression by comparing two hemispheres in the same animal to eliminate variations in genetic and cognitive factors among individuals and in manual processing from experiment to experiment. All monkeys used their right hand when using the tool and their left hand to retrieve the food on most trials, and so the strength of neuronal signals related to visuomotor control in the two hemispheres did not significantly differ. We also compared tissues taken from two groups of monkeys, from one group during tool use learning and from the other group well after the acquisition of tool use ability. The expression of the relevant genes was higher for the monkeys learning tool use than for the monkeys with acquired tool use ability (Fig. 28.4). Because we suctioned brain tissue immediately after training in both groups of monkeys, the strength of neuronal signals related to visuomotor control in the two groups of animals did not significantly differ. Therefore, the induced gene expression should reflect the role of neurotrophins in tool use learning. Neurotrophins secreted

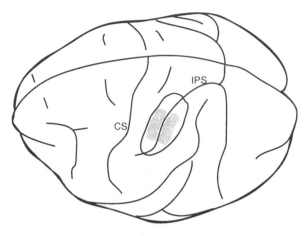

FIGURE 28.4 Tool use–induced gene expression. Brain areas showing induced gene expression are shaded.

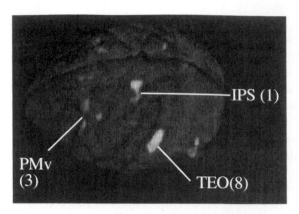

FIGURE 28.5 Tool use–induced monkey brain activities (compared with control task): left oblique 50-degree view.

at the IPS region may attract the neural projection from the vision-related cerebral cortex when a monkey is learning the use of a tool. Further localization analysis revealed that the highest expression of BDNF was seen in the region of the anterior bank of IPS posteriorly adjacent to the somatosensory forearm and shoulder region in area 3b (Ishibashi et al., 2002a). These results are consistent with our introspection that repeatedly used tools become a part of or an extension of the body part (the arm or shoulder, in this case). However, the mechanism by which the visual property is integrated into a body image that includes the tool to create the new map and the mechanism underlying the switching between the two maps remain to be examined.

Brain imaging studies to demonstrate altered body image

Neuroimaging techniques, such as functional magnetic resonance imaging (fMRI) and positron emission tomography (PET), provide us with a better opportunity to test our hypothesis by means of statistical analysis. Our recent monkey PET study, using the $H_2^{15}O$ method, in which regional cerebral blood flow is measured and used as an index of brain activity, revealed brain activation during the tool use of two Japanese monkeys (Obayashi et al., 2001). Tool use–related activity occurred, relative to the corresponding control task, in the intraparietal cortex (in the IPS; corresponding to the recording sites of bimodal neurons showing tool use–induced visual response modification), the higher-order motor cortex (such as the presupplementary motor area [pre-SMA] and premotor cortex [PM]), the basal ganglia, the inferotemporal cortex (IT), and the cerebellum during the single-tool-use task (Fig. 28.5). The control task consisted of repetitive simple-stick

manipulation in which the delivery of reachable pellets was used to condition the monkeys to wave the stick beforehand in their preferred direction with the same hand as under the test condition. As well as being involved in memory retrieval of the acquired skill, estimation of the optimal tool-hand path toward the target, and execution of autonomous tool action, all of these regions might also be involved in learning-related cortical reorganization. Those circuits may be related to the continuous updating of spatial representation needed for the precise guidance of the rake onto the reward by means of organizing motor-sensory acts.

Behavioral evidence of "generalization"

Only a few studies have been reported on the flexible and adaptive application of tool use skill, once that skill has been acquired by monkeys. Ueno and Fujita reported flexible and adaptive tool use by a pet Tonkean macaque that was chained to a tree (Ueno & Fujita, 1998). The subject always used a long stick when the food bowl was placed far away, but used either a long or a short stick when the bowl was placed nearby. When the food was moved away, the monkey quickly exchanged the shorter stick for the longer one. There are two possible interpretations of this behavior. One interpretation is that the subject simply learned to relate the use of the different kind of tools and the distance to the food bowl based on repeated experience. Another interpretation is that the subject not only "knew" how he should solve the problem before he actually started to tackle it, he also flexibly changed his strategy according to the change in the situation. To clarify this issue, we replicated the experimental condition. After repeated use of the stick, we presented Japanese monkeys with a novel, longer tool. They did not show much hesitation in using the unfamiliar long stick when the familiar short stick was not long enough to reach the food (Hihara, Obayashi, & Iriki, in press; Ishibashi et al., 2000). Further, monkeys used multiple tools sequentially without much training; when given two tools of different length, they retrieved the distant long tool with the short tool and then used the long tool to retrieve the food, which suggests that monkeys can coordinate and manage learned motor acts that are not immediately related to the previous experience (Hihara et al., 2003).

Self and others

People have long been interested in how nonhuman animals might conceive of themselves as separate from others. The mark test, developed by Gallup in 1970, offers a way to explore such a question (Gallup, 1970). In the original mark test procedure, each subject was first exposed to a mirror. Social gestures made to the mirror image, as if the image were a companion, disappeared three days after the first exposure to the mirror. Chimpanzees showed an avid interest in the mirror as measured by viewing time, but with the development of self-directed behavior, this interest diminished. When the chimpanzees' faces and ears were painted with dye (under anesthesia), the chimpanzees showed mark-directed responses, indicating that chimpanzees are capable of self-recognition that can be learned through exposure to the mirror. However, three chimpanzees reared in isolation did not show mirror-mediated self-directed responses on the mark test (Gallup, McClure, Hill, & Bundy, 1971). Two were then reared with conspecifics (other individuals of the same species) and showed self-directed responses on the follow-up mark test. The one chimpanzee that continued to be reared in isolation failed the follow-up mark test. These results suggest that the existence of the conspecifics helped the chimpanzees develop an internal representation of the chimpanzee; that is, the brain seemed to become capable of creating an image of the self in relation to others.

How can the concepts of self and other be formed? Human infants' failed attempts to reach and grasp a target or their gaze alternation between a target and another nearby individual that is followed by the retrieval of the target by that individual might trigger the generation of human communication, which in turn develops into language acquisition (Bruner, 1983) or theory of mind (Baron-Cohen, 1991). Although the gestures are imperative in nature at first, they develop into communicative gestures, and this development might be accelerated by the caregiver's rejection of the infant's request. We have trained a monkey to use eye gaze and pointing to indicate her intended target and to comprehend what target a human intends by eye gaze or pointing. After learning how to produce and comprehend the use of eye gaze and pointing, the monkey used those gestures to draw a human's attention to nonfood objects when the experimenter pretended not to notice the objects (Kumashiro, Ishibashi, Itakura, & Iriki, 2002). This persuaded us that bidirectional communication based on the concepts of self and other can be generated between a monkey and a human. Furthermore, two of three monkeys that acquired the joint attention behavior showed imitation, which we define here as performing an act after perceiving it, of human actions (Kumashiro, Ishibashi, Itakura, & Iriki, 2002).

Neural connections from the STS to the IPS region contain data on visual properties of another individual. According to Fogassi and Gallese (Chap. 26, this volume), motor representation exists in the IPS region as well as in the premotor cortex. Data on the visual properties of another individual are combined with somatosensory (touch and proprioception) and some motor information in the IPS region. Thus, the IPS region may be important in constructing one's own body schema or body image and in processing visual information about another individual. This information is sent to the premotor cortex, where it is combined with motor information and processed for actual motor planning. Thus, this circuit may play a crucial role in imitation, although this hypothesis remains to be examined (Fig. 28.6).

Conclusion

We have outlined what the body image consists of and how it can be related to higher intelligence of the self. A monkey's natural intelligence is qualitatively different from that of apes or humans. However, with the use of training-reinforced monkeys, efforts to neuroscientifically study the nature of self-awareness have achieved some realistic grounding. It is possible that the body image in monkeys is more rudimentary than in humans because of poor visual projection onto the somatosensory pathway related to body image creation and maintenance. By reinforcing the capabilities of monkeys by means of tool use and monitor use, we have shown that it is possible to alter the visual responses that form around the real body and around the ikonic body (an image of the hand on the video monitor). Training aimed at enabling imitation or nonverbal communication, such as communication by eye gaze and pointing, offers another approach to studying the body image and how it can be modified in the course of the behavioral development of communication. To understand the neural basis for self-awareness, however, we also need to examine the body image and how it is

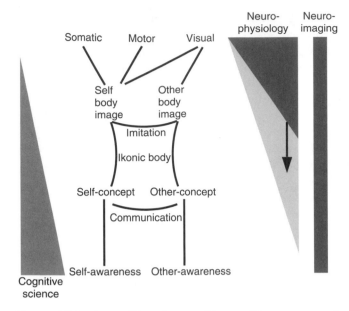

FIGURE 28.6 A possible schema of how self-awareness and other-awareness are constructed. Body image, consisting of somatosensory and visual information and motor efferent copy, is required for the capacity to imitate. Repeated imitation helps create the body image of both self and other, and may also facilitate more abstract representation of the body. The distinction of self from other individuals is made possible after the formation of the representation of ikonic body. Through communication, organisms develop the capacity for self-awareness, mind, and sympathy. The cognitive science approach focuses on elements arrayed in the lower portion of this construct. Functional neuroimaging can focus on a broad range of fields depicted in the figure. Neurophysiology, including various fields such as electrophysiology and biochemistry, is a powerful tool and offers concrete evidence in clarifying the neural basis for the brain's function, but is limited to the field in the upper part of the figure. We will have a better understanding of self once the neurophysiological approach is able to encompass the elements arrayed in the middle portion of this construct, as indicated by the descending arrow.

altered with regard to invisible body parts, such as the face, as well as with regard to visible parts, such as the hands.

REFERENCES

Andersen, R. A., Snyder, L. H., Bradley, D. C., & Xing, J. (1997). Multimodal representation of space in the posterior parietal cortex and its use in planning movements. *Annual Review of Neuroscience, 20,* 303–330.

Baron-Cohen, S. (1991). Precursors to a theory of mind: Understanding attention in others. In A. Whiten (ed.), *Natural theories of mind* (pp. 233–251). Oxford, England: Basil Blackwell.

Beck, B. B. (1980). *Animal tool behavior: The use and manufacture of tools by animals.* New York: Garland Press.

Berti, A., & Frassinetti, F. (2000). When far becomes near: Remapping of space by tool use. *Journal of Cognitive Neuroscience, 12,* 415–420.

Bruner, J. S. (1983). *Child's talk.* Oxford, England: Oxford University Press.

Bruner, J. S., Oliver, R. R., & Greenfield, P. M. (1966). *Studies in cognitive growth.* New York: Wiley.

Cabelli, R. J., Hohn, A., & Shatz, C. J. (1995). Inhibition of ocular dominance column formation by infusion of NT-4/5 or BDNF. *Science, 267,* 1662–1666.

Cabelli, R. J., Shelton, D. L., Segal, R. A., & Shatz, C. J. (1997). Blockade of endogenous ligands of trkB inhibits formation of ocular dominance columns. *Neuron, 19,* 63–76.

Cohen, Y. E., & Andersen, R. A. (2002). A common reference frame for movement plans in the posterior parietal cortex. *Nature Reviews: Neuroscience, 3,* 553–562.

Colby, C. L., Gattass, R., Olson, C. R., & Gross, C. G. (1988). Topographic organization of cortical afferents to extrastriate visual area PO in the macaque: A dual tracer study. *Journal of Comparative Neurology, 269,* 392–413.

Denes, G. (1989). Disorders of body awareness and body knowledge. In F. Boller & J. Grafman (Eds.), *Handbook of neuropsychology* (pp. 207–229). Amsterdam: Elsevier.

Domenici, L., Berardi, N., Carmignoto, G., Vantini, G., & Maffei, L. (1991). Nerve growth factor prevents the amblyopic effects of monocular deprivation. *Proceedings of the National Academy of Sciences, USA, 88,* 8811–8815.

Emery, N. J., & Perrett, D. I. (2000). How can studies of the monkey brain help us to understand "theory of mind" and autism in humans? In S. Baron-Cohen, H. Tager-Flusberg, & D. J. Cohen (Eds.), *Understanding other minds* (pp. 274–305). New York: Oxford University Press.

Fadiga, L., Fogassi, L., Pavesi, G., & Rizzolatti, G. (1995). Motor facilitation during action observation: A magnetic stimulation study. *Journal of Neurophysiology, 73,* 2608–2611.

Farnè, A., & Làdavas, E. (2000). Dynamic size-change of hand peripersonal space following tool use. *NeuroReport, 11,* 1645–1649.

Fogassi, L., Gallese, V., Fadiga, L., & Rizzolatti, G. (1998). Neurons responding to the sight of goal-directed hand/arm actions in the parietal area PF (7b) of the macaque monkey. *Society of Neuroscience Abstracts, 24,* 257.

Fredriks, J. A. M. (1985). Disorders of the body schema. In J. A. M. Fredriks (ed.), *Handbook of clinical neurology* (pp. 373–393). Amsterdam: Elsevier.

Gallese, V., Fadiga, L., Fogassi, L., & Rizzolatti, G. (1996). Action recognition in the premotor cortex. *Brain, 119,* 593–609.

Gallese, V., & Goldman, A. (1998). Mirror neurons and the simulation theory of mind-reading. *Trends in Cognitive Sciences, 2,* 493–501.

Gallup, G. G., Jr. (1970). Chimpanzees: Self-recognition. *Science, 167,* 86–87.

Gallup, G. G., Jr., McClure, M. K., Hill, S. D., & Bundy, R. A. (1971). Capacity for self-recognition in differentially reared chimpanzees. *Psychological Record, 21,* 69–74.

Grafton, S. T., Arbib, M. A., Fadiga, L., & Rizzolatti, G. (1996). Localization of grasp representations in humans by positron emission tomography. 2. Observation compared with imagination. *Experimental Brain Research, 112,* 103–111.

Graziano, M. S. A. (2001). Is reaching eye-centered, body-centered, hand-centered, or a combination? *Reviews in the Neurosciences, 12,* 175–185.

Graziano, M. S. A., Cooke, D. F., & Taylor, C. S. (2000). Coding the location of the arm by sight. *Science, 290,* 1782–1786.

Grossman, E., Donnelly, M., Price, R., Pickens, D., Morgan, V., Neighbor, G., & Blake, R. (2000). Brain areas involved in perception of biological motion. *Journal of Cognitive Neuroscience, 12,* 711–720.

Guariglia, C., & Antonucci, G. (1992). Personal and extrapersonal space: A case of neglect dissociation. *Neuropsychologia, 30,* 1001–1009.

Hall, J., Thomas, K. L., & Everitt, B. J. (2000). Rapid and selective induction of BDNF expression in the hippocampus during contextual learning. *Nature Neuroscience, 3,* 533–535.

Halligan, P. W., & Marshall, J. C. (1991). Left neglect for near but not far space in man. *Nature, 350,* 498–500.

Head, H., & Holmes, G. (1911). Sensory disturbances from cerebral lesions. *Brain, 34,* 102–254.

Hihara, S., Obayashi, S., & Iriki, A. (2003). Rapid learning of multiple-tool usages by macaque monkeys. *Physiology and Behavior, 78,* 427–434.

Iacoboni, M., Woods, R. P., Brass, M., Bekkering, H., Mazziotta, J. C., & Rizzolatti, G. (1999). Cortical mechanisms of human imitation. *Science, 286,* 2526–2528.

Iriki, A., Tanaka, M., & Iwamura, Y. (1996). Coding of modified body schema during tool use by macaque postcentral neurones. *NeuroReport, 7,* 2325–2330.

Iriki, A., Tanaka, M., Obayashi, S., & Iwamura, Y. (2001). Self-images in the video monitor coded by monkey intraparietal neurons. *Neuroscience Research, 40,* 163–173.

Isaac, J. T., Nicoll, R. A., & Malenka, R. C. (1995). Evidence for silent synapses: Implications for the expression of LTP. *Neuron, 15,* 427–434.

Ishibashi, H., Hihara, S., & Iriki, A. (2000). Acquisition and development of monkey tool-use: Behavioral and kinematic analyses. *Canadian Journal of Physiology and Pharmacology, 78,* 958–966.

Ishibashi, H., Hihara, S., Takahashi, M., Heike, T., Yokota, T., & Iriki, A. (2002a). Tool-use learning induces BDNF expression in a selective portion of monkey anterior parietal cortex. *Molecular Brain Research, 102,* 110–112.

Ishibashi, H., Hihara, S., Takahashi, M., Heike, T., Yokota, T., & Iriki, A. (2002b). Tool-use learning selectively induces expression of brain-derived neurotrophic factor, its receptor *trk*B, and neurotrophin 3 in the intraparietal multisensory cortex of monkeys. *Brain Research: Cognitive Brain Research, 14,* 3–9.

Iwamura, Y., Tanaka, M., Sakamoto, M., & Hikosaka, O. (1993). Rostrocaudal gradients in the neuronal receptive field complexity in the finger region of the alert monkey's postcentral gyrus. *Experimental Brain Research, 92,* 360–368.

Jellema, T., Baker, C. I., Wicker, B., & Perrett, D. I. (2000). Neural representation for the perception of the intentionality of actions. *Brain and Cognition, 44,* 280–302.

Johansson, G. (1973). Visual perception of biological motion and a model for its analysis. *Perception & Psychophysics, 14,* 201–211.

Jones, E. G., & Powell, T. P. (1970). An anatomical study of converging sensory pathways within the cerebral cortex of the monkey. *Brain, 93,* 793–820.

Korte, M., Staiger, V., Griesbeck, O., Thoenen, H., & Bonhoeffer, T. (1996). The involvement of brain-derived neurotrophic factor in hippocampal long-term potentiation revealed by gene targeting experiments. *Journal of Physiology (Paris), 90,* 157–164.

Kumashiro, M., Ishibashi, H., Itakura, S., & Iriki, A. (2002). Bidirectional communication between a Japanese monkey and a human through eye gaze and pointing. *Current Psychology of Cognition, 21,* 3–32.

Lohof, A. M., Ip, N. Y., & Poo, M. M. (1993). Potentiation of developing neuromuscular synapses by the neurotrophins NT-3 and BDNF. *Nature, 363,* 350–353.

Maffei, L., Berardi, N., Domenici, L., Parisi, V., & Pizzorusso, T. (1992). Nerve growth factor (NGF) prevents the shift in ocular dominance distribution of visual cortical neurons in monocularly deprived rats. *Journal of Neuroscience, 12,* 4651–4662.

Maravita, A., Husain, M., Clarke, K., & Driver, J. (2001). Reaching with a tool extends visual-tactile interactions into far space: Evidence from cross-modal extinction. *Neuropsychologia, 39,* 580–585.

Matelli, M., Camarda, R., Glickstein, M., & Rizzolatti, G. (1986). Afferent and efferent projections of the inferior area 6 in the macaque monkey. *Journal of Comparative Neurology, 251,* 281–298.

McAllister, A. K., Katz, L. C., & Lo, D. C. (1996). Neurotrophin regulation of cortical dendritic growth requires activity. *Neuron, 17,* 1057–1064.

McAllister, A. K., Katz, L. C., & Lo, D. C. (1997). Opposing roles for endogenous BDNF and NT-3 in regulating cortical dendritic growth. *Neuron, 18,* 767–778.

McAllister, A. K., Lo, D. C., & Katz, L. C. (1995). Neurotrophins regulate dendritic growth in developing visual cortex. *Neuron, 15,* 791–803.

Obayashi, S., Suhara, T., Kawabe, K., Okauchi, T., Maeda, J., Akine, Y., et al. (2001). Functional brain mapping of monkey tool use. *NeuroImage, 14,* 853–861.

Obayashi, S., Tanaka, M., & Iriki, A. (1998). Parietal neurons coding the image of the invisible forearm. *Society of Neuroscience Abstracts, 24,* 435.

Obayashi, S., Tanaka, M., & Iriki, A. (2000). Subjective image of invisible hand coded by monkey intraparietal neurons. *NeuroReport, 11,* 3499–3505.

Piaget, J. (1953). *Origins of intelligence in children.* New York: Routledge.

Poo, M. M. (2001). Neurotrophins as synaptic modulators. *Nature Reviews: Neuroscience, 2,* 24–32.

Prakash, N., Cohen-Cory, S., & Frostig, R. D. (1996). Rapid and opposite effects of BDNF and NGF on the functional organization of the adult cortex in vivo. *Nature, 381,* 702–706.

Reed, C. L., & Farah, M. J. (1995). The psychological reality of the body schema: A test with normal participants. *Journal of Experimental Psychology: Human Perception and Performance, 21,* 334–343.

Rizzolatti, G., & Arbib, M. A. (1998). Language within our grasp. *Trends in Neurosciences, 21,* 188–194.

Rizzolatti, G., Fadiga, L., Gallese, V., & Fogassi, L. (1996). Premotor cortex and the recognition of motor actions. *Brain Research: Cognitive Brain Research, 3,* 131–141.

Rizzolatti, G., Fogassi, L., & Gallese, V. (2001). Neurophysiological mechanisms underlying the understanding and imitation of action. *Nature Reviews: Neuroscience, 2,* 661–670.

Stoop, R., & Poo, M. M. (1996). Synaptic modulation by neurotrophic factors: Differential and synergistic effects of brain-derived neurotrophic factor and ciliary neurotrophic factor. *Journal of Neuroscience, 16,* 3256–3264.

Tokuyama, W., Okuno, H., Hashimoto, T., Xin Li, Y., & Miyashita, Y. (2000). BDNF upregulation during declarative memory formation in monkey inferior temporal cortex. *Nature Neuroscience, 3,* 1134–1142.

Ueno, Y., & Fujita, K. (1998). Spontaneous tool use by a Tonkean macaque (*Macaca tonkeana*). *Folia Primatologica, 69,* 318–324.

Ungerleider, L. G., & Mishkin, M. (1982). Two cortical visual systems. In D. Ingle, M. A. Goodale, & R. J. W. Mansfield (Eds.), *Analysis of visual behavior* (pp. 549–586). Cambridge, MA: MIT Press.

Wang, X. H., & Poo, M. M. (1997). Potentiation of developing synapses by postsynaptic release of neurotrophin-4. *Neuron, 19,* 825–835.

Xie, K., Wang, T., Olafsson, P., Mizuno, K., & Lu, B. (1997). Activity-dependent expression of NT-3 in muscle cells in culture: Implications in the development of neuromuscular junctions. *Journal of Neuroscience, 17,* 2947–2958.

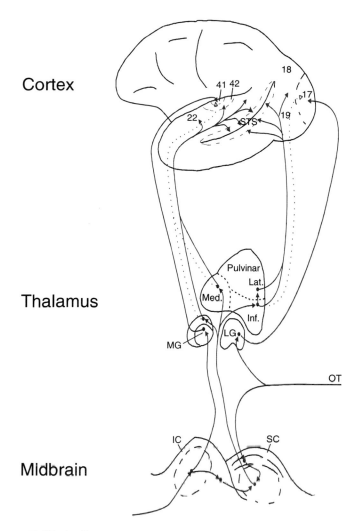

Cortex

Thalamus

Midbrain

PLATE 1   Cerebrum of the macaque, illustrating sensory pathways revealed by tract tracing studies in monkeys.

Shown in green, visual input from the retina by way of the optic tract (OT) innervates the primary visual nucleus of the thalamus, the lateral geniculate (LG). The lateral geniculate in turn densely innervates the primary visual cortex (area 17). A collateral pathway from the optic tract goes to the superficial layers of the superior colliculus (SC) in the midbrain, and from there to the deeper layers of the superior colliculus.

Shown in blue, the auditory pathway ascends through the brainstem to the central nucleus of the inferior colliculus (IC). From this midbrain center, axons project to the primary auditory nucleus of the thalamus, the medial geniculate (MG). The medial geniculate in turn innervates the primary or core auditory cortex (area 41). A collateral branch of the auditory pathway extends to the external region of the inferior colliculus, and from there to the deep layers of the adjacent superior colliculus.

Shown in red, individual neurons in the deep superior colliculus that receive convergent visual and auditory information project to nonprimary thalamic nuclei, including the medial, lateral, and inferior pulvinar and the ancillary nuclei of the medial geniculate. From those nuclei, two types of projections are formed to sensory cortex. Shown in solid red lines, the lateral and inferior pulvinar nuclei project to layer 4 of higher levels of visual cortex (areas 18 and 19), while the medial pulvinar and ancillary medial geniculate nuclei project to higher-level auditory cortex (areas 42 and 22). Shown in dotted red lines, the same pathways form tangential axons in layer 1 of primary visual cortex (area 17) and core auditory cortex (area 41). (See Chapter 13.)

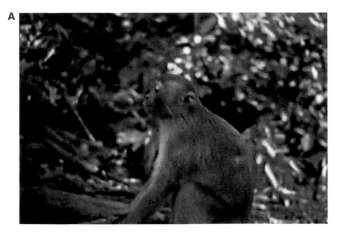

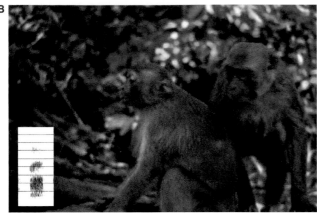

PLATE 2 (*A*) Silent threat expression by juvenile female rhesus macaque, *Macaca mulatta* (Z63), including a *stare, raised eyebrows,* and *ears back.* (*B*) Vocal threat by same female a moment later, including identical visual components with added *bark.* Inset in *B* shows spectrogram of typical bark, with bars from 1 to 8 kHz. Images were digitized from videotape by the author. Monkeys were filmed with permission from the University of Puerto Rico and the Caribbean Primate Research Center. (See Chapter 14.)

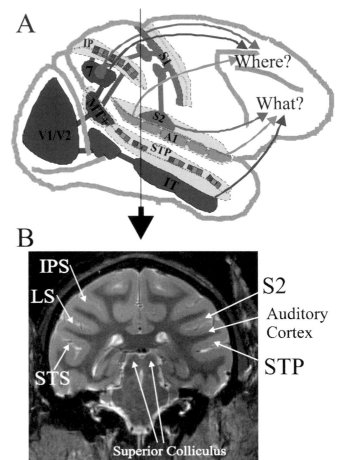

PLATE 3 (*A*) The major sensory and multisensory regions of posterior sensory neocortex. The classic multisensory areas of the superior temporal polysensory (STP) and those in the intraparietal (IP) sulcus are indicated by tricolor patches and shown in relation to the proposed "where" and "what" divisions of the visual (red), auditory (blue), and somatosensory (olive) systems. Sulcal regions are depicted with dashed lines and gray shading. (*B*) Coronal MRI section through a macaque monkey brain at the level indicated by the cut line in *A*, illustrating the anatomical location of several important multisensory regions of posterior sensory neocortex. Also indicated is the position of the superior colliculus. The section is a T2-weighted image taken at 7.0 Tesla, with a section thickness of 2 mm and in-plane resolution of 0.5 × 0.5 mm. Abbreviations: IPS, intraparietal sulcus; LS, lateral sulcus; STS, superior temporal sulcus; STP, superior temporal polysensory area. (Adapted from Schroeder et al., in press.) (See Chapter 18.)

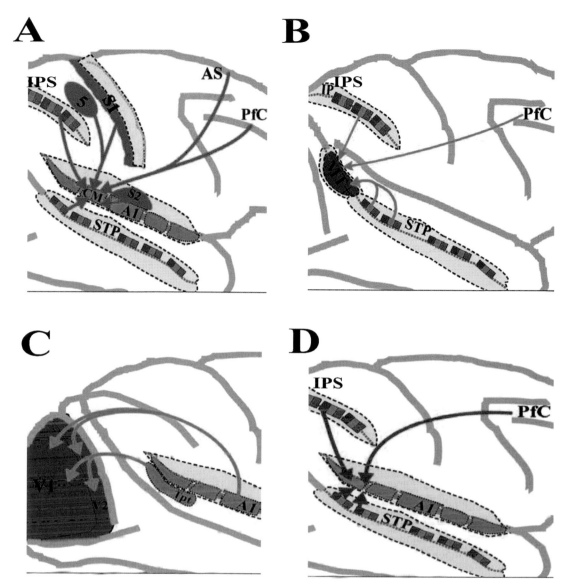

PLATE 4   Schematic diagrams of known projections that are potential substrates for multisensory convergence at early stages of auditory and visual processing. (*A*) Potential sources of somatosensory input to auditory area CM. Abbreviations: IPS, intraparietal sulcus; 5, area 5; S1, somatosensory areas 3a, 3b, 1, and 2; AS, anterior cingulate cortex; PfC, prefrontal cortex; S2, areas "S2" and posteroventral somatosensory cortex; A1, primary auditory cortex; CM, caudomedial auditory cortex; STP, superior temporal polysensory area. (*B*) Potential sources of auditory feedback input into MT+ (MT plus MST). (*C*) Sources of auditory input to V1 (primary visual cortex) and V2 (secondary visual cortex), as identified by Falchier et al. (2001) and Rockland and Ojima (2001). (*D*) Potential sources of visual feedback input into posterior auditory association cortex. (Adapted from Schroeder et al., in press.) (See Chapter 18.)

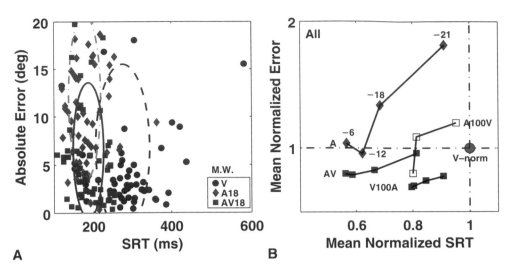

A **B**

PLATE 5 (*A*) First-saccade reaction time versus absolute error of the saccade end-point for V-only (red circles), A-only (−18 dB S/N; green diamonds) and synchronous AV saccades (blue squares). The latter capture the best of both modalities: AV saccades are as fast as A-only saccades and as accurate as V-only saccades, and have less end-point scatter (ellipses). (*B*) Summary of the results averaged and normalized in relation to V-only across subjects. All AV conditions show signs of integration, because none of the AV results coincide with the unimodal conditions. See text for explanation. (Modified from Corneil, Van Wanrooij, et al., 2002.) (See Chapter 23.)

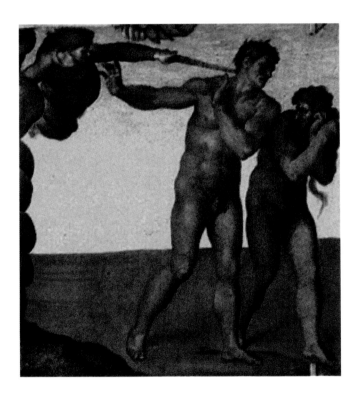

PLATE 6 Detail from Michelangelo's *Fall and Expulsion from Eden*. Both Adam and Eve are in classic defensive poses, with the head turned and the hands raised to defend the face. (See Chapter 27.)

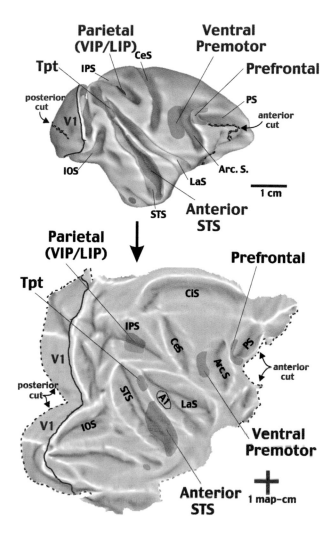

PLATE 7   Approximate locations of cortical sites for audiovisual convergence (green) in the macaque monkey. The location of primary visual cortex (blue line) and an estimate of primary auditory cortex (yellow outline) are also indicated. Red dashed lines depict two of the cuts introduced to flatten the cortical model, which also aid orienting to the flat map format (adapted from Drury et al., 1996). Arc. S., arcuate sulcus; CeS, central sulcus; CiS, cingulate sulcus; IOS, inferior occipital sulcus; IPS, intraparietal sulcus; LaS, lateral (sylvian) sulcus; PS, principal sulcus; STS, superior temporal sulcus. (Adapted from Drury et al., 1996.) (See Chapter 30.)

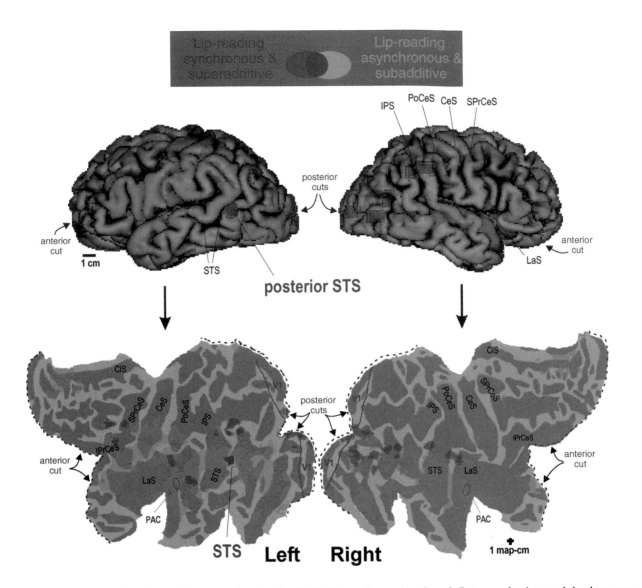

PLATE 8   Cross-modal facilitation and suppression in the STS. Three-dimensional and flat map brain models show group-averaged data (n = 10) obtained during an fMRI study of cross-modal audiovisual speech. Brain areas exhibiting superadditive responses to matched audiovisual speech stimuli (yellow) are superimposed on areas showing subadditive responses to mismatched speech cues (blue). Green highlights areas meeting both criteria. (Adapted from Calvert et al., 2000.) (See Chapter 30.)

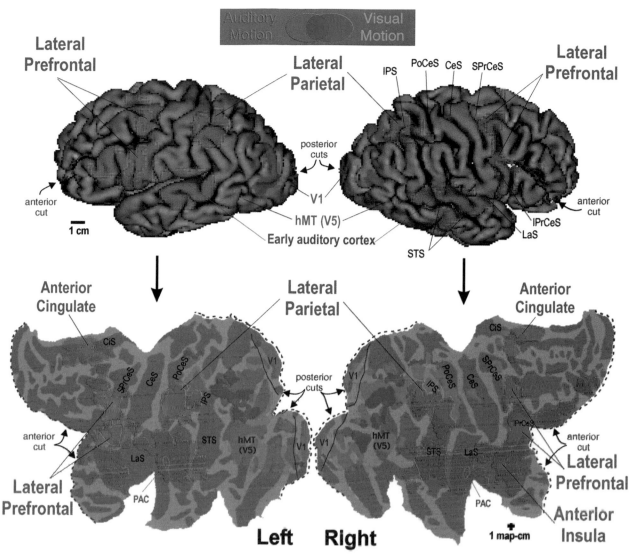

PLATE 9   Cortical overlap of auditory and visual spatial motion processing pathways. Three-dimensional and flat map brain models show group-averaged (n = 9) fMRI activation patterns from an auditory motion paradigm (yellow) and a separate visual motion paradigm (blue plus purple), together with regions of overlap (green). Purple indicates visually responsive regions deactivated during the auditory motion task. The approximate locations of primary auditory cortex (PAC, yellow ovals) and primary visual cortex (V1, dark blue lines) are indicated (Bonferroni corrected $P < 0.001$). Anatomical underlay is the visible human male (Van Essen et al., 1998), and red dashed lines depict two of the cuts introduced to flatten the cortical model. HG, Heschl's gyrus; IPrCeS, inferior precentral sulcus. See text and Figure 30.1 for other details. (Adapted from Lewis et al., 2000.) (See Chapter 30.)

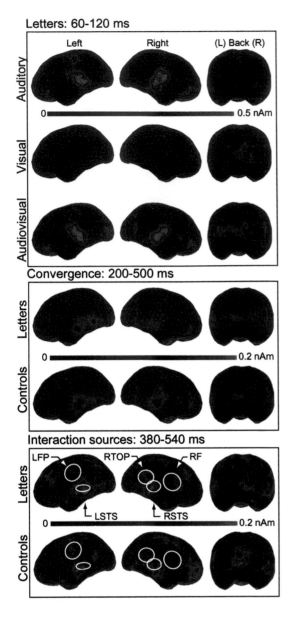

Letters: 60-120 ms

Convergence: 200-500 ms

Interaction sources: 380-540 ms

PLATE 10 MCE source analysis for audiovisual integration of single letters. Upper panel shows early activations (60–120 ms) for auditory, visual, and audiovisual letters. In the middle panel, convergence was calculated as the minimum of the auditory and visual unimodal activations. The Boolean AND operator between unimodal auditory and visual activations corresponding to multiplying the values could have been used as well, but this approach was rejected because of possible noise amplification. In the lower panel, interaction was calculated as the difference between the sum of unimodal auditory and visual activations (A+V) compared with the activity evoked by bimodal audiovisual (AV) stimulus presentation. (Adapted from Raij et al., 2000.) (See Chapter 32.)

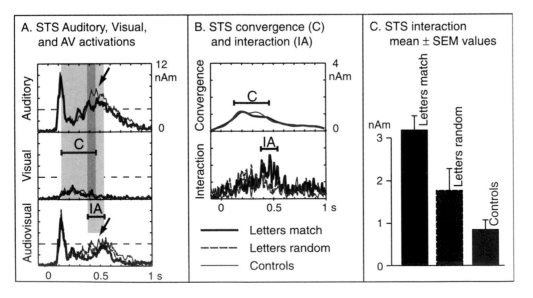

A. STS Auditory, Visual, and AV activations

B. STS convergence (C) and interaction (IA)

C. STS interaction mean ± SEM values

Letters match
Letters random
Controls

PLATE 11 Audiovisual properties of left superior temporal sulcus (STS) activation for letter stimuli. Left panel shows the STS time courses of auditory, visual, and audiovisual activations. Middle panel shows convergence and interaction. Right panel shows the differences in the strength of interaction between matching letters, nonmatching letters, and control stimuli. (Adapted from Raij et al., 2000.) (See Chapter 32.)

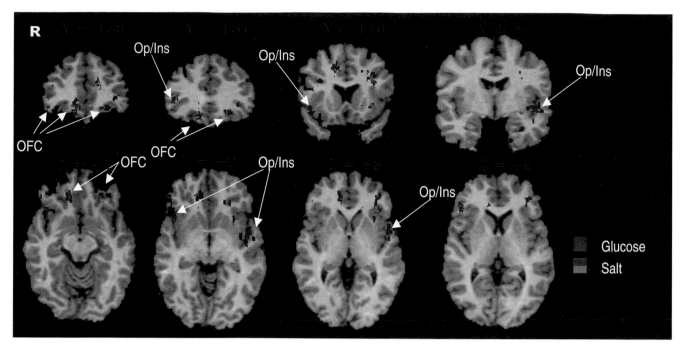

PLATE 12   Group map showing regions of the human brain activated by a pleasant taste (glucose) and an aversive taste (salt). The z-maps from individual subjects were thresholded at $P < 0.01$ (uncorrected) and transformed into Talairach space. Voxels that were commonly activated in a minimum of six out of seven subjects were included in the group combination image (although clusters of less than three contiguous voxels were excluded). Glucose activations are depicted in blue (voxels common to six subjects) and light blue (voxels common to seven subjects). Salt activations are depicted in orange (voxels common to six subjects) and yellow (voxels common to seven subjects). Areas of overlap between the two tastes are shown in green. Coronal sections through regions of interest such as the orbitofrontal cortex and operculum/insula are shown in the top row, and transverse sections are shown in the bottom row, at the Talairach levels indicated. Arrows with labels point to some of the activated regions. OFC, orbitofrontal cortex; Op/Ins, frontal operculum/insula. (From O'Doherty, Rolls, et al., 2001.) (See Chapter 35.)

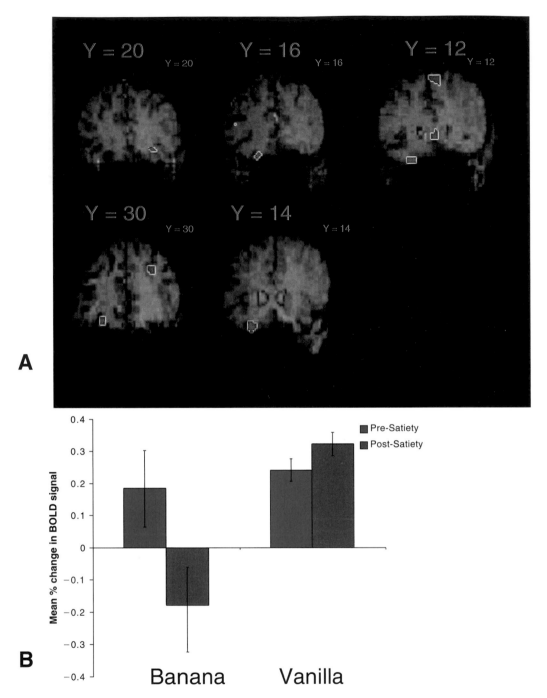

PLATE 13   Olfactory sensory-specific satiety. The figure shows regions of orbitofrontal cortex in which the BOLD signal produced by the presentation of banana and vanilla odor was modulated by sensory-specific satiety by feeding to satiety with one of the two foods (banana). Coronal sections at the anterior (*y*) levels shown through the orbitofrontal cortex are shown for five separate subjects. The threshold is set at $P < 0.05$ corrected for multiple comparisons. (From O'Doherty et al., 2000.) (See Chapter 35.)

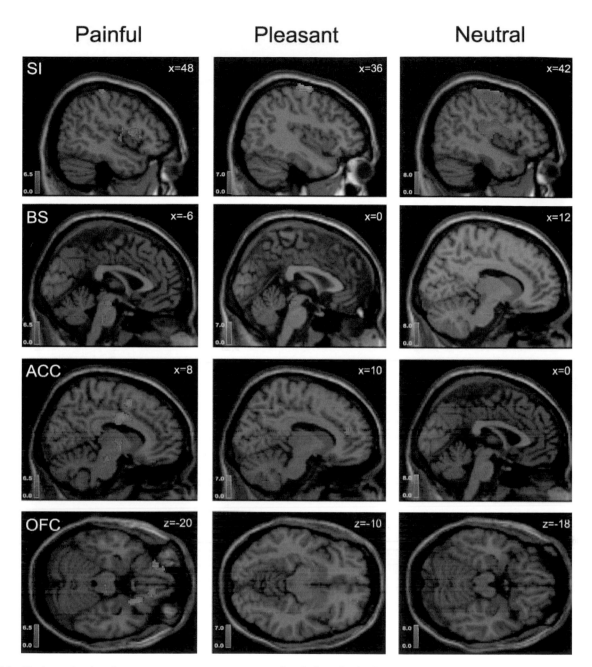

PLATE 14 Brain activation in response to somatosensory stimulation. Sagittal sections are shown for each of the three conditions, painful, pleasant, and neutral, with the group activation significant at $P < 0.05$ (corrected) for multiple comparisons of the contralateral (right) somatosensory cortex (SI), and sagittal sections are shown for activation in brainstem (BS). For the painful and pleasant conditions, sagittal section of activations in the anterior cingulate cortex (ACC) and axial sections of activations in the orbitofrontal cortex are shown. The activations have been thresholded at $P < 0.0001$ to show the extent of activation. (From Rolls et al., 2002.) (See Chapter 35.)

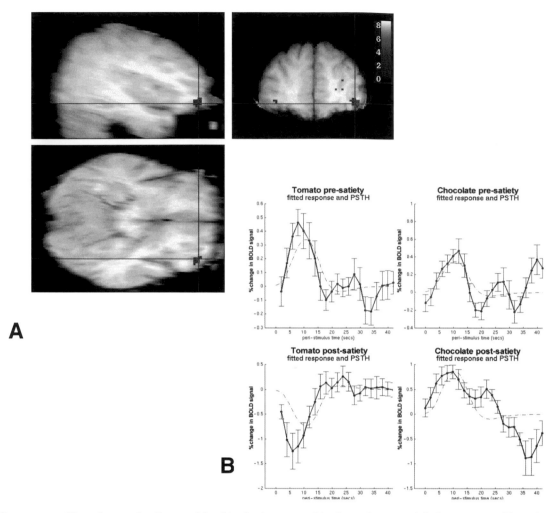

PLATE 15   Sensory-specific satiety to the flavor of food in the human orbitofrontal cortex. (*A*) Sensory-specific satiety-related activation in right mediolateral orbitofrontal cortex to the flavor of food in a single subject fed to satiety on tomato juice. The threshold is set at $P < 0.001$ (uncorrected). (*B*) A plot of the time course of the BOLD response in orbitofrontal cortex is shown for the same subject. Following satiety, the response to the food eaten (tomato juice) is greatly decreased relative to the response to the food not eaten (chocolate milk). This decrease in activation occurred concomitantly with a decrease in the subjective pleasantness of the food. (See Chapter 35.)

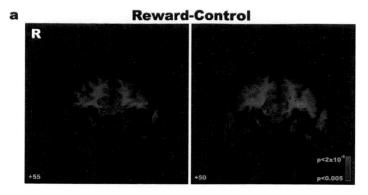

Reward-Control

R

+55   +50

p<2x10⁻⁵
p<0.005

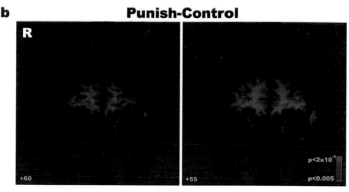

Punish-Control

R

+60   +55

p<2x10⁻⁵
p<0.005

PLATE 16   Comparison of monetary rewards and punishments with a control condition. (*A*) A region of bilateral medial orbitofrontal cortex and medial prefrontal cortex is significantly activated relative to a neutral baseline in the Reward-Control contrast. (*B*) A region of bilateral lateral orbitofrontal cortex is significantly activated relative to a neutral baseline in the Punish-Control contrast. (From O'Doherty, Kringelbach, et al., 2001.) (See Chapter 35.)

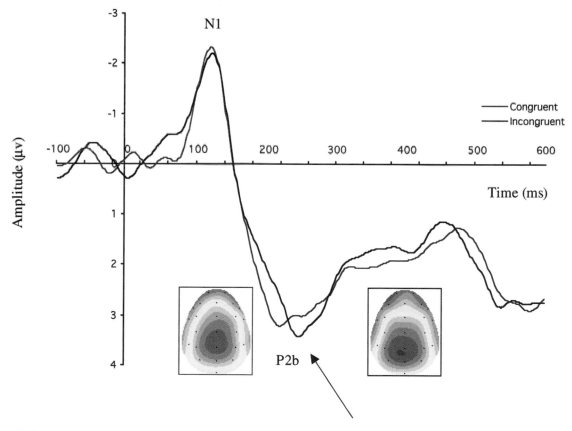

PLATE 17   EEG results. Grand averaged auditory waveforms at the CPz electrode measured during the presentation of congruent and incongruent audiovisual stimulus pairs (and corresponding topographies at 224 ms and 242 ms in the congruent and incongruent condition, respectively). Auditory processing is delayed in time by around 220 ms when realized under an incongruent visual context. (See Chapter 36.)

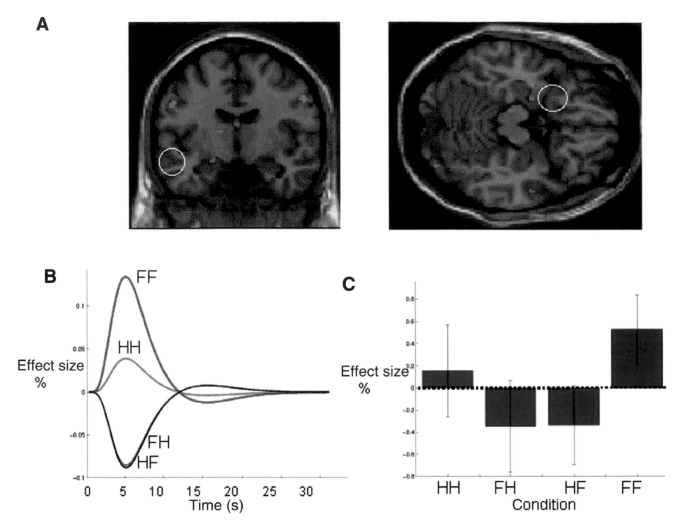

PLATE 18   fMRI results. A statistical parametric map shows an enhanced response in the left amygdala in response to congruent fearful faces plus fearful voices. Condition: H, happy; F, fearful. (See Chapter 36.)

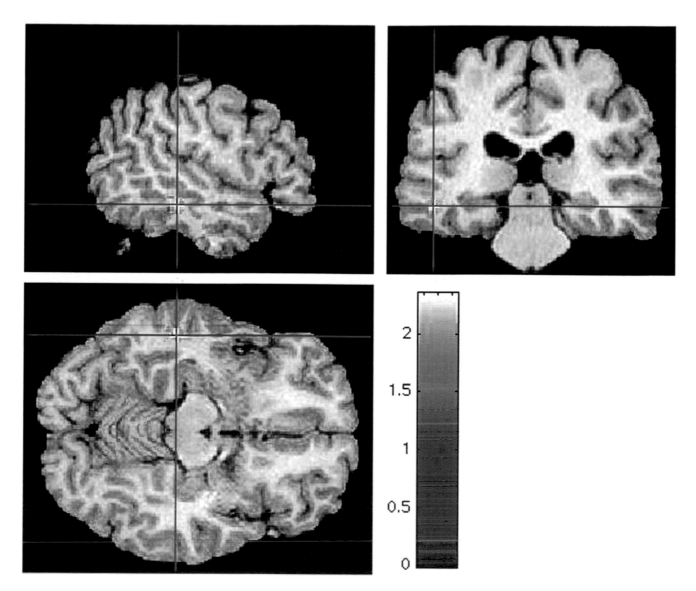

PLATE 19   PET results. Coronal, axial, and sagittal PET sections showing significant activation of a multisensory region in the left middle temporal gyrus ($-52x$, $-30y$, $-12x$) in eight normal subjects during audiovisual trials (happy and fearful emotions) compared with unimodal trials (Visual + Auditory). (See Chapter 36.)

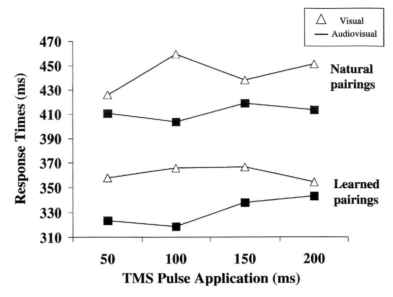

PLATE 20 Results of the TMS experiment. Response times are plotted as a function of the SOA between stimulus presentation and pulse deliverance (a single pulse was delivered 50, 100, 150, or 200 ms after stimulus presentation) when TMS is applied over the left posterior parietal cortex. In the Learned condition (burst tone paired with geometrical figure), there was significant interaction between Modality × SOA, indicating that audiovisual trials are not faster than visual trials at 200 ms. In the Natural condition (tone of voice paired with facial expression), the interaction Modality × SOA is not significant. (See Chapter 36.)

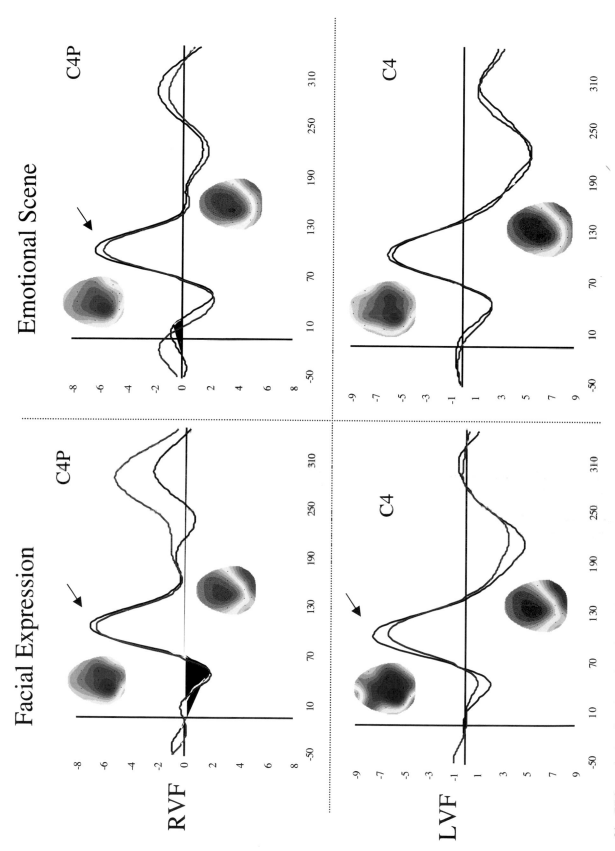

PLATE 21 EEG results in a hemianopic patient with a complete unilateral lesion of the primary visual cortex. Shown are grand averaged auditory waveforms and corresponding topographies (horizontal axis) obtained at central electrodes in each visual condition (congruent pairs in black, incongruent pairs in red) and for each visual hemifield (left/blind vs. right/intact). Congruent pairs elicited a higher auditory N1 component than incongruent pairs for visual presentations (facial expressions or emotional scenes) in the intact field but, only for facial expressions in the blind field. For each topographic map (N1 and P2 components), the time interval is 20 ms and the amplitude scale goes from $-6\ \mu V$ (in blue) to $+6\ \mu V$ (in red). (See Chapter 36.)

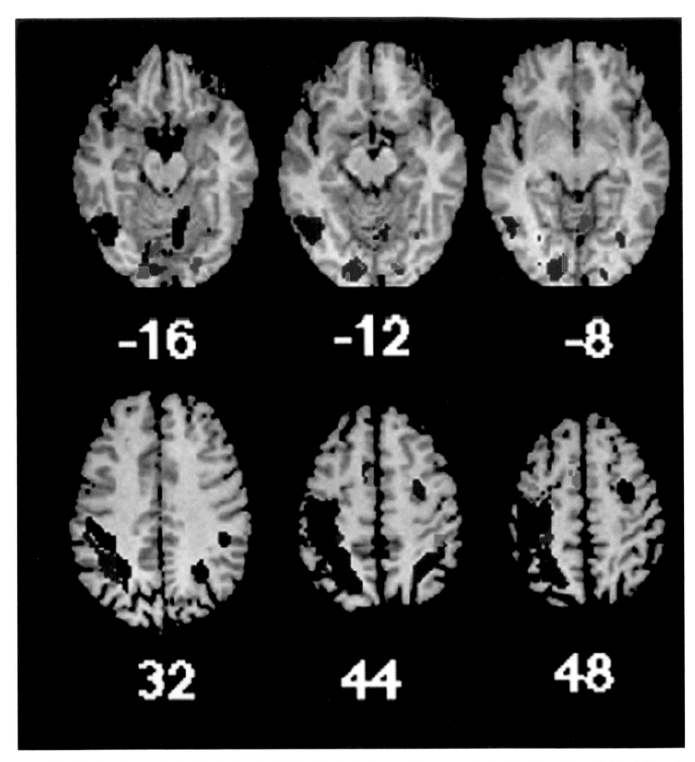

PLATE 22   Conjunction analysis of activation by Braille discrimination task by congenitally blind ($n = 4$), early-blind ($n = 4$), and late-blind ($n = 4$) groups, superimposed on typical MR images unrelated to the study's subjects. Transaxial images 4–16 mm below and 32–52 mm above the anteroposterior commissural line are shown. The pixels show levels of statistical significance above $P < 0.05$ with correction for multiple comparisons at voxel level. Areas commonly activated in congenitally blind, early-blind, and late-blind subjects (violet), congenitally blind and early-blind but not late-blind individuals (red), congenitally blind and late-blind but not early-blind individuals (yellow), early-blind and late-blind but not congenitally blind individuals (green), early-blind individuals only (light blue), and late-blind individuals only (pink) are shown. The primary visual cortex is commonly activated in congenitally blind and early-blind individuals but not in late-blind individuals. (Modified from Cohen et al., 1999.) (See Chapter 45.)

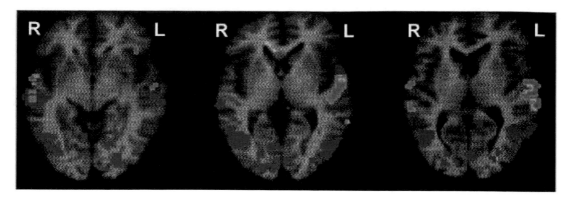

PLATE 23 Speech-reading and listening to speech. Shown are group median activation maps for hearing subjects in three contiguous transaxial scans (n = 7). Blue indicates regions activated by hearing speech; pink indicates regions activated by watching silent speech. Yellow regions are activated both by heard and seen speech. The overlap areas are in auditory cortex on the superior surface of the temporal lobe (From Calvert et al., 1997.) (See Chapter 48.)

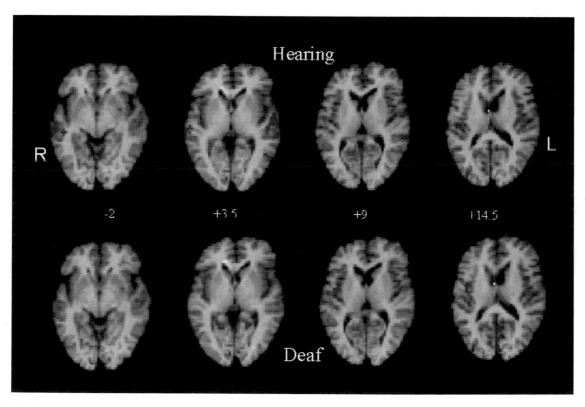

PLATE 24 Activation by speech-reading in hearing and deaf subjects. *Top:* Four contiguous axial images showing median activation by silent speech-reading in hearing subjects (n = 6). Superior temporal gyri were activated bilaterally, extending into auditory cortex. *Bottom:* Corresponding sections for deaf subjects (n = 6). Activation in the deaf subjects is in the right insular/frontal regions, the parahippocampal gyri bilaterally, and the posterior cingulate. There is no activation in auditory cortex-analogous regions. (Adapted from MacSweeney et al., 2001.) (See Chapter 48.)

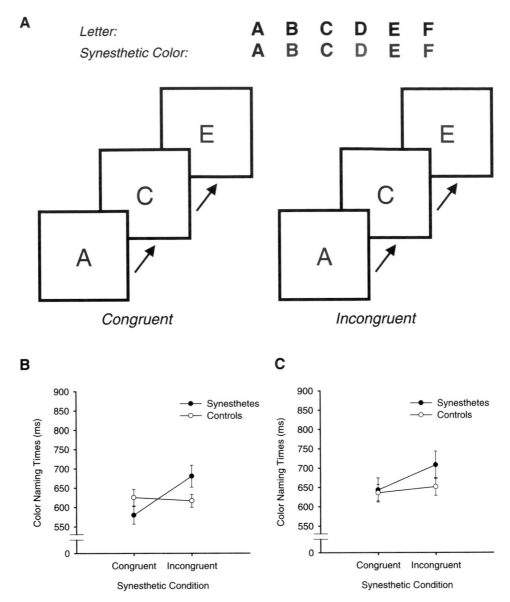

PLATE 25   The synesthetic Stroop task. (*A*) Alphanumeric characters printed in colors that either match ("congruent") or do not match ("incongruent") the synesthetic color experiences of synesthete T.S. (*B*) Mean correct color naming times for 15 synesthetes and 15 nonsynesthetic controls, performing the synesthetic Stroop task—blocked presentation of congruent and incongruent trials. (*C*) Randomized presentation of congruent and incongruent trials. (*A* adapted with permission from Rich and Mattingley, 2002. *B* and *C* reproduced with permission from Mattingley et al., 2001a.) (See Chapter 53.)

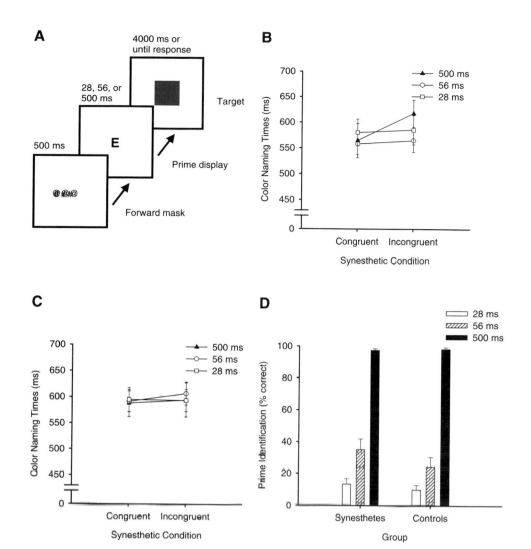

PLATE 26   The synesthetic priming task. (*A*) Sequence of events in a typical trial. The task was to name the target color as quickly as possible. (*B*) Mean correct color naming times for congruent and incongruent trials at prime durations of 28, 56, and 500 ms for synesthetes. (*C*) Nonsynesthetic controls. (*D*) Mean percent correct prime identification for synesthetes and controls. (*B–D* reproduced with permission from Mattingley et al., 2001a.) (See Chapter 53.)

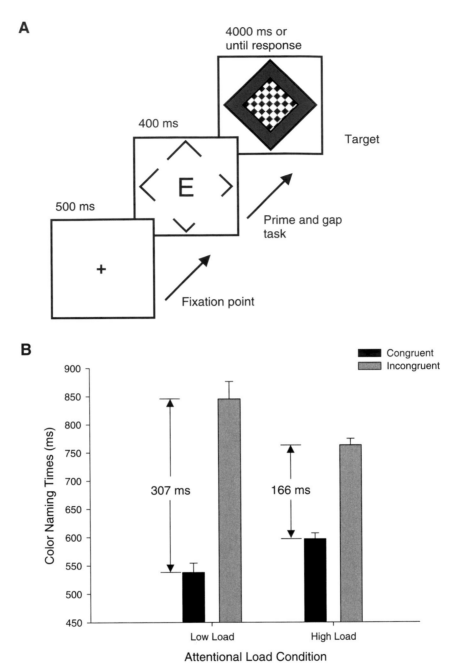

PLATE 27   The effects of priming with a concurrent attentional load on color naming in a variant of the synesthetic priming task. (*A*) Sequence of events in a typical trial of the attentional load paradigm. The primary task was to name the target color as quickly as possible; the secondary task in the low- and high-load conditions was to discriminate the larger of two gaps on diagonally opposite sides of the diamond in the prime display. (*B*) Mean correct color naming times in the low- and high-load conditions for a representative synesthete, with separate bars showing data from congruent and incongruent trials. (See Chapter 53.)

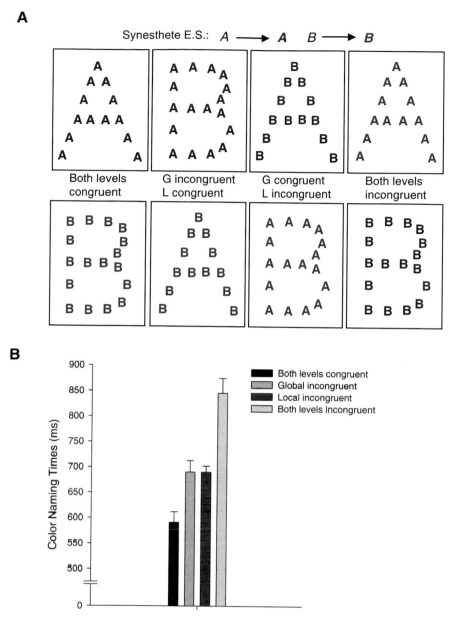

PLATE 28   Synesthetic rivalry induced by global alphanumeric characters composed of local characters. (*A*) Examples of the four stimulus types used to study the effect of rivalry between synesthetic inducers. The task was to name the stimulus color as quickly as possible. Participants never had to name the alphanumeric characters, which were irrelevant and nonpredictive with respect to the display color. (*B*) Mean correct color naming times for each of the four local-global stimulus types, which were randomly intermingled. Data shown are from a single representative synesthete. (G, global; L, local.) (See Chapter 53.)

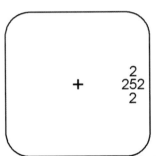

PLATE 29 Schematic representation of displays used to test whether synesthetically induced colors lead to pop-out. (*A*) When presented with a matrix of 5s with a triangle composed of 2s embedded in it, control subjects find it difficult to find the triangle. (*B*) However, because they see the 5s (say) green and the 2s as red, our synesthetic subjects were able to easily find the embedded shape. (See Chapter 54.)

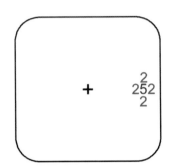

PLATE 30 Demonstration of the crowding effect. A single grapheme presented in the periphery is easily identifiable. However, when it is flanked by other graphemes, the target grapheme becomes much harder to detect. Synesthetic colors are effective (as are real colors) in overcoming this effect. (See Chapter 54.)

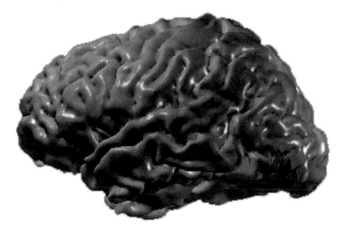

PLATE 31 Schematic showing that cross-wiring in the fusiform might be the neural basis of grapheme-color synesthesia. The left hemisphere of one author's brain (EMH) is shown with area V4 indicated in red and the number-grapheme area indicated in green. (See Chapter 54.)

29 Multisensory Representations of Space in the Posterior Parietal Cortex

YALE E. COHEN AND RICHARD A. ANDERSEN

Introduction

Actions are often directed toward the location of sensory stimuli. It can be argued that a large component of our mental repertoire is dedicated toward directing motor effectors toward the location of a sensory stimulus (Snyder, 2000). The diverse computations underlying this capacity are often grouped under the rubric of the sensorimotor transformation.

In this chapter, we focus on the importance of one component of the sensorimotor transformation, reference-frame (coordinate) transformations. Reference-frame transformations are not trivial, because the location of a sensory stimulus is often coded in a reference frame that is different from the one used by the eventual motor effector. In particular, we examine the role of the posterior parietal cortex (PPC) in reference-frame transformations. We introduce evidence that an aspect of the reference-frame transformation is to represent target locations in a common reference frame in a significant population of neurons in two areas of the PPC. This common reference frame is an eye-centered representation that is "gain" modulated by such factors as eye, head, body, or initial hand position. The advantage of this representation is that it allows the PPC to maintain representations of many different reference frames that can be read out depending on the cognitive and computational needs of the ongoing task. In the next section we introduce the concept of a reference frame and reference-frame transformations, and then discuss the role of the PPC in movement planning and reference-frame transformations.

Reference frames and reference-frame transformations

A reference frame can be defined as a set of axes that describes the location of an object. Many different reference frames can be used to describe the location of the same object. For instance, imagine that you are sitting in the park and looking at a flower in a field. The location of the flower can be described based on the pattern of light that falls on your eyes and retinas. The location of the flower can also be described relative to your head or body position. It is also possible to describe the flower's location in an extrinsic reference frame, one that is based on objects in the world. For example, the flower's location can be described relative to its position in the field or the location of the bench on which you are sitting.

Describing the location of an object in different frames of reference is not simply an academic exercise. Instead, it is a critical computation that underlies our capacity to engage in different types of goal-directed behaviors (Andersen, Snyder, Bradley, & Xing, 1997; Colby, 1998; Graziano, 2001; Pouget & Snyder, 2000). For instance, if you want to look at the flower, it is important to know the location of the flower relative to your eyes and head. In contrast, if you want to pick the flower, it is important to be able to compute the location of the flower relative to your arm and hand.

Although we have focused our description of reference frames on visual stimuli, we can also describe the location of other modality stimuli. However, the computations underlying this capacity initially depend on modality-specific mechanisms. Describing the location of a visual stimulus depends initially on the pattern of light that falls on the retinas and the resulting activation of photoreceptors. In contrast, describing the location of an auditory stimulus depends initially on the brain's capacity to compute interaural level and timing differences and monaural spectral cues (Blauert, 1997; Cohen & Knudsen, 1999; Middlebrooks & Green, 1991). Locating a tactile stimulus uses a third mechanism that is based on the pattern of activity in the array of tactile receptors that lie beneath the skin's surface. This mechanism is akin to that used by the visual system in that both code the location of a stimulus based on the activity in a topographic array of receptors.

The motor system also codes the movement of effectors in particular reference frames (Klier, Wang, & Crawford, 2001; Soechting & Flanders, 1995; Sparks, 1989; Sparks & Mays, 1990). Arm movements are coded based on the difference between initial and final hand position (a limb-centered reference frame; Soechting & Flanders, 1992, 1995). Similarly, eye movements are coded based on the difference between current and desired eye position (an eye-centered reference frame; Sparks, 1989; Sparks & Mays, 1990).

Given these descriptions of motor and sensory reference frames, a computational issue becomes immediately evident. Namely, how can sensory information that is collected in one reference frame guide motor acts that are calculated in a different reference frame? For instance, how can an arm movement that is calculated in a limb-centered reference frame be directed toward a sound whose location is calculated in a head-centered reference frame? The solution to this reference-frame problem is to transform the representation of a sensory stimulus into one that is appropriate for the eventual motor act (Flanders, Tillery, & Soechting, 1992; Ghilardi, Gordon, & Ghez, 1995; Kalaska & Crammond, 1992; Soechting & Flanders, 1989a, 1989b). The PPC plays an important role in this reference-frame transformation. In the next section we highlight the role of the PPC in movement planning and present evidence that, as one element of this reference-frame transformation, the PPC represents target locations that are used in movement planning in a common reference frame.

Role of the PPC in movement planning

A large component of PPC activity appears to be dedicated to the coordination of different movement plans. Although we will stress here the role of the PPC in movement planning, neurons in areas of the PPC are modulated by other cognitive intermediates of sensorimotor transformation. An analysis of these different signals is outside the scope of this discussion but can be found elsewhere (see, e.g., Andersen & Buneo, 2002; Colby & Goldberg, 1999; Kusunoki, Gottlieb, & Goldberg, 2000).

Three functionally distinct movement-planning regions have been identified so far: the lateral intraparietal area (area LIP), the parietal reach region (PRR), and the anterior intraparietal area (area AIP). LIP neurons are modulated preferentially by sensory targets that indicate the future location of an eye movement (Platt & Glimcher, 1997; Snyder, Batista, & Andersen,

1997, 1998, 2000). The PRR, which overlaps with the medial intraparietal area and parieto-occipital cortex, codes reaches (Battaglia-Mayer et al., 2000; Calton, Dickinson, & Snyder, 2002; Colby & Duhamel, 1991; Eskandar & Assad, 1999; Galletti, Battaglini, & Fattori, 1993, 1995; Galletti et al., 1996, 1997, 1999, 2001; Johnson, Ferraina, Bianchi, & Caminiti, 1996; Snyder, Batista, et al., 1997, 1998, 2000). AIP neurons are modulated preferentially by the size, shape, and orientation of objects that specify a particular grasp (Gallese, Murata, Kaseda, Niki, & Sakata, 1994; Murata, Gallese, Kaseda, & Sakata, 1996; Murata, Gallese, Luppino, Kaseda, & Sakata, 2000; Sakata, Taira, Kusunoki, Murata, & Tanaka, 1997).

The different roles of area LIP and PRR in movement planning have been demonstrated in delayed eye-movement and delayed reach tasks in monkeys (Snyder et al., 1997). In the delayed eye-movement task, monkeys made saccades (rapid eye movements) to the location of remembered visual targets. In the delayed reach task, monkeys made reaches to the location of remembered visual targets. Data were analyzed during the period that followed visual-target offset but before any movements were made to the remembered targets. Delay-period activity was examined, because it is not confounded by the presence of the visual stimulus or by the movement itself (Gnadt & Andersen, 1988).

An analysis of the neural activity during this delay period indicated that LIP neurons responded significantly more during the delayed eye-movement task than during the delayed reach task. The response pattern of PRR neurons was the opposite: PRR neurons responded significantly more during the delayed reach task than during the delayed eye-movement task. These two results are consistent with the hypothesis that LIP neurons are preferentially involved in coordinating eye-movement plans, whereas PRR neurons are preferentially involved in coordinating reach plans.

The third identified movement planning area, area AIP, appears to be specialized for grasp planning (Sakata et al., 1997). Reversible inactivations of area AIP produce deficits in a monkey's ability to make the precise finger movements that are required to shape his hand to appropriately grasp an object (Gallese et al., 1994). Supporting this behavioral finding, a neurophysiological study demonstrated that AIP neurons respond preferentially to (1) specifically shaped and oriented objects and (2) the specific hand configurations that are required to properly grasp an object (Murata et al., 1996). These behavioral and neurophysiological studies, as well as other studies (Murata et al., 2000; Nakamura et al., 2001; Sakata, Taira, Murata, & Mine, 1995; Sakata et al., 1999), are consistent with the hypothesis that area AIP plays a role in the coordination of grasp plans.

This parceling of the PPC into functionally distinct regions is not limited to non-human primates. Functional-imaging and patient studies indicate a similar organizational schema for the human PPC (Binkofski et al., 1998; Connolly, Goodale, DeSouza, Menon, & Vilis, 2000; DeSouza et al., 2000; Jancke, Kleinschmidt, Mirzazde, Shah, & Freund, 2001; Karnath, Ferber, & Himmelback, 2001; Kawashima et al., 1996; Luna et al., 1998; Rushworth, Paus, & Sipila, 2001). These studies have identified functional regions in the human PPC that are specialized for eye movements, reaches, and grasps.

Insofar as regions of the PPC are involved in movement planning, it is reasonable to predict that PPC neurons are involved in the coordination of movement plans to targets of different sensory modalities, and this proposition has been borne out in several recent experiments. LIP and PRR neurons respond to auditory and visual stimuli that indicate the future location of a movement (Cohen & Andersen, 2000; Cohen, Batista, & Andersen, 2002; Grunewald, Linden, & Andersen, 1999; Linden, Grunewald, & Andersen, 1999; Mazzoni, Bracewell, Barash, & Andersen, 1996; Stricanne, Andersen, & Mazzoni, 1996). Figure 29.1A shows a PRR response profile that was generated while a monkey made reaches to the remembered location of auditory stimuli. Figure 29.1B shows the response profile from a different PRR neuron that was generated while a monkey made reaches to the remembered location of visual stimuli. All aspects of the task modulated both neurons, since they responded during the presentation of the sensory target, during a delay period that followed the offset of the sensory cue, and during the reach period itself. Functional imaging studies in humans also suggest that the PPC contributes to tasks that use auditory and visual stimuli (Bremmer et al., 2001; Bushara et al., 1999; Griffiths et al., 1998).

Although PPC neurons respond to both auditory and visual targets, they do not appear to code these sensory modalities in a completely similar manner. For example, auditory responses in area LIP appear to be the result of behavioral training in which a monkey has been trained to associate the auditory stimulus with a future eye movement (Grunewald et al., 1999; Linden et al., 1999). In contrast, in untrained or even anesthetized animals, LIP neurons respond robustly to visual stimuli (Grunewald et al., 1999; Blatt, Andersen, & Stoner, 1990). Another difference is that the spatial selectivity of PPC neurons for auditory-target and visual-target locations is different (Cohen et al., 2002; Grunewald et al., 1999; Linden et al., 1999). This difference can be

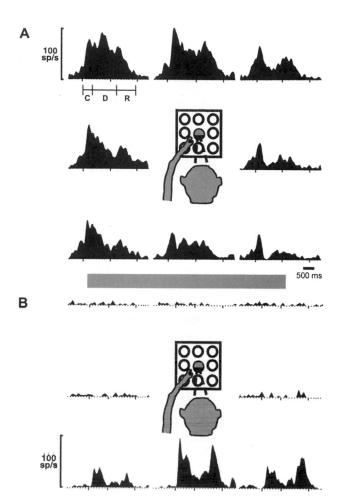

FIGURE 29.1   (A) Response of a PRR neuron during reaches to the remembered location of an auditory stimulus. (B) Response of a PRR neuron during reaches to the remembered location of a visual stimulus. Shown in each case are a schematic of the monkey's initial hand and eye position and a PRR response profile. Circles indicate the relative position of a touch-sensitive button assembly. Each assembly contained light-emitting diodes, which produced visual stimuli, and a speaker, which produced an auditory stimulus. The gray circle in the assembly indicates the button that the monkey pressed initially, and the black circle indicates the button that the monkey fixated; the converging lines indicate the direction of the monkey's gaze. Following presentation of a sensory stimulus from one of the assemblies, monkeys reached and pressed the button in which the stimulus originated. The response profiles are arranged as a function of target location, and neural activity is represented by spike-density histograms. The histograms are aligned relative to the onset of the sensory cue. The gray bar indicates the time of cue onset and the duration of the cue. Tic interval = 100 ms. In A, C, D, and R indicate the times of the cue, delay, and reach periods, respectively. (Modified with permission from Cohen et al., 2002.)

seen in Figure 29.1 by comparing the response profile of a PRR neuron generated during the auditory task (Fig. 29.1A) with one generated during the visual task (Fig. 29.1B). To quantify these differences, we calculated the amount of information related to target location that is conveyed in the firing rate of PRR neurons during different epochs of the delayed reach task (Cohen et al., 2002). The advantage of this information analysis is that it provides a continuous measure (Cover & Thomas, 1991) of the relationship between neural activity and stimulus-target location. We found that during delayed reaches to visual targets, the firing rate of PRR neurons contained the same amount of information, with respect to target location, throughout the task. In contrast, the amount of information contained in the firing rate of PRR neurons during delayed reaches to auditory targets was initially less than that seen during delayed reaches to visual targets. However, as the trial evolved, the amount of information increased, by the reach period becoming equivalent to the amount coded during visual trials (Fig. 29.2). We interpret these data to suggest that the quantity being encoded in the firing rate of PRR neurons is dynamic and changes as the sensory, cognitive, or motor demands of the task change (Cohen et al., 2002).

This form of dynamic coding of different aspects of a task has been seen in other PPC studies. For instance, in one study, a location on a visual object was cued briefly, the object was then rotated, and the monkey then saccaded to the remembered location of the cue (Sabes, Breznen, & Andersen, 2002). LIP neurons initially coded aspects of the visual stimulus, but as the task evolved, LIP activity became more correlated with the direction of the planned saccade. Similarly, during a saccade task in which the reward and target probabilities were altered, LIP neurons initially coded the monkey's expectancy regarding reward amount or target location, but during later periods of the task, LIP activity became more correlated with the location of the saccade target itself (Platt & Glimcher, 1999). In a recent study, monkeys were trained to judge the motion of moving dots on a visual display and to saccade in the direction of the motion (Shadlen & Newsome, 1996, 2001). LIP activity was initially modulated by the monkey's judgment of motion direction but not in later epochs of the task, when the monkeys had selected a saccadic target.

A common spatial representation in areas LIP and PRR

The reference frame of LIP and PRR activity has been studied by asking monkeys to make movements (saccades or reaches) from different initial starting positions. If neural activity is coded in the reference frame of the body part that is shifted, then the target location that elicits the maximal response from a neuron should shift as the initial starting position of the body part is

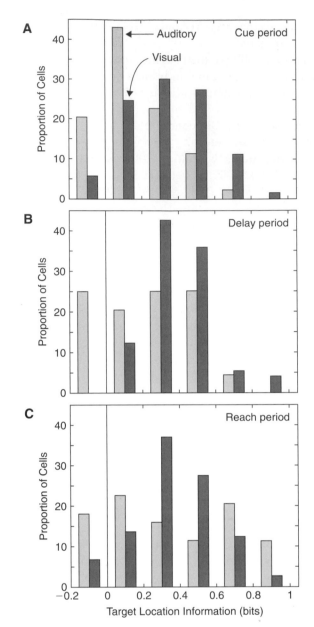

FIGURE 29.2 Distribution of target-location information for 44 PRR neurons that were recorded during delayed reaches to auditory targets and 67 PRR neurons that were recorded during delayed reaches to visual targets. Target-location information is shown for the cue (A), delay (B), and reach (C) periods. Target-location information is a non-parametric index of a neuron's spatial selectivity (Cohen et al., 2002; Cover & Thomas, 1991; Gnadt & Breznen, 1996; Grunewald et al., 1999). The gray bars indicate the distribution of target-location information for auditory-tested PRR neurons and the black bars indicate the distribution for visually-tested PRR neurons. (Modified with permission from Cohen et al., 2002.)

changed. If activity is not coded in that particular reference frame, then the responses of the neurons should be invariant to the shifts in body position.

For instance, LIP neurons code the location of a visual target in an eye-centered reference frame

(Andersen, Bracewell, Barash, Gnadt, & Fogassi, 1990; Brotchie, Andersen, Snyder, & Goodman, 1995; Snyder, Grieve, Brotchie, & Andersen, 1998). In this eye-centered reference frame, the location of a visual stimulus that maximally excites a LIP neuron changes as the monkey's eye position changes (Fig. 29.3A). Do LIP neurons that are responsive to auditory stimuli also code the location of auditory targets in an eye-centered reference frame? Because LIP neurons are involved in the planning of saccades to both auditory and visual stimuli (Grunewald et al., 1999; Linden et al., 1999; Mazzoni et al., 1996; Stricanne et al., 1996), a reasonable hypothesis would be that LIP neurons code the location of an auditory target in the same reference frame as visual targets, an eye-centered reference frame. To test this hypothesis, monkeys were placed in a darkened room and taught to saccade to the remembered locations of auditory stimuli from different initial fixation points (Stricanne et al., 1996). We examined LIP activity during the delay period that followed auditory-stimulus offset but preceded the eye movement. A general linear model tested whether the pattern of neural activity could be attributed to (1) the effect of auditory-target location relative to the monkey's initial eye position or (2) the effect of auditory-target location relative to the monkey's head. If the first variable was significant ($P < 0.05$), that would indicate that LIP activity coded auditory-target location in an eye-centered reference frame (Fig. 29.3A). In contrast, if the second variable was significant, that would suggest that LIP activity was coded in the original head-centered reference frame (Fig. 29.3B) (Blauert, 1997; Cohen & Knudsen, 1999; Middlebrooks & Green, 1991). This possibility, however, is also consistent with the hypothesis that LIP activity codes auditory-target location in a body- or world-centered reference frame; future experiments are needed to address this issue directly. Finally, if both variables were significant, that result would be consistent with the hypothesis that LIP activity codes auditory-target location in a reference frame that is intermediate between a head-centered and an eye-centered reference frame (Fig. 29.3C).

Consistent with the role of LIP in eye-movement planning, we found that a significant population (44%) of LIP neurons codes the location of an auditory target in an eye-centered reference frame. Also, 33% of the neurons coded auditory-target location in a head-centered reference frame. The remaining neurons appeared to code auditory-target location in an intermediate reference frame. The observation that some LIP neurons code auditory-target locations in head-centered and intermediate coordinates is important and suggests that area LIP, and perhaps the PPC in

general, may be directly involved in reference-frame transformations; this concept is discussed in more detail later in the chapter.

We have also examined the reference frame in which PRR neurons code reaches to visual targets (Batista, Buneo, Snyder, & Andersen, 1999). In this study, we examined two alternative hypotheses. First, since PRR neurons code reaches (Battaglia-Mayer et al., 2000; Calton et al., 2002; Eskandar & Assad, 1999; Galletti et al., 1993, 1995, 1996, 1997, 1999, 2001; Johnson et al., 1996; Snyder, Batista, et al., 1998; Snyder et al., 1997, 2000), a likely hypothesis would be that they code the location of visual targets in the reference frame of the motor effector, a reference frame that is based on the difference between initial and final hand position (a limb-centered reference frame; Fig. 29.3E). The second hypothesis that we explored was that PRR neurons code visual reach targets in an eye-centered reference frame (Fig. 29.3A). We explored this reference frame to test the hypothesis that if movement-planning areas in the PPC code in a similar reference frame, PRR activity should be in the same eye-centered reference frame as LIP activity.

These two hypotheses were examined by having monkeys participate in variants of a delayed-reach task to visual targets (see Fig. 29.4). In one variant, monkeys made delayed reaches from different initial-hand positions but maintained the same fixation point. If PRR activity is coded in a limb-centered reference frame (Fig. 29.3E), then the location that maximally excites PRR neurons should shift with changes in initial-hand position. In the second variant, monkeys made delayed reaches from different fixation points but maintained the same initial-hand position. If PRR activity is coded in an eye-centered reference frame (Fig. 29.3A), then the location that maximally excites PRR neurons should shift with changes in initial-eye position.

An example of a PRR neuron that was tested using this paradigm is shown in Figure 29.4. As can be seen, when the monkey made reaches to visual targets from different initial-hand positions, the peak location of the response profile of the neuron was unaltered. In contrast, when the monkey made identical reaches from different fixation points, the peak location of the response profile shifted with eye position. This neuron is typical of the vast majority of PRR neurons and, along with the remaining neurons studied, indicates that PRR neurons code in a format consistent with an eye-centered reference frame for reaches to visually cued locations.

In a separate study, we examined the reference frame of PRR neurons during delayed reaches to auditory targets. Based on the aforementioned results, we

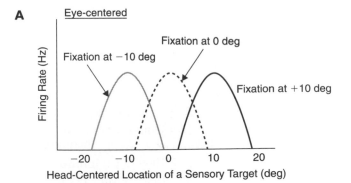

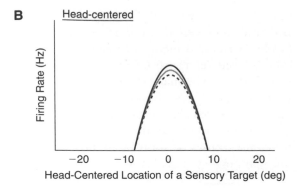

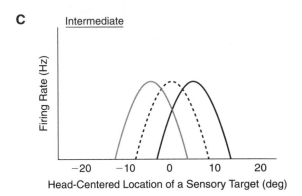

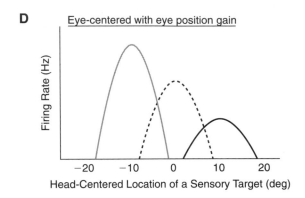

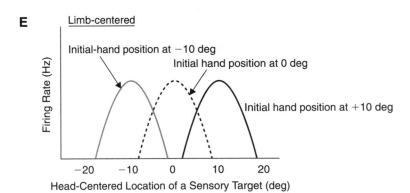

FIGURE 29.3 Schematic of different reference frames. The locations of sensory targets along the abscissa are plotted relative to the observer's head. Hypothetical response profiles in each plot are represented by the bell-shaped curves. (A) If a neuron codes the location of a sensory target in an eye-centered reference frame, then the peak location of the response profile shifts with eye position. For example, a +10-degree shift of eye position would shift the peak of the response profile by +10 degrees. (B) If a neuron codes the location of a sensory target in a head-centered reference frame, then the peak location of the response profile does not shift with eye position. The positions of the three response profiles are offset slightly for visual clarity. (C) If a neuron codes the location of a sensory target in an intermediate reference frame, the peak location of the response profile shifts with eye position. However, the magnitude of the shift is less than the change in eye position. In the hypothetical example shown, a +10-degree shift of eye position shifts the peak of the response profile by only +5 degrees. (D) If a neuron codes the location of a sensory target in an eye-centered reference frame that is modulated by eye position gain, then the peak of the response profile shifts with eye position. Additionally, the magnitude of the response should change with eye position. So, in the hypothetical example shown, a +10-degree shift of eye position shifts the response profile by +10 degrees and decreases the magnitude of the response by 50%. In contrast, a −10-degree shift in eye position shifts the peak response by −10 degrees and increases the magnitude of the response by 50%. For panels A–D, the hypothetical response profile obtained at a fixation point of −10 degrees is plotted in gray, the one at a fixation point of 0 degrees is represented by a dashed line, and the one at a fixation point of +10 degrees is plotted in black. (E) If a neuron codes the location of a sensory target in a limb-centered reference frame, then the peak location of the response profile shifts with initial-hand position. The hypothetical response profile obtained at an initial-hand position of −10 degrees is plotted in gray, the one at an initial-hand position of 0 degrees is represented by a dashed line, and the one obtained at an initial-hand position of +10 degrees is plotted in black.

Different Initial-Hand Positions   Different Eye Positions

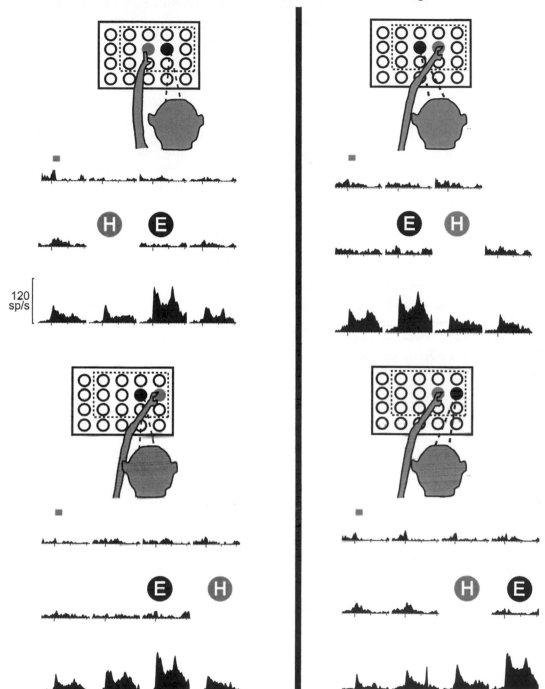

FIGURE 29.4   Example of a PRR neuron that codes reaches to visual targets in an eye-centered reference frame. Each panel in the figure contains a schematic of the monkey's four different variations of initial-hand and eye positions that were employed during this reach task. In each schematic, the circles indicate the relative position of a button assembly that contained two LEDs and a touch-sensitive button, and the dotted square outlines a grid of potential sensory-target locations. Black circle indicates the button that the monkey fixated; the converging line indicates the direction of the monkey's gaze. Gray button indicates the button that the monkey initially pressed. Beneath each schematic is a PRR response profile that was generated from data obtained when the monkey was participating in the variant of the reach task shown in the schematic. The response profiles are arranged as a function of target location, and neural activity is represented by spike density histograms. The histograms are aligned relative to the onset of the sensory cue. The circled E and circled H above the spike-density histograms indicate the location of the monkey's eye position and initial-hand position, respectively. Gray bar indicates the time of cue onset and the duration of the cue. On the left are shown two response profiles generated with the same eye position but different initial-hand positions. On the right are shown two response profiles generated with the same initial-hand position but different eye positions. When eye position varied, the peak of the response profiled shifted. In contrast, when initial-hand position varied, the response profiles did not shift. Tic interval = 100 ms.

predicted that during this auditory reaching task, PRR neurons should also code the location of a sound in an eye-centered reference frame. To test this prediction, we placed monkeys in a darkened room and trained them to make delayed reaches to the remembered locations of auditory stimuli from different initial-hand positions and from different fixation points (Cohen & Andersen, 2000). If PRR auditory activity occurs in a limb-centered reference frame (Fig. 29.3E), then the peak of a PRR response profile should shift with changes in initial hand position. If PRR activity occurs in an eye-centered reference frame (Fig. 29.3A), then the peak of a PRR response profile should shift with changes in the monkey's fixation point.

Figure 29.5 shows the response profiles of a PRR neuron that were obtained while a monkey participated in this delayed-reach task to auditory targets. Much as for the neuron illustrated in Figure 29.4, the peak of this neuron's response profile shifted with changes in eye position and was invariant to changes in initial-hand position, suggesting that this neuron coded the location of an auditory target in an eye-centered reference frame.

Interestingly, in some PRR neurons the eye and initial-hand position affected PRR activity in a complex manner. An example of a complex interaction between eye and initial-hand position is shown in Figure 29.6. When the monkey shifted eye position from left to right, the peak of the response profile shifted from the right of the monkey's initial-hand position to the left of the animal's initial hand position. In contrast, when the monkey shifted initial-hand position from left to right, the peak of the response profile shifted moderately to the right.

To quantify the effect that initial-hand and eye position had on PRR activity during reaches to auditory targets, we examined the firing rate during the delay period. Activity during this period was examined because there was no auditory stimulus present and the monkey was not executing a reach. In a first analysis, we correlated the response profiles that were generated when the monkey made reaches from different eye positions and the response profiles that were generated when the monkey made reaches from different initial-hand positions. We found that, in a significant number of PRR neurons, the correlation coefficient between the response profiles generated from the different eye positions was less than the correlation coefficient between the response profiles generated from the different initial hand positions. In other words, PRR activity was significantly more sensitive to changes in eye position than to changes in initial-hand position.

A second analysis examined directly whether this sensitivity to eye position was equivalent to the hypothesis that PRR neurons coded in an eye-centered reference frame. To test this hypothesis, we calculated the cross-correlation coefficient between the two response profiles generated with different eye positions. The cross-correlation coefficient was generated by calculating the correlation coefficient between the two response profiles when one response profile was held constant and the other was shifted horizontally, relative to the first response profile; the curves were shifted horizontally because the two eye positions used in this study varied along the horizontal dimension. Since the two eye positions were located 18 degrees to the left and 18 degrees to the right of the central fixation position, the response profiles were shifted either by −36 degrees, −18 degrees, 0 degrees, +18 degrees, and +36 degrees. After shifting the response profiles, we correlated them in the region of overlap. The optimal shift was the one with the maximum correlation coefficient. In this analysis, the two response profiles were aligned, relative to eye position, when one response profile was shifted by −36 degrees. Thus, if a cell had an optimal shift of −36 degrees, it aligned best in an eye-centered reference frame. In contrast, a 0-degree optimal shift suggested that the activity of a PRR neuron was insensitive to eye position. Neurons with this optimal-shift value may be in another reference frame, such as head-centered. Intermediate shift values indicated alignment in intermediate frames of reference. We found that a significant proportion (42%) of PRR neurons coded the location of an auditory stimulus in an eye-centered reference frame. For 45% of PRR neurons, changes in initial-hand position and changes in eye position did not affect the location of the peak response. These neurons most likely coded auditory-target location in a head-centered reference frame (Fig. 29.3B), although, as with LIP auditory activity, this proposition needs to be addressed directly. The remaining population of neurons (13%) appeared to code auditory-target location in a reference frame that was intermediate between a head-centered and an eye-centered reference frame (Fig. 29.3C). As with our observations in area LIP, the observation that there are PRR neurons with head and intermediate reference frames is indicative of a direct role for the PPC in reference frame transformations, as will be discussed in greater detail later in this chapter.

We have highlighted analyses of neural activity during the delay period of saccade and reach tasks. However, our observations are not dependent on analyses of delay-period activity. We have found that, during the presentation of the auditory target and during the reach, a significant number of PRR neurons code in a format that is more consistent with eye-centered coordinates

Different Initial-Hand Positions   Different Eye Positions

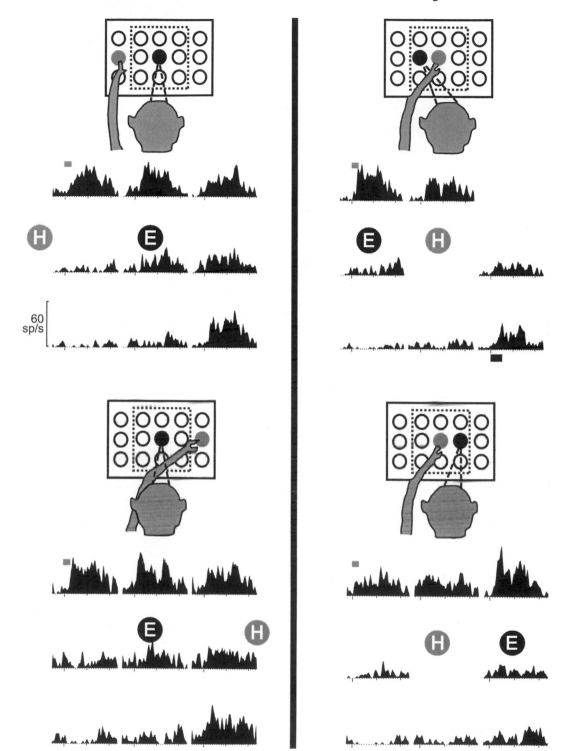

FIGURE 29.5   Example of a PRR neuron that codes reaches to auditory targets in an eye-centered reference frame. Same conventions as those described in Figure 29.4, except that auditory rather than visual targets were used. When eye position varied, the peak of the response profile shifted. In contrast, when initial-hand position varied, the response profiles did not shift. Tic interval = 100 ms.

Different Initial-Hand Positions　　Different Eye Positions

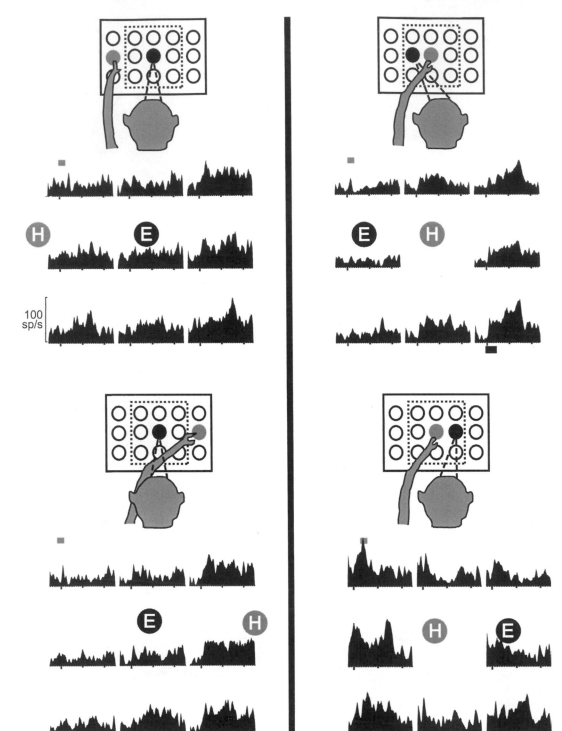

FIGURE 29.6　Example of a PRR neuron that codes reaches to auditory targets in a reference frame that is dependent on both eye position and initial-hand position. Same conventions as those described in Figure 29.4, except that auditory rather than visual targets were used. When eye position varied, the peak of the response profile shifted. In contrast, when initial-hand position varied, the response profiles did not shift. Tic interval = 100 ms.

than arm-centered coordinates (Y. E. Cohen & R. A. Andersen, unpublished observations).

We interpret these reference-frame studies to suggest that a significant proportion of LIP and PRR activity codes the location of a sensory target in a common eye-centered reference frame. This reference frame is considered abstract, insofar as it is (1) not directly linked to the reference frame of the sensory target and (2) not linked to the eventual motor effector. Because the aforementioned studies examined only how PPC neurons code the locations of auditory or visual targets, it will be important to determine whether LIP and PRR neurons that respond to both auditory and visual targets code these sensory targets in the same reference frame.

LIP and PRR activity is further modulated by such factors as head, eye, body, initial hand, and body position (see Fig. 29.3D) (Battaglia-Mayer et al., 2000; Brotchie et al., 1995; Buneo, Jarvis, Batista, & Andersen, 2002; Cohen & Andersen, 1998; Duhamel, Bremmer, BenHamed, & Graf, 1997; Galletti et al., 1995; Snyder, Grieve, et al., 1998). An example of a PRR neuron that is gain modulated is shown in Figure 29.7. The response profiles in this figure were generated from data obtained when a monkey made delayed auditory reaches. The overall response or gain of the neuron was significantly modulated by changes in the monkey's fixation point. When the monkey's fixation point was to the left, the neuron's response was robust, but when the monkey's fixation point was to the right, the response of the neuron was minimal. In contrast, changes in initial-hand position did not substantially change the level of responsiveness of the neuron.

What is the function of these gain fields? Several independent computational studies indicate that gain fields and eye-centered representations form a distributed representation of target locations in different reference frames (Bremmer, Pouget, & Hoffmann, 1998; Deneve, Latham, & Pouget, 2001; Xing & Andersen, 2000a, 2000b; Zipser & Andersen, 1988). As a result, cortical areas that receive input from the PPC are thought to be capable of "reading out" target locations in a reference frame that is appropriate for the computations mediated by that area. For instance, the head-centered location of a sensory target can be computed by convergent inputs from cells that codes the eye-centered location of the target with eye-position gain. This convergence may occur in ventral intraparietal area, a PPC region that contains a substantial population of neurons that code visual targets in a head-centered reference frame (Duhamel et al., 1997), or in a small population of parieto-occipital neurons (Galletti et al., 1993). Combining the eye-centered location of a sensory target with signals about initial-hand position can create a limb-centered reference frame. This computation may occur in area 5, a region of the superior parietal cortex that is involved in programming reaches (Kalaska, 1996). Neurons in this parietal area code the location of visual targets in coordinates intermediate between eye and limb coordinates (Buneo et al., 2002).

These observations at the level of single neurons in area LIP and PRR appear not to be limited to the monkey PPC. Functional homologies of eye-centered representations have been reported in the human PPC (Sereno, Pitzalis, & Martinez, 2001). Also, imaging studies have indicated that neural activity in the human PPC is also gain modulated (Baker, Donoghue, & Sanes, 1999; DeSouza et al., 2000). Finally, psychophysical studies have demonstrated that humans code reaches to auditory, visual, and proprioceptive stimuli in eye-centered coordinates (Bock, 1986; Enright, 1995; Henriques, Klier, Smith, Lowy, & Crawford, 1998; Pouget, Ducom, Torri, & Bavelier, 2002).

Are eye-centered representations of auditory stimuli created in the PPC?

Are eye-centered representations of auditory targets created in the PPC? Or are they generated in areas that project to the PPC? One way to address this issue is to examine the reference frame of auditory activity from brain areas that project either directly to the PPC, such as area Tpt in the superior temporal sulcus, or indirectly to the PPC, such as core regions of the auditory cortex or the inferior colliculus (Andersen, Asanuma, Essick, & Siegel, 1990; Kaas & Hackett, 1998; Leinonen, Hyvärinen, & Sovijarvi, 1980; Lewis & Van Essen, 2000; Pandya & Sanides, 1973; Seltzer & Pandya, 1984, 1994; Sparks & Hartwich-Young, 1989). In all three of these brain areas, auditory neurons code the location of a sound in a head-centered reference frame that is also modulated by changes in eye position (Groh, Trause, Underhill, Clark, & Inati, 2001; Trause, Werner-Reiss, Underhill, & Groh, 2000; Wu & Andersen, 2001). The results of the Tpt study are particularly telling, since this area is the primary source of auditory input to the PPC (Kaas & Hackett, 1998; Leinonen et al., 1980; Lewis & Van Essen, 2000; Pandya & Sanides, 1973; Seltzer & Pandya, 1984, 1994). Insofar as the auditory areas that lead to the PCC represent sensory-target locations in a head-centered reference frame, the PPC may be a locus for transforming head-centered representations of auditory targets into eye-centered representations.

A caveat to this interpretation is that the reference frame of the neurons in these three auditory areas was determined through behavioral tasks that were

Different Initial-Hand Positions

Different Eye Positions

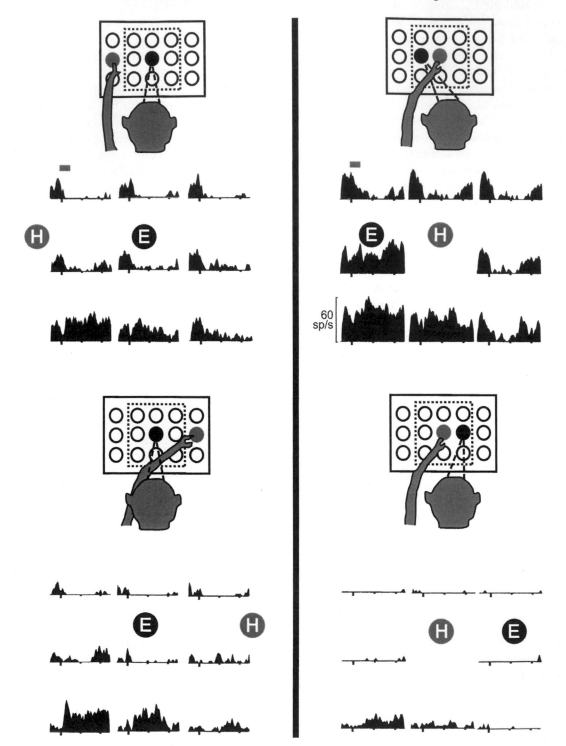

FIGURE 29.7 Example of a PRR neuron that codes reaches to auditory targets in a head-centered reference frame and is substantially gain-modulated by eye position. Same conventions as those described in Figure 29.4. When eye position varied, the magnitude or gain of the response varied substantially. In contrast, when initial-hand position varied, the gain of the response was essentially constant.

somewhat different from those used in the PPC studies. In the inferior colliculus (Groh et al., 2001), auditory cortex (Trause et al., 2000), and Tpt (Wu & Andersen, 2001) studies, monkeys were not required to execute any movements toward the location of the auditory targets. Instead, they listened passively to band-limited noise while maintaining their gaze at different locations. The degree to which a neuron's reference frame depends on the behavioral task is not clear. It is not inconceivable that the reference frame of neurons is task dependent and reflects the needs of the ongoing task (Colby, 1998). If so, then the reference frame of neurons in these auditory areas may be eye-centered during saccade or reach tasks. Direct experimental work in the future should address this interesting issue.

Computational studies also point to the PPC as being a locus for the transformation of head-centered representations of auditory stimuli into eye-centered representations (Deneve et al., 2001; Xing & Andersen, 2000a, 2000b). These studies used three-layer neural networks to probe the mechanisms underlying reference-frame transformations. In the Xing and Andersen model, the first layer, or the input layer, contained a map of visual-target location in an eye-centered reference frame, a map of auditory-target location in a head-centered reference frame, and a representation of head and eye position. The second, "hidden" layer of the network received input from the first input layer and sent connections to the third (output) layer. The output layer was trained to represent target locations in a variety of reference frames, such as eye-centered, head-centered, and/or body-centered.

An analysis of the computational units in the hidden layer of the network following training revealed important insights. First, these units often represented target locations in an intermediate reference frame. For instance, when the network was trained to convert the head-centered representation of an auditory target into an eye-centered representation, a proportion of the units represented auditory-target location in a reference frame intermediate between head and eye. Second, they often coded target location in an eye-centered (or intermediate) reference frame that was modulated by eye and head position. For instance, if the network was trained to code target location in a body-centered reference frame, the units in the hidden layer would code the target location in an eye-centered reference frame that was modulated by eye-position and head-position gain signals. These two observations suggest that cortical areas involved in coordinate transformations utilize both gain fields and intermediate reference frames as mechanisms to convert sensory representations from one reference frame to another.

At least two factors seem likely to contribute to the construction of intermediate reference frames in our network. First, the auditory response fields of the units in the hidden layer were relatively large and asymmetrically shaped, much like the auditory response fields seen in LIP and PRR neurons (Cohen & Andersen, 2000; Stricanne et al., 1996). The second factor was the nonlinear sigmoidal interaction between the eye-position signals and the representations of target location. The combination of these two factors resulted in a partially shifted response field, one that had an intermediate reference frame.

Other modeling studies also illustrated the importance of intermediate reference frames in coordinate transformations (Deneve & Pouget, 2003; Deneve et al., 2001). These studies, like the one mentioned earlier, used a three-layer neural network. However, unlike our network, they allowed for both feed-forward and feedback connections between adjacent layers and lateral connections within a layer and coded target position with a different formulation, namely, a basis set of Gaussian functions. Despite the differences, the computational units in the hidden layer also had gain fields and represented information in an intermediate reference frame.

The finding that gain modulation and intermediate reference frames are seen in PPC neurons (Battaglia-Mayer et al., 2000; Brotchie et al., 1995; Buneo et al., 2002; Cohen & Andersen, 1998; Duhamel et al., 1997; Galletti et al., 1995; Snyder, Grieve, et al., 1998; Stricanne et al., 1996) and in computational models of reference frame transformations (Deneve et al., 2001; Xing & Andersen, 2000a, 2000b; Zipser & Andersen, 1988) supports the notion that the PPC is part of a network for reference-frame transformations. However, there is no direct neurophysiological evidence linking these computational mechanisms with reference-frame transformations. It is important to establish a causal neurophysiological link between gain modulation, intermediate frames of reference, and coordinate transformations to determine directly whether the PPC uses these mechanisms in coordinate transformations.

Advantages of a common reference frame

Although an eye-centered representation of target location in the PPC may represent an intermediate stage of a network devoted to reference-frame transformations, it is also possible that it may be a prerequisite stage in transforming representations of sensory stimuli from sensory-based coordinates into motor-based coordinates that are useful for programming a movement (Flanders et al., 1992; Ghilardi et al., 1995; Kalaska &

Crammond, 1992; Snyder, 2000; Soechting & Flanders, 1989a, 1989b). Another possibility is that it coexists in parallel with these other processes (Graziano, 2001; Snyder, 2000) and is used for specific functions or tasks, such as hand-eye coordination. For example, a common reference frame for encoding the locations of sensory targets may be an efficient manner in which to represent target locations. Since the world contains stimuli of different modalities, a common representation (Batista et al., 1999; Sabes & Jordan, 1997) may facilitate the process by which the brain represents their location and computes the motor plans that are needed to direct an effector toward them. Also, during natural behaviors, we often direct multiple effectors toward a common location. For instance, we often direct our gaze and reach to a common location. Given this, it is reasonable to predict that both area LIP and PRR would be involved in such a task, and a common reference frame may facilitate the coordination and communication between these two areas.

Why, though, is there an eye-centered representation? Because this reference frame is abstract and not tied to stimulus modality or motor effector, it can, in principle, occur in any of a number of different reference frames. We speculate that an eye-centered representation is used because the sensory modality with the highest spatial acuity is vision. Many aspects of auditory perception are modulated by eye position or the location of a visual stimulus (Lewald, 1997, 1998; Lewald & Ehrenstein, 1996; Pouget et al., 2002; Shams, Kamitani, & Shimojo, 2000), and vision plays a key role in calibrating the auditory system's capacity to localize a sound source (King, Schnupp, & Doubell, 2001; Knudsen, 1999; Zwiers, Van Opstal, & Cruysberg, 2001).

Conclusions

The PPC appears to be central to computations that underlie coordinate transformations. Many area LIP and PRR neurons code auditory targets in eye-centered coordinates, similar to the visual representations in these areas. These eye-centered response fields are gain modulated by eye and head position signals (LIP) and eye and limb position signals (PRR). These gain effects allow the population to be read out in a variety of coordinate frames; that is, it can be considered a distributed representation, simultaneously representing locations in many reference frames. The observation of PPC neurons with intermediate reference frames also suggests that the PPC is a locus for coordinate transformations. The common representation in PRR and LIP may be used to facilitate different aspects of goal-oriented behavior. The studies reviewed in this chapter emphasize the role of the PPC as an interface between sensation and action and as an area in which cognitive intermediates of the sensorimotor transformation, such as reference-frame transformations, occur.

Several lines of research are opened by these studies. For instance, is this common reference frame found only in area LIP and PRR, or is it utilized by other cortical areas involved in goal-orientated behavior? Another important question to consider is whether this common reference frame can be extended to other stimulus modalities and other types of movement plans. For instance, might LIP and PRR neurons code somatosensory targets in the same common reference frame as auditory and visual targets? Also, the computational models suggest that neurons with intermediate frames of reference and gain fields are in the middle layer of a network, whereas those with eye-centered representations are in the output layer. How do these observations map onto the anatomical architecture of the PPC? Do PPC neurons with intermediate frames of reference project to those with eye-centered representations? Is there a laminar specificity for neurons with different frames of reference? Examinations of the functional connectivity of the PPC with respect to its intrinsic connectivity and its pattern of afferent and efferent connections are important to further elucidate the specific role of the PPC in reference-frame transformations. Finally, how dynamic is this common reference frame? Is this eye-centered representation obligatory, or can it be changed as the demands of the task change? It is possible that tasks that require hand-eye coordination might be more likely to use a common coordinate frame. However, other tasks may not require such a reference frame, and consequently, target locations may be represented in a different manner.

REFERENCES

Andersen, R. A., Asanuma, C., Essick, G., & Siegel, R. M. (1990). Corticocortical connections of anatomically and physiologically defined subdivisions within the inferior parietal lobule. *Journal of Comparative Neurology, 296,* 65–113.

Andersen, R. A., Bracewell, R. M., Barash, S., Gnadt, J. W., & Fogassi, L. (1990). Eye position effects on visual, memory, and saccade-related activity in areas LIP and 7a of macaque. *Journal of Neuroscience, 10,* 1176–1196.

Andersen, R. A., & Buneo, C. A. (2002). Intentional maps in posterior parietal cortex. *Annual Review of Neuroscience, 25,* 189–220.

Andersen, R. A., Snyder, L. H., Bradley, D. C., & Xing, J. (1997). Multimodal representation of space in the posterior parietal cortex and its use in planning movements. *Annual Review of Neuroscience, 20,* 303–330.

Baker, J. T., Donoghue, J. P., & Sanes, J. N. (1999). Gaze direction modulates finger movement activation patterns in human cerebral cortex. *Journal of Neuroscience, 19,* 10044–10052.

Batista, A. P., Buneo, C. A., Snyder, L. H., & Andersen, R. A. (1999). Reach plans in eye-centered coordinates. *Science, 285,* 257–260.

Battaglia-Mayer, A., Ferraina, S., Mitsuda, T., Marconi, B., Genovesio, A., Onorati, P., et al. (2000). Early coding of reaching in the parietooccipital cortex. *Journal of Neurophysiology, 83,* 2374–2391.

Binkofski, F., Dohle, C., Posse, S., Stephan, K. M., Hefter, H., Seitz, R. J., et al. (1998). Human anterior intraparietal area subserves prehension: A combined lesion and functional MRI activation study. *Neurology, 50,* 1253–1259.

Blatt, G. J., Andersen, R. A., & Stoner, G. R. (1990). Visual receptive field organization and cortico-cortical connections of the lateral intraparietal area (area LIP) in the macaque. *Journal of Comparative Neurology, 299,* 421–445.

Blauert, J. (1997). *Spatial hearing: The psychophysics of human sound localization.* Cambridge, MA: MIT Press.

Bock, O. (1986). Contribution of retinal versus extraretinal signals towards visual localization in goal-directed movements. *Experimental Brain Research, 64,* 476–482.

Bremmer, F., Pouget, A., & Hoffmann, K. P. (1998). Eye position encoding in the macaque posterior parietal cortex. *European Journal of Neuroscience, 10,* 153–160.

Bremmer, F., Schlack, A., Shah, N. J., Zafiris, O., Kubischik, M., Hoffmann, K., et al. (2001). Polymodal motion processing in posterior parietal and premotor cortex: A human fMRI study strongly implies equivalencies between humans and monkeys. *Neuron, 29,* 287–296.

Brotchie, P. R., Andersen, R. A., Snyder, L. H., & Goodman, S. J. (1995). Head position signals used by parietal neurons to encode locations of visual stimuli. *Nature, 375,* 232–235.

Buneo, C. A., Jarvis, M. R., Batista, A. P., & Andersen, R. A. (2002). Direct visuomotor transformations for reaching. *Nature, 416,* 632–636.

Bushara, K. O., Weeks, R. A., Ishii, K., Catalan, M. J., Tian, B., Rauschecker, J. P., et al. (1999). Modality-specific frontal and parietal areas for auditory and visual spatial localization in humans. *Nature Neuroscience, 2,* 759–766.

Calton, J. L., Dickinson, A. R., & Snyder, L. H. (2002). Nonspatial, motor-specific activation in posterior parietal cortex. *Nature Neuroscience, 5,* 580–588.

Cohen, Y. E., & Andersen, R. A. (1998). The parietal reach region (PRR) encodes reaches to auditory targets in an eye-centered reference frame. *Society for Neuroscience Abstracts, 24,* 162.

Cohen, Y. E., & Andersen, R. A. (2000). Reaches to sounds encoded in an eye-centered reference frame. *Neuron, 27,* 647–652.

Cohen, Y. E., Batista, A. P., & Andersen, R. A. (2002). Comparison of neural activity preceding reaches to auditory and visual stimuli in the parietal reach region. *Neuroreport, 13,* 891–894.

Cohen, Y. E., & Knudsen, E. I. (1999). Maps versus clusters: Different representations of auditory space in the midbrain and forebrain. *Trends in Neurosciences, 22,* 128–135.

Colby, C. L. (1998). Action-oriented spatial reference frames in cortex. *Neuron, 20,* 15–24.

Colby, C. L., & Duhamel, J. R. (1991). Heterogeneity of extrastriate visual areas and multiple parietal areas in the macaque monkey. *Neuropsychologia, 29,* 517–537.

Colby, C. L., & Goldberg, M. E. (1999). Space and attention in parietal cortex. *Annual Review of Neuroscience, 22,* 319–349.

Connolly, J. D., Goodale, M. A., DeSouza, J. F., Menon, R. S., & Vilis, T. (2000). A comparison of frontoparietal fMRI activation during anti-saccades and anti-pointing. *Journal of Neurophysiology, 84,* 1645–1655.

Cover, T. M., & Thomas, J. A. (1991). *Elements of information theory.* New York: Wiley.

Deneve, S., Latham, P. E., & Pouget, A. (2001). Efficient computation and cue integration with noisy population codes. *Nature Neuroscience, 4,* 826–831.

Deneve, S., & Pouget, A. (2003). Basis functions for object-centered representations. *Neuron, 37,* 347–359.

DeSouza, J. F. X., Dukelow, S. P., Gati, J. S., Menon, R. S., Andersen, R. A., & Vilis, T. (2000). Eye position signal modulates a human parietal pointing region during memory-guided movements. *Journal of Neuroscience, 20,* 5835–5840.

Duhamel, J. R., Bremmer, F., BenHamed, S., & Graf, W. (1997). Spatial invariance of visual receptive fields in parietal cortex neurons. *Nature, 389,* 845–848.

Enright, J. T. (1995). The non-visual impact of eye orientation on eye-hand coordination. *Vision Research, 35,* 1611–1618.

Eskandar, E. N., & Assad, J. A. (1999). Dissociation of visual, motor and predictive signals in parietal cortex during visual guidance. *Nature Neuroscience, 2,* 88–93.

Flanders, M., Tillery, S. I. H., & Soechting, J. F. (1992). Early stages in a sensorimotor transformation. *Behavior and Brain Science, 15,* 309–362.

Gallese, V., Murata, A., Kaseda, M., Niki, N., & Sakata, H. (1994). Deficit of hand preshaping after muscimol injection in monkey parietal cortex. *Neuroreport, 5,* 1525–1529.

Galletti, C., Battaglini, P. P., & Fattori, P. (1993). Parietal neurons encoding spatial locations in craniotopic coordinates. *Experimental Brain Research, 96,* 221–229.

Galletti, C., Battaglini, P. P., & Fattori, P. (1995). Eye position influence on the parieto-occipital area PO (V6) of the macaque monkey. *European Journal of Neuroscience, 7,* 2486–2501.

Galletti, C., Fattori, P., Battaglini, P. P., Shipp, S., & Zeki, S. (1996). Functional demarcation of a border between areas V6 and V6A in the superior parietal gyrus of the macaque monkey. *European Journal of Neuroscience, 8,* 30–52.

Galletti, C., Fattori, P., Gamberini, M., & Kutz, D. F. (1999). The cortical visual area V6: Brain location and visual topography. *European Journal of Neuroscience, 11,* 3922–3936.

Galletti, C., Fattori, P., Kutz, D. F., & Battaglini, P. P. (1997). Arm movement-related neurons in the visual area V6A of the macaque superior parietal lobule. *European Journal of Neuroscience, 9,* 410–413.

Galletti, C., Gamberini, M., Kutz, D. F., Fattori, P., Luppino, G., & Matelli, M. (2001). The cortical connections of area V6: An occipito-parietal network processing visual information. *European Journal of Neuroscience, 13,* 1572–1588.

Ghilardi, M. F., Gordon, J., & Ghez, C. (1995). Learning a visuomotor transformation in a local area of work space produces directional biases in other areas. *Journal of Neurophysiology, 73,* 2535–2539.

Gnadt, J. W., & Andersen, R. A. (1988). Memory related motor planning activity in posterior parietal cortex of macaque. *Experimental Brain Research, 70,* 216–220.

Gnadt, J. W., & Breznen, B. (1996). Statistical analysis of the information content in the activity of cortical neurons. *Vision Research, 36,* 3525–3537.

Graziano, M. S. (2001). Is reaching eye-centered, body-centered, hand-centered, or a combination? *Review of Neuroscience, 12,* 175–185.

Griffiths, T. D., Rees, G., Rees, A., Green, G. G. R., Witton, C., Rowe, D., et al. (1998). Right parietal cortex is involved in the perception of sound movement in humans. *Nature Neuroscience, 1,* 74–79.

Groh, J. M., Trause, A. S., Underhill, A. M., Clark, K. R., & Inati, S. (2001). Eye position influences auditory responses in primate inferior colliculus. *Neuron, 29,* 509–518.

Grunewald, A., Linden, J. F., & Andersen, R. A. (1999). Responses to auditory stimuli in macaque lateral intraparietal area: I. Effects of training. *Journal of Neurophysiology, 82,* 330–342.

Henriques, D. Y., Klier, E. M., Smith, M. A., Lowy, D., & Crawford, J. D. (1998). Gaze-centered remapping of remembered visual space in an open-loop pointing task. *Journal of Neuroscience, 18,* 1583–1594.

Jancke, L., Kleinschmidt, A., Mirzazde, S., Shah, N. J., & Freund, H. J. (2001). The role of the inferior parietal cortex in linking tactile perception and manual construction of object shapes. *Cerebral Cortex, 11,* 114–121.

Johnson, P. B., Ferraina, S., Bianchi, L., & Caminiti, R. (1996). Cortical networks for visual reaching: Physiological and anatomical organization of frontal and parietal lobe arm regions. *Cerebral Cortex, 6,* 102–119.

Kaas, J. H., & Hackett, T. A. (1998). Subdivisions of auditory cortex and levels of processing in primates. *Audiology & Neurootology, 3,* 73–85.

Kalaska, J. F. (1996). Parietal cortex area 5 and visuomotor behavior. *Canadian Journal of Physiology and Pharmacology, 74,* 483–498.

Kalaska, J. F., & Crammond, D. J. (1992). Cerebral cortical mechanisms of reaching movements. *Science, 255,* 1517–1523.

Karnath, H. O., Ferber, S., & Himmelbach, M. (2001). Spatial awareness is a function of the temporal not the posterior parietal lobe. *Nature, 411,* 950–953.

Kawashima, R., Naitoh, E., Matsumura, M., Itoh, H., Ono, S., Satoh, K., et al. (1996). Topographic representation in human intraparietal sulcus of reaching and saccade. *Neuroreport, 7,* 1253–1256.

King, A. J., Schnupp, J. W., & Doubell, T. P. (2001). The shape of ears to come: Dynamic coding of auditory space. *Trends in Cognitive Sciences, 5,* 261–270.

Klier, E. M., Wang, H., & Crawford, J. D. (2001). The superior colliculus encodes gaze commands in retinal coordinates. *Nature Neuroscience, 4,* 627–632.

Knudsen, E. I. (1999). Mechanisms of experience-dependent plasticity in the auditory localization pathway of the barn owl. *Journal of Comparative Physiology: A Sensory, Neural, and Behavioral Physiology, 185,* 305–321.

Kusunoki, M., Gottlieb, J., & Goldberg, M. E. (2000). The lateral intraparietal area as a salience map: The representation of abrupt onset, stimulus motion, and task relevance. *Vision Research, 40,* 1459–1468.

Leinonen, L., Hyvärinen, J., & Sovijarvi, A. R. (1980). Functional properties of neurons in the temporo-parietal association cortex of awake monkey. *Experimental Brain Research, 39,* 203–215.

Lewald, J. (1997). Eye-position effects in directional hearing. *Behavioural Brain Research, 87,* 35–48.

Lewald, J. (1998). The effect of gaze eccentricity on perceived sound direction and its relation to visual localization. *Hearing Research, 115,* 206–216.

Lewald, J., & Ehrenstein, W. H. (1996). The effect of eye position on auditory lateralization. *Experimental Brain Research, 108,* 473–485.

Lewis, J. W., & Van Essen, D. C. (2000). Corticocortical connections of visual, sensorimotor, and multimodal processing areas in the parietal lobe of the macaque monkey. *Journal of Comparative Neurology, 428,* 112–137.

Linden, J. F., Grunewald, A., & Andersen, R. A. (1999). Responses to auditory stimuli in macaque lateral intraparietal area: II. Behavioral modulation. *Journal of Neurophysiology, 82,* 343–358.

Luna, B., Thulborn, K. R., Strojwas, M. H., McCurtain, B. J., Berman, R. A., Genovese, C. R., et al. (1998). Dorsal cortical regions subserving visually guided saccades in humans: An fMRI study. *Cerebral Cortex, 8,* 40–47.

Mazzoni, P., Bracewell, R. M., Barash, S., & Andersen, R. A. (1996). Spatially tuned auditory responses in area LIP of macaques performing delayed memory saccades to acoustic targets. *Journal of Neurophysiology, 75,* 1233–1241.

Middlebrooks, J. C., & Green, D. M. (1991). Sound localization by human listeners. *Annual Review of Psychology, 42,* 135–159.

Murata, A., Gallese, V., Kaseda, M., & Sakata, H. (1996). Parietal neurons related to memory-guided hand manipulation. *Journal of Neurophysiology, 75,* 2180–2186.

Murata, A., Gallese, V., Luppino, G., Kaseda, M., & Sakata, H. (2000). Selectivity for the shape, size, and orientation of objects for grasping in neurons of monkey parietal area AIP. *Journal of Neurophysiology, 83,* 2580–2601.

Nakamura, H., Kuroda, T., Wakita, M., Kusunoki, M., Kato, A., Mikami, A., et al. (2001). From three-dimensional space vision to prehensile hand movements: The lateral intraparietal area links the area V3A and the anterior intraparietal area in macaques. *Journal of Neuroscience, 21,* 8174–8187.

Pandya, D. N., & Sanides, F. (1973). Architectonic parcellation of the temporal operculum in rhesus monkey and its projection pattern. *Zeitschrift für Anatomie und Entwicklungsgeschichte, 139,* 127–161.

Platt, M. L., & Glimcher, P. W. (1997). Responses of intraparietal neurons to saccadic targets and visual distractors. *Journal of Neurophysiology, 78,* 1574–1589.

Platt, M. L., & Glimcher, P. W. (1999). Neural correlates of decision variables in parietal cortex. *Nature, 400,* 233–238.

Pouget, A., & Snyder, L. H. (2000). Computational approaches to sensorimotor transformations. *Nature Neuroscience, 3*(Suppl.), 1192–1198.

Pouget, A., Ducom, J. C., Torri, J., & Bavelier, D. (2002). Multisensory spatial representations in eye-centered coordinates for reaching. *Cognition, 83,* B1–B11.

Rushworth, M. F., Paus, T., & Sipila, P. K. (2001). Attention systems and the organization of the human parietal cortex. *Journal of Neuroscience, 21,* 5262–5271.

Sabes, P. N., & Jordan, M. I. (1997). Obstacle avoidance and a perturbation sensitivity model for motor planning. *Journal of Neuroscience, 17,* 7119–7128.

Sabes, P. N., Breznen, B., & Andersen, R. A. (2002). Parietal representation of object-based saccades. *Journal of Neurophysiology, 88,* 1815–1829.

Sakata, H., Taira, M., Kusunoki, M., Murata, A., & Tanaka, Y. (1997). The TINS Lecture. The parietal association cortex in depth perception and visual control of hand action. *Trends in Neurosciences, 20*, 350–357.

Sakata, H., Taira, M., Kusunoki, M., Murata, A., Tsutsui, K., Tanaka, Y., et al. (1999). Neural representation of three-dimensional features of manipulation objects with stereopsis. *Experimental Brain Research, 128*, 160–169.

Sakata, H., Taira, M., Murata, A., & Mine, S. (1995). Neural mechanisms of visual guidance of hand action in the parietal cortex of the monkey. *Cerebral Cortex, 5*, 429–438.

Seltzer, B., & Pandya, D. N. (1984). Further observations on parieto-temporal connections in the rhesus monkey. *Experimental Brain Research, 55*, 301–312.

Seltzer, B., & Pandya, D. N. (1994). Parietal, temporal, and occipital projections to cortex of the superior temporal sulcus in the rhesus monkey: A retrograde tracer study. *Journal of Comparative Neurology, 343*, 445–463.

Sereno, M. I., Pitzalis, S., & Martinez, A. (2001). Mapping of contralateral space in retinotopic coordinates by a parietal cortical area in humans. *Science, 294*, 1350–1354.

Shadlen, M. N., & Newsome, W. T. (1996). Motion perception: Seeing and deciding. *Proceedings of the National Academy of Sciences, USA, 93*, 628–633.

Shadlen, M. N., & Newsome, W. T. (2001). Neural basis of a perceptual decision in the parietal cortex (area LIP) of the rhesus monkey. *Journal of Neurophysiology, 86*, 1916–1936.

Shams, L., Kamitani, Y., & Shimojo, S. (2000). What you see is what you hear. *Nature, 408*, 788.

Snyder, L. H. (2000). Coordinate transformations for eye and arm movements in the brain. *Current Opinion in Neurobiology, 10*, 747–754.

Snyder, L. H., Batista, A. P., & Andersen, R. A. (1997). Coding of intention in the posterior parietal cortex. *Nature, 386*, 167–170.

Snyder, L. H., Batista, A. P., & Andersen, R. A. (1998). Change in motor plan, without a change in the spatial locus of attention, modulates activity in posterior parietal cortex. *Journal of Neurophysiology, 79*, 2814–2819.

Snyder, L. H., Batista, A. P., & Andersen, R. A. (2000). Intention-related activity in the posterior parietal cortex: A review. *Vision Research, 40*, 1433–1441.

Snyder, L. H., Grieve, K. L., Brotchie, P., & Andersen, R. A. (1998). Separate body- and world-referenced representations of visual space in parietal cortex. *Nature, 394*, 887–891.

Soechting, J. F., & Flanders, M. (1989a). Errors in pointing are due to approximations in sensorimotor transformations. *Journal of Neurophysiology, 62*, 595–608.

Soechting, J. F., & Flanders, M. (1989b). Sensorimotor representations for pointing to targets in three-dimensional space. *Journal of Neurophysiology, 62*, 582–594.

Soechting, J. F., & Flanders, M. (1992). Moving in three-dimensional space: Frames of reference, vectors, and coordinate systems. *Annual Review of Neuroscience, 15*, 167–191.

Soechting, J. F., & Flanders, M. (1995). Psychophysical approaches to motor control. *Current Opinion in Neurobiology, 5*, 742–748.

Sparks, D. L. (1989). The neural encoding of the location of targets for saccadic eye movements. *Journal of Experimental Biology, 146*, 195–207.

Sparks, D. L., & Hartwich-Young, R. (1989). The deep layers of the superior colliculus. *Review of Oculomotor Research, 3*, 213–255.

Sparks, D. L., & Mays, L. E. (1990). Signal transformations required for the generation of saccadic eye movements. *Annual Review of Neuroscience, 13*, 309–336.

Stricanne, B., Andersen, R. A., & Mazzoni, P. (1996). Eye-centered, head-centered, and intermediate coding of remembered sound locations in area LIP. *Journal of Neurophysiology, 76*, 2071–2076.

Trause, A. S., Werner-Reiss, U., Underhill, A. M., & Groh, J. M. (2000). Effects of eye position on auditory signals in primate auditory cortex. *Society for Neuroscience Abstracts, 26*, 1977.

Wu, S.-M., & Andersen, R. A, (2001). The representation of auditory space in temporoparietal cortex. *Society for Neuroscience Abstracts, 27*, 147.

Xing, J., & Andersen, R. A. (2000a). Memory activity of LIP neurons for sequential eye movements simulated with neural networks. *Journal of Neurophysiology, 84*, 615–665.

Xing, J., & Andersen, R. A. (2000b). Models of the posterior parietal cortex which perform multimodal integration and represent space in several coordinate frames. *Journal of Cognitive Neuroscience, 12*, 601–614.

Zipser, D., & Andersen, R. A. (1988). A back-propagation programmed network that simulates response properties of a subset of posterior parietal neurons. *Nature, 331*, 679–684.

Zwiers, M. P., Van Opstal, A. J., & Cruysberg, J. R. (2001). A spatial hearing deficit in early-blind humans. *Journal of Neuroscience, 21, RC142*, 141–145.

V HUMAN BRAIN STUDIES OF MULTISENSORY PROCESSES

30 Hemodynamic Studies of Audiovisual Interactions

GEMMA A. CALVERT AND JAMES W. LEWIS

Introduction

Over the past decade, neuroimaging of metabolic activity related to brain function has advanced our understanding of how the human brain combines what we see and hear. This chapter examines studies designed to reveal human brain regions and mechanisms underlying audiovisual interactions using functional magnetic resonance imaging (fMRI) and positron emission tomography (PET). Our knowledge of the nature and location of audiovisual interactions and the neural mechanisms underlying such processing is inferred largely from animal experiments, for which we present a brief background. Extending these mechanisms and concepts to human hemodyamic neuroimaging, we then examine a variety of studies designed to expose sites of integration for different parameters shared between auditory and visual stimuli.

BACKGROUND Much of our current understanding of cross-modal interactions is derived from animal studies, as described in earlier chapters of this handbook. Briefly, neuroanatomical and electrophysiological studies in nonhuman primates have identified several cortical regions, depicted in Figure 30.1 (Color Plate 7), where afferents from the auditory and visual cortices converge and/or that contain cells responsive to auditory and visual stimuli. These regions include anterior portions of the superior temporal sulcus (STS) (Baylis, Rolls, & Leonard, 1987; Benevento, Fallon, Davis, & Rezak, 1977; Bruce, Desimone, & Gross, 1981; Desimone & Gross, 1979; Neal, Pearson, & Powell, 1990; Watanabe & Iwai, 1991), posterior portions of the STS, including the temporoparietal association cortex (Tpt) (Desimone & Ungerleider, 1986; Leinonen, Hyvärinen, & Sovijarvi, 1980), parietal cortex, including the ventral (VIP) and lateral (LIP) intraparietal areas (Linden, Grunewald, & Andersen, 1999; Lewis & Van Essen, 2000; Bremmer, Schlack, Duhamel, Graf, & Fink, 2001), and premotor and prefrontal cortex (Graziano, Reiss, & Gross, 1999; Watanabe, 1992). Audiovisual convergence zones have also been identified in subcortical structures, including

the superior colliculus (Fries, 1984), the claustrum (Pearson, Brodal, Gatter, & Powell, 1982), the supra-geniculate and medial pulvinar nuclei of the thalamus (Mesulam & Mufson, 1982; Mufson & Mesulam, 1984), and within the amygdaloid complex (Turner, Mishkin, & Knapp, 1980). Together, this constellation of brain regions represents a network that is involved in various aspects of audiovisual integration.

Investigation of the neuronal mechanisms by which cross-modal interactions are achieved and the rules that govern this process have been confined largely to the superior colliculus (SC), a structure involved in mediating orientation and attentive behaviors. Multisensory neurons in this structure possess overlapping sensory receptive fields, one for each modality—visual, auditory, tactile—to which they respond. Many are also capable of transforming the cross-modal cues into an integrated product, a phenomenon referred to as *multisensory integration*. When auditory and visual stimuli occur in close temporal and spatial proximity, the firing rate of these integrative cells can increase dramatically, sometimes exceeding 12-fold increases in firing rate beyond that expected by summing the impulses exhibited by each unimodal input in isolation (Stein, Meredith, & Wallace, 1993). This cross-modal facilitation appears maximal when the responses to the individual inputs are weakest, a principle referred to as *inverse effectiveness* (Stein & Meredith, 1993). In contrast, cross-modal stimuli that are spatially and/or temporally disparate can induce a profound response depression (or *suppression*). In this case, a vigorous response to a unimodal stimulus can be substantially lessened or even eliminated by the presence of an incongruent stimulus from another modality (Kadunce, Vaughan, Wallace, Benedek, & Stein, 1997). These features of multisensory processing identified at the cellular level in the SC have also been shown to apply to the cross-modal orientation and attentive behaviors mediated by this structure (Stein, Huneycutt, & Meredith, 1988; Stein, Meredith, Huneycutt, & McDade, 1989).

Neurons exhibiting overlapping multisensory receptive fields have also been identified in the cerebral

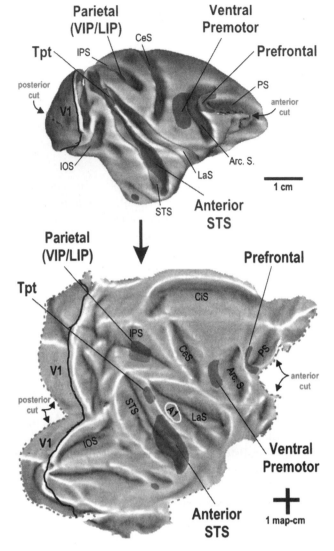

FIGURE 30.1 Approximate locations of cortical sites for audiovisual convergence (green) in the macaque monkey. The location of primary visual cortex (blue line) and an estimate of primary auditory cortex (yellow outline) are also indicated. Red dashed lines depict two of the cuts introduced to flatten the cortical model, which also aid orienting to the flat map format (adapted from Drury et al., 1996). Arc. S., arcuate sulcus; CeS, central sulcus; CiS, cingulate sulcus; IOS, inferior occipital sulcus; IPS, intraparietal sulcus; LaS, lateral (sylvian) sulcus; PS, principal sulcus; STS, superior temporal sulcus. (Adapted from Drury et al., 1996.) (See Color Plate 7.)

cortex of the monkey (Duhamel, Colby, & Goldberg, 1991, 1998; Graziano & Gross, 1998; Mistlin & Perrett, 1990), cat (Wallace, Meredith, & Stein, 1992; Wilkinson, Meredith, & Stein, 1996), and rat (Barth, Goldberg, Brett, & Di, 1995). However, only a few studies have detailed the actual multisensory response properties. In the cat, multisensory integration responses in cells of the anterior ectosylvian fissure and lateral sulcus were found to be relatively less constrained by the precise temporal or spatial correspondence of multisensory

inputs than in the SC (Wallace et al., 1992). This suggests that cross-modal mechanisms in the cerebral cortex may subserve a wider range of roles, although the different functions remain to be explored. Nonetheless, the rudimentary principles of multisensory interactions, such as neural sensitivity to temporal and spatial correspondence, response facilitation and suppression, and inverse effectiveness, at least serve as starting points and are principles amenable to examination in humans using hemodynamic neuroimaging methods.

HUMAN IMAGING APPROACHES Several different strategies have been used to identify brain areas involved in cross-modal interactions in humans. These strategies can perhaps most usefully be divided by task and by paradigmatic or analytic approach. For example, some researchers have employed *cross-modal matching* tasks that involve the explicit comparison of information received through different modalities and pertaining to two distinct objects. Another simple approach has been to compare brain activity evoked during the presentation of information in one modality (e.g., auditory) with that evoked by the same (or related) task carried out in another modality (e.g., visual), where a *superimposition* of the two maps reveals areas of common (or coresponsive) activation. Others have utilized paradigms explicitly designed to tap *cross-modal integration*. In these studies, information from two different modalities perceived as emanating from a common event is fused into an integrated percept (Radeau, 1994; Stein & Meredith, 1993). Other studies have focused on establishing how a sensory cue presented in one modality can speed the response to a stimulus subsequently presented in another modality despite a lag in time between the prime and presentation of the target. This is referred to as *cross-modal priming*.

Experiments examining audiovisual interactions can also be discriminated based on the information being combined. Whereas some experiments have focused on the mechanisms involved in synthesizing inputs relating to stimulus content (i.e., "what"), others have concentrated on those involved in integrating spatial coordinate information (i.e., "where") or even temporal correspondence (i.e., "when"). That the integration of different stimulus parameters may involve different mechanisms and sites of integration is supported by psychophysical data showing that these processes are subject to somewhat different spatial and cognitive constraints for binding (for a review, see Colin, Radeau, Deltenre, & Morais, 2001). Temporal synchrony and spatial location are just two examples of *intermodal invariances*. In other words, the information is analogous, irrespective of the sensory modality in which it is perceived (Lewkowicz, 2000). On the other hand, the appearance of a dog and the sound of its bark are examples of modality-specific features that can also be integrated across modalities. Thus, the cross-modal synthesis of intermodal invariant information and modality-specific cues may also make use of distinct integrative mechanisms.

Despite the distinctions in both task and analytic strategy, a consistent picture of the possible brain areas involved in different facets of audiovisual processing is beginning to emerge. This information has been divided into five areas for discussion in this chapter. First, we address linguistic audiovisual interactions separately, because the language system of humans may potentially incorporate a distinct or specialized organization (see Section II of this handbook). Next we review nonlinguistic aspects of audiovisual interactions, including studies examining the correspondence of multisensory inputs in time and space, and cross-modal mechanisms involved in detecting changes in the sensory environment. This is followed by an examination of the integration of emotional cues from auditory and visual channels. We then briefly discuss studies that have investigated the mechanisms involved in the acquisition or learning of audiovisual associations. The last area of audiovisual processing discussed has to do with cross-modal plasticity in the deaf and blind, and the breakdown of integrative mechanisms in certain patient groups. We then address some methodological issues pertinent to the previous issues, and the possible functional roles of blood-oxygen-level-dependent (BOLD) deactivation signals in cross-modal processing. In this section we also consider the strengths and weaknesses of hemodynamic imaging methods. In conclusion, we present highlights of what has been learned about audiovisual interactions and summarize some of the unresolved questions to be addressed in future studies.

Human imaging studies

LINGUISTIC INTERACTIONS More than three decades ago, nonhuman primate physiological research provided some of the first indications that sensory-specific cortices (e.g., early visual areas) could actually be modulated by nonvisual stimuli, including electric shock, painful tactile stimuli, and a range of frequency-specific or broadband auditory stimuli (Fishman & Michael, 1973; Horn, 1965; Jung, Kornhuber, & Da Fonseca, 1963; Lomo & Mollica, 1962; Morrell, 1972; Murata, Kramer, & Bach-y-Rita, 1965; Spinelli, Starr, & Barrett, 1968). These studies, although few in number, were

extremely provocative and provided an impetus for similar investigations of unisensory areas in humans following the introduction of PET and fMRI. One cognitive process that seemed particularly likely to recruit cortex dedicated to another modality was the perception of seen speech (lipreading), since the visible instantiations of speech were known to have a powerful impact on the perception of the (usually) accompanying auditory speech signals (e.g., McGurk & MacDonald, 1976; Sumby & Polack, 1954).

This prediction was borne out by an early fMRI study showing activation of auditory cortex during silent lipreading in normal listeners (Calvert et al., 1997). Several replications of this finding suggest that this effect is particularly robust in the case of seen speech (e.g., Callan, Callan, & Vatikiotis-Bateson, 2001; MacSweeney et al., 2000, 2001). Furthermore, other fMRI studies have reported activation of auditory cortex during the visual perception of some forms of biological motion (R. J. Howard et al., 1996) as well as during the passive perception of written words (Haist et al., 2001).

These findings raised further questions regarding the route by which visual cues might access auditory cortex (or vice versa), and how information from both modalities is synthesized under the usual circumstances in which the auditory and visual signals co-occur, as in normal face-to-face conversation. Studies using fMRI and PET that have attempted to tackle some of these questions within the language domain can broadly be categorized into two groups. One set of studies has examined the mechanisms involved in the synthesis of audiovisual speech, which has been hypothesized to occur at an early stage of processing, potentially at or before phonetic classification (Summerfield, 1992). Audiovisual speech integration is one example of the synthesis of intermodal invariant information because the audible correlates of a phoneme are determined by, and thus intrinsically correlated with, the accompanying lip and mouth movements. The other school of inquiry has focused on how the brain combines semantic information, which presumably occurs at a later stage of processing, following elaboration of the speech sounds into lexical items. In this case, the extraction of meaning is often based on prior learned associations between arbitrary modality-specific cues (e.g., the acoustic representation of a word or the noise that an animal makes and the corresponding graphical form or visual manifestation). Related to these experiments are studies of audiovisual linguistic priming that have sought to identify the neuronal mechanisms underpinning the improvement in response to one stimulus after previous exposure to a semantically related prime.

Integration of phonetic information Psychophysical studies have long documented the marked, often superadditive improvement in auditory speech comprehension when the speaker can be seen as well as heard (e.g., Sumby & Polack, 1954). On the other hand, incongruent lip and mouth movements can impair the perception of even a clean auditory speech signal, such as when viewing a dubbed foreign movie.

In an initial attempt to investigate the neural bases of these cross-modal gains, Calvert et al. (1997) used fMRI to localize the brain areas involved in silent lipreading and superimposed the resulting activation map onto that generated when the same individuals listened to speech in the absence of visual cues. Speech stimuli consisted of spoken numbers from 1 to 10, which subjects were asked to silently rehearse after each presentation. This strategy revealed several regions of overlap between the auditory and visual tasks in temporal cortex extending superiorly and bilaterally from association regions in the STS (Brodmann's area [BA] 21/22) to the planum temporale (BA 42) and lateral tip of Heschl's gyrus (BA 41). Although the superimposition of activation maps from two different sensory tasks can identify areas responsive to both modalities, this strategy gives no clear indication of the precise sites of convergence under normal bimodal circumstances in which the speaker can be both heard and seen.

In two further fMRI experiments employing the same stimuli and task instructions, bimodal audiovisual speech was contrasted to either heard or seen speech (Calvert et al., 1999). Conjunction analysis of the two resulting data sets permitted isolation of any brain areas that might have a specific role in audiovisual speech, over and above any involvement in perceiving speech unimodally. When subjects perceived speech from both channels, activity in putatively sensory-specific regions of auditory and visual cortex was substantially enhanced. This observation suggested a possible physiological basis underlying the sensory perceptual gains associated with bimodal speech perception and possibly reflected reciprocal propagation of activation. In the absence of any bimodal enhancement in regions of polysensory cortex, the data initially appeared to support a model of "early" cross-modal integration in sensory-specific cortices. This hypothesis is consistent with event-related potential (ERP) data demonstrating multisensory interaction effects at very early stages of processing (i.e., prior to 100 ms post-stimulus onset) in secondary auditory (Foxe et al., 2000; Giard & Peronnet, 1999) and visual (Saron, Schroeder, Foxe, & Vaughan, 2001) cortices. Furthermore, recent neuroanatomical data obtained in the macaque showing direct projections from several auditory parabelt regions to visual areas V1 and V2 (Falchier, Clavagnier, Barone, & Kennedy, 2002; Rockland & Ojima, 2003) have provided a putative substrate for the early synthesis (i.e., prior to convergence in polysensory areas) of cross-modal inputs. However, an alternative and equally plausible explanation for the failure to implicate polysensory areas in audiovisual speech integration was that the design and analytic strategy employed in the study by Calvert et al. (1999) may have precluded the detection of specific interaction events.

To address this issue, Calvert, Campbell, and Brammer (2000) turned to electrophysiological studies of multisensory neurons to guide the design and analysis of their next fMRI experiment. Subjects were scanned while they listened to excerpts from George Orwell's *1984* in the presence of matched or mismatched lip and mouth movements, and to excerpts that were either seen or heard independently. This design permitted the identification of brain areas that exhibited positive interaction effects in the presence of congruent audiovisual speech (AV > A + V) and negative interactions (AV < A + V) or response suppression (AV < A or V, whichever is the greatest) to incongruent combinations. These criteria are consistent with indices of multisensory integration observed at the cellular level in the presence of spatially congruent and incongruent audiovisual inputs. This strategy identified an area, depicted in Figure 30.2 (Color Plate 8), along the ventral bank of the left STS, putatively involved in the integration of audiovisual speech. In contrast to their earlier studies, this experiment used speech streams rather than single words. Although it is entirely possible that this region has a generic involvement in cross-modal speech synthesis regardless of whether the phonetic information is embedded in syllables, words, or sentences, it should be noted that the processing of words in sentences involves phonetic processing across a larger temporal span (e.g., stress feet, phrase and intonational structure), and thus slightly different mechanisms or brain areas may be recruited for words or syllables.

Other brain areas also exhibited positive or negative bimodal interactions, but not both. For example, bimodal response enhancements were again detected in primary and secondary auditory zones and in parts of the visual cortex sensitive to dynamic stimuli (V5 or hMT), replicating the results of their earlier study (Calvert et al., 1999). However, neither of these areas exhibited a statistically significant response depression. This is perhaps not surprising, given that at the cellular level, response depression is less commonly detected in multisensory cells than is response enhancement (Stein & Meredith, 1993). The finding that both phenomena were so clearly observable in the STS suggests

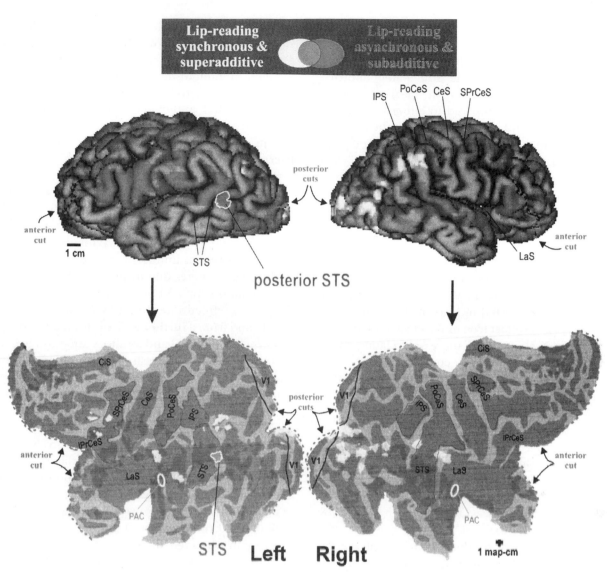

FIGURE 30.2 Cross-modal facilitation and suppression in the STS. Three-dimensional and flat map brain models show group-averaged data (n = 10) obtained during an fMRI study of cross-modal audiovisual speech. Brain areas exhibiting superadditive responses to matched audiovisual speech stimuli (yellow) are superimposed on areas showing subadditive responses to mismatched speech cues (blue). Green highlights areas meeting both criteria. (Adapted from Calvert et al., 2000.) (See Color Plate 8.)

that it is the primary site of convergence for auditory and visual phonetic signals. Indeed, studies investigating the neuroanatomical correlates of auditory language processing have implicated the STS in the processing of phonetic material (Binder, 1997). Enhancement of the BOLD response in other brain regions, including the auditory and visual cortices, may therefore reflect the downstream consequences of convergence in the STS, with modulatory effects being mediated via back-projections from the STS to these sensory-specific areas. Cross-modal interactions were also identified in other polysensory areas, including the inferior temporal (parts of BA 44/45 and 6) and middle temporal (BA 6/8) (MTG), the anterior cingulate (AC; BA 32), and the inferior parietal lobule (BA 40).

This fMRI study highlighted a network of brain areas putatively involved in the synthesis of audiovisual speech. At present, however, the precise function of these areas remains to be clarified. Answers to this question may require data concerning the time course of information flow through this network. Although fMRI lacks the temporal resolution required to shed light on this issue, the combination of data from hemodynamic methods with high temporal resolution techniques, such as ERPs or magnetoencephalography (MEG), may be the route forward.

Callan, Callan, and Vatikiotis-Bateson (2001) have used fMRI to explore cross-modal neural mechanisms underlying the visual enhancement of auditory speech intelligibility in the presence of acoustic noise. Subjects were exposed to audiovisual speech in the presence or absence of auditory noise (multispeaker babble) and to auditory or visual speech in isolation. Behavioral testing prior to scanning revealed the anticipated improvement in word recognition when the speaker could be seen as well as heard (compared to either listening or lipreading speech) and especially so when the auditory channel was unimpaired. Although the behavioral gains afforded by visual cues were most marked in clear acoustic conditions, activity in temporal cortical regions (including the STS and primary auditory cortex—BA 41/42/22/21) was maximally enhanced when audiovisual speech was presented with acoustic noise. Greater augmentation of the BOLD response in the presence of the least perceptible stimuli is reminiscent of the principle of inverse effectiveness identified at the cellular level. This adds credence to the conclusion that the cross-modal gains detected in prior imaging studies of audiovisual speech reflect true multisensory integration responses rather than signal increases relating to increases in attention and/or comprehension when speech is perceived from two sensory modalities rather than one. These findings are consistent with the results of a prior EEG experiment conducted by the same laboratory which showed that, despite predictably better performance when audiovisual speech was presented in clear acoustic conditions, the largest interaction effects in the EEG signal were observed in the left superior temporal gyrus when the identical stimuli were presented in acoustic noise (Callan, Callan, Kroos, & Vatikiotis-Bateson, 2001).

Another strategy used to identify sites of integration during audiovisual speech focused on manipulation of the temporal rather than phonetic correspondence between the two sensory channels (Olson, Gatenby, & Gore, 2002). Subjects were scanned using PET while audiovisual syllables were presented synchronously to induce a McGurk effect, or sufficiently far apart in time as to preclude cross-modal binding. Subtraction of the asynchronous presentations from synchronized audiovisual stimuli revealed a large cluster of differential activation covering the left claustrum and putamen. Additional analysis revealed greater signal changes in the left insula and claustrum and left STS for synchronized versus asynchronous stimuli. However, as these areas were activated in both conditions, the authors hypothesized that they may have a more generic involvement in bimodal speech perception rather than cross-modal integration per se.

One explanation for the discrepancy in results between this study and those by Calvert et al., described earlier, may relate to a difference in emphasis on the parameters on which binding was manipulated (i.e.,

temporal versus phonetic correspondence). The insula/claustrum has been shown by other researchers to be especially sensitive to the temporal correspondence between nonlinguistic audiovisual inputs (Bushara, Grafman, & Hallett, 2001; Calvert, Hansen, Iversen, & Brammer, 2001), and damage to the putamen can cause impairments in discriminating the onset between two stimuli, including across modalities (Artieda, Pastor, Lacruz, & Obeso, 1992; Hosokawa, Nakamura, & Shibuya, 1981).

In sum, there now seems to be considerable evidence from hemodynamic studies that the left STS plays a prominent role in the synthesis of auditory and visual speech signals. That the statistical interactions reported in this area reflect multisensory integration responses rather than changes due to possible fluctuations in attention gains support both from the demonstration of the inverse effectiveness rule by Callan, Callan, et al. (2001) and from a further PET study focusing on the effect of selective visual and auditory attention to audiovisual speech stimuli (Kawashima et al., 1999). When subjects were specifically instructed to attend to either the auditory or the visual components of speech, activity was modulated in sensory-specific cortices but not in the STS. The absence of an attentional effect (but the presence of an interaction effect) in the STS prompted the authors to conclude that "the human superior temporal region plays a role in speech sound perception that involves intermodality integration." Furthermore, in an MEG study examining sites of integration between auditory and visual (written) letters, interaction effects were again observed in the left STS (Raij, Uutela, & Hari, 2001). These data suggest that the STS may be involved in the synthesis of phonetic material even when the visual information (letters) is arbitrary with respect to the corresponding sounds. At present, convergence of phonetic information seems to occur primarily in polysensory areas, including the left STS, although it may also involve or modulate some portions of earlier auditory and visual cortices. The study by Olson et al. (2002) raises the additional possibility that the particular pattern of brain areas recruited during the synthesis of cross-modal inputs may depend on the most persuasive point of correspondence—temporal, spatial, and/or featural—between the different stimuli in any given situation or on the task demands, or both.

Integration at the semantic level An alternative approach to the question of how linguistic information is shared between the auditory and visual modalities has been to identify brain areas involved in the perception and storage of spoken or visually presented words or pictures (or both). This represents a stage beyond that for phonological processing and thus would presumably incorporate "higher-level" association cortices, though this remains to be elucidated. The studies described in this section have highlighted some clear distinctions in terms of neuroanatomical convergence zones.

Early PET studies suggested that semantic information might be stored in a network of brain areas that were largely but not entirely insensitive to input modality. Comparison of the brain areas activated during the visual and auditory processing of single words revealed regions of common activation as well as modality-specific sites. For example, one study that contrasted the repetition of visually or acoustically presented words revealed areas of left temporal activation evoked by both tasks that were distinguishable but very close to each other (Howard et al., 1992). In a later study, Petersen, Fox, Posner, Mintun, and Raichle (1989) examined brain activations when subjects generated an associated verb to a visually versus acoustically presented noun, and observed partially overlapping foci in the left inferior frontal gyrus. The representation of semantic information has also been studied at higher resolution using fMRI. Chee, O'Craven, Bergida, Rosen, and Savoy (1999) contrasted brain areas activated during the determination of whether acoustically or graphically presented words were concrete or abstract (semantic task) to those areas stimulated during a condition in which subjects were instructed to decide whether the words contained one or two syllables (nonsemantic task). Superimposition of the brain activation maps resulting from the auditory and visual semantic tasks revealed areas of coactivation in left inferior frontal cortex (BA 45), consistent with the previous study. Additionally, coactivation was evident in other anterior brain regions, including the anterior prefrontal cortex (BA 10/46) bilaterally, left premotor regions (BA 6), and the anterior supplementary motor area (BA 6/8).

In another fMRI study designed to examine sites of common activation during auditory and visual sentence processing (Michael, Keller, Carpenter, & Just, 2001), subjects were asked to read or listen to a sentence and to answer a question by pressing one of two buttons to indicate whether a subsequently presented probe sentence (read or heard) was a true statement about the initial sentence. Although both tasks recruited classic language areas in the inferior frontal and temporal lobes, there were also slight differences in the degree and extent of activation, the exact locations of the foci, and the pattern of lateralization, depending on whether sentences were heard or seen. These distinctions notwithstanding, similar increases in activation were observed with increasing sentence complexity, regardless of the modality of the input. The authors suggest that whereas earlier stages of language processing

may be sculpted by the modality of input, the higher linguistic functions are computed by mechanisms insensitive to processing modality, and thus reflect processing at hierarchically later stages (i.e., supporting models of late integration).

Other investigators have explicitly probed the role of sensory-specific cortices in the formation or storage of arbitrary semantic symbols. Bookheimer et al. (1998) acquired PET images as subjects performed an auditory responsive naming task (an analogue to visual object naming) while blindfolded. Despite the absence of any visual input, when subjects heard brief phrases describing concrete nouns and were asked to name the object, activation was detected in traditional language centers as well as in parts of the visual cortex, including the primary visual areas and the fusiform gyrus. The location of these activations were identical to those observed in a previous study using visual stimuli of matched semantic content (Bookheimer et al., 1995), suggesting that when subjects hear descriptors of objects, visual images of these items or visually associated knowledge are evoked automatically. Together with data showing activation of primary auditory cortex during passive word reading (Haist et al., 2001), these findings suggest that reciprocal activation of parallel sensory pathways could serve in part to mediate recognition or facilitate retrieval of semantic information by activating a broader network of item-specific knowledge, thereby increasing task efficiency.

Although most studies examining the cross-modal synthesis of semantic information have used linguistic stimuli, a recent fMRI study of environmental sound processing suggests that somewhat different portions of the MTG may be involved in the storage and synthesis of nonlinguistic material. For example, identifying environmental (nonverbal) sounds has also been shown to activate portions of the MTG, which might relate to audiovisual processing. In a study by Lewis et al. (2002), subjects listened (with eyes closed) to a wide array of readily identifiable environmental sounds, including those produced by tools, animals, liquids, and dropped objects. The identifiable sounds (as opposed to the unidentifiable backward played controls) evoked activity in several language-related areas in the left hemisphere, a finding consistent with subjects subvocally naming the sounds they heard. However, activity also included foci in posterior portions of the MTG (pMTG) bilaterally that were distinct from the classic language-related cortex. The left pMTG partially overlapped the left STS focus depicted in Figure 30.2 (green), which is associated with cross-modal speech recognition. Surprisingly, posterior portions of the pMTG foci also partially overlapped cortex previously implicated in high-level visual processing of tools and biological motion. One proposed explanation was that the pMTG foci might be involved in learning or mediating cross-modal associations (cf. Ettlinger & Wilson, 1990). Consistent with this idea, people with normal sight and hearing generally learn of environmental sounds while simultaneously viewing the characteristic movements of (and/or while manipulating) the sound source itself, such as pounding with a hammer or opening a can of soda. Consequently, hearing a familiar sound in isolation may evoke activity in the pMTG, eliciting a sense of recognition of the sound source and its immediate cross-modal (i.e., visual) associations, which appears to occur just prior to or at an early stage of semantic processing.

At present, several studies have identified brain areas involved in the extraction and retrieval of meaning from auditory and visual "objects" (including words). These have consistently implicated the existence of a common semantic network in the left temporal lobe (including MTG), left inferior frontal gyrus, and other anterior brain regions (see Binder & Price, 2001, for a review). Overlap of the auditory and visual semantic information in the left MTG suggests that the arbitrary representations of meaning converge in regions distinct from those implicated in phonetic integration. However, unlike studies of audiovisual speech, the above "semantic-related" studies did not present the auditory and visual material simultaneously. Therefore, it remains to be determined whether the MTG plays a specific role in the synthesis of semantic information from different modalities, or whether it may instead be a repository of modality-specific features. However, both cross-modal integrative systems appear to make additional use of sensory-specific cortices. Whether these areas have a role in cross-modal integration or instead are involved in the storage of the modality-specific features associated with an object also requires further investigation.

Audiovisual priming studies A somewhat different approach to the investigation of cross-modal mechanisms using linguistic material has made use of priming paradigms. *Priming* refers to a change in the ability to identify or produce an item as a consequence of a specific prior encounter with it (Tulving & Schachter, 1990). The relationship between cross-modal priming and integration is currently the topic of some debate (McDonald, Teder-Sälejärvi, & Ward, 2001), but one obvious distinction lies in the relative timing of presentation of the two sensory inputs. Although most studies investigating cross-modal integration present multisensory cues simultaneously or close in time (within a second or so), priming studies usually introduce a substantial time gap (on the order of minutes) between presentation of the cue and presentation of the target. To the extent that information presented in one modality can speed responses to related material subsequently presented in another modality despite marked asynchrony in onset times suggests the possible involvement of multisensory integration sites in the mediation of these effects. Indeed, cross-modal conditioning studies in rats have shown that although temporal synchrony is sufficient to learn cross-modal conjunctions, it may not be essential (see Lewkowicz & Kraebel, Chap. 41, this volume).

To date, the mechanisms involved in human audiovisual priming have only been explored in the context of word stem completion tasks using PET. This entails the presentation of a list of words in one modality (e.g., acoustically), half of which are targets, the remainder fillers. Several minutes later, subjects are scanned while the initial syllables of either previously presented target words or novel syllables are presented in another modality (e.g., visually), and asked to provide completions to the word stems. Compared to the presentation of primes and targets within the same modality, cross-modal visual-to-auditory (Badgaiyan, Schachter, & Alpert, 1999) and auditory-to-visual (Schacter, Badgaiyan, & Alpert, 1999) priming was associated with increased blood flow in the prefrontal cortex and a corresponding decrease in the left angular gyrus.

In a subsequent experiment by the same authors, encoding of the initial targets was performed under conditions of full or divided attention (Badgaiyan, Schachter, & Alpert, 2001). This strategy allowed discrimination of the brain areas involved in the priming effects from those involved in explicit retrieval of the target words. Increased regional cerebral blood flow (rCBF) in the anterior prefrontal cortex was observed in the full attention but not in the divided attention condition, implicating this structure in explicit retrieval. Regardless of the initial encoding conditions, decreased activation was reported in the superior temporal gyrus (BA 39/40). Cognitive studies have argued that cross-modal priming is mediated by some form of abstract lexical representation involved in phonological input or output processing (e.g., Curran, Schachter, & Galluccio, 1999). In the light of these data, the authors suggest that the suppression of activity in areas near to or overlapping those implicated in the cross-modal integration of phonetic and semantic material may reflect a reduction in demand for cross-modal binding for the primed items compared to the nonprimed baseline stems. Although the relationship between cross-modal integration and priming clearly requires further examination, the results of the above studies suggest that at least the neuronal mechanisms underpinning these two phenomena may be closely linked (Munhall & Tohkura, 1998; Sams et al., 1991).

NONLINGUISTIC INTERACTIONS   In this section, we present an overview of studies involving nonlinguistic audiovisual interactions, addressing topics such as shared temporal onset, spatial correspondence, and the mechanisms involved in the detection of meaningful sensory changes in the environment. Although it may transpire that the critical distinction between different cross-modal studies has less to do with differences between linguistic and nonlinguistic information than the basis on which inputs are combined, we have chosen this distinction to try and impose some order on our discussion. Comparison of the brain areas implicated across these different studies may, in due course, lead us to a more accurate description of the relevant integrative parameters.

Temporal correspondence   One sensory attribute critical for binding audiovisual inputs is timing, or intersensory temporal synchrony (Radeau, 1994). A well-recognized cross-modal phenomenon in the speech domain is the ventriloquist's illusion. A comparable nonlinguistic illusion involving perceptual timing is evident in the form of computer or video games. Video images or cartoons (e.g., Pac-Man or a Doom character) and their actions are combined with sounds that arise from spatially disparate locations (i.e., the monitor versus the speakers) and, when timed properly, can give rise to a unified percept of a "cross-modal" object.

Calvert et al. (2001) examined audiovisual temporal correspondence, testing for sites demonstrating facilitation and suppression effects based on the stringent electrophysiological criteria from animal studies. In their study, the visual stimulus consisted of an 8-Hz reversing black-and-white checkerboard that alternated every 30 s with a blank screen. The auditory stimulus consisted of 1 s bursts of white noise that either were timed to coincide precisely with the reversal rate of the visual checkerboard (matched experiment) or were randomly shifted out of synchrony (mismatched experiment). Subjects were instructed to passively attend to the stimuli. The structure exhibiting the most significant cross-modal facilitation and suppression to synchronous and asynchronous bimodal inputs, respectively, was the SC. Weaker cross-modal interactions were identified in a network of brain areas that included the insula/claustrum bilaterally, the left STS, the right IPS, and several frontal regions, including the superior and ventromedial frontal gyri.

Similar results have been reported in a PET study by Bushara et al. (2001) in which subjects were required to detect whether an auditory tone and a visually presented colored circle were presented synchronously or not. Onset asynchrony was varied parametrically, resulting in three levels of difficulty. As a control condition, subjects were asked to decide whether the visual stimulus was green or yellow and to respond only when the auditory stimulus was present (which was always synchronized with the visual stimuli). Subtracting activations from the two conditions revealed a network of heteromodal brain areas involved in audiovisual temporal synchrony detection; this network included the right insular, posterior parietal, and prefrontal regions. Moreover, regression analysis identifying voxels with rCBF responses that correlated positively with increasing task demand (i.e., decreasing asynchrony) revealed a cluster within the right insula, suggesting that this region plays the most prominent role in this process. Interregional covariance analysis also identified task-related functional interactions between the insula and the posterior thalamus and SC. The authors suggested that these findings demonstrate that intersensory temporal processing is mediated via subcortical tecto-thalamo-insula pathways.

Together, these data support a prominent role for the SC and insula in the synthesis of cross-modal cues on the basis of their temporal correspondence. Both studies also implicate regions of polysensory cortex (especially parietal and frontal cortices) in these cross-modal timing experiments. The functional significance of these areas is not yet confirmed, but one possibility is that they may have been sensitive to the apparent spatial coherence of the auditory and visual inputs. Although both studies focus on the temporal correspondence of the auditory and visual information, temporal synchrony can induce the illusion of spatial correspondence despite actual separation of the inputs in space. This is the basis of the ventriloquist's illusion and highlights the requirement for separate and systematic manipulation of the parameters of time and space in order to discriminate the mechanisms involved in synthesizing these distinct attributes.

Spatial concordance   The neural bases underlying the cross-modal construction of auditory and visual external space have been investigated from two different perspectives. The first is from the point of view of exogenous attention. In these studies the subject's attention is engaged by the sensory input (input mechanisms), which can lead to an involuntary integration of invariant cross-modal features, such as the spatial coordinates and timing of a visual object and the sound it produces. The second is from the perspective of endogenous attention, in which the subject's willful attention is required to assess cross-modal sensory information for purposeful behavior (output mechanisms). As attention-related questions have yet to be disentangled from theoretically "lower-level" cross-modal spatial interactions, the neuroanatomical implications for both processes will be considered together. Behavioral and brain lesion studies have given rise to two contrasting theoretical models that address the mechanisms of auditory and visual spatial attention. In one, a supramodal, a single system is considered responsible for directing attention to spatial locations, regardless of the stimulus modality; the other is a modality-specific model (Farah, Wong, Monheit, & Morrow, 1989; Ward, 1994). Neuroimaging studies provide some support for both models.

Support for supramodal systems involved in both the endogenous and exogenous control of attention to space stems from several recent studies. Lewis, Beauchamp, and DeYoe (2000) investigated brain areas involved in the cross-modal synthesis of dynamic spatial information using fMRI. As subjects were instructed to track and respond to the dynamic stimuli, this paradigm entailed endogenous control over attention. In an initial experiment, subjects performed separately a visual and an auditory motion discrimination task that involved determining the speed of coherently moving dots relative to random motion or moving sounds relative to silence. The aim of this approach was simply to activate visual and auditory motion pathways separately, and then superimpose these patterns to reveal potential sites for cross-modal interaction. The results are illustrated in Figure 30.3, where yellow corresponds to activation of auditory motion pathways, blue (and purple) for visual motion, and green for regions of overlap. Purple indicates cortex activated during the visual motion task that was "deactivated" during the auditory task (discussed later under Neuroimaging Methodology and Analysis).

In Figure 30.3 (Color Plate 9), each unimodal motion task evoked a unique pattern of activation of cortical areas extending from the respective primary sensory area to parietal cortex. Regions common to both auditory and visual spatial attention included the lateral parietal cortex, overlapping the intraparietal sulcus (IPS) and postcentral sulcus (PoCeS); lateral frontal cortex, including superior and inferior precentral sulci (SPrCeS and IPrCeS); anterior cingulate (AC) cortex plus medial superior frontal gyri (SFG); and the right anterior insula. The precentral and parietal regions in Figure 30.3 are representative of the commonly reported "frontoparietal" network involved in cross-modal spatial interactions and/or the control of spatial attention that is observed in both unimodal and cross-modal studies (cf. Driver & Spence, 1998; Mesulam, 1998).

To discriminate regions of common activation (or coresponsivity) from areas involved in cross-modal integration (i.e., those exhibiting cross-modal interaction effects), subjects in the study of Lewis et al. (2000) were also scanned while performing an explicit cross-modal speed comparison task. In this experiment, the

visual stimulus consisted of a square grating that moved at speeds approximating those of the moving auditory stimulus (a 300-Hz tone). Visual and auditory stimuli were presented simultaneously, and subjects were instructed to decide whether the visual target was moving faster or slower than the auditory target. In two contrasting conditions, subjects were required to ignore the visual stimuli and compare speeds in the auditory domain, or vice versa. Within individuals, comparison of the cross-modal condition with the combined unimodal tasks revealed audiovisual superadditive responses predominantly in the IPS (left > right), in the anterior insula, and within the anterior midline (SFG and AC). Positive interaction effects were also detected in the STS in some individuals, but these effects were typically weak and scattered. These data suggest that brain areas explicitly involved in the integration of moving auditory and visual stimuli, or the control of attention to space between the two modalities, represent a subset of the regions exhibiting coresponsive behavior depicted in Figure 30.3 (in green). In that study, the auditory and visual information was perceived to be moving not only in roughly coincident trajectories in space but also simultaneously. Thus, it is interesting to note the involvement across modalities of the insular cortex, which was previously suggested to have a role in the processing of time (Bushara et al., 2001; Calvert et al., 2001).

A study by Bremmer, Schlack, Shah, et al. (2001) also revealed bilateral parietal foci (overlapping the IPS sites in Fig. 30.3) as sites responsive to auditory and visual motion, but additionally found activity evoked by tactile motion processing (air moving across the face). This evidence further supported the idea that the cross-modal parietal foci may have homologous functions to the VIP of the macaque monkey (cf. Figs. 30.1 and 30.3). Area VIP is known to receive inputs from visual, tactile, and auditory-related cortex (Lewis & Van Essen, 2000), and contain cells responsive to the direction of motion of visual, tactile, and auditory stimuli (Bremmer, Schlack, Duhamel, et al., 2001; Duhamel et al., 1998). In contrast to the results depicted in Figure 30.3, cross-modal coactivation in the study by Bremmer et al. (2001) was nearly absent or limited in extent to precentral and AC cortex. One explanation may lie in the distinction between the extent of endogenous and exogenous attentional mechanisms. When subjects are explicitly required to direct their attention to a specific spatial location or stimulus attribute (endogenous attention) and to make response decisions by pressing a button, this may require a greater involvement of top-down frontal areas acting on the IPS via back-projections (see Iacoboni, Woods, & Mazziotta, 1998). In contrast, during "passive" observation

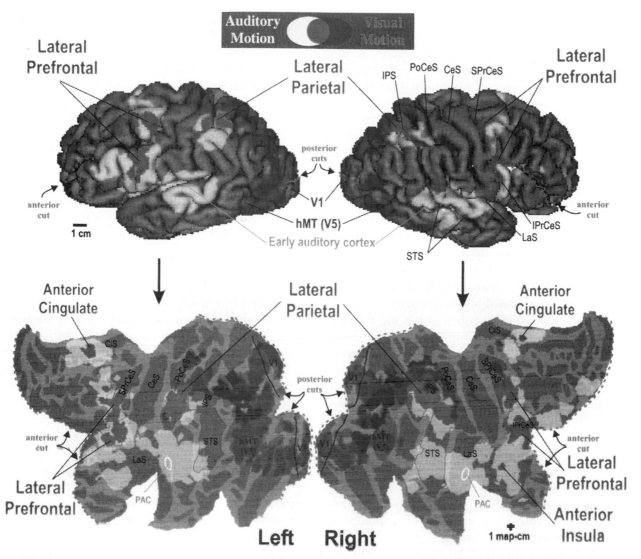

FIGURE 30.3   Cortical overlap of auditory and visual spatial motion processing pathways. Three-dimensional and flat map brain models show group-averaged (n = 9) fMRI activation patterns from an auditory motion paradigm (yellow) and a separate visual motion paradigm (blue plus purple), together with regions of overlap (green). Purple indicates visually responsive regions deactivated during the auditory motion task. The approximate locations of primary auditory cortex (PAC, yellow ovals) and primary visual cortex (V1, dark blue lines) are indicated (Bonferroni corrected P < 0.001). Anatomical underlay is the visible human male (Van Essen et al., 1998), and red dashed lines depict two of the cuts introduced to flatten the cortical model. HG, Heschl's gyrus; IPrCeS, inferior precentral sulcus. See text and Figure 30.1 for other details. (Adapted from Lewis et al., 2000.) (See Color Plate 9.)

conditions (predominantly exogenous attention), as in the study by Bremmer, Schlack, Shah, et al. (2001), fewer top-down influences would be expected.

The issue of task-related output was addressed in a PET study of endogenous spatial localization by Bushara et al. (1999). Subjects performed two spatial localization tasks separately for each modality. The first task was a delayed match-to-sample task in which each stimulus location was matched to that of the preceding one. The second task required the immediate motor response of moving a joystick to indicate the stimulus location. The visual stimuli consisted of flashed LEDs

along a horizontal array. The auditory stimuli consisted of noise bursts, which were also presented along a horizontal array in virtual three-dimensional (3D) space via headphones. This paradigm allowed for subtraction and conjunction analysis methods so that brain regions associated with the processing of auditory or visual spatial localization per se could be identified independent of the task performed.

Consistent with the studies outlined above, the strategy used by Bushara et al. (1999) revealed partially overlapping foci in lateral parietal cortex associated with the visual and auditory localization pathways.

Activation was also detected in foci along precentral cortex and medial frontal cortex, among other regions. In contrast to the studies previously described, the visual- and auditory-related precentral and anterior midline foci were not overlapping. This led the authors to conclude that separate portions of prefrontal (and posterior parietal cortex) are individually specialized for auditory or visual spatial processing. Consistent with the human lesion literature, they further proposed that the auditory and visual foci in the superior parietal lobule (SPL) relays modality-specific input (pertaining to early spatial processing) to areas of the inferior parietal lobule (IPL). The IPL then represents both spatial and nonspatial supramodal (or amodal) aspects of perception for additional processing. However, as neither of these tasks required integration per se, it is not possible to conclude that these areas are critical for the synthesis of auditory and visual spatial information.

In summary, heteromodal zones within the inferior parietal lobe are increasingly implicated in the cross-modal construction of space, which is consistent with the primate literature. That these regions may be controlled by top-down frontal mechanisms when attention is internally rather than externally controlled is suggested by studies conducted thus far. Depending on the task, this frontoparietal network may modulate activity in earlier modality-specific pathways to achieve cross-modal interactions. Whether the posited distinction between "cross-modal spatial attention" and "cross-modal integration of spatial coordinate information" has neurophysiological validity or is simply a terminological distinction remains to be elucidated.

Detection of changes in sensory events In addition to the possibility of a cross-modal network being involved in spatial attention, other studies using both auditory and visual stimuli are beginning to suggest that similar multisensory mechanisms may be involved in attention to the detection of salient and novel stimuli within the environment. In a series of fMRI studies, Downar and colleagues examined areas responsive to transitions in visual, auditory, or tactile stimulation. In their first paradigm (Downar, Crawley, Mikulis, & Davis, 2000), stimuli in all three modalities were continuously present. In a random order they toggled one modality at a time between two states: croaking frogs versus running water, circular brushing versus rapid tapping of the leg, and blue versus red abstract figure. Brain regions commonly activated by transitions within all three modalities during passive observation included AC, SMA, IFG, and insula, similar to the network shown in Figure 30.3. However, the largest region of activation was identified in the right temporoparietal junction (TPJ), the peak focus of which lies in the dorsal bank of the posterior

STS. The authors concluded that the right TPJ, together with frontal, insula, and cingulate cortex, plays an important role in the detection of salient stimuli across different modalities, perhaps mediating involuntary attention to events in the sensory environment.

In a subsequent study, Downar et al. (2001) investigated whether the same network was involved in the capture of attention to changing stimuli across modalities regardless of whether these changes were task relevant or irrelevant. To manipulate task relevance, subjects were instructed across different blocks of event-related trials to attend and respond to transients in either the visual or auditory streams. Visual changes were accomplished by rotating a square box containing a diagonal box 10 degrees clockwise or counterclockwise. Auditory changes involved increasing or decreasing the pitch of the auditory stimulus, a steady buzzing sound, by 5%. The detection of stimulus changes in the task-relevant conditions stimulated a wide network of areas, including the right and left TPJ, left precuneus, anterior insula and AC, and right lateralized thalamus. Independent of the task, activations to changes in auditory or visual sensory events recruited a network encompassing a large sector of the left SMA and cingulate motor areas, right IFG, the precuneus and inferior temporal gyrus bilaterally, the right anterior insula, and the left posterior cingulate cortex.

The results of these two studies have implicated a large network of brain areas in the detection of change in the environment, regardless of modality. The roles of the various components identified in these experiments remain to be determined, but many of the same regions have been implicated in the cross-modal integration of spatial, temporal, or featural cues. Given that changes occur in time and space, the involvement of brain areas sensitive to such attributes is to be expected. The one area most consistently implicated in the detection of sensory changes regardless of modality was the TPJ (posterior STS). Damage in or near this region can result in neglect of multiple sensory cues in the (typically) left side of space (Pizzamiglio et al., 1998), adding neuropsychological evidence to data from human brain imaging studies implicating this region in the cross-modal construction of (and attention to) auditory and visual space.

AUDIOVISUAL INTERACTIONS RELATING TO EMOTION Several authors have begun to examine the cross-modal integration of information relating to emotional material. Royet et al. (2000) used PET to identify areas of coincident activation to emotional stimuli presented in the auditory, visual, and olfactory modalities. Subjects were scanned while pleasant, unpleasant, or neutral stimuli were presented in each sensory modality. During the emotionally valenced conditions, subjects were instructed to perform forced-choice pleasant and unpleasant judgments. During the neutral conditions, subjects were asked to select at random one of two key-press buttons. Superimposition of the brain activation maps in response to emotionally valenced stimuli across all three sensory modalities led to increased rCBF in the orbitofrontal cortex, the temporal pole, and the superior frontal gyrus in the left hemisphere. Activation of the amygdala was observed solely for emotionally valenced olfactory stimuli. The orbitofrontal cortex has also been implicated in the representation of the rewarding properties of tactile, gustatory, and olfactory stimuli in both monkey (see Rolls, 2001) and human imaging (Francis et al., 1999) studies. Together, these data indicate a prominent role for the amygdala plus the orbitofrontal region and related structures in the synthesis of information relating to the hedonic value of information presented in the auditory and visual modalities.

More recently, Dolan, Morris, and de Gelder (2001) used fMRI to investigate cross-modal integration of emotional cues from the voice and face. Subjects were exposed to fearful or happy faces presented together with a sentence spoken either in a happy or fearful tone. By calculating interaction terms among the four possible combinations, the authors found that the presentation of congruent fearful stimuli enhanced activation in the amygdala and fusiform gyrus, compared with pairing of the fearful face with a happy voice. Similar response enhancements were not observed when subjects perceived happy face-voice combinations, suggesting that the amygdala is specifically involved in the synthesis of fear-related audiovisual cues. The output of this cross-modal integration may then feed back to earlier visual areas to modulate the response in face-processing areas in the fusiform gyrus.

Studies of this type are too few to make any firm conclusions, but to date there is evidence that integration of emotional cues emanating from auditory and visual streams may converge or interact in the orbitofrontal cortex and amygdala. The precise involvement of these structures may depend on the positive or negative valence of the stimuli.

AUDIOVISUAL ASSOCIATIVE LEARNING   Imaging studies investigating the neural mechanisms mediating the development of cross-modal associations in adult subjects have concentrated on the acquisition of arbitrary associations between simple auditory and visual stimuli. The emphasis on modality-specific associations is largely due to the fact that sensitivity to modality-invariant information is acquired early in development (see Lewkowicz & Kraebel, Chap. 41, this volume). Using PET, McIntosh,

Cabeza, and Lobaugh (1998) demonstrated that after a learning period in which a visual stimulus was consistently paired with an audible tone, presentation of the tone in isolation induced activation in visual cortex. The reverse association was later studied using fMRI (Rosenfeld, 1999). By repeatedly pairing one of two audible tones with a simultaneously presented visual stimulus, subsequent presentation of the visual stimulus alone triggered activation of the primary auditory cortex. The results of these studies are interesting and may provide a physiological basis to explain reports of "hallucinating" the sound or appearance of a stimulus previously paired with a stimulus from another modality, even though the stimuli are no longer concurrent (Howells, 1944). Neither study investigated whether these effects were transient or extended beyond the period of the experiment, so we cannot rule out the possibility that these activations reflect a general effect of expectation instead. For example, Kastner et al. (1999) showed that activation in visual cortex could be induced when a visual stimulus was expected (based on the timing of other visual stimuli) but did not materialize. Moreover, since both studies concentrated solely on the postlearning phase, they may have failed to identify mechanisms involved in the acquisition of the cross-modal association per se.

More recently, Gonzalo, Shallice, and Dolan (2000) attempted to identify time-dependent neural changes related to associative learning across sensory modalities. Subjects were studied during three separate training sessions in which they were exposed to consistently and inconsistently paired audiovisual inputs and to single visual and auditory stimuli. The participants were instructed to learn which audiovisual pairs were consistent over the training period. Time-dependent effects during the acquisition of this cross-modal association were identified in posterior hippocampus and SFG. Additional activations specific to the learning of consistent pairings included medial parietal and right dorsolateral prefrontal cortices. The acquisition of data at different stages of the learning process clearly represents an advance on the earlier studies. However, as there were no intramodal (auditory-auditory and visual-visual) associative learning comparison conditions, it is not yet known to what extent the areas identified by these investigators are specific to cross-modal associative processes or simply reflect generic stimulus-stimulus associative learning operations.

CROSS-MODAL PLASTICITY AND CROSS-MODAL INTEGRATION IN PATHOLOGICAL STATES   Not only is the brain capable of synthesizing multisensory cues to facilitate performance, it can use this information interchangeably.

For example, tactile and auditory cues can supplant vision in darkness or when blindness occurs. The mechanisms by which sensory systems dedicated to one modality can compensate for impaired sensation in another modality are the subject of cross-modal plasticity studies. Because several chapters in this handbook explore this topic, we will describe only a few representative studies that have begun to investigate the neural bases of enhanced vision or audition in the deaf and blind.

Finney, Fine, and Dobkins (2001) used fMRI to measure evoked activity in the auditory cortex of both early-deafened and normal-hearing individuals during relatively simple visual tasks (detecting dimming of a moving-dot array or of the central fixation spot). In contrast to hearing subjects, deaf subjects exhibited activation in a region of the right auditory cortex corresponding to BA 42 and 22, as well as in BA 41 (primary auditory cortex), suggesting that early deafness can lead to the "processing" of visual stimuli in auditory cortex, although the functional significance of such activity remains unclear. Reciprocal recruitment of visual cortex for auditory processing has been shown in blind subjects. Using PET, Weeks et al. (2000) scanned sighted and congenitally blind subjects while the subjects performed auditory localization tasks. Both the sighted and blind subjects activated posterior parietal areas. The blind subjects, however, also activated association areas in the right occipital cortex, the foci of which were similar to areas previously identified in visual location and motion-detection experiments in sighted subjects. The blind subjects therefore demonstrated visual-to-auditory cross-modal plasticity in which auditory localization activated occipital association areas that in normally sighted individuals are involved in dorsal stream visual ("where") processing. These studies are part of a growing literature demonstrating that sensory cortex dedicated to one modality can be recruited by another following sensory deprivation. Whether or not these plastic changes are mediated by other brain areas might only be uncovered by studies that track the concomitant changes in brain activity with slow perceptual deterioration over time.

Understanding the way in which cross-modal integration systems break down in pathological states may also provide useful insights into the normal workings of these processes. For example, deficits in cross-modal coincidence detection have been reported following damage to the putamen in some patients with Parkinson's disease (Hosokawa et al., 1981), highlighting a role for this structure in binding multisensory inputs on the basis of their temporal correspondence. This might explain the unexpected involvement of this structure in an fMRI study of audiovisual speech inte-gration (Olson et al., 2002). Unlike previous studies, which manipulated the phonetic correspondence of the auditory and visual inputs in such a way as to cause or preclude integration, the study by Olson and colleagues attempted to achieve a similar effect by altering the temporal onsets of the two stimuli. Given the known involvement of the putamen in the detection of stimulus coincidence, the authors were able to interpret the role of this structure in synthesizing phonetic inputs based on their temporal correspondence.

Deficits in cross-modal integration mechanisms have also been posited to underlie certain schizophrenic symptoms (e.g., Nayani & David, 1996). To investigate these claims, Surguladze et al. (2001) scanned schizophrenic patients using fMRI while they perceived auditory or visual speech and nonspeech gurning movements. Despite apparently normal audiovisual integration as assessed by McGurk fusions, schizophrenic patients with psychotic symptoms, but not the patients in remission, showed a distinct pattern of activation in response to the perception of nonspeech gurning movements. Specifically, greater activation was observed in insula-striatal structures than was seen in controls (or the subgroup in remission). The authors suggest that such activations may reflect an abnormal tendency to activate polysensory structures in perceptually ambiguous conditions. Furthermore, secondary to deficits in the processing of dynamic visual stimuli, there may be compensatory top-down processing strategies driven by the search for meaning mediated by multisensory mechanisms.

Studies of cross-modal integration in pathological states are still in their infancy. Although the current findings must therefore be interpreted cautiously, it is clear such studies offer considerable potential for providing insights into the normal integrative mechanisms that may not be easily gleaned by studying healthy people.

Neuroimaging methodology and analysis

The studies described in the previous sections used a wide range of paradigms and analytic strategies to identify brain areas putatively involved in coordinating audiovisual processing. In this section we assess some of the strengths and weaknesses of several general methods and issues pertaining to interpretation of blood flow decreases, or "deactivation," as a potential form of cross-modal interaction.

Intersection and conjunction designs The simplest approach to identifying putative intersensory integration sites has been to carry out separate experiments using different unimodal stimuli relating to the same object (e.g., the sound of a cat versus the image of a cat) and then seek to identify areas of the brain commonly activated across the experiments, A ∩ V, using intersection or conjunction analysis (e.g., Calvert et al., 1997; Chee et al., 1999; Lewis et al., 2000). To compute an intersection, one determines those areas that overlap across the separate unimodal activation maps. A slightly different approach to analyzing such data is by implementing a conjunction analysis, which is a statistical method for determining brain areas that show "context-free" activation (i.e., those areas commonly activated across a range of experiments). Friston et al. (1997) have summarized this approach as testing the hypothesis "that activations across a range of tasks are jointly significant." In essence, it consists of combining the data from the separate experiments and identifying those areas that show significant activation in the combined data. The statistical inference is therefore performed on the combined data and not on the individual experiments prior to a simple overlapping of maps. The necessary condition is that both "active" tasks should contain the component of interest; i.e., in AV − A and AV − V, the idea is to find context-free regions responding to AV, regardless of the unimodal contrast condition (A or V).

One problem with intersection or conjunction designs, however, relates to the fact that a single voxel in a functional imaging experiment samples a very large number of neurons (many tens of millions in a typical $3.75 \times 3.75 \times 6 \, mm^3$ voxel). At the neuronal level, "multisensory integration" has been defined as an enhancement of the response induced by a stimulus from one sensory modality by input from a different modality (Stein et al., 1993). However, bimodal enhancement need not be multiplicative to demonstrate integration. In the context of a neuroimaging experiment, anything less than a superadditive cross-modal response observed in a given brain voxel could simply reflect the linear summation of the activity from two separate populations of sensory-specific neurons present within that space. This strategy may therefore erroneously identify an area as being putatively involved in cross-modal integration (Type I error). A second problem is that this strategy may also preclude the detection of true multisensory integration sites (Type II errors) due to weak unimodal responses. For example, one or both of the unimodal stimuli presented in isolation may fail to reach a statistical criterion for significance, as has been shown of some multisensory cells in the SC (Stein & Meredith, 1993). Attempts to overcome this problem by relaxing the statistical threshold for response detection would immediately run into the problem of Type I errors, especially if applied to whole-brain analysis.

An improvement on this strategy would seem to be (at least on the face of it) to contrast unimodal stimuli with true bimodal stimuli and attempt to identify areas where bimodal stimulation gives a greater response than either modality presented in isolation (e.g., Calvert et al., 1999). Here the idea is to expose subjects to bimodal stimulation, auditory and visual stimulation and then compute (AV − V) ∩ (AV − A). However, if AV is simply the linear sum of A and V, and if the differences are both significant, conjunction analysis may simply detect voxels in which unimodal auditory-responsive and unimodal visual-responsive neurons coexist. Thus, this strategy may not afford any real improvement over computing the simple intersection, A ∩ V.

Activation interaction designs A more robust method for identifying integration responses involves the inclusion of a reference ("rest") condition in which rest, A, V, and AV conditions are presented, permitting the computation of the interaction effect (AV-rest) − ([A-rest] + [V-rest]). Interaction effects are commonly used in statistical analysis to identify changes that occur when two factors are simultaneously altered that would not be predicted from the results of altering each factor in isolation. In the context of multisensory integration, the use of interaction effects therefore permits the clear demonstration that the bimodal response cannot simply be predicted from the sum of the unimodal responses.

This approach has a number of advantages over the other analytic techniques discussed. First, the strategy is based on the known electrophysiological behavior of cells carrying out signal integration. Second, it provides a de facto demonstration that some form of interaction has occurred, as the output signal is significantly different from the sum of the inputs, overcoming the problem that a response to two unimodal inputs could simply be due to different populations of sensory-specific neurons. Third, it allows integrative behavior to be detected when unimodal responses are weak. For studies of cross-modal integration at least, as opposed to cross-modal matching, these conditions will necessarily ensure that the paradigm meets criteria for binding, such that the two or more temporally proximal sensory inputs are perceived as emanating from a common event (Radeau, 1994).

The use of different analytic strategies has inevitably contributed to differences in results across imaging experiments (e.g., see Calvert, 2001, for a discussion of these issues). As with any other statistical approach, however, results from interaction designs must be interpreted with caution. For example, superadditive effects to bimodal stimuli may be difficult to detect in the event that the BOLD responses to the unimodal stimuli are at or near ceiling. It may therefore be advisable to study interaction effects within a parametric design in which the intensity of the unimodal stimuli is systematically varied. Serendipitously, the principle of inverse effectiveness may help to counter the problem of BOLD ceiling responses, as the largest cross-modal enhancements occur when the unimodal stimuli are minimally effective. Another point of caution concerning the above designs is in regard to the analysis of decreased blood flow signals (also termed cortical deactivation, suppression, or suspension), which are often more difficult to interpret.

Deactivation interactions   In fMRI studies, increases in blood flow signals (BOLD signals) evoked by a stimulus or task are known to directly reflect increases in neuronal activity, particularly local field potentials (Logothetis, Pauls, Augath, Trinath, & Oeltermann, 2001). However, interpreting decreases in blood flow signals has been more controversial. Several auditory, visual, and cross-modal studies have revealed blood flow decreases in a variety of brain regions that may be indicative of cross-modal interactions. For example, visual tasks can lead to depressed responses in auditory cortex (e.g., Haxby et al., 1994; Laurienti et al., 2002), and auditory tasks can lead to depressed responses in visual cortex (e.g., Laurienti et al., 2002; Lewis et al., 2000). Earlier accounts of such decreases in blood flow suggested that decreases may represent a general suppression of the unattended modality, or perhaps a simple blood-stealing artifact in which an increase in blood flow to one brain region causes a relative decrease in blood flow to another region. An alternative view is that blood flow decreases may be explained by a synchronous reduction in activity of groups of tonically active neurons (Binder et al., 1999; Waldvogel et al., 2000), thereby representing a reduction in the "baseline" level of synaptic activity. Using this interpretation, cortical deactivation patterns have been ascribed to both task-irrelevant and task-relevant factors.

One likely source for some cortical deactivation pertains to task-irrelevant factors. Studies that include a "rest" condition together with nonlinguistic auditory and/or visual stimuli (as with the interaction designs) often reveal deactivation in midline structures, including nonclassic language areas in posterior cingulate and medial prefrontal cortex, and in parieto-occipital cortex (Binder et al., 1999; McKiernan et al., 2002; Raichle et al., 2001). This apparent deactivation can be explained by considering the behavioral shift in switching from the control to the active task. During the control (rest) task, the subject is free to engage in uncontrolled cognitive activity (e.g., monitoring for novel inputs, semantic monitoring, daydreaming, etc.). During the attention-demanding task, such cognitive activities are disrupted. Thus, the activity associated with uncontrolled activity (rest) manifests as deactivation during the task phase.

However, this explanation can only account for some of the deactivation patterns reported.

Another source of deactivation may relate specifically to cross-modal interactions. For instance, Lewis et al. (2000) observed deactivation in regions of visual motion-responsive cortex during an auditory motion task, as illustrated in Figure 30.3 (purple), which were topographically distinct from those relating to the task-irrelevant factors described above. (The deactivation of auditory cortex by the visual paradigms was less evident in the study by Lewis et al., as visual stimuli were also present in the control condition, thereby subtracting out most of the deactivation responses). To address the possibility that some cortical deactivations might relate to inadvertent eye movements, they examined the magnitude of deactivation signals (below a 20-s resting baseline level measured at the beginning of each scan) under different viewing conditions (eyes closed, open and fixated, or open and tracking the sound source). Their results suggested that the visual cortex deactivation was not a simple artifact due to poor visual fixation or image slip while attending to the sound stimuli but rather may have been related to aspects of eye fixation control and/or suppression of visually tracking the virtual sound source. One possibility, therefore, is that deactivation in these regions may reflect attenuated activity in mechanisms that might otherwise attempt to visually locate and track a salient sound source.

An in-depth study of cortical deactivations in the context of cross-modal experiments and the implications of such for interpreting interaction effects has recently been undertaken using fMRI by Laurienti et al. (2002). In this study, test periods consisted of 30 s blocks of visual stimuli (flashes of a checkerboard), auditory (white noise bursts), or bimodal (synchronized presentation of both stimuli) conditions interleaved with 30 s rest periods. During auditory blocks they observed decreased signals in some sensory-specific visual areas (bilateral lingual and fusiform gyri and right cuneus). A corresponding pattern of deactivation in auditory areas (superior and middle temporal gyri, BA 21/22) was observed during the visual condition. The locations of these foci were also topographically distinct from those related to task-irrelevant deactivation patterns described above (e.g., semantic monitoring during rest periods). The relative responses in auditory cortex evoked by the auditory-only and bimodal conditions were comparable, as were the responses in visual cortex evoked by the visual-only and bimodal conditions. Additionally, no deactivation responses were apparent in the bimodal condition. Thus, they argued that the magnitude of the bimodal activation was significantly greater than the predicted sum of the individual auditory and visual responses (superadditivity) if the deactivation responses were factored in. The main point here is that one may underestimate integration sites if looking for superadditivity solely on the basis of positive interaction effects using the strict criterion of $AV > A + V$, if there is a deactivation in visual cortex with A alone or in auditory cortex with V alone. It may not be necessary that the individual unimodal responses reach significance (above baseline) for interaction effects to be identified in response to the bimodal inputs. However, it may be important to determine if either of them fall below baseline. At present, the specific experimental tasks, attentional demands, and other related factors that affect the deactivation signal have yet to be critically examined. Consequently, the interpretation of task-specific deactivations due to sensory stimulation from a single modality remains controversial.

Summary

The past several years have produced a wealth of audiovisual imaging data. Although it has not been possible to review all the material in this chapter, a framework of human brain regions involved in audiovisual interactions is beginning to emerge, with highlights on where and how many putatively distinct integration sites exist. Their relative involvement in dynamic temporal processing in any one task remains to be determined by other techniques. Some of the principles characterizing multisensory processing at the cellular level have now been identified in the context of imaging experiments. This suggests that the cellular indices of cross-modal integration are detectable at the level of cell populations. Given the caveats regarding BOLD ceiling effects, cross-modal cortical deactivations, and the possible modulatory effects of attention, validation of these BOLD signal changes must be made, perhaps by combining electrophysiology and fMRI studies in both human and nonhuman primates.

A growing body of evidence suggests that the left STS is involved in synthesizing the auditory and visual components of speech, although it may have a broader role in the more general integration of audiovisual signals. The MTG has been implicated in processing semantic information from the auditory and visual modalities, but so far there has been no explicit investigation of cross-modal interactions in this region. It may transpire that convergence of such higher-order representations may not rely on the same type of mechanism (multisensory cells) as that observed for lower-level integration.

Beyond the domain of speech, in both involuntary and directed attention situations, audiovisual interaction effects have been consistently reported in the IPS during the integration of cross-modal spatial coordinate information. The additional involvement of frontal regions may be rather specific to circumstances in which attention is endogenously controlled. Tasks that have explicitly focused on cross-modal synchrony of audiovisual inputs are beginning to implicate subcortical structures, including the SC and putamen, as well as the insula/claustrum, in the binding of multisensory inputs on the basis of their shared temporal onset. The challenge now will be to investigate the consequences of task, context, and the persuasiveness of the relative parameters of time, space, and identity on these binding mechanisms. Systematic manipulation of these parameters using the same stimuli and within the same subject group may provide some answers.

REFERENCES

Artieda, J., Pastor, M. A., Lacruz, F., & Obeso, J. A. (1992). Temporal discrimination is abnormal in Parkinson's disease. *Brain, 115,* 199–210.

Badgaiyan, R. D., Schacter, D. L., & Alpert, N. M. (1999). Auditory priming within and across modalities: Evidence from positron emission tomography. *Journal of Cognitive Neuroscience, 11,* 337–348.

Badgaiyan, R. D., Schacter, D. L., & Alpert, N. M. (2001). Priming within and across modalities: Exploring the nature of rCBF increases and decreases. *NeuroImage, 13,* 272–282.

Barth, D. S., Goldberg, N., Brett, B., & Di, S. (1995). The spatiotemporal organization of auditory, visual, and auditory-visual evoked potentials in rat cortex. *Brain Research, 678,* 177–190.

Baylis, G. C., Rolls, E. T., & Leonard, C. M. (1987). Functional subdivisions of the temporal lobe neocortex. *Journal of Neuroscience, 7,* 330–342.

Benevento, L. A., Fallon, J., Davis, B. J., & Rezak, M. (1977). Auditory-visual interaction in single cells in the cortex of the superior temporal sulcus and the orbital frontal cortex of the macaque monkey. *Experimental Neurology, 57,* 849–872.

Binder, J. R. (1997). Neuroanatomy of language processing studied with functional MRI. *Clinical Neuroscience, 4,* 87–94.

Binder, J. R., Frost, J. A., Hammeke, T. A., Bellgowan, P. S., Rao, S. M., & Cox, R. W. (1999). Conceptual processing during the conscious resting state: A functional MRI study. *Journal of Cognitive Neuroscience, 11,* 80–93.

Binder, J. R., & Price, C. J. (2001). Functional neuroimaging of language. In R. Cabeza & A. Kingstone (Eds.), *Handbook of functional neuroimaging of cognition* (pp. 187–251). Cambridge, MA: MIT Press.

Bookheimer, S. Y., Zeffiro, T. A., Blaxton, T. A., Gaillard, W. D., Malow, B., & Theodore, W. H. (1998). Regional cerebral blood flow during auditory responsive naming: Evidence for cross-modality neural activation. *Neuroreport, 9,* 2409–2413.

Bruce, C., Desimone, R., & Gross, C. G. (1981). Visual properties of neurons in a polysensory area in superior temporal sulcus of the macaque. *Journal of Neurophysiology, 46,* 369–384.

Bremmer, F., Schlack, A., Duhamel, J. R., Graf, W., & Fink, G. R. (2001). Space coding in primate posterior parietal cortex. *NeuroImage, 14*(1 Pt. 2), S46–S51.

Bremmer, F., Schlack, A., Shah, N. J., Zafiris, O., Kubischik, M., Hoffmann, K., et al. (2001). Polymodal motion processing in posterior parietal and premotor cortex: A human fMRI study strongly implies equivalencies between humans and monkeys. *Neuron, 29,* 287–296.

Bushara, K. O., Grafman, J., & Hallett, M. (2001). Neural correlates of auditory-visual stimulus onset asynchrony detection. *Journal of Neuroscience, 21,* 300–304.

Bushara, K. O., Weeks, R. A., Ishii, K., Catalan, M. J., Tian, B., Rauschecker, J. P., et al. (1999). Modality-specific frontal and parietal areas for auditory and visual spatial localization in humans. *Nature Neuroscience, 2,* 759–766.

Callan, D. E., Callan, A. M., Kroos, C., & Vatikiotis-Bateson, E. (2001). Multimodal contribution to speech perception revealed by independent component analysis: A single-sweep EEG case study. *Cognitive Brain Research, 10,* 349–353.

Callan, D. E., Callan, A. M., & Vatikiotis-Bateson, E. (2001). Neural areas underlying the processing of visual speech information under conditions of degraded auditory information. *Proceedings of the AVSP,* pp. 45–49.

Calvert, G. A. (2001). Crossmodal processing in the human brain: Insights from functional neuroimaging studies. *Cerebral Cortex, 11,* 1110–1123.

Calvert, G. A., Brammer, M. J., Bullmore, E. T., Campbell, R., Iversen, S. D., & David, A. S. (1999). Response amplification in sensory-specific cortices during cross-modal binding. *Neuroreport, 10,* 2619–2623.

Calvert, G. A., Campbell, R., & Brammer, M. J. (2000). Evidence from functional magnetic resonance imaging of cross-modal binding in the human heteromodal cortex. *Current Biology, 10,* 649–657.

Calvert, G. A., Bullmore, E. T., Brammer, M. J., Campbell, R., Williams, S. C., McGuire, P. K., et al. (1997). Activation of auditory cortex during silent lipreading. *Science, 276,* 593–596.

Calvert, G. A., Hansen, P. C., Iversen, S. D., & Brammer, M. J. (2001). Detection of audiovisual integration sites in humans by application of electrophysiological criteria to the BOLD effect. *NeuroImage, 14,* 427–438.

Chee, M. W., O'Craven, K. M., Bergida, R., Rosen, B. R., & Savoy, R. L. (1999). Auditory and visual word processing studied with fMRI. *Human Brain Mapping, 7,* 15–28.

Colin, C., Radeau, M., Deltenre, P., & Morais, J. (2001). Rules of intersensory integration in spatial scene analysis and speechreading. *Psychologica Belgica, 41,* 131–144.

Curran, T., Schacter, D. L., & Galluccio, L. (1999). Cross-modal priming and explicit memory in patients with verbal production deficits. *Brain and Cognition, 39,* 133–146.

Desimone, R., & Gross, C. G. (1979). Visual areas in the temporal cortex of the macaque. *Brain Research, 178,* 363–380.

Desimone, R., & Ungerleider, L. G. (1986). Multiple visual areas in the caudal superior temporal sulcus of the macaque. *Journal of Comparative Neurology, 248,* 164–189.

Dolan, R. J., Morris, J. S., & de Gelder, B. (2001). Crossmodal binding of fear in voice and face. *Proceedings of the National Academy of Sciences, USA, 98,* 10006–10010.

Downar, J., Crawley, A. P., Mikulis, D. J., & Davis, K. D. (2000). A multimodal cortical network for the detection of changes in the sensory environment. *Nature Neuroscience, 3,* 277–283.

Downar, J., Crawley, A. P., Mikulis, D. J., & Davis, K. D. (2001). The effect of task relevance on the cortical response to changes in visual and auditory stimuli: An event-related fMRI study. *NeuroImage, 14,* 1256–1267.

Driver, J., & Spence, C. (1998). Attention and the crossmodal construction of space. *Trends in Cognitive Sciences, 2,* 254–262.

Drury, H. A., Van Essen, D. C., & Anderson, C. H. (1996). Computerized mappings of the cerebral cortex: A multiresolution flattening method and a surface-based coordinate system. *Journal of Cognitive Neuroscience, 8,* 1–28.

Duhamel, J. R., Colby, C. L., & Goldberg, M. E. (1991). In J. Paillard (Ed.), *Brain and space* (pp. 223–236). New York: Oxford University Press.

Duhamel, J. R., Colby, C. L., & Goldberg, M. E. (1998). Ventral intraparietal area of the macaque: Congruent visual and somatic response properties. *Journal of Neurophysiology, 79,* 126–136.

Ettlinger, G., & Wilson, W. A. (1990). Cross-modal performance: Behavioural processes, phylogenetic considerations and neural mechanisms. *Behavioural Brain Research, 40,* 169–192.

Falchier, A., Clavagnier, S., Barone, P., & Kennedy, H. (2002). Anatomical evidence of multimodal integration in primate striate cortex. *Journal of Neuroscience, 22,* 5749–5759.

Farah, M. J., Wong, A. B., Monheit, M. A., & Morrow, L. A. (1989). Parietal lobe mechanisms of spatial attention: Modality-specific or supramodal? *Neuropsychologia, 27,* 461–470.

Finney, E. M., Fine, I., & Dobkins, K. R. (2001). Visual stimuli activate auditory cortex in the deaf. *Nature Neuroscience, 4,* 1171–1173.

Fishman, M. C., & Michael, P. (1973). Integration of auditory information in the cat's visual cortex. *Vision Research, 13,* 1415–1419.

Foxe, J. J., Morocz, I. A., Murray, M. M., Higgins, B. A., Javitt, D. C., & Schroeder, C. E. (2000). Multisensory auditory-somatosensory interactions in early cortical processing revealed by high-density electrical mapping. *Cognitive Brain Research, 10,* 77–83.

Francis, S., Rolls, E. T., Bowtell, R., McGlone, F., O'Doherty, J., Browning, A., et al. (1999). The representation of pleasant touch in the brain and its relationship with taste and olfactory areas. *Neuroreport, 10,* 453–459.

Fries, W. (1984). Cortical projections to the superior colliculus in the macaque monkey: A retrograde study using horseradish peroxidase. *Journal of Comparative Neurology, 230,* 55–76.

Friston, K. J., Buechel, C., Fink, G. R., Morris, J., Rolls, E., & Dolan, R. J. (1997). Psychophysiological and modulatory interactions in neuroimaging. *NeuroImage, 6,* 218–229.

Giard, M. H., & Peronnet, F. (1999). Auditory-visual integration during multimodal object recognition in humans: A behavioral and electrophysiological study. *Journal of Cognitive Neuroscience, 11,* 473–490.

Gonzalo, D., Shallice, T., & Dolan, R. (2000). Time-dependent changes in learning audio-visual associations: A single-trial fMRI study. *NeuroImage, 11,* 243–255.

Graziano, M. S. A., & Gross, C. G. (1998). Spatial maps for the control of movement. *Current Opinion in Neurobiology, 8,* 195–201.

Graziano, M. S. A., Reiss, L. A., & Gross, C. G. (1999). A neuronal representation of the location of nearby sounds. *Nature, 397,* 428–430.

Haist, F., Song, A. W., Wild, K., Faber, T. L., Popp, C. A., & Morris, R. D. (2001). Linking sight and sound: fMRI evidence of primary auditory cortex activation during visual word recognition. *Brain and Language, 76,* 340–350.

Haxby, J. V., Horwitz, B., Ungerleider, L. G., Maisog, J. M., Pietrini, P., & Grady, C. L. (1994). The functional organization of human extrastriate cortex: A PET-rCBF study of selective attention to faces and locations. *Journal of Neuroscience, 14* (11 Pt. 1), 6336–6353.

Horn, G. (1965). The effect of somaesthetic and photic stimuli on the activity of units in the striate cortex of unanesthetized, unrestrained cats. *Journal of Physiology, 179,* 263–277.

Hosokawa, T., Nakamura, R., & Shibuya, N. (1981). Monotic and dichotic fusion thresholds in patients with unilateral subcortical lesions. *Neuropsychologia, 19,* 241–248.

Howard, D., Patterson, K., Wise, R., Brown, W. D., Friston, K., Weiller, C., et al. (1992). The cortical localization of the lexicons: Positron emission tomography evidence. *Brain, 115,* (Pt. 6), 1769–1782.

Howard, R. J., Brammer, M., Wright, I., Woodruff, P. W., Bullmore, E. T., & Zeki, S. (1996). A direct demonstration of functional specialization within motion-related visual and auditory cortex of the human brain. *Current Biology, 6,* 1015–1019.

Howells, T. (1944). The experimental development of color-tone synesthesia. *Journal of Experimental Psychology, 34,* 87–103.

Iacoboni, M., Woods, R. P., & Mazziotta, J. C. (1998). Bimodal (auditory and visual) left frontoparietal circuitry for sensorimotor integration and sensorimotor learning. *Brain, 121,* 2135–2143.

Jung, R., Kornhuber, H. H., & Da Fonseca, J. S. (1963). Multisensory convergence on cortical neurons: Neuronal effects of visual, acoustic and vestibular stimuli in the superior convolutions of the cat's cortex. In G. Moruzzi, A. Fessard, & H. H. Jasper (Eds.), *Progress in brain research* (pp. 207–240), Amsterdam: Elsevier.

Kadunce, D. C., Vaughan, J. W., Wallace, M. T., Benedek, G., & Stein, B. E. (1997). Mechanisms of within- and cross-modality suppression in the superior colliculus. *Journal of Neurophysiology, 78,* 2834–2847.

Kastner, S., Pinsk, M. A., De Weerd, P., Desimone, R., & Ungerleider, L. G. (1999). Increased activity in human visual cortex during directed attention in the absence of visual stimulation. *Neuron, 22,* 751–761.

Kawashima, R., Imaizumi, S., Mori, K., Okada, K., Goto, R., Kiritani, S., et al. (1999). Selective visual and auditory attention toward utterances: A PET study. *NeuroImage, 10,* 209–215.

Laurienti, P. J., Burdette, J. H., Wallace, M. T., Yen, Y.-F., Field, A. S., & Stein, B. E. (2002). Deactivation of sensory-specific cortex by cross-modal stimuli. *Journal of Cognitive Neuroscience, 14,* 420–429.

Leinonen, L., Hyvärinen, J., & Sovijarvi, A. R. (1980). Functional properties of neurons in the temporo-parietal association cortex of awake monkey. *Experimental Brain Research, 39,* 203–215.

Lewis, J. W., Beauchamp, M. S., & DeYoe, E. A. (2000). A comparison of visual and auditory motion processing in human cerebral cortex. *Cerebral Cortex, 10,* 873–888.

Lewis, J. W., & Van Essen, D. C. (2000). Corticocortical connections of visual, sensorimotor, and multimodal processing areas in the parietal lobe of the macaque monkey. *Journal of Comparative Neurology, 428,* 112–137.

Lewis, J. W., Wightman, F. L., Brefczynski, J. A., Phinney, R. E., Binder, J. R., & DeYoe, E. A. (2002). *Human brain regions involved in recognizing environmental sounds.* Manuscript submitted for publication.

Lewkowicz, D. J.(2000). The development of intersensory temporal perception: An epigenetic systems/limitations view. *Psychological Bulletin, 126,* 281–308.

Linden, J. F., Grunewald, A., & Andersen, R. A. (1999). Responses to auditory stimuli in macaque lateral intraparietal area: II. Behavioral modulation. *Journal of Neurophysiology, 82,* 343–358.

Logothetis, N. K., Pauls, J., Augath, M., Trinath, T., & Oeltermann, A. (2001). Neurophysiological investigation of the basis of the fMRI signal. *Nature, 412,* 150–157.

Lomo, T., & Mollica, A. (1962). Activity of single units in the primary optic cortex in the unanesthetized rabbit during visual, acoustic, olfactory and painful stimulation. *Archives Italiennes de Biologie, 100,* 86–120.

MacSweeney, M., Amaro, E., Calvert, G. A., Campbell, R., David, A. S., McGuire, P., et al. (2000). Activation of auditory cortex by silent speechreading in the absence of scanner noise: An event-related fMRI study. *Neuroreport, 11,* 1729–1733.

MacSweeney, M., Campbell, R., Calvert, G. A., McGuire, P. K., David, A. S., Suckling, J. D., et al. (2001). Dispersed activation in the left temporal cortex for speech-reading in congenitally deaf people. *Proceedings of the Royal Society (London), 268,* 451–457.

McDonald, J. J., Teder-Sälejärvi, W. A., & Ward, L. M. (2001). Multisensory integration and cross-modal attention effects in the human brain. *Science, 292,* 1791.

McGurk, H., & MacDonald, J. W. (1976). Hearing lips and seeing voices. *Nature, 264,* 746–748.

McIntosh, A. R., Cabeza, R. E., & Lobaugh, N. J. (1998). Analysis of neural interactions explains the activation of occipital cortex by an auditory stimulus. *Journal of Neurophysiology, 80,* 2790–2796.

McKiernan, K. A., Kaufman, J. N., Kucera-Thompson, J., & Binder, J. R. (2002). *A parametric manipulation of factors affecting task-induced deactivation in functional neuroimaging.* Unpublished manuscript.

Mesulam, M.-M. (1998). From sensation to cognition. *Brain, 121,* 1013–1052.

Mesulam, M.-M., & Mufson, E. J. (1982). Insula of the old world monkey: III Efferent cortical output and comments on function. *Journal of Comparative Neurology, 212,* 38–52.

Michael, E. B., Keller, T. A., Carpenter, P. A., & Just, M. A. (2001). FMRI investigation of sentence comprehension by eye and by ear: Modality fingerprints on cognitive processes. *Human Brain Mapping, 13,* 239–252.

Mistlin, A. J., & Perrett, D. I. (1990). Visual and somatosensory processing in the macaque temporal cortex: The role of "expectation." *Experimental Brain Research, 82,* 437–450.

Morrell, F. (1972). Visual system's view of acoustic space. *Nature, 238,* 44–46.

Mufson, E. J., & Mesulam, M.-M. (1984). Thalamic connections of the insula in the rhesus monkey and comments on the paralimbic connectivity of the medial pulvinar nucleus. *Journal of Comparative Neurology, 227,* 109–120.

Munhall, K. G., & Tohkura, Y. (1998). Audiovisual gating and the time course of speech perception. *Journal of Acoustical Society of America, 104,* 530–539.

Murata, K., Cramer, H., & Bach-y-Rita, P. (1965). Neuronal convergence of noxious, acoustic, and visual stimuli in the visual cortex of the cat. *Journal of Neurophysiology, 28,* 1223–1239.

Nayani, T. H., & David, A. S. (1996). The auditory hallucination: A phenomenological survey. *Psychology and Medicine, 26,* 177–189.

Neal, J. W., Pearson, R. C. A., & Powell, T. P. S. (1990). The connections of area PG, 7a, with cortex in the parietal, occipital and temporal lobes of the monkey. *Brain Research, 532,* 249–264.

O'Leary, D. S., Andreasen, N. C., Hurtig, R. R., Torres, I. J., Flashman, L. A., Kesler, M. L., et al. (1997). Auditory and visual attention assessed with PET. *Human Brain Mapping, 5,* 422–436.

Olson, I. R., Gatenby, J. C., & Gore, J. C. (2002). A comparison of bound and unbound audio-visual information processing in the human cerebral cortex. *Cognitive Brain Research, 14,* 129–138.

Pearson, R. C., Brodal, P., Gatter, K. C., Powell, T. P. (1982). The organization of the connections between the cortex and the claustrum in the monkey. *Brain Research, 234,* 435–441.

Petersen, S. E., Fox, P. T., Posner, M. I., Mintun, M., & Raichle, M. E. (1988). Positron emission tomographic studies of the cortical anatomy of single-word processing. *Nature, 331,* 585–589.

Pizzamiglio, L., Perani, D., Cappa, S. F., Vallar, G., Paolucci, S., Grassi, F., et al. (1998). Recovery of neglect after right hemispheric damage: H$_2$(15)O positron emission tomographic activation study. *Archives of Neurology, 55,* 561–568.

Radeau, M. (1994). Auditory-visual spatial interaction and modularity. *Current Psychology of Cognition, 13,* 3–51.

Raichle, M. E., MacLeod, A. M., Snyder, A. Z., Powers, W. J., Gusnard, D. A., & Shulman, G. L. (2001). A default mode of brain function. *Proceedings of the National Academy of Sciences, USA, 98,* 676–682.

Raij, T., Uutela, K., & Hari, R. (2001). Audio-visual integration of letters in the human brain. *Neuron, 28,* 617–625.

Rockland, K. S., & Ojima, H. (2003). Multisensory convergence in calcarine visual areas in macaque monkey. *International Journal of Psychophysiology, 50,* 19–26.

Rolls, E. T. (2001). The rules of formation of the olfactory representations found in the orbitofrontal cortex olfactory areas in primates. *Chemical Senses, 26,* 595–604.

Rosenfeld, J. (1999). *An fMRI study of the neural mechanisms involved in audio-visual association learning.* Unpublished master's thesis, University of Oxford.

Royet, J. P., Zald, D., Versace, R., Costes, N., Lavenne, F., Koenig, O., et al. (2000). Emotional responses to pleasant and unpleasant olfactory, visual, and auditory stimuli: A positron emission tomography study. *Journal of Neuroscience, 20,* 7752–7759.

Sams, M., Aulanko, R., Hamalanin, M., Hari, R., Lounasmaa, O., Lu, S., et al. (1991). Seeing speech: Visual information from lip movements modifies activity in the human auditory cortex. *Neuroscience Letters, 127,* 141–145.

Saron, C. D., Schroeder, C. E., Foxe, J. J., & Vaughan, H. G., Jr. (2001). Visual activation of frontal cortex: Segregation from occipital activity. *Brain Research and Cognition, 12,* 75–88.

Schacter, D. L., Badgaiyan, R. D., & Alpert, N. M. (1999). Visual word stem completion priming within and across modalities: A PET study. *Neuroreport, 10,* 2061–2065.

Spinelli, D. N., Starr, A., & Barrett, T. W. (1968). Auditory specificity in unit recordings from cat's visual cortex. *Experimental Neurology, 22,* 75–84.

Stein, B. E., & Meredith, M. A. (1993). *Merging of the senses.* Cambridge, MA: MIT Press.

Stein, B. E., Meredith, M. A., & Wallace, M. T. (1993). The visually responsive neuron and beyond: Multisensory integration in cat and monkey. *Progress in Brain Research, 95,* 79–90.

Stein, B. E., Huneycutt, W. S., & Meredith, M. A. (1988). Neurons and behavior: The same rules of multisensory integration apply. *Brain Research, 448,* 355–358.

Stein, B. E., Meredith, M. A., Huneycutt, W. S., & McDade, L. (1989). Behavioural indices of multisensory integration: Orientation to visual cues is affected by auditory stimuli. *Journal of Cognitive Neuroscience, 1,* 12–24.

Sumby, W. H., & Pollack, I. (1954). Visual contribution to speech intelligibility in noise. *Journal of the Acoustical Society of America, 26,* 212–215.

Summerfield, Q. (1992). Lipreading and audio-visual speech perception. *Philosophical Transactions of the Royal Society of London, Series B: Biological Sciences, 335,* 71–78.

Surguladze, S. A., Calvert, G. A., Brammer, M. J., Campbell, R., Bullmore, E. T., Giampietro, V., et al. (2001). Audio-visual speech perception in schizophrenia: An fMRI study. *Psychiatry Research, 106,* 1–14.

Tulving, E., & Schacter, D. L. (1990). Priming and human memory systems. *Science, 247,* 301–306.

Turner, B. H., Mishkin, M., & Knapp, M. (1980). Organization of the amygdalopetal projections from modality-specific cortical association areas in the monkey. *Journal of Comparative Neurology, 191,* 515–543.

Van Essen, D. C., Drury, H. A., Joshi, S., & Miller, M. I. (1998). Functional and structural mapping of human cerebral cortex: Solutions are in the surfaces. *Proceedings of the National Academy of Sciences, USA, 95,* 788–795.

Waldvogel, D., van Gelderen, P., Muellbacher, W., Ziemann, U., Immisch, I., & Hallett, M. (2000). The relative metabolic demand of inhibition and excitation. *Nature, 406,* 995–998.

Wallace, M. T., Meredith, M. A., & Stein, B. E. (1992). Integration of multiple sensory modalities in cat cortex. *Experimental Brain Research, 91,* 484–488.

Ward, L. M. (1994). Supramodal and modality-specific mechanisms for stimulus-driven shifts of auditory and visual attention. *Canadian Journal of Experimental Psychology, 48,* 242–259.

Watanabe, J., & Iwai, E. (1991). Neuronal activity in visual, auditory and polysensory areas in the monkey temporal cortex during visual fixation task. *Brain Research Bulletin, 26,* 583–592.

Weeks, R., Horwitz, B., Aziz-Sultan, A., Tian, B., Wessinger, C. M., Cohen, L. G., et al. (2000). A positron emission tomographic study of auditory localization in the congenitally blind. *Journal of Neuroscience, 20,* 2664–2672.

Wilkinson, L. K., Meredith, M. A., & Stein, B. E. (1996). The role of anterior ectosylvian cortex in cross-modality orientation and approach behavior. *Experimental Brain Research, 112,* 1–10.

31 Multiple Electrophysiological Mechanisms of Audiovisual Integration in Human Perception

ALEXANDRA FORT AND MARIE-HÉLÈNE GIARD

Introduction

A fundamental issue to neuroscientists engaged in the study of multisensory phenomena is understanding the neurophysiological mechanisms by which the brain combines and integrates information from different sensory channels to form a unified percept.

This question can be approached in multiple ways. Animal studies over the past two decades have shown the existence of multisensory cells in the deep layers of the superior colliculus (SC), a midbrain structure involved in attentive and orienting behaviors, and in various cortical areas in primates and many other mammals (reviewed in Stein & Meredith, 1993; see also Barth, Goldberg, Brett, & Di, 1995; Bruce, Desimone, & Gross, 1981; Hikosaka, Iwai, Saito, & Tanaka, 1988; Wallace, Wilkinson, & Stein, 1996). In addition, the Stein group has shown that the integrative properties of multisensory neurons depend on a set of neural "principles." The *spatial* and *temporal* principles predict that the firing rate of these neurons increases in a superadditive way when two or more stimuli of different modalities are presented in the same location and at the same time; in contrast, spatially or temporally disparate stimuli trigger inhibitory mechanisms that can suppress the responses to either unimodal cue. The principle of *inverse effectiveness* stipulates that the magnitude of the interaction inversely depends on the effectiveness of the unimodal inputs (Stein & Meredith, 1993). These integration principles devised at the cell level in the SC have also been found to apply to the attentive and orienting behaviors mediated by this structure (Stein, Huneycutt, & Meredith, 1988), and globally to multisensory neurons in the neocortex (Stein & Wallace, 1996).

It is important to note, however, that the collicular and cortical multisensory neurons appear to belong to separate neural circuits, because they are not directly connected to each other (Wallace, Meredith, & Stein, 1993), and they are sensitive in different ways to the spatial factors, the multisensory neurons in the SC being more strictly dependent on the *spatial rule* of integration than the cortical neurons (Stein & Wallace, 1996). These features suggest that different integration mechanisms may exist for orienting processes ("where" information), mainly governed by the SC and for higher-level perceptual processes ("what" information), mediated by the cortex (Calvert, Hansen, Iversen, & Brammer, 2001; Hughes, Reuter-Lorenz, Nozawa, & Fendrich, 1994; Stein, London, Wilkinson, & Price, 1996).

Although human research on the neurophysiological bases of multisensory integration is much more recent, the rapidly growing number of neuroimaging studies has already provided an impressive number of results (reviewed in Calvert, 2001). Although the data are difficult to compare because of the different sensitivities of the methods—hemodynamic (positron emission tomography [PET] and functional magnetic resonance imaging [fMRI]) versus electromagnetic (electroencephalographic [EEG] and magnetoencephalographic [MEG]) approaches—and the variability of the experimental paradigms used, they already indicate that the physiological mechanisms of multisensory integration are complex and multiple. For example, they depend on the modalities of the sensory inputs (e.g., Calvert et al., 1999; Foxe et al., 2000; Giard & Peronnet, 1999; Macaluso, Frith, & Driver, 2000; Sams et al., 1991) or on the nature (speech/nonspeech) of the information to be combined (Callan, Callan, Kroos, & Vatikiotis-Bateson, 2001; Calvert et al., 2001; Raij, Uutela, & Hari, 2000). Yet when the *principles of integration* were considered in these studies, they were found to apply both to the magnitude of the physiological effects (Calvert et al., 2001; Widmann, Schröger, Shimojo, & Munka, 2000) and to related behavioral indices (see, however, Stein et al., 1996).

Within the large categories enumerated above (sensory modalities involved, spatial or nonspatial content of information to be bound, speech or nonspeech signals), however, it is tempting to consider multisensory integration as a particular brain function mediated by a specific chain of cross-modal operations; that is, for a given set of sensory inputs, the combination of the unimodal signals would be achieved by "standard" means through roughly invariant neurophysiological processes (Ettlinger & Wilson, 1990).

In this chapter we show, using event-related potentials (ERPs), that the neural mechanisms of multisensory integration in humans cannot be described in terms of hardwired cross-modal operations depending only on the input category. We argue that these mechanisms instead rely on dynamic neural systems with a spatiotemporal organization that depends on exogenous parameters (experimental conditions and tasks) as well as on endogenous factors (expertise of the subject for the task, attention). In addition, some of the neural operations related to multisensory integration may not follow the enhancement/depression rule that characterizes the integrative properties of multisensory cells, and, more generally, some neural principles of multisensory integration may not apply similarly at the cellular level, at the cortical population level, and at the behavioral level.

To this end, we will first discuss some general properties of ERPs and the particular advantages and limits of their use in investigating the physiological processes underlying multisensory integration. Then we present a set of data from three ERP experiments that used the same physical (nonspeech) stimuli but required a different perceptual task for these stimuli. Finally, we discuss these data, taking advantage of the high temporal resolution of the electrophysiological approach, and more broadly with respect to other neuroimaging findings in humans and to the neural principles of multisensory integration that apply at the single-cell level in animals.

ERPs for studying cross-modal interactions: General considerations

POLARITY Scalp ERPs are recorded as sequences of positive and negative waveforms. Their polarity depends on complex excitatory and inhibitory mechanisms at the synaptic level but has no direct implication for the functional processes with which the ERPs are associated.

SPATIOTEMPORAL INFORMATION ERPs carry double—temporal and spatial—information. Although their time resolution is excellent, on the order of a millisecond, their spatial distribution on the scalp reflects, at any given instant, the summed activities of possibly several intracerebral current "generators" (local sets of synchronously active neurons), which may have been distorted through the different conductive volumes formed by the brain structures, skull, and scalp. Surface potential maps (obtained by interpolation of the voltage values recorded at a large number of electrodes) are therefore difficult to interpret in terms of source localization. Finer spatial information can be provided by radial scalp current densities (SCDs), estimated by computing the second spatial derivatives of the interpolated potential distributions (Perrin, Pernier, Bertrand, & Echallier, 1989; Perrin, Pernier, Bertrand, & Giard, 1987). SCD maps are reference-free and have several interesting properties that can help disentangle the contribution of multiple sources that may overlap in surface potential maps. They have sharper peaks and troughs than potential maps, allowing better source separation, and SCD amplitudes at the scalp decrease more rapidly with the depth of the source in the brain than do potential amplitudes. Therefore, SCD maps emphasize the activity of shallow, cortical generators and are blind to deep, subcortical sources (Pernier, Perrin, & Bertrand, 1988).

THE ADDITIVE MODEL A procedure commonly used for studying cross-modal interactions in EEG and MEG recordings is to compare the response to a bimodal (e.g., audiovisual, AV) stimulus with the sum of the responses elicited by the unimodal cues presented in isolation (Au, Vi) (Fort, Delpuech, Pernier, & Giard, 2002a, 2002b; Foxe et al., 2000; Giard & Peronnet, 1999; Schröger & Widmann, 1998; MEG: Raij et al., 2000). The rationale is that, at early stages of stimulus analysis, the neural activities induced by the audiovisual stimulus are equal to the sum of activities induced separately by the auditory and visual stimuli plus the putative activities specifically elicited by the bimodal stimulation (auditory-visual interactions). Over this period, we may therefore use the summative model to estimate the AV interactions:

$$\text{ERP (AV)} = \text{ERP (Au)} + \text{ERP (Vi)}$$
$$+ \text{ERP (Au} \times \text{Vi interactions)}$$

This procedure relies on the law of superposition of electric fields and applies whatever the nature (number, configuration, geometry) of the intracerebral generators. Audiovisual interactions may therefore be quantified in the difference wave, AV − (Au + Vi), obtained by subtracting the sum of the responses to the unimodal stimuli from the response to multisensory stimuli (see Barth et al., 1995). It is important to note that the validity of this additive model depends on a number of conditions. Indeed, any activities that are common to all (unimodal and bimodal) stimulus types will not be eliminated in the difference waveform and may therefore be confounded with actual cross-modal interactions.

These common activities may be of several types. First, they include general task-related neural activities that may follow the sensory analysis of the stimulus (e.g., N2b, P3, or motor-related processes). These activities usually arise after about 200 ms post-stimulus. Therefore, sub-additive effects occurring after this period could be strongly contaminated by these nonspecific potentials being subtracted twice and not eliminated in the model. It should be noted that these activities may signal processes in multisensory *convergence* sites, but not necessarily *integration* mechanisms.

Second, in paradigms requiring speeded responses with rapidly presented stimuli, "anticipatory" slow potentials may arise before each stimulus and continue for a time after stimulus onset (Teder-Sälejärvi, McDonald, Di Russo, & Hillyard, 2002). These anticipatory potentials, usually ramplike negativities such as the *contingent negative variation,* appear, when present, as a negative-going shift in the prestimulus period and give rise to spurious effects in the difference waveforms that may be confused with early cross-modal interactions (Teder-Sälejärvi et al., 2002). This phenomenon can be controlled by visual inspection of the ERP morphology in the prestimulus baseline period and by verifying the stability of the early cross-modal effects (whenever present) when the latency of the prestimulus reference baseline period is modified or when the data are high-pass filtered with a 2-Hz cut-off frequency (Teder-Sälejärvi et al., 2002). This last solution, however, may also decrease the amplitudes of genuine cross-modal interactions.

Three experiments using the same physical stimuli

We used this additive model to compare the cross-modal interactions during three different nonspatial perceptual tasks performed on the same physical stimuli. The stimuli were two objects, A and B, defined either by unimodal visual or auditory features alone or by a combination of the visual and auditory features (Fig. 31.1). Object A consisted of either the deformation of a basic circle to a horizontal ellipse (V1), or a tone burst (A1), or the conjunction of the two features (A1V1). Object B was designed similarly as the deformation of a circle to a vertical ellipse (V2), or a slightly different tone burst (A2), or the conjunction of the two features (A2V2). The six stimuli were presented randomly with equal probability in a central position to the subjects. (A detailed description of the stimuli and procedure is available in Giard & Peronnet, 1999.)

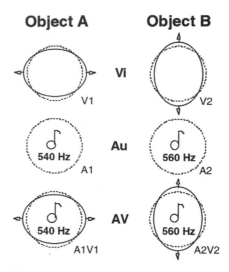

FIGURE 31.1   Two objects, A and B, were used. Each of them could be presented either in an auditory condition alone (object A: 540-Hz tone burst; object B: 560-Hz) or in a visual condition alone (transient deformation of a circle into a horizontal [object A] or vertical [object B] ellipse), or in a bimodal condition that combined auditory and visual features. The duration of each stimulus was 240 ms.

In the first experiment, the task was to identify, at each trial, which object (A or B) was presented by pressing one of two keys. In this object recognition task, therefore, the bimodal stimuli were characterized by *redundant* (auditory and visual) information. This experiment will be referred to as a *redundant-cue identification task.*

In the second experiment, subjects again had to identify the objects A and B, but the bimodal stimuli were now defined by *nonredundant* information. For that, we introduced a third object C, defined by either auditory features alone (A3 tone burst) or visual features alone (V3: deformation of the basic circle into a slightly larger circle), or, in its bimodal form by the combination of the unimodal components of objects A and B (A1V2, A2V1). All ten stimuli (A1, V1, A1V1; A2, V2, A2V2; A3, V3, A1V2, A2V1) were presented randomly; the task was to identify, in each trial, object A, B, or C by pressing one of three keys. The subjects therefore had to process both unimodal cues in the bimodal stimulus condition to execute the task correctly. Only the responses to objects A and B were analyzed to compare the interactions induced by strictly the same stimuli. This experiment will be referred to as *nonredundant-cue identification task.*

The third experiment entailed a simple *detection task.* Objects A and B were presented as in the first experiment, but the subjects had to press one key upon detecting any stimulus, whatever its nature. In this condition, therefore, no object identification was necessary, and the unimodal components may be considered redundant for bimodal stimulus detection.

In all three experiments, the stimuli were presented at relatively long and variable interstimulus intervals (reaction time period plus a delay of 1100–2900 ms) to avoid anticipatory effects.

Behavioral measures

Figure 31.2 displays the mean reaction times (averaged across objects A and B) according to the input modalities (Au, Vi, AV) in the three experiments. In Experiment 1, as expected from behavioral studies on the *redundant target effect* (Miller, 1982, 1986), the objects were identified more rapidly when they were presented in the bimodal condition (562 ms) than in either of the unimodal conditions (621 ms for the auditory presentation and 631 ms for the visual presentation).

In contrast, in the nonredundant-cue identification task (Experiment 2), recognition of the bimodal objects (966 ms) was not facilitated compared with recognition of either of the unimodal objects (Au: 938 ms; Vi: 950 ms), because both unimodal cues in the AV stimulus had to be identified before response selection. Rather, the similarity of the response times in the three conditions suggests that the auditory and visual features may have been processed in parallel in the bimodal condition.

In Experiment 3 (detection task), subjects responded more rapidly to bimodal stimuli (247 ms) than to either of the unimodal stimuli, and, in accordance with previous behavioral observations (Hershenson, 1962; Welch & Warren, 1986), they were faster to respond to auditory stimuli (276 ms) than to visual stimuli (310 ms).

Therefore, behavioral facilitation effects for bimodal processing were seen only in Experiments 1 and 3, manipulating redundant sensory inputs, yet ERP cross-modal interaction patterns were found in all three tasks.

Cross-modal interactions before 200 ms latency

As described earlier, the cross-modal interactions were measured as the differences between the responses to the bimodal stimuli and the sum of the unimodal responses within the first 200 ms of stimulus analysis and were assessed using Student t tests comparing the amplitude of the [AV − (Au + Vi)] difference wave against zero at each electrode and time sample. Sequential t maps could then indicate the spatiotemporal regions (scalp areas and timing of activation) of significant effects. We considered as cross-modal interactions those scalp areas with significant [AV − (Au + Vi)] amplitudes for at least 15 consecutive time samples (15 ms) (Thorpe, Fize, & Marlot, 1996). Detailed descriptions of these interaction patterns have been reported elsewhere (Fort et al., 2002a, 2002b; Giard & Peronnet, 1999), and only their main features will be summarized here. We will examine the main effects in sensory-specific areas, in deep brain structures (SC), and in the right temporofrontal regions.

INTERACTIONS IN SENSORY-SPECIFIC AREAS Figure 31.3 displays, for each experiment, the topographies and statistical significances of [AV − (Au + Vi)] on posterior scalp areas in three latency ranges (50–100 ms, 100–150 ms, and 150–200 ms). Several important differences can already be noted:

• In the two *redundant-cue* conditions (Experiments 1 and 3), significant [AV − (Au + Vi)] amplitudes were found already by 50 ms post-stimulus at occipital sites with scalp distributions typical of activities in visual cortex (Fig. 31.3, lines 1 and 3, column 1).

• Between 100 and 150 ms (Fig. 31.3, second column), significant interactions were still found in Experiments 1 and 3, but they strongly differed from each other, with a positive potential field at occipital visual sites on the identification task (Experiment 1)

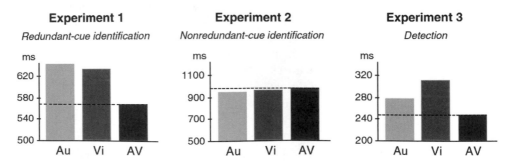

FIGURE 31.2 Mean reaction times (averaged over objects A and B) for unimodal auditory (Au), visual (Vi), or bimodal (AV) inputs in the three experiments (redundant-cue identification, nonredundant-cue identification, and detection tasks). A facilitation effect for bimodal processing was observed only in Experiments 1 and 3.

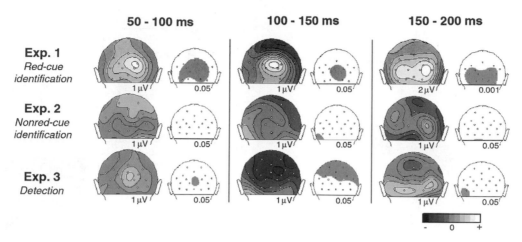

50 - 100 ms   **100 - 150 ms**   **150 - 200 ms**

Exp. 1
Red-cue identification
1 μV   0.05   1 μV   0.05   2 μV   0.001

Exp. 2
Nonred-cue identification
1 μV   0.05   1 μV   0.05   1 μV   0.05

Exp. 3
Detection
1 μV   0.05   1 μV   0.05   1 μV   0.05

FIGURE 31.3   Potential maps (left columns) and statistical Student *t* maps (right columns) of cross-modal interactions on posterior visual scalp areas in three latency windows (50–100 ms, 100–150 ms, and 150–200 ms post-stimulus) in the three experiments. Significant early effects (50–100 ms) were found only on the redundant-cue identification and detection tasks.

and negative potentials widely distributed over centro-parietal sites on the detection task (Experiment 3). This last effect will be analyzed in detail later.

• Between 150 and 200 ms latency (Fig. 31.3, third column), significant effects were observed only on the redundant-cue identification task (Experiment 1). In addition, Figure 31.4 shows that this interaction pattern has the same topography and latency as the unimodal visual N185 component, known to be generated in extrastriate visual cortex (Mangun, 1995). Thus, this cross-modal pattern probably indicates that the N185 generator activities in extrastriate cortex are modulated when an auditory cue is added to the visual stimulus. Interestingly, this modulation is a *decrease* in the unimodal N185 visual response. This amplitude decrease is not observed for the two other tasks (Fig. 31.3, lines 2 and 3, column 3).

In sum, identification of bimodal objects containing redundant information (Experiment 1) induces complex cross-modal effects in visual areas between

about 40 and 150 ms post-stimulus and decreases the amplitude of the unimodal visual response in extrastriate cortex at around 185 ms, whereas on a simple detection task (Experiment 3), only early interactions (45–85 ms) are observed in visual regions. No significant effects on posterior sites were found on the nonredundant-cue identification task (Experiment 2).

These cross-modal effects can be analyzed more finely if one takes into account the fact that in the first experiment, some subjects found it easier to categorize the objects on the basis of the objects' visual features than their auditory features, while others, generally those having some training in singing or music, found the reverse to be true. Therefore, on the two identification tasks (Experiments 1 and 2), subjects were divided into two groups according to the modality of their shortest reaction time in unimodal object recognition: subjects who identified auditory objects faster than visual objects were called auditory dominant, while those who identified visual objects faster than auditory objects were denoted visually dominant subjects. (Note that according to this criterion, all the subjects were auditory-dominant for the detection task and are classified as such in the following discussion.)

Reanalyzing the data separately for the two groups of subjects led to somewhat different results in sensory-specific areas, as shown in Figure 31.5. First, in all the experiments (both identification and detection tasks), auditory dominant subjects presented significant cross-modal interactions in visual cortex below 150 ms, while visually dominant subjects showed no or only marginal effects on the two identification tasks (Experiments 1 and 2). Conversely, on these two identification tasks the visually dominant subjects presented interaction patterns at around 100–150 ms, typical of activities in

Exp. 1   *Redundant-cue identification*

185 ms

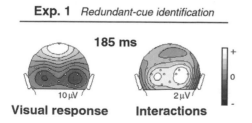

10 μV   2 μV

Visual response   **Interactions**

FIGURE 31.4   In Experiment 1, cross-modal interactions (right image) were found with the same spatiotemporal distribution as the unimodal visual N185 response (left image), suggesting that discrimination of redundant bimodal objects *decreases* the amplitude of the unimodal N185 component in extrastriate cortex.

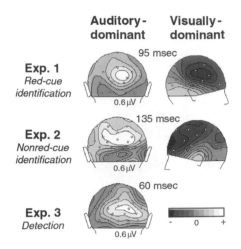

Auditory-dominant   **Visually-dominant**

Exp. 1
Red-cue identification
95 msec
0.6 µV

Exp. 2
Nonred-cue identification
135 msec
0.6 µV

Exp. 3
Detection
60 msec
0.6 µV
− 0 +

FIGURE 31.5 Patterns of cross-modal interactions analyzed separately in auditory-dominant and visually dominant subjects on the two identification tasks (Experiments 1 and 2). Although the latency of the effects could vary within the conditions, auditory-dominant subjects presented clear interaction patterns in posterior visual areas (also verified in Experiment 3, where all the subjects were auditory-dominant for the detection task), whereas visually dominant subjects displayed topographical patterns typical of activities in the auditory cortex.

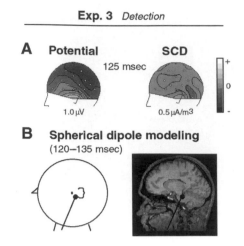

Exp. 3 *Detection*

A   **Potential**   **SCD**
125 msec
1.0 µV   0.5 µA/m3
+
0
−

B   **Spherical dipole modeling**
(120–135 msec)

FIGURE 31.6 (*A*) Scalp potential (left) and current density (right) distributions of AV − (Au + Vi) at around 120–135 ms post-stimulus. The very weak SCD amplitudes associated with the wide voltage pattern strongly suggests multisensory activities in deep brain structures. (*B*) Spatiotemporal dipole modeling of the interactions. One equivalent current dipole (ECD) accounts for more than 80% of the total experimental variance. Its projection onto the closest sagittal MRI section of one subject was found within 15 mm of the SC.

auditory cortex (negative potential fields on frontal scalp areas reversing polarity at inferotemporal mastoid sites). In other words, the audiovisual interactions before 150 ms latency were more important in the cortex of the *nondominant* modality (visual cortex for auditory-dominant subjects, and vice versa).

SUPERIOR COLLICULUS? Figure 31.3 (line 3, column 2) shows that the detection task (Experiment 3) induces, at around 100–150 ms, significant interactions, with a scalp distribution strongly differing from that found during the identification of the same bimodal stimuli. Figure 31.6*A* (left image) presents in more detail this interaction pattern, which is characterized by a negative potential field widely distributed over the frontal, central, and parietal scalp regions. This pattern was not present in either unimodal response. Interestingly, SCD analysis of [AV − (Au + Vi)] at around the same latency revealed only very weak current distributions (Fig. 31.6*A*, right image). Given that the amplitude of SCDs decreases more rapidly at the scalp surface as the source of the intracerebral generators deepens in the brain than potential amplitudes do (Pernier et al., 1988; Perrin et al., 1987), the morphological differences between the potential and SCD [AV − (Au + Vi)] distributions at the scalp strongly suggest that the underlying neural activities are localized in deep (subcortical) brain structures, possibly the SC, which is known to be a major site of multisensory integration. This hypothesis

is strengthened by spatiotemporal source modeling (Scherg, 1990). We used a spherical head model and a single equivalent current dipole to model the interaction pattern within the 120–135 ms period, during which the topography of the effects was stable. The best-fitting dipole explained the potential distributions with a goodness of fit of 81.7%. The dipole projection onto the MRI of one subject (Fig. 31.6*B*) by means of automatic adjustment of the sphere model to the subject's head (Fort et al., 2002b) was found within 15 mm of the SC, a distance on the same order of precision as the spherical head dipole modeling (Yvert, Bertrand, Thevenet, Echallier, & Pernier, 1997).

RIGHT TEMPOROFRONTAL SCALP REGIONS In all three experiments and in both auditory-dominant and visually dominant subjects, similar cross-modal interaction patterns were found over the right temporofrontal scalp regions at around 140–185 ms latencies (Fig. 31.7). Such activities were not observed on the left hemiscalp or in the unimodal responses in either experiment, indicating that the effect was due to neuronal populations in the anterior part of the right hemisphere responding only to bimodal inputs. Although a precise localization is not possible with ERPs, the topography of this effect is consistent with sources in the right insula, the right prefrontal cortex, and/or the temporopolar cortex (Benevento, Fallon, Davis, & Rezak, 1977; Füster, Bodner, & Kroger, 2000; Jones & Powell, 1970).

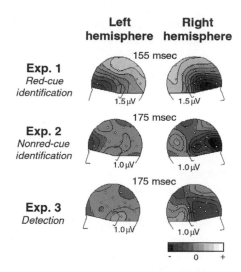

Left **Right**
hemisphere **hemisphere**

Exp. 1
*Red-cue
identification*
155 msec
1.5 µV   1.5 µV

Exp. 2
*Nonred-cue
identification*
175 msec
1.0 µV   1.0 µV

Exp. 3
Detection
175 msec
1.0 µV   1.0 µV

- 0 +

FIGURE 31.7   In all three experiments, similar cross-modal effects were found over the right temporofrontal scalp regions, strongly suggesting involvement of the same nonspecific brain areas (right insula?) on the three perceptual tasks.

A particularly interesting candidate is the right insula, which has repeatedly been found to be active when two stimuli of different modalities are presented in temporal synchrony (Bushara, Grafman, & Hallett, 2001; Calvert et al., 2001; Downar, Crawley, Mikulis, & Davis, 2000; Hadjikhani & Roland, 1998; Paulesu et al., 1995).

Implications for the physiological mechanisms of multisensory integration

The data presented so far show that, despite their poor spatial resolution, human scalp ERPs can provide important insight into the brain mechanisms of multisensory integration. Detailed discussion and comparison of the interaction patterns generated in the three experiments have been reported elsewhere (Fort et al., 2002a, 2002b; Giard & Peronnet, 1999). Here we will focus on the implications of the data for the spatiotemporal organization and functional properties of the neural systems involved in multisensory integration.

TEMPORAL DYNAMICS OF CROSS-MODAL PROCESSES   A fundamental interest in using an ERP approach is to obtain timing information on the mechanisms of intersensory synthesis. The data presented in this chapter show that the responses to bimodal stimuli may differ from the sum of the unimodal responses very early, from 40–50 ms post-stimulation (Experiments 1 and 3), that is, already around the latencies of the very first cortical activations. Although anticipatory activities, which are not eliminated in the additive model, could generate similar spurious effects in [AV − (Au + Vi)] (see the

Introduction), several arguments strongly suggest that the early interactions in our data reflect genuine cross-modal operations. First, in all our experiments, the objects were presented at slow rates (interstimulus intervals varying within 1350–2850 ms and 1100–3200 ms in Experiments 1 and 3, respectively), which probably makes subjects' anticipation needless to achieve the task. Second, as expected in the absence of anticipatory slow potentials, the 100 ms prestimulus baselines in these two studies were remarkably flat and stable around zero (Giard & Peronnet, 1999, Fig. 4; Fort et al., 2002b, Fig. 2); additional controls for slow wave effects showed that using the 100–50 ms prestimulus period for baseline correction or high-pass filtering the data with a 2-Hz cut-off frequency (Teder-Sälejärvi et al., 2002) did not fundamentally change the latency or configuration of the early interactions (Fort et al., 2002b). In addition, these early effects are similar to those found with a paradigm that did not require any task (therefore expectation) from the subjects (Foxe et al., 2000). Therefore, the surprisingly early latencies of cross-modal effects in posterior visual areas would indicate that unisensory analysis of two simultaneous inputs of different modalities and cross-modal synthesis of these inputs can operate in parallel (in time) and interact intimately at the very first cortical stages.

These observations are still difficult to explain in light of our current knowledge on transmission of information flow through the sensory pathways. Indeed, the precocity of the earliest effects is hardly compatible with the hypothesis of neural projections from polysensory areas to sensory-specific cortices (Calvert et al., 2001), although this phenomenon could well account for later cross-modal enhancements in auditory and visual cortices. Another explanation can be drawn from the results of two very recent studies in monkeys that showed the existence of direct projections from the primary auditory cortex (usually already activated at 20–30 ms post-stimulation) to low-level areas (V1) of the visual cortex (Falchier, Clavagnier, Barone, & Kennedy, 2002; Rockland & Ojima, 2001). Similar projections from visual to auditory cortex have already been reported in monkey studies (Schroeder et al., 1995), as have somatosensory inputs to auditory cortex (Fu et al., 2001; Schroeder et al., 2001). Although the functional role of such connections is not known, they could increase the efficiency of bimodal processing under top-down control in appropriate perceptual or attentional contexts.

MULTIPLICITY AND FLEXIBILITY OF THE NEURAL MECHANISMS FOR AUDIOVISUAL INTEGRATION   Three features show that synthesis of the same audiovisual inputs can be achieved through different neural operations. First, in all three experiments, we repeatedly found that when subjects were separated into visually dominant and auditory-dominant groups for the considered task, the effects in sensory-specific areas were stronger in the cortex of the nondominant modality (visual cortex for auditory-dominant subjects, and vice versa). These observations have implications at two levels. They show that the integrative operations can finely adapt to the individual sensory expertise; on the other hand, they may be directly related to the inverse effectiveness principle of multisensory integration and may show that this principle applies at the integrated level of sensory cortex activity in humans, with multisensory enhancement being dependent on the *subjective* effectiveness of the unimodal cues (since the same physical objects were used for all the subjects).

A second feature is the task dependency of integration effects in sensory-specific areas. Indeed, a modulation of the unimodal visual N1 response (185 ms latency) was found in the first experiment only (redundant-cue identification task). It has recently been shown that the visual N1 component generated in extrastriate cortex (Mangun, 1995) has a particular role in discrimination within the focus of attention (Vogel & Luck, 2000). Interestingly, although this component was elicited in the unimodal visual conditions in all three experiments, no modulation of its amplitude was found when discrimination was not relevant to the task (simple detection in Experiment 3) or when discrimination was not facilitated because of the nonredundant character of bimodal stimuli (Experiment 2). We will return to these effects later; taken together with the major effects in the nondominant sensory cortex at earlier latencies, however, they already emphasize the high complexity and flexibility of the integrative processes within the brain regions traditionally held to be unisensory.

A third finding is the observation of bimodal interactions in deep brain structures (probably the SC) at around 105–140 ms post-stimulus on the detection task (Experiment 3) without similar effects on the other tasks (Experiments 1 and 2). This finding suggests that deep brain structures may be involved in nonspatial aspects of bimodal integration. More important, these results highlight an important feature of multisensory mechanisms. Indeed, identification and discrimination may be considered as higher-level perceptual processes, compared with simple detection of the same stimuli. One may therefore expect, if detection precedes identification in the sensory processing hierarchy, that the low-level neural operations necessary for detection are

also activated during identification and discrimination of the same bimodal stimuli. The data observed here do not support this hypothesis, or at least clearly show that there is no cross-modal facilitation at these low levels of sensory processing when finer stimulus analysis is necessary. This result again underlines the exquisite flexibility of the integrative processes, which probably adapt for the most efficient result at the lowest energy cost.

Besides the subject- and task-dependent character of cross-modal operations, it was found that the bimodal stimuli in all experiments and subjects activated the right temporofrontal brain region within 140–185 ms. In our first study, we had proposed that these brain sites "could carry out more general integration functions" (Giard & Peronnet, 1999) than the operations carried out in sensory-specific cortices. This interpretation is strengthened by the generalization of this finding across the three experiments. As discussed above, however, the topography of the effect is compatible with an activation, at least in part, of the right insula, and could also reflect the detection of temporally coincident sensory inputs (Bushara et al., 2001), a brain process common to all three tasks.

BEHAVIORAL AND PHYSIOLOGICAL INDICES OF INTEGRATION MAY DIFFER   The presence of cross-modal interactions in the nonredundant-cue identification task (Experiment 3) indicates that the relationships between the behavioral and physiological indices of multisensory integration are not as straightforward as previously thought. Indeed, it has been shown that multisensory integration at the single-neuron level in animals is associated with facilitation effects on behavioral measures (Stein et al., 1988, 1989). Conversely, psychological models in humans have proposed that the behavioral facilitation indexed by shorter reaction times to process redundant bimodal stimuli (redundant target effect) is associated with cross-modal interactions, either during sensory analysis ("interactive coactivation model"; Miller, 1986) or at later stages of processing (Fournier & Eriksen, 1990; Hughes et al., 1994; Schmidt, Giele, & van den Heuvel, 1984), or even could be explained without interaction of unimodal information (Raab, 1962).

ERP data provide unequivocal evidence for coactivation models with cross-modal interactions at early stages of stimulus analysis, but they also show that sensory information processing interacts even when the bimodal character of the stimulus does not induce behavioral facilitation. Although these results could not be predicted by any of the theories cited above, they are in accordance with the neural principles that govern multisensory integration at the single-cell level in animals: namely, cross-modal neural synergy may be induced whenever two inputs of different modalities occur in spatial and temporal coincidence (Stein & Meredith, 1993; Stein & Wallace, 1996; see also Bushara et al., 2001).

Neural Depression May Also Signal Cross-Modal Facilitation   Animal studies have shown that the integrative character of multisensory neurons (responding to spatially and temporally coincident bimodal inputs) is manifested as vigorous increases in their firing rate at a level much exceeding that predicted by summing the unimodal responses, whereas the responses to spatially or temporally disparate stimuli can produce profound response depression (Kadunce, Vaughan, Wallace, Benedek, & Stein, 1997). Such indices of response enhancement and depression have been taken as criteria in BOLD signals for detecting sites of multisensory integration during human fMRI experiments (Calvert, 2001). Yet our data show that multisensory integration may be manifested by a decreased amplitude of the visual N1 response (185 ms latency) in extrastriate cortex. As discussed earlier, this ERP component has been associated with visual discrimination processes. A decrease in N1 amplitude may therefore reflect a lesser energy demand (neural facilitation) from the visual system to discriminate stimuli made more salient by the addition of an auditory cue. Similar depression effects have been found in early ERP studies (e.g., Davis, Osterhammel, Wier, & Gjerdingen, 1972) and MEG recordings (Busch, Wilson, Orr, & Papanicolaou, 1989; Raij et al., 2000). In this latter study, however, response depression was reported in the left posterior superior temporal sulcus, "a part of Wernicke's area," when subjects had to categorize target letters presented in auditory and visual modalities. The latency of the effects (380 ms) makes it unclear whether these effects reflect genuine cross-modal interactions, or common activities in Wernicke's area related to the verbal nature of all (unimodal and bimodal) stimuli and not eliminated in the difference operation, [AV − (Au + Vi)]. In any case, many examples exist as learning situations in which processing facilitation is manifested not only in ERP/MEG signals, but also in PET and fMRI recordings, by suppressive responses (e.g., Kok & de Jong, 1980; Raichle et al., 1994). That cross-modal facilitation at a behavioral level might also be signaled by neural depression is therefore not surprising and emphasizes the variety of neural mechanisms participating in multisensory integration.

Conclusion

Overall, the ERP data reported in this chapter indicate that the neural mechanisms of intersensory synthesis are more complex than was first expected. Specifically, the ERP data show that the routes of multisensory integration are multiple even for the synthesis of the same input material (here, nonspatial, nonlinguistic, audiovisual information). If one keeps in mind that the functional role of multisensory integration is to facilitate the processing of bimodal inputs *for a specific goal* (depending on the task requirement), our findings would indicate that cross-modal interactions operate preferentially at the level of the brain processes that most efficiently meet the task demands (SC for simple detection, nondominant sensory cortex for sensory analysis, N1 amplitude decrease for discrimination). This neural facilitation for particular brain processes may occur in sensory-specific as well as nonspecific cortices, and may manifest as both depression and enhancement of the sensory signals. Conversely, the right temporofrontal integration sites could signal more general activities, adding to the different task-related cross-modal operations to increase the functional efficiency of multisensory integration.

REFERENCES

Barth, D. S., Goldberg, N., Brett, B., & Di, S. (1995). The spatiotemporal organization of auditory, visual and auditory-visual evoked potentials in rat cortex. *Brain Research, 678,* 177–190.

Benevento, L. A., Fallon, J., Davis, B. J., & Rezak, M. (1977). Auditory-visual interaction in single cells in the cortex of the superior temporal sulcus and the orbital frontal cortex of the macaque monkey. *Experimental Neurology, 57,* 849–872.

Bruce, C., Desimone, R., & Gross, C. G. (1981). Visual properties of neurons in a polysensory area in superior temporal sulcus of the macaque. *Journal of Neurophysiology, 46,* 369–383.

Busch, C., Wilson, G., Orr, C., & Papanicolaou, A. C. (1989). Cross-modal interactions of auditory stimulus presentation on the visual evoked magnetic response. In S. J. Williamson (Ed.), *Advances in biomagnetism* (pp. 221–224). New York: Plenum Press.

Bushara, K. O., Grafman, J., & Hallett, M. (2001). Neural correlates of auditory-visual stimulus onset asynchrony detection. *Journal of Neuroscience, 21,* 300–304.

Callan, D. E., Callan, A. M., Kroos, C., & Vatikiotis-Bateson, E. (2001). Multimodal contribution to speech perception revealed by independent component analysis: A single-sweep EEG case study. *Cognitive Brain Research, 10,* 349–353.

Calvert, G. A. (2001). Crossmodal processing in the human brain: Insights from functional neuroimaging studies. *Cerebral Cortex, 11,* 1110–1123.

Calvert, G. A., Brammer, M. J., Bullmore, E. T., Campbell, R., Iversen, S. D., & David, A. S. (1999). Response amplification in sensory-specific cortices during crossmodal binding. *NeuroReport, 10,* 2619–2623.

Calvert, G. A., Hansen, P. C., Iversen, S. D., & Brammer, M. J. (2001). Detection of audio-visual integration sites in humans by application of electrophysiological criteria to the BOLD effect. *NeuroImage, 14,* 427–438.

Davis, H., Osterhammel, P. A., Wier, C. C., & Gjerdingen, D. B. (1972). Slow vertex potentials: Interactions among auditory, tactile, electric and visual stimuli. *Electroencephalography and Clinical Neurophysiology, 33,* 537–545.

Downar, J., Crawley, A. P., Mikulis, D. J., & Davis, K. D. (2000). A multimodal cortical network for the detection of changes in the sensory environment. *Nature Neuroscience, 3,* 277–283.

Ettlinger, G., & Wilson, W. A. (1990). Cross-modal performance: Behavioural processes, phylogenetic considerations and neural mechanisms. *Behavioural Brain Research, 40,* 169–192.

Falchier, A., Clavagnier, S., Barone, P., & Kennedy, H. (2002). Anatomical evidence of multimodal integration in primate striate cortex. *Journal of Neuroscience, 22,* 5749–5759.

Fort, A., Delpuech, C., Pernier, J., & Giard, M. H. (2002a). Early auditory-visual interactions in human cortex during nonredundant target identification. *Cognitive Brain Research, 14,* 20–30.

Fort, A., Delpuech, C., Pernier, J., & Giard, M. H. (2002b). Dynamics of cortico-subcortical crossmodal operations involved in audio-visual object detection in humans. *Cerebral Cortex, 12,* 1031–1039.

Fournier, L. R., & Eriksen, C. W. (1990). Coactivation in the perception of redundant targets. *Journal of Experimental Psychology: Human Perception and Performance, 16,* 538–550.

Foxe, J. J., Morocz, I. A., Murray, M. M., Higgins, B. A., Javitt, D. C., & Schroeder, C. E. (2000). Multisensory auditory-somatosensory interactions in early cortical processing revealed by high-density electrical mapping. *Cognitive Brain Research, 10,* 77–83.

Fu, K. G., Johnston, T. A., Shah, A. S., Arnold, L., Smiley, J., Hackett, T. A., et al. (2001). Characterization of somatosensory input to auditory association cortex in macaques. *Society for Neuroscience Abstracts, 27,* 681.3.

Füster, J. M., Bodner, M., & Kroger, J. K. (2000). Cross-modal and cross-temporal association in neurons of frontal cortex. *Nature, 405,* 347–351.

Giard, M. H., & Peronnet, F. (1999). Auditory-visual integration during multimodal object recognition in humans: A behavioral and electrophysiological study. *Journal of Cognitive Neuroscience, 11,* 473–490.

Hadjikhani, N., & Roland, P. E. (1998). Cross-modal transfer of information between the tactile and the visual representations in the human brain: A positron emission tomographic study. *Journal of Neuroscience, 18,* 1072–1084.

Hershenson, M. (1962). Reaction time as a measure of intersensory facilitation. *Journal of Experimental Psychology, 63,* 289–293.

Hikosaka, K., Iwai, E., Saito, H., & Tanaka, K. (1988). Polysensory properties of neurons in the anterior bank of the caudal superior temporal sulcus of the macaque monkey. *Journal of Neurophysiology, 60,* 1615–1637.

Hughes, H. C., Reuter-Lorenz, P. A., Nozawa, G., & Fendrich, R. (1994). Visual-auditory interactions in sensorimotor processing: Saccades versus manual responses. *Journal of Experimental Psychology: Human Perception and Performance, 20,* 131–153.

Jones, E. G., & Powell, T. P. S. (1970). An anatomical study of converging sensory pathways within the cerebral cortex of the monkey. *Brain, 93,* 793–820.

Kadunce, D. C., Vaughan, J. W., Wallace, M. T., Benedek, G., & Stein, B. E. (1997). Mechanisms of within- and cross-modality supression in the superior colliculus. *Journal of Neurophysiology, 78,* 2834–2847.

Kok, A., & de Jong, H. L. (1980). The effect of repetition of infrequent familiar and infamiliar visual patterns on components of the event-related brain potential. *Biological Psychology, 10,* 167–188.

Macaluso, E., Frith, C., & Driver, J. (2000). Modulation of human visual cortex by crossmodal spatial attention. *Science, 289,* 1206–1208.

Mangun, G. R. (1995). Neural mechanisms of visual selective attention. *Psychophysiology, 32,* 4–18.

Miller, J. O. (1982). Divided attention: Evidence for coactivation with redundant signals. *Cognitive Psychology, 14,* 247–279.

Miller, J. O. (1986). Time course of coactivation in bimodal divided attention. *Perception & Psychophysics, 40,* 331–343.

Paulesu, E., Harrison, J., Baron Cohen, S., Watson, J. D. G., Goldstein, L., Heather, J., et al. (1995). The physiology of coloured hearing: A PET activation study of colour-word synaesthesia. *Brain, 118,* 661–676.

Pernier, J., Perrin, F., & Bertrand, O. (1988). Scalp current density fields: Concept and properties. *Electroencephalography and Clinical Neurophysiology, 69,* 385–389.

Perrin, F., Pernier, J., Bertrand, O., & Echallier, J. F. (1989). Spherical splines for scalp potential and current density mapping. *Electroencephalography and Clinical Neurophysiology, 72,* 184–187.

Perrin, F., Pernier, J., Bertrand, O., & Giard, M. H. (1987). Mapping of scalp potentials by surface spline interpolation. *Electroencephalography and Clinical Neurophysiology, 66,* 75–81.

Raab, D. H. (1962). Statistical facilitation of simple reaction times. *Transactions of the New York Academy of Sciences, 24,* 574–590.

Raichle, M. E., Fiez, J. A., Videen, T. O., McLeod, A. M., Pardo, J. V., Fox, P. T., et al. (1994). Practice-related changes in human brain functional anatomy during nonmotor learning. *Cerebral Cortex, 4,* 8–26.

Raij, T., Uutela, K., & Hari, R. (2000). Audiovisual integration of letters in the human brain. *Neuron, 28,* 617–625.

Rockland, K. S., & Ojima, H. (2001). Calcarine area V1 as a multimodal convergence area. *Society for Neuroscience Abstracts, 27,* 511.20.

Sams, M., Aulanko, R., Hamalainen, H., Hari, R., Lounasmaa, O. V., Lu, S. T., et al. (1991). Seeing speech: Visual information from lip movements modifie activitiy in the human auditory cortex. *Neuroscience Letters, 127,* 141–145.

Scherg, M. (1990). Fundamentals of dipole source potential analysis. In F. Grandori, M. Hoke, & G. L. Romani (Eds.), *Auditory evoked magnetic fields and electric potentials. Advances in Audiology, 5,* 40–69.

Schmidt, R. A., Giele, S. C., & van den Heuvel, P. J. M. (1984). The locus of intersensory facilitation of reaction time. *Acta Psychologia, 57,* 145–164.

Schroeder, C. E., Lindsley, R. W., Specht, C., Marcovici, A., Smiley, J. F., & Javitt, D. C. (2001). Somatosensory input to auditory association cortex in the macaque monkey. *Journal of Neurophysiology, 85,* 1322–1327.

Schroeder, C. E., Mehta, A. D., Ulbert, I., Steinschneider, M., & Vaughan, H. G. (1995). Visual responses in auditory cortex and their modulation by attention. *Society for Neuroscience Abstracts, 21,* 694.

Schröger, E., & Widmann, A. (1998). Speeded responses to audiovisual signal changes result from bimodal integration. *Psychophysiology, 35,* 755–759.

Stein, B. E., Huneycutt, W. S., & Meredith, M. A. (1988). Neurons and behavior: The same rules of multisensory integration apply. *Brain Research, 448,* 355–358.

Stein, B. E., London, N., Wilkinson, L. K., & Price, D. D. (1996). Enhancement of perceived visual intensity by auditory stimuli: A psychophysical analysis. *Journal of Cognitive Neuroscience, 8,* 497–506.

Stein, B. E., & Meredith, M. A. (1993). *The merging of the senses.* Cambridge, MA: MIT Press.

Stein, B. E., Meredith, M. A., Huneycutt, W. S., & McDade, L. (1989). Behavioral indices of multisensory integration: Orientation to visual cues is affected by auditory stimuli. *Journal of Cognitive Neuroscience, 1,* 12–24.

Stein, B. E., & Wallace, M. T. (1996). Comparison of cross-modality integration in midbrain and cortex. *Progress in Brain Research, 112,* 289–299.

Teder-Sälejärvi, W. A., McDonald, J. J., Di Russo, F., & Hillyard, S. A. (2002). An analysis of audio-visual cross-modal integration by means of potential (ERP) recordings. *Cognitive Brain Research, 14,* 106–114.

Thorpe, S., Fize, D., & Marlot, C. (1996). Speed of processing in the human visual system. *Nature, 381,* 520–522.

Vogel, E. K., & Luck, S. J. (2000). The visual N1 component as an index of a discrimination process. *Psychophysiology, 37,* 190–203.

Wallace, M. T., Meredith, M. A., & Stein, B. E. (1993). Converging influences from visual, auditory, and somatosensory cortices onto output neurons of the superior colliculus. *Journal of Neurophysiology, 69,* 1797–1809.

Wallace, M. T., Wilkinson, L. K., & Stein, B. E. (1996). Representation and integration of multiple sensory inputs in primate superior colliculus. *Journal of Neurophysiology, 76,* 1246–1266.

Welch, R. B., & Warren, D. H. (1986). Intersensory interactions. In K. R. Boff, L. Kaufman, & J. P. Thomas (Eds.), *Handbook of perception and human performance: Vol. 1. Sensory processes and perception* (pp. 25-1–25-36). New York: Wiley.

Widmann, A., Schröger, E., Shimojo, S., & Munka, L. (2000). Does the "spatial rule" of audiovisual integration hold in humans? *Psychophysiology, 37*(Suppl. 1), S104.

Yvert, B., Bertrand, O., Thevenet, M., Echallier, J. F., & Pernier, J. (1997). A systematic evaluation of the spherical model accuracy in EEG dipole localization. *Electroencephalography and Clinical Neurophysiology, 102,* 452–459.

32 MEG Studies of Cross-Modal Integration and Plasticity

TOMMI RAIJ AND VEIKKO JOUSMÄKI

Introduction

The brain is an almost real-time processor that receives a constant flow of sensory information through several parallel sensory channels, binds the information from different senses, compares the stimuli with previous experience and current goals, and produces motor output to best fit the current circumstances. The sensory-specific cortices and the motor cortices have been studied in detail even in humans, whereas the processes that integrate various senses with each other as well as with the motor output are still largely unexplored. Given the technical challenges, this lack of knowledge is hardly surprising: multisensory processes involve several brain areas with widespread serial and parallel connections and with rapidly changing weights of activity in these neural networks (see, e.g., Goldman-Rakic, 1995; McClelland, Rumelhart, & Clinton, 1986; Mesulam, 1998). To unravel the neural mechanisms contributing to multisensory processing it is necessary to follow the spread of activations and interactions between various brain areas with high temporal and spatial accuracy.

Each research tool excels in revealing specific aspects of brain functions. Functional brain imaging methods based on changes in metabolism, energy consumption, or blood flow, such as positron emission tomography (PET) or functional magnetic resonance imaging (fMRI), have excellent spatial accuracy but poor temporal resolution because of the slow time course of hemodynamic and metabolic changes. Electrophysiological measures, on the other hand, have excellent temporal resolution, but accurate identification of the involved brain areas (source configurations) can be complicated because of the nonunique *electromagnetic inverse problem.* However, magnetoencephalography (MEG) offers several advantages in studying multisensory processing mechanisms of the human brain, allowing characterization of large-scale neurocognitive cortical networks both in time and in space. The hitherto small overlap in experimental designs of multisensory MEG versus EEG studies discourages extensive comparison across multisensory MEG and EEG results; the reader is therefore referred to other chapters in this handbook for multisensory EEG studies.

This chapter begins with a short description of the MEG method, followed by a review of results obtained by using MEG to evaluate multisensory brain functions. We have divided multisensory processing in two main categories. *Real-time processing* refers to integration of different sensory modalities from the constant flow of sensory information that occurs almost automatically, and in which the stimuli are naturally associated through spatiotemporal coincidence. *Learning-dependent multisensory processing* refers to situations in which association between different stimuli requires extensive previous experience, and the stimulus combinations can be entirely arbitrary; such processes are essential for high-level human cognition. The chapter concludes with a discussion of the plasticity of the brain from a multisensory point of view.

Magnetoencephalography

Figure 32.1 shows the principles and instrumentation of MEG. Electric currents generate magnetic and electric fields according to principles formalized in Maxwell's equations. MEG records weak magnetic fields generated by neural currents (for reviews, see Hämäläinen & Hari, 2002; Hämäläinen, Hari, Ilmoniemi, Knuutila, & Lounasmaa, 1993). The measured fields are mainly associated with intracellular postsynaptic currents of cortical pyramidal neurons. The upper left panel in Figure 32.1 illustrates a simplified genesis of the MEG signal in a histological section through the cerebral cortex (the cortical surface is to the right). Activation of the apical dendrites of pyramidal cells results in a flow of intracellular electric current, in this case toward the soma (white arrowhead). The current generates a magnetic field around the dendrite (black ovals). When thousands of dendrites act in concert, the signals become strong enough to be detectable outside the head.

The lower left panel of Figure 32.1 shows a modern helmet-shaped array of MEG sensors that allows recording of the magnetic field simultaneously over the whole

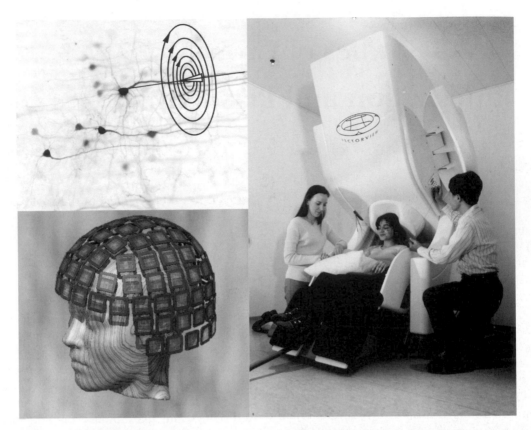

FIGURE 32.1   MEG principles and instrumentation. The upper left panel illustrates, in simplified form, the genesis of neuromagnetic signals. A histological section through the cerebral cortex is illustrated, with cortical surface to the right (histological slide courtesy of Dr. Lutz Slomianka). The cell bodies and dendrites of pyramidal neurons are shown. When the apical dendrite (to the right) is activated, the postsynaptic potentials result in a net electrical current, in this case toward the soma (white arrowhead), thus generating a magnetic field around the dendrite (black ovals; the arrowheads show the direction of the flux). Other neural structures, such as basal dendrites of pyramidal neurons, also generate magnetic fields, but their orientation is too random and/or symmetrical to generate fields that could be recorded from a distance. Action potentials in the brain are typically not seen with MEG, because their duration is much shorter than that of postsynaptic potentials, and the patterns of axonal currents during an action potential largely cancel each other out (see, e.g., Hämäläinen & Hari, 2002). However, somatosensory MEG recordings have shown rapid bursts in the 600-Hz range that have been suggested to reflect action potentials (Curio et al., 1994; Hashimoto et al., 1996).

At lower left is a helmet-shaped array of 306 sensors from Vectorview™ (Elekta Neuromag, Finland). Each of the 102 measurement locations contains two planar gradiometers and one axial gradiometer. Large arrays allow sampling of the whole brain in a single session. At right a subject is being prepared for an MEG measurement with a Vectorview™ (Elekta Neuromag, Finland) neuromagnetometer.

brain. The first neuromagnetometers covering the whole scalp were introduced in 1992 (Ahonen et al., 1993; Vrba et al., 1993). Whole-scalp coverage has greatly increased the applicability of MEG to basic research and clinical studies.

The right panel of Figure 32.1 shows a subject being prepared for an MEG study performed using the 306-channel Vectorview™ (Elekta Neuromag, Finland) neuromagnetometer. In modern MEG systems, neuromagnetic fields are detected with extremely sensitive superconducting quantum interference devices (SQUIDs). The SQUIDs are functional only at low temperatures, typically reached by immersing the sensors in liquid helium bath at −269°C (4°K) in a special vacuum-insulated dewar.

Localization of the activated brain areas from MEG (or from electroencephalography, EEG) data is not straightforward because of the electromagnetic inverse problem: the primary current distribution (i.e., the activated brain areas) underlying a measured signal distribution (i.e., the MEG or EEG responses) has an infinite number of possible configurations. However, some configurations are more probable than others, and the uncertainty can be further reduced by introducing constraints based on the anatomy and physiology of the brain into source analysis. For example, the conductivity distribution of the head can be modeled by a sphere covering the intracranial space or by a more realistic head model based on magnetic resonance (MR) images. There are several methods for estimating the source locations. The current distribution in the head can be modeled with equivalent current dipoles (ECDs; Tuomisto, Hari, Katila, Poutanen, & Varpula, 1983) and with extended/distributed-source estimation techniques such as magnetic-field tomography (Ioannides, Bolton, & Clarke, 1990), minimum norm estimates (Hämäläinen & Ilmoniemi, 1994), and low-resolution electromagnetic tomography (Pascual-Marqui, Michel, & Lehmann, 1994). In addition, focal estimation techniques such as minimum current estimates have been applied (Matsuura & Okabe, 1995; Uutela, Hämäläinen, & Somersalo, 1999). If necessary, even more information can be injected into MEG source analysis from other imaging modalities such as fMRI (Dale et al., 2000). Once the sources have been identified, the dynamics of their activations can be determined with millisecond temporal accuracy.

MEG recordings have been widely used in basic research on the human brain since the 1970s, specifically in the study of auditory functions (e.g., Hari, 1990; Hari, Aittoniemi, Järvinen, Katila, & Varpula, 1980), visual processing (Ahlfors, Ilmoniemi, & Hämäläinen, 1992; Aine, Bodis-Wollner, & George, 1990; Cohen, 1968, 1972; ffytche, Guy, & Zeki, 1995; Halgren, Raij, Marinkovic, Jousmäki, & Hari, 2000; Uusitalo, Williamson, & Seppä, 1996), somatosensory processing (Hari & Forss, 1999; Hari et al., 1984), motor functions (Gross et al., 2000; Hari & Salenius, 1999; Salenius, Portin, Kajola, Salmelin, & Hari, 1997), spontaneous oscillations (Hari & Salmelin, 1997), and cognitive neuroscience (Hari, Levänen, & Raij, 2001; Lounasmaa, Hämäläinen, Hari, & Salmelin, 1996; Näätänen, Ilmoniemi, & Alho, 1994; Pulvermüller, 1999). MEG is also gaining an increasingly important role in clinical neurophysiology (Hari, 1999) and neurosurgery (Mäkelä et al., 2001; Simos et al., 2000).

MEG has several properties that make it particularly suitable for studying multisensory brain functions:

• Excellent submillisecond temporal resolution. Brain functions can best be understood with accurate data on brain temporal dynamics. This is particularly important in multisensory processing, where signals from various sensory organs arrive within a short time window at multiple sensory projection cortices and multisensory association areas in widely separate parts of the brain. The order and strength of activations in various brain areas across different stimuli and experimental conditions reveal important information about their functional significance. This property of MEG is also useful in determining neural activation trace lifetimes. The sensory projection cortices clearly show faster decay of the effect of previous stimuli than do high-order association

cortices in the auditory (Lü, Williamson, & Kaufman, 1992), visual (Uusitalo et al., 1996), and somatosensory (Hamada et al., 2002) pathways. Consequently, transient activation of a multisensory association area would be expected to affect the processing of future incoming stimuli from other modalities in a time window of several seconds. This might facilitate establishing multisensory associations between cross-modal stimuli even with relatively large temporal asynchrony in multisensory association cortices.

• Reasonable (a few millimeters) spatial resolution for cortical sources in sulci. Magnetic fields pass through biological tissue (such as cerebrospinal fluid, skull, and skin) without distortion. Thus, these tissues are practically transparent to MEG. In contrast, the electric inhomogeneities of extracerebral tissues distort the electric (EEG) signals significantly. For this reason it is more straightforward and accurate to analyze sources of MEG than of EEG (Leahy, Mosher, Spencer, Huang, & Lewine, 1998), and MEG sources colocalize extremely well with intracranial recordings (Gharib et al., 1995). MEG can also pick up signals from deep brain regions (e.g., Erne & Hoke, 1990; Lütkenhöner, Lammertmann, Ross, & Pantev, 2000; Parkkonen & Mäkelä, 2002; Tesche, 1996; Tesche, Karhu, & Tissari, 1996), but its localization accuracy decreases as a function of depth.

• Sensitivity to current orientation. MEG is mainly sensitive to currents that are oriented tangentially with respect to the curvature of the head, i.e., activity in the fissural cortex. Interpretation and source analysis of MEG responses are thus easier than interpretation of EEG signals, to which both radial and tangential sources contribute; however, the greater ease comes at the cost of decreased sensitivity of MEG to activity in the crests of cortical gyri (Hillebrand & Barnes, 2002).

• No need for a reference electrode. In MEG recordings, no reference similar to the reference electrode in EEG recordings is needed, and thus interpretation of the obtained field patterns is rather straightforward.

• Noninvasiveness. No tracer substances or injections are needed, and the subjects are not exposed to radiation or strong external magnetic fields. This makes MEG applicable to healthy humans without any risk.

• Population dynamics instead of single cells. MEG reflects mass activity of at least thousands of neurons, and modern whole-head neuromagnetometers allow sampling of the whole brain at once. This characteristic makes MEG particularly suitable for studying activations of large-scale neural networks and dynamic properties and frequency power/coherence across distant parts of the brain (e.g., Gross et al., 2001; Jensen & Vanni, 2002; Jousmäki, 2000).

Real-time multisensory processing

Real-time multisensory processing here refers to cross-modal integration of the constant flow of sensory information in which the stimuli from different senses are naturally associated through spatiotemporal coincidence (i.e., the stimuli originate in the same spatial location at the same time).

As described elsewhere in this book, real-time multisensory integration starts in several midbrain structures, including the inferior (Groh, Trause, Underhill, Clark, & Inati, 2001) and superior colliculi, where the multisensory information is also combined with a motor map (Stein & Meredith, 1993). These processes extend to cortex as well (Stein & Wallace, 1996), and the cortical and subcortical multisensory processes interact (Jiang, Wallace, Vaughan, & Stein, 2001). A wide variety of species use such "on-line" mechanisms while roaming in and interacting with a natural environment (Stein, 1998).

AUDIOVISUAL INTEGRATION Lipreading occurs when subjects look at the face of a person speaking. Behavioral studies suggest that when the auditory and visual stimuli are in synchrony within a time window of about 200–250 ms, this facilitates comprehension, especially in noisy surroundings (McGrath & Summerfield, 1985; Munhall, Gribble, Sacco, & Ward, 1996); Massaro, Cohen, and Smeele (1996) have suggested even longer time windows. The well-known McGurk effect arises experimentally when subjects monitor a videotaped face articulating short syllables and an incongruent syllable is occasionally presented on the audio track. In such situations the perceived sound can change to something that does not represent the visual or the auditory stimulus (McGurk & MacDonald, 1976). The neural mechanisms of this phenomenon have been studied with MEG (Sams et al., 1991). When the illusion was perceived, the responses in the supratemporal auditory cortex were modulated starting at about 180 ms. In a related MEG study, infrequently presented incongruent audiovisual speech stimuli activated the supratemporal auditory cortices more strongly than frequently presented congruent audiovisual stimuli at 140–160 and 200–300 ms in the left hemisphere and 205–315 and 345–375 ms in the right hemisphere (Möttönen, Krause, Tiippana, & Sams, 2002). Thus, during lipreading, visual input has access to auditory processing in supratemporal auditory cortex. The location and timing of the changes would be in accord with the modulation occurring in association auditory cortical areas surrounding the unimodal primary auditory cortex. The McGurk effect has recently been investi-gated with MEG in the frequency domain as well (Krause et al., 2002). Calvert, Campbell, and Brammer (2000) in an fMRI study expanded on these results by showing with fMRI that temporally congruent audiovisual speech activates the left superior temporal sulcus (STS), suggesting that multisensory association areas also participate in integration of auditory and visual input during lipreading.

AUDIOTACTILE INTEGRATION Audiovisual interactions have been studied much more extensively than audio-tactile interactions, which often go unnoticed in real-life situations. Audiotactile and visuotactile interactions are of great functional importance, however, as they link remote senses (audition and vision) to the body. In addition, both audition and the tactile system are capable of detecting low-frequency sounds and vibrations, which are common in our natural environment; thus, audiotactile interactions are very likely. Sensory dominance (see, e.g., Giard & Peronnet, 1999; Lederman, Thorne, & Jones, 1986) determines the perception, although audition and tactile systems are linked together. The exploration of different textures is associated with concomitant sounds that typically do not attract our attention because the tactile stimulus easily dominates the perception. Nevertheless, if the auditory part is modified, for example by artificially accentuating the high frequencies of sounds elicited by rubbing the palms together, the tactile percept will change (*parchment skin illusion;* Guest, Catmur, Lloyd, & Spence, 2002; Jousmäki & Hari, 1998). Perceptually such a multimodal integration persists even with tens of milliseconds' asynchrony between the auditory and tactile stimuli.

To reveal the neural correlates of audiotactile interactions, a recent MEG study compared the responses to unimodal auditory (A, binaural tone pips) or somatosensory (S, pressure pulses to the right thumb) stimuli with responses to bimodal (AS) audiotactile stimulation (Lütkenhöner, Lammertmann, Simões, & Hari, 2002). Interaction was estimated as the difference between the sum of unimodal activations and the bimodal activation ([A + S] − AS). Interactions were found more often in the left than in the right hemisphere, with two peaks at about 140 ms and 220 ms. In a majority of subjects, the interactions originated in the secondary somatosensory cortex (SII), with possible contributions from temporal auditory cortex. A previous combined EEG/MEG study searched for audiotactile interactions using tone bursts and median nerve electrical stimuli (Huttunen, Hari, & Vanni, 1987). This study employed a four-channel neuromagnetometer and an EEG electrode at the vertex. The MEG responses

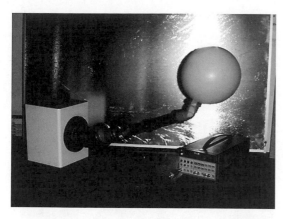

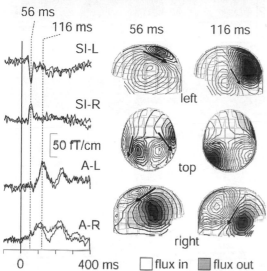

FIGURE 32.2 MEG audiotactile stimulation experiment. Upper panel shows an audiotactile stimulator, consisting of a loudspeaker, a tube, a balloon, and a function generator. Lower panel shows the waveforms from four gradiometer channels picking up the maximal signal just above a dipolar source located over the left and right somatosensory (two upper curves) and auditory (two lower curves) cortices. The black vertical line shows the time of the stimulus onset. The two overlying curves for each source demonstrate excellent replicability of the procedure. The magnetic field patterns and the equivalent current dipoles (ECDs) are shown at 56 ms (middle column) and 116 ms (right column), viewed from the left (top), above (middle), and the right (bottom). Isocontour step is 20 fT, with shaded areas showing magnetic flux out of the head and blank areas into the head. (Adapted from Jousmäki & Hari, 1999.)

that were recorded only over the right hemisphere did not show interactions, but the vertex potential did. This is in accord with the recent findings of Lütkenhöner et al. (2002) showing with a whole-head 306-channel neuromagnetometer that the processing is left hemisphere dominant.

Figure 32.2 shows the potential of MEG to identify the locations and time courses of neuronal events in a multimodal stimulation experiment (Jousmäki & Hari, 1999).

The stimuli were presented using a loudspeaker and a balloon that vibrated at the same frequency (upper panel). The subjects held the ball between their palms, thus receiving combined and congruent somatosensory and auditory stimulation from the same source. The lower panel shows the activated areas and their time courses in a single subject; the left column shows MEG signals over the left (upper) and right (lower) somatosensory and auditory cortices. The time courses were extracted by searching for sources at 56 ms for somatosensory cortices and at 116 ms for auditory cortices; the corresponding field patterns are shown in the middle and right columns. The corresponding ECDs were then used to predict the measured response waveforms while their locations and orientations were kept fixed. The prediction was calculated for each time point separately, thus producing the activation strengths of the four brain areas as a function of time. Although this study did not directly address multisensory questions, it shows that MEG can separate simultaneously activated multisensory sources bilaterally. In addition, Jousmäki and Hari (1999) used very natural stimuli, which may be very important in multisensory experiments. A simple multisensory experiment could have been generated by changing the congruent input to incongruent (by delivering auditory stimuli of a different frequency than somatosensory stimulation) or by comparing results obtained by bimodal versus unimodal stimulation.

VISUOTACTILE INTEGRATION The visual and tactile systems interact frequently during, for example, adjusting limb position and manipulation and identification of objects at hand (see, e.g., Cohen & Andersen, 2002; Graziano & Gross, 1998; Haggard, 2001; Newport, Hindle, & Jackson, 2001). Lam et al. (1999, 2001) reported that continuous visual stimulation affects somatosensory-evoked MEG responses at around 33–133 ms and suggested that these interactions occur in proximity to the primary (SI) and secondary (SII) somatosensory cortices. However, the continuous mode of visual stimulation employed in these studies makes it difficult to compare the results with the results of the other MEG studies discussed here.

Learning-dependent multisensory processing

Many environmental stimuli are related to human-made artifacts, in which different stimuli can be unnaturally associated in a culture-dependent way. Learning-dependent multisensory processing here refers to such situations in which associating different stimuli with each other requires extensive previous experience. Such processes form the neural basis for associative learning across various sensory systems. The stimulus combinations can be entirely arbitrary (e.g., a visual form *A* and an auditory sound *a*), which allows the formation of concepts (the "letter" *A*). Thus, one stimulus can come to represent another—the cornerstone of language and other forms of symbolic representations. Because concepts break the normal rules of spatiotemporal coincidence for multisensory integration, they allow such symbols to rise above the actual stimuli. The world of abstract thought is built on these mechanisms.

AUDIOVISUAL ASSOCIATIVE LEARNING The learned associations between visual letters of the alphabet and the "corresponding" auditory phonemes are an example of learning-dependent multisensory processes. Raij, Uutela, and Hari (2000) recorded neuromagnetic signals to unimodal auditory and visual and bimodal audiovisually presented letters and control stimuli. As expected, the reaction times to target letters were significantly shorter for audiovisual presentations than for unimodal auditory or visual presentations (Hershenson, 1962; Miller, 1986; Schröger & Widmann, 1998). The locations and time behavior of the activated neuronal sources (to nontarget stimuli) were estimated with minimum current estimates (MCEs).

Figure 32.3 shows the brain activations (see also Color Plate 10). The upper panel shows the early modality-specific activations in response to auditory, visual, and audiovisual presentations of letters and control stimuli. After this, the auditory and visual brain activations converged (i.e., certain areas were activated by both unimodal auditory and visual stimuli) maximally at around 225 ms after stimulus onset, especially in the temporal lobes. Convergence was remarkably similar for letters and control stimuli (middle panel). Convergence was followed by interaction (lower panel) predominantly in the right temporo-occipito-parietal junction (280–345 ms) and the left (380–540 ms) and right (450–535 ms) STS. These multisensory brain areas, which play a role in audiovisual convergence and interaction of phonemes and graphemes, participate in the neural network supporting the supramodal concept of a letter.

Figure 32.4 shows the left STS time courses of activations to auditory, visual, and audiovisual stimuli, convergence, and interaction (see also Color Plate 11). The left STS differentiated not only letters from control stimuli, but also matching (e.g., visual *A* with an auditory *a*) from nonmatching (e.g., visual *A* with an auditory *k*) audiovisual letters. The observed interaction was suppressive: the audiovisual activations were weaker than the sum of the unimodal activations. The orientations of net currents were similar for auditory, visual, and audiovisual stimuli, and thus the suppressive inter-

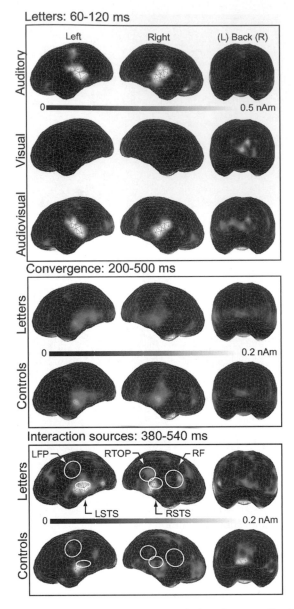

Figure 32.3 MCE source analysis for audiovisual integration of single letters. Upper panel shows early activations (60–120 ms) for auditory, visual, and audiovisual letters. In the middle panel, convergence was calculated as the minimum of the auditory and visual unimodal activations. The Boolean AND operator between unimodal auditory and visual activations corresponding to multiplying the values could have been used as well, but this approach was rejected because of possible noise amplification. In the lower panel, interaction was calculated as the difference between the sum of unimodal auditory and visual activations (A+V) compared with the activity evoked by bimodal audiovisual (AV) stimulus presentation. (Adapted from Raij et al., 2000.) (See Color Plate 10.)

action appears to rise from local neuronal interactions. The possible causes and significance of multisensory suppression are discussed below.

Several studies have argued that when two spatiotemporally congruent stimuli (e.g., auditory and visual)

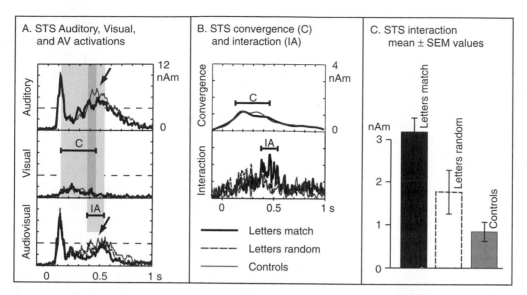

FIGURE 32.4   Audiovisual properties of left superior temporal sulcus (STS) activation for letter stimuli. Left panel shows the STS time courses of auditory, visual, and audiovisual activations. Middle panel shows convergence and interaction. Right panel shows the differences in the strength of interaction between matching letters, nonmatching letters, and control stimuli. (Adapted from Raij et al., 2000.) (See Color Plate 11.)

interact, this results in a nonlinearly strong potentiation of the activity of bimodal neurons; similarly, when the two stimuli are spatiotemporally incongruent, a suppression should be expected (e.g., Kadunce et al., 1997, 2001). This has been repeatedly demonstrated in single-cell recordings and PET/fMRI studies. However, multisensory MEG and EEG studies have typically shown both or mainly suppressive interactions instead of potentiative interactions at most latencies and over most brain areas (Busch, Wilson, Orr, & Papanicolau, 1989; Davis, Osterhammel, Wier, & Gjerdingen, 1972; Fort, Delpuech, Pernier, & Giard, 2002; Foxe et al., 2000; Giard & Peronnet, 1999; Lütkenhöner et al., 2002; Molholm et al., 2002; Morrell, 1968; Raij et al., 2000; Schröger & Widmann, 1998; Squires, Donchin, Squires, & Grossberg, 1977; Teder-Sälejärvi, McDonald, Di Russo, & Hillyard, 2002; see also Fort & Giard, Chap. 31, this volume). This apparent discrepancy could reveal important information about the neural mechanisms supporting multisensory interactions (Raij et al., 2000; Meredith, 2002). On the other hand, many of these multisensory studies have employed stimulus intensities that elicit maximal neuronal responses. Based on single-cell recordings and the rule of inverse effectiveness (Stein & Meredith, 1993), weak stimulus intensities may be more suitable to elicit multisensory potentiation.

Cortical intralaminar recordings in macaques have shown both suppressive and potentiative multisensory interactions, probably through cross-modal modulation of postsynaptic potentials locally (Schroeder & Foxe,

2002). Further, cortical recordings in cats have shown patterns of excitatory-inhibitory multisensory interactions (Meredith, 2002). Thus, there is little doubt that both multisensory potentiation and suppression exist. Different stimulus types and tasks could give rise to opposite effects: most early cross-modal studies used stimuli and stimulus combinations that were not ecologically valid (e.g., light flashes and auditory clicks), and more recent studies have mainly focused on stimuli that naturally occur together (such as auditory speech and moving faces or lips during lipreading). Raij et al. (2000) used stimuli that were not naturally associated (auditory phonemes and visual letters) but required learning, during which stimuli from multiple sensory channels become combined. Learning can lead to decreased signal amplitudes in electrophysiological, PET, and fMRI recordings (Büchel, Coull, & Friston, 1999; Kok & de Jong, 1980; Raichle et al., 1994; for reviews, see Desimone, 1996; Wiggs & Martin, 1998), apparently because learning leads to optimization of activation in the local network. The process could be compared with sharpening of neuronal tuning, resulting in suppressed net responses (Hurlbert, 2000). Audiovisual learning effects could thus reflect multisensory suppression rather than potentiation (Meredith, 2002; Raij et al., 2000).

From a technical point of view, the difference between results of unit recordings and MEG/EEG studies could lie in the fact that unit recordings measure the activity of a small number of neurons, whereas MEG/EEG recordings reflect the activation of large populations of neurons. On the other hand, the difference between fMRI/PET recordings and MEG/EEG studies could reflect the fact that the former measure energy consumption and/or local blood flow, and both potentiation and suppression of neural activity can be energy-consuming processes, whereas electrophysiological methods record net electric currents, where suppression would be expected to result in diminished responses. Hypothetically, the observed multisensory suppression could reflect a "lateral inhibition" cortical activation pattern in which a small area of cortex showing multisensory potentiation is surrounded by a larger zone of multisensory suppression: if the net currents at the center and in the surrounding zone flowed to opposite directions and only partially canceled each other out, the net effect of such a configuration would be expected to be suppressive.

CROSS-MODAL MENTAL IMAGERY In a visual imagery task, the instructions *what* and *when* to imagine typically are given verbally. Because the input is verbal, the auditory (especially language-related) areas would be expected to be activated first. Some areas that are also activated in similar tasks with real visual stimuli become activated during visual imagery; thus, visual imagery appears to be at least partly a function of visual brain areas. Some activations would thus be expected to support the audiovisual transformation of the verbal instructions to the visual image, making this a cross-modal issue.

Raij (1999) presented subjects with an auditory sequence consisting of single letters of the alphabet and tone pips. The subjects were instructed to visually imagine the lowercase letters corresponding to the auditory stimuli and to examine their visuospatial properties; the associated brain activity was compared with activity evoked by the same stimuli when the subjects just detected the intervening tones. This allowed extracting activations specific to the imagery task. After initial activation of the auditory cortices, the earliest imagery-related responses originated in the left prerolandic area 320 ms after the voice onset. They were followed within 70 ms by signals originating in the posterior parietal lobe close to midline (precuneus) and, 100 ms later, in the posterior STS, predominantly in the left hemisphere. The activations were sustained and partially overlapping in time. The precuneus was apparently activated due to the visuospatial load of the task (the subjects had to evaluate the imagined letter forms). Most important, the same area in the left STS that was mainly responsible for the interaction of auditory and visual letters (Raij et al., 2000) was again activated, and this imagery-specific activation started at exactly the same time as the audiovisual interaction.

In a related MEG study, auditory imagery evoked by visual notes was studied (Schürmann, Raij, Fujiki, & Hari, 2002). Musicians were presented with a sequence of notes (single notes on a staff line) and asked to imagine hearing the corresponding sounds. In a control condition, the subjects were shown similar stimuli with intermittently appearing faces instead of the notes, with the instruction to ignore the notes and focus on the faces. In another control condition, we showed black dots similar to the notes but without the staff lines, with the instruction to look at the dots. Some brain activations were enhanced by or specific to the auditory imagery task requiring visual-to-auditory transformation. First, enhanced activity of left and right occipital areas (onset at 120–150 ms) was observed. The activations then spread to the precuneus (again, the subjects had to visuospatially evaluate the position of the note with respect to the staff lines) and to such extraoccipital areas that were not at all activated during the control tasks (e.g., left STS and left and right premotor cortices). Thus, a complex temporospatial activation sequence of multiple cortical areas was observed when musicians recalled firmly established audiovisual associations, and the left STS, along with a few other activations in association cortex, apparently reflected a visual-to-auditory conversion process.

Cross-modal plasticity due to sensory deprivation or brain defects

LACK OF SENSORY INPUT: BLINDNESS AND DEAFNESS When adults lose a limb or part of a limb, their somatosensory cortex reorganizes in a matter of days (Elbert et al., 1994; Merzenich et al., 1984; Weiss et al., 2000; Yang et al., 1994). The changes reverse after replantation (Wiech et al., 2000). This can be interpreted as a form of learning in which the lack of or addition of sensory input results in a brain organizational chance. Such effects can also be observed in less dramatic situations. For example, learning to play a violin increases the somatosensory response strength representing the left (fingering) hand, possibly reflecting an increase in the size of the cortical projection area (Elbert et al., 1995). Musicians also develop abnormally large auditory cortical representations for processing certain sound characteristics (Pantev, Roberts, Schulz, Engelien, & Ross, 2001). An important factor in determining the size and stability of the brain changes is the age at which the individual starts to adjust to the new situation (Elbert et al., 1995; Pantev & Lütkenhöner, 2000).

Extreme examples of changed input leading to profound brain organizational changes are blindness and deafness. Such changes, when they occur early in

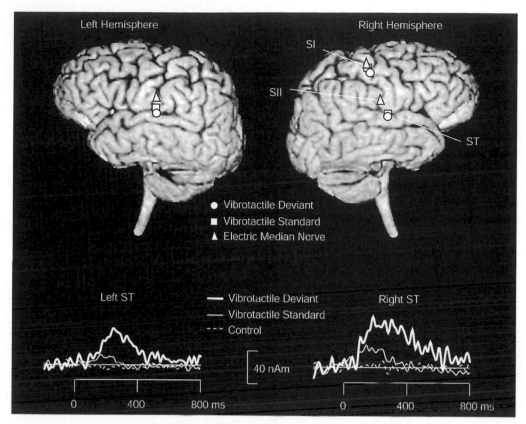

FIGURE 32.5 Auditory cortex activation in response to vibrotactile stimulation in a congenitally deaf subject. The vibrotactile stimuli were delivered to the left palm of the subject using an oddball paradigm (standards, 250 Hz, 85%; deviants, 180 Hz, 15%; duration, 100 ms); electrical stimulation of the left median nerve was used as well. At top, the locations of the activations are projected on the surface reconstruction of the subject's MR images. Below, the time courses of the activations in the left and right supratemporal sources for different types of vibrotactile stimulation are shown. A control condition in which the stimuli were presented normally but without the deaf subject touching the vibrotactile stimulator did not result in any activation, thus eliminating any residual hearing as a potential source of contamination. (Adapted from Levänen, Jousmäki, & Hari, 1998.)

ontogenesis, coincide with a period of maturation of neural connections. Consequently, the resulting organizational brain changes during this period can be profound. Sensory deprivation occurring later in life can also lead to functional changes, but these changes are more attributable to the plasticity associated with learning and sensory dominance.

Similar rules seem to apply for multisensory as for unisensory changes in the presence of changed input. In congenitally deaf subjects, perceptual accuracy for vibrotactile stimuli is increased (Levänen & Hamdorf, 2001). Figure 32.5 shows that in a congenitally deaf subject, vibrotactile stimuli can activate the supratemporal area normally occupied by the auditory cortex (Levänen, Jousmäki, & Hari, 1998). In normal-hearing control subjects, the supratemporal cortices were not activated by the same vibrotactile stimuli. The lack of auditory input from an early age can apparently lead to other functions or modalities taking over the unoccupied part of cortex (for fMRI data showing correspond-

ing occupation of the auditory cortex by visual functions, see Finney, Fine, & Dobkins, 2001).

In primates with early visual deprivation, integration of visuospatial information with spatial information from other senses (and the motor system) cannot develop normally in the parietal lobe; consequently, parietal association cortex is recruited by other tasks (Carlson, Pertovaara, & Tanila, 1987; Hyvärinen, Hyvärinen, & Linnankoski, 1981). Similar findings have been reported in other vertebrates (Yaka, Yinon, & Wollberg, 1999). Corresponding EEG results in humans suggest that association cortices can learn to process sensory input differently even when sensory deprivation occurs in adulthood (Kujala et al., 1997); some recent fMRI studies offer corroborating evidence (Kauffman, Theoret, & Pascual-Leone, 2002). Based on MEG recordings in humans with early-onset blindness, occipital areas that would normally be predominantly visual become activated during sound discrimination (Kujala et al., 1995; for a review, see Kujala et al., 2000).

Further, in the blind, the supratemporal auditory cortex is apparently increased in size and even appears to increase its processing speed, compared with what occurs in subjects with normal vision (Elbert et al., 2002).

BRAIN DEFECTS MEG has also revealed widespread reorganization of normal functional anatomy in, for example, the linguistic functions of patients with brain structural abnormalities. Normal subjects show convergence of activations evoked by auditorily and visually presented words in the superior temporal lobes, predominantly in the left hemisphere. In agreement with the timing of convergence for single letters, temporal lobe convergence for words occurs at about 150–250 ms (Papanicolaou et al., 2001; Simos et al., 2000; in these studies, interactions were not studied). Patients with brain structural anomalies such as tumors or arteriovenous malformations show changed patterns of language convergence, either in a way that shifts the convergence area away from the lesion or in a way that rearranges the distribution of convergence between the left and right hemispheres (Papanicolau et al., 2001; Simos et al., 2000).

Conclusions

Information about the dynamical aspects of brain function is of great importance for understanding the neural mechanisms of multisensory integration. MEG allows noninvasive brain recordings to be made with submillisecond temporal accuracy, thus making it possible to follow patterns of cortical activity supporting multisensory processing.

The number of multisensory MEG studies reported so far is small, but some patterns have begun to emerge. Audiovisual speech is integrated at least partially in the supratemporal auditory cortices at about 140–375 ms, probably in areas surrounding the core auditory projection areas (Möttönen et al., 2002; Sams et al., 1991). Audiovisually presented letters, on the other hand, are integrated in a widely distributed neural network in which left STS activity at around 380–540 ms appears to play a key role (Raij et al., 2000). Audiotactile interactions have been shown at around 140–180 ms, originating in the secondary somatosensory cortices and possibly also in the supratemporal auditory cortices (Lütkenhöner et al., 2002). Visuotactile integration has been suggested to modulate activity in the primary and secondary somatosensory cortices at around 33–133 ms (Lam et al., 1999, 2001).

MEG studies have thus provided evidence for multisensory integration close to the sensory projection cortices, in higher-order sensory cortices, and in multisensory association cortices. In most of the MEG studies discussed here, cross-modal modulation of neural activity near the sensory cortices, at least for real-time multisensory integration, has been suggested to occur relatively early, starting at about 140 ms (or even much earlier), whereas for learning-dependent audiovisual integration, multisensory association cortices clearly seem to participate later. If multisensory processing actually starts in lower-order sensory cortices and only later recruits multisensory association cortices, this would have important implications for theories regarding convergence versus association and binding as a neural basis for cross-modal integration (for a review of these theories, see Bernstein, Auer, & Moore, Chap. 13, this volume). However, so far no single MEG study has shown multisensory effects occurring both in lower-order sensory cortices and in multisensory association cortices. Also, because the multisensory loci and latencies are sensitive to the particular sensory systems, type of stimuli, and tasks, it is too early to draw other than preliminary conclusions.

ACKNOWLEDGMENTS The authors are most grateful to Academy Professor Riitta Hari for insightful comments. This work was supported by the Sigrid Juselius Foundation, the Academy of Finland, and the Finnish Medical Foundation.

REFERENCES

Ahlfors, S. P., Ilmoniemi, R. J., & Hämäläinen, M. S. (1992). Estimates of visually evoked cortical currents. *Electroencephalography and Clinical Neurophysiology, 82,* 225–236.

Ahonen, A. I., Hämäläinen, M. S., Kajola, M. J., Knuutila, J. E. T., Laine, P. P., Lounasmaa, O. V., et al. (1993). 122-channel SQUID instrument for investigating the magnetic signals from the human brain. *Physica Scripta, T49,* 198–205.

Aine, C. J., Bodis-Wollner, I., & George, J. S. (1990). Generators of visually evoked neuromagnetic responses: Spatial-frequency segregation and evidence for multiple sources. *Advances in Neurology, 54,* 141–155.

Büchel, C., Coull, J. T., & Friston, K. J. (1999). The predictive value of changes in effective connectivity for human learning. *Science, 283,* 1538–1541.

Busch, C., Wilson, G., Orr, C., & Papanicolau, A. (1989). Crossmodal interactions of auditory stimulus presentation on the visual evoked magnetic response. In S. J. Williamson, M. Hoke, G. Stroink, & M. Kotani (Eds.), *Advances in biomagnetism* (pp. 221–224). New York: Plenum Press.

Calvert, G. A., Campbell, R., & Brammer, M. J. (2000). Evidence from functional magnetic resonance imaging of crossmodal binding in the human heteromodal cortex. *Current Biology, 10,* 649–657.

Carlson, S., Pertovaara, A., & Tanila, H. (1987). Late effects of early binocular visual deprivation on the function of Brodmann's area 7 of monkeys (*Macaca arctoides*). *Brain Research, 430,* 101–111.

Cohen, D. (1968). Magnetoencephalography: Evidence of magnetic field produced by alpha-rhythm currents. *Science, 161,* 784–786.

Cohen, D. (1972). Magnetoencephalography: Detection of the brain's electrical activity with a superconducting magnetometer. *Science, 175,* 664–666.

Cohen, Y. E., & Andersen, R. A. (2002). A common reference frame for movement plans in the posterior parietal cortex. *Nature Reviews in Neuroscience, 3,* 553–562.

Curio, G., Mackert, B. M., Burghoff, M., Koetitz, R., Abraham-Fuchs, K., & Harer, W. (1994). Localization of evoked neuromagnetic 600 Hz activity in the cerebral somatosensory system. *Electroencephalography and Clinical Neurophysiology, 91,* 483–487.

Dale, A. M., Liu, A. K., Fischl, B. R., Buckner, R. L., Belliveau, J. W., Lewine, J. D., et al. (2000). Dynamic statistical parametric mapping: Combining fMRI and MEG for high-resolution imaging of cortical activity. *Neuron, 26,* 55–67.

Davis, H., Osterhammel, P. A., Wier, C. C., & Gjerdingen, D. B. (1972). Slow vertex potentials: Interactions among auditory, tactile, electric and visual stimuli. *Electroencephalography and Clinical Neurophysiology, 33,* 537–545.

Desimone, R. (1996). Neural mechanisms for visual memory and the role of attention. *Proceedings of the National Academy of Sciences, USA, 93,* 13494–13499.

Elbert, T., Flor, H., Birbaumer, N., Knecht, S., Hampson, S., Larbig, W., et al. (1994). Extensive reorganization of the somatosensory cortex in adult humans after nervous system injury. *Neuroreport, 5,* 2593–2597.

Elbert, T., Pantev, C., Wienbruch, C., Rockstroh, B., & Taub, E. (1995). Increased cortical representation of the fingers of the left hand in string players. *Science, 270,* 305–307.

Elbert, T., Sterr, A., Rockstroh, B., Pantev, C., Muller, M. M., & Taub, E. (2002). Expansion of the tonotopic area in the auditory cortex of the blind. *Journal of Neuroscience, 22,* 9941–9944.

Erne, S. N., & Hoke, M. (1990). Short-latency evoked magnetic fields from the human auditory brainstem. *Advances in Neurology, 54,* 167–176.

ffytche, D. H., Guy, C. N., & Zeki, S. (1995). The parallel visual motion inputs into areas V1 and V5 of human cerebral cortex. *Brain, 118,* 1375–1394.

Finney, E. M., Fine, I., & Dobkins, K. (2001). Visual stimuli activate auditory cortex in the deaf. *Nature Neuroscience, 4,* 1171–1173.

Fort, A., Delpuech, C., Pernier, J., & Giard, M.-H. (2002). Early auditory-visual interactions in human cortex during nonredundant target identification. *Brain Research: Cognitive Brain Research, 14,* 20–30.

Foxe, J. J., Morocz, I. A., Murray, M. M., Higgins, B. A., Javitt, D. C., & Schroeder, C. E. (2000). Multisensory auditory-somatosensory interactions in early cortical processing revealed by high-density electrical mapping. *Brain Research: Cognitive Brain Research, 10,* 77–83.

Gharib, S., Sutherling, W. W., Nakasato, N., Barth, S. D., Baumgartner, C., Alexopoulos, N., et al. (1995). MEG and EcoG localization accuracy test. *Electroencephalography and Clinical Neurophysiology, 94,* 109–114.

Giard, M. H., & Peronnet, F. (1999). Auditory-visual integration during multimodal object recognition in humans: A behavioral and electrophysiological study. *Journal of Cognitive Neuroscience, 11,* 473–490.

Goldman-Rakic, P. S. (1995). Changing concepts of cortical connectivity: Parallel distributed cortical networks. In P. Rakic & W. Singer (Eds.), *Neurobiology of neocortex* (pp. 177–202). Chichester: Wiley.

Graziano, M. S. A., & Gross, C. G. (1998). Spatial maps for the control of movement. *Current Opinion in Neurobiology, 8,* 195–201.

Groh, J. M., Trause, A. S., Underhill, A. M., Clark, K. R., & Inati, S. (2001). Eye position influences auditory responses in primate inferior colliculus. *Neuron, 29,* 509–518.

Gross, J., Kujala, J., Hämäläinen, M., Timmermann, L., Schnitzler, A., & Salmelin, R. (2001). Dynamic imaging of coherent sources: Studying neural interactions in the human brain. *Proc. Natl. Acad. Sci. USA, 98,* 694–699.

Gross, J., Tass, P. A., Salenius, S., Hari, R., Freund, H. J., & Schnitzler, A. (2000). Cortico-muscular synchronization during isometric muscle contraction in humans as revealed by magnetoencephalography. *Journal of Physiology, 527,* 623–631.

Guest, S., Catmur, C., Lloyd, D., & Spence, C. (2002). Audiotactile interactions in roughness perception. *Experimental Brain Research, 146,* 161–171.

Haggard, P. (2001). Look and feel. *Trends in Cognitive Sciences, 5,* 462–463.

Halgren, E., Raij, T., Marinkovic, K., Jousmäki, V., & Hari, R. (2000). Cognitive response profile of the human fusiform face area as determined by MEG. *Cerebral Cortex, 10,* 69–81.

Hamada, Y., Otsuka, S., Okamoto, T., & Suzuki, R. (2002). The profile of the recovery cycle in human primary and secondary somatosensory cortex: A magnetoencephalography study. *Clinical Neurophysiology, 113,* 1787–1793.

Hämäläinen, M., Hari, R., Ilmoniemi, R. J., Knuutila, J., & Lounasmaa, O. V. (1993). Magnetoencephalography: Theory, instrumentation, and applications to noninvasive studies of the working human brain. *Reviews in Modern Physics, 65,* 413–497.

Hämäläinen, M., & Ilmoniemi, R. (1994). Interpreting magnetic fields of the brain: Minimum norm estimates. *Medical and Biological Engineering and Computing, 32,* 35–42.

Hämäläinen, M., & Hari, R. (2002). Magnetoencephalographic characterization of dynamic brain activation: Basic principles and methods of data collection and source analysis. In A. W. Toga & J. C. Mazziotta (Eds.), *Brain mapping: The methods* (2nd ed., pp. 227–253). New York: Academic Press.

Hari, R. (1990). The neuromagnetic method in the study of the human auditory cortex. In F. Grandori, M. Hoke, & G. L. Romani (Eds.), *Auditory evoked magnetic fields and potentials. Advances in Audiology, 6,* 222–282.

Hari, R. (1999). Magnetoencephalography as a tool of clinical neurophysiology. In E. Niedermeyer & F. Lopes Da Silva (Eds.), *Electroencephalography: Basic principles, clinical applications, and related fields* (4th ed., pp. 1107–1134). Baltimore: Williams & Wilkins.

Hari, R., Aittoniemi, K., Järvinen, M.-L., Katila, T., & Varpula, T. (1980). Auditory evoked transient and sustained magnetic fields of the human brain. *Experimental Brain Research, 40,* 237–240.

Hari, R., Levänen, S., & Raij, T. (2001). Neuromagnetic monitoring of human cortical activation sequences during cognitive functions. *Trends in Cognitive Sciences, 4,* 455–462.

Hari, R., & Forss, N. (1999). Magnetoencephalography in the study of human somatosensory cortical processing.

Philosophical Transactions of the Royal Society of London, Series B: Biological Sciences, 354, 1145–1154.

Hari, R., Reinikainen, K., Kaukoranta, E., Hämäläinen, M., Ilmoniemi, R., Penttinen, A., et al. (1984). Somatosensory evoked cerebral magnetic fields from SI and SII in man. *Electroencephalography and Clinical Neurophysiology, 57,* 254–263.

Hari, R., & Salenius, S. (1999). Rhythmical corticomotor communication. *Neuroreport, 10,* R1–10.

Hari, R., & Salmelin, R. (1997). Human cortical rhythms: A neuromagnetic view through the skull. *Trends in Neurosciences, 20,* 44–49.

Hashimoto, I., Mashiko, T., & Imada, T. (1996). Somatic evoked high-frequency magnetic oscillations reflect activity of inhibitory interneurons in the human somatosensory cortex. *Electroencephalography and Clinical Neurophysiology, 100,* 189–203.

Hershenson, M. (1962). Reaction time as a measure of intersensory facilitation. *Journal of Experimental Psychology, 63,* 289–293.

Hillebrand, A., & Barnes, G. R. (2002). A quantitative assessment of the sensitivity of whole-head MEG to activity in the adult human cortex. *NeuroImage, 16,* 638–650.

Hurlbert, A. (2000). Visual perception: Learning to see through noise. *Current Biology, 10,* R231–233.

Huttunen, J., Hari, R., & Vanni, S. (1987). Crossmodal interaction is reflected in vertex potentials but not in evoked magnetic fields. *Acta Neurologica Scandinavica, 75,* 410–416.

Hyvärinen, J., Hyvärinen, L., & Linnankoski, I. (1981). Modification of parietal association cortex and functional blindness after binocular deprivation in young monkeys. *Experimental Brain Research, 42,* 1–8.

Ioannides, A. A., Bolton, J. P. R., & Clarke, C. J. S. (1990). Continuous probabilistic solutions to the biomagnetic inverse problem. *Inverse Problems, 6,* 523–542.

Jensen, O., & Vanni, S. (2002). A new method to identify multiple sources of oscillatory activity from magnetoencephalographic data. *NeuroImage, 15,* 568–574.

Jiang, W., Wallace, M. T., Vaughan, J. W., & Stein, B. E. (2001). Two cortical areas mediate multisensory integration in superior colliculus neurons. *Journal of Neurophysiology, 85,* 506–522.

Jousmäki, V. (2000). Tracking functions of cortical networks on a millisecond timescale. *Neural Networks, 13,* 883–889.

Jousmäki, V., & Hari, R. (1998). Parchment-skin illusion: Sound-biased touch. *Current Biology, 8,* R190.

Jousmäki, V., & Hari, R. (1999). Somatosensory evoked fields to large-area vibrotactile stimuli. *Clinical Neurophysiology, 110,* 905–909.

Kadunce, D. C., Vaughan, J. W., Wallace, M. T., Benedek, G., & Stein, B. E. (1997). Mechanisms of within- and cross-modality suppression in the superior colliculus. *Journal of Neurophysiology, 78,* 2834–2847.

Kadunce, D. C., Vaughan, J. W., Wallace, M. T., & Stein, B. E. (2001). The influence of visual and auditory receptive field organization on multisensory integration in the superior colliculus. *Experimental Brain Research, 139,* 303–310.

Kauffman, T., Theoret, H., & Pascual-Leone, A. (2002). Braille character discrimination in blindfolded human subjects. *Neuroreport, 13,* 571–574.

Kok, A., & de Jong, H. L. (1980). The effect of repetition on infrequent familiar and infamiliar visual patterns on com-

ponents of the event-related brain potential. *Biological Psychology, 10,* 167–188.

Krause, C., Möttönen, R., Jensen, O., Auranen, T., Tiippana, K., Lampinen, J., et al. (2002). Brain oscillatory responses during an audiovisual memory task: An MEG study. *Abstracts of the International Multisensory Research Forum, 3rd Annual Meeting, 55.*

Kujala, T., Huotilainen, M., Sinkkonen, J., Ahonen, A. I., Alho, K., Hämäläinen, M. S., et al. (1995). Visual cortex activation in blind humans during sound discrimination. *Neuroscience Letters, 183,* 143–146.

Kujala, T., Alho, K., Huotilainen, M., Ilmoniemi, R. J., Lehtokoski, A., Leinonen, A., et al. (1997). Electrophysiological evidence for cross-modal plasticity in humans with early- and late-onset blindness. *Psychophysiology, 34,* 213–216.

Kujala, T., Alho, K., & Näätänen, R. (2000). Cross-modal reorganization of human cortical functions. *Trends in Neurosciences, 23,* 115–120.

Lam, K., Kakigi, R., Kaneoke, Y., Naka, D., Maeda, K., & Suzuki, H. (1999). Effect of visual and auditory stimulation on somatosensory evoked magnetic fields. *Clinical Neurophysiology, 110,* 295–304.

Lam, K., Kakigi, R., Mukai, T., & Yamasaki, H. (2001). Attention and visual interference stimulation affect somatosensory processing: A magnetoencephalographic study. *Neuroscience, 104,* 689–703.

Leahy, R. M., Mosher, J. C., Spencer, M. E., Huang, M. X., & Lewine, J. D. (1998). A study of dipole localization accuracy for MEG and EEG using a human skull phantom. *Electroencephalography and Clinical Neurophysiology, 107,* 159–173.

Lederman, S. J., Thorne, G., & Jones, B. (1986). Perception of texture by vision and touch: Multidimensionality and intersensory integration. *Journal of Experimental Psychology: Human Perception and Performance, 12,* 169–180.

Levänen, S., & Hamdorf, D. (2001). Feeling vibrations: Enhanced tactile sensitivity in congenitally deaf humans. *Neuroscience Letters, 301,* 75–77.

Levänen, S., Jousmäki, V., & Hari, R. (1998). Vibration-induced auditory-cortex activation in a congenitally deaf adult. *Current Biology, 8,* 869–872.

Lounasmaa, O. H., Hämäläinen, M., Hari, R., & Salmelin, R. (1996). Information processing in the human brain: Magnetoencephalographic approach. *Proceedings of the National Academy of Sciences, USA, 93,* 8809–8815.

Lü, Z.-L., Williamson, S., & Kaufman, L. (1992). Human auditory primary and association cortex have differing lifetimes for activation traces. *Brain Research, 572,* 236–241.

Lütkenhöner, B., Lammertmann, C., Ross, B., & Pantev, C. (2000). Brainstem auditory evoked fields in response to clicks. *Neuroreport, 11,* 913–918.

Lütkenhöner, B., Lammertmann, C., Simões, C., & Hari, R. (2002). Magnetoencephalographic correlates of audiotactile interaction. *NeuroImage, 15,* 509–522.

Mäkelä, J. P., Kirveskari, E., Seppä, M., Hämäläinen, M., Forss, N., Avikainen, S., Salonen, O., et al. (2001). Three-dimensional integration of brain anatomy and function to facilitate intraoperative navigation around the sensorimotor strip. *Human Brain Mapping, 12,* 180–192.

Massaro, D. W., Cohen, M. M., & Smeele, P. M. T. (1996). Perception of asynchronous and conflicting visual and auditory speech. *Journal of the Acoustical Society of America, 100,* 1777–1786.

Matsuura, K., & Okabe, U. (1995). Selective minimum-norm solution of the biomagnetic inverse problem. *IEEE Transactions on Bio-medical Engineering, 42,* 608–615.

McClelland, J. L., Rumelhart, D. E., & Hinton, G. E. (1986). The appeal of parallel distributed processing. In D. E. Rumelhart & J. L. McClelland (Eds.), *Parallel distributed processing* (pp. 4–44). Cambridge, MA: MIT Press.

McGrath, M., & Summefield, Q. (1985). Intermodal timing relations and audio-visual speech recognition by normal-hearing adults. *Journal of the Acoustical Society of America, 77,* 678–685.

McGurk, H., & MacDonald, J. (1976). Hearing lips and seeing voices. *Nature, 264,* 746–748.

Meredith, M. A. (2002). On the neuronal basis for multisensory convergence: A brief overview. *Brain Research: Cognitive Brain Research, 14,* 31–40.

Merzenich, M. M., Nelson, R. J., Stryker, M. P., Cynader, M. S., Schoppmann, A., & Zook, J. M. (1984). Somatosensory cortical map changes following digit amputation in adult monkeys. *Journal of Comparative Neurology, 224,* 591–605.

Mesulam, M.-M. (1998). From sensation to cognition. *Brain, 121,* 1013–1052.

Miller, J. (1986). Timecourse of coactivation in bimodal divided attention. *Perception & Psychophysics, 40,* 331–343.

Molholm, S., Ritter, W., Murray, M. M., Javitt, D. C., Schroeder, C. E., & Foxe, J. J. (2002). Multisensory auditory-visual interactions during early sensory processing in humans: A high-density electrical mapping study. *Brain Research: Cognitive Brain Research, 14,* 115–128.

Morrell, L. K. (1968). Sensory interaction: Evoked potential observations in man. *Experimental Brain Research, 6,* 146–155.

Möttönen, R., Krause, C. M., Tiippana, K., & Sams, M. (2002). Processing of changes in visual speech in the human auditory cortex. *Brain Research: Cognitive Brain Research, 13,* 417–425.

Munhall, K. G., Gribble, P., Sacco, L., & Ward, M. (1996). Temporal constraints on the McGurk effect. *Perception & Psychophysics, 58,* 351–362.

Näätänen, R., Ilmoniemi, R., & Alho, K. (1994.) Magneto-encephalography in studies of human cognitive brain function. *Trends in Neurosciences, 17,* 389–395.

Newport, R., Hindle, J. V., & Jackson, S. R. (2001). Links between vision and somatosensation: Vision can improve the felt position of the unseen hand. *Current Biology, 11,* 975–980.

Pantev, C., & Lütkenhöner, B. (2000). Magnetoencephalographic studies of functional organization and plasticity of the human auditory cortex. *Journal of Clinical Neurophysiology, 17,* 130–142.

Pantev, C., Roberts, L. E., Schulz, M., Engelien, A., & Ross, B. (2001). Timbre-specific enhancement of auditory cortical representations in musicians. *Neuroreport, 12,* 169–174.

Papanicolaou, A. C., Simos, P. G., Breier, J. I., Wheless, J. W., Mancias, P., Baumgartner, J. E., et al. (2001). Brain plasticity for sensory and linguistic functions: A functional imaging study using magnetoencephalography with children and young adults. *Journal of Child Neurology, 16,* 241–252.

Parkkonen, L., & Mäkelä, J. (2002). MEG sees deep sources: Measuring and modeling brainstem auditory evoked fields. In H. Nowak, J. Haueisen, F. Giessler, & R. Huonker (Eds.), *Proceedings of the 13th International Conference on Biomagnetism* (pp. 107–109). Berlin: VDE Verlag.

Pascual-Marqui, R. D., Michel, C. M., & Lehmann, D. (1994). Low resolution electromagnetic tomography: A new method for localizing electrical activity in the brain. *International Journal of Psychophysiology, 18,* 49–65.

Pulvermüller, F. (1999). Words in the brain's language. *Behavioural Brain Science, 22,* 253–279 [discussion 280–336].

Raichle, M. E., Fiez, J. A., Videen, T. O., MacLeod, A. M., Pardo, J. V., et al. (1994). Practice-related changes in human brain functional anatomy during nonmotor learning. *Cerebral Cortex, 4,* 8–26.

Raij, T. (1999). Patterns of brain activity during visual imagery of letters. *Journal of Cognitive Neuroscience, 11,* 282–299.

Raij, T., Uutela, K., & Hari, R. (2000). Audiovisual integration of letters in the human brain. *Neuron, 28,* 617–625.

Salenius, S., Portin, K., Kajola, M., Salmelin, R., & Hari, R. (1997). Cortical control of human motoneuron firing during isometric contraction. *Journal of Neurophysiology, 77,* 3401–3405.

Sams, M., Aulanko, R., Hämäläinen, M., Hari, R., Lounasmaa, O. V., Lu, S.-T., et al. (1991). Seeing speech: Visual information from lip movements modifies activity in the human auditory cortex. *Neuroscience Letters, 127,* 141–145.

Schroeder, C. E., & Foxe, J. J. (2002). The timing of laminar profile of converging inputs to multisensory areas of the macaque neocortex. *Brain Research: Cognitive Brain Research, 14,* 187–198.

Schröger, E., & Widmann, A. (1998). Speeded responses to audiovisual signal changes result from bimodal integration. *Psychophysiology, 35,* 755–759.

Schürmann, M., Raij, T., Fujiki, N., & Hari, R. (2002). Mind's ear in a musician: Where and when in the brain. *NeuroImage, 16,* 434–440.

Simos, P. G., Papanicolaou, A. C., Breier, J. I., Wheless, J. W., Constantinou, J. E., Gormley, W., et al. (1999). Localization of language specific cortex by using magnetic source imaging and electrical stimulation mapping. *Journal of Neurosurgery, 91,* 787–796.

Simos, P. G., Papanicolaou, A. C., Breier, J. I., Fletcher, J. M., Wheless, J. W., Maggio, W. W., et al. (2000). Insights into brain function and neural plasticity using magnetic source imaging. *Journal of Clinical Neurophysiology, 17,* 143–162.

Squires, N. K., Donchin, E., Squires, K. C., & Grossberg, S. (1977). Bisensory stimulation: Inferring decision-related processes from P300 component. *Journal of Experimental Psychology: Human Perception and Performance, 3,* 299–315.

Stein, B. E. (1998). Neural mechanisms for synthesizing sensory information and producing adaptive behaviors. *Experimental Brain Research, 123,* 124–135.

Stein, B. E., & Meredith, M. A. (1993). The merging of the senses. Cambridge, MA: MIT Press.

Stein, B. E., & Wallace, M. T. (1996). Comparisons of cross-modality integration in midbrain and cortex. *Progress in Brain Research, 112,* 289–299.

Teder-Sälejärvi, W. A., McDonald, J. J., Di Russo, F., & Hillyard, S. A. (2002). An analysis of audio-visual cross-modal integration by means of event-related potential (ERP) recordings. *Brain Research: Cognitive Brain Research, 14,* 106–114.

Tesche, C. D. (1996). Non-invasive imaging of neuronal population dynamics in the human thalamus. *Brain Research, 112,* 289–299.

Tesche, C. D., Karhu, J., & Tissari, S. O. (1996). Non-invasive detection of neuronal population activity in human hippocampus. *Brain Research: Cognitive Brain Research, 4,* 39–47.

Tuomisto, T., Hari, R., Katila, T., Poutanen, T., & Varpula, T. (1983). Studies of auditory evoked magnetic and electric responses: Modality specificity and modelling. *Nuovo Cimento, 2D,* 471–494.

Uusitalo, M. A., Williamson, S. J., & Seppä, M. T. (1996). Dynamical organisation of the human visual system revealed by lifetimes of activation traces. *Neuroscience Letters, 213,* 149–152.

Uutela, K., Hämäläinen, M., & Somersalo, E. (1999). Visualization of magnetoencephalographic data using minimum current estimates. *NeuroImage, 10,* 173–180.

Vrba, J., Betts, K., Burbank, M., Cheung, T., Fife, A. A., Haid, G., et al. (1993). Whole-cortex, 64 channel SQUID biomagnetometer system. *IEEE Transactions on Applied Superconductivity, 3,* 1878–1882.

Weiss, T., Miltner, W. H., Huonker, R., Friedel, R., Schmidt, I., & Taub, E. (2000). Rapid functional plasticity of the somatosensory cortex after finger amputation. *Experimental Brain Research, 134,* 199–203.

Wiech, K., Preissl, H., Lutzenberger, W., Kiefer, R. T., Topfner, S., Haerle M., et al. (2000). Cortical reorganization after digit-to-hand replantation. *Journal of Neurosurgery, 93,* 876–883.

Wiggs, C. L., & Martin, A. (1998). Properties and mechanisms of perceptual priming. *Current Opinion Neurobiology, 8,* 227–233.

Yaka, R., Yinon, U., & Wollberg, Z. (1999). Auditory activation of cortical visual areas in cats after early visual deprivation. *European Journal of Neuroscience, 11,* 1301–1312.

Yang, T. T., Gallen, C. C., Ramachandran, V. S., Cobb, S., Schwartz, B. J., & Bloom, F. E. (1994). Noninvasive detection of cerebral plasticity in adult human somatosensory cortex. *Neuroreport, 5,* 701–704.

33 Functional Imaging Evidence for Multisensory Spatial Representations and Cross-Modal Attentional Interactions in the Human Brain

EMILIANO MACALUSO AND JON DRIVER

Introduction

Many of the external events that we experience in everyday life produce multiple signals, each stimulating different sensory modalities. The multimodal nature of these signals can enrich our perceptual experience, but it also raises the issue of how coherent neuronal representations are formed for such different signals in the brain. Although the origin of a set of multisensory signals might correspond to a single external event, the initial processing of signals to different senses will occur in anatomically distant areas. This raises the question of how the unity of the original event is reconstructed in the brain via multisensory integration. In this chapter we review several recent findings from human functional imaging studies that address these issues, with a focus on spatial multisensory representations and attentional selection of spatial locations. We show that several neural mechanisms might underlie the integration of spatial representations across sensory modalities. These mechanisms include feed-forward convergence of signals from early sensory-specific areas to higher-level brain regions, forming multimodal spatial representations, and also cross-modal spatial influences on relatively early (apparently unimodal) sensory-specific areas, which may involve feedback influences from multimodal attentional control structures.

Mapping unimodal and multimodal brain areas with functional imaging

Signals to different sensory modalities are initially processed, at the cortical level, in anatomically distant sensory-specific (unimodal) brain areas. For example,

an object that can be both seen and felt should activate visual areas located in the occipital cortex and somatosensory areas in the postcentral gyrus. It has long been thought that such sensory-specific areas for processing information received through different modalities are not directly interconnected (but see Falchier, Clavagnier, Barone, & Kennedy, 2002), with occipital cortex not responding directly to tactile stimulation and somatosensory areas not responding directly to visual stimulation in the normal adult brain (but see Buchel, Price, Frackowiak, & Friston, 1998; Burton et al., 2002; Cohen et al., 1997; and Sathian & Zangaladzeb, 2002, for evidence from various clinical populations). This presumed lack of a direct connection raises the question of how signals conveyed in different modalities but concerning the same event could interact to provide a coherent representation of the external world.

Although some sensory-specific brain areas for different modalities may not be directly connected with each other, they nevertheless do project to common multimodal brain areas, such as higher-order association areas in parietal, frontal, and temporal regions, at the cortical level. Electrophysiological studies have shown that single neurons in the latter areas can respond to stimulation of different sensory modalities (for ventral intraparietal sulcus [VIP] see, e.g., Duhamel, Colby, & Goldberg, 1998; for area 7b: Graziano & Gross, 1995; for posterior temporal regions: Bruce, Desimone, & Gross, 1981; for ventral premotor cortex: Fogassi et al., 1996). Multimodal responses can also be found in certain subcortical sites (e.g., for the superior colliculus [SC]: Stein & Meredith, 1993). Moreover, at all these sites, the convergence of information from different senses appears to be spatially organized, so that each neuron has receptive fields (RFs) for roughly corresponding regions of space in each of the modalities that can drive it (e.g., Duhamel et al., 1998; Graziano & Gross, 1995; Stein & Meredith, 1993). Multimodal neurons of this general type suggest one possible mechanism for multisensory integration: unimodal areas processing stimuli in different sensory modalities send signals to common multimodal areas via feed-forward projections. Signals from different modalities might then interact in the multimodal regions.

Recent imaging studies indicate that a basic separation between apparently unimodal (early) and multimodal (later) stages of cortical processing can also be introduced for the human brain. For example, Bremmer et al. (2001) used visual, tactile, or auditory stimulation during functional magnetic resonance imaging (fMRI). When they compared each of these unimodal stimulations with baseline conditions, they found that the intraparietal sulcus (IPS), ventral premotor areas, and anterior regions of the inferior parietal lobule could be activated, and activation was independent of the modality of stimulation. Figure 33.1A shows similar results from an fMRI study of our own, which used visual or tactile stimulation to reveal areas responding to stimulation from both modalities (i.e., candidate multimodal brain regions). These results are all in good agreement with previous electrophysiological work in nonhuman primates (Bruce et al., 1981; Duhamel et al., 1998; Graziano & Gross, 1995) that found multimodal neurons in all of the higher-level cortical areas that were activated multimodally with fMRI. Because of the limited spatial resolution of imaging techniques, however, apparent colocalization of brain activation for several different modalities might also be consistent with closely neighboring or interdigitated neural populations for the different senses, rather than areas containing multimodal neurons in which the different senses directly interact (see Calvert, 2001, for related arguments).

Other recent imaging studies have used more sophisticated paradigms to highlight cross-modal *interactions*. The principle behind such experiments is that cross-modal interactions are demonstrated if activity during certain pairwise combinations of multimodal stimulation cannot be accounted for by simple summation of activity during the two unimodal stimulations (i.e., superadditive or subadditive interactions). Pioneering electrophysiological studies that first employed analogous methods have shown that, at the single-cell level, such cross-modal interactions can depend on the relative location and timing of the two inputs (see Stein & Meredith, 1993, for a review of such work on the SC). It should be noted that temporal or spatial coincidences between different modalities are likely to provide useful cues as to whether the stimulation in the different modalities relates to the same external event (and so should be integrated), or not.

Calvert, Campbell, and Bremmer (2000) provide one example of an fMRI study examining possible audiovisual interactions during speech perception (see also Calvert, 2001, for nonspeech examples). In different blocks, the subjects either listened to a story (auditory-only condition), viewed the lip movements of a speaker reading the same story (visual-only condition), or were presented with a bimodal version of the story (in which auditory and visual signals were in their usual synchrony). In another experiment, the auditory and visual signals in the bimodal condition concerned different stories and thus did not have systematic synchrony or any systematic phonemic relation. The results showed that both unimodal auditory and unimodal visual conditions (compared to rest without stimulation) activated a candidate multimodal region in the superior temporal sulcus (STS). Critically, the left STS also showed a superadditive interaction for the matching audiovisual inputs in the bimodal condition and a subadditive interaction for the mismatching audiovisual inputs compared with the unimodal conditions, suggesting an influence of multisensory integration here (see also Calvert & Lewis, Chap. 30, this volume).

Spatial representations within and across modalities

Location is a property that can be extracted by different sensory modalities and thus can provide a useful cue for multisensory integration. Representations of space, in the form of neurons that respond to stimuli only when delivered at specific locations (i.e., within the neuron's RF), are widespread in the brain. For the case of vision, early cortical areas show higher spatial specificity than later areas. The retinotopic organization of early occipital visual areas, previously shown in nonhuman primates (e.g., Tootell, Silverman, Switkes, & De Valois, 1982), has since been confirmed for the human brain with fMRI (e.g., DeYoe et al., 1996; Tootell et al., 1997). By contrast, somatosensory cortex, in postcentral areas, is organized in terms of somatotopic space. Given the large anatomical separation between such visual and somatosensory regions and the different nature of their spatial organization, one may ask how the spatial unity of a single, multimodal, tactile-visual event at the same location could be represented. In light of the hierarchical organization of the sensory pathways introduced earlier, it might be suggested that higher-level multimodal areas show spatially specific responses for stimuli

A. NON-SPATIAL <u>bimodal</u> effects for Vision AND Touch

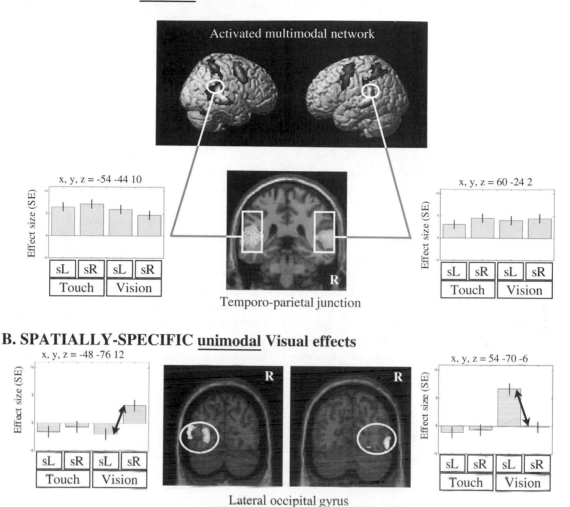

Activated multimodal network

x, y, z = -54 -44 10

Effect size (SE)

sL	sR	sL	sR
Touch		Vision	

Temporo-parietal junction

x, y, z = 60 -24 2

Effect size (SE)

sL	sR	sL	sR
Touch		Vision	

B. SPATIALLY-SPECIFIC <u>unimodal</u> Visual effects

x, y, z = -48 -76 12

Effect size (SE)

sL	sR	sL	sR
Touch		Vision	

Lateral occipital gyrus

x, y, z = 54 -70 -6

Effect size (SE)

sL	sR	sL	sR
Touch		Vision	

C. SPATIALLY-SPECIFIC <u>bimodal</u> effects for Vision AND Touch

x, y, z = -50 -24 54

Effect size (SE)

sL	sR	sL	sR
Touch		Vision	

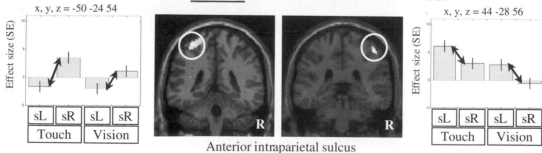

Anterior intraparietal sulcus

x, y, z = 44 -28 56

Effect size (SE)

sL	sR	sL	sR
Touch		Vision	

FIGURE 33.1   Responses to peripheral stimulation in vision and touch. (*A*) Lateral views showing brain regions responding to both visual and tactile stimulation, irrespective of stimulated hemifield. The coronal section shows activation at the temporoparietal junction, with plots of activity for the four stimulation conditions (left or right hemifield, vision or touch) against a no-stimulation baseline condition (see Macaluso & Driver, 2001). (*B*) Differential activation of occipital visual areas depending on the stimulated hemifield. Both inferior and lateral occipital regions responded more to contralateral than to ipsilateral visual stimulation (see arrows in each plot) but did not show effects of tactile stimulation (first two bars in each plot). (*C*) Spatially specific effects in the anterior part of the intraparietal sulcus. This area responded more to stimulation in the contralateral hemifield than to stimulation in the ipsilateral hemifield. Critically, these spatial effects were independent of the sensory modality (tactile or visual) of the stimulation (arrows in each plot). Effect sizes are expressed in standard error (SE) units. SPM thresholds are set to *P* (uncorrected) = 0.001. sL/sR, stimulation of the left or right hemifield.

presented at a given location (or locations), and that these responses are independent of the modality of the stimuli. As briefly mentioned earlier, this phenomenon has already been found for several areas at the level of single-cell recording.

This general idea can also be assessed with functional imaging of the human brain. A recent fMRI study of our own (Macaluso & Driver, 2001) provides one simple example. We presented subjects with tactile stimuli on either hand or visual stimuli (near either hand) in either the left or right hemifield during fMRI. The use of stimuli in two different positions, left or right, allowed us to test for brain areas with spatially specific responses, in the sense of responding more to stimuli presented in one hemifield than to stimuli presented in the other hemifield. By using visual or tactile stimuli, we could differentiate between brain areas displaying such a spatially specific response only when one particular modality was stimulated (i.e., "unimodal" spatial effects) and areas showing an analogous spatially specific response (as a function of stimulus side) that was independent of the stimulated modality (i.e., "multimodal" spatial effects). The latter type of response would be expected in brain regions that code space multimodally.

The four blocked conditions of unilateral sensory stimulation (i.e., vision-left, vision-right, touch-left, and touch-right) were alternated with a rest condition (no stimulation). Unimodal spatial effects (i.e., differential responses depending on the hemifield stimulated, but applicable to one modality only) were found in contralateral occipital areas for vision and in contralateral postcentral regions for touch. Figure 33.1B shows the modality-specific effects in occipital visual cortex. The arrows in the plots indicate the critical effects, with a difference between left and right stimulation found only during visual stimulation.

More important, a comparison of left and right stimulation across both sensory modalities revealed multimodal spatial activations in the IPS contralateral to the stimulated side. Peak activation was found in the anterior part of the sulcus at the interception of the IPS and the postcentral sulcus. As shown in Figure 33.1C, activity in this area was higher during contralateral stimulation than during ipsilateral stimulation, for both visual and tactile stimulation (see arrows on plots). This observation suggests that this region of the IPS might represent the contralateral side of space, irrespective of the modality of stimulation there (i.e., for both vision and touch), a proposal consistent with the multimodal spatial representations here in the human brain, which might arise via feed-forward convergence from unimodal spatial representations (see also Grefkes, Weiss,

Zilles, & Fink, 2002, showing multimodal effects in a similar parietal region during visuotactile object discrimination).

The anterior IPS was the only region to show this pattern in our study for the stimuli used. It might seem surprising that only a single area showed multimodal spatial responses as we defined them. However, it bears emphasis that the responses in the anterior IPS were not only multimodal but also spatially specific, in the sense that they were activated by stimulation in one hemifield more than by stimulation in the other hemifield. By comparing results with a baseline condition, we could also test for multimodal responses that did not have to be spatially specific in this manner (as in Bremmer et al., 2001; see also Fig. 33.1A, the plots for the temporoparietal junction). This comparison revealed activation of additional intraparietal regions, the temporoparietal junction (TPJ) and premotor areas. These results are in agreement with those of Bremmer et al. (2001) and with electrophysiological recordings that found neurons showing multimodal responses in all these areas (Bruce et al., 1981; Duhamel et al., 1998; Graziano & Gross, 1995). However, any nonspatial multimodal activations found when simply comparing stimulation in different modalities versus rest (see Bremmer et al., 2001; Macaluso & Driver, 2001) might in principle involve further processes, such as expectation or attention. In the following sections we address these issues and explicitly investigate the role of spatial attention in multisensory processing.

Endogenous spatial attention: Unimodal and multimodal modulations

The data presented in the previous section and summarized in Figure 33.1 can be easily reconciled with the traditional concept that cortical sensory processing is organized hierarchically, with unimodal areas feeding into higher-level multimodal areas. However, that most of the experimental paradigms described thus far did not involve any task, just passive stimulation. Although recording responses to passive stimulation might be a good starting point for mapping unimodal versus multimodal areas in the human brain and related spatial representations, it obscures the fact that brain activity is not determined solely by the stimuli presented but is also affected by the current relevance of these stimuli to the subject, as determined by selective attention. Moreover, in many situations in daily life, we receive multiple stimulation in every modality, a phenomenon that raises the question of how task-relevant locations and modalities are selected from among irrelevant competing stimulation?

ENDOGENOUS SELECTION OF RELEVANT LOCATIONS
There has been considerable research on how endogenous covert attention to a particular location might affect sensory processing and perceptual judgments (see Driver & Frackowiak, 2001, for an overview). Although much of this research has considered just a single modality at a time, recent work using behavioral (Spence & Driver, 1996; Spence, Pavani, & Driver, 2000) or ERP (Eimer & Driver, 2000) methods has found that directing endogenous attention to a particular location to judge one modality can have consequences for processing at that location in other modalities also. This finding suggests that endogenous selection of a particular spatial location might arise at a level where locations are represented multimodally.

There have been many recent functional imaging studies of how endogenous covert spatial attention may affect brain activity, with the majority of these studies considering just a single modality, usually vision (see Kanwisher & Wojciulik, 2000, for a review). In a prototypical study, subjects are presented with two streams of stimuli, one in each hemifield. During scanning, subjects covertly attend to one side to perform some judgment for the attended stimuli there while ignoring all stimuli presented in the opposite hemifield (e.g., Heinze et al., 1994). In different blocks or trials, subjects attend to the other hemifield. Brain activity during the two types of block or trial is compared in order to highlight regional differences characteristic for attention toward one side or the other. In the visual modality, this type of experiment has shown that attention toward one hemifield can result in increased activity in contralateral occipital cortex (Heinze et al., 1994; Hopfinger, Buonocore, & Mangun, 2000). This observation fits naturally with the fact that occipital areas represent the contralateral side of visual space, and suggests that these representations can be modulated endogenously. Thus, it appears that endogenous selection of specific visual locations involves modulation of relatively early, sensory-specific areas.

How might such findings of endogenous spatial attention affecting relatively early, modality-appropriate regions be reconciled with the behavioral evidence briefly introduced above (Spence & Driver, 1996; Spence, Pavani, et al., 2000), demonstrating that there are cross-modal links in endogenous spatial attention? We addressed this issue with a positron emission tomograph (PET) experiment that used a method analogous to that used previously in purely visual studies (Heinze et al., 1994), but with stimulation in two different modalities (Macaluso, Frith, & Driver, 2000a). Subjects received unimodal stimuli *bilaterally,* with either visual or tactile stimulation in different blocks. The study used a 2 × 2 factorial design, with the endogenously attended side (left or right) and the modality of the stimulation (vision or touch) as orthogonal factors. The effects of spatial attention were investigated by directly comparing attention to one side versus attention to the other side. Critically, the use of two different sensory modalities within the same experiment allowed us to examine whether any effects of spatial attention were modality-specific (i.e., observed during stimulation of one modality only) or multimodal (i.e., observed independently of the stimulated modality). Moreover, the visual stimuli were presented near the hands (where any tactile stimuli were delivered), so that stimulation in both modalities was delivered at approximately the same external locations, although in separate blocks.

Unimodal effects of spatial selective attention were found in occipital visual cortex during visual stimulation only, and in somatosensory postcentral regions during tactile stimulation only. Both of these effects consisted of increased blood flow in the hemisphere contralateral to the attended side. Hence, spatial attention modulated activity in brain regions thought to represent the attended location in the modality that was stimulated. This result replicated findings previously reported for the visual modality (e.g., Heinze et al., 1994; Hopfinger et al., 2000), but it also extended the effect of spatially selective attention on early sensory-specific areas to the tactile modality. In relation to the multimodal issue and to possible neural substrates for the selection of external locations across sensory modalities, the critical comparisons concerned effects of spatial selection that were independent of the stimulated modality. These effects included activation of the anterior part of the IPS, contralateral to the attended side. This multimodal modulation of the IPS by spatial attention appears consistent with our demonstration (see Fig. 33.1C) that this region may provide a multimodal representation of the contralateral side of space (Macaluso & Driver, 2001). Our attentional PET data (Macaluso et al., 2000a) extend this observation by showing that the representations in IPS can be modulated endogenously by spatial attention in a similar way to the modulation found for unimodal regions.

The multimodal attentional effects in the IPS fit with the hierarchical organization of the sensory pathways described previously and might in principle relate to the cross-modal links observed in behavioral studies (e.g., Spence & Driver, 1996; Spence, Pavani, et al., 2000). However, this PET study also showed some multimodal effects of spatially selective attention in areas traditionally regarded as unimodal visual cortex. In particular, we found that both lateral and superior occipital areas showed a significant effect of attention to the contralateral side of space even during blocks of tactile stimulation. Although this particular PET experiment (Macaluso et al., 2000a) did not allow us to determine directly in the same study whether these occipital areas responded to visual stimulation only, their anatomical location, and a strong main effect of visual stimulation versus tactile stimulation there (see Macaluso et al., 2000a), suggest that these areas are indeed unimodal visual areas. Moreover, the fMRI experiment we described earlier (Macaluso & Driver, 2001) also indicated that occipital areas do not respond to tactile stimulation, and showed unimodal effects on the stimulated side that were specific to visual stimulation (see Fig. 33.1*B*). Therefore, visual areas that apparently respond only to visual stimulation of the contralateral hemifield (i.e., unimodal areas) can be affected by attention to the contralateral hemifield during a purely tactile task, revealing a spatially specific cross-modal effect on "unimodal" cortex. This PET finding is consistent with several event-related potential (ERP) results (e.g., Eimer & Driver, 2000) that also demonstrate that attending to one side for a tactile task can modulate components traditionally regarded as sensory-specific for vision.

Such findings of multimodal effects of spatial attention in apparently unimodal visual areas raise several new questions. First, in the PET experiment just described (Macaluso et al., 2000a), there may have been no penalty for subjects merely choosing to direct both tactile and visual attention toward the instructed side during the tactile task (cf. Spence & Driver, 1996). It was therefore possible that the multimodal effects found in visual cortex simply reflected an optional choice by the subjects to shift both visual and tactile attention toward one side of space. However, this is unlikely to be the sole explanation for cross-modal links in spatial attention, in light of behavioral (Spence, Ranson, & Driver, 2000) and ERP (Eimer, 1999) evidence that deployment of visual and tactile attention toward the same side is difficult to suppress voluntarily. Because tactile attention can boost contralateral visual areas, a second issue that arises concerns how subjects could correctly select just a tactile target on one side, in a situation where visual distracters were also presented there. Finally, because no direct projection from tactile areas to visual occipital cortex is known as yet, what possible mechanisms could underlie these apparently tactile influences (i.e., concerning which side is relevant for the tactile task) on occipital visual cortex?

We addressed some of these issues with a second PET experiment (Macaluso, Frith, & Driver, 2002a). Again, we used a selective spatial attention paradigm involving both vision and touch in the same experiment. The effects of endogenous spatial attention were again investigated by presenting bilateral stimulation and comparing covert attention toward one side with attention toward the other side. However, unlike in the previous PET experiment (Macaluso et al., 2000a), we now delivered bimodal, visuotactile stimulation to both sides during all conditions of attention to one or other side (Macaluso et al., 2002a). Thus, subjects received four independent streams of stimuli: visual in the left and right visual fields, and tactile to the left and right hand. As before, visual and tactile stimuli on the same side were delivered in close spatial proximity (i.e., the visual stimuli were near either hand). During each block, the subjects were asked to attend endogenously to just one side and just one modality, to detect infrequent targets on the relevant side and in the relevant modality. All stimuli on the opposite side, or on the same side but in the irrelevant modality, had to be ignored, as otherwise they would intrude on performance.

The design can again be considered as a 2×2 factorial, with attended side as one factor. Unlike in the previous PET experiment, which had used the modality of stimulation as second factor, the second factor was now the attended modality (vision or touch), with both modalities now being stimulated throughout the attentional conditions. This use of bimodal stimulation introduces an important conceptual change in the paradigm. Although in the previous experiment, subjects could choose to shift both their visual and tactile attention toward the same side without any penalty, in the subsequent experiment any deployment of visual attention to the same location as tactile attention should have brought visual distracters there within the focus of attention. Thus, the design was expected to discourage subjects from voluntarily shifting both visual and tactile attention to the same side as a strategic option.

As in the previous PET experiment (Macaluso et al., 2000a), our analysis aimed at separating unimodal and multimodal effects of spatial covert attention. During tactile attention only, signal increases were again detected in the postcentral gyrus contralateral to the attended side, whereas during visual attention only, the contralateral superior occipital gyrus was activated. As in the previous PET experiment, multimodal spatial effects were detected in the anterior part of the IPS contralateral to the attended side, and these effects were independent of the attended modality (Fig. 33.2*A*). The multimodal effects of spatial attention on areas in unimodal occipital cortex were also replicated. Both the lateral occipital gyrus and portions of the superior occipital gyrus showed higher activity during attention toward the contralateral hemifield, irrespective of whether vision or touch was relevant. These multimodal spatial

A. Multimodal effect of attention in <u>multimodal</u> association cortex

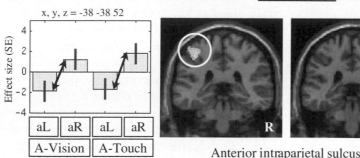

Effect of attended
side not significant
for this hemisphere
in this study

Anterior intraparietal sulcus

B. Multimodal effect of attention in <u>unimodal</u> visual cortex

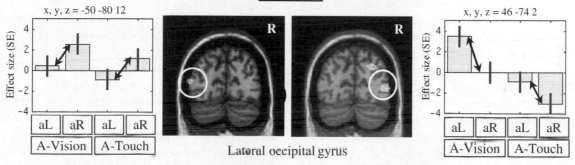

Lateral occipital gyrus

FIGURE 33.2   Multimodal spatial effects (i.e., independent of the attended modality) of endogenous attention during bimodal and bilateral stimulation (Macaluso et al., 2002a) in the intraparietal sulcus (IPS) and part of the superior occipital gyrus. Although the multimodal attentional effects in IPS could be predicted on the basis of the multimodal, spatially specific responses of this region (see Fig. 33.1*C*), the multimodal effect in occipital cortex highlighted a new example of cross-modal influences on unimodal visual areas. Activity in the various conditions is plotted with respect to a baseline in which subjects directed attention centrally, so that the bimodal bilateral stimulation was then unattended (see Macaluso et al., 2002a, for details). SPM thresholds for the main effect of attended side were set to P (uncorrected) = 0.001. aL/aR, attend left, attend right; a-Vision/a-Touch, attend-vision, attend-touch conditions.

effects on visual cortex are shown in Figure 33.2*B*. Activity in the left lateral occipital gyrus is plotted in the leftmost panel for the four experimental conditions. The effect of spatial attention (right minus left) was present not only during the attend-vision blocks (second versus first bar), but also during the attend-touch blocks (compare fourth versus third bar). In the right hemisphere (rightmost panel in Fig. 33.2*B*) analogous effects were found, with spatial attention again modulating activity in occipital cortex during both visual and tactile blocks (now with a higher signal for attention to the left side). Thus, directing attention toward one side of space not only results in the modulation of sensory-specific areas processing the target stimuli (e.g., somatosensory cortex for the selection of tactile targets), it also seems to trigger spatial biases in activation for remote brain areas that represent the attended location for another modality. This comodulation of activity in anatomically distant brain areas might constitute one mechanism for linking sensory signals in different modalities on the basis of their position in external space.

As in the previous PET experiment (Macaluso et al., 2000a) no multimodal effect was found in somatosensory postcentral areas, which were modulated only according to the direction of tactile attention. The reason for this might lie in the different spatial acuity of the two sensory systems, with visual cortex providing a more accurate representation of external space. Alternatively, some difference in the perceptual salience of the stimuli that we used in the two different modalities (an aspect difficult to quantify or equate perfectly across sensory modalities) might also have contributed to the asymmetry observed here and in other visuo-tactile studies. Generally, it appears that cross-modal effects specific for attention to one or another location can be found more reliably in visual cortex than in somatosensory cortex (but see Eimer & Driver, 2000).

The observed activation of visual areas during selection of tactile stimuli (even though visual distracters were now presented at the same location) raises the question of how subjects are able to select the correct tactile targets for response, rather than the visual distracters presented at the same location. Some additional mechanism may be needed to select just the relevant tactile stimuli for further processing and to determine overt responses. A comparison of visual attention versus tactile attention in this PET experiment (Macaluso et al., 2002a) suggests two possible mechanisms. First, occipital visual areas that were modulated according to the direction of tactile attention (i.e., cross-modal spatial effects on visual cortex) also showed an effect of *inter-modal* attention, with lower regional cerebral blood flow (rCBF) when touch was attended rather than vision (see also Laurienti et al., 2002, showing potentially related nonspatial intermodal effects in unimodal areas). This result effectively means that activity in visual occipital cortex was at its maximum when subjects attended to contralateral visual stimuli. This can be seen in Figure 33.2*B*, where maximal activity in the left occipital cortex was found for attention to the right hemifield during visual blocks (second bar in the leftmost panel). In the right occipital cortex, maximal activity was found for attention to the left, again during visual blocks (first bar in the rightmost panel). This overlap between multimodal spatial effects and intermodal attention at the same cortical sites might resolve the ambiguity of whether vision or touch should be selected, resulting in maximal activity for attended contralateral stimuli in the relevant modality. A second finding that might explain correct selection of the currently relevant modality at the attended location was the activation of additional brain regions, specifically for visual or tactile attention. Activity in posterior parietal cortex selectively increased during visual blocks, while the parietal operculum was activated for attention to touch. These regions did not show any effect of attended side, and are located "later" along the sensory pathways with respect to those regions that showed spatially specific attentional effects (i.e., occipital and postcentral areas).

POSSIBLE CONTROL STRUCTURES FOR ENDOGENOUS COVERT SPATIAL ATTENTION The finding of spatially specific multimodal attentional effects in "unimodal" visual cortex raises the important question of how information concerning the tactile modality (i.e., which hand to attend to endogenously for tactile judgments) could reach visual cortex. As already discussed, visual occipital areas are not thought to receive direct projections from the somatosensory system, and apparently do not respond to tactile stimulation (see Fig. 33.1*B*). The two PET experiments discussed in the previous section (Macaluso et al., 2000a, 2002a) indicated that tactile influences on visual areas may be determined by the deployment of spatial attention. Any supramodal control process for directing attention (see, e.g., Mesulam, 1998) might thus in principle explain the cross-modal influences on unimodal cortices.

In imaging research on purely visual attention, a distinction has been drawn between the *site* of observed sensory modulations and the *source* (or control process) that imposes those modulations (e.g., Driver & Frackowiak, 2001; Hopfinger et al., 2000; Kastner et al., 1999; see also Corbetta & Shulman, 2002, for a review). Several different approaches have been taken in an effort to identify the sources of attentional modulation. In one line of research, blocks involving many shifts of spatial visual attention are compared with blocks (ideally with similar stimulation and responses) in which attention is maintained at one location (e.g., Corbetta, Miezin, Shulman, & Petersen, 1993; Gitelman et al., 1999). Such comparisons in purely visual studies have typically implicated an extensive frontoparietal network in the control of visuospatial attention (see also Rosen et al., 1999). In more recent visual research, event-related designs have been used. For example, Hopfinger et al. (2000) cued subjects via a central symbol to attend to one or the other visual hemifield, on a trial-by-trial basis. After a variable delay, bilateral visual stimulation was briefly flashed. The results not only showed the expected attentional modulation of sensory activity induced by the bilateral visual stimulation (with contralateral enhancement) but also identified a network of frontoparietal areas that was activated by the attention-directing cue.

Such visual studies have led to the view that a distributed network of frontoparietal areas (including the TPJ) may be involved in controlling the deployment of visuospatial attention (e.g., Corbetta & Shulman, 2002; Hopfinger et al., 2000; Kastner et al., 1999; Rosen et al., 1999; Shulman et al., 2002). Moreover, as we saw earlier in this chapter, several frontal and parietal regions also show multimodal responses (e.g., Fig. 33.1*A*; see also Bremmer et al., 2001). This observation provides an initial hint that some of the areas involved in controlling endogenous spatial attention for the visual modality might also play a multimodal role (see also Mesulam, 1990, 1998).

We have addressed the hypothesis that similar brain regions might be involved in the control of attention across different sensory modalities (i.e., a shared

A. Attention sustained to peripheral locations

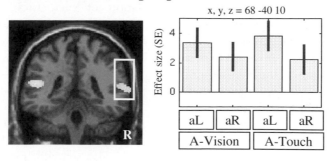

x, y, z = 68 -40 10

B. Low rate of attention shifting

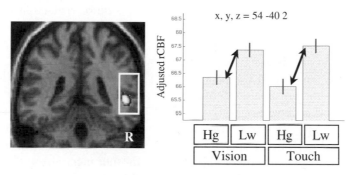

x, y, z = 54 -40 2

FIGURE 33.3   Activation of temporoparietal areas for control of *endogenous* spatial attention. (*A*) Activation of the superior/posterior temporal lobe for sustained attention to peripheral locations during bimodal-bilateral stimulation (Macaluso et al., 2002a). Activation was detected irrespective of attended modality and side (all bars above zero, i.e., greater activity than during central attention with identical bimodal-bilateral stimulation). (*B*) Brain responses depended on the rate of attention shifting (Macaluso et al., 2001). The signal in this area increased when attention to the same peripheral location was sustained for longer periods of time and was then suddenly switched to the opposite hemifield. Critically, this effect was again independent of the sensory modality used. H/L, high rate, low rate. All SPM thresholds were set to *P* = 0.001.

attentional control network), using several types of comparisons. The first comparison was implemented in the second of the two PET experiments already described (i.e., with bimodal stimulation presented bilaterally and attention directed toward one of the four sensory streams; Macaluso et al., 2002a). The design included a control condition consisting of a central detection task. During this control condition, subjects responded to subtle brightening of the central fixation point while ignoring the visual and tactile stimulations that were still presented in both the left and right hemifields. The central task ensured that the number of overt responses during the control condition matched the number of responses during covert attention to peripheral locations, while the stimulation presented was also the same. A comparison of covert attention to any peripheral location with the control central task showed activation of the inferior part of the TPJ (i.e., STS) plus the superior premotor cortex. Critically, both of these areas were activated by all conditions of peripheral attention, irrespective of attended modality and attended

side (although the premotor region was somewhat more active during the visual task than during the tactile task). Figure 33.3*A* shows the anatomical location and the pattern of activity in the STS (with the signal changes expressed in relation to the central-task control condition). Interestingly, both STS (see lateral views plus the section in Fig. 33.1*A*) and also premotor cortex (see lateral view in Fig. 33.1*A*) were also activated multimodally in our passive stimulation fMRI experiment (see also Macaluso & Driver, 2001), so their multimodal involvement during covert peripheral attention may not come as a surprise. Moreover, both areas have previously been associated with spatial covert orienting in vision. For example, Hopfinger et al. (2000) reported activation of TPJ regions and premotor areas on presentation of central visual cues that instructed subjects to direct visual attention endogenously to either the left or right visual hemifield (see also Corbetta et al., 1993; Rosen et al., 1999). Our results extend these findings, indicating that the network that directs endogenous spatial attention might operate multimodally.

A second experiment providing further evidence for multimodal control mechanisms of endogenous spatial attention was another PET study that again used vision and touch (Macaluso, Frith, & Driver, 2001). The aim of this study was to identify brain areas involved in regular shifts of spatial attention between the two hemifields versus areas activated during periods of sustained attention toward one side followed by a sudden shift. During scanning blocks, subjects were presented with unimodal, unilateral tactile or visual stimuli that were switched from one hemifield to the other at different rates. In different blocks, the position of the stimuli either alternated on every trial (regular high rate of attentional shifts) or was maintained for several consecutive trials (low rate of attention shifting, with longer periods of sustained spatial attention followed by a sudden shift). The advantage of this design was that all target discriminations were performed for peripheral locations. This should avoid any possible confounds between covert attention and the detection of targets at peripheral locations that might otherwise arise when conditions of attention to peripheral locations are compared with central tasks (see Corbetta et al., 1993; Gitelman et al., 1999; Rosen et al., 1999; see also Macaluso et al., 2002a). Critically, our study (Macaluso et al., 2001) used either visual or tactile stimuli within the same design, allowing us to test whether any attention-related activity was specific to a single modality or was modality independent. The direct comparison of a low versus a high rate of shifting of attention (i.e., long versus short periods of attention sustained toward one side) showed activation of the posterior part of the STS (i.e., in the inferior part of the TPJ junction). The response pattern of the STS in this experiment is shown in Figure 33.3B. The differential activation depending on the rate of attention shifting was independent of the modality of the stimuli (see arrows in the plots), highlighting again the multimodal role of this region in voluntary covert orienting.

To summarize this section, imaging studies on endogenous spatial attention have revealed three basic findings that might relate to the attention-related integration of spatial representations in different sensory modalities (here, vision and touch). First, a multimodal area in the anterior part of the IPS was modulated according to the region of space that was attended. The signal here increased when attention was directed toward the contralateral side of space, and this modulation was independent of the sensory modality (vision or touch) that was attended (see Fig. 33.2A). This result is consistent with the notion that this area represents spatial locations supramodally (see also Fig. 33.1C). Cross-modal links in attention associated with the selection of specific spatial locations may involve modulation of such multimodal spatial representations. This could accord with the view that cross-modal integration of spatial representations involves feed-forward convergence of signals from different modalities to common—multimodal—representations in higher association areas (e.g., Mesulam, 1998). However, a second important finding was that activity in occipital visual areas can also be affected by the direction of endogenous attention for a tactile task. These effects were also spatially specific: when tactile attention was voluntarily directed toward one side, regions in the contralateral visual cortex that represent the corresponding side of visual space showed increased activity (see Fig. 33.2B). These cross-modal influences of tactile attention on visual cortex effectively mean that somatosensory cortex and occipital areas became "focused" on the same location. That is, the activation pattern in anatomically distant areas reflected the current relevance of one specific location and was independent of the stimulated or attended modality. This coordinated activation pattern might constitute another mechanism by which spatial representations in different sensory modalities could be integrated. According to this view, not only might multisensory integration arise via sensory convergence from fully independent unimodal areas to common multimodal higher-order structures, but spatial information may also be shared between anatomically distant unimodal areas that represent the same portion of space for different senses.

The third type of result concerns the possible existence of supramodal systems for controlling the distribution of endogenous spatial attention. In two different experiments, we showed that the inferior part of the TPJ (and possibly also some premotor regions) may be involved in the control of endogenous spatial attention for both vision and touch (see Fig. 33.3). Previous visual studies have suggested that one possible function of such attentional control centers may be to bias activity in early sensory-specific areas (e.g., Hopfinger et al., 2000; Kastner et al., 1999). Combining this concept of top-down modulatory signals and our own finding of multimodal activations for attentional control may offer an explanation of how the distribution of tactile attention can affect activity in visual areas. One possibility is that voluntary selection of a given location occurs in high-order multimodal control structures. Here anticipatory spatial biases would be generated and then fed back to lower-level unimodal spatial representations, via back-projections (top-down effects). Because the control structures operate multimodally, spatial biases would also be transferred to unimodal areas for other modalities, potentially leading to the observed coherence between activity in anatomically distant spatial representations.

Cross-modal interactions in exogenous spatial attention

The data presented so far have addressed the issue of multimodal spatial representations either in relation to passive stimulation of vision alone or touch alone in one or the other hemifield (Fig. 33.1C), or in relation to the effects of endogenously directing attention toward one or other side for a visual or tactile task (Figs. 33.2 and 33.3). Perhaps the most remarkable result was the finding of spatially specific effects from tactile attention on unimodal visual cortex (see also Eimer & Driver, 2000, for related ERP evidence). We tentatively associated these cross-modal effects on unimodal areas with the existence of possible supramodal systems for the control of spatial attention. However, the experiments we discussed were strictly concerned with endogenous spatial attention. The next question we address is whether cross-modal modulations of visual areas can also be observed in situations of stimulus-driven covert orienting (i.e., *exogenous* attention), and whether the systems engaged in the control of such exogenous spatial attention might also operate supramodally.

STIMULUS-DRIVEN CROSS-MODAL INTERACTIONS: SPATIAL SPECIFICITY Behavioral evidence for cross-modal links in exogenous spatial attention has been found in a variety of paradigms in both normal subjects (e.g., McDonald, Teder-Sälejärvi, & Hillyard, 2000; Spence & Driver, 1997; Spence, Nicholls, Gillespie, & Driver, 1998) and neurologically impaired subjects (e.g., Farah, Wong, Monheit, & Morrow, 1989; Làdavas, de Pellegrino, Farnè, & Zeloni, 1998; Mattingley, Driver, Beschin, & Robertson, 1997). A classic paradigm involves delivering spatially nonpredictive peripheral cues in one modality, followed by target stimuli in a different modality. The general finding is that when cue and target are delivered at the same location, the judgment of the target stimulus can improve (e.g., in perceptual sensitivity; McDonald et al., 2000) compared to when the cue and the target are presented in opposite hemifields.

Interestingly, the manipulation of spatial (and temporal) relationships between stimuli in different modalities for such cuing studies has some analogies with the pioneering electrophysiological paradigms used to study multisensory integration at a single-cell level. For instance, as described by Stein and colleagues (see Chap. 15, this volume), multisensory integration by neurons in the SC not only depends on approximate temporal coincidence for inputs from the different modalities but is also critically affected by the spatial relation of the multimodal stimuli. In particular, stimuli presented in different modalities but at the same external location can lead to increases in firing rate, while stimulation presented at different locations can lead to decreases (see Stein & Meredith, 1993, for a review).

Our findings of cross-modal effects on visual cortex for cases of endogenous (or voluntary) covert orienting (e.g., Macaluso et al., 2001, 2002a), reviewed in the previous section, raise the possibility that stimulus-driven cross-modal interactions might likewise affect activity in unimodal visual cortex. We investigated this possibility with an event-related fMRI study (Macaluso, Frith, & Driver, 2000b). On a trial-by-trial basis, subjects received visual stimulation in either the right or left hemifield. Unpredictably, on half of the trials unseen tactile stimulation was delivered to one hand (the left hand in one group of subjects, the right hand in another group). Subjects responded to all visual stimuli (by pressing a button with the unseen and never stimulated hand) while ignoring any tactile stimulation. The visual stimulus on the same side as the stimulated hand was placed in close spatial proximity to the finger that could be tactually stimulated. Thus, for the right-hand group, when touch was delivered together with right visual targets, the multimodal stimulation was spatially congruent (as opposed to the spatially incongruent situation that occurred when right-hand touch was coupled with a left visual target). For the other group, which received tactile stimulation to the left hand, spatially congruent multimodal stimulation occurred when touch was coupled with left visual targets. The crucial characteristic of this design was that it allowed us to investigate how the spatial relation of stimuli in different modalities can affect brain activity.

The main results of this study are shown in Figure 33.4. Figure 33.4A shows the results for the group receiving tactile stimulation to the right hand, with multimodal spatial correspondence occurring for right visual targets combined with touch. As the signal plot shows, activity in contralateral left visual cortex was modulated by the presence of touch. The left lingual gyrus responded preferentially to visual stimulation of the right hemifield (compare bars 2 and 4 with 1 and 3), indicating spatial specificity for stimulation of the right visual field, as would be expected for this contralateral visual area. Of importance, this spatial specificity was modulated by the presence of task-irrelevant tactile stimulation: responses to visual stimuli increased when vision and touch were combined at the same contralateral

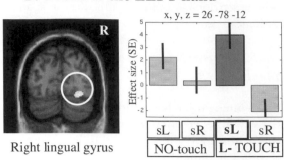

A. Touch to the RIGHT hand

x, y, z = -18 -82 -6

Effect size (SE)

sL	sR	sL	**sR**
NO-touch		**R- TOUCH**	

Left lingual gyrus

B. Touch to the LEFT hand

x, y, z = 26 -78 -12

Effect size (SE)

Right lingual gyrus

sL	sR	**sL**	sR
NO-touch		**L- TOUCH**	

FIGURE 33.4   Stimulus-driven cross-modal spatial interactions in visual cortex (Macaluso et al., 2000b). Brief flashes of light were delivered either to the left (sL) or to the right (sR) visual hemifield. In two different groups, the visual stimuli were sometimes coupled with tactile stimulation to the right hand (A) or the left hand (B). When a visual stimulus in the contralateral hemifield was coupled with tactile stimulation at the same location, visual responses in visual cortex were amplified (darker bar in each plot). SPM thresholds were set to P (uncorrected) = 0.05.

location (i.e., the difference between bar 4 minus bar 3 is larger than the difference between bar 2 minus bar 1, for the left plot in Fig. 33.4A). Figure 33.4B shows cross-modal effects observed for the group that received tactile stimulation to the left hand. Now cross-modal interactions were found in the right occipital visual cortex, again contralateral to the location where multimodal spatial correspondence occurred (i.e., in the left hemifield for this group). Thus, cross-modal spatial interactions between vision and touch can modulate responses in "unimodal" visual areas for the case of stimulus-driven exogenous effects, analogous to what was seen previously for endogenous attention effects. Once again, these cross-modal effects are spatially specific. The increased visual responses did not simply reflect the addition of tactile stimulation but were dependent on vision and touch being presented at the same location. This finding of cross-modal effects in unimodal visual areas for exogenous attention is important because, unlike the endogenous case, it now points to a stimulus-driven system that governs cross-modal spatial interactions in unimodal cortices (see Kennett, Eimer, Spence, & Driver, 2001; see also McDonald & Ward, 2000, for related ERP findings).

Why should cross-modal effects influence unimodal cortex? One speculative explanation may be that unimodal areas possess neural machinery better suited to analyse certain aspects of incoming sensory signals. For example, whereas a tactile signal might provide an early warning that something has approached a part of the body, the visual system might be better suited to recognize and classify the nature of that object. Touch at one location may automatically attract "visual" attention to the same location, to promote analysis of any visual signals (e.g., concerning color or form) that originate from the same position. As argued extensively elsewhere

in this volume (see, e.g., Stein et al., Chap. 15), cross-modal interactions in multimodal regions may be able to render one location particularly salient. This salience may then be fed back to unimodal regions to facilitate further processing of modality-specific properties at that location.

As we suggested earlier for the case of endogenous attention, such an architecture might provide an additional mechanism for the integration of spatial representations across different sensory modalities. Brain areas that represent the same external location but in different modalities could have mutual influences that would allow a coherent but distributed representation of salient (exogenous case) or task-relevant (endogenous case) spatial locations to arise across anatomically distant brain regions. For the case of endogenous spatial attention, we suggested that cross-modal effects in visual areas might be mediated by spatial attention. We showed that the system that controls voluntary deployment of spatial attention may operate supramodally (see Fig. 33.3). On the assumption that attentional control areas generate spatial biases to modulate unimodal brain areas (e.g., Hopfinger et al., 2000; Kastner et al., 1999), we proposed that signals concerning the distribution of tactile attention can influence activity in visual cortex via this shared attentional control system. The finding of cross-modal effects in visual areas during exogenous *stimulus-driven* attention also suggests that such an architecture might generally account for cross-modal links in spatial attention, rather than being specific to the endogenous case.

POSSIBLE MULTIMODAL CONTROL PROCESSES FOR STIMULUS-DRIVEN SHIFTS OF ATTENTION   We have further examined two very different kinds of imaging evidence to address the issue of possible multimodal control processes for stimulus-driven shifts of attention. In the first study (Macaluso et al., 2002b), we used event-related fMRI to examine the situation in which subjects expected a target to appear on one side of space, but on a minority of trials the target actually appeared on the other side (see also Corbetta et al., 2000; Posner, 1980). A symbolic central auditory cue indicated the most likely location for a subsequent target. On a trial-by-trial basis, either the left or the right side was cued. On 80% of the trials the target appeared at the cued location (valid trials), while on the remaining 20% of the trials the target was unpredictably presented in the opposite hemifield (invalid trials). In order to address the multimodal issue, targets were either visual or tactile in our study (with the modality of the target unpredictably randomized). It should be noted that although the initial covert orienting prompted by the symbolic cue was endogenous, invalid trials with targets presented at the unattended location should trigger a stimulus-driven shift of attention from the cued side to the target side, with this shift being triggered only when a target was presented in one particular modality on the uncued side. Thus, brain activations associated with invalid trials (as compared with valid trials) may reveal the neural substrate involved in stimulus-driven spatial reorienting (see also Corbetta et al., 2000, for a purely visual analogue of this study). By presenting targets in either of two different modalities, vision or touch, we could assess whether the activations for invalid trials were unimodal (i.e., associated with attentional reorienting only for targets of one specific modality) or multimodal (i.e., independent of the modality of the target).

The results showed specific activation of the TPJ and inferior premotor cortex for the invalid trials (see also Corbetta et al., 2000, for closely related visual data). Figure 33.5A shows the pattern of activity in the inferior parietal lobule (comprising the dorsal part of the TPJ) for all trial types. The critical result was that differential activation, depending on the validity of the cue (invalid greater than valid), was independent of the modality of the targets. The presentation of a target on the invalid side fully specified the modality of the trial, and so modality-specific effects could in principle be expected. However, none was found, with only multimodal effects being observed. These results indicate that during stimulus-triggered reorienting of spatial attention, a common brain system is engaged, independent of the modality of the stimuli used to trigger the shift of spatial attention (see also Downar, Crawley, Mikulis, & Davis, 2000). Finding such a multimodal or supramodal system supports our hypothesis that, in the case of exogenous attention, just as previously argued for endogenous attention, sensory information about the location of tactile stimuli might be transferred to unimodal visual areas via common higher-order attentional control structures.

A link between spatially specific cross-modal effects on unimodal visual areas and the common activation of multimodal areas by vision and touch receives further support from an analysis of effective connectivity (Friston et al., 1997). Using the data of Macaluso et al. (2000b), with peripheral visual targets and task-irrelevant tactile stimuli presented either at the same or at different locations as the visual target, we examined the coupling of the posterior visual area that was modulated cross-modally (i.e., lingual gyrus) with any other brain areas. Because touch modulated visual responses only when presented at the same location as the visual target, we tested whether any brain region changed its pattern of connectivity with the lingual gyrus in a manner that depended specifically on the spatial congruence of the multimodal stimulation. Our analysis showed that a region of the inferior parietal lobule (the dorsal part of the TPJ) changed its coupling with the lingual gyrus according to the relative positions of the multimodal stimuli, with higher coupling specifically for vision and touch presented at the same location. Curiously, this result was observed only in the hemisphere ipsilateral to the location of the spatially congruent stimulation. That is, the right TPJ was involved in the group that received tactile stimulation on the right hand (Fig. 33.5B, left panel), and the left TPJ was involved in the left-hand group (Fig. 33.5B, right panel). This result does not simply reflect the hand used to respond, because the result was specific to the presentation of stimuli at the same external location.

An interplay between TPJ and the lingual gyrus in producing cross-modal effects of touch on visual cortex makes sense in terms of the other findings we presented earlier in this chapter for a role of the TPJ in multimodal control of spatial attention. However, the exact reason for the unexpected laterality of the connectivity findings remains to be determined. One possibility is that the relevance of one location versus another is determined according to the salience (in our study, simply the presence or absence) of sensory input at both contralateral and ipsilateral locations. Competition between tactile and visual stimuli on opposite sides of space may have been particularly important in changing the effective connectivity observed.

To summarize this section, the two basic phenomena that we observed for endogenous spatial attention were found to apply analogously for stimulus-driven (exogenous) attention also. First, the location of task-irrelevant tactile stimulations was found to affect processing in visual cortex, thus producing cross-modal

A. Shifts of spatial attention

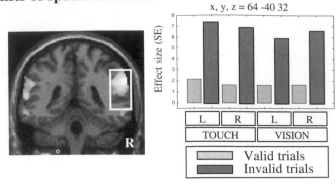

x, y, z = 64 -40 32

B. Changes in effective connectivity

Increased coupling with the left lingual gyrus

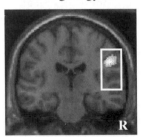

Right IPL

Increased coupling with the right lingual gyrus

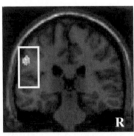

Left IPL

FIGURE 33.5   Activation of temporoparietal areas for control of *exogenous* spatial attention. Plots are shown for the right hemisphere. (*A*) Invalid versus valid trials on a spatial cuing task that used either visual or tactile targets (Macaluso et al., 2002b). This region activated when attention had to be shifted from the cued location to the opposite hemifield (i.e., invalid trials), and activation was independent of modality or side (sL/sR) of the target. (*B*) Increased coupling between parietal and visual areas during spatially congruent visuotactile stimulation versus spatially incongruent stimulation (analysis of the data from Macaluso et al., 2000b). We found increased coupling between the lingual gyrus contralateral to the visual stimulus and the inferior parietal lobule (IPL) in the opposite hemisphere. Thus, for the group of subjects that received spatially congruent bimodal stimulation in the right hemifield (with modulation of the left lingual gurus, see Fig. 33.4A) the increased coupling was detected with the right IPL (left panel in *B*). The group that received spatially congruent bimodal stimulation in the left hemifield (with modulation of the right lingual gurus, see Fig. 33.4B) showed increased coupling in the left IPL (right panel in *B*). All SPM thresholds were set to *P* = 0.001.

effects on apparently unimodal visual regions. Critically, these effects were again spatially specific, with touch boosting visual responses only when presented at the same location as visual targets. Second, higher-order association areas (in particular the TPJ) were found to be involved in the control of stimulus-driven spatial attention, independently of the modality of the stimuli used. This finding may support the notion of a supramodal attentional control system for exogenous attention as well as for endogenous attention. Finally, an analysis of effective connectivity indicated a possible link between these two findings, suggesting that spatially specific tactile effects on visual cortex might involve multimodal attentional structures in the TPJ.

Spatial frames of reference for cross-modal interactions

A final issue that we will briefly address concerns the possible frames of reference that govern cross-modal spatial interactions. All of the "spatially specific" cross-modal effects that we have discussed so far in this chapter (in particular, the influence of tactile manipulations on visual areas for both endogenous and exogenous spatial attention) were identified by comparing attention or stimulation to one or the other hemifield. This design provided a simple method to ensure that cross-modal effects were not simply due, for example, to stimulation of two modalities rather than one, but instead depended on the locations concerned. However, in addressing issues of spatial representations, it is important to consider the frames of reference in which any spatially specific effects may arise. Our findings of tactile influences on apparently unimodal visual areas raises the question of how somatotopic tactile signals could affect responses in visual areas thought to code space retinotopically. In all of the studies presented thus far, the spatial relation of the visual and tactile stimuli was fixed. Stimulation of the right hand always occurred in the right visual field, and stimulation of the left hand always occurred in the left visual field. This fixed relation is somewhat unnatural, given that in daily life, the eyes move around continuously and arm posture is often changed. These posture changes can occur independently, thus continuously altering the spatial alignment of visual and tactile representations.

Problems relating to the realignment of different spatial representations have been extensively studied in the context of visuomotor transformations, in which visual input in retinocentric coordinates must ultimately be transformed into, for instance, hand-centered motor coordinates in the case of reaching (for reviews, see Andersen, Snyder, Bradley, & Xing, 1997; Colby & Goldberg, 1999; Snyder, 2000). Single-unit recordings in awake monkeys have suggested that modulatory influences (gain fields) conveying information about eye or arm posture can influence the neural response to retinocentric visual signals, as stimulus processing proceeds from occipital visual areas to higher-order areas in the parietal lobe (Andersen, Essick, & Siegel, 1985; Snyder, Batista, & Andersen, 2000). With regard to the present issue of multisensory spatial representations and spatial integration between sensory modalities, most existing electrophysiological data concern multimodal neurons in parietal and premotor cortex. For example, in recordings from ventral premotor cortex, Graziano (1999) showed that multimodal neurons responding to both visual and tactile stimuli may code locations with respect to the body part on which the tactile RF lies (e.g., hand-centered frame of reference). Accordingly, the visual RF of these neurons can shift on the retina when the arm of the monkey is moved from one position to another, thus maintaining to some extent the spatial alignment of tactile and visual RFs in relation to external space.

Our findings of spatially specific tactile effects on unimodal visual areas raise related issues. If a multimodal visuotactile event takes place at a fixed location in the external world, the retinal location of that event would shift if the direction of gaze was changed, whereas the somatotopic location would remain unchanged. Given that we find cross-modal influences in visual areas that

are thought to be organized retinotopically, some additional mechanism would have to take into account the realignment of somatotopic and retinocentric representations when the eyes move, if the effects are to be determined by alignment in external space. Alternatively, it might be that the "spatially specific" cross-modal effects that we have observed thus far in visual areas (e.g., Macaluso, Frith, & Driver, 2000b) do not really depend on a common origin for the multimodal signals in external space. For instance, models of spatial attention based on hemispheric competition would suggest that cross-modal amplifications for vision and touch presented in the same hemifield might simply reflect the multiple (bimodal) stimulation of a common hemisphere (see Kinsbourne, 1970).

We recently addressed these issues in an event-related fMRI study (Macaluso, Frith, & Driver, 2002c) that investigated the consequences of changing the retinal location of spatially congruent multimodal events. On a trial-by-trial basis, subjects responded to visual targets presented in either the left or the right visual field. To trigger cross-modal interactions, on half of the trials task-irrelevant tactile stimulation was delivered to the right hand (placed at the subject's body midline; see Fig. 33.6A). We manipulated the spatial alignment between retinal and somatotopic frames of reference by changing just the direction of gaze, while head position was fixed facing directly forward. In different blocks, fixation was maintained either to the left or to the right of the stimulated right hand (Fig. 33.6A). During leftward fixation, multimodal spatial congruence in external space occurred for right-hand touch combined with right visual field targets (i.e., both vision and touch presented in position 2), while during rightward fixation spatial congruence occurred when right-hand touch was coupled with left visual field targets (again with both stimuli at position 2, but now right touch coupled with left visual stimulation). Accordingly, we predicted that the anatomical locus for cross-modal amplification of visual responses by touch at a common (external) location should shift from one hemisphere to the other (i.e., contralateral to the retinal position of the visual stimulation), to account for the change in gaze direction. The change of gaze direction, it should be noted, did not affect the somatotopic location of the tactile stimulation (right-hand touch will always initially project to the left hemisphere). Therefore, a simple model based on hemispheric competition (e.g., Kinsbourne, 1970) would predict that regardless of the direction of gaze, tactile stimulation on the right hand should always boost visual responses in the left hemisphere.

The result of this experiment (Fig. 33.6B) showed that cross-modal influences of touch on unimodal visual

A. EXPERIMENTAL SETUP

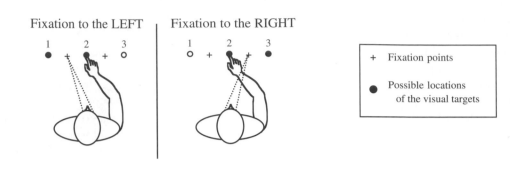

B. IMAGING RESULTS

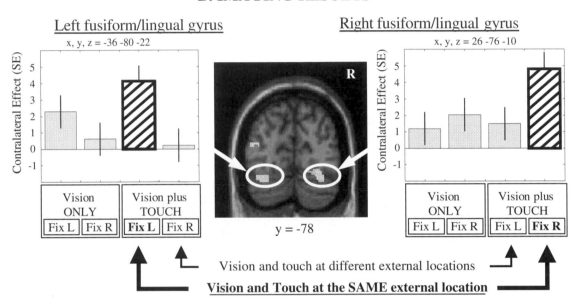

Vision and touch at different external locations

Vision and Touch at the SAME external location

FIGURE 33.6   Remapping of cross-modal interactions in visual cortex (Macaluso et al., 2002c). (*A*) The experimental setup. In different blocks, participants fixated either leftward or rightward of the centrally placed right hand. During leftward fixation, visual stimuli could be delivered in either position 1 or position 2. When a visual stimulus in position 2 was coupled with tactile stimulation of the right hand, the multimodal stimulation was spatially congruent. However, because both stimuli projected to the same (left) hemisphere, any amplification of brain responses for this condition might have been due to intrahemispheric effects rather than to the spatial relation of the stimuli in external space. The inclusion of the conditions of rightward fixation allowed us to disambiguate these two alternatives. During rightward fixation, multimodal spatial congruency occurred for simultaneous stimulation of the *left* visual field plus *right* hand touch (both stimuli in position 2), with the two stimuli now projecting to different hemispheres. If cross-modal effects in visual cortex remap to account for changes in posture (i.e., they are determined by the spatial relation of stimuli in external space), cross-modal amplification of visual responses should now occur in the right hemisphere, contralateral to the visual location of the multimodal stimulation, but ipsilateral to the stimulated right hand. This is exactly what was found (see Fig. 33.4*B*). (*B*) Activity in ventral visual cortex for the different stimulation conditions and directions of gaze. Signal plots show the activity in the two hemispheres expressed as the difference between visual stimulation of the contralateral minus ipsilateral visual hemifield (i.e., contralateral effect, in standard error [SE] units). As predicted, maximal effects were detected when the contralateral visual stimulus was coupled with touch (crosshatched bar) in the hemisphere contralateral to the external location of the multimodal event (i.e., left hemisphere for leftward fixation [left panel] and right hemisphere for rightward fixation [right panel]). SPM thresholds were set to P (uncorrected) = 0.01.

areas depended on the relative position of the stimuli in external space, and were not simply due to initial hemispheric projections. During leftward fixation, maximal activity was found in the left lingual/fusiform gyrus for trials in which visual targets in the right visual field were

coupled with tactile stimulation to the right hand. Critically, when fixation was shifted to the right of the tactually stimulated right hand, the anatomical locus of the cross-modal effect now switched to the right hemisphere. Maximal activity was now observed here when right-hand touch was combined with left visual field targets, at the same external location. This result was found regardless of whether the right hand was visible or occluded. This observation suggests that postural information (here the direction of gaze) is taken into account in order to determine whether multimodal events are congruent in external space, even though such events can exert an influence on areas that represent space in retinocentric coordinates. The implication is again that tactile information exerts an influence on visual responses via areas that form multimodal representations of space (involving eye position signals also, in this particular example).

Summary and conclusions

In this chapter, we have summarized several studies investigating possible neural mechanisms for multisensory spatial integration in the human brain, as measured with functional imaging. We examined the spatial specificity of cross-modal interactions from several perspectives. First, we determined brain areas showing different levels of activation for passive stimulation as a function of stimulus location (left versus right hemispace), testing whether these spatial effects were specific to stimulation of one modality (unimodal spatial effects) or occurred independently of the stimulated modality (multimodal spatial effects). The results showed that spatially specific responses follow the expected hierarchical organization of the sensory systems. Early visual areas in the occipital lobe and somatosensory regions in the postcentral gyrus showed unimodal spatial contralaterality (see Fig. 33.1B), while a region in the anterior part of the intraparietal sulcus showed multimodal spatially specific responses for stimulation on the contralateral side (see Fig. 33.1C). These results appear consistent with multimodal spatial representations being constructed via feed-forward convergence from unimodal areas to common multimodal areas in parietal cortex. Accordingly, multisensory integration may rely in part on the interaction of signals concerning different sensory modalities in such higher-order multimodal convergence zones.

However, experiments that manipulated voluntary (endogenous) spatial attention found cross-modal effects in unimodal areas also. In particular, the direction of tactile attention was found to affect activity not only in somatosensory and intraparietal cortex but also in "unimodal" visual cortex. Visual areas showing such cross-modal effects included both the middle and the superior occipital gyrus, possibly corresponding to areas V5/hMT and V3, respectively (see Fig. 33.2B), as well as ventral occipital regions that might correspond

to area VP or V4v (see Figs. 33.4 and 33.6). Although in each single experiment only one or another portion of occipital cortex reached our conservative criteria for statistically significant cross-modal effects, in fact similar activation trends could often be observed in other occipital regions within the same hemisphere. Critically, all these cross-modal attentional modulations were spatially specific: tactile attention toward one side modulated occipital areas that represent the same side of space but for vision (e.g., Fig. 33.2B). This result indicates that anatomically distant unimodal areas might become "focused" on signals conveyed via different modalities but originating from the same external position. Such a mechanism could provide one way of boosting signals relating to a single multimodal event in the external world and presented at a common location. Moreover, this mechanism could also provide some functional link between anatomically distant unimodal spatial representations and so may constitute another form of multisensory integration, complementary to convergence of unimodal signals to multimodal areas.

It might be argued that tactile effects on visual cortex in the endogenous attention experiments arose only because subjects voluntarily chose to direct visual attention to the same location that was currently relevant for touch (but see Eimer, 1999; Spence, Ranson, et al., 2000). This criticism becomes less plausible in light of the results of further studies that used task-irrelevant tactile stimulations during purely visual tasks to study stimulus-driven (exogenous) cross-modal effects (Macaluso et al., 2000b). In such situations, we also found spatially specific cross-modal interactions in visual cortex. When task-irrelevant tactile stimulation was delivered at the same location as a visual target, responses in visual cortex contralateral to the multimodal event were increased (see Fig. 33.4). This result was not an unspecific effect of merely adding any tactile stimulation, because touch at one location combined with a visual target at a different location did not cause any such amplification of responses in visual cortex. The results of these stimulus-driven experiments indicate that the links between spatial representations in different modalities do not merely depend on some strategic option by the subjects, but rather may reflect a more general mechanism for cross-modal integration.

The finding of spatially specific tactile effects on unimodal visual areas raises two important issues. First, by definition, neurons in unimodal visual cortex should not respond directly to touch, so how can information about the location of tactile stimuli or attention reach visual cortex? Second, in somatosensory cortex locations are represented according to a somatotopic frame of reference that is different from and independent of the retinocentric system found in unimodal visual cortex. If these two systems use incompatible frames of reference, how can touch affect visual responses in a spatially specific manner? One insight into the latter issue was gained from an experiment that independently manipulated the spatial congruence of multimodal stimuli and the retinal location of these multimodal events (by shifting gaze but not the hand). The results showed that despite affecting regions of visual cortex thought to code space retinotopically, the critical factor for cross-modal interaction was the common location of visual and tactile stimuli in external space, with current eye position taken into account (Fig. 33.6). This implies that postural signals concerning the current alignment of somatotopic and retinocentric spatial representations are also integrated, to accommodate the different reference frames used initially by vision and touch.

With regard to possible mechanisms that might allow tactile information to influence unimodal visual cortex, experiments on both endogenous and exogenous attention point to a possible link between the cross-modal effects on visual cortex and the existence of supramodal attentional control systems. We found activation of the posterior STS for sustained periods of voluntary attention to peripheral locations (see Fig. 33.3A) and activation in the inferior parietal lobule when sudden stimulus onsets on an unexpected side automatically triggered shifts of exogenous spatial attention (Fig. 33.5A). The posterior STS is anatomically adjacent to the inferior parietal lobule, so here we have referred to these activations as jointly involving the TPJ. Because our manipulations of endogenous and exogenous attention have to date been conducted in different experiments (using different imaging techniques and different subjects), it would be premature for us to speculate on whether or not exactly the same multimodal regions are involved during both endogenous and exogenous spatial attention for vision and touch. The critical point is that, in both cases, the activation was found to be independent of the modality of the stimuli or task. Moreover, the multimodal engagement of this general temporoparietal region during spatial attention fits with the finding of multimodal responses here when a single modality was stimulated at a time, in either vision or touch (see Fig. 33.1A; see also Bremmer et al., 2001).

We further linked the activation of supramodal systems for the control of spatial attention to our observed tactile effects on visual areas, on the basis of two additional arguments. First, many recent unimodal visual studies have suggested that spatially specific modulations of visual responses during attention to the contralateral visual hemifield are controlled by frontoparietal circuits (involved in top-down control) in structures that appear to be multimodal, as our own data show. Second, our own results show that, even for the case of stimulus-driven attentional orienting, modulatory influences of touch on visual processing may involve higher-order multimodal areas (see Fig. 33.5B). It thus seems physiologically plausible not only that signals are relayed from lower unimodal areas to higher multimodal regions (feed-forward processing), but also that information can be transmitted from multimodal regions to unimodal regions via back-projections.

These considerations lead to the following proposal. Unimodal inputs converge from sensory-specific areas to common multimodal control areas (e.g., the TPJ) by feed-forward connections. Here a first type of cross-modal interaction may occur, resulting in multisensory integration by sensory convergence. At such a level, signals concerning the current alignments between the different coordinate systems for the various modalities might also be involved (e.g., signals regarding gaze direction or arm posture). Voluntary attention may generate anticipatory spatial biases at such a multimodal level of spatial representation. The output from such attentional control areas (sources) would then produce spatially specific modulatory signals, to influence appropriate unimodal spatial representations (sites), via back-projections. Critically, the multimodal nature of the processes occurring at the control level would result in modulatory signals that carry information concerning different sensory modalities. This could lead to the observed cross-modal effects in anatomically distant unimodal areas, providing a distributed—but integrated—system for the representation of space across sensory modalities.

REFERENCES

Andersen, R. A., Essick, G. K., & Siegel, R. M. (1985). Encoding of spatial location by posterior parietal neurons. *Science, 230,* 456–458.

Andersen, R. A., Snyder, L. H., Bradley, D. C., & Xing, J. (1997). Multimodal representation of space in the posterior parietal cortex and its use in planning movements. *Annual Review of Neuroscience, 20,* 303–330.

Bremmer, F., Schlack, A., Shah, N. J., Zafiris, O., Kubischik, M., Hoffmann, K., et al. (2001). Polymodal motion processing in posterior parietal and premotor cortex: A human fMRI study strongly implies equivalencies between humans and monkeys. *Neuron, 29,* 287–296.

Bruce, C., Desimone, R., & Gross, C. G. (1981). Visual properties of neurons in a polysensory area in superior temporal sulcus of the macaque. *Journal of Neurophysiology, 46,* 369–384.

Buchel, C., Price, C., Frackowiak, R. S., & Friston, K. (1998). Different activation patterns in the visual cortex of late and congenitally blind subjects. *Brain, 121,* 409–419.

Burton, H., Snyder, A. Z., Conturo, T. E., Akbudak, E., Ollinger, J. M., & Raichle, M. E. (2002). Adaptive changes in early and late blind: A fMRI study of Braille reading. *Journal of Neurophysiology, 87,* 589–607.

Calvert, G. A. (2001). Crossmodal processing in the human brain: Insights from functional neuroimaging studies. *Cerebral Cortex, 11,* 1110–1123.

Calvert, G. A., Campbell, R., & Brammer, M. J. (2000). Evidence from functional magnetic resonance imaging of crossmodal binding in the human heteromodal cortex. *Current Biology, 10,* 649–657.

Cohen, L. G., Celnik, P., Pascual-Leone, A., Corwell, B., Falz, L., Dambrosia, J., et al. (1997). Functional relevance of cross-modal plasticity in blind humans. *Nature, 389,* 180–183.

Colby, C. L., & Goldberg, M. E. (1999). Space and attention in parietal cortex. *Annual Review of Neuroscience, 22,* 319–349.

Corbetta, M., Kincade, J. M., Ollinger, J. M., McAvoy, M. P., & Shulman, G. L. (2000). Voluntary orienting is dissociated from target detection in human posterior parietal cortex. *Nature Neuroscience, 3,* 292–297.

Corbetta, M., Miezin, F. M., Shulman, G. L., & Petersen, S. E. (1993). A PET study of visuospatial attention. *Journal of Neuroscience, 13,* 1202–1226.

Corbetta, M., & Shulman, G. L. (2002). Control of goal-directed and stimulus-driven attention in the brain. *Nature Reviews: Neuroscience, 3,* 215–229.

DeYoe, E. A., Carman, G. J., Bandettini, P., Glickman, S., Wieser, J., Cox, R., et al. (1996). Mapping striate and extrastriate visual areas in human cerebral cortex. *Proceedings of the National Academy of Sciences, USA, 93,* 2382–2386.

Downar, J., Crawley, A. P., Mikulis, D. J., & Davis, K. D. (2000). A multimodal cortical network for the detection of changes in the sensory environment. *Nature Neuroscience, 3,* 277–283.

Driver, J., & Frackowiak, R. S. (2001). Neurobiological measures of human selective attention. *Neuropsychologia, 39,* 1257–1262.

Duhamel, J. R., Colby, C. L., & Goldberg, M. E. (1998). Ventral intraparietal area of the macaque: Congruent visual and somatic response properties. *Journal of Neurophysiology, 79,* 126–136.

Eimer, M. (1999). Can attention be directed to opposite locations in different modalities? An ERP study. *Clinical Neurophysiology, 110,* 1252–1259.

Eimer, M., & Driver, J. (2000). An event-related brain potential study of cross-modal links in spatial attention between vision and touch. *Psychophysiology, 37,* 697–705.

Falchier, A., Clavagnier, S., P. Barone, P., & Kennedy, H. (2002). Anatomical evidence of multimodal integration in primate striate cortex. *Journal of Neuroscience, 22,* 5749–5759.

Farah, M. J., Wong, A. B., Monheit, M. A., & Morrow, L. A. (1989). Parietal lobe mechanisms of spatial attention: Modality-specific or supramodal? *Neuropsychologia, 27,* 461–470.

Fogassi, L., Gallese, V., Fadiga, L., Luppino, G., Matelli, M., & Rizzolatti, G. (1996). Coding of peripersonal space in inferior premotor cortex (area F4). *Journal of Neurophysiology, 76,* 141–157.

Friston, K. J., Buechel, C., Fink, G. R., Morris, J., Rolls, E., & Dolan, R. J. (1997). Psychophysiological and modulatory interactions in neuroimaging. *NeuroImage, 6,* 218–229.

Gitelman, D. R., Nobre, A. C., Parrish, T. B., LaBar, K. S., Kim, Y. H., Meyer, J. R., et al. (1999). A large-scale distributed network for covert spatial attention: Further anatomical delineation based on stringent behavioural and cognitive controls. *Brain, 122,* 1093–1106.

Graziano, M. S. (1999). Where is my arm? The relative role of vision and proprioception in the neuronal representation of limb position. *Proceedings of the National Academy of Sciences, USA, 96,* 10418–10421.

Graziano, M. S., & Gross, C. G. (1995). The representation of extrapersonal space: A possible role for bimodal, visuotactile neurons. In M. S. Gazzaniga (Ed.), *The cognitive neurosciences* (pp. 1021–1034). Cambridge, MA: MIT Press.

Grefkes, C., Weiss, P. H., Zilles, K., & Fink, G. R. (2002). Crossmodal processing of object features in human anterior intraparietal cortex: An fMRI study implies equivalencies between humans and monkeys. *Neuron, 35,* 173–184.

Heinze, H. J., Mangun, G. R., Burchert, W., Hinrichs, H., Scholz, M., Munte, T. F., et al. (1994). Combined spatial and temporal imaging of brain activity during visual selective attention in humans. *Nature, 372,* 543–546.

Hopfinger, J. B., Buonocore, M. H., & Mangun, G. R. (2000). The neural mechanisms of top-down attentional control. *Nature Neuroscience, 3,* 284–291.

Kanwisher, N., & Wojciulik, E. (2000). Visual attention: Insights from brain imaging. *Nature Reviews: Neuroscience, 1,* 91–100.

Kastner, S., Pinsk, M. A., De Weerd, P., Desimone, R., & Ungerleider, L. G. (1999). Increased activity in human visual cortex during directed attention in the absence of visual stimulation. *Neuron, 22,* 751–761.

Kennett, S., Eimer, M., Spence, C., & Driver, J. (2001). Tactile-visual links in exogenous spatial attention under different postures: Convergent evidence from psychophysics and ERPs. *Journal of Cognitive Neuroscience, 13,* 462–478.

Kinsbourne, M. (1970). A model for the mechanism of unilateral neglect of space. *Transactions of the American Neurological Association, 95,* 143–146.

Làdavas, E., di Pellegrino, G., Farnè, A., & Zeloni, G. (1998). Neuropsychological evidence of an integrated visuotactile representation of peripersonal space in humans. *Journal of Cognitive Neuroscience, 10,* 581–589.

Laurienti, P. J., Burdette, J. H., Wallace, M. T., Yen, Y. F., Field, A. S., & Stein, B. E. (2002). Deactivation of sensory-specific cortex by cross-modal stimuli. *Journal of Cognitive Neuroscience, 14,* 420–429.

Macaluso, E., & Driver, J. (2001). Spatial attention and cross-modal interactions between vision and touch. *Neuropsychologia, 39,* 1304–1316.

Macaluso, E., Frith, C., & Driver, J. (2000a). Selective spatial attention in vision and touch: Unimodal and multimodal mechanisms revealed by PET. *Journal of Neurophysiology, 83,* 3062–3075.

Macaluso, E., Frith, C. D., & Driver, J. (2000b). Modulation of human visual cortex by crossmodal spatial attention. *Science, 289,* 1206–1208.

Macaluso, E., Frith, C. D., & Driver, J. (2001). Multimodal mechanisms of attention related to rates of spatial shifting in vision and touch. *Experimental Brain Research, 137,* 445–454.

Macaluso, E., Frith, C. D., & Driver, J. (2002a). Directing attention to locations and to sensory modalities: Multiple levels of selective processing revealed with PET. *Cerebral Cortex, 12,* 357–368.

Macaluso, E., Frith, C. D., & Driver, J. (2002b). Supramodal effects of covert spatial orienting triggered by visual or tactile events. *Journal of Cognitive Neuroscience, 14,* 389–401.

Macaluso, E., Frith, C. D., & Driver, J. (2002c). Crossmodal spatial influences of touch on extrastriate visual areas take current gaze direction into account. *Neuron, 34,* 647–658.

Mattingley, J. B., Driver, J., Beschin, N., & Robertson, I. H. (1997). Attentional competition between modalities: Extinction between touch and vision after right hemisphere damage. *Neuropsychologia, 35,* 867–880.

McDonald, J. J., Teder-Sälejärvi, W. A., & Hillyard, S. A. (2000). Involuntary orienting to sound improves visual perception. *Nature, 407,* 906–908.

McDonald, J. J., & Ward, L. M. (2000). Involuntary listening aids seeing: Evidence from human electrophysiology. *Psychological Science, 11,* 167–171.

Mesulam, M. M. (1990). Large-scale neurocognitive networks and distributed processing for attention, language, and memory. *Annals of Neurology, 28,* 597–613.

Mesulam, M. M. (1998). From sensation to cognition. *Brain, 121,* 1013–1052.

Posner, M. I. (1980). Orienting of attention. *Quarterly Journal of Experimental Psychology, 32,* 3–25.

Rosen, A. C., Rao, S. M., Caffarra, P., Scaglioni, A., Bobholz, J. A., Woodley, S. J., et al. (1999). Neural basis of endogenous and exogenous spatial orienting: A functional MRI study. *Journal of Cognitive Neuroscience, 11,* 135–152.

Sathian, K., & Zangaladzeb, A. (2002). Feeling with the mind's eye: Contribution of visual cortex to tactile perception. *Behavioural Brain Research, 135,* 127–132.

Shulman, G. L., Tansy, A. P., Kincade, M., Petersen, S. E., McAvoy, M. P., & Corbetta, M. (2002). Reactivation of networks involved in preparatory states. *Cerebral Cortex, 12,* 590–600.

Snyder, L. H. (2000). Coordinate transformations for eye and arm movements in the brain. *Current Opinion in Neurobiology, 10,* 747–754.

Snyder, L. H., Batista, A. P., & Andersen, R. A. (2000). Saccade-related activity in the parietal reach region. *Journal of Neurophysiology, 83,* 1099–1102.

Spence, C., & Driver, J. (1996). Audiovisual links in endogenous covert spatial attention. *Journal of Experimental Psychology: Human Perception and Performance, 22,* 1005–1030.

Spence, C., & Driver, J. (1997). Audiovisual links in exogenous covert spatial orienting. *Perception & Psychophysics, 59,* 1–22.

Spence, C., Nicholls, M. E., Gillespie, N., & Driver, J. (1998). Cross-modal links in exogenous covert spatial orienting between touch, audition, and vision. *Perception & Psychophysics, 60,* 544–557.

Spence, C., Pavani, F., & Driver, J. (2000). Crossmodal links between vision and touch in covert endogenous spatial attention. *Journal of Experimental Psychology: Human Perception and Performance, 26,* 1298–1319.

Spence, C., Ranson, J., & Driver, J. (2000). Cross-modal selective attention: On the difficulty of ignoring sounds at the locus of visual attention. *Perception & Psychophysics, 62,* 410–424.

Stein, B. E., & Meredith, M. A. (1993). *The merging of the senses.* Cambridge, MA: MIT Press.

Tootell, R. B., Mendola, J. D., Hadjikhani, N. K., Ledden, P. J., Liu, A. K., Reppas, J. B., et al. (1997). Functional analysis of V3A and related areas in human visual cortex. *Journal of Neuroscience, 17,* 7060–7078.

Tootell, R. B., Silverman, M. S., Switkes, E., & De Valois, R. L. (1982). Deoxyglucose analysis of retinotopic organization in primate striate cortex. *Science, 218,* 902–904.

34 Electrophysiological Studies of Multisensory Attention

MARTIN EIMER

Introduction

To adaptively control its behavior, an organism requires information about the location of external objects and events. This information is conveyed simultaneously and independently by different sensory systems, which initially represent object properties within modality-specific coordinate systems (retinotopic in vision, somatotopic in touch, tonotopic in audition). In order to localize and identify relevant stimuli or events, spatial information delivered by different input systems needs to be integrated. Although the neural mechanisms underlying intersensory integration have been extensively studied (see Stein & Meredith, 1993), the question of how attention can be directed to objects and events when these are initially represented in different sensory modalities has only recently begun to be addressed (see Driver & Spence, 1998, for an overview). Directing attention to specific locations enhances the processing of sensory information originating from attended locations relative to other locations. To select visual, auditory, and tactile information originating from the same object, spatial attention must be coordinated across different sensory modalities. This cross-sensory coordination may have important implications for mechanisms of selective attention, which could involve spatial synergies (cross-modal links) in the attentional processing of information across sensory modalities.

Until recently, experimental investigations of spatial attention were confined to the study of spatially selective processing within single sensory modalities (see Parasuraman, 1998, for a recent review). Numerous studies have shown that shifts of attention can be triggered both involuntarily (stimulus-driven or exogenous attention) and voluntarily (intentional or endogenous attention). In the former case, attention is attracted to the location of salient but spatially nonpredictive peripheral events. In the latter case, attention is directed to the expected location of relevant stimuli, as when this location is indicated by a spatially predictive symbolic cue. Both exogenous and endogenous attention result in faster and more accurate responses when visual, auditory, or tactile stimuli are presented at attended locations.

Because research on attentional selectivity has traditionally focused almost entirely on unimodal attention, issues related to multisensory spatial attention have not yet been investigated systematically. Very few experiments have studied whether there are any cross-modal links in spatial attention between and among vision, audition, and touch, and which mechanisms are responsible for such links. Does directing attention to the expected location of a visual event affect the processing of auditory or tactile stimuli at visually attended versus unattended locations? Does the automatic capture of attention by an irrelevant peripheral sound or touch have any spatially selective impact on the processing of subsequently presented visual stimuli?

Results from several recent behavioral studies (e.g., Butter, Buchtel, & Santucci, 1989; Spence & Driver, 1996; Spence, Pavani, & Driver, 2000) have suggested that there are cross-modal links in endogenous spatial attention between and among vision, audition, and touch. In these experiments, participants directed attention to the expected location of target stimuli within one primary modality. On a minority of trials, stimuli of a different (secondary) modality were presented, which were equally likely (or even more likely) to appear on the side opposite to the expected location in the primary modality. Performance benefits for stimuli at the location attended in the primary modality were observed not only for that primary modality, but also for secondary modality stimuli, thus demonstrating that the locus of attention within one modality (that is, a spatial expectancy specific to a particular modality) affects the processing of information in other modalities.

Along similar lines, other recent studies have demonstrated that involuntary shifts of spatial attention triggered by stimuli in one modality can affect performance in response to subsequently presented stimuli in a different modality, thereby reflecting cross-modal links in exogenous spatial attention. Responses to visual stimuli are faster or more accurate (or both) when these stimuli are presented on the same side as a previous

549

uninformative auditory event (Spence & Driver, 1997; McDonald & Ward, 2000), and responses to auditory stimuli can be facilitated by previous visual events at the same location (Ward, 1994; Ward, McDonald, & Lin, 2000). Irrelevant auditory events influence not only the speed of responses to subsequent visual targets but also signal detection performance, as masked visual stimuli are detected more accurately when preceded by an auditory event at the same location (McDonald, Teder-Sälejärvi, & Hillyard, 2000).

Although such observations from behavioral studies demonstrate cross-modal links in endogenous and exogenous spatial attention, they do not provide any direct insight into the neural processes underlying such links. For example, performance benefits for secondary modality stimuli at attended locations could result from the effects of cross-modal endogenous attention on perceptual processes or from attentional modulations of postperceptual stages (see Spence & McDonald, Chap. 1, this volume, for further discussion). Do cross-modal links in spatial attention affect modality-specific sensory-perceptual processes, or are the effects of such links restricted to later, postperceptual processing stages? In addition, the existence of cross-modal links in endogenous attention may also have implications for our understanding of covert processes involved in the control of attentional shifts. Such attentional control processes are activated in anticipation of and in preparation for stimuli expected at a specific location. The presence of cross-modal links in spatial attention could indicate that endogenous attentional orienting processes are controlled by a single supramodal system that directs spatial attention to the location of relevant external stimuli, regardless of their modality (Farah, Wong, Monheit, & Morrow, 1989). Alternatively, shifts of spatial attention may primarily be controlled by modality-specific mechanisms, although the effects of such attentional shifts will spread to other sensory modalities (Spence & Driver, 1996).

To obtain further insights into the neural basis of cross-modal attention, measures of behavioral performance need to be combined with different brain imaging methods. This chapter reviews recent electrophysiological studies investigating multisensory spatial attention with event-related brain potential (ERP) measures. ERPs reflect phasic modulations of brain activity that are time-locked to the onset of external or internal events. They can be obtained by averaging the EEG activity measured in response to such events over a number of recording epochs. ERP waveforms consist of positive- and negative-going deflections that are assumed to be generated at least partially by synchronous postsynaptic activities at the apical dendrites of pyramidal cells in cortical layer IV. ERP components are labeled with respect to their polarity (positive or negative) and latency, and are assumed to reflect different stages in the processing of external or internal events. In contrast to other measures of brain activity, such as single-cell recordings, ERPs provide a noninvasive method of monitoring brain events that take place during cognitive processing. ERPs can thus be obtained in normal voluntary subjects under standard experimental conditions. Compared with functional brain imaging measures such as positron emission tomography (PET) and functional magnetic resonance imaging (fMRI), the spatial resolution of ERP recordings is relatively poor, but their temporal resolution is excellent. ERPs provide a continuous on-line measure of cerebral activities, and so are especially useful as markers of the time course of information processing.

This chapter discusses ERP studies investigating a number of questions and issues related to cross-modal links in endogenous and exogenous spatial attention. The next section considers how cross-modal links in endogenous attention affect the processing of visual, auditory, and tactile information. Do such links modulate modality-specific sensory processing stages, or are cross-modal effects primarily located at later postperceptual stages? The third section discusses which spatial coordinates frames are involved in cross-modal links in endogenous spatial attention. In the fourth section, we consider whether cross-modal links in endogenous spatial attention are strategy dependent or reflect genuine constraints on the processing of sensory information within and across modalities. The fifth section reviews ERP studies investigating effects of cross-modal links in exogenous (involuntary) attention. The final section discusses whether covert attentional control processes active during shifts of endogenous spatial attention are supramodal or modality-specific.

Cross-modal links in endogenous spatial attention affect early stages of visual, auditory, and somatosensory processing

Although behavioral studies have already provided evidence of the existence of cross-modal links in endogenous spatial attention between and among vision, audition, and touch, these studies cannot answer the important question of whether such links primarily affect early sensory-perceptual processing or whether their impact is confined to subsequent, postperceptual processing stages. Several recent studies have investigated this question by studying how components of ERP waveforms are modulated by cross-modal attention. Short-latency ERP components are elicited over modality-specific brain regions and are sensitive to variations in basic physical stimulus parameters. Such early components are assumed to reflect modality-specific perceptual processes in the visual, auditory, or somatosensory systems. In contrast, longer-latency ERP components usually have a modality-nonspecific scalp distribution and are not directly affected by variations in physical stimulus attributes. These late components have been linked to postperceptual processing stages such as stimulus identification and categorization, response selection, and activation (Donchin, Ritter, & McCallum, 1978). If early and late ERP components reflect sensory-perceptual processing and postperceptual processing stages, respectively, studying how these components are affected by cross-modal links in spatial attention should help to distinguish perceptual effects from postperceptual effects of cross-modal attention.

In a pioneering ERP study on cross-modal links in spatial attention between vision and audition, Hillyard, Simpson, Woods, Van Voorhis, and Münte (1984) presented a stream of single brief flashes and tone bursts to the left or right of fixation. Participants had to attend either to the tones or to the flashes, and were requested to press a button whenever an infrequent, longer-duration stimulus in the relevant modality (vision or audition) was presented at a relevant location (left or right side). Relevant locations were specified at the beginning of each block, and relevant modalities were varied among groups of participants. For the participant group attending to visual stimuli, visual ERPs elicited by flashes at relevant locations revealed an enhanced negativity starting about 150 ms after stimulus presentation, compared with ERPs elicited by flashes at irrelevant locations. Of note, this spatial attention effect on visual ERPs was also present for the participant group attending to auditory stimuli, although it was considerably smaller than for the visual group. For the group attending to tones, auditory spatial attention resulted in a broad ERP negativity elicited by sounds at attended relative to unattended locations beyond 100 ms. This effect of spatial attention on auditory ERPs was smaller but still reliable for participants who directed attention to relevant locations of visual stimuli. These results provided initial electrophysiological evidence for the existence of cross-modal links in spatial attention between vision and audition. Directing attention to the location of relevant auditory events resulted in a spatially selective modulation of ERPs elicited by irrelevant visual stimuli, and directing attention to the location of relevant visual events similarly affected ERPs in response to sounds at visually attended versus unattended locations. In other words, there were systematic differences between ERPs elicited by stimuli at attended versus unattended locations, even when a given modality could be entirely ignored.

Similar results have been obtained in more recent ERP studies of cross-modal visual/auditory links (Eimer & Schröger, 1998). The design of this experiment was similar to that used by Hillyard et al. (1984) except that the direction of spatial attention was now indicated by arrow cues presented at fixation at the beginning of each trial. In one experimental half (Vision Relevant), participants were instructed to respond to infrequent visual targets on the side specified by the cue, and to ignore all auditory stimuli. In the other half (Audition Relevant), infrequent auditory targets at cued locations had to be detected, and visual stimuli were to be ignored. Visual stimuli were delivered via light-emitting diodes (LEDs), and auditory stimuli were presented via loudspeakers. Visual and auditory targets were slightly longer than nontargets, and all stimuli were presented one at a time on the left or right side at closely aligned locations for the two different modalities. Participants had to maintain central fixation and had to direct their attention covertly to the left or right side within the relevant modality in order to detect and respond to infrequent target stimuli in only the currently relevant modality at the cued location. They were instructed to ignore relevant modality stimuli at unattended locations, as well as all irrelevant modality stimuli regardless of their position.

Figure 34.1 illustrates the effects of cross-modal links in spatial attention between vision and audition obtained in this study. On the left side, visual ERPs obtained at occipital electrodes contralateral to the visual field of stimulus presentation in response to visual nontarget stimuli at attended and unattended locations are shown. ERPs are displayed separately for the Vision Relevant condition (top) and for the Audition Relevant condition, where visual stimuli could be entirely ignored (bottom). When vision was relevant, enhanced visual N1 components were elicited by visual stimuli at attended locations, thus confirming findings from previous unimodal ERP studies on visual-spatial attention (e.g., Eimer, 1994; Mangun & Hillyard, 1991). There was no reliable attentional modulation of the earlier occipital P1. P1 and N1 are modality-specific components thought to be generated in ventrolateral extrastriate occipital cortex (P1) or in lateral occipitotemporal areas (occipitotemporal N1; Mangun, Hillyard, & Luck, 1993). Attentional modulations of these components thus reflect the effects of spatial attention on relatively

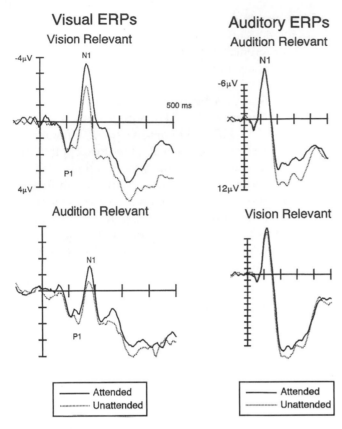

Visual ERPs

Vision Relevant

-4µV

N1

500 ms

P1

4µV

Audition Relevant

N1

P1

Auditory ERPs

Audition Relevant

N1

-6µV

12µV

Vision Relevant

N1

——— Attended
·············· Unattended

——— Attended
·············· Unattended

FIGURE 34.1 *Left:* Grand averaged event-related potentials (ERPs) elicited at occipital electrodes (OL, OR) contralateral to the visual field of stimulus presentation in response to visual nontarget stimuli at attended locations (solid lines) and unattended locations (dashed lines) when attention was directed to one side within vision (Vision Relevant, top), or within audition (Audition Relevant, bottom). *Right:* Grand averaged ERPs elicited at Cz in response to auditory nontarget stimuli at attended locations (solid lines) and unattended locations (dashed lines) when attention was directed to one side within audition (Audition Relevant, top), or within vision (Vision Relevant, bottom). (Data from Eimer & Schröger, 1998.)

early stages of visual-perceptual processing. Most important, attentional modulations of occipital N1 elicited by visual stimuli were also found when audition was task-relevant and all visual stimuli could simply be ignored. N1 was significantly larger in response to visual stimuli at cued locations (Fig. 34.1, bottom left). This finding not only reflects the existence of cross-modal links in spatial attention from audition to vision, but also suggests that such links may affect modality-specific perceptual stages of visual processing.

Figure 34.1 (right) shows ERPs elicited at midline electrode Cz by auditory stimuli at attended and unattended locations, separately for the Audition Relevant and Vision Relevant conditions. Similar to previous unimodal auditory ERP studies (e.g., Alho, 1992),

auditory-spatial attention was reflected in an enhanced negativity for sounds at cued locations that started on the descending flank of the auditory N1 component and remained present for several hundred milliseconds. The early phase of this negative difference ("early Nd") between attended and unattended auditory stimuli is thought to originate from auditory cortex in the superior temporal lobe, whereas later portions of this effect have been linked to subsequent processing stages, such as the maintenance of stimuli in auditory memory (Näätänen, 1982). As can be seen from Figure 34.1 (right), an early Nd effect was present not only when audition was task-relevant but also in the Vision Relevant condition, where auditory stimuli could be completely ignored. This finding suggests cross-modal links in spatial attention from vision to audition, and indicates that the current focus of visual-spatial attention can modulate sensory-specific auditory processing (see also Teder-Sälejärvi, Münte, Sperlich, & Hillyard, 1999, for similar results and for topographical evidence that these effects might be generated in auditory cortex).

The effects obtained by Eimer and Schröger (1998), as well as similar results found in other ERP studies investigating cross-modal links in spatial attention between vision and audition (Hillyard et al., 1984; Teder-Sälejärvi et al., 1999), demonstrate electrophysiological effects of such links, thus supporting and extending behavioral evidence (Spence & Driver, 1996). The fact that cross-modal attention modulates sensory-specific components in the currently irrelevant modality suggests that cross-modal links can affect modality-specific perceptual processing stages. Directing attention within audition modulates the sensory processing of visual stimuli, and directing attention within vision modulates the modality-specific processing of auditory stimuli. However, attentional ERP modulations tended to be larger for the currently relevant modality than for the modality that could be entirely ignored. This result indicates that task relevance does play a role in the spatially selective processing of stimuli within different modalities (this issue is discussed further later in the chapter).

In a recent study (Eimer & Driver, 2000), we used ERPs to investigate the effects of cross-modal links of spatial attention between vision and touch. Experimental procedures were similar to those used in the previous visual/auditory study (Eimer & Schröger, 1998), except that attention now had to be maintained at one specific location for an entire experimental block (as in the visual/auditory experiments by Hillyard et al., 1984, and Teder-Sälejärvi et al., 1999) and auditory stimuli were replaced by tactile stimuli. Participants were instructed at the beginning of each block to direct their attention to the left or right side within the currently relevant modality (vision or touch) in order to detect infrequent targets at the attended location in that modality only. Thus, they had to respond to visual targets at attended locations in the Vision Relevant condition and to tactile targets at attended locations in the Touch Relevant condition while ignoring all irrelevant modality stimuli, regardless of their location. Visual and tactile target stimuli contained a gap, when the continuous stimulation was briefly interrupted by an empty interval. Visual stimuli were again delivered via LEDs, while tactile stimuli were delivered by punctators attached to the left and right index finger, close to the location of the LED on the same side.

Attentional modulations of visual ERPs at occipital electrodes contralateral to the visual field of stimulus presentation that were obtained when attention was directed within touch (Touch Relevant) are shown in Figure 34.2 (top). Visual stimuli at tactually attended locations elicited larger P1 and N1 components than did visual stimuli at unattended locations, even though touch was relevant and visual stimuli could be entirely ignored. The finding that cross-modal attentional effects on visual ERPs in the Touch Relevant condition started about 100 ms after stimulus presentation provides strong evidence that cross-modal links in spatial attention from touch to vision can affect early perceptual stages of visual processing. Figure 34.2 (bottom) shows attentional modulations of somatosensory ERPs at electrodes located over somatosensory areas contralateral to the stimulated hand under conditions in which attention had to be directed to the location of potentially relevant visual stimuli (Vision Relevant). Tactile stimuli at visually attended locations elicited an enhanced negativity that overlapped with the modality-specific somatosensory N140 component. This result is similar to observations from previous unimodal ERP studies on tactile attention (e.g., Michie, Bearpark, Crawford, & Glue, 1987). Because the N140 component is assumed to be generated in secondary somatosensory cortex (SII; Frot, Rambaud, Guénot, & Maugière, 1999), the attentional modulation of this component indicates that visual-spatial attention can modulate sensory-specific stages of somatosensory processing.

It should be noted that the effects of visual-spatial attention on somatosensory ERPs as shown in Figure 34.2 (bottom) were only obtained under conditions in which participants could not completely ignore touch, because they were instructed to respond to rare tactile targets (delivered on only six out of 96 trials per block), regardless of their location. In another task condition in which all tactile stimuli were task-irrelevant, no attentional

Visual ERPs
Touch Relevant

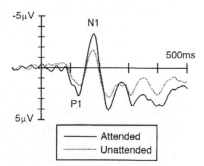

Somatosensory ERPs
Vision Relevant

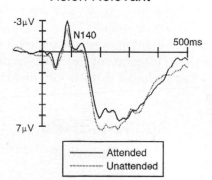

FIGURE 34.2 *Top:* Grand averaged ERPs elicited at occipital electrodes (OL, OR) contralateral to the visual field of stimulus presentation in response to visual nontarget stimuli at attended locations (solid lines) and unattended locations (dashed lines) when attention was directed to one side within touch (Touch Relevant). *Bottom:* Grand averaged ERPs elicited at central electrodes (C3, C4) contralateral to the stimulated hand in response to tactile nontarget stimuli at attended locations (solid lines) and unattended locations (dashed lines) when attention was directed to one side within vision (Vision Relevant). In this condition, rare tactile targets were delivered with equal probability to the left and right hand. (Data from Eimer & Driver, 2000.)

modulations of somatosensory ERPs were elicited (Eimer & Driver, 2000). This result suggests that unlike vision and audition, somatosensory processing can be decoupled from spatial attention within other sensory modalities when tactile stimuli can be completely ignored. Overall, the results obtained by Eimer and Driver (2000) demonstrate cross-modal links in spatial attention between touch and vision, and vice versa, and indicate that these links can affect relatively early perceptual stages of visual and somatosensory processing. However, somatosensory processing may be decoupled from spatially selective processes within vision when tactile stimuli are task-irrelevant throughout and thus can be entirely ignored.

Cross-modal links between audition and touch have not yet been investigated systematically. Initial results from the only behavioral study to date (Lloyd, Spence, Merat, & McGlone, 2003) suggest that attentional spatial synergies between audition and touch may be considerably weaker than cross-modal links between vision and audition and between vision and touch. This question was further studied in a recent ERP experiment investigating cross-modal links in spatial attention between audition and touch (Eimer, Van Velzen, & Driver, 2002). As before, task-relevant versus task-irrelevant modalities (audition or touch) were blocked in successive experimental halves, and irrelevant-modality stimuli could be entirely ignored. Attended locations were cued on a trial-by-trial basis. Figure 34.3 shows ERPs elicited by auditory stimuli at midline electrode Cz under condition in which attention had to be directed to the location of relevant tactile events (Touch Relevant). Similar to the results observed in the

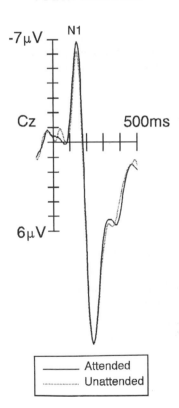

Auditory ERPs
Touch Relevant

FIGURE 34.3 Grand averaged ERPs elicited at Cz in response to auditory stimuli at attended locations (solid lines) and unattended locations (dashed lines) when attention was directed to one side within touch (Touch Relevant). (Data from Eimer, Van Velzen, & Driver, 2003.)

visual/auditory study (Eimer & Schröger, 1998; see Fig. 34.1), an enhanced negativity was elicited for auditory stimuli at tactually attended locations, and this negativity overlapped with the auditory N1 component. This result suggests that there are cross-modal links in spatial attention from touch to audition, and that their effects on auditory processing are very similar to the effects of visual attention on audition (see also Hötting, Röder, & Rösler, 2003, for similar findings). In contrast, no reliable attentional modulations of somatosensory ERP waveforms were found when audition was relevant and tactile stimuli could be completely ignored, suggesting again that touch may be decoupled from attentional orienting within another modality when entirely task-irrelevant.

The ERP experiments discussed in this section provide electrophysiological evidence for the existence of cross-modal links in spatial attention. Effects of spatial attention were found for ERPs elicited by stimuli in a currently irrelevant modality (with the possible exception of touch, which may be decoupled from spatial attention in other modalities when tactile stimuli can be entirely ignored). The latencies and scalp distributions of these ERP effects also provide some evidence as to which processing stages are affected by cross-modal attention. Cross-modal links in spatial attention were reflected by amplitude modulations of early sensory-specific ERP components between 100 and 200 ms after stimulus presentation. In vision, occipital P1 and/or N1 components were modulated when attention was directed within audition or within touch. Likewise, the auditory N1 was affected when attention was directed to the location of relevant visual events, and the somatosensory N140 component was modulated by visual-spatial attention. These amplitude modulations of exogenous ERP components suggest an attentional gating of sensory-specific perceptual processing, indicating that cross-modal links in spatial attention can affect sensory-perceptual processes within modality-specific cortical regions. In contrast, cross-modal ERP effects of spatial attention beyond 200 ms post-stimulus were small or entirely absent, suggesting that these links may have less impact on postperceptual processing stages.

Cross-modal links in endogenous spatial attention are mediated by coordinates of external space

One issue central to understanding cross-modal interactions in spatial attention concerns the spatial coordinate systems involved in cross-modal attention. Integrating spatial information across modalities is a nontrivial problem, not only because spatial representations are initially modality-specific, but also because eyes, head, and body move independently, so that spatial mappings between sensory modalities have to be updated with each posture change. In the experiments discussed in the previous section, head and eyes were fixed straight ahead, and hands rested in their usual position. Under these conditions, visual and tactile stimuli on the same side are initially projected to the same contralateral hemisphere. Cross-modal links in spatial attention between vision and touch could therefore be explained in terms of systematic differences in the activation levels of both hemispheres. According to Kinsbourne (1993), the activation of control structures in the left hemisphere results in a rightward shift of spatial attention, while right hemisphere activation produces an attentional shift to the left side. If attentional shifts were controlled by a differential level of activation between both hemispheres, cross-modal links in spatial attention could result from a spread of this activation to modality-specific areas within the same hemisphere. An alternative to this hemispheric activation account is the hypothesis that cross-modal links in spatial attention are based on representations of common locations in external space across modalities, regardless of initial hemispheric projections.

These two hypotheses can be distinguished by studying cross-modal links in spatial attention when hand posture is varied. With crossed hands, the left hand is located on the right side of external space, but still projects to the anatomically contralateral (right) hemisphere. If directing attention to one hand was achieved by activating control structures in the contralateral hemisphere, attending to the hand located on the left should result in attentional benefits on the left side of visual space with uncrossed hands, but in benefits for the opposite visual field when hands are crossed. However, if cross-modal links depend on common external locations instead of hemispheric projections, the position of an attended hand relative to the body midline should determine cross-modal attentional effects on the processing of visual stimuli. Attending to the hand on the left side should result in processing benefits for the left side of visual space, regardless of hand posture.

We tested whether cross-modal links in spatial attention from touch to vision are determined by external spatial reference frames or by differences in hemispheric activation levels in an ERP study (Eimer, Cockburn, Smedley, & Driver, 2001) in which participants directed tactile attention to the left or right side in order to detect infrequent tactile targets delivered to the hand located on that side. Tactile stimulation of the other hand and visual stimuli on either side were to be

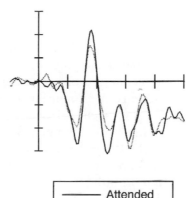

FIGURE 34.4   Grand averaged ERPs elicited at occipital electrodes (OL, OR) contralateral to the visual field of stimulus presentation in response to visual nontarget stimuli at the same external location as attended tactile events (attended; solid lines) or at external locations opposite to the side attended within touch (unattended; dashed lines). Attention was directed to one side within touch (Touch Relevant), and hands were either uncrossed (top panel) or crossed (bottom panel). (Data from Eimer et al., 2001.)

ignored. The crucial additional manipulation concerned hand posture. In separate experimental blocks, hands were either uncrossed or crossed. Figure 34.4 shows ERPs elicited at occipital electrodes contralateral to the side of visual stimulation by visual stimuli presented on the tactually attended or unattended side of external space, separately for blocks where hands were uncrossed (top) and for blocks where hands were crossed (bottom). The effects of spatial attention on ERPs elicited by irrelevant visual stimuli at tactually attended and unattended locations did not differ systematically between the two hand postures, when considered in terms of their external locations. Visual stimuli presented at the same external location as the attended hand elicited enhanced P1, N1, and P2 components, and this effect was present when hands were uncrossed as well as crossed. This finding is inconsistent with the hemispheric activation account. This account clearly predicts a reversal of cross-modal attentional effects on ERPs elicited by visual stimuli at tactually attended and unattended positions to reverse when hands are crossed.

The pattern of results shown in Figure 34.4 indicates that cross-modal links in endogenous spatial attention between touch and vision are mediated by the proximity of visual stimuli to the current location of an attended hand in external space, and not by fixed hemispheric projections. When hand posture changes, the spatial mapping between vision and touch will be updated, and this remapping is based on coordinates of external space (see also Spence et al., 2000, for corresponding findings from behavioral studies). At the single-cell level, such tactile-visual remapping processes could be mediated by multimodal neurons responding to both visual and tactile events. Such neurons have been observed in cortical regions such as parietal and premotor areas (cf. Andersen, Snyder, Bradley, & Xing, 1997; Graziano & Gross, 1998), and many of these neurons show a degree of remapping across changes in posture. For example, a neuron with a tactile receptive field on one hand will typically respond to visual events near that hand in such a manner that its visual field shifts across the retina if the hand posture is changed.

Cross-modal links in endogenous spatial attention do not reflect optional processing strategies

One could argue that the ERP results discussed in the two previous sections do not reflect any hard-wired links between spatial attention across sensory modalities but are the result of a specific processing strategy adopted by the participants in these experiments. In most ERP studies described so far, responses were required only to relevant modality targets at attended locations. Because irrelevant-modality stimuli could be ignored regardless of their location, directing attention to a specific location within the currently irrelevant modality was therefore unlikely to disrupt task performance. Thus, participants might have chosen the default strategy of shifting attention simultaneously to identical locations in currently relevant and irrelevant modalities, because this could be done without behavioral costs. If this was the case, effects of cross-modal attention described in the previous section should be seen as the result of an optional processing strategy, and not as a reflection of fixed, task-independent links between attentional processes across modalities.

One way to investigate this possibility is to study the effects of spatial attention across modalities under conditions that require attention to be simultaneously directed to opposite directions within different modalities. If the effects of cross-modal attention discussed previously were just a reflection of participants' adopting a specific strategy, it should be possible to split spatial selectivity between modalities when this is required by the demands of an experimental task. In contrast, if the cross-modal effects of spatial attention reflected fixed and strategy-independent links, visual, auditory, and tactile attention should shift together regardless of task requirements. In this case, directing attention to opposite locations within different modalities should be difficult if not impossible.

These alternative possibilities were tested in an ERP experiment (Eimer, 1999) in which visual or auditory stimuli were presented on the left or right side in an unpredictable sequence. Participants had to detect infrequent visual as well as auditory target stimuli from among nontargets at one side, which was specified prior to an experimental block. In the Attend Same Side condition, this relevant location (left or right) was identical for both modalities. In the Attend Opposite Sides condition, participants had to detect visual targets on the left side and auditory targets on the right, or vice versa. If spatial synergies in attentional processing across modalities were independent of specific processing strategies, the ERP effects of spatial attention should be largely eliminated under conditions in which attention has to be directed to opposite locations in vision and audition. In contrast, if cross-modal effects in spatial attention primarily result from an optional choice to direct attention to common locations in different modalities, splitting the attentional focus between modalities should be possible. In this case, having to attend to identical or to opposite locations within different modalities should have little or no effect on attentional ERP modulations observed for each modality.

Figure 34.5 (upper panel) shows ERPs elicited at posterior parietal electrodes contralateral to the visual field of stimulus presentation by visual stimuli at visually attended and unattended locations. As expected, spatial attention resulted in a modulation of sensory-specific components in the Attend Same Side condition (left), with enhanced P1 and N1 amplitudes elicited by visual stimuli at attended locations. In contrast, attentional P1 and N1 effects were completely eliminated under Attend Opposite Sides instructions (right). However, an enhanced negativity elicited by visual stimuli at attended locations in the N2 time range (200–300 ms post-stimulus) in the Attend Same Side condition remained present, albeit in an attenuated fashion, in the Attend Opposite Sides condition. A very similar pattern

Visual ERPs

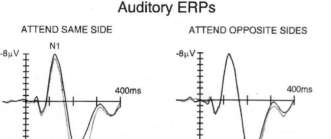

ATTEND SAME SIDE

-5μV
N1
N2
P1
3μV
400ms

ATTEND OPPOSITE SIDES

-5μV
3μV
400ms

— Attended
······ Unattended

Auditory ERPs

ATTEND SAME SIDE

-8μV
N1
8μV
400ms

ATTEND OPPOSITE SIDES

-8μV
8μV
400ms

— Attended
······ Unattended

FIGURE 34.5   *Top:* Grand averaged ERPs elicited at parietal electrodes (PL, PR) contralateral to the visual field of stimulus presentation in response to visual stimuli at attended locations (solid lines) and unattended locations (dashed lines) under conditions in which attention had to be directed to identical locations within vision and audition (Attend Same Side, left), or to opposite sides within vision and audition (Attend Opposite Sides, right). *Bottom:* Grand averaged ERPs elicited at Cz in response to auditory stimuli presented at attended locations (solid lines) and unattended locations (dashed lines) when attention had to be directed to identical locations within vision and audition (Attend Same Side, left) or to opposite sides within vision and audition (Attend Opposite Sides, right). (Data from Eimer, 1999.)

of results was found for auditory stimuli. Figure 34.5 (lower panel) shows auditory ERPs at midline electrode Cz under Attend Same Side (left) and Attend Opposite Sides (right) instructions. Although an early attentional negativity overlapping with the auditory N1 was elicited when attention was directed to identical locations in both modalities during Attend Same Side blocks (left), this effect was completely eliminated in the Attend Opposite Sides condition (right). Here, enhanced negativities for auditory stimuli at attended locations emerged only about 200 ms after stimulus onset, and this effect was considerably smaller than in the Attend Same Side condition.

This pattern of results is inconsistent with the idea that the effects of cross-modal links in spatial attention

merely reflect an optional strategic decision to direct attention to common locations in different modalities. If this was the case, participants should have been able to adopt a different processing strategy when this strategy was required by task demands. The results shown in Figure 34.5 reveal not only that spatially selective modulations of perceptual processes in vision and audition are linked when directing attention to the same location in different modalities is unlikely to interfere with task performance, but also that they remain linked even when experimental instructions require attention to be split between modalities.

Cross-modal links between vision, audition, and touch in exogenous (involuntary) spatial attention

The experiments reviewed in the previous sections investigated the effects of cross-modal links in endogenous (voluntary) spatial attention. However, attention can also be attracted reflexively and involuntarily by salient external objects and events. For example, visual stimuli that appear abruptly in the visual field will automatically summon attention to their location, resulting in superior performance in response to subsequent visual stimuli presented at that location (e.g., Jonides, 1981). If there were cross-modal links in exogenous spatial attention, the processing of visual stimuli should also be affected by reflexive attention shifts elicited by auditory events, and this should be reflected in systematic modulations of visual ERP waveforms. ERP effects of cross-modal links in exogenous spatial attention from audition to vision were found in a recent study (McDonald & Ward, 2000) in which uninformative auditory events on the left or right side were followed after 100 or 300 ms by visual targets at the same or the opposite location. Responses to visual targets were faster when they appeared on the same side as the preceding auditory event, thus reflecting behavioral effects of cross-modal links in exogenous spatial attention. An enhanced negativity was found for visual ERPs at contralateral occipital sites between 200 and 400 ms after stimulus onset in trials in which auditory and visual stimuli appeared at identical locations, relative to trials in which auditory and visual stimuli were presented on opposite sides. This observation provides initial electrophysiological evidence for cross-modal links in exogenous spatial attention. Although no attentional effects on P1 and N1 components were observed in this study, cross-modal attentional negativities were assumed to be generated in lateral occipital areas, thus representing attentional modulations of perceptual processes (see Spence & McDonald, Chap. 1, this volume, for further discussion).

Along similar lines, we have recently investigated ERP correlates of cross-modal links in exogenous spatial attention from touch to vision in a study in which single visual stimuli presented on the left or right side were preceded by spatially nonpredictive tactile events (Kennett, Eimer, Spence, & Driver, 2001). Visual stimuli were presented with equal probability on the same or the opposite side relative to the preceding tactile stimulus. Participants had to ignore all tactile stimuli, and to respond to infrequent visual targets regardless of their location. In separate experimental blocks, the interval between the onset of tactile and visual stimuli was 150 ms or 300 ms. In addition, hand posture was also varied in separate blocks (uncrossed hands versus crossed hands) to investigate spatial coordinate systems underlying cross-modal links in exogenous spatial attention.

Figure 34.6 shows ERPs elicited at lateral occipital electrodes in response to visual nontarget stimuli at tactually cued and uncued locations with short cue-target intervals (150 ms), displayed separately for uncrossed hands (left) and for crossed hands (right). ERP waveforms are time-locked to the onset of the tactile cue stimuli, and the onset of subsequent visual stimuli is indicated by dashed vertical lines. Although no reliable effects of cross-modal attentional cuing were obtained for the P1 component, subsequent visual ERP components were modulated by

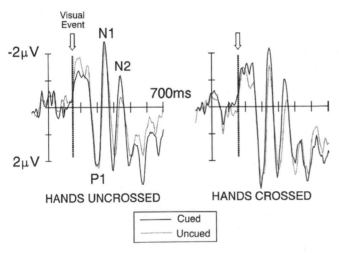

FIGURE 34.6 Grand averaged ERPs elicited in response to visual nontarget stimuli at tactually cued (solid lines) and uncued (dashed lines) locations. Tactile cues were uninformative with respect to the location of subsequent visual events, and the interval separating the onset of tactile and subsequent visual events was 150 ms. ERPs are plotted with the y-axes at the onset of the tactile cue. The onset of the subsequent visual stimulus is indicated by dashed vertical lines. ERP data are collapsed across right and left occipital electrodes (OL, OR) and visual stimulus positions. Waveforms are shown separately for uncrossed hands (left) and crossed hands (right). (Data from Kennett et al., 2001.)

the location of the tactile cue. Most important, the N1 component was reliably enhanced in response to visual stimuli at tactually cued relative to uncued positions (see Fig. 34.6), which suggests effects of cross-modal exogenous attention on the modality-specific processing of visual stimuli. The only exception to this general pattern was the crossed hands/long cue-target interval condition, which failed to produce any significant cross-modal exogenous attention effects (not shown in Fig. 34.6).

These ERP effects of cross-modal exogenous spatial attention were mirrored by the results of a parallel behavioral experiment included in the same study (Kennett et al., 2001). Here, participants made elevation judgments with respect to visual stimuli presented near tactually cued or uncued locations. Judgments were better for visual stimuli on the tactually cued side, and this effect was absent in the crossed hands/long interval condition. The observation that both behavioral and ERP effects of cross-modal attention were observed not only with uncrossed hands but also when hands were crossed indicates that similar to endogenous attention, cross-modal links in exogenous attention operate in a reference frame based on coordinates of external space, in which posture changes are taken into account.

The results of this tactile/visual experiment (Kennett et al., 2001), as well as the findings from the auditory/visual study (McDonald & Ward, 2000), provide electrophysiological evidence of cross-modal links in exogenous spatial attention from touch and audition to vision. The fact that cross-modal links from touch to vision influenced modality-specific brain responses as early as occipital N1 suggests that similar to endogenous spatial attention, exogenous shifts of spatial attention triggered by salient events within one modality can affect sensory-perceptual processing stages within other modalities. At the single-cell level, such effects of cross-modal exogenous attention may be mediated by the activity of multimodal neurons, which were found in several brain regions, including the superior colliculus, parietal lobe, and superior temporal sulcus (see Stein & Meredith, 1993). The receptive fields of these neurons are typically organized in close spatial register across modalities, so that visual, auditory, or tactile stimuli originating from a common region of external space are able to activate the same neurons. Activation of such multimodal neurons by auditory or tactile information may lower their threshold for responding to a subsequent visual event presented at the same location, thus producing behavioral and ERP effects of cross-modal exogenous attention.

Cross-modal links in endogenous spatial attention reflect the activity of supramodal attentional control mechanisms

The ERP studies discussed in the previous sections investigated effects of cross-modal links in spatial attention on the processing of stimulus events at currently attended versus unattended locations within different sensory modalities. In addition to studying such cross-modal effects across modalities, research on cross-modal endogenous attention also needs to investigate covert attentional control processes that are initiated in anticipation of upcoming relevant information at a specific location. Such attentional control processes might be mediated by a unitary supramodal mechanism that controls attentional shifts within different modalities (Farah et al., 1989). Here, cross-modal links in spatial attention are seen as immediate consequences of the supramodal control of attentional orienting. Alternatively, attention shifts in vision, audition, and touch may be controlled by separate modality-specific mechanisms. According to this view, cross-modal attentional effects reflect spatial synergies between separate attentional control processes (Spence & Driver, 1996).

ERP measures can be an important tool to investigate directly whether control processes involved in shifts of spatial attention are supramodal or modality-specific. Not only are ERPs sensitive to the processing of sensory events, they also reflect covert cognitive processes that may occur in the absence of sensory stimulation or behavioral output. Recording ERPs during anticipatory shifts of spatial attention that are elicited in preparation for visual, auditory, or tactile stimuli at specific locations may thus provide important insights into the nature of attentional control processes involved in cross-modal links in spatial attention. Different accounts of the nature of attentional control processes make different predictions for ERP correlates of covert attentional shifts observed while attention is directed to specific locations within different modalities in anticipation of expected target events. If shifts of spatial attention in vision, audition, and touch were controlled by a unitary supramodal system, one should find similar ERP patterns for preparatory attention shifts in all these modalities. In contrast, if separate modality-specific control systems were involved, this should be reflected in systematic differences between ERPs recorded during anticipatory attentional shifts within different modalities.

Although several studies have investigated ERP correlates of attentional control in the interval between a cue stimulus indicating the direction of an attentional shift and a subsequent target stimulus, all these studies have been unimodal, focusing exclusively on visual-spatial orienting. For example, Harter, Miller, Price, LaLonde, and Keyes (1989) measured ERPs during leftward versus rightward shifts of visual attention, triggered by central arrow cues that indicated the side of an upcoming visual event. An early negative deflection at posterior electrodes contralateral to the direction of the induced attentional shift ("early directing attention negativity," or EDAN) was followed by a posterior contralateral positivity ("late directing attention positivity," or LDAP). Other studies (Mangun, 1994; Nobre, Sebestyen, & Miniussi, 2000) have also observed enhanced negativities at frontal electrodes contralateral to the direction of attentional shifts ("anterior directing attention negativity," or ADAN). These effects are thought to reflect successive phases in the control of covert visual-spatial orienting. The EDAN has been linked to the encoding of spatial information provided by the cue and the initiation of an attentional shift (Harter et al., 1989). The ADAN may reflect the activation of frontal structures involved in the control of attentional shifts (Nobre et al., 2000), and the LDAP has been interpreted as indicating preparatory modulations in the excitability of visual sensory areas in anticipation of an expected visual stimulus at a specific location (Harter et al., 1989).

Because these earlier studies of covert spatial orienting focused exclusively on processes underlying the control of visual-spatial attention, they do not provide any information as to whether attentional shifts are controlled by supramodal or modality-specific mechanisms. To investigate whether similar ERP effects can be observed during anticipatory shifts of auditory or tactile attention (as predicted by the view that attentional orienting is controlled supramodally), we recently recorded ERPs in response to attentional cues that directed attention to the location of task-relevant auditory or tactile events (Eimer et al., 2002). Participants had to detect infrequent auditory or tactile target stimuli at a cued location, and responses were required for just one currently relevant modality (either audition or touch in different experimental halves). Cues were visual arrow stimuli presented at the beginning of each trial at fixation, and these cues preceded subsequent peripheral auditory or tactile stimuli by 700 ms.

ERP modulations time-locked to the central cue and sensitive to the direction of a covert attentional shift were strikingly similar when attention was directed within audition or touch, and also closely resembled the effects previously found in unimodal visual studies. Figure 34.7 (top and middle panels) shows ERPs elicited at lateral occipital electrodes OL and OR in the 800 ms interval following the onset of the attentional

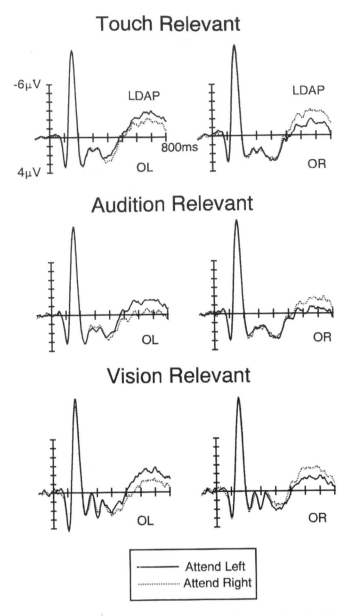

Touch Relevant

LDAP

-6µV

LDAP

800ms

OL

OR

4µV

Audition Relevant

OL

OR

Vision Relevant

OL

OR

——— Attend Left

················· Attend Right

FIGURE 34.7   Grand averaged ERPs elicited at lateral occipital electrodes OL and OR in the 800 ms interval following the onset of a central symbolic cue directing attention to the left side (solid lines) or right side (dashed lines). *Top and middle:* ERPs elicited when the cue indicated the relevant location of tactile events (top) or auditory events (middle). (Data from Eimer, Van Velzen, & Driver, 2002.) *Bottom:* ERPs elicited when the cue indicated the relevant location of visual events (unpublished data). In all three conditions, an enhanced positivity contralateral to the direction of an attentional shift ("late directing attention positivity," or LDAP) was elicited.

cue directing attention either to the left or to the right side. The top panel displays results obtained in the Touch Relevant condition, and the middle panel shows the results from the Audition Relevant condition. An occipital positivity contralateral to the direction of an attentional shift, starting about 500 ms after the onset of

the attentional cue, was elicited during shifts of attention to the location of relevant tactile events as well as during shifts of attention to the side where a relevant auditory event was expected. This LDAP was very similar in terms of latencies and scalp distributions to the LDAP effect observed in previous unimodal studies of visual-spatial orienting (e.g., Harter et al., 1989). To illustrate the similarity of LDAP effects during shifts of tactile, auditory, and visual attention, Figure 34.7 (bottom panel) shows ERPs obtained in an unpublished study in response to central precues specifying the relevant location of upcoming visual events. An LDAP was clearly present during shifts of visual attention, and this effect closely resembled the ERP pattern observed for attention shifts within touch and audition.

In addition to the LDAP, the same study (Eimer et al., 2002) also revealed an earlier frontocentral negativity that was elicited during the cue-target interval contralateral to the direction of an attentional shift. This effect was similar to the ADAN reported in previous unimodal studies of visual-spatial attention (Mangun, 1994; Nobre et al., 2000) and was present regardless of whether attention was directed to the location of relevant tactile or auditory events. This ADAN could reflect supramodal control processes within an anterior attention system, which may determine spatial parameters of attentional shifts regardless of the modality of an expected sensory event. The LDAP may reflect supramodal attentional control processes in posterior parietal areas involved in the control of visual-spatial attention and in the integration of information from different sense modalities. The observation that the frontal ADAN preceded the posterior LDAP is in line with the idea that anterior circuits may control more posterior spatial attention circuits (Posner & Petersen, 1990).

Although these results appear to support the hypothesis that supramodal mechanisms regulate shifts of spatial attention for different stimulus modalities, alternative interpretations are possible. For example, it has previously been suggested that the LDAP is related to the preparatory activation of modality-specific visual areas (Harter et al., 1989). Initially, this hypothesis seems inconsistent with the fact that an LDAP is elicited not only when attention is directed in anticipation of relevant visual events on one side or the other, but also during shifts of tactile or auditory attention (Fig. 34.7). There is no reason to assume that visual areas should be selectively activated in anticipation of auditory or tactile events at specific locations. However, one could argue that multimodal spatial attention will often be dominated by visual representations of space, because vision has better spatial acuity than audition or touch

(Ward, 1994). It is also possible that attentional shifts within visual space are facilitated whenever important visual sources of spatial information (such as visual cues, visual fixation, the visible position of hands and arms, the visible locations of loudspeakers and tactile stimulators) are continuously available. Under these conditions, visual information may be used to guide spatial selection, even when attention is directed to relevant auditory or tactile events.

In a recent experiment (Eimer, Van Velzen, Forster, & Driver, 2003), we tested whether ERP modulations sensitive to the direction of an attentional shift are still elicited under conditions in which these potentially confounding factors are removed. In this study, single visual or tactile stimuli were presented on the left or right side, and attention had to be directed to one side in order to detect infrequent tactile targets at that location. All visual stimuli could be ignored. Relevant locations were indicated by auditory rather than visual cues (to control for potential effects of cue modality), and all stimuli were delivered in complete darkness (to eliminate continuously available visual sources of information about stimulus locations). An LDAP was reliably elicited under these conditions, suggesting that this effect is elicited independently of the modality of an attentional cue and does not require the presence of additional visual sources of spatial information.

The observation that ERP modulations sensitive to the direction of anticipatory attentional shifts elicited in response to cues indicating the side of upcoming task-relevant visual, auditory, or tactile events are highly similar across modalities and are not contingent on the modality of the cue or on the availability of additional visual sources of spatial information supports the hypothesis that shifts of spatial attention are controlled by supramodal processes (Farah et al., 1989). However, the fact that effects of spatial attention tend to be larger within a relevant modality than for a modality that is currently task-irrelevant seems more in line with the idea that attentional control processes within different modalities are at least partially independent than with a fully supramodal account. If attentional shifts were controlled by an entirely supramodal system, one should expect to find equivalent attentional effects within different modalities, regardless of whether a specific modality is currently relevant or irrelevant. The attenuation of attentional effects for currently irrelevant modalities indicates that some aspect of attentional control is affected by the task relevance of one specific sensory modality, even though ERP correlates of anticipatory attentional orienting are virtually indistinguishable when attention is directed to the location of relevant auditory, tactile, or visual events.

These apparently inconsistent findings might be reconciled by assuming that although the selection of relevant locations typically operates in a supramodal manner, effects of spatial selection on stimulus processing within a particular sensory modality also depend on the tonic state of activity within that modality. Instructing participants to attend to one relevant modality and to simultaneously ignore irrelevant modality stimuli may result in systematic tonic differences in the overall activation level of modality-specific visual, auditory, or somatosensory areas. Attentional effects may be attenuated within currently irrelevant modalities as a result of such tonic baseline shifts of modality-specific activation levels, which are determined by the task relevance of a modality.

Overall, the study of ERP modulations sensitive to the direction of anticipatory endogenous attentional shifts elicited by symbolic cues directing attention to the location of relevant visual, auditory, or tactile events has revealed findings that are relevant for our understanding of attentional control processes. The observation that highly similar ERP patterns were elicited during shifts of auditory, tactile, and visual attention is in line with the idea that attentional shifts within different sensory modalities are mediated by a unitary supramodal attentional control system. These results are still preliminary and need to be confirmed by further experiments, including studies using functional imaging measures. If future research were to confirm the conclusions drawn from these initial findings, the existence of cross-modal links in spatial attention between and among vision, audition, and touch and their effects on visual, auditory, and somatosensory processing may come to be seen as a natural and immediate consequence of the fact that shifts of spatial attention are controlled supramodally.

REFERENCES

Alho, K. (1992). Selective attention in auditory processing as revealed by event-related brain potentials. *Psychophysiologia, 29,* 247–263.

Andersen, R. A., Snyder, L. H., Bradley, D. C., & Xing, J. (1997). Multimodal representations of space in the posterior parietal cortex and its use in planning movements. *Annual Review of Neuroscience, 20,* 303–330.

Butter, C. M., Buchtel, H. A., & Santucci, R. (1989). Spatial attentional shifts: Further evidence for the role of polysensory mechanisms using visual and tactile stimuli. *Neuropsychologia, 27,* 1231–1240.

Donchin, E., Ritter, W., & McCallum, C. (1978). Cognitive psychophysiology: The endogenous components of the ERP. In E. Callaway, P. Tueting, & S. H. Koslow (Eds.), *Event-related brain potentials in man* (pp. 349–411). New York: Academic Press.

Driver, J., & Spence, C. (1998). Attention and the crossmodal construction of space. *Trends in Cognitive Sciences, 2,* 254–262.

Eimer, M. (1994). "Sensory gating" as a mechanism for visual-spatial orienting: Electrophysiological evidence from trial-by-trial cueing experiments. *Perception & Psychophysics, 55,* 667–675.

Eimer, M. (1999). Can attention be directed to opposite locations in different modalities? An ERP study. *Clinical Neurophysiology, 110,* 1252–1259.

Eimer, M., Cockburn, D., Smedley, B., & Driver, J. (2001). Cross-modal links in endogenous spatial attention are mediated by common external locations: Evidence from event-related brain potentials. *Experimental Brain Research, 139,* 398–411.

Eimer, M., & Driver, J. (2000). An event-related brain potential study of cross-modal links in spatial attention between vision and touch. *Psychophysiologia, 37,* 697–705.

Eimer, M., & Schröger, E. (1998). ERP effects of intermodal attention and cross-modal links in spatial attention. *Psychophysiologia, 35,* 313–327.

Eimer, M., Van Velzen, J., & Driver, J. (2002). Crossmodal interactions between audition, touch and vision in endogenous spatial attention: ERP evidence on preparatory states and sensory modulations. *Journal of Cognitive Neuroscience, 14,* 254–271.

Eimer, M., Van Velzen, J., Forster, B., & Driver, J. (2003). Shifts of attention in light and in darkness: An ERP study of supramodal attentional control and crossmodal links in spatial attention. *Cognitive Brain Research, 15,* 308–323.

Farah, M. J., Wong, A. B., Monheit, M. A., & Morrow, L. A. (1989). Parietal lobe mechanisms of spatial attention: Modality-specific or supramodal? *Neuropsychologia, 27,* 461–470.

Frot, M., Rambaud, L., Guénot, M., & Maugière, F. (1999). Intracortical recordings of early pain-related CO_2-laser evoked potentials in human second somatosensory (SII) area. *Clinical Neurophysiology, 110,* 133–145.

Graziano, M. S. A., & Gross, C. G. (1998). Spatial maps for the control of movement. *Current Opinion in Neurobiology, 8,* 195–201.

Harter, M. R., Miller, S. L., Price, N. J., LaLonde, M. E., & Keyes, A. L. (1989). Neural processes involved in directing attention. *Journal of Cognitive Neuroscience, 1,* 223–237.

Hillyard, S. A., Simpson, G. V., Woods, D. L., Van Voorhis, S., & Münte, T. F. (1984). Event-related brain potentials and selective attention to different modalities. In F. Reinoso-Suarez & C. Ajmone-Marsan (Eds.), *Cortical integration* (pp. 395–414). New York: Raven Press.

Hötting, K., Röder, B., & Rösler, F. (2003). Crossmodal and intermodal attention modulates event-related brain potentials to tactile and auditory stimuli. *Experimental Brain Research, 148,* 26–37.

Jonides, J. (1981). Voluntary versus automatic control over the mind's eye's movement. In J. B. Long & A. B. Baddeley (Eds.), *Attention and performance IX* (pp. 187–203). Hillsdale, NJ: Erlbaum.

Kennett, S., Eimer, M., Spence, C., & Driver, J. (2001). Tactile-visual links in exogenous spatial attention under different postures: Convergent evidence from psychophysics and ERPs. *Journal of Cognitive Neuroscience, 13,* 462–478.

Kinsbourne, M. (1993). Orientational model of unilateral neglect: Evidence from attentional gradients within hemi-space. In I. H. Robertson & J. C. Marshall (Eds.), *Unilateral neglect: Clinical and experimental studies* (pp. 63–86). Hillsdale, NJ: Erlbaum.

Lloyd, D. M., Merat, N., McGlone, F., & Spence, C. (2003). Crossmodal links between audition and touch in covert endogenous spatial attention. *Perception and Psychophysics, 65,* 901–924.

Mangun, G. R. (1994). Orienting attention in the visual fields: An electrophysiological analysis. In H. J. Heinze, T. F. Münte, & G. R. Mangun (Eds.), *Cognitive electrophysiology* (pp. 81–101). Boston: Birkhäuser.

Mangun, G. R., & Hillyard, S. A. (1991). Modulations of sensory-evoked brain potentials indicate changes in perceptual processing during visual-spatial priming. *Journal of Experimental Psychology: Human Perception and Performance, 17,* 1057–1074.

Mangun, G. R., Hillyard, S. A., & Luck, S. J. (1993). Electrocortical substrates of visual selective attention. In D. E. Meyer & S. Kornblum (Eds.), *Attention and performance XIV* (pp. 219–243). Cambridge, MA: MIT Press.

McDonald, J. J., Teder-Sälejärvi, W. A., & Hillyard, S. A. (2000). Involuntary orienting to sound improves visual perception. *Nature, 407,* 906–908.

McDonald, J. J., & Ward, L. M. (2000). Involuntary listening aids seeing: Evidence from human electrophysiology. *Psychological Science, 11,* 167–171.

Michie, P. T., Bearpark, H. M., Crawford, J. M., & Glue, L. C. T. (1987). The effects of spatial selective attention on the somatosensory event-related potential. *Psychophysiologia, 24,* 449–463.

Näätänen, R. (1982). Processing negativity: An evoked-potential reflection of selective attention. *Psychological Bulletin, 92,* 605–640.

Nobre, A. C., Sebestyen, G. N., & Miniussi, C. (2000). The dynamics of shifting visuospatial attention revealed by event-related brain potentials. *Neuropsychologia, 38,* 964–974.

Parasuraman, R. (Ed.). (1998). *The attentive brain.* Cambridge, MA: MIT Press.

Posner, M. I., & Petersen, S. E. (1990). The attention system of the human brain. *Annual Review of Neuroscience, 13,* 25–42.

Spence, C., & Driver, J. (1996). Audiovisual links in endogenous covert spatial attention. *Journal of Experimental Psychology: Human Perception and Performance, 22,* 1005–1030.

Spence, C., & Driver, J. (1997). Audiovisual links in exogenous covert spatial orienting. *Perception & Psychophysics, 59,* 1–22.

Spence, C., Pavani, F., & Driver, J. (2000). Crossmodal links between vision and touch in covert endogenous spatial attention. *Journal of Experimental Psychology: Human Perception and Performance, 26,* 1298–1319.

Stein, B. E., & Meredith, M. A. (1993). *The merging of the senses.* Cambridge, MA: MIT Press.

Teder-Sälejärvi, W. A., Münte, T. F., Sperlich, F. J., & Hillyard, S. A. (1999). Intra-modal and cross-modal spatial attention to auditory and visual stimuli: An event-related brain potential (ERP) study. *Cognitive Brain Research, 8,* 327–343.

Ward, L. M. (1994). Supramodal and modality-specific mechanisms for stimulus-driven shifts of auditory and visual attention. *Canadian Journal of Experimental Psychology, 48,* 242–259.

Ward, L. M., McDonald, J. J., & Lin, D. (2000). On asymmetries in cross-modal spatial attention orienting. *Perception & Psychophysics, 62,* 1258–1264.

35 Neuroimaging Studies of Cross-Modal Integration for Emotion

JOHN O'DOHERTY, EDMUND T. ROLLS, AND MORTEN KRINGELBACH

Introduction

In this chapter the contributions of two multimodal brain areas, the orbitofrontal cortex and amygdala, to affective processing are evaluated in the light of evidence from human neuroimaging. Neuroimaging studies are reviewed that are consistent with at least two functions for these regions: first, in representing the affective value of stimuli in different modalities, and second, in stimulus-reinforcer learning, where associations are learned between arbitrary neutral stimuli and reinforcing stimuli (with affective value). Although processing in these regions can be confined to a single modality, in many cases the stimulus representations can be considered to be multimodal, and stimulus-reinforcer learning is usually, though not exclusively, concerned with cross-modal associations.

The orbitofrontal cortex is located on the ventral surface of the frontal lobes and may be defined as the area that receives afferent input from the mediodorsal nucleus of the thalamus (Fuster, 1997). The amygdala is a almond-shaped structure in the anterior portion of the medial temporal lobes, adjacent and anterior to the hippocampus. Both of these regions can be considered to be multimodal association areas, as they receive inputs from each sensory modality as well as from polymodal areas in the temporal lobe (Amaral & Price, 1984; Cavada, Company, Tejedor, Cruz Rizzolo, & Reinoso Suarez, 2000). There is considerable evidence from animal studies and human lesion studies to implicate the orbitofrontal cortex and amygdala in several functions. First, these regions appear to be important in representing the affective value of stimuli in many different sensory modalities (Rolls, 1999, 2000). Evidence from single-neuron neurophysiology studies (see Chap. 12) indicates that in nonhuman primates, the reward value of taste, olfactory, and visual stimuli is represented in orbitofrontal cortex, as neurons in this region respond to the taste and/or odor and/or the sight of

food when an animal is hungry but decrease their responses once the animal has eaten that food to satiety (Rolls, Sienkiewicz, & Yaxley, 1989). Neurons in the primate orbitofrontal cortex have been found to code for the relative preference of a reward in that they gradually reduce their responses to a food consumed to satiety as a preference for it relative to other foods, to which the neurons continue to respond, diminishes (Rolls, 2002; Rolls et al., 1989), and respond more to a preferred reinforcer presented in a block of trials with a less preferred reinforcer (Tremblay & Schultz, 1999). Crossed unilateral lesions of the orbitofrontal cortex and amygdala impair the ability of an animal to alter its goal-directed responses toward a reward, once the value of that reward has been altered by feeding the animal to satiety on that reward (Baxter, Parker, Lindner, Izquierdo, & Murray, 2000).

A second function in which the orbitofrontal cortex is involved is that of learning to predict which events or objects in the environment are associated with reinforcement and which are not (Everitt et al., 1999; LeDoux, 1995; Rolls, 1990, 1999, 2000). Evidence for this function comes from single-neuron neurophysiological studies in nonhuman primates in which neurons in orbitofrontal cortex respond to a stimulus that has been associated with a reward or punishment but stop responding to that stimulus following a change in the reinforcement contingencies (Thorpe, Rolls, & Madison, 1983). This is an example of stimulus-reinforcer association learning in which the previously neutral stimulus may be a visual or olfactory stimulus and the primary (unlearned or innate) reinforcer may be a stimulus such as taste or touch. This learning is an example of stimulus-stimulus association learning, and typically the stimuli are in different sensory modalities. The process thus describes one way in which cross-modal neuronal responses are built in the brain. Neurons in the orbitofrontal cortex have been found to respond to cue stimuli that are predictive of subsequent reinforcement,

563

or during a delay period in which a reward is expected (Hikosaka & Watanabe, 2000; Schoenbaum, Chiba, & Gallagher, 1998; Schultz, Tremblay, & Hollerman, 2000). Humans and nonhuman primates with orbitofrontal cortex lesions have difficulty reversing their choice of stimulus when a stimulus that was previously associated with a reward is no longer rewarded (Dias, Robbins, & Roberts, 1996; Iversen & Mishkin, 1970; Rolls, Hornak, Wade, & McGrath, 1994).

The amygdala has also been found to be involved in learning to predict subsequent reinforcement. Lesions of the amygdala abolish fear-conditioned responses to the presentation of a cue that is predictive of a subsequent aversive event (Davis, 2000). Lesions of the amygdala also impair stimulus-reward learning in rats (Everitt et al., 1999; Parkinson, Robbins, & Everitt, 2000). Neurons in the rat amygdala have been found to respond during expectation of rewards and punishments (Schoenbaum, Chiba, & Gallagher, 1999). In relation to multisensory integration, the underlying hypothesis is that the orbitofrontal cortex and amygdala are involved in implementing a particular form of cross-modal association learning in which learned associations are formed between a stimulus in one sensory modality and a primary reinforcer (a stimulus with innate affective value) in another (or the same) sensory modality (Rolls, 1990, 2000).

In this chapter, evidence from human neuroimaging of a role for the orbitofrontal cortex and amygdala in representing the affective value of stimuli in different sensory modalities, as well as in stimulus-reinforcer association learning and reversal, is presented. The first part of the chapter outlines evidence that these regions are involved in unimodal processing for several different sensory modalities, with a representation of affective or reinforcing value in each case. The involvement of these regions in multimodal processing is then discussed. Before considering this evidence, we will first discuss the imaging methods used in these studies.

Imaging methods for the human orbitofrontal cortex and amygdala

Two imaging techniques have been used to detect activation in the human orbitofrontal cortex and amygdala: Positron emission tomography (PET) and functional magnetic resonance imaging (fMRI). PET entails measuring regional cerebral blood flow (rCBF) following injection of a radioactive tracer (such as $H_2^{15}O$). Measurements are typically recorded during a time window of approximately 60–90 s, and brain activity in a given task is summed over that period. The poor temporal resolution of this method has obvious disad-

vantages for the study of cognitive processes (of which affective processing is an example), which are likely to involve transient or time-dependent neuronal activity. However, one relative advantage of PET is that in contrast to fMRI, there is no signal loss in the vicinity of the orbitofrontal cortex or amygdala.

fMRI entails the acquisition of brain images using a rapid MRI protocol (echoplanar imaging is typically used). The images are optimized to detect transient local changes in magnetic susceptibility induced by alterations in blood oxygenation caused by neuronal activity. The rapid acquisition of these images (leading to whole-brain coverage, typically in less than 3 s) allows a much greater temporal resolution than that afforded by PET, although it is somewhat limited by the slow time course of the hemodynamic response. Nevertheless, fMRI provides sufficient temporal resolution to detect evoked responses corresponding to a single stimulus event (e.g., the receipt of a rewarding stimulus). Unfortunately, there is one major disadvantage to fMRI for regions of interest encompassing the orbitofrontal cortex and medial temporal lobes, including the amygdala. In these areas, prominent differences in intrinsic magnetic susceptibility between the brain and adjoining tissue (such as the air-filled sinuses in the frontal bone) may result in substantial magnetic field inhomogeneities over these areas. The result is twofold. First, signal loss occurs that can result in signal dropout in the image in the orbitofrontal cortex and/or medial temporal lobe regions, and second, geometric distortion may be produced. These problems increase with magnetic field strength, being considerably worse at 3 Tesla than at 1.5 Tesla, for example. Despite these difficulties, a number of strategies and imaging protocols have been developed that enable signal recovery in those regions, and methods also exist to correct geometric distortions (Deichmann, Josephs, Hutton, Corfield, & Turner, 2002; Ojemann et al., 1997; Wilson et al., 2002). Consequently, although it is challenging to correct for signal loss and distortion in those regions with fMRI, it is worthwhile doing so in order to take advantage of the increased spatial and temporal resolution that this technique affords.

Role of the orbitofrontal cortex and amygdala in representing the affective value of stimuli in different sensory modalities

GUSTATORY STIMULI The cortical taste system in nonhuman primates has been localized to two main brain regions: the primary taste cortex, located in the rostral insula and the adjoining frontal operculum, which receives afferents directly from the taste thalamus (parvocellular component of the ventral posteromedial thalamic nucleus), and the secondary taste cortex, which is found rostral to the insula in the caudolateral orbitofrontal cortex (Baylis, Rolls, & Baylis, 1994; Rolls, Yaxley, & Sienkiewicz, 1990).

The emergence of human neuroimaging techniques has enabled the localization of gustatory areas in the human brain. Initial PET studies using simple gustatory stimulation methods (such as applying taste stimuli to the tongue using filter paper) revealed variable activation in both the frontal operculum/insula and the orbitofrontal cortex (Kinomura et al., 1994; Small et al., 1997a, 1997b; see also review by Small et al., 1999). The location of the activations within these regions was found to be quite variable, but the finding that these regions were activated by gustatory stimuli was broadly consistent with the hypothesis that the frontal operculum/insula and orbitofrontal cortex have roughly homologous gustatory functions in the human brain to those analyzed in the macaque.

Neuroimaging studies of gustation present unique methodological challenges arising from the fact that in addition to chemosensory stimulation, delivery of a gustatory stimulus is also associated with orofacial somatomotor effects, such as somatosensory stimulation of the tongue, tongue and mouth movements, and swallowing. In order to control for these additional effects it is important to employ an adequate baseline comparison condition that incorporates the somatomotor components without producing chemosensory stimulation. The approach used in many of the early PET studies to control for these non-taste-related effects was to use water as a control stimulus. In such studies, areas involved in gustatory responses were sought by subtracting the scans obtained during stimulation with water from the scans obtained during stimulation with one or a combination of taste stimuli. However, the use of water as a control stimulus turned out to be problematic, for at least two reasons. First, water can produce neuronal responses in the primary and secondary cortical gustatory areas in nonhuman primates (Rolls et al., 1989). This may arise partly from somatosensory effects, but it may also be due to a change in the ionic concentration of saliva in the mouth. Second, water can be considered to be an appetitive stimulus, so that, depending on a subject's motivational state (degree of thirst), water may be perceived as pleasant. Indeed, in the nonhuman primate orbitofrontal cortex, neurons that respond to water when an animal is thirsty have been found to decrease their responses if the animal drinks water to satiety (Rolls et al., 1989). A subtraction between another taste stimulus and water could therefore result in the sensory or affective responses to the taste stimulus being masked by the effects of the water or misidentified. Indeed, in some experiments reported by Small et al. (1999) and in a study by Frey and Petrides (1999), the effects of water as a taste stimulus in its own right were assessed using a variety of comparison conditions. In one study reported by Small et al. (1999), Zald and colleagues showed that a variety of areas in the insular cortex could be activated by water when compared with a passive rest condition (a design that clearly provides no control for nonspecific somatomotor effects). Frey and Petrides (1999) asked subjects to actively move their tongues and in another condition to move their mouths without receiving any tastes, as a means of producing a set of control conditions for tongue and mouth movement, respectively. When water was used as a taste stimulus, the primary taste cortex was found to be activated. Zald and Pardo (2000) have also reported responses in primary taste cortex to stimulation with water when compared with a baseline resting state or with a voluntary swallowing condition. As a consequence, water may not be an appropriate control stimulus for neuroimaging studies of gustation, particularly where the affective aspects of taste are being investigated.

Another approach to controlling for non-taste-related activation was developed by Francis et al. (1999). This study used a tasteless control solution that was composed of the main ionic components of saliva (consisting of 25mM KCl and 2.5mM NaHCO$_3$). The rationale for using this stimulus was that it was designed to be equivalent in its ionic constituents to natural saliva, and thus was expected to induce much less of a change in ionic concentrations in the mouth than water. Employing an ON/OFF block design, and in this case with fMRI rather than PET as the imaging modality, 0.5 mL of 1M glucose was delivered to each subject's mouth at the start of an 8 s ON period. This was followed by delivery of 0.5 mL of the tasteless control solution. In both the ON and OFF conditions, the subjects were instructed to move their mouths and to swallow once. This design thus enabled all of the somatosensory, swallowing, and movement effects to be subtracted out. Activation was consistently produced in the insula/operculum and orbitofrontal cortex across subjects, adding further support to the idea that these areas in humans are homologous of the macaque primary and secondary taste cortices, respectively.

Evidence that aversive taste is represented in the human orbitofrontal cortex was found by Zald, Lee, Fluegel, and Pardo (1998). In a PET study, subjects were scanned while participating in three taste-stimulation conditions: aversive taste (using 5% saline solution), pleasant flavor (using chocolate dissolved on the tongue) and neutral taste (using water, which can be regarded as an appetitive stimulus). A region of left orbitofrontal cortex was found to respond to the aversive gustatory stimulation when compared with both the neutral or pleasant taste conditions. No responses were reported in either of these regions in the pleasant flavor condition, which may relate to the fact that water was used as a control stimulus.

Further evidence that pleasant as well as unpleasant taste can activate the human orbitofrontal cortex was obtained by O'Doherty, Rolls, Francis, Bowtell, and McGlone (2001). In this fMRI study, saline was used as the aversive stimulus. Responses to the aversive stimulus were compared with the responses produced by a tasteless control solution identical to that used by Francis et al. (1999) and described earlier. In addition to the aversive and neutral stimuli, a pleasant taste stimulus was also used (1M glucose). Activation of the orbitofrontal cortex was produced by the pleasant and the unpleasant stimulus, indicating that this region of the human brain is involved in processing both pleasant and aversive tastes. Notably, when compared with the neutral baseline condition, the pleasant and aversive tastes produced activation in adjacent but separate regions of the orbitofrontal

cortex (Fig. 35.1; Color Plate 12.). This observation is compatible with the possibility that the regions of the orbitofrontal cortex that respond to pleasant and aversive tastes are at least partly separable. This possibility was explored in a further study of the representation of pleasant and aversive tastes by O'Doherty, Deichmann, Critchley, & Dolan (2002). In this study, activation of the orbitofrontal cortex in response to both pleasant and aversive taste was again observed. As in the previous study by O'Doherty, Rolls, et al. (2001), in separate contrasts between the pleasant and aversive taste conditions and the neutral taste, activation was found in nearby but separate regions of orbitofrontal cortex at the statistical threshold used. However, direct comparisons between the salt and glucose conditions revealed no significant differences, indicating that although the activation peaks were in slightly different locations when contrasted with the neutral baseline, the areas activated by the pleasant and aversive tastes did not differ significantly from each other. However, the difference in findings between the two studies may be due to the fact that O'Doherty, Deichman, et al. (2002) based their analysis on group average statistics, whereas in the study by

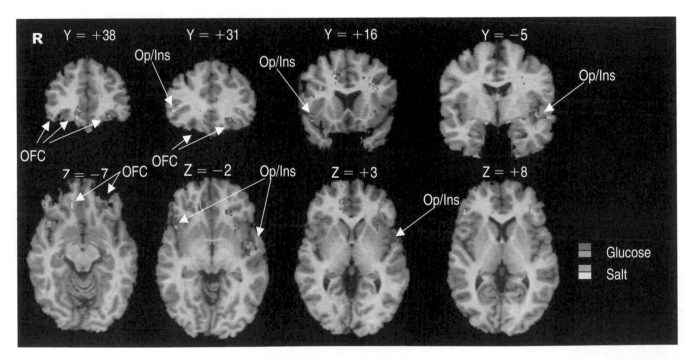

FIGURE 35.1 Group map showing regions of the human brain activated by a pleasant taste (glucose) and an aversive taste (salt). The z-maps from individual subjects were thresholded at $P < 0.01$ (uncorrected) and transformed into Talairach space. Voxels that were commonly activated in a minimum of six out of seven subjects were included in the group combination image (although clusters of less than three contiguous voxels were excluded). Glucose activations are depicted in blue (voxels common to six subjects) and light blue (voxels common to seven subjects). Salt activations are depicted in orange (voxels common to six subjects) and yellow (voxels common to seven subjects). Areas of overlap between the two tastes are shown in green. Coronal sections through regions of interest such as the orbitofrontal cortex and operculum/insula are shown in the top row, and transverse sections are shown in the bottom row, at the Talairach levels indicated. Arrows with labels point to some of the activated regions. OFC, orbitofrontal cortex; Op/Ins, frontal operculum/insula. (From O'Doherty, Rolls, et al., 2001.) (See Color Plate 12.)

O'Doherty, Rolls, et al. (2001), the analysis showed that there was often more marked separation between the regions involved in responding to pleasant and aversive tastes within individual subjects, which tended to be less clear when a group average was used because the exact region that represents tastes may not correspond precisely across subjects. Of course, the difference between different tastes is exquisitely represented at the level of single neurons in the orbitofrontal cortex (Rolls et al., 1990), and it is convenient for functional neuroimaging studies, which necessarily have rather low spatial resolution, if some self-organizing map-forming process has placed neurons with similar responses close together topologically (Rolls & Deco, 2002; Rolls & Treves, 1998).

Taken together, these findings indicate that the human orbitofrontal cortex is involved in representing both pleasant and aversive taste, and they are consistent with the idea that the secondary human gustatory cortex is located in this region. (See further De Araujo, Kringelbach, Rolls, & McGlone, 2003, and De Araujo, Kringelbach, Rolls, & Hobden, 2003.)

Activation of the Human Amygdala by Aversive and Pleasant Tastes   In the PET study by Zald, Lee, et al. (1998) described earlier, activation was also reported in the right amygdala in response to aversive taste, and the activation was reported as being greater in the subset of subjects who found the taste to be highly aversive than in those who reported the stimulus to be moderately aversive. As we will see later in this chapter, evidence from both animal studies and human neuroimaging and lesion studies implicates the amygdala in processing aversive and in particular fear-related stimuli (Adolphs, Tranel, Damasio, & Damasio, 1994; LeDoux, 1995; Morris et al., 1996). In neuroimaging studies of facial expression processing, the amygdala has been found to be consistently activated by facial expressions of fear, but not by other expressions such as happy faces (Morris et al., 1996; Phillips et al., 1997). In humans lesions of the amygdala can produce relatively selective impairment in identifying facial expressions of fear (Adolphs, Damasio, Tranel, & Damasio, 1996; Adolphs et al., 1999). This finding has led to the tacit assumption that the human amygdala is exclusively involved in processing aversive stimuli. However, in the animal literature, the amygdala has been shown to be involved in appetitive as well as aversive processing. For instance, there is evidence from single-cell recordings in nonhuman primates that some amygdala neurons are responsive to the taste or sight of food (Ono & Nishijo, 2000; Sanghera, Rolls, & Roper-Hall, 1979; Scott et al., 1993). Further, lesions of the amygdala cause impairment in reinforcer devaluation (Malkova, Gaffan,

& Murray, 1997), as well as disrupting Pavlovian and instrumental appetitive conditioning (Everitt et al., 1999; Parkinson et al., 2000). Evidence that the human amygdala is involved in responding to pleasant as well as aversive stimuli was provided by O'Doherty, Rolls, et al. (2001) in a study in which amygdala activation occurred in response to stimulation with a pleasant taste (1M glucose) and in response to an aversive taste, relative to an affectively neutral baseline taste. These findings provide clear evidence that the human amygdala is sensitive to stimuli of both positive and negative valence. Consistent with this finding, Zald et al. (2002) in a PET study reported activation of the amygdala in response to an aversive quinine solution when compared with response to water, and also observed amygdala activation relative to a resting baseline (which did not control for non-taste-related oral inputs) to sucrose and to water, both of which are appetitive stimuli. Further evidence for this function of the amygdala is discussed subsequently in the context of its function in stimulus-reinforcer learning.

Olfactory Stimuli   In nonhuman primates, the primary olfactory cortex is located at the border of the anterior temporal lobes and the ventral frontal lobes. The primary olfactory cortex consists of the piriform cortex, the anterior olfactory nucleus, the periamygdaloid cortex, and the lateral entorhinal area. The primary olfactory cortex receives connections directly from the olfactory bulb, and thus olfaction is the only sensory modality whose primary cortical representation is not relayed via the thalamus (Carmichael, Clugnet, & Price, 1994). Neurons with olfactory responses in the macaque posterior orbitofrontal cortex were reported by Tanabe, Yarita, Iino, Ooshima, and Takagi (1975). Direct connections have been reported from the primary olfactory area to the orbitofrontal cortex, terminating in agranular insular transition cortex and a caudomedial part of area 13 (13a) (Carmichael et al., 1994). It has been suggested that this region constitutes the secondary olfactory cortex (Rolls, 1997). Olfactory connections have also been reported to areas 14 and 25 (Carmichael et al., 1994).

Zatorre, Jones-Gotman, Evans, and Meyer (1992) investigated human olfaction with functional neuroimaging (PET). Eight different odors were presented to subjects during a 60 s scanning period. The odors were presented on a cotton wand birhinally. Subjects inhaled during each presentation. The PET scans obtained during this period were compared with scans obtained when subjects were presented with an odorless cotton wand. Activation of the piriform cortex at the junction of the frontal and temporal lobes was found bilaterally, as well as activation of a region of the right mediolateral orbitofrontal cortex. The authors suggested that these regions correspond to the human primary and secondary olfactory cortices, respectively. A number of other PET studies have confirmed activation of the piriform area in response to olfactory stimulation (Dade, Jones-Gotman, Zatorre, & Evans, 1998; Small et al., 1997b). Francis et al. (1999) also found piriform activation in response to the odor of vanillin in an fMRI study. However, activation in the piriform area in response to odors has proved elusive to demonstrate in a number of other studies (O'Doherty et al., 2000; Sobel et al., 1997; Yousem et al., 1997; Zald & Pardo, 1997). This difficulty has provoked interest into the reasons for the inconsistency in piriform activity across studies. A plausible characterization of olfactory responses in piriform cortex was proposed by Sobel et al. (2000). In this study, which used a block fMRI design, the profile of the blood-oxygen-level-dependent (BOLD) response in the piriform cortex was examined for time-dependent responses. It was found that activity was produced in the piriform cortex to odor, but that this occurred within the first 30–40 s of olfactory stimulation and then showed rapid habituation. When time-dependent responses in the piriform cortex were modeled, activation was found consistently across subjects. This finding provides a reasonable explanation for the failure to obtain activation in some previous fMRI and PET studies. It suggests that in order to observe piriform cortex activation, the temporal dynamics of the response must be taken into account.

Activity in the orbitofrontal cortex in response to odor, by contrast, appears to be much less susceptible to habituation effects (Zald & Pardo, 2000). Consequently, activity in this region has been much more commonly reported (Francis et al., 1999; O'Doherty et al., 2000; Small et al., 1997b; Sobel et al., 1998, 2000; Yousem et al., 1997; Zald & Pardo, 1997). The original finding of Zatorre et al. (1992) of a right laterality effect in the orbitofrontal cortex has been borne out in subsequent studies, with activation being reported most consistently on the right. However, some studies have also reported activity in response to olfactory stimuli in the left orbitofrontal cortex (Francis et al., 1999; Yousem et al., 1997; Zald & Pardo, 1997).

A small number of studies to date have explicitly investigated the representation of the affective aspects of odor in the human brain. Zald and Pardo (1997) used PET to investigate the representation of aversive odor. The odor used in the study consisted of a mix of sulfide compounds. Signal changes were observed in the left orbitofrontal cortex and left amygdala in response to the aversive odor. Correlations were observed between the mean aversiveness ratings and the magnitude of the rCBF changes in both the left orbitofrontal cortex and the left amygdala across subjects. In a subsequent publication, Zald, Donndelinger, and Pardo (1998) presented the results of a functional connectivity analysis that investigated the covariance in activation between the orbitofrontal cortex and amygdala during a number of conditions, including aversive odor stimulation (the imaging data used were the same as those reported in the previous study). A significant correlation was found between activity in the left orbitofrontal cortex and amygdala during aversive odor stimulation, indicating that these areas may be coupled in their neural activity during the processing of aversive odors. Rolls, Kringelbach and De Araujo (2003) found that pleasant odors activate the medial orbitofrontal cortex.

In a study by O'Doherty et al. (2000), the phenomenon of sensory-specific satiety was used to investigate whether orbitofrontal cortex and other regions are involved in representing the reward value of an olfactory stimulus. Sensory-specific satiety refers to the effect whereby the pleasantness of the taste or odor of a food can decrease markedly after that food is eaten to satiety in a meal, whereas the pleasantness of other foods not eaten in the meal shows much less of a decrease (Rolls, 1999). The elegance of the use of sensory-specific satiety to study the affective representation of odors is that the design is very well controlled because the same stimulus is used in the comparison between the two affective states. If a different odor were used as the affectively neutral or aversive stimulus, the study design would not have controlled completely for the possibility that the results obtained pertained to differences between stimulus attributes other than the hedonic value. The presence of another stimulus that does not undergo the same hedonic modulation yet is presented in both pre- and postsatiety conditions also acts as a control for a number of other potential confounds, such as order effects and fMRI session effects. Hungry subjects were scanned while being presented with two different food-related odors, vanilla and banana essence. Subjects were then fed to satiety with bananas for lunch, and then scanned again with the two different odor conditions, enabling the areas modulated by sensory-specific satiety to the banana odor to be identified. A region of the caudal orbitofrontal cortex (predominantly on the right), most probably corresponding to the location of the human secondary olfactory cortex, showed a profile of activation consistent with the behavioral effect of sensory-specific satiety. Activation was produced in the region in response to both odors before satiety, but activation in response to the odor of the food that had been eaten to satiety showed a selective decrease relative to the odor of the food that had not been eaten to satiety (Fig. 35.2; Color Plate 13.). This investigation

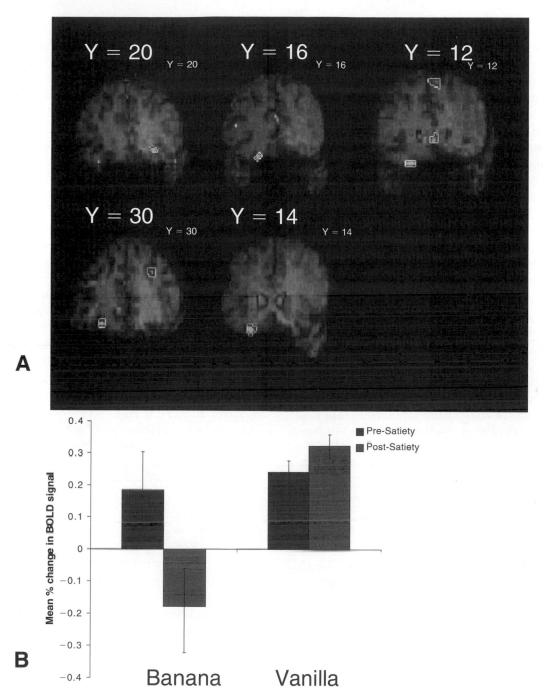

FIGURE 35.2   Olfactory sensory-specific satiety. The figure shows regions of orbitofrontal cortex in which the BOLD signal produced by the presentation of banana and vanilla odor was modulated by sensory-specific satiety by feeding to satiety with one of the two foods (banana). Coronal sections at the anterior (*y*) levels shown through the orbitofrontal cortex are shown for five separate subjects. The threshold is set at *P* < 0.05 corrected for multiple comparisons. (From O'Doherty et al., 2000.) (See Color Plate 13.)

provides evidence that the pleasantness or reward value of an olfactory stimulus is represented in the human caudal orbitofrontal cortex. (See further Rolls, Kringelbach, & De Araujo, 2003.)

SOMATOSENSORY STIMULI Somatosensory afferents reach the orbitofrontal cortex from areas 1 and 2 in the primary somatosensory cortex, from area SII in the inferior parietal lobule, from areas 7a and 7b, and from caudal insula (Barbas, 1988, 1993; Carmichael & Price, 1995; Friedman, Murray, O'Neill, & Mishkin, 1986; Morecraft, Geula, & Mesulam, 1992). The role of the orbitofrontal cortex in representing the pleasantness of a somatosensory stimulus was investigated in an fMRI experiment by Francis et al. (1999). The study design compared the activations of different brain regions in response to a soft and pleasant touch to the hand (using velvet) with the activations produced by an affectively neutral but more intense touch to the hand using the smooth end of a wooden dowel. Stimulation with the pleasant stimulus produced significantly more activation of the orbitofrontal cortex than the neutral stimulus, indicating that the orbitofrontal cortex is involved in representing the pleasantness of the stimulus. By contrast, the more intense neutral stimulus produced stronger activation of somatosensory cortex, indicating that this region is more involved in representing the intensity of a stimulus. In order to determine whether aversive or painful touch produces activation of orbitofrontal cortex, a further study (Rolls et al., 2002) was carried out in which painful stimulation applied to the hand with a pointed stylus was compared with the neutral and pleasant touch conditions. Contralateral (to the hand of stimulation) orbitofrontal cortex was found to be significantly more activated by both the painful and pleasant touch conditions relative to the neutral touch conditions (Fig. 35.3; Color Plate 14.). Activation in the human orbitofrontal cortex has also been reported in other neuroimaging studies of pain (Gyulai, Firestone, Mintun, & Winter, 1997; Hsieh, Belfrage, Stone Elander, Hansson, & Ingvar, 1995; Petrovic, Petersson, Ghatan, Stone Elander, & Ingvar, 2000; Rainville et al., 1999). These findings indicate that the orbitofrontal cortex is involved in representing the affective aspects of somatosensory stimuli of both positive and negative valence.

VISCERAL AND SOMATIC REPRESENTATION Another "modality" that may be especially important in the context of affect and emotion is input from the viscera, consisting of somatic sensation from the internal organs, as well as feedback relating to the body's state of autonomic arousal, such as heart rate, blood pressure, and so on. Visceral input enters the insular transition area in the far caudal orbitofrontal cortex from a region of the ventrolateral posteromedial nucleus of the thalamus (Carmichael & Price, 1995; Ongur & Price, 2000). The part of the VPMpc that projects to this region is distinct from that which projects to primary gustatory cortex. This component of VPMpc receives input from a part of the NTS in the brainstem implicated in visceral sensation, which in turn receives input from the vagus nerve (Beckstead, Morse, & Norgren, 1980; Carmichael & Price, 1995; Price, Carmichael, & Drevets, 1996). Consistent with this arrangement, a number of neuroimaging studies have reported activation in human orbitofrontal cortex following visceral stimulation. Responses have been found in this area following

anorectal stimulation (Hobday et al., 2001; Lotze et al., 2001). Further, stimulation of baroreceptors leading to alterations in blood pressure sensation was found to produce activation in a region of inferior lateral prefrontal cortex bordering the orbitofrontal cortex (Weisz et al., 2001). Critchley, Elliott, Mathias, and Dolan (2000) measured skin conductance responses when subjects were performing a gambling task while simultaneously undergoing fMRI scanning. These authors reported that responses in a region of posterolateral orbitofrontal cortex correlated with changes in autonomic arousal as indexed by galvanic skin conductance. These preliminary data suggest that the human orbitofrontal cortex is involved in visceral representation as well as in the central representation of autonomic arousal.

ORBITOFRONTAL CORTEX ACTIVATION BY VISUAL STIMULI Visual information reaches the orbitofrontal cortex and amygdala from the end of the ventral stream from areas in inferior temporal cortex (Barbas, 1988, 1993). Auditory information arrives from superior temporal cortex (Aggleton, Burton, & Passingham, 1980). Face expressions are probably the most frequently studied of all affective stimuli in functional neuroimaging. This may be in part because of the ease with which such stimuli can be presented to subjects in an imaging laboratory, as well as the degree to which such stimuli can be easily manipulated to address specific experimental questions. A role for the human orbitofrontal cortex in processing facial expressions of emotion was proposed by Hornak, Rolls, and Wade (1996) and Hornak, Bramham, Rolls, et al. (2003), who found that patients with lesions of the ventral prefrontal cortex, including the orbital surface, were impaired at identifying facial expressions. Consistent with this neuropsychological evidence, neuroimaging studies have found activation in the orbitofrontal cortex and adjoining ventral prefrontal cortex in response to the presentation of emotional facial expressions (Blair, Morris, Frith, Perrett, & Dolan, 1999; Gorno-Tempini et al., 2001; Kringelbach, Araujo, & Rolls, 2001; Nakamura et al., 1999; Sprengelmeyer, Rausch, Eysel, & Przuntek, 1998). Aside from expression, another facial attribute that can elicit a strong affective response is the attractiveness or beauty of a face, and there is evidence to suggest that the orbitofrontal cortex is involved in responding to this attribute. Aharon et al. (2001) showed in a block design fMRI study that regions of orbitofrontal cortex were activated during a blocked presentation of attractive faces. In an event-related fMRI study, O'Doherty, Winston, et al. (2002), showed that a region of anterior medial orbitofrontal cortex responded specifically to the presentation of faces with high attractiveness, and

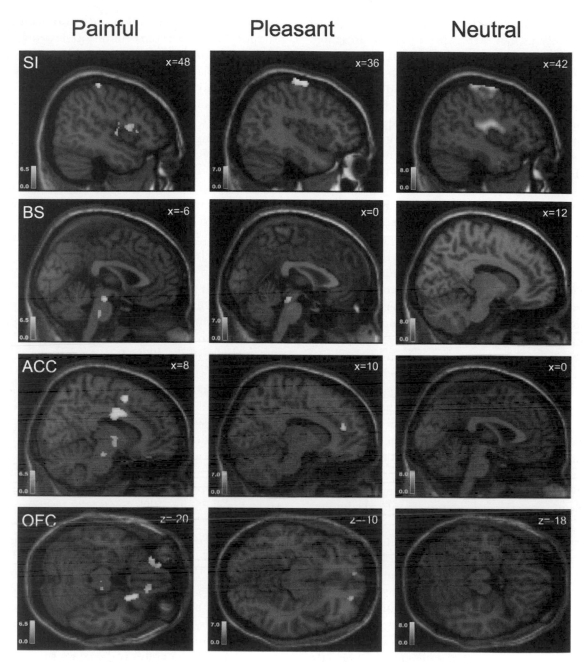

Painful **Pleasant** **Neutral**

FIGURE 35.3 Brain activation in response to somatosensory stimulation. Sagittal sections are shown for each of the three conditions, painful, pleasant, and neutral, with the group activation significant at $P < 0.05$ (corrected) for multiple comparisons of the contralateral (right) somatosensory cortex (SI), and sagittal sections are shown for activation in brainstem (BS). For the painful and pleasant conditions, sagittal section of activations in the anterior cingulate cortex (ACC) and axial sections of activations in the orbitofrontal cortex are shown. The activations have been thresholded at $P < 0.0001$ to show the extent of activation. (From Rolls et al., 2002.) (See Color Plate 14.)

that the responses in that region were modulated by the presence or absence of a perceiver-directed smile. Although most of the studies of visual affect to date have used facial stimuli, there is at least some evidence that the orbitofrontal cortex may also be involved in responding to affective visual stimuli other than facial. For instance, orbitofrontal cortex activation has been reported in response to complex visual stimuli of posi-

tive and negative valence from the International Affective Picture series (Lang, Greenwald, Bradley, & Hamm, 1993; Paradiso et al., 1999).

AMYGDALA RESPONSES TO VISUAL REINFORCERS The human amygdala has also been implicated in responding to emotional facial expressions, particularly of fear (Breiter et al., 1996; Morris et al., 1996). Indeed, amygdala responses have been found to fearful facial expressions even when such expressions are presented outside of conscious awareness, as in a backward masking procedure (Morris, Ohman, Dolan, 1999). The amygdala may also be involved in responding to at least some other facial expressions. Blair et al. (1999) presented subjects with angry and sad expressions and found amygdala activation to sad faces when compared with the angry face condition. Although there is little evidence of a response in the amygdala to the one affectively positive emotional expression stimulus, "happy" faces (though see Breiter et al., 1996), it may be premature to conclude that the amygdala is involved solely in processing aversive facial expressions. To date, a rather limited set of facial stimuli has typically been used in imaging studies of facial expression processing (e.g., the Ekman faces; Ekman & Friesen, 1975), and the reward value of a happy face may well be determined by an interaction with other factors, such as familiarity, facial attractiveness, and so on. These factors will probably need to be explored in order to evaluate whether the amygdala is also sensitive to rewarding facial stimuli.

There is, however, evidence to suggest that the human amygdala is involved in responding to at least one class of pleasant visual stimulus—pictures of food items. LaBar et al. (2001) scanned subjects in both a hungry and a satiated state and showed that pictures of food items elicited responses in the human amygdala in a hungry state relative to a satiated state, whereas this was not found for affectively neutral nonfood stimuli.

ORBITOFRONTAL CORTEX ACTIVATION BY AUDITORY STIMULI
Auditory information arrives in the orbitofrontal cortex and amygdala from the superior temporal cortex (Aggleton et al., 1980). Brain regions involved in processing affective aspects of auditory stimuli were evaluated in a PET study by Blood, Zatorre, Bermudez, and Evans (1999). In an elegant design, these authors used a sequence of musical notes and systematically varied the consonance between the notes. The higher the degree of consonance, the more pleasant the music was perceived by the subjects. Subjects were scanned while listening to six different versions of the music ranging from high to low consonance. A positive correlation was found between activity in the medial orbitofrontal cortex and the degree of consonance of the music, indicating that the more pleasant the music, the greater the activity in this region. Activity has also been reported in the caudolateral orbitofrontal cortex in response to aversive music. In a PET study by Frey, Kostopoulos, and Petrides (2000), aversive sound stimuli (loud car crashes) were found to activate orbitofrontal cortex when compared with sounds that were rated by the subjects as pleasant.

Vocal expressions of emotion have also been found to produce activation in the orbitofrontal cortex, a finding consistent with neuropsychological evidence that orbitofrontal cortex lesions result in impairment in recognition of vocal emotion (Hornak et al., 1996; Morris, Scott, & Dolan, 1999). Consequently, there is at least some evidence that the orbitofrontal cortex is involved in representing the affective value of auditory stimuli (Rolls, 2002; see also Rolls, Chap. 19, this volume).

AMYGDALA AND AUDITORY REINFORCERS Although the amygdala has robustly been shown to be involved in responding to facial emotion (specifically of fear), the role of this region in processing vocal emotion remains unresolved. Phillips et al. (1998) performed an fMRI experiment in which subjects were presented in separate runs with facial and vocal expressions of fear and disgust. Vocal expressions of fear were found to activate a region of hippocampus that the authors reported as extending into the amygdala. However, a PET study by Morris, Scott, et al. (1999) found contradictory results, in that vocal expressions of fear produced a deactivation rather than an activation in the amygdala. These ambiguous neuroimaging findings are also reflected in the human lesion literature: in one study, a patient with a bilateral lesion of the amygdala was found to be impaired at vocal emotion recognition, whereas other studies have described patients with bilateral amygdala lesions that are unimpaired (Adolphs & Tranel, 1999; Anderson & Phelps, 1998; Scott et al., 1997).

Cross-modal integration of auditory and visual emotion in the amygdala

In spite of the ambiguity concerning the role of the amygdala in unimodal representations of vocal affect, Dolan, Morris, and de Gelder (2001) investigated the role of the human amygdala in responding during the conjoint presentation of facial and vocal emotion. The task involved the presentation of facial and vocal emotion stimuli corresponding to two emotions, happy and fearful. Each trial consisted of the presentation of either congruent (i.e., both happy or fearful) or incongruent (i.e., one happy and the other fearful) facial and vocal emotion pairs. Amygdala activity was found to increase during the congruent presentation of vocal and facial emotions of fear relative to the incongruent presentation of either facial or vocal emotions of fear. This result provides evidence for cross-modal processing in the amygdala in the visual and auditory domain, in that amygdala responses to an emotional stimulus in one modality were modulated as a function of the congruence of an emotional stimulus in the other modality.

Cross-modal integration in the human orbitofrontal cortex: The representation of flavor

The orbitofrontal cortex receives gustatory, olfactory, and texture inputs (Barbas, 1993; Baylis et al., 1994; Morecraft et al., 1992). In nonhuman primates, olfactory and taste inputs converge rostral to the secondary olfactory and gustatory cortex in area 13 of the orbitofrontal cortex. In this area of the orbitofrontal cortex, bimodal neurons have been found to respond to both gustatory and olfactory stimuli, often with correspondence of tuning between the two modalities (Baylis et al., 1994). For example some neurons respond to the taste of glucose and odor of banana, while other neurons respond to salty taste and savory odors. It is probably here that these two modalities converge to produce the representation of flavor (Rolls & Baylis, 1994).

Small, Zatorre, Dagher, Evans, and Jones-Gotman (2001) showed in a PET study that orbitofrontal cortex activation altered while a whole-food stimulus was eaten to satiety, and altered from being subjectively pleasant to aversive. The authors found that signal in medial orbitofrontal cortex decreased as the subject was fed to satiety, and on the basis of this result the authors suggested that the pleasantness of the chocolate food was represented in this region. Conversely, a part of caudolateral orbitofrontal cortex was found to increase in signal as subjects ate the chocolate to satiety, and this increase in signal was concomitant with an increase in the aversiveness of the chocolate. However, it should be noted that in addition to changes in subjective pleasantness of the food eaten, some of the observed effects in this study may also be related to changes in the subjects' overall level of satiety.

As described in a previous section, sensory-specific satiety is the phenomenon whereby the pleasantness of a food eaten to satiety decreases selectively to a food eaten in the meal, whereas the pleasantness of a food not eaten in the meal shows much less of a decrease and may even increase in pleasantness (Rolls, Rolls, Rowe, & Sweeney, 1981). In a follow-up of the study by O'Doherty et al. (2000) in which sensory-specific satiety-related effects in response to a food odor were shown in the orbitofrontal cortex, Kringelbach, O'Doherty, Rolls, and Andrews (2003) used a similar paradigm to investigate the neural basis of sensory-specific satiety-related responses to a whole-food stimulus. Subjects were scanned when hungry while being presented with two food flavors, chocolate milk and tomato juice. The stimuli were delivered in 0.75 mL aliquots at the beginning of a 16 s block, and subjects were cued to swallow 10 s after the stimulus delivery. A control condition was also included in which subjects were presented with a neutral, tasteless

solution. Subjects were then removed from the scanner and fed to satiety with one of the two foods. The food eaten to satiety was counterbalanced so that half the subjects ingested to satiety chocolate milk and the other half ingested tomato juice. The subjects were then placed back into the scanner and the protocol was repeated. Subjective pleasantness ratings were obtained during each scanning session for each food. Consistent with the previous results for pure olfactory stimuli, activation in a part of mediolateral orbitofrontal cortex showed sensory-specific satiety-related responses to the food flavors, with activation in response to the food eaten decreasing selectively in this region following satiety but no such decrease being evident for the food not eaten to satiety (Fig. 35.4; Color Plate 15.). This evidence indicates that the reward value of a whole-food stimulus with olfactory, gustatory, and texture components is represented in orbitofrontal cortex. (See further De Araujo, Rolls, Kringelbach, et al., 2003.)

Stimulus-reinforcer association learning in the amygdala and orbitofrontal cortex

One way in which amygdala and orbitofrontal cortex can be considered to be involved in cross-modal processing is through their role in stimulus-reinforcer learning. In this case, an arbitrary affectively neutral stimulus (often called the conditioned stimulus, or CS) in one modality can by temporal contiguity become associated with a reinforcing stimulus (often called the unconditioned stimulus, or UCS) in another or the same modality. This is a form of stimulus-stimulus learning, and is usually cross-modal (Rolls, 1999).

Classical fear conditioning can be thought of as an instance of stimulus-reinforcer learning in which the learning takes place between an arbitrary affectively neutral stimulus and an unconditioned (primary reinforcing) stimulus, such as a loud noise or electric shock, that elicits an aversive fear response. Through temporal pairing of CS and UCS presentations, the CS also comes to be associated with the aversive consequences of the UCS and comes to elicit fear responses. Fear responses are often indexed in human studies by a measure of autonomic arousal, such as galvanic skin conductance. It is known that lesions of the medial temporal lobe or more discrete lesions of the amygdala produce impairments in fear conditioning acquisition in humans (Bechara, Damasio, Damasio, & Lee, 1999; Bechara et al., 1995; LaBar, LeDoux, Spence, & Phelps, 1995). Using an event-related fMRI paradigm, the role of the amygdala in human fear conditioning was investigated by Buchel, Morris, Dolan, and Friston (1998). Subjects were scanned while they were being

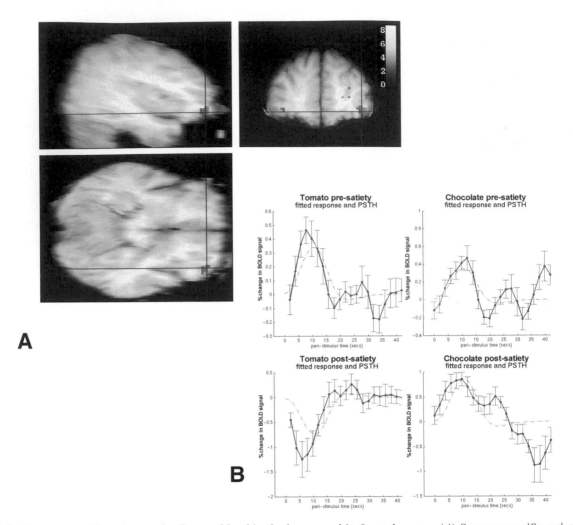

FIGURE 35.4 Sensory-specific satiety to the flavor of food in the human orbitofrontal cortex. (*A*) Sensory-specific satiety-related activation in right mediolateral orbitofrontal cortex to the flavor of food in a single subject fed to satiety on tomato juice. The threshold is set at $P < 0.001$ (uncorrected). (*B*) A plot of the time course of the BOLD response in orbitofrontal cortex is shown for the same subject. Following satiety, the response to the food eaten (tomato juice) is greatly decreased relative to the response to the food not eaten (chocolate milk). This decrease in activation occurred concomitantly with a decrease in the subjective pleasantness of the food. (See Color Plate 15.)

conditioned to a face stimulus (CS+) that was paired using a 50% reinforcement schedule with an aversive loud bang. Responses to the CS+ were assessed by comparing unpaired presentations of the CS+ to trials in which a CS− was presented (another face that was not paired with an aversive loud bang). The amygdala was shown to respond to the CS+ during the early stages of conditioning, yet the responses were found to habituate over time. Similar time-dependent responses were observed in the amygdala in a fear conditioning study by LaBar, Gatenby, Gore, LeDoux, and Phelps (1998). These results are compatible with a role for the human amygdala in fear conditioning, although the time-dependent nature of the responses suggests that increased amygdala metabolism (which is what fMRI reflects) may be particularly involved in the early

stages of conditioning when CS-UCS associations are being established.

In contrast to the amygdala, the orbitofrontal cortex may not be essential for the acquisition of fear conditioning, as patients with lesions of ventromedial prefrontal cortex that includes bilateral medial orbitofrontal cortex are unimpaired at acquiring fear-conditioned responses (Bechara et al., 1999). However, in the case of fMRI studies of fear conditioning, an absence of reported activations in this area could also be accounted for by the fact that studies to date have not focused on the orbitofrontal cortex, and thus have not used techniques designed to maximize signal in this area. Although the human orbitofrontal cortex may not be necessary for the acquisition of fear conditioning, the region may be involved in the extinction or reversal of stimulus-reinforcer associations (Rolls et al., 1994).

Aversive learning aside, there is evidence to implicate the human amygdala and orbitofrontal cortex in cross-modal associative learning for rewarding stimuli. O'Doherty, Deichmann, et al. (2002) scanned subjects who were, on each trial, presented with one of three arbitrary visual stimuli associated with the subsequent delivery of either a pleasant sweet taste (1M glucose), a mildly aversive salt taste (0.2M NaCl), or an affectively neutral taste control (a tasteless control solution). This design enabled the responses to a predictive visual stimulus to be dissociated from the responses to receipt of taste reward. Responses were found in human amygdala and orbitofrontal cortex to the visual stimulus that signaled reward expectation, suggesting that these brain areas are involved in predictive coding of subsequent reinforcement for rewards. Indeed, the orbitofrontal cortex was found to respond not only during reward expectation but also following reward receipt, indicating that this region can be considered to be involved in multimodal convergence for reward, responding to both a visual stimulus that is predictive of subsequent taste reward and to receipt of the taste reward itself.

Evidence from single-cell neurophysiology and lesion studies indicates that the orbitofrontal cortex is especially involved in rapidly altering stimulus-reinforcer associations following a reversal of the reinforcement contingencies (Rolls, 1999; Thorpe et al., 1983). The role of the human orbitofrontal cortex in stimulus-reward reversal learning was investigated in an fMRI study by O'Doherty, Kringelbach, et al. (2001), as follows. In this study, subjects were presented with a choice of two arbitrary visual stimuli, each of which was associated with a monetary outcome, and had to choose between the stimuli in order to maximize their monetary gain. Both stimuli were associated with monetary rewards and punishments, but the stimuli differed in the probability of obtaining a reward and in the magnitudes of the rewards and punishments that could be obtained. One stimulus, designated S+, was associated with a greater likelihood of obtaining a monetary reward, and the magnitude of the reward was larger than that associated with the alternative stimulus (S−). S− was associated with a greater probability of obtaining a monetary loss which was much larger in magnitude than the probabilistically low monetary loss associated with S+. Consequently, subjects learned to consistently

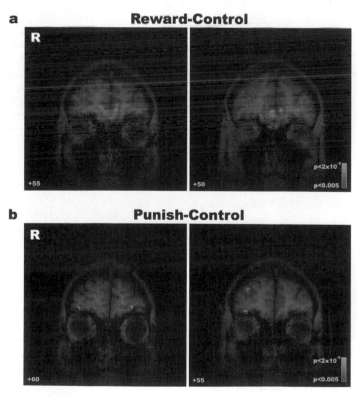

FIGURE 35.5   Comparison of monetary rewards and punishments with a control condition. (A) A region of bilateral medial orbitofrontal cortex and medial prefrontal cortex is significantly activated relative to a neutral baseline in the Reward-Control contrast. (B) A region of bilateral lateral orbitofrontal cortex is significantly activated relative to a neutral baseline in the Punish-Control contrast. (From O'Doherty, Kringelbach, et al., 2001.) (See Color Plate 16.)

choose S+ and avoid S−. Once learning was established, the contingencies were reversed so that subjects had to update stimulus-reinforcer associations and alter their responses in order to keep track of the contingencies. Subjects were scanned while performing the reversal task, and neural responses in the orbitofrontal cortex and other brain regions to the receipt of the monetary feedback were analyzed. Responses were found in medial orbitofrontal cortex during receipt of the monetary reward that correlated with the magnitude of the monetary reward received. By contrast, the lateral orbitofrontal cortex was found to respond to the receipt of the monetary punishment, and indeed the signal was proportional to the magnitude of the punishment received. These results showed that the orbitofrontal cortex was sensitive to the receipt of abstract reinforcers, and that during reversal learning, medial and lateral orbitofrontal cortex were differentially engaged during the receipt of positive and negative reinforcement (Fig. 35.5; Color Plate 16.). In this case the association was between an arbitrary visual stimulus and a reinforcer that was abstract, money, and in a sense also a secondary (learned) reinforcer. This study thus extends the notion of orbitofrontal cortex involvement in associations between stimuli and primary (unlearned) reinforcers such as taste and touch to its involvement in learning, and particularly in reversing associations between previously neutral (e.g., visual) stimuli and abstract stimuli such as monetary reward and loss that might be considered amodal, abstract concepts, though of course ultimately associated with primary reinforcers.

Conclusions

This chapter has presented evidence from functional neuroimaging that each of the sensory modalities, taste, touch, vision, smell, and audition, activates the orbitofrontal cortex, and most also activate the amygdala. In most cases the activation is related to the reward or punishment (subjectively affective) value of the stimuli. In cases where the stimulus is not a primary (unlearned) reinforcer, such as vision, the implication is that stimulus-reinforcement (sensory-sensory) association learning builds the correct multimodal representations.

Multimodal information serves at least two important functions. First, the orbitofrontal cortex and amygdala appear to be important in the representation and evaluation of the reward value of primary and secondary reinforcers. Second, the orbitofrontal cortex and amygdala are important in the learning of reinforcement associations, and in reversing those associations. These two functions are key functions for brain areas involved in emotion. The neuroimaging evidence presented in

this chapter is consistent with a role of the orbitofrontal cortex and the amygdala in human emotion and motivation, as proposed by Rolls (1999).

REFERENCES

Adolphs, R., Damasio, H., Tranel, D., & Damasio, A. R. (1996). Cortical systems for the recognition of emotion in facial expressions. *Journal of Neuroscience, 16,* 7678–7687.

Adolphs, R., & Tranel, D. (1999). Intact recognition of emotional prosody following amygdala damage. *Neuropsychologia, 37,* 1285–1292.

Adolphs, R., Tranel, D., Damasio, H., & Damasio, A. (1994). Impaired recognition of emotion in facial expressions following bilateral damage to the human amygdala. *Nature, 372,* 669–672.

Adolphs, R., Tranel, D., Hamann, S., Young, A. W., Calder, A. J., Phelps, E. A., et al. (1999). Recognition of facial emotion in nine individuals with bilateral amygdala damage. *Neuropsychologia, 37,* 1111–1117.

Aggleton, J. P., Burton, M. J., & Passingham, R. E. (1980). Cortical and subcortical afferents to the amygdala in the rhesus monkey (*Macaca mulatta*). *Brain Research, 190,* 347–368.

Aharon, I., Etcoff, N., Ariely, D., Chabris, C. F., O'Connor, E., & Breiter, H. C. (2001). Beautiful faces have variable reward value: fMRI and behavioral evidence. *Neuron, 32,* 537–551.

Amaral, D. G., & Price, J. L. (1984). Amygdalo-cortical projections in the monkey (*Macaca fascicularis*). *Journal of Comparative Neurology, 230,* 465–496.

Anderson, A. K., & Phelps, E. A. (1998). Intact recognition of vocal expressions of fear following bilateral lesions of the human amygdala. *Neuroreport, 9,* 3607–3613.

Barbas, H. (1988). Anatomic organization of basoventral and mediodorsal visual recipient prefrontal regions in the rhesus monkey. *Journal of Comparative Neurology, 276,* 313–342.

Barbas, H. (1993). Organization of cortical afferent input to the orbitofrontal area in the rhesus monkey. *Neuroscience, 56,* 841–864.

Baxter, M. G., Parker, A., Lindner, C. C., Izquierdo, A. D., & Murray, E. A. (2000). Control of response selection by reinforcer value requires interaction of amygdala and orbital prefrontal cortex. *Journal of Neuroscience, 20,* 4311–4319.

Baylis, L. L., Rolls, E. T., & Baylis, G. C. (1994). Afferent connections of the orbitofrontal cortex taste area of the primate. *Neuroscience, 64,* 801–812.

Bechara, A., Damasio, H., Damasio, A. R., & Lee, G. P. (1999). Different contributions of the human amygdala and ventromedial prefrontal cortex to decision-making. *Journal of Neuroscience, 19,* 5473–5481.

Bechara, A., Tranel, D., Damasio, H., Adolphs, R., Rockland, C., & Damasio, A. R. (1995). Double dissociation of conditioning and declarative knowledge relative to the amygdala and hippocampus in humans. *Science, 269,* 1115–1118.

Beckstead, R. M., Morse, J. R., & Norgren, R. (1980). The nucleus of the solitary tract in the monkey: Projections to the thalamus and brainstem nuclei. *Journal of Comparative Neurology, 190,* 259–282.

Blair, R. J., Morris, J. S., Frith, C. D., Perrett, D. I., & Dolan, R. J. (1999). Dissociable neural responses to facial expressions of sadness and anger. *Brain, 122*(Pt. 5), 883–893.

Blood, A. J., Zatorre, R. J., Bermudez, P., & Evans, A. C. (1999). Emotional responses to pleasant and unpleasant music correlate with activity in paralimbic brain regions. *Nature Neuroscience, 2,* 382–387.

Breiter, H. C., Etcoff, N. L., Whalen, P. J., Kennedy, W. A., Rauch, S. L., Buckner, R. L., et al. (1996). Response and habituation of the human amygdala during visual processing of facial expression. *Neuron, 17,* 875–887.

Buchel, C., Morris, J., Dolan, R. J., & Friston, K. J. (1998). Brain systems mediating aversive conditioning: An event-related fMRI study. *Neuron, 20,* 947–957.

Carmichael, S. T., Clugnet, M. C., & Price, J. L. (1994). Central olfactory connections in the macaque monkey. *Journal of Comparative Neurology, 346,* 403–434.

Carmichael, S. T., & Price, J. L. (1995). Sensory and premotor connections of the orbital and medial prefrontal cortex of macaque monkeys. *Journal of Comparative Neurology, 363,* 642–664.

Cavada, C., Company, T., Tejedor, J., Cruz Rizzolo, R. J., & Reinoso Suarez, F. (2000). The anatomical connections of the macaque monkey orbitofrontal cortex: A review. *Cerebral Cortex, 10,* 220–242.

Critchley, H. D., Elliott, R., Mathias, C. J., & Dolan, R. J. (2000). Neural activity relating to generation and representation of galvanic skin conductance responses: A functional magnetic resonance imaging study. *Journal of Neuroscience, 20,* 3033–3040.

Dade, L. A., Jones-Gotman, M., Zatorre, R., & Evans, A. C. (1998). Human brain function during odor encoding and recognition: A PET activation study. In C. Murphy (Ed.), *Olfaction and Taste XII: An International Symposium. Annals of the New York Academy of Sciences, 855,* 572–575.

Davis, M. (2000). The role of the amygdala in conditioned and unconditioned fear and anxiety. In J. Aggleton (Ed.), *The amygdala: A functional analysis* (2nd ed., pp. 213–288). Oxford, England: Oxford University Press.

De Araujo, I. E. T., Kringelbach, M. L., Rolls, E. T., & Hobden, P. (2003). Representation of umami taste in the human brain. *Journal of Neurophysiology, 90,* 313–319.

De Araujo, I. E. T., Kringelbach, M. L., Rolls, E. T., & McGlone, F. (2003). Human cortical responses to water in the mouth, and the effects of thirst. *Journal of Neurophysiology, 90,* 1865–1876.

De Araujo, I. E. T., Rolls, E. T., Kringelbach, M. L., McGlone, F., & Phillips, N. (2003). Taste-olfactory convergence, and the representation of the pleasantness of flavour, in the human brain. *European Journal of Neuroscience, 18,* 2059–2068.

Deichmann, R., Josephs, O., Hutton, C., Corfield, D. R., & Turner, R. (2002). Compensation of susceptibility-induced BOLD sensitivity losses in echo-planar fMRI imaging. *NeuroImage, 15,* 120–135.

Dias, R., Robbins, T. W., & Roberts, A. C. (1996). Dissociation in prefrontal cortex of affective and attentional shifts. *Nature, 380,* 69–72.

Dolan, R. J., Morris, J. S., & de Gelder, B. (2001). Crossmodal binding of fear in voice and face. *Proceedings of the National Academy of Sciences, USA, 98,* 10006–10010.

Ekman, P., & Friesen, W. V. (1975). *Unmasking the face.* Englewood Heights, NJ: Prentice-Hall.

Everitt, B. J., Parkinson, J. A., Olmstead, M. C., Arroyo, M., Robledo, P., & Robbins, T. W. (1999). Associative processes in addiction and reward: The role of amygdala-ventral stri-atal subsystems. *Annals of the New York Academy of Sciences, 877,* 412–438.

Francis, S., Rolls, E. T., Bowtell, R., McGlone, F., O'Doherty, J., Browning, A., et al. (1999). The representation of pleasant touch in the brain and its relationship with taste and olfactory areas. *Neuroreport, 10,* 453–459.

Frey, S., Kostopoulos, P., & Petrides, M. (2000). Orbitofrontal involvement in the processing of unpleasant auditory information. *European Journal of Neuroscience, 12,* 3709–3712.

Frey, S., & Petrides, M. (1999). Re-examination of the human taste region: A positron emission tomography study. *European Journal of Neuroscience, 11,* 2985–2988.

Friedman, D. P., Murray, E. A., O'Neill, J. B., & Mishkin, M. (1986). Cortical connections of the somatosensory fields of the lateral sulcus of macaques: Evidence for a corticolimbic pathway for touch. *Journal of Comparative Neurology, 252,* 323–347.

Fuster, J. M. (1997). *The prefrontal cortex.* New York: Raven Press.

Gorno-Tempini, M. L., Pradelli, S., Serafini, M., Pagnoni, G., Baraldi, P., Porro, C., et al. (2001). Explicit and incidental facial expression processing: An fMRI study. *NeuroImage, 14,* 465–473.

Gyulai, F. E., Firestone, L. L., Mintun, M. A., & Winter, P. M. (1997). In vivo imaging of nitrous oxide–induced changes in cerebral activation during noxious heat stimuli. *Anesthesiology, 86,* 538–548.

Hikosaka, K., & Watanabe, M. (2000). Delay activity of orbital and lateral prefrontal neurons of the monkey varying with different rewards. *Cerebral Cortex, 10,* 263–271.

Hobday, D. I., Aziz, Q., Thacker, N., Hollander, I., Jackson, A., et al. (2001). A study of the cortical processing of ano-rectal sensation using functional MRI. *Brain, 124*(Pt. 2), 361–368.

Hornak, J., Bramham, J., Rolls, E. T., Morris, R. G., O'Doherty, J., Bullock, P. R., & Polkey, C. E. (2003). Changes in emotion after circumscribed surgical lesions of the orbitofrontal and cingulate cortices. *Brain, 126,* 1691–1712.

Hornak, J., Rolls, E. T., & Wade, D. (1996). Face and voice expression identification in patients with emotional and behavioural changes following ventral frontal lobe damage. *Neuropsychologia, 34,* 247–261.

Hsieh, J. C., Belfrage, M., Stone Elander, S., Hansson, P., & Ingvar, M. (1995). Central representation of chronic ongoing neuropathic pain studied by positron emission tomography. *Pain, 63,* 225–236.

Iversen, S. D., & Mishkin, M. (1970). Perseverative interference in monkeys following selective lesions of the inferior prefrontal convexity. *Experimental Brain Research, 11,* 376–386.

Kinomura, S., Kawashima, R., Yamada, K., Ono, S., Itoh, M., Yoshioka, S., et al. (1994). Functional anatomy of taste perception in the human brain studied with positron emission tomography. *Brain Research, 659,* 263–266.

Kringelbach, M., Araujo, I., & Rolls, E. T. (2001). Face expression as a reinforcer activates the orbitofrontal cortex in an emotion-related reversal task. *NeuroImage, 13,* S433.

Kringelbach, M. L., O'Doherty, J., Rolls, E. T., & Andrews, C. (2003). Activation of the human orbitofrontal cortex to a liquid food stimulus is correlated with its subjective pleasantness. *Cerebral Cortex, 13,* 1064–1071.

Kringelbach, M. L., & Rolls, E. T. (2003). Neural correlates of rapid reversal learning in a simple model of human social interaction. *NeuroImage, 20,* 1371–1383.

LaBar, K. S., Gatenby, J. C., Gore, J. C., LeDoux, J. E., & Phelps, E. A. (1998). Human amygdala activation during conditioned fear acquisition and extinction: A mixed-trial fMRI study. *Neuron, 20,* 937–945.

LaBar, K. S., LeDoux, J. E., Spencer, D. D., & Phelps, E. A. (1995). Impaired fear conditioning following unilateral temporal lobectomy in humans. *Journal of Neuroscience, 15,* 6846–6855.

LaBar, K. S., Gitelman, D. R., Parrish, T. B., Kim, Y. H., Nobre, A. C., & Mesulam, M. M. (2001). Hunger selectivity modulates corticolimbic activation to food stimuli in humans. *Behavioral Neuroscience, 115,* 493–500.

Lang, P. J., Greenwald, M. K., Bradley, M. M., & Hamm, A. O. (1993). Looking at pictures: Affective, facial, visceral, and behavioral reactions. *Psychophysiology, 30,* 261–273.

LeDoux, J. E. (1995). Emotion: Clues from the brain. *Annual Review of Psychology, 46,* 209–235.

Lotze, M., Wietek, B., Birbaumer, N., Ehrhardt, J., Grodd, W., & Enck, P. (2001). Cerebral activation during anal and rectal stimulation. *NeuroImage, 14,* 1027–1034.

Malkova, L., Gaffan, D., & Murray, E. A. (1997). Excitotoxic lesions of the amygdala fail to produce impairment in visual learning for auditory secondary reinforcement but interfere with reinforcer devaluation effects in rhesus monkeys. *Journal of Neuroscience, 17,* 6011–6020.

Morecraft, R. J., Geula, C., & Mesulam, M.-M. (1992). Cytoarchitecture and neural afferents of orbitofrontal cortex in the brain of the monkey. *Journal of Comparative Neurology, 232,* 341–358.

Morris, J. S., Frith, C. D., Perrett, D. I., Rowland, D., Young, A. W., Calder, A. J., et al. (1996). A differential neural response in the human amygdala to fearful and happy facial expressions. *Nature, 383,* 812–815.

Morris, J. S., Ohman, A., & Dolan, R. J. (1999). A subcortical pathway to the right amygdala mediating "unseen" fear. *Proceedings of the National Academy of Sciences, USA, 96,* 1680–1685.

Morris, J. S., Scott, S. K., & Dolan, R. J. (1999). Saying it with feeling: Neural responses to emotional vocalizations. *Neuropsychologia, 37,* 1155–1163.

Nakamura, K., Kawashima, R., Ito, K., Sugiura, M., Kato, T., Nakamura, A., et al. (1999). Activation of the right inferior frontal cortex during assessment of facial emotion. *Journal of Neurophysiology, 82,* 1610–1614.

O'Doherty, J., Deichmann, R., Critchley, H. D., & Dolan, R. J. (2002). Neural responses during anticipation of a primary taste reward. *Neuron, 33,* 815–826.

O'Doherty, J., Kringelbach, M. L., Rolls, E. T., Hornak, J., & Andrews, C. (2001). Abstract reward and punishment representations in the human orbitofrontal cortex. *Nature Neuroscience, 4,* 95–102.

O'Doherty, J., Rolls, E. T., Francis, S., Bowtell, R., & McGlone, F. (2001). Representation of pleasant and aversive taste in the human brain. *Journal of Neurophysiology, 85,* 1315–1321.

O'Doherty, J., Rolls, E. T., Francis, S., Bowtell, R., McGlone, F., Kobal, G., et al. (2000). Sensory-specific satiety-related olfactory activation of the human orbitofrontal cortex. *Neuroreport, 11,* 893–897.

O'Doherty, J., Winston, J., Critchley, H. D., Perrett, D. I., Burt, D. M., & Dolan, R. J. (2002). Beauty in a smile: The role of medial orbitofrontal cortex in facial attractiveness. *Neuropsychologia, 41,* 147–155.

Ojemann, J. G., Akbudak, E., Snyder, A. Z., McKinstry, R. C., Raichle, M. E., & Conturo, T. E. (1997). Anatomic localization and quantitative analysis of gradient refocused echoplanar fMRI susceptibility artifacts. *NeuroImage, 6,* 156–167.

Ongur, D., & Price, J. L. (2000). The organization of networks within the orbital and medial prefrontal cortex of rats, monkeys and humans. *Cerebral Cortex, 10,* 206–219.

Ono, T., & Nishijo, H. (2000). Neurophysiological basis of emotion in primates: Neuronal responses in the monkey amygdala and anterior cingulate cortex. In M. S. Gazzaniga (Ed.), *The new cognitive neurosciences.* Cambridge, MA: MIT Press.

Paradiso, S., Johnson, D. L., Andreasen, N. C., O'Leary, D. S., Watkins, G. L., Ponto, L. L., et al. (1999). Cerebral blood flow changes associated with attribution of emotional valence to pleasant, unpleasant, and neutral visual stimuli in a PET study of normal subjects. *American Journal of Psychiatry, 156,* 1618–1629.

Parkinson, J. A., Robbins, T. W., & Everitt, B. J. (2000). Dissociable roles of the central and basolateral amygdala in appetitive emotional learning. *European Journal of Neuroscience, 12,* 405–413.

Petrovic, P., Petersson, K. M., Ghatan, P. H., Stone Elander, S., & Ingvar, M. (2000). Pain-related cerebral activation is altered by a distracting cognitive task. *Pain, 85,* 19–30.

Phillips, M. L., Young, A. W., Scott, S. K., Calder, A. J., Andrew, C., Giampietro, V., et al. (1998). Neural responses to facial and vocal expressions of fear and disgust. *Proceedings of the Royal Society of London, Series B: Biological Sciences, 265,* 1809–1817.

Phillips, M. L., Young, A. W., Senior, C., Brammer, M., Andrew, C., Calder, A. J., et al. (1997). A specific neural substrate for perceiving facial expressions of disgust. *Nature, 389,* 495–498.

Price, J. L., Carmichael, S. T., & Drevets, W. C. (1996). Networks related to the orbital and medial prefrontal cortex: A substrate for emotional behavior? *Progress in Brain Research, 107,* 523–536.

Rainville, P., Hofbauer, R. K., Paus, T., Duncan, G. H., Bushnell, M. C., & Price, D. D. (1999). Cerebral mechanisms of hypnotic induction and suggestion. *Journal of Cognitive Neuroscience, 11,* 110–125.

Rolls, B. J., Rolls, E. T., Rowe, E. A., & Sweeney, K. (1981). Sensory specific satiety in man. *Physiology and Behavior, 27,* 137–142.

Rolls, E. T. (1990). A theory of emotion, and its application to understanding the neural basis of emotion. *Cognition and Emotion, 4,* 161–190.

Rolls, E. T. (1997). Taste and olfactory processing in the brain and its relation to the control of eating. *Critical Reviews in Neurobiology, 11,* 263–287.

Rolls, E. T. (1999). *The brain and emotion.* Oxford, England: Oxford University Press.

Rolls, E. T. (2000). The orbitofrontal cortex and reward. *Cerebral Cortex, 10,* 284–294.

Rolls, E. T. (2002). The functions of the orbitofrontal cortex. In D. T. Stuss & R. T. Knight (Eds.), *Principles of frontal lobe function* (pp. 354–375). Oxford, England: Oxford University Press.

Rolls, E. T., & Baylis, L. L. (1994). Gustatory, olfactory, and visual convergence within the primate orbitofrontal cortex. *Journal of Neuroscience, 14,* 5437–5452.

Rolls, E. T., & Deco, G. (2002). *Computational neuroscience of vision*. Oxford, England: Oxford University Press.

Rolls, E. T., Hornak, J., Wade, D., & McGrath, J. (1994). Emotion-related learning in patients with social and emotional changes associated with frontal lobe damage. *Journal of Neurology, Neurosurgery and Psychiatry, 57,* 1518–1524.

Rolls, E. T., Kringelbach, M. L., & De Araujo, I. E. T. (2003). Different representations of pleasant and unpleasant odors in the human brain. *European Journal of Neuroscience, 18,* 695–703.

Rolls, E. T., O'Doherty, J., Kringelbach, M., Francis, S., Bowtell, R., & McGlone, F. (2002). Representations of pleasant and painful touch in the human orbitofrontal and cingulate cortices. *Cerebral Cortex, 13,* 308–317.

Rolls, E. T., Sienkiewicz, Z. J., & Yaxley, S. (1989). Hunger modulates the responses to gustatory stimuli of single neurons in the caudolateral orbitofrontal cortex of the macaque monkey. *European Journal of Neuroscience, 1,* 53–60.

Rolls, E. T., & Treves, A. (1998). *Neural networks and brain function*. Oxford, England: Oxford University Press.

Rolls, E. T., Yaxley, S., & Sienkiewicz, Z. J. (1990). Gustatory responses of single neurons in the caudolateral orbitofrontal cortex of the macaque monkey. *Journal of Neurophysiology, 64,* 1055–1066.

Sanghera, M. K., Rolls, E. T., & Roper-Hall, A. (1979). Visual responses of neurons in the dorsolateral amygdala of the alert monkey. *Experimental Neurology, 63,* 610–626.

Schoenbaum, G., Chiba, A. A., & Gallagher, M. (1998). Orbitofrontal cortex and basolateral amygdala encode expected outcomes during learning. *Nature Neuroscience, 1,* 155–159.

Schoenbaum, G., Chiba, A. A., & Gallagher, M. (1999). Neural encoding in orbitofrontal cortex and basolateral amygdala during olfactory discrimination learning. *Journal of Neuroscience, 19,* 1876–1884.

Schultz, W., Tremblay, L., & Hollerman, J. R. (2000). Reward processing in primate orbitofrontal cortex and basal ganglia. *Cerebral Cortex, 10,* 272–284.

Scott, T. R., Karadi, Z., Oomura, Y., Nishino, H., Plata-Salaman, C. R., Lenard, L., et al. (1993). Gustatory neural coding in the amygdala of the alert macaque monkey. *Journal of Neurophysiology, 69,* 1810–1820.

Scott, S. K., Young, A. W., Calder, A. J., Hellawell, D. J., Aggleton, J. P., & Johnson, M. (1997). Impaired auditory recognition of fear and anger following bilateral amygdala lesions. *Nature, 385,* 254–257.

Small, D. M., Jones-Gotman, M., Zatorre, R. J., Petrides, M., & Evans, A. C. (1997a). A role for the right anterior temporal lobe in taste quality recognition. *Journal of Neuroscience, 17,* 5136–5142.

Small, D. M., Jones-Gotman, M., Zatorre, R. J., Petrides, M., & Evans, A. C. (1997b). Flavor processing: More than the sum of its parts. *Neuroreport, 8,* 3913–3917.

Small, D. M., Zald, D. H., Jones-Gotman, M., Zatorre, R. J., Pardo, J. V., Frey, S., et al. (1999). Human cortical gustatory areas: A review of functional neuroimaging data. *Neuroreport, 10,* 7–14.

Small, D. M., Zatorre, R. J., Dagher, A., Evans, A. C., & Jones-Gotman, M. (2001). Changes in brain activity related to eating chocolate: From pleasure to aversion. *Brain, 124*(Pt. 9), 1720–1733.

Sobel, N., Prabhakaran, V., Desmond, J. E., Glover, G. H., Goode, R. L., Sullivan, E. V., et al. (1998). Sniffing and smelling: Separate subsystems in the human olfactory cortex. *Nature, 392,* 282–286.

Sobel, N., Prabhakaran, V., Desmond, J. E., Glover, G. H., Sullivan, E. V., & Gabrieli, J. D. (1997). A method for functional magnetic resonance imaging of olfaction. *Journal of Neuroscience Methods, 78,* 115–123.

Sobel, N., Prabhakaran, V., Zhao, Z., Desmond, J. E., Glover, G. H., Sullivan, E. V., et al. (2000). Time course of odorant-induced activation in the human primary olfactory cortex. *Journal of Neurophysiology, 83,* 537–551.

Sprengelmeyer, R., Rausch, M., Eysel, U. T., & Przuntek, H. (1998). Neural structures associated with recognition of facial expressions of basic emotions. *Proceedings of the Royal Society of London, Series B: Biological Sciences, 265,* 1927–1931.

Tanabe, T., Yarita, H., Iino, M., Ooshima, Y., & Takagi, S. F. (1975). An olfactory projection area in orbitofrontal cortex of the monkey. *Journal of Neurophysiology, 38,* 1269–1283.

Thorpe, S. J., Rolls, E. T., & Maddison, S. (1983). Neuronal activity in the orbitofrontal cortex of the behaving monkey. *Experimental Brain Research, 49,* 93–115.

Tremblay, L., & Schultz, W. (1999). Relative reward preference in primate orbitofrontal cortex. *Nature, 398,* 704–708.

Weisz, J., Emri, M., Fent, J., Lengyel, Z., Marian, T., Horvath, G., et al. (2001). Right prefrontal activation produced by arterial baroreceptor stimulation: A PET study. *Neuroreport, 12,* 3233–3238.

Wilson, J. L., Jenkinson, M., de Araujo, I., Kringelbach, M. L., Rolls, E. T., & Jezzard, P. (2002). Fast, fully automated global and local magnetic field optimisation for fMRI of the human brain. *NeuroImage, 17,* 967–976.

Yousem, D. M., Williams, S. C., Howard, R. O., Andrew, C., Simmons, A., Allin, M., et al. (1997). Functional MR imaging during odor stimulation: Preliminary data. *Radiology, 204,* 833–888.

Zald, D. H., Donndelinger, M. J., & Pardo, J. V. (1998). Elucidating dynamic brain interactions with across-subjects correlational analyses of positron emission tomographic data: The functional connectivity of the amygdala and orbitofrontal cortex during olfactory tasks. *Journal of Cerebral Blood Flow and Metabolism, 18,* 896–905.

Zald, D. H., Lee, J. T., Fluegel, K. W., & Pardo, J. V. (1998). Aversive gustatory stimulation activates limbic circuits in humans. *Brain, 121*(Pt. 6), 1143–1154.

Zald, D. H., & Pardo, J. V. (1997). Emotion, olfaction, and the human amygdala: Amygdala activation during aversive olfactory stimulation. *Proceedings of the National Academy of Sciences, USA, 94,* 4119–4124.

Zald, D. H., & Pardo, J. V. (2000). Functional neuroimaging of the olfactory system in humans. *International Journal of Psychophysiology, 36,* 165–181.

Zatorre, R. J., Jones-Gotman, M., Evans, A. C., & Meyer, E. (1992). Functional localization of human olfactory cortex. *Nature, 360,* 339–340.

36 Multisensory Perception of Emotion, Its Time Course, and Its Neural Basis

BEATRICE DE GELDER, JEAN VROOMEN, AND GILLES POURTOIS

Introduction

Our senses provide information that often appears to arrive simultaneously from the same spatial location but via different modalities, such as when we *observe* a noisily bouncing ball, *hear* a laughing face, or *see* a burning fire and *smell* smoke. To the observer, spatial and temporal contiguity offers a strong incentive to draw together sensory cues as deriving from a single object or event. Cross-talk between the senses is probably adaptive. By reducing stimulus ambiguity and by insulating the organism from the effects of environmental noise, cross-talk between the senses improves performance. At the level of subjective experience, multisensory integration contributes to a sense of self and an intensified presence of the perceiver in his or her world. This aspect of multisensory integration is particularly relevant for multisensory perception of emotion, which is the focus of this chapter. Indeed, disorders of sensory integration have been associated with loss of the sense of self, as has been documented in schizophrenia (Bleuber, 1911; de Gelder, Vroomen, Annen, Masthof, & Hodiamont, 2003; de Gelder, Vroomen, & Hodiamont, 2003).

Audiovisual emotion perception: A new case of pairing based on event identity pairings

Facial expressions and emotional voice expressions are complex visual and auditory stimuli, whereas multisensory research has traditionally addressed very simple phenomena, such as the combined processing of a light flash and a sound beep. It was found that in such combinations, the presentation of a weak light flash enhanced localization of a weak auditory stimulus presented simultaneously. Many researchers in the field of multisensory perception have argued, either implicitly or explicitly, that focusing on simple stimuli is the safest route to understanding more complex stimuli. One

well-known exception to this bias in favor of physically simple stimuli is audiovisual speech. Another is the audiovisual perception of emotion, which we present here.

Complex cases are inherently of greater interest because they concern situations that are more typical of the rich environment in which the brain operates. Perhaps of more importance, complex cases are also more likely to correspond to environmental situations that resemble constraints the brain faced in the course of evolution. The simplicity of a stimulus as defined in physical terms is not the same as simplicity as defined from an evolutionary point of view. For example, a square is physically a less complex stimulus than a face, yet the latter is evolutionarily more functional and thus "simpler" than the former. Of course, the overall goal is to apply to the study of complex cases methodological imperatives similar to those applied to the study of simple stimulus combinations in the past. Conversely, the investigation of more complex cases may illuminate important issues that await discussion for the simple cases. One such issue is the need to avoid interference from perceptual strategies of the observer; and this concern is equally relevant for the simple and the more complex cases.

We can approach the issue of constraints by asking what makes the more complex cases different from the better known, simpler ones. For this purpose we introduce a distinction between pairings based on *space-time coordinates* and those primarily based on *event identity* (Bertelson & de Gelder, 2003; de Gelder & Bertelson, 2003). The phenomenon of audiovisual pairing of emotion is one example of audiovisual phenomena where pairing seems to be based on event identity, similar to audiovisual speech pairings. When event identity is at stake, cross-talk between the senses is induced not so much by the requirement that the information arrives within the same space-time window, as is typically the case in laboratory experiments with simple stimulus pairings, but by the fact that each modality contributes to event identification. Recognition of event identity is thus an important ingredient of multisensory perception of complex stimulus pairings. Of course, dependence on time makes good functional sense, even when identity plays an important role. For example, synchrony plays a role in audiovisual speech integration (Bertelson, Vroomen, & de Gelder, 1997; Massaro & Egan, 1996; Munhall, Gribble, Sacco, & Ward, 1996). How temporal and spatial factors interact with contraints on pairing that have their basis in recognition of meaningful events is a topic for future research (de Gelder, 2000; de Gelder & Bertelson, 2003; Frissen & de Gelder, 2002).

A mention of the processes involved in recognition of event identity brings to the foreground higher cognitive processes, which play a more important role in complex event recognition. The multisensory perception of event identity depends to some extent on the perceiver's cognitive and emotional state. For instance, integration might depend on the viewer's beliefs about the likelihood that stimuli originated in a single object, or might even be related to the broader cognitive or motivational context in which the stimuli are presented. Such subjective biases would conflict with a major motivation for studying audiovisual integration, which is that it reflects truly perceptual, automatic, and mandatory processes that are not influenced by an observer's strategies or task settings (for recent discussions see Bertelson, 1999; Bertelson & de Gelder, 2003; Pylyshyn, 1999).

Fortunately, a wealth of recent empirical data supports the notion that stimuli that carry emotional information are perceived nonconsciously. Of course, this perceptual kernel can be integrated in later, more cognitive elaborations (LeDoux, 1996), and according to some definitions, emotions do indeed reflect higher cognitive states. This relation indicates that recognition of emotion has a perceptual basis that is insulated from subjective experience, just as, for example, the perception of color has a perceptual basis. For example, we now know that recognition of emotional stimuli proceeds in the absence of awareness (e.g., Morris, Ohman, & Dolan, 1999; Whalen et al., 1998) and, even more radically, in the absence of primary visual cortex (de Gelder, Pourtois, van Raamsdonk, Vroomen, & Weiskrantz, 2001; de Gelder, Vroomen, Pourtois, & Weiskrantz, 1999). The fact that facial expressions are perceived in a mandatory way is thus a good starting point for investigating whether presenting a facial expression together with an affective tone of voice will have an automatic and mandatory effect on perceptual processes in the auditory modality.

To summarize our discussion to this point, from the perspective of the brain's evolutionary history, auditory and visual expressions of emotion are simple stimuli that can be processed independently of subjective consciousness. Against this background it appears plausible that audiovisual pairing of emotional stimuli proceeds in an automatic and mandatory way even if identity plays an important role in this kind of multisensory event.

Before reviewing the research on this phenomenon, we wish to clarify the distinction between the multisensory perception of emotion, on the one hand, and on the other, similarities in the perception of emotion in visual and auditory modalities. As a first approach, we contrast the specific issues related to the perception of multisensory affect with studies that have investigated similarities between perceiving emotion in either the auditory or the visual modality.

Correspondences between perceiving emotion in faces and voices

The overwhelming majority or studies on human emotion recognition have used facial expressions (for a recent overview, see Adolphs, 2002; see also Adolphs, Damasio, Tranel, & Damasio, 1996), but only a few studies have studied how emotion in the voice is perceived (see Ross, 2000, for a review). Researchers have been interested in finding similarities between face and voice recognition and in acquiring empirical evidence for the existence of a common, abstract processing locus that would be shared by visual and auditory affective processes alike (Borod et al., 2000; Van Lancker & Canter, 1982). In support of this perspective, patients with visual impairments were tested for residual auditory abilities, and vice versa. For some time this research was also conducted within a framework of hemispheric differences, and evidence was adduced for right hemispheric involvement in the perception of facial and vocal expressions. More specific questions targeting individual emotions came to the fore as it became increasingly clear that different types (positive vs. negative) and different kinds of emotions (e.g., fear vs. happiness) are subserved by different subsystems of the brain (Adolphs et al., 1996).

It is fair to say that at present, there is no consensus on the existence of a dedicated functional and neuroanatomical locus where both facial and vocal expressions might be processed. A strong case was initially made for a role of the amygdala in recognizing facial as well as vocal expressions of fear, but so far studies have not yielded consistent results (Scott et al., 1997; but see Adolphs & Tranel, 1999; Anderson & Phelps, 1998).

Moreover, researchers have usually approached the issue of a common functional and possibly neuro-anatomical basis for recognition of vocal and facial expressions by looking for correlations (Borod et al., 2000). But such data are not directly useful to understanding how, when both the face and the voice are present (as is often the case in natural conditions), the two information streams are actually integrated. Whether or not amodal or abstract representation systems exist that use representations that transcend either modality (but that can be shared by both, and thereby play a role in processing auditory as well as visual information) is at present an empirical question. It is also worth noting that the issue of a common basis reappears in a very different context, as we will see when discussing models of audiovisual integration.

Behavioral experiments measuring cross-modal bias between facial and vocal expressions: A first review and some methodological issues

In our first behavioral studies of intersensory perception of affect, we adapted a paradigm frequently used in studies of audiovisual speech (Massaro, 1998). We combined a facial expression with a short auditory vocal segment and instructed participants to attend to and categorize either the face or the voice, depending on the condition. These experiments provided clear evidence that an emotional voice expression that is irrelevant for the task at hand can influence the categorization of a facial expression presented simultaneously (de Gelder, Vroomen, & Teunisse, 1995). Specifically, participants categorizing a happy or fearful facial expression were systematically influenced by the expression of the voice (e.g., the face was judged as less fearful if the voice sounded happy) (Fig. 36.1). Massaro and Egan (1996) obtained similar results using a synthetic facial expression paired with a vocal expression. Subsequently we explored the situation in which participants were asked to ignore the face but had to rate the expression of the voice. A very similar cross-modal effect was observed for recognition of the emotional expression in the voice (de Gelder & Vroomen, 2000, Experiment 3). The effect of the face on voice recognition disappeared when facial images were presented upside down, adding further proof that the facial expression was the critical variable (de Gelder, Vroomen, & Bertelson, 1998). It is worth noting that these bias effects were obtained with stimulus pairs consisting of a static face and a vocal expression. With the exception of one behavioral study done in a cortically blind patient, in which we used short video clips with mismatched voice fragments (de Gelder, Pourtois, Vroomen, & Weiskrantz, 1999), all effects were obtained

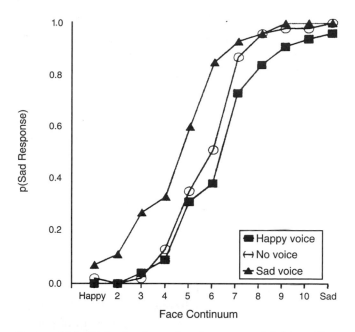

FIGURE 36.1 Behavioral results. A cross-modal bias effect from the voice to the face is indicated by a systematic response bias toward the concurrent tone of voice when participants were asked to judge the emotion in the face.

with static facial images. One might object that such pairs are not entirely ecological, because in naturalistic situations the voice one hears belongs to a moving face. But support for the use of static stimuli is provided by studies indicating that the perception of emotion in faces is linked to processes inducing imitation (Dimberg, Thunberg, & Elmehed, 2000) and experiencing of the emotion (Adolphs, Damasio, Tranel, Cooper, & Damasio, 2000).

In the behavioral experiments, we used the paradigm of *cross-modal bias*, one of the few classical paradigms known to provide evidence for intersensory integration. (Other useful paradigms include the study of aftereffects and of intersensory fusion; for a discussion, see Bertelson, 1999; Bertelson & de Gelder, 2003.) Cross-modal bias measures the on-line effect of intersensory conflict on the task-relevant input modality; in other words, it measures how processing in the task-relevant modality is biased in the direction of the information presented in the other modality. As such, it is a measure of on-line conflict resolution. In contrast, studies of aftereffects investigate the consequences of intersensory conflict resolution by observing how perception in one modality is more or less permanently changed as a consequence of intersensory conflict. A major advantage of this approach is its robustness in the light of possible confounds. When measuring aftereffects one need be much less concerned with the possibility that the results are contaminated by the perceiver's perceptual bias.

Until now, aftereffects were exclusively measured in studies of spatial and temporal aspects of intersensory conflict. Only recently was the methodology applied successfully to the study of conflict at the level of stimulus identity for speech (Bertelson, Vroomen, & de Gelder, 2003). Because of its robustness, it is also a good tool for studying other situations of cross-talk between the senses due to presumed event identity effects. We are currently exploring the aftereffects of exposure to audiovisual conflict in affective pairs.

In cross-modal bias paradigms, the behavioral measures are accuracy and latency (see Massaro, 1999, for a full discussion). These measures can be influenced by factors such as attention, task demands, or subjective response bias. The situation of multisensory paradigms is quite similar to that used in studies of the redundant target effect (Miller, 1982, 1986). In both cases the experimenter measures the impact of a task-irrelevant secondary stimulus on the accuracy and latency of performance. By themselves, differences in either measure are not sufficient to demonstrate that multisensory integration has occurred and that performance primarily reflects the observer's experience of a single percept. Moreover, the typical effects on behavior of the presentation of a secondary stimulus as manifested in latency and accuracy are also observed when two stimuli are presented simultaneously and the secondary stimulus is presented in the same modality as the target. This is typically the case when a secondary visual stimulus is presented together with a primary visual stimulus. It is difficult to decide whether the observed behavioral effects reflect multisensory perceptual integration or instead are due to the influence of the secondary stimulus on how the task is performed. Unfortunately, such matters cannot be resolved by showing that the data fit a mathematical model, such as the FMLP (Massaro & Egan, 1996). More generally, such models do not distinguish well between effects that result from early integration and late decision-based ones (de Gelder & Vroomen, 2000). Behavioral methods need to be applied in concert with neurophysiological methods to make progress here.

A role for attention in audiovisual emotion perception

Cognitive theories of attention, like the one defended by Treisman (1996), predict that attention plays a critical role in combining isolated cues present in different modalities, thus making attention the prime candidate for bringing about intersensory integration. In other words, if attention plays a critical role, we would no longer observe a cross-modal bias when subjects are entirely focused on the task related to one modality and not paying attention to information in the other modality that is irrelevant to the task at hand. When this is indeed the case, it follows that for some intersensory processes, which one would then want to qualify as genuinely perceptual, attention does not play a critical role in bringing about integration or explaining its effects. In other words, if cross-modal integration of affective information is a truly automatic process, it should take place regardless of the demands of an additional task. Indeed, independence from demands on attentional capacity has long been one of the defining characteristics of "automatic" processes (see Shiffrin & Schneider, 1977). For example, we considered the role of either exogenous (reflexive, involuntary) or endogenous (voluntary) attention in ventriloquism. We found no evidence that either played a role in sound to visual location attraction (Bertelson, Vroomen, de Gelder, & Driver, 2000; Vroomen, Bertelson, & de Gelder, 2001).

To address whether attention plays a causal role in bringing about multisensory integration, one should really ask whether, if participants had to judge the voice, there would be a cross-modal effect from the facial to the vocal judgments if the face were not attended to. Recent research on attention has shown that irrelevant visual stimuli may be particularly hard to ignore under "low-load" attention conditions, yet they can be successfully ignored under higher-load conditions in which the specified task consumes more attentional capacity (e.g., Lavie, 1995, 2000). The facial expression in de Gelder and Vroomen's study (2000, Experiment 3), although irrelevant for the task, in which participants were required to judge emotion in the voice, might therefore have been unusually hard to ignore, due to the low-load attention of the task situation (the face was the only visual stimulus present, and the only task requirement was categorization of the voice). It is thus possible that the influence of the seen facial expression on judgments of the emotional tone of a heard voice would be eliminated under conditions of higher attentional load (e.g., with additional visual stimuli present and with a demanding additional task).

Attention as a possible binding factor was studied in a dual-task format in which we asked whether cross-modal integration of affective information would suffer when a demanding task had to be performed concurrently (Vroomen, Driver, & de Gelder, 2001). A positive result, meaning an effect of attentional load on the degree of integration taking place, would suggest that attentional resources are required for cross-modal integration of emotion to occur. If, on the other hand, a competing task did not influence performance, it is reasonably safe to assume that cross-modal interactions do not require attentional resources (Kahneman, 1973). Thus, we measured the influence of a visible static facial expression on judgments of the emotional tone of a voice (as in de Gelder & Vroomen, 2000) while varying attentional demands by presenting participants with an additional attention-capturing task.

A general concern in applying the dual-task method is whether tasks compete for the same pool of resources or whether there are multiple resource pools each of which deals separately with the various cognitive and perceptual aspects of the two tasks (Wickens, 1984). When tasks do not interfere, it may be that one of the tasks (or both) does not require any attentional resources (i.e., they are performed automatically), or it may be that they draw on different resource pools. To distinguish between these alternatives, we varied the nature of the additional task. If none of the different tasks interfered with the cross-modal interactions, this result would suggest that the cross-modal effect itself does not require attention. Participants judged whether a voice expressed happiness or fear while trying to ignore a concurrently presented static facial expression. As an additional task, participants were instructed to add two numbers together rapidly (Experiment 1), or to count the occurrences of a target digit in a rapid serial visual presentation (Experiment 2), or judge the pitch of a tone as high or low (Experiment 3). The face had an impact on judgments of the heard voice emotion in all experiments. This cross-modal effect was independent of whether or not subjects performed a demanding additional task. This result indicates that the integration of visual and auditory information about emotions is a mandatory process, unconstrained by attentional resources. It is also worth pointing out at this stage that in order to rule out response bias in later studies, we used an orthogonal task, for example sex classification, which did not require attending to the emotional content.

Recent neurophysiological techniques provide means of looking at intersensory fusion before its effects are manifest in behavior. Each of these methods has its limits. Theoretical conclusions that strive to be general and to transcend particular techniques, whether behavioral or neurophysiological, about multisensory perception require convergence from different methods. (For example, it is still difficult to relate a measure such as a gain in latency observed in behavioral studies and an increase in blood-oxygen-level-dependent [BOLD] signal measured on functional magnetic resonance imaging (fMRI), or the degree of cell firing and degree of BOLD signal.) Our first studies used electroencephalographic (EEG) recordings to acquire insight into the time course of integration. Our goal was to reduce the role of attention and of stimulus awareness through the use of indirect tasks. The focus on early effects and the selective study of clinical populations with specific deficits helped to clarify some central aspects of automatic multisensory perception of affect.

Electrophysiological studies of the time course of multisensory affect perception

To investigate the time course of face-voice integration of emotion, we exploited the high temporal resolution provided by event-related brain potentials (ERPs) and explored its neuroanatomical location using source localization models. Electrophysiological studies (either EEG or MEG) of multisensory perception have indicated large amplitude effects, sometimes consisting in an increase and at other times in a decrease of early exogenous components such as the auditory N1 or the visual P1 component (each generated around 100 ms for stimulus presentation in their respective modality) during presentation of multisensory stimuli (Foxe et al., 2000; Giard & Peronnet, 1999; Raij, Uutela, & Hari, 2000; Rockland & Ojima, 2003; Sams et al., 1991). Amplification of the neural signal in modality-specific cortex is thought to reflect an electrophysiological correlate of intersensory integration and has been observed when responses to multisensory presentations are compared with responses to the single-modality presentations individually. On the other hand, a decrease in amplitude is sometimes observed when the comparison focuses specifically on the contrast between congruent versus incongruent bimodal conditions (de Gelder, Pourtois, & Weiskrantz, 2002).

In our first study we used the phenomenon of *mismatch negativity* (MMN; Näätänen, 1992) as a means of tracing the time course of the combination of the affective tone of voice with information provided by the expression of the face (de Gelder, Böcker, Tuomainen, Hensen, & Vroomen, 1999). In the standard condition subjects were presented with concurrent voice and face stimuli with identical affective content (a fearful face paired with a fearful voice). On the anomalous trials the vocal expression was accompanied by a face with an incongruent expression. We reasoned that if the system was tuned to combine these inputs, as was suggested by our behavioral experiments, and if integration is reflected by an influence of the face on how the voice is processed, this would be apparent in some auditory ERP components. Our results indicated that when presentations of a voice-face pair with the same expression were followed by presentation of a pair in which the voice stimulus was the same but the facial expression was different, an early (170 ms) deviant response with

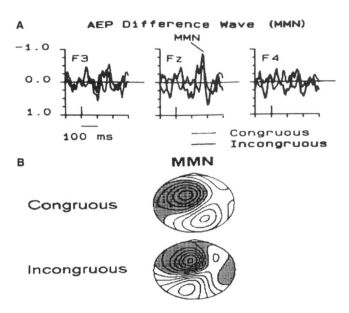

MMN

Congruous

Incongruous

FIGURE 36.2   EEG results. (A) The grand averaged deviant −
standard difference wave of the auditory brain potential for
both congruent (thin line) and incongruent (thick line) face-
voice pairs. Surplus negativity evoked by the deviant stimulus
pair is plotted upward. The vertical bar on the x-axis indicates
the onset of the auditory stimulus. Amplitude (μV) is plotted
on the y-axis. (B) The isopotential map (0.1 μV between lines;
shaded area negative) at 178 ms, showing the scalp distribution of the mismatch negativity (MMN) for voices with congruent and incongruent faces.

frontal topography was elicited (Fig. 36.2). This response strongly resembles the MMN, which is typically
associated with a change (whether in intensity, duration or location) in a train of standard, repetitive auditory stimuli (Näätänen, 1992). Our results are consistent with previous EEG results (Surakka, Tenhunen-
Eskelinen, Hietanen, & Sams, 1998) showing that pitch
MMN may be influenced by the simultaneous presentation of positive nonfacial stimuli (colored light
flashes).

Converging evidence for the integrated perception
of facial expressions and spoken sentence fragments
was provided in a follow-up EEG study (Pourtois, de
Gelder, Vroomen, Rossion, & Crommelinck, 2000) in
which we measured the early effects of adding a facial
expression to a sentence fragment spoken in an emotional tone of voice. Significant increases in the amplitude of P1 and auditory N200 were obtained for congruent face-voice pairs but not for incongruent ones, or
for pairs in which the face was presented upside down.
In a subsequent study (Pourtois, Debatisse, Despland, &
de Gelder, 2002), we showed that congruent face-voice
pairs elicited an earlier P2b component (the P2b component follows the auditory P2 exogenous component
with a more posterior topography) than incongruent

pairs (Fig. 36.3; Color Plate 17). This result suggests
that the processing of affective prosody is delayed in the
presence of an incongruent facial context. The temporal and topographical properties of the P2b component
suggest that this component does not overlap with EEG
components (e.g., the N2-P3 complex) known to be involved in cognitive processes at later decisional stages.
Source localization carried out on the time window of
the P2b component disclosed a single dipole solution in
anterior cingulate cortex, an area selectively implicated
in processing congruency or conflict between stimuli
(MacLeod & MacDonald, 2000). The contribution of
anterior cingulate cortex in dealing with perceptual
and cognitive congruency has been shown in many previous brain imaging studies (Cabeza & Nyberg, 2000).
The anterior cingulate is also one of the areas strongly
associated with human motivational and emotion
processes (Mesulam, 1998).

*Neuroanatomy of audiovisual perception
of emotion*

There are as yet only few general theoretical suggestions
in the literature concerning the neuroanatomical correlates of multisensory integration (e.g., Damasio, 1989;
Ettlinger & Wilson, 1990; Mesulam, 1998). Recent studies have considered a variety of audiovisual situations,
including arbitrarily associated pairs (Fuster, Bodner, &
Kroger, 2000; Giard & Peronnet, 1999; Schröger &
Widmann, 1998), naturalistic pairs, such as audiovisual
speech pairs (Calvert et al., 1999; Raij et al., 2000), and
audiovisual affect pairs (de Gelder, Böcker, et al., 1999;
Dolan, Morris, & de Gelder, 2001; Pourtois et al., 2000).

Our first study directly addressing the audiovisual integration of emotion with brain imaging methods
(fMRI) suggested that an important element of a mechanism for such cross-modal binding in the case of fearful face-voice pairs is be found in the amygdala (Dolan
et al., 2001). In this study, subjects heard auditory fragments paired with either a congruent or an incongruent facial expression (happiness or fearfulness) and
were instructed to judge the emotion from the face.
When fearful faces were accompanied by short sentence fragments spoken in a fearful tone of voice, an
increase in activation was observed in the amygdala
(Fig. 36.4; Color Plate 18) and the fusiform gyrus. The
increased amygdala activation suggests binding of face
and voice expressions (Goulet & Murray, 2001), but further research is needed to investigate the underlying
mechanism. Unlike in our behavioral studies, no advantage was observed for happy pairs. This could suggest
that the rapid integration across modalities is not as automatic for happy expressions as it is for fear signals.

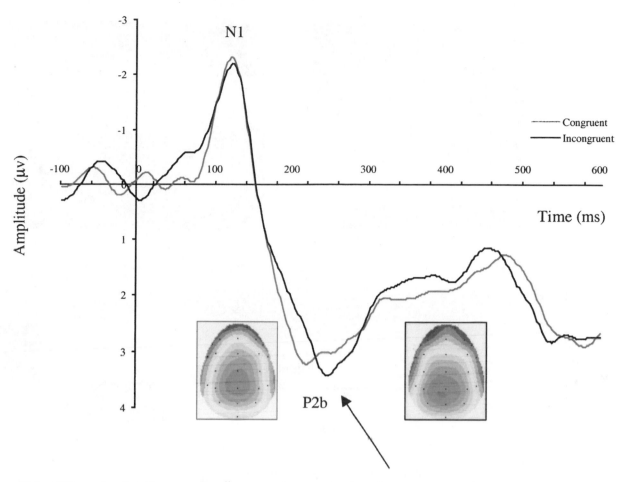

FIGURE 36.3 EEG results. Grand averaged auditory waveforms at the CPz electrode measured during the presentation of congruent and incongruent audiovisual stimulus pairs (and corresponding topographies at 224 ms and 242 ms in the congruent and incongruent condition, respectively). Auditory processing is delayed in time by around 220 ms when realized under an incongruent visual context. (See Color Plate 17.)

More generally, such a finding is consistent with increasing awareness of the neurobiological specificity of each emotion.

In a follow-up study (Pourtois, de Gelder, Bol, & Crommelinck, 2003) performed using $H_2^{15}O$ PET, we compared activations to unimodal stimuli and to bimodal pairs in order to find areas specifically involved in audiovisual integration. We also investigated whether activation in heteromodal areas would be accompanied by increased activation in modality-specific cortices (such as the primary auditory cortex or primary visual cortex). The latter phenomenon has been reported previously and can tentatively be viewed as a downstream consequence in modality-specific cortex of multisensory integration (see Calvert, Campbell, & Brammer, 2000; de Gelder, 2000; Dolan et al., 2001; Driver & Spence, 2000; Macaluso, Frith, & Driver, 2000). Such feedback or top-down modulations could be the correlate of the well-known cross-modal bias effects typically observed in behavioral studies of audiovisual

perception (Bertelson, 1999; Bertelson & de Gelder, 2003). But some of these effects might in part depend on attention to the task-related modality. The fact that attentional demands can modulate the effects of multisensory integration is still entirely consistent with the notion that attention itself is not the basis of intersensory integration (for discussion, see Bertelson et al., 2000; de Gelder, 2000; McDonald, Teder-Sälejärvi, & Ward, 2001; Vroomen, Bertelson, et al., 2001, for a discussion). To avoid attentional modulation, we used a gender decision task that does not require attention to the emotion expressed, whether in the voice, the face, or both. Our main results suggest that the perception of audiovisual emotions activates a cortical region situated in the left middle temporal gyrus (MTG) and the left anterior fusiform gyrus (Fig. 36.5; Color Plate 19). The MTG has already been shown to be involved in multisensory integration (Streicher & Ettlinger, 1987) and has been described as a convergence region between multiple modalities (Damasio, 1989; Mesulam, 1998).

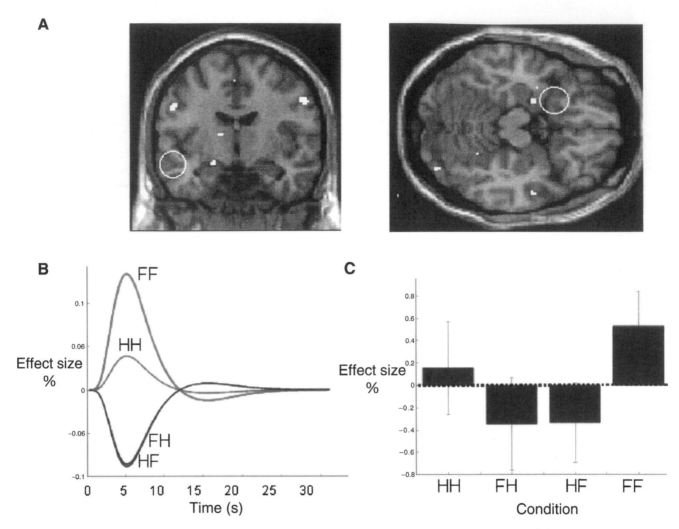

FIGURE 36.4 fMRI results. A statistical parametric map shows an enhanced response in the left amygdala in response to congruent fearful faces plus fearful voices. Condition: H, happy; F, fearful. (See Color Plate 18.)

Activation of the fusiform gyrus is consistent with the results of our previous fMRI study (Dolan et al., 2001) of recognition of facial expression paired with tones of voice. Interestingly, our results showed that within the left MTG (BA 21), there was no difference between visual and auditory levels of activation, but instead there was a significant increase for the audiovisual condition compared with the unimodal conditions. Of note, activation in the left MTG did not correspond to an increase in regional cerebral blood flow (rCBF) in regions that are modality-specific. Moreover, activations were also observed separately for the two emotions when visual and auditory stimuli were presented concurrently. "Happy" audiovisual trials activate different frontal and prefrontal regions (BA 8, 9, 10, and 46) that are all lateralized in the left hemisphere, while audiovisual "fear" activates the superior temporal gyrus in the right hemisphere, confirming strong hemispheric asymmetries in the processing of positively (pleasant) versus negatively (unpleasant) valenced stimuli (see Davidson & Irwin, 1999, for a review).

An intriguing possibility is that presentation in one modality activates areas typically associated with stimulation in the other modality. For example, using fMRI we investigated auditory sadness and observed strong and specific orbitofrontal activity. Moreover, in line with the possibility just raised, among the observed foci there was strong activation of the left fusiform gyrus, an area typically devoted to face processing, following presentation of sad voices (Malik, de Gelder, & Breiter, in prep.). A similar effect was observed by Calvert and collaborators studying audiovisual speech. They found activation of auditory cortex following presentation of silent speech movements (Calvert et al., 1997). For the case of emotion, such effects also make sense when one takes into account that sensorimotor cortex plays a role in the perception of emotional expressions of the face (Adolphs, 2002).

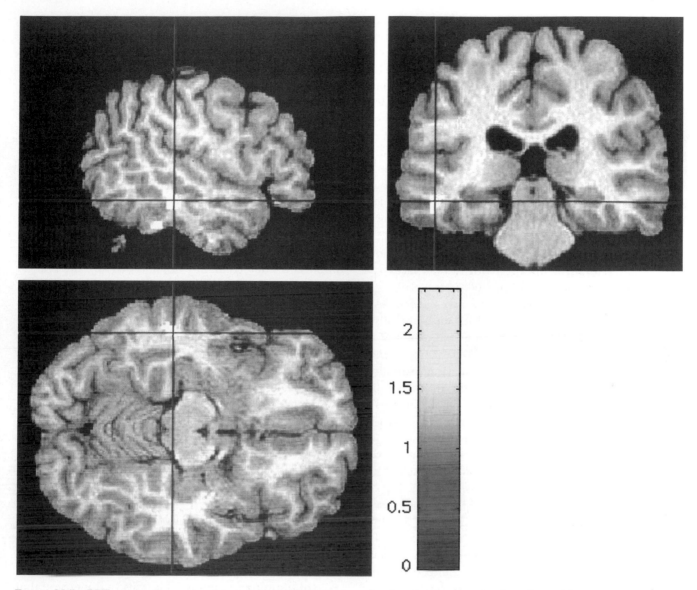

FIGURE 36.5 PET results. Coronal, axial, and sagittal PET sections showing significant activation of a multisensory region in the left middle temporal gyrus ($-52x$, $-30y$, $-12z$) in eight normal subjects during audiovisual trials (happy and fearful emotions) compared with unimodal trials (Visual + Auditory). (See Color Plate 19.)

Much more research is needed before we can begin to understand what is common to the different instances of audiovisual integration. A small number of candidate areas for audiovisual integration have been reported so far, but it is difficult to generalize from the available evidence. Comparisons are also complicated by differences in paradigms, in the choice of baseline, and in the use of different control conditions in each of these studies. For example, arbitrary audiovisual pairs have been used as a control condition for audiovisual speech pairs (Raij et al., 2000; Sams et al., 1991), but other studies have used meaningless grimaces (Calvert et al., 1997). In other studies the sum of unimodal activation in each modality has been used as a baseline (Calvert et al., 2000). Also, different analytic strategies

are available, such as strategies that contrast unimodal versus multimodal situations or bimodal congruent situations with bimodal incongruent ones.

Selectivity in audiovisual affect pairing

How selective is the pairing mechanism underlying pairings in which event identity plays a critical role? So far we have mentioned studies of audiovisual affect in which the visual stimuli consisted of facial expressions. Such pairings are based on congruence in stimulus identity—that is, emotional meaning—across the two input modalities. However, other visual stimuli, such as objects and pictures of visual scenes, also carry affective information and are equally conspicuous in the daily environment.

Similarly, there are other sources of auditory affect information besides affective prosody, the most obvious candidates being word meaning and nonverbal auditory signals. If semantic relationship were the only determinant of identity-based pairings, either of those visual inputs should combine with either of those two alternative auditory messages. Selectivity is an important issue for identity pairings, and learning more about it should reveal important insights into the biological basis of multisensory perception. On the other hand, we do not know to what extent the familiar boundaries of our own species are the limits of our biological endowment. For example, for human observers, the facial expressions of higher apes might bind more easily with vocalizations than visual scenes do because vocalizations share more biologically relevant properties with human faces (de Gelder, van Ommeren, & Frissen, 2003).

The matter of selectivity has recently been investigated in a number of ways. In one ERP study, the possible biological basis of identity pairings was explored by contrasting two kinds of auditory components, prosodic and semantic, for the same visual stimulus. Our goal was to find indicators for the difference between the two kinds of auditory stimuli combined with the same visual stimulus. We contrasted the impact of affective prosody (Prosodic condition) versus word meaning (Semantic condition) of a spoken word on the way a facial expression was processed. To test for the presence of specific audiovisual responses in the EEG at the level of the scalp, we compared ERPs to audiovisual trials (AV) with brain responses for visual plus auditory stimuli trials (A + V) (Barth, Goldberg, Brett, & Di, 1995). Subjects performed a gender discrimination task chosen because it was unrelated to the effects studied. In both conditions, ERPs for AV trials were higher in amplitude than ERPs for A + V trials. This amplification effect was manifested for early peaks with a central topography, such as N1 (at 110 ms), P2 (at 200 ms), and N2 (at 250 ms). However, our results indicated that the time course of responses face-voice pairings differs from that of responses to face-word pairings. The important finding was that the amplification effect observed for AV trials occurred earlier for face-voice pairings than for face-word parings. The amplification effect associated with AV presentations and manifested at the level of the scalp was already observed at around 110 ms in the Prosodic condition, whereas this effect was at its maximum later (around 200 ms) in the Semantic condition. These results suggest different nonoverlapping time courses for affective prosodic pairing versus semantic word pairing.

We subsequently addressed the same issue using a different technique, single-pulse transcranial magnetic stimulation (TMS) (Pourtois & de Gelder, 2002). Two types of stimulus pairs were compared, one consisting of arbitrary paired stimuli in which the pairing was learned, and the other consisting of natural pairings as described above. Participants were trained on the two types of pairs to ensure that the same level of performance was obtained for both. Our hypothesis was that TMS would interfere with cross-modal bias obtained with meaningless shape-tone pairs (Learned condition) but not with the cross-modal bias effect of voice-face pairs (Natural condition). Single-pulse TMS applied over the left posterior parietal cortex at 50, 100, 150, and 200 ms disrupted integration at 150 ms and later, but only for the learned pairs. Our results suggest that content specificity as manipulated here could be an important determinant of audiovisual integration (Fig. 36.6; Color Plate 20). Such a position is consistent with some recent results indicating domain specific sites of intersensory integration. Content is likely to represent an important constraint on audiovisual integration.

A different way of investigating selectivity is by looking at possible contrasts between pairings that are presented under conditions of normal stimulus awareness and outside the scope of visual consciousness. This approach might be particularly sensitive to the contrast between facial expressions and emotional scenes, given the special evolutionary status of faces. We comment on this research line in the next section, in a discussion on consciousness.

Qualitative differences between conscious and nonconscious audiovisual perception

An important aspect of audiovisual integration is the role of stimulus awareness. This is also a dimension that has so far rarely been considered but that appears important in light of findings about the unconscious processing of facial expressions (de Gelder, Vroomen, et al., 1999; Morris et al., 1999; Whalen et al., 1998). If we can obtain evidence that unseen stimuli, or at least stimuli the observer is not aware of, still exert a cross-modal bias, then the case for an automatic, mandatory perceptual phenomenon is even stronger. By the same token, the requirement that audiovisual bias should be studied in situations that are minimally transparent to the observer is met equally well when observers are unaware of the second element of the stimulus pair. Patients with visual agnosia that includes an inability to recognize facial expressions pose a unique opportunity for investigating this issue. We studied a patient with visual agnosia and severe facial recognition problems due to bilateral occipitotemporal damage (Bartolomeo et al., 1998; de Gelder, Pourtois, Vroomen, & Bachoud-Levi, 2000; Peterson,

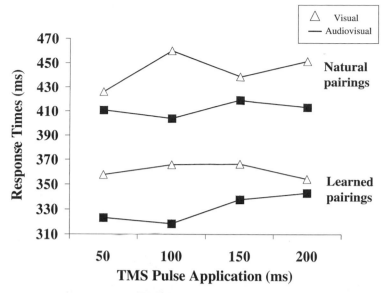

FIGURE 36.6   Results of the TMS experiment. Response times are plotted as a function of the SOA between stimulus presentation and pulse deliverance (a single pulse was delivered 50, 100, 150, or 200 ms after stimulus presentation) when TMS is applied over the left posterior parietal cortex. In the Learned condition (burst tone paired with geometrical figure), there was significant interaction between Modality × SOA, indicating that audiovisual trials are not faster than visual trials at 200 ms. In the Natural condition (tone of voice paired with facial expression), the interaction Modality × SOA is not significant. (See Color Plate 20.)

de Gelder, Rapcsak, Gerhardstein, & Bachoud-Levi, 2000). Her recognition of facial expressions is almost completely lost, although recognition of emotions in voices is intact. This combination allowed us to look at spared covert recognition of facial expressions, as we could use a cross-modal bias paradigm. With this indirect testing method we found clear evidence of covert recognition, as her recognition of emotions in the voice was systematically affected by the facial expression that accompanied the voice fragment she was rating (de Gelder et al., 2000).

Patients with hemianopia but who have retained some residual visual abilities (see Weiskrantz, 1986, 1997) offer an even more radical opportunity to study audiovisual integration under conditions in which there was no awareness of the stimuli presented. Moreover, such cases offer a window onto the neuroanatomy of nonconscious visual processes and the role of striate cortex in visual awareness. Phenomenologically, these patients manifest the same pattern as patients with visual agnosia, because in both cases, conscious recognition of the facial expression is impaired. In the hemianopic patient G. Y. we found behavioral and electrophysiological evidence for a cross-modal bias of unseen facial expressions on processing of the emotion in the voice (de Gelder, Vroomen, & Pourtois, 2001). More recently we looked at a possible interaction between awareness and type of audiovisual pairing (de Gelder et al., 2002). For this purpose we designed two types of pairs, each with a different visual component. One type

of pair consisted of facial expression/voice pairs and the other type consisted of emotional scene/voice pairs. In this study, the face/voice pairs figured as the natural pairings and the scene/voice pairs as the semantic ones. Intersensory integration was studied in two hemianopic patients with a complete unilateral lesion of the primary visual cortex. ERPs were measured in these two patients, and we compared the pattern obtained in the intact hemisphere, with patients conscious of the visual stimuli, with that obtained in the blind hemisphere, where there was no visual awareness. We explored the hypothesis that unlike natural pairings, semantic pairings might require conscious perception and mediation by intact visual cortex (possibly based on feedback to primary cortex from higher cognitive processes). Our results indicate that adding visual affective information to the voice results in an amplitude increase of auditory-evoked potentials, an effect that obtains for both natural and semantic pairings in the intact field but is limited to the natural pairings in the blind field (Fig. 36.7; Color Plate 21). These results are in line with previous studies that have provided evidence in favor of qualitatively different processing systems for conscious and nonconscious perception (LeDoux, 1996; Weiskrantz, 1997).

With the possibility of different systems for conscious and nonconscious processes, some novel and intriguing possibilities arise. First, it is in principle possible that conflicts between the two systems could arise when two different stimuli are simultaneously presented in the

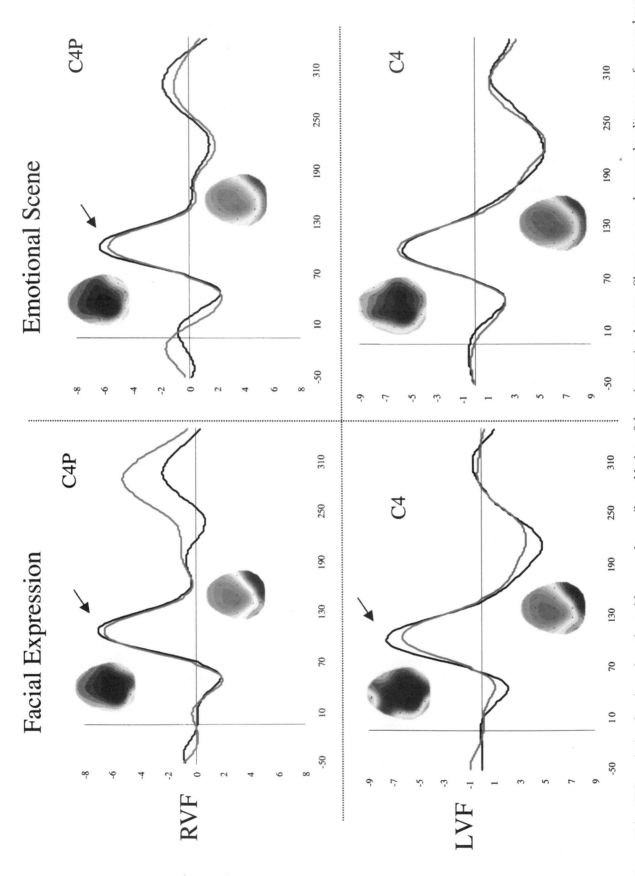

FIGURE 36.7 EEG results in a hemianopic patient with a complete unilateral lesion of the primary visual cortex. Shown are grand averaged auditory waveforms and corresponding topographies (horizontal axis) obtained at central electrodes in each visual condition (congruent pairs in black, incongruent pairs in red) and for each visual hemifield (left/blind vs. right/intact). Congruent pairs elicited a higher auditory N1 component than incongruent pairs for visual presentations (facial expressions or emotional scenes) in the intact field but, only for facial expressions in the blind field. For each topographic map (N1 and P2 components), the time interval is 20 ms and the amplitude scale goes from −6 μV (in blue) to +6 μV (in red). (See Color Plate 21.)

blind field and in the intact field. Second, different integration effects might obtain for conscious and nonconscious presentation of visual stimuli, and integration effects might obtain for the former but not for the latter. We began to explore such situations by taking advantage of the blindsight phenomenon. Participants were presented with visual stimuli (either faces or scenes) and auditory stimuli. Only amygdala responses to faces (and not scenes) are enhanced by congruent voices (in either the intact or the blind field). There are enhanced fusiform responses to faces (but not to scenes) with congruent voices (as in de Gelder et al., 2002). When looking at blind versus intact differences there are activations of superior colliculus (SC) for blind fearful faces (but not for blind fearful scenes). Fusiform responses are enhanced more by congruent voice-face pairings in the intact field than in the blind field. But the SC activation in response to fearful faces is enhanced by congruency between voices and faces, and the enhancement is greater for presentation in the blind field than for presentation in the intact field (de Gelder, Morris, & Dolan, in prep.). These results indicate that awareness of the stimulus plays an important role in the pairings obtained. This aspect warrants more attention in other areas of multisensory research.

Models for multisensory perception of affect

So far, our studies have explored the perceptual dimension of multisensory affect perception mainly by trying to rule out postperceptual biases. If we take audiovisual speech as the closest example at hand, it is fair to say that at present, a number of different models of integration can be envisaged (Summerfield, 1987), without any compelling arguments in favor of any of them. More research is needed before some theoretical models offered for audiovisual speech can be completely ruled out for the case of audiovisual emotion. For example, we have distinguished between the traditional problem of finding parallels between facial and vocal expression deficits. Although these are two different issues, we do not rule out that emotional face- and voice-recognition processes might have a lot in common. Nor can one rule out at present a second theoretical possibility, which assumes recoding of one of the input representations into the format of the other (e.g., visual representations recoded into auditory ones). Likewise, we must still consider that both sensory representations are recoded into a supramodal abstract representation system (Farah, Wong, Monheit, & Morrow, 1989). A complicating factor that is specific to the case of audiovisual affect is that the integration mechanism might be sensitive to the specific affective content, such that the

mechanism for fear integration might actually be different from that for sad or happy pairings. For example, we observed an increase in amygdala activation for fearful voice-face combinations but not for happy ones (Dolan et al., 2001). Converging evidence from different methods is needed to make some progress in understanding these complex issues.

One reason why we became interested in the issue of selectivity of pairings is that it might provide cues as to the underpinnings of emotional perception. Would a special status of voice-face pairs indicate that there exists a specific functional underpinning for this kind of pair? According to this view, scene-voice pairs, scene-word pairings, or face-word pairs would have different characteristics than face-voice pairs. One possible interpretation, although a rather speculative one, for the special status of the voice prosody-face pairings is that they are mediated by action schemes (de Gelder & Bertelson, 2003). The analogy that comes to mind here is that of articulatory representation or phonetic gestures, in the sense of abstract representations that figure in the description of auditorily transmitted as well as visually transmitted speech. Ultimately, a notion of motor schemes could be developed along similar lines as was done for the motor theory of speech perception (Liberman & Mattingly, 1985). This action framework suggests an interesting interpretation for the special status of some kinds of audiovisual pairings. Some stimulus combinations make pairings that are always congruent when they occur in naturalistic circumstances. They are so tightly linked that a special effort is needed in the laboratory to separate them and to rearrange the pairings into incongruent combinations for the purpose of experiments. We have used the notion of biologically determined (de Gelder & Bertelson, 2003) or of naturalistic pairings (Pourtois & de Gelder, 2002) to characterize that type of pairing. Which pairings are naturalistic is obviously a significant issue for future empirical research. Evolutionary arguments by themselves are too general and too open-ended to provide specific constraints on the action repertoire of an organism.

Conclusions

Our overview of audiovisual emotion perception has brought together different topics of interest in this new field. Various themes have emerged in the course of this discussion. Some themes are methodological. An example is the need to base conclusions on converging lines of evidence obtained with different methods, such as behavioral and brain imaging studies, because these methods use different metrics. Comparing data is hard, but with progress in multimodal imaging methods, such comparisons should become easier. Other themes that have been addressed in this chapter are more theoretical. We asked whether attention is the glue of audiovisual emotion perception, and we have described some data pointing to a negative answer. We made a beginning by distinguishing different types of audiovisual pairs as we contrasted arbitrary and natural pairs. In the category of natural emotion pairs, and in particular with respect to the auditory component, the difference between semantic and prosodic components turned out to be important. We questioned whether awareness was an important factor in audiovisual integration of emotions, and we found that in fact it was, at least in some cases. Moreover, awareness needs to be considered a critical variable for understanding the kinds of pairings obtained under different circumstances. All of these themes are important for future research on audiovisual emotion, yet none is specific to this domain. Instead, we are dealing with a phenomenon that is basic to our understanding of multisensory integration and important for the study of emotion.

REFERENCES

Adolphs, R. (2002). Recognizing emotion from facial expressions: Psychological and neurological mechanisms. *Behavioral and Cognitive Neuroscience Reviews, 1,* 21–61.

Adolphs, R., Damasio, H., Tranel, D., Cooper, G., & Damasio, A. D. (2000). A role for somatosensory cortices in the visual recognition of emotion as revealed by three-dimensional lesion mapping. *Journal of Neuroscience, 20,* 2683–2690.

Adolphs, R., Damasio, H., Tranel, D., & Damasio, A. R. (1996). Cortical systems for the recognition of emotion in facial expressions. *Journal of Neuroscience, 16,* 7678–7687.

Adolphs, R., & Tranel, D. (1999). Preferences for visual stimuli following amygdala damage. *Journal of Cognitive Neuroscience, 6,* 610–616.

Anderson, A. K., & Phelps, E. A. (1998). Intact recognition of vocal expressions of fear following bilateral lesions of the human amygdala. *Neuroreport, 9,* 3607–3613.

Barth, D. S., Goldberg, N., Brett, B., & Di, S. (1995). The spatiotemporal organization of auditory, visual, and auditory-visual evoked potentials in rat cortex. *Brain Research, 678,* 177–190.

Bartolomeo, P., Bachoud-Levi, A. C., de Gelder, B., Denes, G., Dalla Barba, G., Brugieres, P., et al. (1998). Multiple-domain dissociation between impaired visual perception and preserved mental imagery in a patient with bilateral extrastriate lesions. *Neuropsychologia, 36,* 239–249.

Bertelson, P. (1999). Ventriloquism: A case of crossmodal perceptual grouping. In G. Aschersleben, T. Bachmann, & J. Musseler (Eds.), *Cognitive contributions to the perception of spatial and temporal events* (pp. 347–362). Amsterdam: Elsevier.

Bertelson, P., & de Gelder, B. (2003). The psychology of multisensory perception. In C. Spence & J. Driver (Eds.), *Crossmodal space and crossmodal attention.* Oxford, England: Oxford University Press.

Bertelson, P., Vroomen, J., & de Gelder, B. (1997). Auditory-visual interaction in voice localisation and b-modal speech recognition: The effects of desynchronization. In C. Benoit & R. Campbell (Eds.), *Proceedings of the Workshop on Audiovisual Speech Processing: Cognitive and Computational Approaches* (pp. 97–100). Rhodes.

Bertelson, P., Vroomen, J., & de Gelder, B. (2003). Visual recalibration of auditory speech identification: A McGurk aftereffect. *Psychological Science, 14,* 592–597.

Bertelson, P., Vroomen, J., de Gelder, B., & Driver, J. (2000). The ventriloquist effect does not depend on the direction of deliberate visual attention. *Perception & Psychophysics, 62,* 321–332.

Bleuler, E. (1911). Dementia Praecox oder Gruppe der Schizophrenien [Dementia praecox or the group of schizophrenias]. In: Aschaffenburg Handbuch der Psychiatrie. Leipzig: Deuticke.

Borod, J. C., Pick, L. H., Hall, S., Sliwinski, M., Madigan, N., Obler, L. K., et al. (2000). Relationships among facial, prosodic, and lexical channels of emotional perceptual processing. *Cognition and Emotion, 14,* 193–211.

Cabeza, R., & Nyberg, L. (2000). Imaging cognition: II. An empirical review of 275 PET and fMRI studies. *Journal of Cognitive Neuroscience, 12,* 1–47.

Calvert, G. A., Bullmore, E. T., Brammer, M. J., Campbell, R., Williams, S. C., McGuire, P. K., et al. (1997). Activation of auditory cortex during silent lipreading. *Science, 276,* 593–596.

Calvert, G. A., Brammer, M. J., Bullmore, E. T., Campbell, R., Iversen, S. D., & David, A. S. (1999). Response amplification in sensory-specific cortices during crossmodal binding. *Neuroreport, 10,* 2619–2623.

Calvert, G. A., Campbell, R., & Brammer, M. J. (2000). Evidence from functional magnetic resonance imaging of crossmodal binding in the human heteromodal cortex. *Current Biology, 10,* 649–657.

Damasio, A. R. (1989). Time-locked multiregional retroactivation: A systems-level proposal for the neural substrates of recall and recognition. *Cognition, 33,* 25–62.

Davidson, R. J., & Irwin, W. (1999). The functional neuroanatomy of emotion and affective style. *Trends in Cognitive Sciences, 3,* 11–21.

de Gelder, B. (2000). More to seeing than meets the eye. *Science, 289,* 1148–1149.

de Gelder, B., & Bertelson, P. (2003). Multisensory integration, perception, and ecological validity. *Trends in Cognitive Sciences, 10,* 460–467.

de Gelder, B., Böcker, K. B., Tuomainen, J., Hensen, M., & Vroomen, J. (1999). The combined perception of emotion from voice and face: Early interaction revealed by human electric brain responses. *Neuroscience Letter, 260,* 133–136.

de Gelder, B., Pourtois, G., van Raamsdonk, M., Vroomen, J., & Weiskrantz, L. (2001). Unseen stimuli modulate conscious visual experience: Evidence from interhemispheric summation. *Neuroreport, 12,* 385–391.

de Gelder, B., Pourtois, G. R. C., Vroomen, J. H. M., & Bachoud-Levi, A.-C. (2000). Covert processing of faces in prosopagnosia is restricted to facial expressions: Evidence from cross-modal bias. *Brain and Cognition, 44,* 425–444.

de Gelder, B., Pourtois, G. R. C., & Weiskrantz, L. (2002). Fear recognition in the voice is modulated by unconsciously recognized facial expressions but not by unconsciously recognized affective pictures. *Proceedings of the National Academy of Sciences, 99,* 4121–4126.

de Gelder, B., van Ommeren, B., & Frissen, I. (2003). Feelings are not specious: Recognition of facial expressions and vocalizations of chimpanzees (*Pan troglodytes*) by humans. Presented at the Annual Meeting of the Cognitive Neuroscience Society.

de Gelder, B., & Vroomen, J. (2000). The perception of emotion by ear and by eye. *Cognition & Emotion, 14,* 289–311.

de Gelder, B., Vroomen, J. H. M., Annen, L., Masthof, E., & Hodiamont, P. P. G. (2003). Audiovisual integration in schizophrenia. *Schizophrenia Research, 59,* 211–218.

de Gelder, B., Vroomen, J., & Bertelson, P. (1998). Upright but not inverted faces modify the perception of emotion in the voice. *Current Psychology of Cognition, 17,* 1021–1031.

de Gelder, B., Vroomen, J., & Hodiamont, P. (2003). *Deficits in multisensory perception of affect in schizophrenia.* Manuscript submitted for publication.

de Gelder, B., Vroomen, J., & Pourtois, G. (2001). Covert affective cognition and affective blindsight. In B. de Gelder, E. de Haan, & C. A. Heywood (Eds.), *Out of mind: Varieties of unconscious processing.* Oxford, England: Oxford University Press.

de Gelder, B., Vroomen, J., Pourtois, G., & Weiskrantz, L. (1999). Non-conscious recognition of affect in the absence of striate cortex. *Neuroreport, 10,* 3759–3763.

de Gelder, B., Vroomen, J., & Teunisse, J.-P. (1995). Hearing smiles and seeing cries: The bimodal perception of emotions. *Bulletin of the Psychonomic Society, 30.*

Dimberg, U., Thunberg, M., & Elmehed, K. (2000). Unconscious facial reactions to emotional facial expressions. *Psychological Science, 11,* 86–89.

Dolan, R., Morris, J., & de Gelder, B. (2001). Crossmodal binding of fear in voice and face. *Proceedings of the National Academy of Sciences, USA, 98,* 10006–10010.

Driver, J., & Spence, C. (2000). Multisensory perception: Beyond modularity and convergence. *Current Biology, 10,* 731–735.

Ettlinger, G., & Wilson, W. A. (1990). Cross-modal performance: Behavioural processes, phylogenetic considerations and neural mechanisms. *Behavioral Brain Research, 40,* 169–192.

Farah, M. J., Wong, A. B., Monheit, M. A., & Morrow, L. A. (1989). Parietal lobe mechanisms of spatial attention: Modality-specific or supramodal? *Neuropsychologia, 27,* 461–470.

Foxe, J. J., Morocz, I. A., Murray, M. M., Higgins, B. A., Javitt, D. C., & Schroeder, C. E. (2000). Multisensory auditory-somatosensory interactions in early cortical processing revealed by high-density electrical mapping. *Cognitive Brain Research, 10,* 77–83.

Frissen, I., & de Gelder, B. (2002). Visual bias on sound location modulated by content-based processes. *Journal of the Acoustical Society of America, 112,* 2244.

Fuster, J. M., Bodner, M., & Kroger, J. K. (2000). Cross-modal and cross-temporal association in neurons of frontal cortex. *Nature, 405,* 347–351.

Giard, M. H., & Peronnet, F. (1999). Auditory-visual integration during multisensory object recognition in humans: A behavioral and electrophysiological study. *Journal of Cognitive Neuroscience, 11,* 473–490.

Goulet, S., & Murray, E. A. (2001). Neural substrates of cross-modal association memory in monkeys: The amygdala versus the anterior rhinal cortex. *Behav Neuroscience, 115,* 271–284.

Kahneman, D. (1973). *Attention and effort.* Englewood Cliffs, NJ: Prentice Hall.

Lavie, N. (1995). Perceptual load as a necessary condition for selective attention. *Journal of Experimental Psychology: Human Perception and Performance, 21,* 451–468.

Lavie, N. (2000). Selective attention and cognitive control. In S. Monsell & J. Driver (Eds.), *Control of cognitive processes: Attention and performance XVIII* (pp. 175–194). Cambridge, MA: MIT Press.

LeDoux, J. E. (1996). *The emotional brain.* New York: Simon & Schuster.

Liberman, A. M., & Mattingly, I. G. (1985). The motor theory of speech perception revised. *Cognition, 21,* 1–36.

Macaluso, E., Frith, C. D., & Driver, J. (2000). Modulation of human visual cortex by crossmodal spatial attention. *Science, 289,* 1206–1208.

MacLeod, C. M., & MacDonald, P. A. (2000). Interdimensional interference in the Stroop effect: Uncovering the cognitive and neural anatomy of attention. *Trends in Cognitive Sciences, 4,* 383–391.

Massaro, D. W. (1998). *Perceiving talking faces: From speech perception to a behavioural principle.* Cambridge, MA: MIT Press.

Massaro, D. W. (1999). Speechreading: Illusion or window into pattern recognition? *Trends in Cognitive Sciences, 3,* 310–317.

Massaro, D. W., & Egan, P. B. (1996). Perceiving affect from the voice and the face. *Psychonomic Bulletin and Review, 3,* 215–221.

McDonald, J. J., Teder-Sälejärvi, W. A., & Ward, L. M. (2001). Multisensory integration and crossmodal attention effects in the human brain. *Science, 292,* 1791.

Mesulam, M. M. (1998). From sensation to cognition. *Brain, 121,* 1013–1052.

Miller, J. O. (1982). Divided attention: Evidence for coactivation with redundant signals. *Cognitive Psychology, 14,* 247–279.

Miller, J. O. (1986). Time course of coactivation in bimodal divided attention. *Perception & Psychophysics, 40,* 331–343.

Morris, J. S., Ohman, A., & Dolan, R. J. (1999). A subcortical pathway to the right amygdala mediating "unseen" fear. *Proceedings of the National Academy of Sciences, USA, 96,* 1680–1685.

Munhall, K. G., Gribble, P., Sacco, L., & Ward, M. (1996). Temporal constraints on the McGurk effect. *Perception & Psychophysics, 58,* 351–362.

Näätänen, R. (1992). *Attention and brain function.* Hillsdale, NJ: Erlbaum.

Peterson, M. A., de Gelder, B., Rapcsak, S. Z., Gerhardstein, P. C., & Bachoud-Levi, A. C. (2000). Object memory effects on figure assignment: Conscious object recognition is not necessary or sufficient. *Vision Research, 40,* 1549–1567.

Pourtois, G., Debatisse, D., Despland, P. A., & de Gelder, B. (2002). Facial expressions modulate the time course of long latency auditory brain potentials. *Cognitive Brain Research, 14,* 99–105.

Pourtois, G., & de Gelder, B. (2002). Semantic factors influence multisensory pairing: A transcranial magnetic stimulation study. *Neuroreport, 12,* 1567–1573.

Pourtois, G., de Gelder, B., Bol, A., & Crommelinck, M. (2003). *Convergence of visual and auditory affective information in human multisensory cortex.* Manuscript submitted for publication.

Pourtois, G., de Gelder, B., Vroomen, J., Rossion, B., & Crommelinck, M. (2000). The time-course of intermodal binding between seeing and hearing affective information. *Neuroreport, 11*, 1329–1333.

Pylyshyn, Z. (1999). Is vision continuous with cognition? The case for cognitive impenetrability of visual perception. *Behavioral and Brain Sciences, 22*, 341–365.

Raij, T., Uutela, K., & Hari, R. (2000). Audiovisual integration of letters in the human brain. *Neuron, 28*, 617–625.

Rockland, K. S., & Ojima, H. (2003). Multisensory convergence in calcarine visual areas in macaque monkey. *International Journal of Psychophysiology, 50*, 19–26.

Ross, E. D. (2000). Affective prosody and the aprosodias. In M. M. Mesulam (Ed.), *Principle of behavioral and cognitive neurology* (pp. 316–331). Oxford, England: Oxford University Press.

Sams, M., Aulanko, R., Hamalainen, M., Hari, R., Lounasmaa, O. V., Lu, S. T., et al. (1991). Seeing speech: Visual information from lip movements modifies activity in the human auditory cortex. *Neurosci Letters, 127*, 141–145.

Schröger, E., & Widmann, A. (1998). Speeded responses to audiovisual signal changes result from bimodal integration. *Psychophysiology, 35*, 755–759.

Scott, S. K., Young, A. W., Calder, A. J., Hellawell, D. J., Aggleton, J. P., & Johnson, M. (1997). Impaired auditory recognition of fear and anger following bilateral amygdala lesions. *Nature, 385*, 254–257.

Shiffrin, R. M., & Schneider, W. (1977). Controlled and automatic human information processing: 2. Perceptual learning, automatic attending, and a general theory. *Psychological Review, 84*, 127–190.

Streicher, M., & Ettlinger, G. (1987). Cross-modal recognition of familiar and unfamiliar objects by the monkey: The effects of ablation of polysensory neocortex or of the amygdaloid complex. *Behavioural Brain Research, 23*, 95–107.

Summerfield, Q. (1987). Some preliminaries to a comprehensive account of audio-visual speech perception. In B. Dodd & R. Campbell (Eds.), *Hearing by eye: The psychology of lip-reading* (pp. 3–51). Hillsdale, NJ: Erlbaum.

Surakka, V., Tenhunen-Eskelinen, M., Hietanen, J. K., & Sams, M. (1998). Modulation of human auditory information processing by emotional visual stimuli. *Cognitive Brain Research, 7*, 159–163.

Treisman, A. (1996). The binding problem. *Current Opinions in Neurobiology, 6*, 171–178.

Van Lancker, D. R., & Canter, G. J. (1982). Impairment of voice and face recognition in patients with hemispheric damage. *Brain and Cognition, 1*, 185–195.

Vroomen, J., Bertelson, P., & de Gelder, B. (2001). The ventriloquist effect does not depend on the direction of automatic visual attention. *Perception & Psychophysics, 63*, 651–659.

Vroomen, J., Driver, J., & de Gelder, B. (2001). Is cross-modal integration of emotional expressions independant of attentional resources? *Cognitive and Affective Neurosciences, 1*, 382–387.

Weiskrantz, L. (1986). *Blindsight: A case study and implications.* Oxford, England: Oxford University Press.

Weiskrantz, L. (1997). *Consciousness lost and found.* Oxford, England: Oxford University Press.

Whalen, P. J., Rauch, S. L., Etcoff, N. L., McInerney, S. C., Lee, M. B., & Jenike, M. A. (1998). Masked presentations of emotional facial expressions modulate amygdala activity without explicit knowledge. *Journal of Neuroscience, 18*, 411–418.

Wickens, D. D. (1984). Processing resources in attention. In R. Pararsuraman & D. R. Davies (Eds.), *Varieties of attention* (pp. 63–102). Orlando, FL: Academic Press.

VI THE MATURATION AND PLASTICITY OF MULTISENSORY PROCESSES

37 Epigenetic Factors That Align Visual and Auditory Maps in the Ferret Midbrain

ANDREW J. KING, TIMOTHY P. DOUBELL, AND IRINI SKALIORA

Introduction

Many of the chapters in this volume have highlighted the way in which different sensory systems work together to influence perception and behavior as well as the activity of neurons in different regions of the brain. In order for these cross-modal interactions to be of value, however, the various sensory signals arising from a common source must be coordinated within the brain. This requirement applies both to amodal features, which include the timing, location, and intensity of the stimuli, and to modality-specific properties, such as voice pitch and facial features.

This capacity to combine information across different sensory channels to form a coherent multisensory representation of the world has its origin in the way in which the sensory systems interact during development. Behavioral and neurophysiological studies carried out on a variety of species have highlighted the importance of sensory experience in this process (see Gutfreund & Knudsen, Chap. 38; Wallace, Chap. 39; and Lickliter & Bahrick, Chap. 40, this volume). In particular, experience plays a critical role in matching the neural representations of spatial information provided by the different sensory systems. As in the adult brain, most developmental studies of multisensory processing at the neuronal level have focused on the superior colliculus (SC; see Stein, Jiang, & Stanford, Chap. 15, this volume).

The choice of species in which to investigate the development of multisensory spatial integration is governed by a number of scientific as well as economic and clinical factors. Like many other groups interested in the early development and plasticity of sensory systems (e.g., Chapman, Stryker, & Bonhoeffer, 1996; Dantzker & Callaway, 1998; Henkel & Brunso-Bechtold, 1995; Juliano, Palmer, Sonty, Noctor, & Hill, 1996; Moore, Hutchings, King, & Kowalchuk, 1989; Weliky & Katz, 1999; see also Sur, Chap. 42, this volume), we use the ferret, *Mustela putorius furo*, for our work on the SC. The ferret is a carnivore whose central nervous system is organized much like that of the more extensively studied cat. Both are altricial species, although the ferret is particularly immature at birth. Indeed, evoked-potential measurements show that these animals are unable to hear until near the end of the first postnatal month (Moore & Hine, 1992). Eye opening typically occurs a few days after this, although responses to complex visual stimuli can be recorded in the thalamus and cortex through the closed eyelids as early as 21 days after birth (Krug, Akerman, & Thompson, 2001). Despite their relative immaturity, young ferrets are robust and highly suitable for both in vivo and in vitro electrophysiological recording experiments. Moreover, mature ferrets can be readily trained to make behavioral responses to remotely presented stimuli (e.g., Kelly, Kavanagh, & Dalton, 1986; King, Parsons, & Moore, 2000; Moore, Hine, Jiang, Matsuda, Parsons, & King, 1999; von Melchner, Pallas, & Sur, 2000). This allows the functional significance of experience-driven changes in neuronal response properties to be assessed and provides a valuable link to psychophysical studies in humans.

In this chapter, we examine the development of sensory map registration in the mammalian SC, with an emphasis on the steps that lead to the emergence of spatially tuned auditory responses and their alignment with visual receptive fields (RFs). Many of these studies have been carried out in ferrets, with experimental approaches ranging from measurement of orienting behavior to the response characteristics of individual neurons (see King, 1999; King & Schnupp, 2000; King et al., 2000, for recent reviews).

Sensory representations in the ferret SC

The ferret SC shares the basic vertebrate plan in which different sensory representations are organized topographically to form overlapping maps of sensory space. Most recording studies in this species have focused on

599

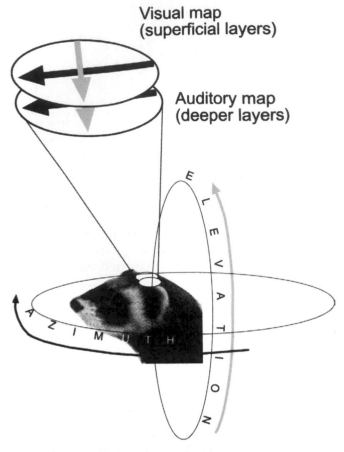

Visual map (superficial layers)

Auditory map (deeper layers)

ELEVATION

AZIMUTH

FIGURE 37.1   Representation of sensory space in the superior colliculus (SC). The superficial layers are exclusively visual, whereas neurons in the deeper layers respond to auditory (as well as visual and tactile) stimuli. Stimulus azimuth is mapped on the rostrocaudal axis (black arrow) and elevation is mapped on the mediolateral (gray arrow) axis of the nucleus. The portion of visual and auditory space represented within the SC is indicated by the arrows around the ferret's head and corresponds approximately to the extent of the visual field of the contralateral eye.

the visual and auditory inputs, which, as expected for a carnivore, appear to dominate the sensory responses of neurons in its intermediate and deep layers (Meredith, Clemo, & Dehneri, 2000). The topographic organization of ferret deep-layer visual responses has not been mapped in any detail, but the map of auditory space is known to be closely aligned with the visual map in the superficial layers (Fig. 37.1). Although the auditory spatial RFs of mammalian SC neurons can be large, sometimes occupying up to or even more than a hemifield, the great majority are spatially tuned in that they respond maximally to a specific sound direction. Comparison of the preferred stimulus direction with that of the much smaller visual RFs recorded in the overlying superficial layers reveals that both maps cover approximately the same region of space, corresponding

to the visual field of the contralateral eye (King & Carlile, 1995; King & Hutchings, 1987). Moreover, for both modalities, a larger region of the SC is devoted to the representation of the area in front of the animal than to more peripheral regions of space.

Many neurons in the deeper layers of the ferret SC respond to stimuli in more than one sensory modality (King & Schnupp, 2000; Meredith et al., 2000). The multisensory properties of these neurons have not been studied in as much detail as in other species (cat: Kadunce, Vaughan, Wallace, Benedek, & Stein, 1997; Meredith & Stein, 1996; guinea pig: King & Palmer, 1985; monkey: Wallace, Wikinson, & Stein, 1996). Nevertheless, as in these earlier studies, neuronal discharge rates can be significantly increased when visual and auditory stimuli are presented together (King & Schnupp, 2000). In cats, the relative location of the individual sensory cues is an important factor in determining whether a given SC neuron gives enhanced or depressed responses to multisensory stimulation. Equivalent effects are also manifest at the behavioral level, suggesting that these interactions contribute to the ability of animals to detect and localize stimuli that are registered by different sense organs (Stein, Meredith, Huneycutt, & McDade, 1989; see also Stein, Jiang, & Stanford, Chap. 15, this volume).

Like cats, ferrets can localize spatially congruent visual-auditory stimuli more accurately than they can localize either stimulus presented by itself, whereas performance is degraded when the visual and auditory targets are separated (Kacelnik, Walton, Parsons, & King, 2002). These cross-modal influences on stimulus localization have been observed when performance is measured by training the animal to approach the source of the stimulus and, to a lesser extent, by measuring the accuracy of the initial head-orienting response (Fig. 37.2). It remains to be seen to what extent the activity of SC neurons contributes to the accuracy with which multisensory targets are localized. However, if visual and auditory signals are to interact in a behaviorally useful manner, it would make sense that the RFs of the neurons involved, whether in the SC or elsewhere in the brain, are in register.

Aligning visual and auditory maps in the SC

Despite the similarity in their organization in the SC, the neural maps of visual and auditory space are constructed according to very different principles. The visual field is projected by the optical components of the eye onto the retina and then represented in the SC and in other visual centers as a direct consequence of the topographically organized pathways that connect these

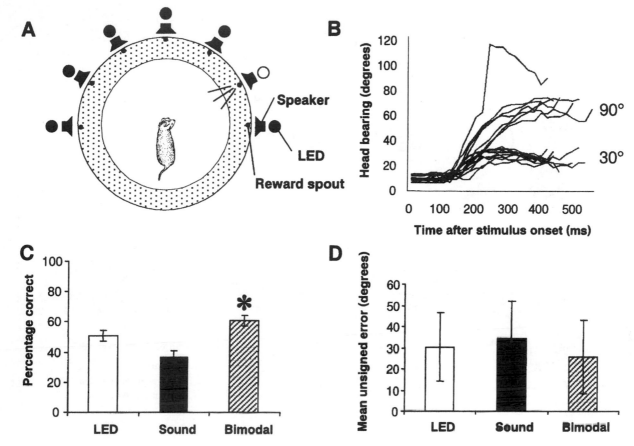

FIGURE 37.2 Behavioral responses to multisensory stimuli. (A) Schematic view of the testing chamber. Ferrets were trained to stand on a platform at the center of the circular testing chamber and initiate a trial by licking a waterspout (not shown). Each trial consisted of an auditory stimulus (20-ms burst of broadband noise at 25 dB SPL), a visual stimulus (20 ms flash from an LED), or both together, presented from one of seven locations in the frontal hemifield. The animal was rewarded for approaching and licking the spout associated with the location of the stimulus that was triggered. (B) Head-orienting responses were measured using a video contrast detection device. These traces show the head turns made by one animal to sounds presented at either 30 degrees or 90 degrees from the midline. (C) The approach-to-target responses show that ferrets localize spatially congruent multisensory stimuli significantly more accurately than either auditory or visual stimuli presented separately. (D) Head-orienting responses to combined visual-auditory cues are also faster and more accurate than those made following unimodal stimulation, although these differences are not significant.

structures. On the other hand, the direction of a sound source has to be computed within the brain through the sensitivity of central neurons to acoustic localization cues that result from interactions with the head and external ears (King, Schnupp, & Doubell, 2001). These cues may be provided by one ear alone, as in the spectral cues that are produced by the directional filtering properties of the external ear, or by differences in the sound between the two ears. Sensitivity to interaural time differences does not appear to underlie the mapping of auditory space in the mammalian SC (Campbell, Doubell, Nodal, Schnupp, & King, 2002; Hirsch, Chan, & Yin, 1985). Instead, these neurons derive their spatial selectivity from a combination of interaural level differences and monaural spectral cues (Carlile & King, 1994; King, Moore, & Hutchings, 1994). The registration of the

visual and auditory maps in the SC is therefore based on a correspondence between particular values of these cues and positions on the retina.

The initial processing of monaural and binaural localization cues takes place in largely independent pathways in the brainstem that converge in the inferior colliculus. A number of different subcortical and cortical auditory areas innervate the deeper layers of the ferret SC (Jiang, King, Moore, & Thompson, 1996; King, Jiang, & Moore, 1998), with the largest inputs originating in the nucleus of the brachium of the inferior colliculus (nBIC) and the external nucleus of the inferior colliculus (ICX). In particular, the nBIC appears to play a key role in the synthesis of the map of auditory space. Its rostral and caudal regions are reciprocally connected with corresponding parts of the SC

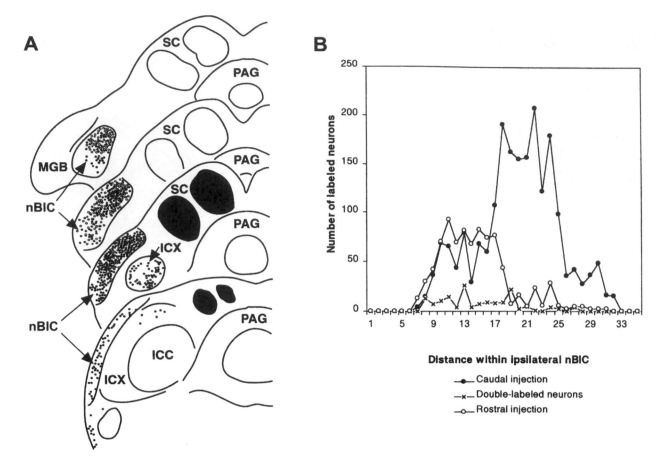

FIGURE 37.3   Auditory inputs to the ferret SC. (A) Distribution of retrograde labeling in subcortical auditory structures after injections of green fluorescent microspheres into rostral SC and red microspheres into caudal SC. The frontal sections are arranged from rostral (top) to caudal (bottom). The open and filled areas in the SC indicate the injection sites of green and red tracers, respectively. The small open and filled circles show the positions of retrogradely red or green labeled cells, respectively. The small asterisks indicate double labeled cells. More limited labeling is also found in the contralateral auditory midbrain and in other auditory brainstem nuclei. nBIC, nucleus of the brachium of the inferior colliculus; MGB, medial geniculate body; ICX, external nucleus of the inferior colliculus; ICC, central nucleus of the inferior colliculus; PAG, periaqueductal gray. (B) Number of single- and double-labeled neurons counted in serial, frontal sections from the rostral to the caudal end of the nBIC. The pattern of labeling indicates that the projection to the SC from the nBIC is spatially ordered along the rostrocaudal axis. (Modified, with permission, from King, Jiang, et al., 1998. Journal of Comparative Neurology. ©1998 Wiley-Liss, Inc., a Wiley Company.)

(Figs. 37.3 and 37.4; Doubell, Baron, Skaliora, & King, 2000; King, Jiang, & Moore, 1998), and in both nuclei these regions contain neurons that are tuned to anterior and posterior areas of space, respectively (Schnupp & King, 1997). However, in terms of the range of preferred sound directions, the representation of sound azimuth in the nBIC is less precise, and in contrast to the SC, neurons in this nucleus lack elevation topography (Schnupp & King, 1997). Thus, additional processing, possibly involving inputs from other auditory structures, is required in order to construct the two-dimensional map that characterizes the auditory responses in the SC.

The capacity of many species, including cats and some primates, to move their eyes and ears independently creates a problem for maintaining the alignment of the sensory maps in the SC. Potential mismatches between the maps appear to be at least partially resolved in these species by shifting auditory (Hartline, Pandey Vimal, King, Kurylo, & Northmore, 1995; Jay & Sparks, 1984; Populin & Yin, 1998) and somatosensory (Groh & Sparks, 1996) RFs whenever the eyes move. Ferrets have immobile pinnae and appear to rely primarily on head turns as a means of effecting a shift in the direction of gaze. Nevertheless, it seems likely that their SC responses may also be influenced by eye position signals.

Developmental emergence of sensory map alignment in the SC

The size, shape, and relative positions of the different sense organs change during the course of development

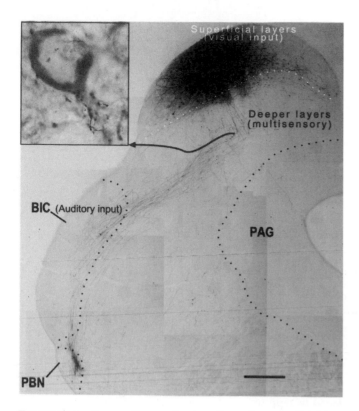

Superficial layers
(visual input)

Deeper layers
(multisensory)

BIC (Auditory input)

PAG

PBN

FIGURE 37.4 Descending projections from the superficial layers of the ferret SC. An injection of biotinylated dextran amine into the superficial layers labeled axons that course ventrally into the deeper layers and then turn laterally to run through or along the medial side of the brachium of the inferior colliculus (BIC) before entering the parabigeminal nucleus (PBN). Axon terminals are formed on NMDA-labeled neurons in both the deep SC and the nucleus of the BIC, as shown at higher magnification in the inset. The white dotted line indicates the border between the superficial layers and the deeper layers of the SC. The black dotted lines delimit the area occupied by the BIC and by the periaqueductal gray (PAG). Scale bar = 500 μm. (Modified, with permission, from Doubell et al., 2000. © 2000 Federation of European Neuroscience Societies.)

(King, Schnupp, et al., 2001). This has important consequences for the maturation of the individual maps and for the emergence of intersensory map alignment in the SC. It has been found in both altricial and precocial species that the visual topography in the superficial layers of the SC is present at the time of eye opening, reflecting the maturity of the retinocollicular projection (Kao, McHaffie, Meredith, & Stein, 1994; King & Carlile, 1995; Wallace, McHaffie, & Stein, 1997). In contrast, visual, auditory, and somatosensory maps in the deeper layers exhibit a much more protracted period of development (King & Carlile, 1995; Wallace & Stein, 1997, 2001; Withington-Wray, Binns, & Keating, 1990a). The representation of visual azimuth in the superficial layers and of auditory azimuth in the deeper layers of the ferret SC at different ages is shown in Figure 37.5.

The registration of the two maps gradually improves over the second postnatal month as the development of the auditory map proceeds.

Age-dependent changes in the spatial RFs may reflect the maturation of the afferent connections and synaptic properties of neurons both in the SC and at earlier stages in the pathway. This is particularly relevant for the map of auditory space, which relies on the preprocessing of auditory localization cues in the brainstem. But another important factor that needs to be considered is the maturity of the sense organs themselves. As the head grows, the values of the monaural and binaural localization cues that correspond to particular directions in space change quite dramatically (Fig. 37.6; King & Carlile, 1995; King, Schnupp, et al., 2001; Schnupp, Booth, & King, 2003). Even if the tuning of the neurons to these cues is adultlike from an early stage, it is highly likely that the spatial RFs will change in size and shape as the acoustic information on which they are based changes. This is supported by the observation that the maturation of the cues follows a similar time course to the emergence of topographic order in the auditory representation (King & Carlile, 1995). Moreover, by presenting sounds via earphones, it is possible to provide juvenile animals with adult "virtual" ears. Recordings from neurons in the auditory cortex of young ferrets show that this procedure produces an immediate and significant sharpening of the spatial RFs, so that they become closer in size to those measured in adult animals (Mrsic-Flogel, Schnupp, & King, 2003).

Compared to recordings in adult ferrets, the peaks and notches that characterize the monaural spectral localization cues are shifted to higher frequencies in young animals (Fig. 37.6). These age-related differences can be reduced, however, by scaling the juvenile amplitude spectra by an amount that corresponds to the intersubject difference in the dimensions of the ears (Schnupp et al., 2003). The implication of this is that, as with certain features of the binaural cues (see Gutfreund & Knudsen, Chap. 38, this volume), the correspondence between the spectral cue values and sound direction is predictable, as is the way in which this relationship changes with age. In principle, neural sensitivity to these cues could therefore be specified genetically. Nevertheless, differences between subjects in the size and shape of the auditory periphery mean that the localization cue values that are naturally available can be quite different from one individual to another. Indeed, the virtual sound source approach has been used to show that adult humans localize more accurately when listening to sounds filtered through their own ears than those of another subject (Middlebrooks, 1999; Wenzel, Arruda, Kistler, & Wightman, 1993). This

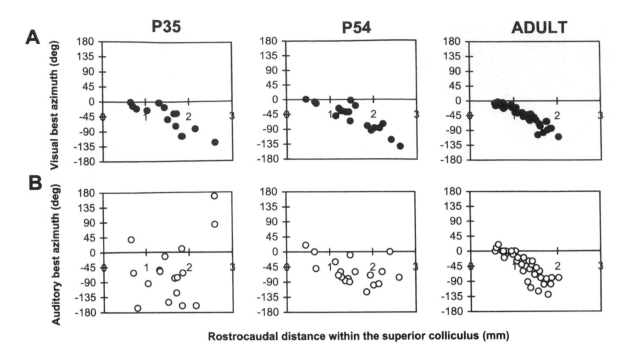

FIGURE 37.5   Development of sensory maps in the ferret SC. The stimulus locations that evoked the strongest response (best azimuth) from visual neurons recorded in the superficial layers (*A*) and from auditory neurons recorded in the deeper layers (*B*) in the same electrode penetrations that passed vertically through the SC are plotted against the rostrocaudal location of each recording site. These data are based on multiunit responses recorded at the approximate postnatal ages indicated at the top of each panel. The visual topography is apparent as soon as the eyes open (which occurs at about 1 month after birth), whereas topographic order in the auditory representation emerges some weeks later.

suggests that the auditory localization system has to be calibrated by experience of the cues available to the individual, which has now been confirmed by studies in which acoustic cue values have been altered experimentally (Hofman, Van Riswick, & Van Opstal, 1998; King, Kacelnik, et al., 2001; King, Schnupp, et al., 2001).

Plasticity of auditory spatial processing in the SC

Given its computational nature, it is not surprising that most of the evidence for a role for experience in shaping the development of the sensory maps in the SC has come from studies of the auditory representation (King, 1999). Plugging one ear during infancy leads to a compensatory change in auditory RFs in the ferret SC, which, despite the abnormal binaural cue values available, are reasonably well aligned with the visual RFs in the superficial layers (King, Hutchings, Moore, & Blakemore, 1988; King et al., 2000). A different result is found, however, if the spectral localization cues are disrupted by surgically reshaping both external ears in infancy. In this instance, recordings from adult animals reveal that the topography of the auditory representation is more seriously disrupted, and so the alignment

with the unchanged visual map breaks down (Schnupp, King, & Carlile, 1998). Corresponding effects on auditory localization behavior are found in each case, since ferrets raised with one ear occluded can learn to localize accurately (King, Kacelnik, et al., 2001), whereas rearing with abnormal spectral cues results in less complete adaptation (Parsons, Lanyon, Schnupp, & King, 1999). Although these findings imply that the capacity of the brain to accommodate abnormal auditory inputs depends on how the cues are altered, there is growing evidence that the amount of experience in using the modified cues may also determine the rate and extent of adaptation (Kacelnik, Parsons, & King, 2004; King, Kacelnik, et al., 2001).

AUDITORY CONSEQUENCES OF ALTERED VISUAL EXPERIENCE Auditory map plasticity can also be induced by depriving animals of a normal visual input or by altering the topography of the visual map. Although it remains topographically organized, abnormalities in the auditory representation are found in barn owls (Knudsen, Esterly, & du Lac, 1991), ferrets (King & Carlile, 1993) and guinea pigs (Withington, 1992) that have been deprived of normal patterned visual experience by binocular eyelid suture. Elimination of all visual experience

604   THE MATURATION AND PLASTICITY OF MULTISENSORY PROCESSES

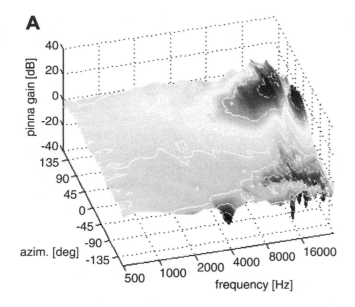

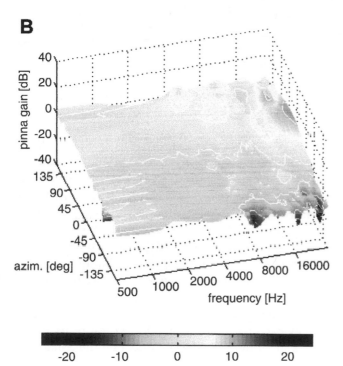

FIGURE 37.6 Maturation of monaural spectral cues for sound location. Direction-dependent filtering of sounds by the head and external ear of an adult ferret (*A*) and a 33-day-old juvenile ferret (*B*). Changes in gain are shown as a function of sound frequency and azimuth. The transfer functions are quite different at these ages. Where equivalent spatial features can be identified, they are shifted to higher frequencies in the younger animal.

by dark rearing has more disruptive effects on auditory spatial tuning (Withington-Wray, Binns, & Keating, 1990b) and appears to remove the capacity of SC

neurons to integrate multisensory inputs (see Wallace, Chap. 39, this volume). The functional significance of these abnormal auditory responses has yet to be determined. Although lid-sutured barn owls localize less well than normal birds (Knudsen et al., 1991), early loss of vision in other species, including ferrets (King & Parsons, 1999), has been reported to lead to superior auditory localization abilities (see Rauschecker, Chap. 43; Röder & Rösler, Chap. 46, this volume).

A guiding influence of vision in aligning the sensory maps in the midbrain has been revealed by raising barn owls with prisms mounted in front of their eyes that displace the visual field to one side. Because of the owl's very limited ocular mobility, the prisms produce a persistent displacement of the visual RFs of neurons in the optic tectum, the avian homologue of the SC, which gradually induces a compensatory shift in auditory spatial tuning (Knudsen & Brainard, 1991; see also Gutfreund & Knudsen, Chap. 38, this volume). An alternative approach for shifting the visual map relative to the head has been adopted in ferrets. Removal of the medial rectus, one of the extraocular muscles, causes the eye to deviate laterally by 15–20 degrees. If this procedure is performed in young ferrets, the preferred sound directions of auditory neurons in the contralateral SC are shifted by a corresponding amount, so that the maps of visual and auditory space remain in register (King et al., 1988; Fig. 37.7). As with the consequences of altering the auditory localization cues available to young ferrets, the capacity to make these adaptive changes appears to be limited by the extent to which the visual map is changed. Thus, section of all six extraocular muscles, followed by rotation of the eye by 180 degrees, results in more scattered auditory spatial tuning, rather than a systematic realignment with the inverted visual field representation. That these changes in the auditory responses are a direct consequence of the altered visual inputs, rather than of eye position signals reaching the SC, is indicated by the much more limited effects of early eye rotation if the animals are visually deprived at the same time (see King & Carlile, 1995).

How do visual signals shape the developing auditory responses?

The results of studies in which developing animals receive altered sensory experience suggest that repeated exposure to correlated visual and auditory activity, arising from objects or events that are both seen and heard, helps to align the sensory maps in the SC, despite individual differences in the relative geometry of the different sense organs. Elucidation of the cellular

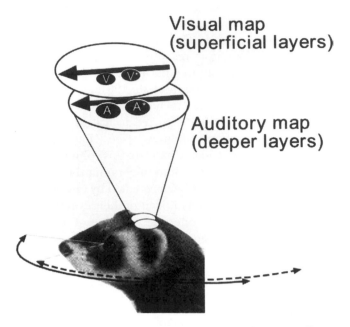

**Visual map
(superficial layers)**

**Auditory map
(deeper layers)**

FIGURE 37.7 Visual calibration of the developing auditory space map in the ferret SC. Removal of the medial rectus muscle just before natural eye opening induces a small outward deviation of the eye. The visual field is therefore shifted laterally relative to the head. This is shown schematically as the RF of a superficial layer neuron in the contralateral SC shifting from position V to V*. Electrophysiological recordings in adult ferrets revealed that the auditory RFs of deep SC neurons are also shifted laterally by a corresponding amount (A→A*). As a result of this adaptive change, the correspondence between the superficial layer visual map and the deep-layer auditory map is preserved.

mechanisms involved requires identification of the site of auditory plasticity, as well as the source and nature of the instructive visual signals.

Anatomical and electrophysiological studies have demonstrated that neurons in the superficial layers project topographically to the deeper, multisensory layers of the SC (Fig. 37.4; Behan & Appell, 1992; Doubell, Skaliora, Baron, & King, 2003; Lee, Helms, Augustine, & Hall, 1997; Meredith & King, 2004). In adult ferrets, the superficial layer axons often terminate on SC projection neurons, suggesting that they contribute to the visuomotor functions of this nucleus (Doubell et al., 2003). However, partial aspiration of the superficial SC layers in neonatal ferrets disrupts the development of the auditory map in the deeper layers, implying an additional function for these interlaminar connections (King, Schnupp, & Thompson, 1998). The auditory responses were affected in this study only in the region of the SC lying below the lesion, suggesting that a topographically organized visual input from the superficial layers is required for the normal develop-

ment of the auditory space map. A similar study in prism-reared barn owls also concluded that the developing auditory space map conforms to a visual template arising from the superficial layers of the optic tectum (Hyde & Knudsen, 2002; see also Gutfreund & Knudsen, Chap. 38, this volume).

The growing evidence that neuronal sensitivity to acoustic localization cues is matched to a map of visual space that matures at an earlier stage of development is consistent with a Hebbian model of synaptic plasticity, in which auditory inputs are selectively stabilized or destabilized according to whether they are active at the same time as visual inputs that converge on the same neuron. Because of their voltage-dependent properties, conductance through NMDA receptor channels relies on the correlation of presynaptic and postsynaptic activity, a key feature of a Hebbian synapse. Studies in which NMDA receptor function has been altered chronically suggest that these excitatory glutamate receptors are widely involved in the developmental refinement of neural connections (Constantine-Paton, Cline, & Debski, 1990; Katz & Shatz, 1996). The contribution of these receptors to the development of the auditory space map has been addressed by placing sheets of the slow-release polymer Elvax onto the dorsal surface of the ferret SC, in order to release an NMDA receptor antagonist over a period of several weeks (Schnupp, King, Smith, & Thompson, 1995). Application of NMDA antagonists during the postnatal period over which the auditory map would normally mature disrupts the topographic order in these responses, whereas this order remains unaltered after chronically implanting adult animals with Elvax. This age-dependent effect is most likely related to a decline in the contribution of NMDA receptors to the synaptic currents of SC neurons in older animals (Hestrin, 1992; King, 1999; Shi, Aamodt, & Constantine-Paton, 1997). As expected, chronic pharmacological blockade of NMDA receptors in either juvenile or adult ferrets has no effect on the visual map in the superficial layers of the SC.

The disruptive effects of chronic NMDA receptor blockade on the development of topographically aligned sensory maps in the SC are consistent with a mechanism for detecting temporal correlations among converging inputs. This process, however, is unlikely to be based solely on excitatory interactions and must also take into account the intrinsic properties of the neurons as well as their inhibitory inputs. Indeed, an alternative explanation for the abnormal auditory topography in animals reared with Elvax implants is that the drug release may have interfered with the visual instructive signals from the superficial layers by reducing

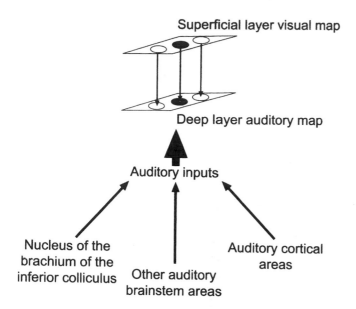

Superficial layer visual map

Deep layer auditory map

Auditory inputs

Nucleus of the brachium of the inferior colliculus

Other auditory brainstem areas

Auditory cortical areas

FIGURE 37.8　Visual and auditory inputs to the deeper layers of the ferret SC. The deeper layers receive converging inputs from several auditory brainstem and cortical areas, including a spatially ordered projection from the nucleus of the brachium of the inferior colliculus. Neurons in the superficial layers of the SC project topographically both to the underlying deeper layers and to the nucleus of the brachium of the inferior colliculus (not shown). The map of visual space in the superficial layers appears to provide an activity template that guides the development and plasticity of the auditory representation.

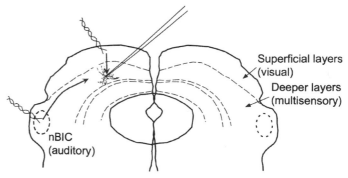

Superficial layers (visual)

Deeper layers (multisensory)

nBIC (auditory)

FIGURE 37.9　Examining visual-auditory interactions in vitro. Schematic drawing of a midbrain slice cut in the coronal plane showing the positions of the recording and stimulation electrodes. Whole-cell patch-clamp recordings were made from cells in the deeper layers of the SC while electric stimulation was applied through bipolar electrodes in the superficial layers and in the nucleus of the brachium of the inferior colliculus (nBIC).

NMDA-mediated synaptic currents. In either case, it is not surprising that changes observed in the auditory representation following long-term application of NMDA receptor antagonists are similar to those produced by neonatal lesions of the superficial layers.

Together, these findings suggest that topographically organized visual signals arising from the superficial layers of the SC may calibrate the developing auditory space map by refining inputs to the deeper layers from the nBIC or other auditory structures (Fig. 37.8). However, it is possible that the site of auditory plasticity lies at an earlier stage, for instance in the nBIC, rather than in the SC itself. In ferrets, both superficial and deeper layers of the SC project topographically to the ipsilateral nBIC (Fig. 37.4). These inputs are excitatory and most likely form the basis for the visual responses that are sometimes recorded from nBIC neurons (Doubell et al., 2000). It is not known whether the development of auditory spatial selectivity in these neurons is influenced by visual experience, but this has to be considered, given that visually guided plasticity in the owl's midbrain is first observed at the level of the ICX (Brainard & Knudsen, 1993; Hyde & Knudsen, 2002).

Studying visual-auditory convergence in vitro

Having characterized the neural pathways involved in the formation and plasticity of the auditory space map (Fig. 37.8), we have started examining these circuits in a slice preparation of the juvenile ferret midbrain. Because of the laminar organization of the SC and the trajectory of its connections with the ipsilateral nBIC (Figs. 37.3 and 37.4), it is possible to cut 400- to 500-μm-thick coronal slices that preserve inputs from both the superficial layers and from the nBIC to neurons in the deeper layers of the SC (Fig. 37.9), as well as projections from both regions of the SC that feed back to the nBIC. Although cortical and other long-range inputs are obviously severed, the slice preparation provides direct access to pre- and postsynaptic components and allows high-resolution intracellular recordings of both excitatory and inhibitory subthreshold responses to be made in order to characterize the inputs onto individual, morphologically identified neurons.

Using this approach, it has been possible to show that many neurons in the deeper layers of the ferret SC receive converging excitatory inputs from both the overlying superficial layers and the nBIC. Examples of the synaptic responses recorded from one intermediate-layer neuron following electric stimulation of either the superficial layers or the nBIC are shown in Figure 37.10. It is possible to infer whether these responses reflect monosynaptic connections or more indirect polysynaptic inputs from measurements of response latency and the variability of these values. From these measurements, we estimated that more than 40% of the recorded neurons received converging monosynaptic

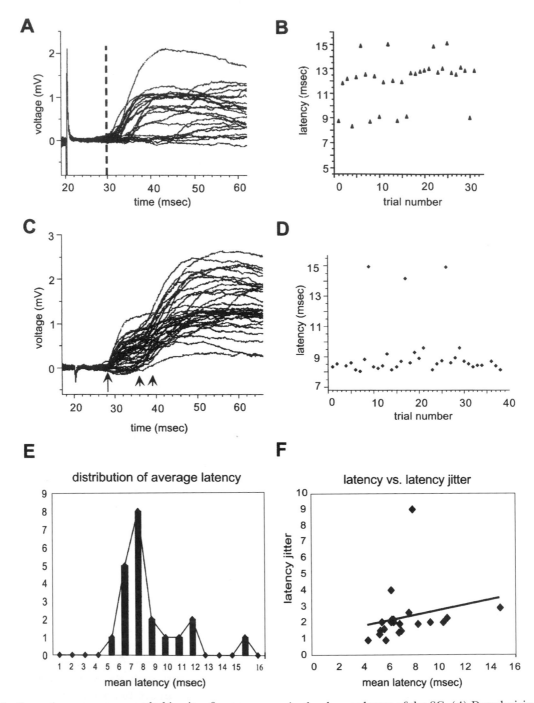

FIGURE 37.10 Synaptic responses recorded in vitro from a neuron in the deeper layers of the SC. (*A*) Depolarizing postsynaptic potentials evoked from a stimulation site in the superficial layers. Two groups of traces can be distinguished, one with a longer and one with a shorter latency. This is better illustrated in (*B*), where the latencies for each evoked response are plotted sequentially. Electric stimulation at this location appears to excite three sets of inputs, with average latencies of 9, 13, and 15 ms, respectively. (*C* and *D*) Depolarizing potentials evoked in the same SC neuron by electrical stimulation in the nBIC. In this case, stimulation elicited responses with two components, a faster one at about 8.5 ms (*large arrow*) and a slower one with a latency of 14–19 ms (*short arrows*). (*E*) Distribution of average response latencies for all recorded deep SC neurons following stimulation of the superficial layers. (*F*) Plots of absolute latency against latency jitter (the difference between the shortest and longest latency value) can be used to infer whether the neurons are activated directly or by polysynaptic connections. Short-latency responses (≤6 ms) tend to have low-latency jitter (≤2 ms), indicating the presence of a monosynaptic input. At longer latencies, this correlation is fairly flat, possibly reflecting variability in the degree of myelination. (Modified, with permission, from Doubell et al., 2003. © 2003 by the Society for Neuroscience.)

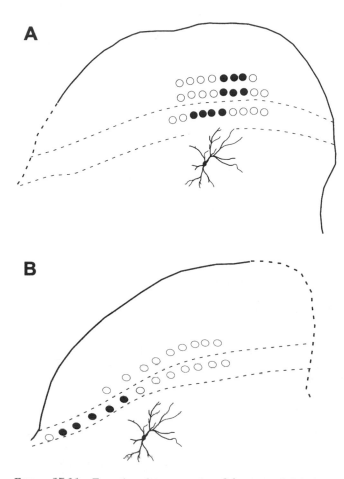

A

B

FIGURE 37.11 Functional topography of the superficial–deep layer projection in the juvenile ferret SC. (*A* and *B*) Examples of recordings from two different midbrain slices. In each case a double-barreled glass stimulating electrode was moved systematically within the superficial layers to assess the area over which a neuron in the intermediate layers could be activated. Open circles indicate sites where stimulation was applied but no response was evoked, whereas gray and black solid circles indicate locations from which polysynaptic and monosynaptic responses were elicited, respectively. (Modified, with permission, from Doubell et al., 2003. © 2003 by the Society for Neuroscience.)

inputs from both sites. Moreover, by systematically varying the location of the stimulating electrode, it was shown that intermediate-layer neurons receive direct excitatory inputs from a fairly restricted area within the superficial layers (Fig. 37.11; Doubell et al., 2003). This is consistent with the anatomical evidence for topographic order in the superficial–deep layer projection and with the effects of superficial layer lesions on the underlying auditory representation.

These in vitro recordings demonstrate that the circuitry by which visual signals could influence the responses of SC neurons to auditory stimuli is functional before the onset of hearing. By examining the effects of activation of the superficial layers on the nBIC inputs,

this preparation offers the potential for investigating the cellular and molecular changes that take place when one network of neurons guides the development of another.

Concluding remarks

The registration of visual, auditory, and tactile maps in the SC provides an efficient way of coordinating and integrating multisensory signals as a means of guiding reflexive orienting behavior. Compared with the visual and somatosensory maps, which mirror the functional organization of each receptor surface, considerable central processing is required in order to synthesize a neural map of auditory space. The generation of intersensory map alignment requires that SC neurons be tuned to acoustic localization cue values corresponding to sound source directions that match positions on the retina and body surface.

Studies in the ferret have shown that the acoustic cue values vary with the size and shape of the head and ears and change during development as these structures grow. The maturation of the cues almost certainly contributes to the protracted period of postnatal life over which the auditory topography in the SC develops. The emergence of sensory map registration is not a purely passive process, however, as activity-dependent mechanisms also play a role in matching the auditory spatial tuning of individual neurons to specific locations in visual space. This has been demonstrated in ferrets and other species by manipulating auditory or visual inputs during infancy. These experiments show that correlated experience in both modalities is used to calibrate the emerging representation of auditory space. In particular, the higher-resolution spatial information supplied by the visual system appears to provide an activity template against which auditory spatial tuning is matched. This template is provided by the map of visual space in the superficial layers of the SC, which matures at a relatively early stage of development. Superficial layer neurons send excitatory, topographically ordered projections both to the deeper layers of the SC and to its principal source of auditory input in the inferior colliculus, and are therefore well placed to influence the subsequent maturation of auditory spatial selectivity.

The cross-modal plasticity observed in the developing SC provides one of the clearest examples of how experience-mediated changes in the properties of neurons and their assemblies can be useful to the animal. This ensures that the registration of multiple sensory maps in the SC is achieved in spite of individual differences in the size and relative positions of the different sense organs. As a consequence, neurons in the deeper layers of the SC can synthesize multisensory signals that are linked in space and time and therefore associated with a common object or event. But it does not necessarily follow that the absence of visual cues will lead to impaired auditory localization. As described in other chapters in this handbook, compensatory changes in the brain may actually enhance auditory spatial hearing in blind individuals. Under normal circumstances, however, cross-modal influences on spatial processing and attention generally reflect a preeminent role for vision over the other senses.

REFERENCES

Behan, M., & Appell, P. P. (1992). Intrinsic circuitry in the cat superior colliculus: Projections from the superficial layers. *Journal of Comparative Neurology, 315,* 230–243.

Brainard, M. S., & Knudsen, E. I., (1993). Experience-dependent plasticity in the inferior colliculus: A site for visual calibration of the neural representation of auditory space in the barn owl. *Journal of Neuroscience, 13,* 4589–4608.

Campbell, R. A. A., Doubell, T. P., Nodal, F. R., Schnupp, J. W. H., & King, A. J. (2002). Responses of ferret superior colliculus neurons to stimuli presented in virtual acoustic space. *International Journal of Audiology, 41,* 244.

Carlile, S., & King, A. J. (1994). Monaural and binaural spectrum level cues in the ferret: Acoustics and the neural representation of auditory space. *Journal of Neurophysiology, 71,* 785–801.

Chapman, B., Stryker, M. P., & Bonhoeffer, T. (1996). Development of orientation preference maps in ferret primary visual cortex. *Journal of Neuroscience, 16,* 6443–6453.

Constantine-Paton, M., Cline, H. T., & Debski, E. (1990). Patterned activity, synaptic convergence, and the NMDA receptor in developing visual pathways. *Annual Review of Neuroscience, 13,* 129–154.

Dantzker, J. L., & Callaway, E. M. (1998). The development of local, layer-specific visual cortical axons in the absence of extrinsic influences and intrinsic activity. *Journal of Neuroscience, 18,* 4145–4154.

Doubell, T. P., Baron, J., Skaliora, I., & King, A. J. (2000). Topographical projection from the superior colliculus to the nucleus of the brachium of the inferior colliculus in the ferret: Convergence of visual and auditory information. *European Journal of Neuroscience, 12,* 4290–4308.

Doubell, T. P., Skaliora, I., Baron, J., & King, A. J. (2003). Functional connectivity between the superficial and deeper layers of the superior colliculus: An anatomical substrate for sensorimotor integration. *Journal of Neuroscience, 23,* 6596–6607.

Groh, J. M., & Sparks, D. L. (1996). Saccades to somatosensory targets: III. Eye-position-dependent somatosensory activity in primate superior colliculus. *Journal of Neurophysiology, 75,* 439–453.

Hartline, P. H., Pandey Vimal, R. L., King, A. J., Kurylo, D. D., & Northmore, D. P. M. (1995). Effects of eye position on auditory localization and neural representation of space in superior colliculus of cats. *Experimental Brain Research, 104,* 402–408.

Henkel, C. K., & Brunso-Bechtold, J. K. (1995). Development of glycinergic cells and puncta in nuclei of the superior olivary complex of the postnatal ferret. *Journal of Comparative Neurology, 354,* 470–480.

Hestrin, S. (1992). Developmental regulation of NMDA receptor-mediated synaptic currents at a central synapse. *Nature, 357,* 686–689.

Hirsch, J. A., Chan, J. C. K., & Yin, T. C. T. (1985). Responses of neurons in the cat's superior colliculus to acoustic stimuli: I. Monaural and binaural response properties. *Journal of Neurophysiology, 53,* 726–745.

Hofman, P. M., Van Riswick, J. G., & Van Opstal, A. J. (1998). Relearning sound localization with new ears. *Nature Neuroscience, 1,* 417–421.

Hyde, P. S., & Knudsen, E. I. (2002). The optic tectum controls visually guided adaptive plasticity in the owl's auditory space map. *Nature, 415,* 73–76.

Jay, M. F., & Sparks, D. L. (1984). Auditory receptive fields in primate superior colliculus shift with changes in eye position. *Nature, 309,* 345–347.

Jiang, Z. D., King, A. J., Moore, D. R., & Thompson, I. D. (1996). Auditory cortical projections to the superior colliculus in the ferret. *British Journal of Audiology, 30,* 109.

Juliano, S. L., Palmer, S. L., Sonty, R. V., Noctor, S., & Hill, G. F., II (1996). Development of local connections in ferret somatosensory cortex. *Journal of Comparative Neurology, 374,* 259–277.

Kacelnik, O., Parsons, C. H., & King, A. J. (2004). Adaptation to altered auditory localization cues in adulthood. Manuscript submitted for publication.

Kacelnik, O., Walton, M. E., Parsons, C. H., & King, A. J. (2002). Visual-auditory interactions in sound localization: From behavior to neural substrate. *Proceedings of the Neural Control of Movement Satellite Meeting,* p. 21.

Kadunce, D. C., Vaughan, J. W., Wallace, M. T., Benedek, G., & Stein, B. E. (1997). Mechanisms of within- and cross-modality suppression in the superior colliculus. *Journal of Neurophysiology, 78,* 2834–2847.

Kao, C. Q., McHaffie, J. G., Meredith, M. A., & Stein, B. E. (1994). Functional development of a central visual map in cat. *Journal of Neurophysiology, 72,* 266–272.

Katz, L. C., & Shatz, C. J. (1996). Synaptic activity and the construction of cortical circuits. *Science, 274,* 1133–1138.

Kelly, J. B., Kavanagh, G. L., & Dalton, J. C. (1986). Hearing in the ferret (*Mustela putorius*): Thresholds for pure tone detection. *Hearing Research, 24,* 269–275.

King, A. J. (1999). Sensory experience and the formation of a computational map of auditory space. *Bioessays, 21,* 900–911.

King, A. J., & Carlile, S. (1993). Changes induced in the representation of auditory space in the superior colliculus by rearing ferrets with binocular eyelid suture. *Experimental Brain Research, 94,* 444–455.

King, A. J., & Carlile, S. (1995). Neural coding for auditory space. In M. S. Gazzaniga (Ed.), *The cognitive neurosciences.* (pp. 279–293). Cambridge, MA: MIT Press.

King, A. J., & Hutchings, M. E. (1987). Spatial response properties of acoustically responsive neurons in the superior colliculus of the ferret: A map of auditory space. *Journal of Neurophysiology, 57,* 596–624.

King, A. J., Hutchings, M. E., Moore, D. R., & Blakemore, C. (1988). Developmental plasticity in the visual and auditory representations in the mammalian superior colliculus. *Nature, 332,* 73–76.

King, A. J., Jiang, Z. D., & Moore, D. R. (1998). Auditory brainstem projections to the ferret superior colliculus: Anatomical contribution to the neural coding of sound azimuth. *Journal of Comparative Neurology, 390*, 342–365.

King, A. J., Kacelnik, O., Mrsic-Flogel, T. D., Schnupp, J. W. H., Parsons, C. H., & Moore, D. R. (2001). How plastic is spatial hearing? *Audiology and Neurootology, 6*, 182–186.

King, A. J., Moore, D. R., & Hutchings, M. E. (1994). Topographic representation of auditory space in the superior colliculus of adult ferrets after monaural deafening in infancy. *Journal of Neurophysiology, 71*, 182–194.

King, A. J., & Palmer, A. R. (1985). Integration of visual and auditory information in bimodal neurones in the guinea-pig superior colliculus. *Experimental Brain Research, 60*, 492–500.

King, A. J., & Parsons, C. H. (1999). Improved auditory spatial acuity in visually deprived ferrets. *European Journal of Neuroscience, 11*, 3945–3956.

King, A. J., Parsons, C. H., & Moore, D. R. (2000). Plasticity in the neural coding of auditory space in the mammalian brain. *Proceedings of the National Academy of Sciences, USA, 97*, 11821–11828.

King, A. J., & Schnupp, J. W. H. (2000). Sensory convergence in neural function and development. In M. S. Gazzaniga (Ed.), *The new cognitive neurosciences* (2nd ed., pp. 437–450). Cambridge, MA: MIT Press.

King, A. J., Schnupp, J. W. H., & Doubell, T. P. (2001). The shape of ears to come: Dynamic coding of auditory space. *Trends in Cognitive Sciences, 5*, 261–270.

King, A. J., Schnupp, J. W. H., & Thompson, I. D. (1998). Signals from the superficial layers of the superior colliculus enable the development of the auditory space map in the deeper layers. *Journal of Neuroscience, 18*, 9394–9408.

Knudsen, E. I., & Brainard, M. S. (1991). Visual instruction of the neural map of auditory space in the developing optic tectum. *Science, 253*, 85–87.

Knudsen, E. I., Esterly, S. D., & du Lac, S. (1991). Stretched and upside-down maps of auditory space in the optic tectum of blind-reared owls: Acoustic basis and behavioral correlates. *Journal of Neuroscience, 11*, 1727–1747.

Krug, K., Akerman, C. J., & Thompson, I. D. (2001). Responses of neurons in neonatal cortex and thalamus to patterned visual stimulation through the naturally closed lids. *Journal of Neurophysiology, 85*, 1436–1443.

Lee, P. H., Helms, M. C., Augustine, G. J., & Hall, W. C. (1997). Role of intrinsic synaptic circuitry in collicular sensorimotor integration. *Proceedings of the National Academy of Sciences, USA, 94*, 13299–13304.

Meredith, M. A., & King, A. J. (2004). Spatial distribution of functional superficial-deep connections in the adult ferret superior colliculus. Manuscript submitted for publication.

Meredith, M. A., Clemo, H. R., & Dehneri, L. R. (2000). Responses to innocuous, but not noxious, somatosensory stimulation by neurons in the ferret superior colliculus. *Somatosensory and Motor Research, 17*, 297–308.

Meredith, M. A., & Stein, B. E. (1996). Spatial determinants of multisensory integration in cat superior colliculus neurons. *Journal of Neurophysiology, 75*, 1843–1857.

Middlebrooks, J. C. (1999). Virtual localization improved by scaling nonindividualized external-ear transfer functions in frequency. *Journal of the Acoustical Society of America, 106*, 1493–1510.

Moore, D. R., & Hine, J. E. (1992). Rapid development of the auditory brainstem response threshold in individual ferrets. *Developmental Brain Research, 66*, 229–235.

Moore, D. R., Hine, J. E., Jiang, Z. D., Matsuda, H., Parsons, C. H., & King, A. J. (1999). Conductive hearing loss produces a reversible binaural hearing impairment. *Journal of Neuroscience, 19*, 8704–8711.

Moore, D. R., Hutchings, M. E., King, A. J., & Kowalchuk, N. E. (1989). Auditory brainstem of the ferret: Some effects of rearing with a unilateral ear plug on the cochlea, cochlear nucleus, and projections to the inferior colliculus. *Journal of Neuroscience, 9*, 1213–1222.

Mrsic-Flogel, T. D., Schnupp, J. W. H., & King, A. J. (2003). Acoustic factors govern developmental sharpening of spatial tuning in the auditory cortex. *Nature Neuroscience, 6*, 981–988.

Parsons, C. H., Lanyon, R. G., Schnupp, J. W. H., & King, A. J. (1999). Effects of altering spectral cues in infancy on horizontal and vertical sound localization by adult ferrets. *Journal of Neurophysiology, 82*, 2294–2309.

Populin, L. C., & Yin, T. C. T. (1998). Sensitivity of auditory cells in the superior colliculus to eye position in the behaving cat. In A. R. Palmer, A. Rees, A. Q. Summerfield, & R. Meddis (Eds.), *Psychophysical and physiological advances in hearing.* (pp. 441–448). London: Whurr.

Schnupp, J. W. H., Booth, J., & King, A. J. (2003). Modeling individual differences in ferret external ear transfer functions. *Journal of the Acoustical Society of America, 113*; 2021–2030.

Schnupp, J. W. H., & King, A. J. (1997). Coding for auditory space in the nucleus of the brachium of the inferior colliculus in the ferret. *Journal of Neurophysiology, 78*, 2717–2731.

Schnupp, J. W. H., King, A. J., & Carlile, S. (1998). Altered spectral localization cues disrupt the development of the auditory space map in the superior colliculus of the ferret. *Journal of Neurophysiology, 79*, 1053–1069.

Schnupp, J. W. H., King, A. J., Smith, A. L., & Thompson, I. D. (1995). NMDA-receptor antagonists disrupt the formation of the auditory space map in the mammalian superior colliculus. *Journal of Neuroscience, 15*, 1516–1531.

Shi, J., Aamodt, S. M., & Constantine-Paton, M. (1997). Temporal correlations between functional and molecular changes in NMDA receptors and GABA neurotransmission in the superior colliculus. *Journal of Neuroscience, 17*, 6264–6276.

Stein, B. E., Meredith, M. A., Huneycutt, W. S., & McDade, L. (1989). Behavioral indices of multisensory integration: Orientation to visual cues is affected by auditory stimuli. *Journal of Cognitive Neuroscience, 1*, 12–24.

von Melchner, L., Pallas, S. L., & Sur, M. (2000). Visual behaviour mediated by retinal projections directed to the auditory pathway. *Nature, 404*, 871–876.

Wallace, M. T., McHaffie, J. G., & Stein, B. E. (1997). Visual response properties and visuotopic representation in the newborn monkey superior colliculus. *Journal of Neurophysiology, 78*, 2732–2741.

Wallace, M. T., & Stein, B. E. (1997). Development of multisensory neurons and multisensory integration in cat superior colliculus. *Journal of Neuroscience, 17*, 2429–2444.

Wallace, M. T., & Stein, B. E. (2001). Sensory and multisensory responses in the newborn monkey superior colliculus. *Journal of Neuroscience, 21*, 8886–8894.

Wallace, M. T., Wilkinson, L. K., & Stein, B. E. (1996). Representation and integration of multiple sensory inputs in primate superior colliculus. *Journal of Neurophysiology, 76,* 1246–1266.

Weliky, M., & Katz, L. C. (1999). Correlational structure of spontaneous neuronal activity in the developing lateral geniculate nucleus in vivo. *Science, 285,* 599–604.

Wenzel, E. M., Arruda, M., Kistler, D. J., & Wightman, F. L. (1993). Localization using nonindividualized head-related transfer functions. *Journal of the Acoustical Society of America, 94,* 111–123.

Withington, D. J. (1992). The effect of binocular lid suture on auditory responses in the guinea-pig superior colliculus. *Neuroscience, Letters, 136,* 153–156.

Withington-Wray, D. J., Binns, K. E., & Keating, M. J. (1990a). The developmental emergence of a map of auditory space in the superior colliculus of the guinea pig. *Developmental Brain Research, 51,* 225–236.

Withington-Wray, D. J., Binns, K. E., & Keating, M. J. (1990b). The maturation of the superior collicular map of auditory space in the guinea pig is disrupted by developmental visual deprivation. *European Journal of Neuroscience, 2,* 682–692.

38 Visual Instruction of the Auditory Space Map in the Midbrain

YORAM GUTFREUND AND ERIC I. KNUDSEN

Introduction

Visual and auditory information about the location of objects is processed and combined in a midbrain nucleus called the optic tectum (also called the superior colliculus [SC] in mammals). A primary function of the optic tectum is to create a multimodal map of space that can be used to orient attention and gaze toward interesting stimuli, regardless of the source of the sensory information (Peck, 1996; Stein & Meredith, 1993).

The optic tectum receives spatial information from the visual and auditory systems that is mutually independent and complementary. Vision provides high-resolution spatial information about the location of distant objects, even though they may be silent. Hearing provides spatial information about objects, even though they may not be visible. When objects can be both seen and heard, the cooperative combination of visual and auditory signals increases the capacity of the optic tectum to detect and locate stimuli under a wide range of difficult conditions (Stein & Meredith, 1993).

Combining spatial information across sensory modalities presents a challenging task to the nervous system, because visual and auditory information is initially encoded in completely different coordinate frames. Visual space is derived from the locus of activity within the topographic projections from the retina. In contrast, auditory space is derived from the evaluation of a variety of localization cues that arise from the interaction of incoming sound with the physical properties of the head and ears (Middlebrooks & Green, 1991). Auditory localization cues consist of interaural time differences (ITDs), which result from a difference in the distance traveled by a sound to reach the left versus the right ear, and interaural level differences (ILDs) and monaural spectral cues, both of which arise from the frequency-dependent directional properties of the external ears.

Visual and auditory spatial information is combined in the optic tectum by translating auditory cues into a topographic representation of space (Knudsen, 1982). The auditory system transforms its representations of cue values into a map of space by integrating information across frequency channels and across cues. This integration helps to resolve spatial ambiguities that are inherent to individual, frequency-specific cues and creates neurons that are broadly tuned for frequency but sharply tuned for space (Brainard, Knudsen, & Esterly, 1992). The auditory map is aligned with the visual map of space in the optic tectum so that tectal neurons respond to either visual or auditory stimuli located in the same region of space (Fig. 38.1).

The mutual alignment of visual and auditory receptive fields (RFs) in the tectum indicates that tectal neurons are tuned to the values of auditory cues that are produced by a sound source at the location of their visual RFs. Establishing and maintaining tuning to the correct values of auditory cues is made complicated by the variation in the correspondence between cue values and locations in the visual field that occurs across sound frequencies, across individuals, and within individuals during growth. Furthermore, the correspondence between encoded cue values and locations in the visual field changes with changes in the relative sensitivities of the ears and with development and aging of the nervous system. It is not surprising, therefore, that the tuning of tectal neurons to auditory localization cues is shaped by experience (King, Hutchings, Moore, & Blakemore, 1988; Knudsen & Knudsen, 1989; Knudsen, Knudsen, & Esterly, 1984).

This chapter discusses how visual experience shapes auditory tuning in the optic tectum. We focus on data from the barn owl because its auditory map exhibits the highest resolution among all species studied, and our knowledge of the effects of experience on the map is most complete for this species. We describe mechanisms of adaptive auditory plasticity and the teaching signals that guide the plasticity. Finally, we present a model that accounts for the plasticity in terms of

613

A   Auditory Receptive Field

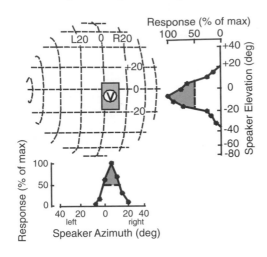

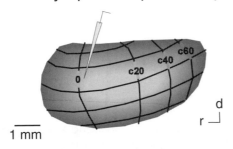

B Auditory Space Map in the Optic Tectum

FIGURE 38.1   Auditory and visual maps in the optic tectum. (*A*) Auditory and visual receptive fields measured from a bimodal unit in the optic tectum are plotted on a globe of space. The coordinates are relative to the visual axes of the owl. The visual receptive field, indicated by the circled V, was mapped by moving a light bar across the visual field. Responses of the unit to sound bursts (100 ms noise burst at 20 dB above threshold) as a function of azimuth and of elevation are shown below and to the right, respectively. The shaded area represents the area from which the sound response was more than 50% of maximum (auditory best area). (*B*) Lateral view of the left optic tectum. The contour lines indicate the locations of units with similar tuning. The approximate location of the recording site in *A* is indicated. C, contralateral; d, dorsal; r, rostral. (Adapted from Knudsen, 1982.)

cellular mechanisms and principles of learning that are likely to apply equally well to other species and to other networks in the brain.

Innate aspects of the auditory space map

Many animals, including humans, can orient in the general direction of an auditory stimulus soon after birth (Ashmead, Clifton, & Reese, 1986; Morrongiello, Fenwick, Hillier, & Chance, 1994). This indicates that certain expectations about the relations between auditory localization cues and locations in space are preprogrammed into the auditory system. For this to happen, the relations must be constant and reliable across evolutionary time. What might those expectations be?

The fact that ears are located on either side of the head leads to a number of predictable relations between binaural cues and locations in space. First, simultaneous sound at the two ears corresponds to a stimulus located near the midline (0-degree azimuth). Second, left-ear-leading ITDs indicate stimuli to the left, and right-ear-leading ITDs indicate stimuli to the right, with the maximum ITD value indicating stimuli presented directly to each side. Third, ITD changes approximately (although not perfectly) as a linear function of azimuth. Analogous predictable relations hold for ILD cues. However, because the spatial patterns of ILD cues are more complicated and more frequency dependent than those of ITD cues, and because they are affected greatly by the position and movement of the external ears, these relations are far less precise. Nevertheless, a map of auditory space, particularly of the horizontal dimension, could be preprogrammed in the auditory system on the basis of these expectations.

Consistent with these predictable aspects of cue-location relations and the ability of animals to identify the general locations of sound sources soon after birth, the auditory space maps in young guinea pigs, ferrets, and barn owls that are raised with both eyelids sutured from birth have a number of normal features: the map of azimuth is approximately normal, with frontal space represented at the rostral end of each tectum and progressively more contralateral locations represented progressively more caudal in the tectum (King & Carlile, 1993; Knudsen, Esterly, & du Lac, 1991; Withington, 1992). The influence of innate patterns of connectivity that anticipate normal relations between auditory cues (especially ITD) and locations in space is evident in the anatomical and functional effects of abnormal experience on the development of the auditory space map, discussed in the following sections.

Visual calibration of the auditory space map

Although auditory maps of space develop in the optic tecta of blind-reared animals, the maps are not entirely normal: in guinea pigs, azimuthal tuning is abnormally broad (Withington, 1992); in ferrets, some units exhibit multiple RFs (King & Carlile, 1993); in owls, elevational tuning is often highly abnormal (Knudsen et al., 1991); and in all species there is a decrease in the precision of alignment between auditory and visual RFs. These data imply that vision helps to shape the development of the auditory space map. This implication is reinforced by the topography of the auditory space map in normal owls. The auditory space map overrepresents frontal space relative to peripheral space in a manner that is not predicted by the spatial patterns of auditory localization cues (Knudsen, 1982). Instead, the overrepresentation of frontal space mimics the expansion of frontal space that exists in the visual space map, which in turn reflects the increased density of photoreceptors in the area centralis of the retina.

The shaping influence of vision on the development of the auditory space map has been demonstrated directly by raising owls with prismatic spectacles that displace the visual field horizontally (Figs. 38.2*A* and *B*). Barn owls cannot move their eyes by more than a few degrees from their resting positions. Therefore, prisms produce a chronic discrepancy between visual and auditory spatial information. The immediate effect of prisms is an optical displacement of visual RFs in the tectum. Sustained experience with the prism spectacles, over a period of 6–8 weeks, leads to a horizontal shift in auditory spatial tuning in the optic tectum that realigns auditory RFs with the optically displaced visual RFs (Knudsen & Brainard, 1991). The basis for the horizontal shift of auditory spatial tuning is a shift in unit tuning to ITD, the dominant localization cue for azimuth (Fig. 38.2*C*). The adjustment of auditory tuning in response to prism experience is adaptive because it realigns the auditory and visual maps in the tectum and it adjusts the auditory-orienting responses mediated by

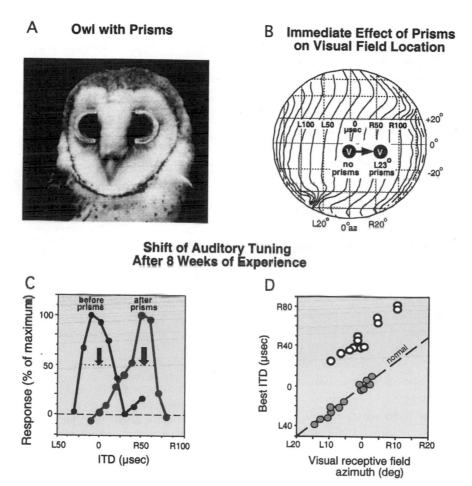

A Owl with Prisms

B Immediate Effect of Prisms on Visual Field Location

Shift of Auditory Tuning After 8 Weeks of Experience

C

D

FIGURE 38.2   Effect of prism experience on the ITD tuning of tectal neurons. (*A*) An owl wearing prismatic spectacles. (*B*) The visual receptive field (RF) of a tectal unit recorded before and after mounting prisms that displace the visual RF by 23 degrees to the left (L23°). The globe represents space relative to the visual axes of the owl. The contours projected onto the globe indicate the locations from which sound produces similar ITD values. The immediate effect of prisms is a shift in visual RFs (indicated by a circled V). (*C*) The ITD tuning of tectal neurons before and after 8 weeks of experience with L23° prisms. Both units had visual RFs centered at 0 degrees azimuth. Before prisms (black line), the unit is tuned to about 0 μs ITD. After 8 weeks of L23° prism experience ITD tuning at this site was shifted to 50 μs right-ear-leading (gray line). The arrows indicate the midpoint of the range of ITD values that elicited more than 50% of the maximum response (best ITD). (*D*) Best ITDs plotted versus the azimuth of the visual RF for tectal units before prism experience (gray circles) and after 8 weeks of wearing L23° prisms. The dashed line indicates the regression of the best ITDs on visual RF azimuth before prisms (normal). A systematic shift in the relation between best ITDs and visual RFs is apparent. (Data from Brainard & Knudsen, 1993.)

the tectum so that the animal foveates an auditory target viewed through the prisms. Analogous results have been reported for young ferrets that have had one eye removed and the other eye chronically deviated: over time, auditory RFs in the optic tectum shift according to the deviation of the remaining eye (King et al., 1988). These experiments demonstrate that visual signals, when available, are the dominant source of instructive information for shaping the auditory space map.

Site of plasticity

The owl's auditory system processes sound localization cues in parallel in the midbrain and forebrain (Cohen & Knudsen, 1999). The midbrain pathway (Fig. 38.3) branches from the main tonotopic pathway at the level of the central nucleus of the inferior colliculus (ICC). In the ICC, auditory cue values are represented in frequency-specific channels (Wagner, Takahashi, & Konishi, 1987). The next structure in the pathway is the external nucleus of the inferior colliculus (ICX). Here, information about cue values is integrated across frequency channels to create neurons that are sharply tuned for space and are organized to form a map of space (Knudsen, 1983). This auditory space map is then conveyed to the optic tectum by a topographic projection (Knudsen & Knudsen, 1983).

A major site of adaptive plasticity is the ICX, where the map is created. In prism-reared owls that acquire a shifted map of ITD in the optic tectum, the map of ITD in the ICX is shifted as well. In contrast, the representation of ITD at the next earlier stage, in the ICC, remains normal (Brainard & Knudsen, 1993).

Associated with the adaptive shift of the ITD map in the ICX is a corresponding change in the anatomy of the axonal projection from the ICC to the ICX (Fig. 38.3B). The ICC-ICX projection in normal owls is topographic. In prism-reared owls that have acquired a shifted map of ITD in the ICX, the ICC-ICX projection is asymmetrically broader than normal, with bouton-laden axons appearing at abnormal locations in the ICX where they could support the newly learned responses to abnormal values of ITD (DeBello, Feldman, & Knudsen, 2001). Interestingly, the normal anatomical projection is also maintained in these owls, even though responses to the normal input are not expressed. Thus, both learned and normal circuitry can coexist in the ICX.

Pharmacological experiments in prism-reared owls also demonstrate that the ICX is a site of plasticity. Excitatory transmission in the ICX is glutamatergic and relies heavily on NMDA receptor currents (Feldman & Knudsen, 1994). Blocking selectively NMDA receptors

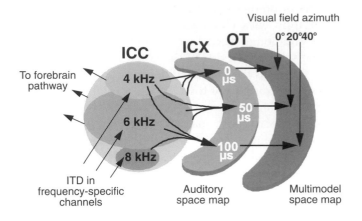

A Normal

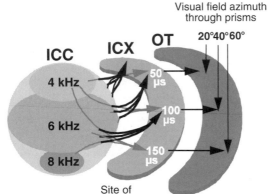

B Prism Experience

FIGURE 38.3 Schematic representation of the midbrain auditory localization pathway. (*A*) Auditory localization cues are initially synthetised in frequency-specific channels. This information ascends to the central nucleus of the inferior colliculus (ICC). From the ICC, auditory information proceeds to the ICX. In the projection from ICC to ICX, information about cue values is combined to produce spatially restricted auditory RFs and a map of space. This map is projected to the optic tectum (OT) through the topographic ICX-OT pathway. In the OT the auditory map merges with a visual map of space. (*B*) Prism experience induces an anatomical change in the ICC-ICX projection. An abnormal rostralward projection appears in one side of the brain and a caudalward projection in the other side. The normal projection remains intact.

in the ICX by focal application of the NMDA receptor blocker AP5 causes a reduction of about 50% of the normal auditory response. However, in owls that have been exposed to prisms, newly learned responses are far more sensitive to NMDA receptor blockade (Feldman, Brainard, & Knudsen, 1996). These data indicate that newly functional synapses in the ICX, supporting learned responses, are richer in NMDA receptors.

The instructive signal

SUPERVISED LEARNING   The adaptive plasticity of the auditory space map is an example of supervised learning. In supervised learning, one system or network serves as the instructor for another. The instructive signal carries information needed for learning and passes it on to a different network, where it guides appropriate changes in the pattern of connectivity (Knudsen, 1994). In the midbrain auditory localization pathway, information from the visual system, which is the most reliable source for determining target location, guides the association of auditory cue values with the locations in the visual field that produced them. But what is the nature of this instructive signal? How does it reach the auditory system, and how does it work?

The instructive signal could be generated in two different ways. It could be derived from a visual assessment of the accuracy of auditory orienting responses. The results of this evaluation could destabilize the auditory network when the stimulus is not successfully foveated, or reinforce the auditory network when the stimulus is acquired by the fovea. We refer to such a nontopographic signal as a foveation-based signal.

Alternatively, a topographic representation of visual space could provide a template for learning. In this case, patterns of auditory activity are compared with the visually based template. Auditory inputs that contribute to a pattern of activity that matches the template are strengthened; those that do not are weakened. This type of signal is referred to as a template-based signal.

PARTIAL OCCLUSION OF THE VISUAL FIELD   A template-based instructive signal and a foveation-based instructive signal lead to very different predictions about the adjustments in the auditory space map that would occur when distinct portions of the visual field are altered differently. In the case of a template-based signal, the adjustments that occur in the auditory space map depend on the visual conditions that exist in each corresponding portion of visual space. Therefore, elimination or alteration of visual input from a specific region of the visual field should only affect adjustments in the corresponding portion of the auditory space map. In contrast, in the case of a foveation-based signal, where adjustments are based on the accuracy of auditory orienting responses as evaluated by the center of gaze, all portions of the auditory map should adjust according to the visual conditions at the center of gaze.

Such an experiment was conducted recently by Hyde and Knudsen (2001). Barn owls wore spectacles that blocked peripheral vision on one side. Because the eyes of owls are essentially immobile in the orbits, this manipulation established different visual conditions in the blocked periphery versus the unblocked center of gaze. These owls were then presented with a prolonged auditory-visual misalignment in the unblocked center of gaze, either by optically displacing the visual field or by removing prisms from owls that had already acquired a shifted map of ITD. After several weeks of experience, the auditory space map in the tectum was examined to determine whether the auditory representation of the center of gaze and of the periphery were altered differently, or whether the entire map was altered as predicted by the visual conditions at the center of gaze.

The results of this experiment are consistent with the hypothesis that the instructive signal is a template-based signal. Occlusion of the visual periphery reduced the adaptive change that occurred in the portion of the auditory space map representing the occluded part of the visual field (Fig. 38.4A). Conversely, occlusion of the center of gaze reduced the adaptive changes in the part of the auditory space map representing the center of gaze, but not in the part representing the periphery (Fig. 38.4B). The results demonstrate that a template-based instructive signal coming from the visual system is involved in the auditory learning process.

THE SOURCE OF THE INSTRUCTIVE SIGNAL TO THE ICX   Since the ICX is a site of plasticity, the instructive signal must enter and act in the ICX, but where does the signal come from? To identify possible sources of instructive input, retrograde tracers were injected into the ICX. As a result, cell bodies in the optic tectum were labeled (Fig. 38.5; Hyde & Knudsen, 2000), indicating that neurons in the optic tectum project to the ICX. Because the primary target of ICX output is the optic tectum, this projection from the optic tectum to the ICX is referred to as a feedback projection.

The optic tectum receives visual spatial information from both the retina and the forebrain (Bravo & Pettigrew, 1981) and therefore is an excellent candidate source of a visual instructive signal to the ICX. Analysis of the locations of labeled somata following injections of tracer into the ICX shows that the distribution of labeled cells in the optic tectum changes systematically with the location of the injection site in ICX (Fig. 38.5B), demonstrating that the optic tectum-ICX feedback connection is topographically organized. Moreover, the point-to-point topography of the optic tectum-ICX projection mirrors that of the feed-forward auditory projection from the ICX to the optic tectum: injections of tracers into the ICX result in anterogradely labeled axons and retrogradely labeled somata at the same location in the optic tectum. Most of the tectal cells that project to the ICX are located in an intermediate

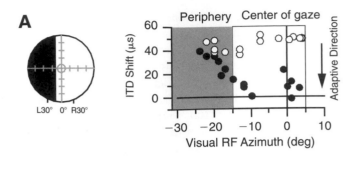

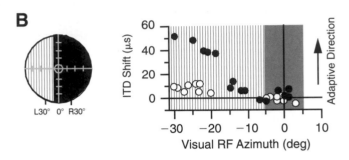

FIGURE 38.4 The effect of partial occlusion of the visual field on auditory map plasticity. The circles on the left represent visual space relative to the owl's center of gaze. The optical conditions in each region of visual space are indicated. Black indicates a region of the field from which light is occluded, white indicates a normal, unaltered region, and the vertical lines indicate a region displaced by prisms. (*A*) Adaptation to normal vision at the center of gaze and occlusion of the left visual periphery. The panel on the right side depicts the shifts in ITD tuning from the predicted normal as a function of the visual RF azimuth. The open circles indicate the ITD shifts obtained after 7 weeks of prism experience. Following this experience, the owl was exposed to the conditions indicated by the circle on the left. Sites with visual RFs in the center of gaze adapted significantly better than sites with visual RFs in the occluded periphery. Shaded box indicates the occluded region of visual space. (*B*) Adaptation to occlusion of the center of gaze and prismatic displacement of the periphery. The panel on the right side depicts the shifts in ITD tuning from the predicted normal as a function of the visual RF azimuth. The open circles indicate the ITD shifts measured before the owl was exposed to the conditions indicated by the circle on the left. After experience with these conditions (gray circles), sites with visual RFs in the periphery adapted significantly better than sites with visual RFs in the occluded center of gaze. The shaded box indicates the occluded region of visual space and the hatched box indicates the region displaced by prisms. (Data from Hyde & Knudsen, 2001.)

layer (Fig. 38.5*C*) and have dendrites that project radially into both the superficial layers, which receive direct input from the retina, and the deep layers, which receive auditory input from the ICX as well as visual input from the forebrain. Therefore, the morphology and location of the feedback cells put them in a position to integrate visual and auditory information from a restricted region of space. This topographically orga-

nized input to the ICX is ideally suited to provide a spatial template for instructing changes in the auditory space map in the ICX.

Strong evidence for a topographic instructive signal originating in the optic tectum comes from lesion experiments (Hyde & Knudsen, 2002). In these experiments, a restricted lesion was made unilaterally in the rostral part of the optic tectum (representing frontal space; Fig. 38.6*A*). Lesions were made in owls that had worn prisms for many weeks and that had acquired shifted auditory maps of space in the optic tectum. After the lesion was made, the prisms were removed, exposing the owls to normal optical conditions. The effect of the lesion on auditory map plasticity was tested in a frontal part of the map on both sides of the brain and, in addition, in a more peripheral part of the map on the lesioned side. Adaptive plasticity was eliminated specifically in the portion of the map that corresponded to the lesion—that is, in the frontal part of the map on the lesioned side (Fig. 38.6*B*). Map adjustments were normal on the intact side of the brain. In the peripheral part of the map on the lesioned side, adaptive adjustments in the auditory map continued to occur, although their magnitude decreased. The decreased magnitude of adjustments on this side of the brain could be due to interference caused by the portion of the map that was rendered nonadjustable by the lesion. This interference could be mediated by lateral inhibition within the map (Zheng & Knudsen, 1999).

Restricted lesions in the optic tectum have a strikingly similar effect to blocking part of the visual field, discussed previously: both manipulations result in the specific elimination of adaptive changes in the corresponding part of the auditory space map. The data demonstrate that a visually based, topographic instructive signal from the optic tectum controls adaptive auditory plasticity in the ICX. Similarly in ferrets, a topographic visual signal from the superficial layers of the SC have been shown to be essential for the normal development of the auditory space map (King, Schnupp, & Thompson, 1998).

GATING OF THE INSTRUCTIVE SIGNAL   For visual activity to provide instructive information to the auditory space map, a stimulus object must be both seen and heard, and the corresponding visual and auditory signals must be treated as though they originated from the same source. Visual activity from objects that do not produce sounds is not useful for instructing the auditory map. Conversely, auditory information about objects that cannot be seen cannot be visually calibrated. Therefore, the instructive visual activity to the auditory space map should be gated. If it were not, then this activity would interfere with the

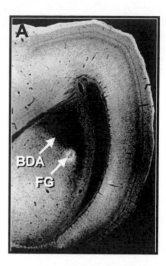
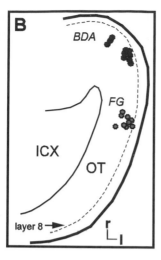
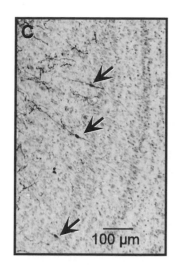

FIGURE 38.5 Topography of the optic tectum-ICX projection. (*A*) Photomicrograph of a horizontal section through the tectal lobe. Injections of biotinylated dextran amine (BDA) and fluoro-gold (FG) were placed in the ICX. Arrows indicate injection sites. The FG injection was more caudal than the BDA injection. (*B*) Composite camera lucida reconstruction of the BDA- and FG-labeled cell bodies in the optic tectum resulting from the injections shown in *A*. Black circles indicate the locations of cell bodies labeled with BDA and gray circles indicate the locations of FG-labeled cell bodies. (*C*) High magnification view of a transverse section through the optic tectum. Retrogradely labeled cells, located in layers 10 and 11, are indicated by arrowheads. Scale bars in *A* = 500 μm, in *B* = 250 μm. (Data from Hyde & Knudsen, 2000.)

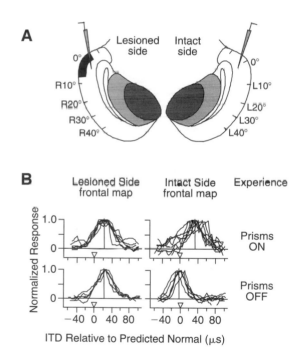

FIGURE 38.6 Effect of a restricted lesion in the optic tectum on auditory map plasticity. (*A*) Schematic representation of the left and right tectal lobes. The lesioned area in the rostral left tectum is indicated by the black region. The sites of recording in the deep layers on both the lesioned and intact sides are indicated. (*B*) Normalized ITD tuning curves measured before (top) and after (bottom) removal of prisms. ITD values are given relative to the predicted normal best ITD. Vertical bars indicate the mean best ITD value relative to normal. Arrowheads indicate the normal ITD tuning. ITD curves measured on the lesioned side (left panels) maintained shifted tuning and did not adapt following the

normal processing of auditory information and might induce plasticity at inappropriate times, leading to maladaptive changes in the auditory network. The system is therefore challenged with the task of selecting those visual objects that produce sounds. Moreover, the nervous system must decide that the visual and auditory signals represent the same stimulus object. A number of studies have shown that auditory and visual stimuli are associated on the basis of common temporal modulations of auditory and visual signals (Hershey & Movellan, 2000; Radeau & Bertelson, 1977), previous knowledge regarding the nature of the stimulus object (Thurlow & Jack, 1973), and possibly attention (Driver & Spence, 1998). All these factors may influence the access of the instructive signal to the ICX.

MAINTENANCE ROLE OF THE INSTRUCTIVE SIGNAL The instructive signal plays a role not only in guiding plasticity, but also in maintaining a shifted auditory map. In prism-reared owls that have a shifted map in the ICX, a lesion of the feedback connection from the optic tectum causes a gradual shift in the adapted auditory map back toward normal, even though the owl continues to wear prisms (Hyde & Knudsen, 2002). This gradual shift occurs only in the region of the auditory map that corresponds with the site of the lesion. This indicates

removal of prisms. In contrast, on the intact side (right panels), ITD tuning shifted back to normal. (Data from Hyde & Knudsen, 2001.)

that instructive input is required to hold the map in its shifted state. It has been noted previously that in an ICX that is expressing a shifted map of space, inputs that support the normal map remain functional, but action potential responses to the normal inputs are differentially suppressed by inhibition (Zheng & Knudsen, 1999). It is not surprising, therefore, that when a visually based instructive signal is eliminated, the map has a tendency to shift back toward an intermediate state between the normal and the shifted maps.

A model of adaptive plasticity in the ICX

INITIAL MAP FORMATION   We hypothesize that an auditory map of space is formed initially by vision-independent mechanisms. This is evident from the presence of a normal auditory map early in development even when visual input is altered or disrupted.

The initial map would reflect genetically determined connections that anticipate the predictable relations of auditory localization cues with locations in space (described in the previous section) and self-organizational processes that strengthen connections that are synchronously activated by natural sounds (Kempter, Leibold, Wagner, & van Hemmen, 2001). However, the auditory space map in the absence of normal visual input does not develop to align precisely with the visual space map in the optic tectum.

NATURE AND MECHANISMS OF THE INSTRUCTIVE SIGNAL IN THE ICX   Precise alignment of the auditory map with the visual map is guided by a topographic instructive signal to the ICX that originates in the tectum. The type of information carried by the instructive signal is not known. Three possible signals are illustrated schematically in Figure 38.7. One possible signal (Fig. 38.7A) is

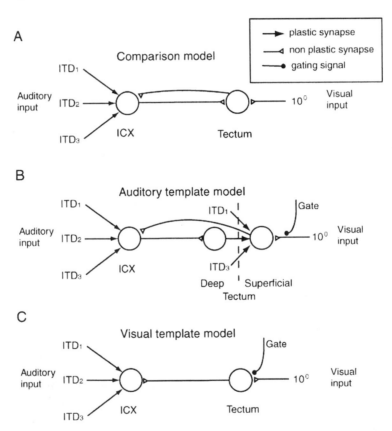

FIGURE 38.7   Three possible models for the instructed plasticity in the ICX. The circles on the left represent neurons in the ICX. The circles on the right represent neurons in optic tectum. A black arrowhead indicates a plastic connection. An empty triangle indicates a connection that is nonplastic during auditory-visual interactions. An ICX neuron receives inputs from various ITD channels (arrows from left). The correct value is selected by a reinforcing instructive signal originating in the tectum (right circle). The different models assume different types of instructive signals. In A, the comparison model, the instructive signal is generated by cells in the tectum that compare auditory spatial information coming from the ICX with visual spatial information. If the spatial information from the two modalities is matched, the cell is activated and a signal is sent back to the optic tectum. In B, the auditory template model, the instructive signal is activated by a specific ITD value for each site. The selection of an ITD value is achieved in the superficial layers of the optic tectum by selecting auditory inputs from the deep layers of the tectum that carry ITD values that match a restricted visual input. In C, the visual template model, the instructive signal is activated by visual stimuli from a restricted region in space. This visual signal reinforces auditory inputs in ICX that are simultaneously activated.

the result of a comparison between visual and auditory spatial information that takes place in the optic tectum. The result of this comparison is sent back to the ICX in a topographic manner to reinforce connections in the ICX that contribute to a correct alignment of the maps or to destabilize the auditory network when the match is not successful. A second possible signal (Fig. 38.7B) is an adjusted auditory template that results from adaptive auditory plasticity in the superficial layers of the optic tectum. This shifted auditory map is sent back to the ICX as an auditory template that instructs auditory plasticity. A third possible signal (Fig. 38.7C) is a topographic representation of the visual field that is sent to the ICX as a visual template for instructing auditory plasticity.

All of these instructive signals require a gate to avoid irrelevant visual activation in the auditory system. In the case of a comparison signal (Fig. 38.7A), the gate can be achieved by a smart mechanism of coincidence detection that allows activation only when visual and auditory activation are likely to rise from a common source. However, if the signal is an auditory or visual template (Fig. 38.7B and C), an external gating mechanism is required. The site of gating differs: in the case of an auditory template signal, the gating must be at the level of the visual input to the site of plasticity in the optic tectum, whereas in the case of a visual template signal, the gating can be either at the level of the visual input or at the level of the cells projecting to the ICX.

To determine which of the signals actually operates in this system, it is essential to record the instructive signal in the ICX. If the signal represents a comparison between auditory and visual signals, ICX units will respond differentially to the alignment of bimodal stimuli. If the signal is an altered auditory template, a delayed adjusted auditory response should appear in the ICX. If the signal is a visual template, ICX units will be activated by visual stimuli originating from a restricted RF that overlaps the normal auditory RF.

The activity of ICX units has been monitored for visual responses. None has been observed, nor has any modulation of auditory responses by visual stimuli been observed. This result might mean that the instructive signal is not visual but rather an adjusted auditory template (Fig. 38.7B). However, the auditory responses in the superficial layers of the OT have long delays, typically 15–20 ms, compared to the 6–8 ms delays typical of ICX units. If the optic tectum-ICX signal is auditory, the time course of auditory responses in the ICX should display a biphasic pattern, representing feed-forward activation and instructive feedback. Examination of poststimulus time histograms measured in the ICX does not disclose any evidence for such a biphasic pattern.

A recent finding, however, strongly implicates a visual template signal in the ICX (Gutfreund, Zheng, & Knudsen, 2002). When bicuculline, a GABA$_A$ antagonist, is focally applied in the optic tectum, ICX units representing the equivalent location in space begin responding to visual stimuli (Fig. 38.8A). Moreover, the visual responses in the ICX have restricted RFs that match the auditory RFs expressed at the same site (Fig. 38.8B). Thus the optic tectum can, under certain conditions, send a visual template signal to the ICX. Such a template could instruct the adjustment of the auditory space map.

Normally the visual signals in the ICX are gated off by GABAergic inhibition in the tectum. It is assumed that under natural conditions, when the animal is interacting with the environment, only visual signals that are associated with auditory signals are permitted to enter the ICX to instruct adjustments in the auditory map.

ALIGNMENT OF THE AUDITORY AND VISUAL MAPS Assuming that the instructive signal is a visual template, auditory map plasticity could be achieved by mechanisms of Hebbian long-term potentiation (LTP) and long-term depression (LTD) (Brown, Chapman, Kairiss, & Keenan, 1988; Mulkey & Malenka, 1992). A single ICX cell receives multiple inputs from the ICC representing a range of values for each cue. When instructive activity enters the ICX, active auditory inputs that synapse on neurons that are activated by the instructive signal are strengthened by LTP, and active auditory inputs that synapse on neurons not activated by the instructive input are weakened by LTD. Axonal remodeling and synaptogenesis may take place to increase the strength of the connections. Such a mechanism ensures that the ICC-ICX projections form an auditory map that matches the topography of the instructive signal.

The instructing synapse must be stable, unaffected by auditory activity. There is no evidence yet that the optic tectum-ICX projection is unaffected by auditory experience; however, it is known that this projection appears early in development, before hatching (Luksch, Gauger, & Wagner, 2000), suggesting that no experience is required for the development of the optic tectum-ICX projection.

TIMING PROBLEM The mechanisms of learning suggested above (LTP and LTD) are based on the correlated activity of pre- and postsynaptic neurons (Stent, 1973). Such mechanisms are suited to support self-organizational plasticity where different inputs compete for control over the activity of the postsynaptic neuron. In supervised learning, however, synapses are

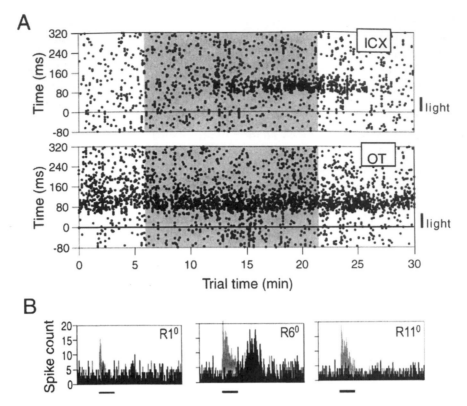

FIGURE 38.8 The effect of bicuculline iontophoresis in optic tectum on visual responses in the ICX. (*A*) Light flashes (50 ms long) were presented every 5 seconds. The multiunit spike response to each presentation is shown by the dots along the vertical axis. The gray area indicates the time during which iontophoretic application of bicuculline was maintained. The horizontal line, at time 0, indicates the onset of light stimulus. In the ICX site (upper raster), units did not respond to light before iontophoresis of bicuculline. However, following 6 minutes of drug application in the optic tectum, clear responses to light appear, with a delay of about 70 ms. In contrast, at the site of drug application (lower raster), light responses are measured before and during bicuculline iontophoresis. (*B*) Light flashes or sound bursts of 50 ms duration were presented from different locations along the horizon (steps of 5 degrees, each location 50 presentations). The poststimulus time histograms of multiunit recording are shown in black for the light stimulus and in gray for the sound stimulus (the auditory response is scaled by 0.5). Responses to light at this site were evident only when the LED was located 6 degrees to the right of the owl's center of gaze. Strongest auditory responses were evoked when the speaker was located at the location that produced visual responses.

selected based on the action of an instructive signal that may arrive long after the synapses that are to be modified are active. This is especially apparent in cases of motor learning. For example, in learning goal-directed movements (Georgopoulos, 1986), movement errors are fed back to the sensorimotor network long after the information is transmitted through the network. For correct adjustments to take place, some trace of the pattern of activation must persist in the network until the instructive signal arrives.

A similar timing problem occurs in the auditory localization system. Visual responses recorded in the ICX appear ~70 ms after the onset of a light stimulus (Fig. 38.8). In contrast, ICX units are activated by an auditory stimulus just 6–8 ms after sound reaches the ear. This implies that by the time a visual instructive signal associated with a short bimodal stimulus activates ICX units, they may have finished processing the auditory stimulus. Whatever learning mechanism is used,

it must be able to accommodate such long delays. Moreover, the relative timing of auditory and visual signals in the ICX depends strongly on the distance of the bimodal stimulus from the animal. Due to the time it takes for sound waves to reach the ears, the delay between auditory and visual activity reaching the ICX decreases with the distance of the object out to about 20 meters, at which point auditory and visual signals arrive simultaneously in the ICX. It is assumed, therefore, that the precise timing of auditory and visual inputs to the ICX is not critical, but rather that auditory synapses can be influenced by an instructive visual activity arriving over a window of time of up to 60 ms following the arrival of auditory activation.

Conclusion

The optic tectum is a structure in the brain in which spatial information from visual and auditory modalities converges into a premotor network that controls gaze direction. In the optic tectum, the auditory and visual modalities form maps of space that are mutually aligned. To achieve alignment, spatial information in the auditory system, which is encoded initially by auditory localization cues such as ILD and ITD, is transformed into a topographic map of space. This transformation is shaped by experience. A major component of the experience-dependent plasticity occurs in the ICX, the nucleus preceding the optic tectum in the midbrain auditory localization pathway. Auditory RFs are synthesized and a map of space is formed in the ICX. The representation of auditory cue values in the auditory maps of space in the ICX and optic tectum is shaped by visual experience.

We are beginning to understand how the visual system instructs auditory map plasticity in the ICX. The instructive signal that controls plasticity is organized topographically: visual-auditory experience in a certain region of space instructs plasticity in the corresponding region of the auditory space map. The source of this signal is the optic tectum, which receives visual information both from the retina and the forebrain. Connections from the optic tectum to the ICX are organized topographically. This anatomical pathway is ideally suited to provide a visually based template to the ICX.

When GABAergic inhibition is blocked in the optic tectum, ICX units respond to visual stimuli. These visual responses have restricted RFs that match the auditory RFs expressed at the same site. Thus, under certain conditions, the optic tectum is capable of sending a topographic representation of the visual field into the ICX. This visual activity could serve as a template for guiding adjustments in the auditory space map. Moreover, the gating of visual activity to the ICX may be the mechanism by which the instructive signal is controlled to prevent interference with normal auditory processing and to avoid changes in the network that are not adaptive.

Unanswered questions about this system include the following: (1) What are the synaptic mechanisms that underlie the instructed modifications of auditory inputs to the ICX? (2) What are the pathways that control the gating of visual signals into the ICX? (3) What are the natural conditions that open the gate and permit visual activity to enter the ICX?

REFERENCES

Ashmead, D. H., Clifton, R. K., & Reese, E. P. (1986). Development of auditory localization in dogs: Single source and precedence effect sounds. *Developmental Psychobiology, 19,* 91–103.

Brainard, M. S., & Knudsen, E. I. (1993). Experience-dependent plasticity in the inferior colliculus: A site for visual calibration of the neural representation of auditory space in the barn owl. *Journal of Neuroscience, 13,* 4589–4608.

Brainard, M. S., Knudsen, E. I., & Esterly, S. D. (1992). Neural derivation of sound source location: Resolution of spatial ambiguities in binaural cues. *Journal of the Acoustical Society of America, 91,* 1015–1027.

Bravo, H., & Pettigrew, J. D. (1981). The distribution of neurons projecting from the retina and visual cortex to the thalamus and tectum opticum of the barn owl, *Tyto alba,* and the burrowing owl, *Speotyto cunicularia. Comparative Neurology, 199,* 419–441.

Brown, T. H., Chapman, P. F., Kairiss, E. W., & Keenan, C. L. (1988). Long-term synaptic potentiation. *Science, 242,* 724–728.

Cohen, Y. E., & Knudsen, E. I. (1999). Maps versus clusters: Different representations of auditory space in the midbrain and forebrain. *Trends in Neurosciences, 22,* 128–135.

DeBello, W. M., Feldman, D. E., & Knudsen, E. I. (2001). Adaptive axonal remodeling in the midbrain auditory space map. *Journal of Neuroscience, 21,* 3161–3174.

Driver, J., & Spence, C. (1998). Crossmodal attention. *Current Opinion in Neurobiology, 8,* 245–253.

Feldman, D. E., Brainard, M. S., & Knudsen, E. I. (1996). Newly learned auditory responses mediated by NMDA receptors in the owl inferior colliculus. *Science, 271,* 525–528.

Feldman, D. E., & Knudsen, E. I. (1994). NMDA and non-NMDA glutamate receptors in auditory transmission in the barn owl inferior colliculus. *Journal of Neuroscience, 14,* 5939–5958.

Georgopoulos, A. P. (1986). On reaching. *Annual Review of Neuroscience, 9,* 147–170.

Gutfreund, Y., Zheng, W., & Knudsen, E. I. (2002). Gated visual input to the central auditory system. *Science, 297,* 1556–1559.

Hershey, J., & Movellan, J. R. (2000). Audio vision: Using audio-visual synchrony to locate sounds. In S. A. Solla, T. K. Leen, & K. R. Muller (Eds.), *Advances in neural information processing systems 12* (pp. 813–819). Cambridge, MA: MIT Press.

Hofman, P. M., Van Riswick, J. G., & Van Opstal, A. J. (1998). Relearning sound localization with new ears. *Nature Neuroscience, 1,* 417–421.

Hyde, P. S., & Knudsen, E. I. (2000). Topographic projection from the optic tectum to the auditory space map in the inferior colliculus of the barn owl. *Journal of Comparative Neurology, 421,* 146–160.

Hyde, P. S., & Knudsen, E. I. (2001). A topographic instructive signal guides the adjustment of the auditory space map in the optic tectum. *Journal of Neuroscience, 21,* 8586–8593.

Hyde, P. S., & Knudsen, E. I. (2002). The optic tectum controls adaptive plasticity of the auditory space map in the inferior colliculus. *Nature, 415,* 73–76.

Kempter, R., Leibold, C., Wagner, H., & van Hemmen, J. L. (2001). Formation of temporal-feature maps by axonal propagation of synaptic learning. *Proceedings of the National Academy of Sciences, USA, 98,* 4166–4171.

King, A. J., & Carlile, S. (1993). Changes induced in the representation of auditory space in the superior colliculus by rearing ferrets with binocular eyelid suture. *Experimental Brain Research, 94,* 444–455.

King, A. J., Hutchings, M. E., Moore, D. R., & Blakemore, C. (1988). Developmental plasticity in the visual and auditory representations in the mammalian superior colliculus. *Nature, 332,* 73–76.

King, A. J., Schnupp, J. W., & Thompson, I. D. (1998). Signals from the superficial layers of the superior colliculus enable the development of the auditory space map in the deeper layers. *Journal of Neuroscience, 18,* 9394–9408.

Knudsen, E. I. (1982). Auditory and visual maps of space in the optic tectum of the owl. *Journal of Neuroscience, 2,* 1177–1194.

Knudsen, E. I. (1983). Subdivisions of the inferior colliculus in the barn owl *(Tyto alba). Journal of Comparative Neurology, 218,* 174–186.

Knudsen, E. I. (1994). Supervised learning in the brain. *Journal of Neuroscience, 14,* 3985–3997.

Knudsen, E. I., & Brainard, M. S. (1991). Visual instruction of the neural map of auditory space in the developing optic tectum. *Science, 253,* 85–87.

Knudsen, E. I., Esterly, S. D., & du Lac, S. (1991). Stretched and upside-down maps of auditory space in the optic tectum of blind-reared owls: Acoustic basis and behavioral correlates. *Journal of Neuroscience, 11,* 1727–1747.

Knudsen, E. I., & Knudsen, P. F. (1983). Space-mapped auditory projections from the inferior colliculus to the optic tectum in the barn owl *(Tyto alba). Journal of Comparative Neurology, 218,* 187–196.

Knudsen, E. I., & Knudsen, P. F. (1989). Vision calibrates sound localization in developing barn owls. *Journal of Neuroscience, 9,* 3306–3313.

Knudsen, E. I., Knudsen, P. F., & Esterly, S. D. (1984). A critical period for the recovery of sound localization accuracy following monaural occlusion in the barn owl. *Journal of Neuroscience, 4,* 1012–1020.

Luksch, H., Gauger, B., & Wagner, H. (2000). A candidate pathway for a visual instructional signal to the barn owl's auditory system. *Journal of Neuroscience, 20,* RC70.

Middlebrooks, J. C., & Green, D. M. (1991). Sound localization by human listeners. *Annual Review of Psychology, 42,* 135–159.

Morrongiello, B. A., Fenwick, K. D., Hillier, L., & Chance, G. (1994). Sound localization in newborn human infants. *Developmental Psychobiology, 27,* 519–538.

Mulkey, R. M., & Malenka, R. C. (1992). Mechanisms underlying induction of homosynaptic long-term depression in area CA1 of the hippocampus. *Neuron, 9,* 967–975.

Peck, C. K. (1996). Visual-auditory integration in cat superior colliculus: Implications for neuronal control of the orienting response. *Progress in Brain Research, 112,* 167–177.

Radeau, M., & Bertelson, P. (1977). Adaptation to auditory-visual discordance and ventriloquism in semirealistic situations. *Perception & Psychophysics, 22,* 137–146.

Stein, B. E. (1998). Neural mechanisms for synthesizing sensory information and producing adaptive behaviors. *Experimental Brain Research, 123,* 124–135.

Stein, B. E., & Meredith, M. A. (1993). *The merging of the senses.* Cambridge, MA: MIT Press.

Stent, G. S. (1973). A physiological mechanism for Hebb's postulate of learning. *Proceedings of the National Academy of Sciences, USA, 70,* 997–1001.

Thurlow, W. R., & Jack, C. E. (1973). Certain determinants of the "ventriloquism effect." *Perceptual and Motor Skills, 36,* 1171–1184.

Wagner, H., Takahashi, T., & Konishi, M. (1987). Representation of interaural time difference in the central nucleus of the barn owl's inferior colliculus. *Journal of Neuroscience, 7,* 3105–3116.

Withington, D. J. (1992). The effect of binocular lid suture on auditory responses in the guinea-pig superior colliculus. *Neuroscience Letters, 136,* 153–156.

Zheng, W., & Knudsen, E. I. (1999). Functional selection of adaptive auditory space map by $GABA_A$-mediated inhibition. *Science, 284,* 962–965.

39 The Development of Multisensory Integration

MARK T. WALLACE

Introduction

We live in a multisensory world in which we are continually bombarded with information conveyed via the different sensory modalities. One important and frequently unappreciated role of the brain is to synthesize this melange of sensory information into an adaptive and coherent perceptual *Gestalt*. Simply stated, information from the different senses that is associated with a single object or event (e.g., the sight and sound of an automobile) must be interpreted as such, whereas information from the different senses that is not associated with an object or event must be interpreted in a very different manner. As indicated by the wealth of literature on cross-modal interactions in human perception (see Stein & Meredith, 1993; Welch & Warren, 1986), this sensory synthesis is a constantly occurring phenomenon that is continually shaping our view of the world. Not surprisingly, not only do these interactions modify our perceptions, they also play an important role in influencing our reactions to sensory stimuli. For example, simple reaction times are often made faster by multisensory stimuli (Andreassi & Greco, 1975; Bernstein, Clark, & Edelstein, 1969; Gielen, Schmidt, & Van den Heuvel, 1983; Hershenson, 1962; Hughes, Reuter-Lorenz, Vozawa, & Fendrich, 1994; Morrell, 1968), and a similar speeding is seen for simple motor acts such as rapid eye movements (i.e., saccades; see Frens, Van Opstal, & Van der Willigen, 1995; Goldring, Dorris, Corneil, Ballantyne, & Munoz, 1996; Harrington & Peck, 1998; Hughes et al., 1994; Nozawa, Reuter-Lorenz, & Hughes, 1994; Perrott, Saberi, Brown, & Strybel, 1990).

Much work has gone into understanding the neural underpinnings of these cross-modal processes. Numerous sites of multisensory convergence and integration have been identified in the brain, and the principles according to which individual multisensory neurons integrate their various inputs have been elucidated in several model populations (see Stein & Meredith, 1993). This work has made clear that the spatial, temporal, and physical characteristics of the stimuli that are combined critically determine how they are synthesized. Thus, multisensory stimuli that are in close physical proximity, that occur at or near the same moment in time, that are weakly effective on their own, and that are contextually similar result in enhanced neural activity. In contrast, stimuli that are spatially or temporally distant or incongruent result in depressed neural activity. Such changes in neuronal response have striking parallels in the behavioral realm, where they likely play an important deterministic role in these overt responses (Stein, Huneycutt, & Meredith, 1988; Stein, Meredith, Huneycutt, & McDade, 1989).

Despite the recent explosion of interest in studying multisensory interactions at the neuronal and behavioral levels, little research effort has been directed toward understanding the ontogeny of these cross-modal processes. This lack is quite surprising, given the long history of research attempting to elucidate the basic principles of sensory development in both humans and animals. The importance of gaining a better understanding of these questions is best framed by two radically different views of human multisensory development (for a more in-depth discussion of this debate, see Lewkowicz & Kraebel, Chap. 41, this volume). On the one side are those who view this process as a chronological progression from the development of modality-specific responsiveness to multisensory responsiveness. According to this view, the young infant has segregated channels for processing information arriving via the different senses, and only develops multisensory capacities with the associations between the senses that occur during postnatal experience. Alternatively, some investigators believe the process moves in the opposite direction, with the young infant being extraordinarily multisensory and only later learning to segregate information on a sense-by-sense basis.

Studies of human sensory development are extremely difficult to conduct and interpret, although their results are fascinating and quite important. A different approach to understanding the genesis of multisensory development is to conduct such studies in animal models, where it is possible to examine the appearance and functional maturation of elements within the nervous system as development progresses.

Sensory and multisensory development in the SC

We begin by reviewing work on multisensory development in the midbrain structure, the superior colliculus (SC), which has become the preeminent model for studying multisensory processes at the neuronal level. This work has largely been done in two species for which there is a substantial database on multisensory neural processing in adults, the cat and the rhesus monkey. These two species, besides having very different behavioral repertoires—one is a carnivore and the other an omnivore—are born at very different points in the maturational process. The cat, an altricial species, is born at a relatively early developmental stage, whereas the monkey, a precocial species, is born relatively late in this process. The neuroethological correlates of this difference are straightforward. The cat is born at a time when its nervous system is so young as to be unable to support much coordinated behavior. Relative to this state, the newborn monkey has a far more sophisticated set of behaviors immediately after birth.

Electrophysiological recordings obtained in the cat in the first several days after birth reveal little sensory activity in what is to become the multisensory (i.e., below the stratum opticum) layers of the SC (Stein, Labos, & Kruger, 1973; Wallace & Stein, 1997). Microelectrodes can traverse long expanses of the structure without encountering a single element responsive to sensory stimuli. What sensory drive is present in these layers at this time is solely responsive to somatosensory (i.e., tactile) cues. Such responses are consistent with the needs and behavioral repertoire of the newborn. Kittens spend their first few days in close proximity to their mother, rarely losing direct tactile contact. The directed behaviors that are present at this stage are quite simple, revolving around finding the nipple in order to feed. Toward the end of the first postnatal week, responses to a second sensory modality, audition, begin to appear in the deep SC. Again, this progression makes sense from a behavioral perspective, insofar as the first orientation responses (typically of the head and body) to auditory cues are seen at about this time (Fox, 1970; Levine, Hull, & Buchwald, 1980; Villablanca & Olmstead, 1979). Following the appearance of these somatosensory- and auditory-responsive neurons, their prevalence gradually increases as postnatal development progresses. With the increasing prevalence of each of these modality-specific neuron types, there is the appearance of the first multisensory SC neurons—those responsive to somatosensory and auditory cues. As discussed later in this chapter, these early multisensory neurons behave very differently from their adult counterparts.

Visual responses can first be elicited in the SC at about the time of eye opening (approximately 7–8 days postnatally; see Kao, McHaffie, Meredith, & Stein, 1994). However, these early visual responses are restricted to the superficial SC layers, layers that will never take on a multisensory character. In contrast to this early appearance of superficial visual responses, neurons in the deep SC remain unresponsive to visual cues until the third postnatal week (Wallace & Stein, 1997). Consistent with the profile for somatosensory and auditory neurons, soon after visual responses appear in these layers, the first visually responsive multisensory neurons are found. Over the ensuing 2–3 months, the prevalence of multisensory neurons in the deep SC gradually rises to adult values (Fig. 39.1). Ultimately, they represent approximately 60%–70% of the deep-layer population.

In the monkey, the developmental timetable is somewhat different. In this species, somatosensory, auditory, and visual responses are present in the deep SC immediately after birth (Wallace & Stein, 2001). As a likely consequence of information from each of these modalities being present at this time, multisensory neurons are also found at birth. Nonetheless, the proportionate representation of multisensory neurons in the newborn monkey is about half of what it will become in the adult (Fig. 39.2). The chronological time frame in which the growth of the multisensory population takes place has yet to be determined for this species.

Maturation of sensory response properties in the SC

The earliest sensory-responsive neurons in the SC have activity profiles very different from those they will acquire as they mature. The degree to which these response characteristics differ from the adult state appears to depend on the developmental chronology of the appearance of that sensory modality in the SC. Thus, at any given age during early development, somatosensory responses are the most mature, auditory responses are intermediate, and visual responses are the most immature and different from the adult. The maturation of these sensory response characteristics appears to proceed in an identical manner for modality-specific (e.g., auditory alone) and multisensory (e.g., visual-auditory) neurons.

For the somatosensory-responsive population, several response characteristics are already indistinguishable from adult responses at birth in both cat and monkey.

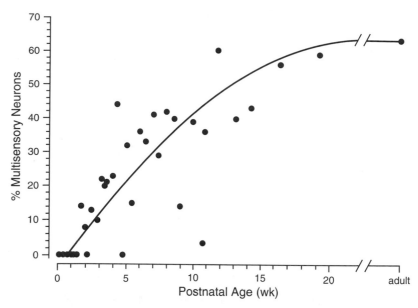

FIGURE 39.1 The population of multisensory SC neurons in the cat grows substantially during postnatal development. Plotted is the proportion of multisensory neurons in the deep layers of the SC as a function of postnatal age. (Adapted from Wallace & Stein, 1997.)

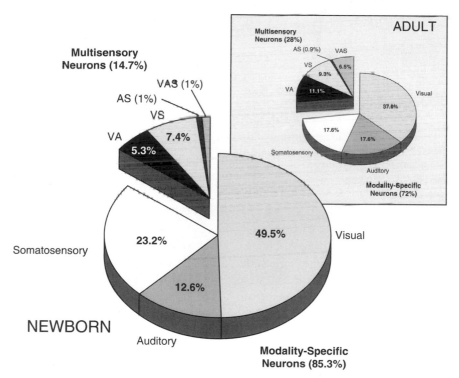

FIGURE 39.2 The distributions of sensory-responsive neurons in the deep layers of the newborn and adult (inset) rhesus monkey. Although of low prevalence, a significant population of multisensory neurons is found in the newborn monkey SC. (Adapted from Wallace & Stein, 2001.)

Little difference can be noted in the relative distribution of receptor types (hair, skin, deep), adaptation class (fast vs. slow), and velocity preference. Nonetheless, early somatosensory responses are weaker, have longer latencies, and have larger receptive fields (RFs) than at later times in postnatal development. In the most readily

measured of these response characteristics, somatosensory response latencies decline precipitously in cat SC over the first 6–8 weeks of postnatal life (Fig. 39.3).

Although later to appear (and less adultlike when they do appear), auditory-responsive SC neurons seem to mature over a similar time period as their

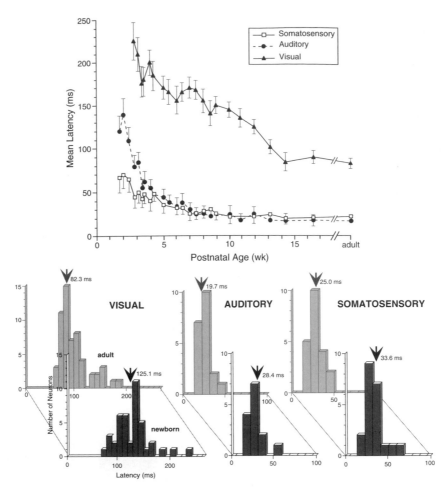

FIGURE 39.3 Response latencies decline during postnatal development in both cat (top) and monkey (bottom). (*Top*) Curves depicting the changes in mean response latencies for somatosensory, auditory, and visual responses as a function of postnatal age in the developing cat SC. (*Bottom*) Histograms depicting the distributions of mean response latencies for visual, auditory, and somatosensory responsive neurons in the newborn (black) and adult (gray) monkey SC. Arrows point to the mean latency for each population. (Adapted from Wallace & Stein, 1997, 2001.)

somatosensory-responsive counterparts. In both cat and monkey, mean auditory thresholds are quite high early in postnatal life and decline to adult levels in the first few postnatal months. For example, in the cat, mean auditory thresholds to broadband sounds are 71 dB SPL (sound pressure level) at 3 postnatal weeks, 58 dB SPL at 6 weeks, and 53 dB SPL at 13 weeks. Similarly, auditory response latencies decline from an average of about 120 ms at 3 postnatal weeks to approximately 20 ms by 8–10 postnatal weeks (Fig. 39.3). The change is less dramatic in the monkey, where auditory latencies in the newborn (mean, 28.4 ms) are approximately 50% longer than in the adult (mean, 19.7 ms) (Fig. 39.3). Although difficult to assess rigorously in a free-field setting, qualitative assessment of binaural inputs to the SC suggests that there is a significant shift in the balance of these inputs during early postnatal maturation. In the cat, the earliest auditory-responsive neurons respond in

an excitatory manner to inputs presented in either contralateral or ipsilateral space. Such an organization fits well with the finding of largely omnidirectional neurons (i.e., no spatial RFs) at this early stage of development. By the fourth postnatal week, neurons appear that lack any response to stimuli presented in ipsilateral space, creating the first population with discrete RFs. A week or so later, the first neurons with inhibitory characteristics are found, thus providing a mechanism to further shape auditory RFs.

As mentioned earlier, visual responses in the multisensory layers of the SC mature later than somatosensory or auditory responses. Not surprisingly, when they do appear, the response properties of these early visual neurons are quite immature. Although the degree of stimulus selectivity in adult SC neurons is relatively poor compared with neurons in the geniculostriate pathway (a difference that likely reflects the spatial rather than

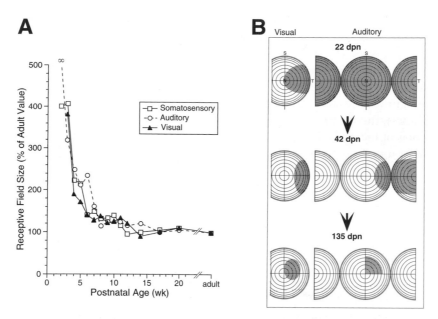

FIGURE 39.4   Receptive fields (RFs) in cat SC neurons decline dramatically in size during postnatal development. (*A*) Plot of RF size standardized to the adult mean as a function of postnatal age. Note the precipitous decline in RF size over the first 6–8 weeks of postnatal life. (*B*) Representative RFs (shading) from visual-auditory neurons at three postnatal time points. In the representation of auditory space, the central hemisphere depicts space in front of the interaural line, and the split hemisphere on either side (folded forward) depicts auditory space caudal to the interaural line. Note the consolidation of RFs, which reveals a good register between them. N, nasal; T, temporal; S, superior; I, inferior. (Adapted from Wallace & Stein, 1997.)

identity-oriented emphasis of the SC), there is still a significant developmental progression in visual responses. For example, although direction selectivity is found in a substantial component of the adult visual population (Wallace & Stein, 1997; see also Hoffmann, 1973; McIlwain & Buser, 1968; Stein & Arigbede, 1972; Sterling & Wickelgren, 1969; Straschill & Hoffmann, 1969), the first directionally selective neuron in the neonatal cat is not found until the postnatal week 7, 3 weeks after the appearance of visual responses. Another property that is characteristic of most adult SC neurons is that they are tuned to a specific range of stimulus speeds. This property is absent in the first visually responsive neurons and appears gradually during postnatal development. Developmental changes are also seen in the degree and prevalence of surround inhibition, spatial summation and inhibition, habituation, and responses to stationary flashed versus moving stimuli. Finally, as with the other modalities, visual response latencies exhibit a precipitous decline during the first several months of postnatal life (Fig. 39.3).

Receptive field consolidation during development

One of the most readily apparent developmental changes in SC neurons is in the size of their RFs. The earliest RFs of multisensory neurons (and of their modality-specific neighbors) are typically very large,

often spanning an entire hemifield or half of the body (and in some instances encompassing all of sensory space; Fig. 39.4) (Wallace & Stein, 1997). This is in stark contrast to the adult state, where SC RFs, although large relative to other sensory representations, still are confined to discrete regions of sensory space (Clemo & Stein, 1991; Meredith, Clemo, & Stein, 1991; Meredith & Stein, 1986a, 1986b; Middlebrooks & Knudsen, 1984; Stein, Magalhaes-Castro, & Kruger, 1976). In the cat, the developmental profile of RF size shows a steep decline in the earliest stages of postnatal development, followed by a more gradual decline until about 3–4 months after birth (Fig. 39.4) (Wallace & Stein, 1997).

As a consequence of this developmental consolidation in RFs, the sensory topographies that characterize the adult SC become increasingly apparent as the animal matures. Thus, whereas in early postnatal stages only a very coarse topography can be demonstrated in the deep SC, as development progresses each of the sensory representations takes on an increasingly finer-grained resolution. Quite strikingly, in individual multisensory neurons, this RF consolidation appears to occur concomitantly for *each* of the neuron's RFs. Such a finding suggests a common mechanistic underpinning to this consolidation, a result we will return to when we consider the developmental role of inputs from cortex in shaping the responses of their SC target neurons.

In the monkey, RF consolidation appears to be very similar, except for the more advanced developmental timetable for this precocial species (Wallace & Stein, 2001). Thus, although not examined at a series of postnatal time points as in the cat, the RFs of neurons in the newborn monkey SC are significantly larger than in the adult (Fig. 39.5). Nonetheless, the intermediate size of these RFs makes the topographic organization of the newborn monkey SC more apparent than that of the newborn cat, as is seen in the single rostrocaudally oriented electrode penetration depicted in Figure 39.5.

Multisensory integration is absent in early developmental stages

As should be clear from the preceding discussion, multisensory neurons appear almost as soon as inputs from two modalities can be observed to converge in the

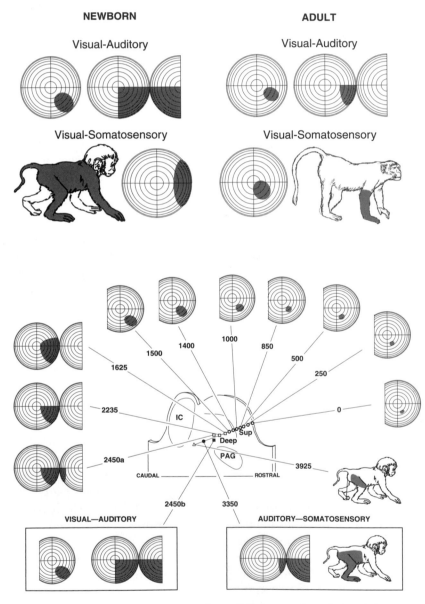

FIGURE 39.5   Receptive fields in the newborn monkey are substantially larger than their adult counterparts, yet a topographic order is readily apparent. At top are shown representative examples of RFs (shaded) in visual-auditory and visual-somatosensory neurons in the newborn (left) and adult (right) monkey SC. Conventions are the same as in Figure 39.4. At bottom are shown RFs mapped during a single electrode penetration through the newborn monkey SC. The penetration is depicted on the drawing of a sagittal section through the SC, with symbols representing locations where individual neurons were isolated. Lines extend out to the RFs recorded at each of these locations, with the depth of the recorded element (in μm) noted on the line. The RFs of multisensory neurons are shown within boxes. Sup, superficial SC layers; Deep, deep SC layers; PAG, periaqueductal gray; IC, inferior colliculus. (From Wallace & Stein, 2001.)

SC. Furthermore, the growth of the multisensory population appears to mirror the relative growth of the different sensory-responsive cell types. For example, as visually responsive elements become increasingly prevalent, there is a concomitant growth in the visually responsive multisensory population.

Simply by nature of the increasing convergence of inputs from multiple modalities, multisensory neurons are created during development at a steadily increasing rate. However, when compared with such neurons in the adult (see Stein, Jiang, & Stanford, Chap. 15, this volume), these early multisensory neurons behave very differently. The most strikingly different feature is the manner in which they respond to combinations of stimuli from multiple modalities (Wallace & Stein, 1997). Early multisensory neurons respond nearly identically to both individual stimuli and to their combination. An example is shown in Figure 39.6A. In this visual-somatosensory neuron (recorded from a 20-days-postnatal cat), a weak response is elicited when the visual stimulus is presented alone, and a similarly weak response is elicited when the somatosensory stimulus is presented alone. Pairing these two stimuli elicits a response that is virtually indistinguishable from either of the modality-specific responses. This pattern of responses is invariant, occurring regardless of the spatial or temporal relationships of the combined stimuli or their physical features. This type of response profile is observed in all multisensory neurons prior to 28 days postnatally, and is dramatically different from the adult response to multisensory stimulus combinations, in which responses significantly different from the component modality-specific responses are the norm.

Although much more mature in many ways, a similar pattern of results is seen in the SC of the newborn monkey. Here, despite the presence of a reasonable multisensory population, the sophisticated integrative features of these neurons have yet to develop (Wallace & Stein, 2001). In many respects, the SC of the newborn monkey can be seen as equivalent to the SC of the 3-week-old cat. Multisensory neurons, including those with a visual component, are present, yet these neurons lack the integrative abilities of the adult.

The appearance of multisensory integration

In the cat, several weeks after the appearance of multisensory neurons in the SC, a change begins to be seen in this population. Now, neurons begin to appear that have very different integrative characteristics than those found just a day or two earlier. Most notably, and somewhat surprisingly, these neurons integrate their multisensory inputs in a fashion very much resembling that seen in the adult. Thus, as can be seen in the example shown in Figure 39.6B, these neurons respond to combined stimulation with fairly dramatic changes in their response profiles.

Both response enhancements and response depressions can be elicited in these early integrating neurons. Furthermore, the magnitude of these changes is very similar to that seen in the adult. This result was surprising and ran counter to the idea that the integrative capacity of a given multisensory neuron developed gradually. The all-or-none nature of the appearance of multisensory integration suggests that this property is developmentally gated, a finding we return to when we discuss the role of cortex in the maturational process.

Despite the all-or-none nature of the appearance of multisensory integration in any given SC neuron, because of the gradual maturational profile of both multisensory neurons and their integrative capacity, the SC as a structure does not reach multisensory maturity until approximately 4 months after birth. At this time, both the proportion of multisensory neurons and the percentage of those neurons that have the capacity to integrate multisensory cues are at adult levels.

The maturation of multisensory integration and receptive fields may be linked

Intriguingly, when examined for factors that might predict the multisensory nature of a given SC neuron (i.e., integrative vs. nonintegrative) in the cat, a single RF property was found to have a strong predictive value. Thus, whereas neurons with large RFs fields were highly unlikely to exhibit adultlike multisensory integration, those with RFs similar in size to adult RFs had a high probability of being classified as integrating (Wallace & Stein, 1997). For example, regardless of the age at which they were found, multisensory neurons with RFs more than double the size of those found in the adult had a less than 15% probability of exhibiting multisensory integration (Fig. 39.7). In contrast, neurons with RFs equivalent in size to those found in the adult had a greater than 80% probability of exhibiting integration. This dichotomy was most dramatically illustrated in recordings from the same animal. In these examples, which were found at ages between 28 and 84 days postnatally, both nonintegrating multisensory neurons with large RFs and integrating neurons with adultlike RFs could be found.

Maturation of integrative properties in multisensory neurons

As already described, in one respect the maturation of multisensory integration appears to take place in a

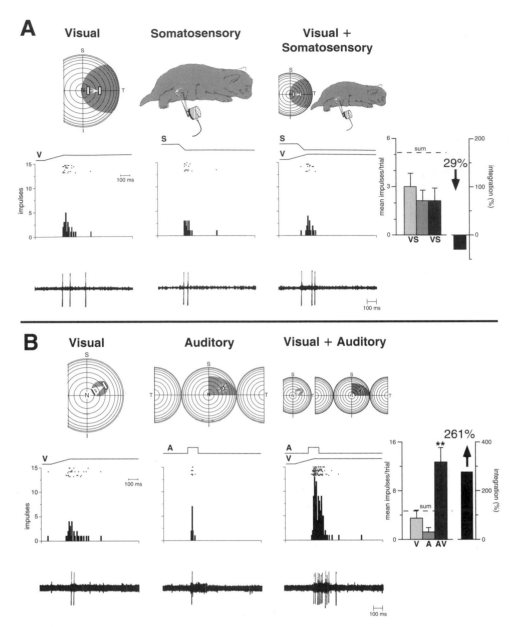

FIGURE 39.6   Multisensory integration is absent in the earliest multisensory neurons and appears during postnatal development. (*A*) Receptive fields (top) and neural responses (bottom) for a visual-somatosensory SC neuron recorded at 21 days postnatally (dpn). Shading depicts the RFs, and icons denote the locations of the stimuli used in quantitative tests. Rasters, peristimulus time histograms, and summary bar graphs illustrate this neuron's response to the visual stimulus alone (left, ramp V represents movement of the visual stimulus shown at the top), the somatosensory stimulus alone (left center, ramp S represents indentation of the skin produced by the tactile probe shown at the top), and the combination of these same stimuli (right center, VS). Summary bar graph (right) shows the mean neural responses and the proportionate change generated by the stimulus combination. Dashed line labeled *sum* shows the predicted multisensory response based on the sum of the two modality-specific responses. For determining multisensory integration, the following formula was used: % interaction = $[(CM - SM_{max})/SM_{max}] \times 100$, where CM is the response to the combined modality presentation and SM_{max} is the response to the best of the modality-specific stimuli. Representative oscillographic traces at the bottom illustrate the neuron's responses to a single stimulus presentation. (*B*) Receptive fields and neuronal responses for a visual-auditory neuron in a 35 dpn animal. Note the smaller RFs and the significant enhancement to the stimulus combination. (Adapted from Wallace & Stein, 1997.)

binary fashion. Thus, when a given neuron can be shown to integrate multisensory cues, the magnitude of the changes that characterize that integration is the same as in the adult. Such a finding raises the question

of whether the other integrative features of developing multisensory neurons are similarly mature, or whether some (or all) of these properties mature at a more gradual rate.

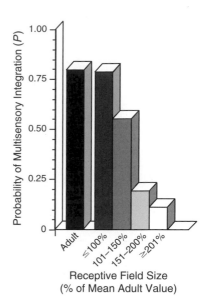

FIGURE 39.7　Receptive field size and the probability of multi-sensory integration are well correlated. In the adult, the probability of multisensory integration in any given SC neuron is approximately 0.8. This value is quite similar for multisensory neurons in the neonate with RFs equivalent in size to the adult (≤100%), and declines progressively for larger RFs. RF sizes were standardized relative to location in the SC. (Adapted from Wallace & Stein, 1997.)

As already discussed in Chapter 15, by Stein and colleagues, adult multisensory neurons abide by a spatial principle that depends on the organization of their RFs. The RFs of these neurons exhibit good overlap, and response enhancements are typically generated when multisensory stimuli are positioned within these RFs. However, when one of the stimuli is positioned outside the excitatory borders of its RF, either no interaction or a response depression is generated. The presence or absence of such depression appears to be a function of inhibitory surrounds (Kadunce, Vaughan, Wallace, Benedek, & Stein, 1997). In neonatal multisensory neurons that have developed the capacity to integrate their cross-modal cues, this principle is much the same (Wallace & Stein, 1997). Thus, within-RF stimulus pairings generally give rise to response enhancements, whereas response depressions or no interaction are generated when one of the stimuli is positioned outside its RF.

Similarly, neonatal integrating neurons appear to abide by the principle of inverse effectiveness first established in the adult. In this principle, the pairing of stimuli that, when presented individually, result in weak responses, gives rise to the greatest proportionate response enhancements. On the other hand, the pairing of more effective stimuli gives rise to progressively smaller enhancements. For example, whereas the pairing of a weak visual and a weak auditory stimulus may

result in a response enhancement of several hundred percent, the pairing of a strong visual and a strong auditory stimulus may result in little or no enhancement. Another principle that appears similar in the earliest integrative neurons and in the adult is the manner in which they respond to within-modality stimulus pairings (e.g., their responses to two visual stimuli). In both instances, the combination of two stimuli within a given modality results in a response little different from the response to one of the stimuli. This is in striking contrast to what is seen when stimuli are paired across different modalities in these same neurons.

Immediately after they have developed their integrative capacity, neonatal multisensory neurons do differ in one important respect from their adult counterparts. Whereas adult multisensory neurons typically have a fairly large window of time (i.e., several hundred milliseconds) within which they can combine their multisensory inputs in order to give an integrated response, this window is substantially smaller in the neonate (Wallace & Stein, 1997). In fact, it appears that the first integrating neurons have no temporal window at all; they show interactions only when stimuli are combined at a single onset asynchrony (Fig. 39.8). As development progresses, this temporal window gradually expands toward the adult range of values (Fig. 39.8).

Although the reason (and physiological mechanism) for this temporal difference between the neonate and the adult remains unknown, one possibility is that it reflects the very different behavioral "working" distances seen at these two ages. Very early in postnatal development, cats have an extremely limited behavioral repertoire, staying close to their mother and their den. Consequently, the range of distances that are of behavioral significance is quite restricted. One can think of the temporal window of multisensory integration as a crude representation of stimulus distance, which is created on the basis of the different speeds at which signals are propagated in the environment (e.g., the differences between the speed of sound and the speed of light) and the different times of arrival of the relevant information at the SC (see Stein & Meredith, 1993). Whereas a constricted temporal window might represent a very limited set of working distances, a more expanded window could represent a broader range of distances.

Except for this temporal difference, the transition from the nonintegrative to the integrative state in any given SC neuron appears to be quite abrupt. Although the exact time needed for this transition awaits the continuous recording from the same multisensory neuron at different ages, these results are very suggestive that the transition occurs as the consequence of the rapid opening of a biological gate.

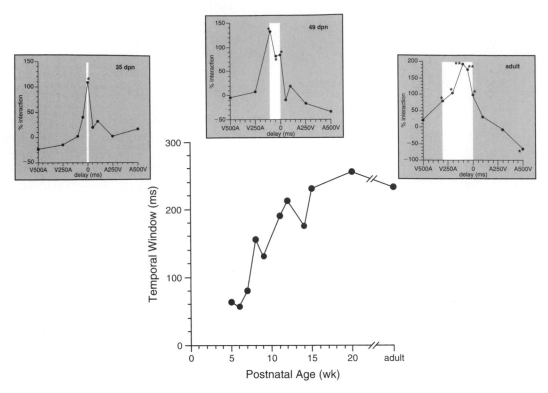

FIGURE 39.8   The temporal window for multisensory integration expands during postnatal development. The center graph plots the growth of this temporal window as a function of age. Insets show representative data from neurons at three different developmental stages. Plotted in each of these examples is the magnitude of the multisensory interaction generated at different stimulus onset asynchronies (delay). In this convention, V500A indicates that the onset of the visual stimulus preceded the onset of the auditory stimulus by 500 ms, V = A indicates simultaneous onsets, and so on. Lighter shading shows the size of the temporal window. *$P < 0.05$; **$P < 0.01$. (Adapted from Wallace & Stein, 1997.)

Role of cortical inputs in multisensory integration in the SC

As we have seen, the SC is the site for the convergence of sensory inputs from multiple modalities, with the end result being the creation of a substantial population of multisensory neurons. Anatomical and physiological studies in cat have shown that these sensory inputs converge on the SC from a broad array of different sources, including inputs from both subcortical and cortical structures (Berson, 1985; Berson & McIlwain, 1982; Edwards, Ginsburgh, Henkel, & Stein, 1979; Huerta & Harting, 1984; Kawamura, Hattori, Higo, & Matsuyama, 1982; Kawamura & Konno, 1979; Meredith & Clemo, 1989; Mize, 1983; Mucke, Norita, Benedek, & Creutzfeldt, 1982; Norita et al., 1986; Olson & Graybiel, 1987; Segal & Beckstead, 1984; Stein, Spencer, & Edwards, 1983; Tortelly, Reinoso-Suarez, & Llamas, 1980). The substantial sensory convergence seen in the SC raises an intriguing question. Are all of the sensory inputs to the SC equivalent for the multisensory processing capabilities exhibited by its neurons? Stated a bit differently, would a visual-auditory neuron that

received its visual input from the retina and its auditory input from the inferior colliculus behave in the same manner as a visual-auditory neuron that received its visual input from extrastriate visual cortex and its auditory input from association auditory cortex?

To answer this question, it was first necessary to detail the pattern of inputs onto individual multisensory SC neurons. To begin this analysis, we examined the projections from those cortical regions shown in anatomical studies to provide the heaviest input to the deep SC, two areas classically described as "association" in function. These areas are the cortex of the anterior ectosylvian sulcus (AES) (which is divided into separate visual, auditory, and somatosensory regions) and the lateral suprasylvian (LS) cortex. Using electrical stimulation techniques, we established that the vast majority of multisensory SC neurons received input from at least one of these cortical regions and that the majority received convergent input from two or more sites within these cortical domains (Wallace, Meredith, & Stein, 1993). The next step in the analysis was to try and dissect out the functional importance of these cortical inputs to the multisensory character of their SC targets.

To do this, we used the technique of cryogenic blockade, in which a given cortical region was selectively and reversibly deactivated by cooling while we examined the multisensory responses of neurons in the SC. These initial studies (Wallace & Stein, 1994), which have now been extended and elaborated (W. Jiang, Wallace, Jiang, Vaughan, & Stein, 2001), produced a striking result. Although during cortical deactivation the multisensory identity of SC neurons was relatively unaffected (i.e., a visual-somatosensory neuron remained visual-somatosensory), the integrative responses of these neurons were dramatically altered. The significant response enhancements and depressions that characterize normal multisensory integration were no longer present; the neurons now responded to the combined stimuli in a manner little different from their response to the most effective of the two modality-specific stimuli. In short, the multisensory integrative capacity of SC neurons was abolished during cortical deactivation. Upon restoration of cortical function (by rewarming the deactivated cortex), multisensory integration returned. Although the initial study focused largely on the contribution of AES to multisensory integration in the SC, more recent work has found a second cortical area, the rostral lateral suprasylvian (r-LS) cortex, to play an important role as well (W. Jiang et al., 2001). In keeping with the results of these physiological studies, an examination of orientation behaviors during cortical deactivation has highlighted the importance of these cortical areas for multisensory processes (W. Jiang, Jiang, & Stein, 2002; Wilkinson, Meredith, & Stein, 1996).

It was interesting to note that during cortical deactivation, multisensory neurons in the adult SC bore a striking resemblance to multisensory neurons recorded from neonatal animals prior to the appearance of their integrative capacity. That is, both sets of neurons responded to the combination of sensory stimuli with responses that were indistinguishable from their responses to the more effective of the two modality-specific stimuli. This similarity led us to hypothesize that the lack of multisensory integration early in development might reflect an absence of functional corticotectal inputs.

Maturation of corticotectal influences

To examine this possibility, we conducted similar deactivation experiments in cats at different developmental stages. As soon as multisensory neurons could be recorded in the developing animal (i.e., during the second postnatal week), we examined their response profiles before, during, and after deactivation of the AES (the r-LS was not examined in these initial studies) (Wallace & Stein, 2000). Consistent with our previous results, the earliest multisensory neurons lacked the capacity to integrate their multisensory inputs. In addition, in keeping with our hypothesis, there was little demonstrable effect on the responses of these neurons during AES deactivation (Fig. 39.9A). However, upon the appearance of a neuron's integrative capacity (for the first neurons, beginning toward the end of the fourth postnatal week), cortical influences were readily apparent (Fig. 39.9B). As in the adult, these influences showed a striking specificity for multisensory integration and relatively little effect on the modality-specific response profile of the recorded neuron.

As development progressed, there was a gradual rise in the proportion of integrative multisensory neurons in the SC, and an almost one-to-one relationship between this integrative capacity and the ability to compromise it by AES deactivation (Fig. 39.10). When examined as a population, these integrative neurons in the neonatal cat appeared identical to nonintegrative neurons (in both the neonate and the adult) during the period of cortical deactivation.

Taken together, these results suggest a multisensory developmental progression that can be divided into three distinct stages (Fig. 39.11). In the first stage, the SC can be considered as an exclusively modality-specific structure, lacking neurons with convergent inputs from multiple modalities. In the second stage, multisensory neurons appear but lack the ability to integrate their cross-modal inputs. It is presumed that at this stage, the corticotectal inputs that are necessary for the elaboration of multisensory integration have yet to reach functional maturity. Finally, in the third and final developmental stage, these corticotectal inputs become functional, resulting in the appearance of a growing population of multisensory integrative neurons.

Multisensory cortical populations and their development

Several association cortical areas have been shown to be of fundamental importance in the development and maintenance of multisensory integration in the brain stem. As we have seen, these areas, consistent with their definition as association cortex, play an integral role in how information from multiple modalities is synthesized at a distant site, the SC. In addition to this role, these areas also appear to play an important role in multisensory processing independent of the SC.

The best examined of these areas is the cortex of the AES. This region, which lies at the junction of the frontal, parietal, and temporal lobes in the cat, is comprised of three neighboring modality-specific

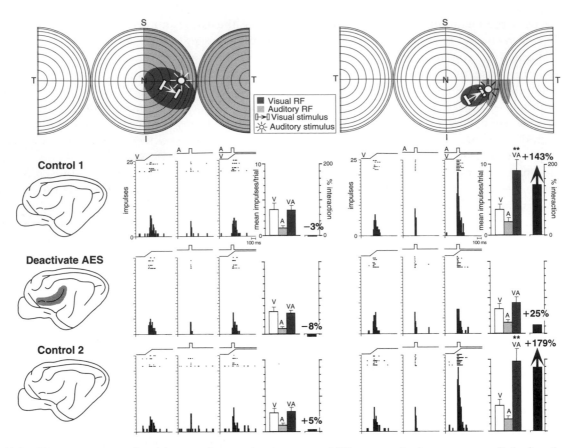

FIGURE 39.9   The appearance of multisensory integration in neonatal SC neurons in the cat appears linked to the appearance of functional corticotectal projections. At the top are shown the receptive fields (shading) and stimulus locations (icons) used for quantitative testing in two visual-auditory SC neurons recorded from animals at 28 (left) and 42 (right) days postnatally (dpn). Note the substantial difference in the sizes of the receptive fields at these two ages. Rasters, histograms, and summary bar graphs (see Fig. 39.6 for conventions) illustrate the responses of these two neurons to visual (V), auditory (A), and combined visual-auditory (VA) stimulation before (Control 1), during (Deactivate AES) and after (Control 2) deactivation of the anterior ectosylvian sulcus (AES) cortex. Note the lack of multisensory interactions and the lack of any demonstrable effect upon deactivating AES in the neuron from the 28 dpn animal (left). In contrast, note the significant multisensory enhancement in the neuron from the 42 dpn animal prior to AES deactivation, the loss of this enhancement during AES deactivation (and the lack of any obvious effect on the modality-specific responses), and its return upon rewarming of the cortex. **P < 0.01. (Adapted from Wallace & Stein, 2001.)

representations. At the rostral pole lies the fourth somatosensory cortex (SIV), a somatotopically ordered area containing a complete representation of the body surface (Burton, Mitchell, & Brent, 1982; Clemo & Stein, 1982, 1983). On the ventral bank of the AES is found the anterior ectosylvian visual area (AEV), an extrastriate area, lacking an obvious topographic order, that has been implicated in visual motion processing and in the control of conjugate eye movements (Benedek, Mucke, Norita, Albowitz, & Creutzfeldt, 1988; Mucke et al., 1982; Norita et al., 1986; Olson & Graybiel, 1987; Scannell et al., 1996; Tamai, Miyashita, & Nakai, 1989). Finally, on the dorsal bank of the caudal AES is field AES (FAES), an auditory area whose functional role remains obscure (Clarey & Irvine, 1986; Meredith & Clemo, 1989) but which may play a role in the distributed coding of sound source location

(Middlebrooks, Xu, Eddins, & Green, 1998; Xu, Furukawa, & Middlebrooks, 1998).

In addition to these three modality-specific representations, the AES contains a substantial population of multisensory neurons (H. Jiang, Lepore, Ptito, & Guillemot, 1994a, 1994b; Wallace, Meredith, & Stein, 1992). Although debate continues as to the exact distribution of these multisensory neurons within AES (see Wallace et al., 1992; H. Jiang et al., 1994a), an analysis of their response properties suggests that they share a number of similarities with subcortical multisensory neurons (Stein & Wallace, 1996; Wallace et al., 1992). Thus, and somewhat surprisingly, given the lack of obvious topography in the visual and auditory representations in AES, multisensory neurons here exhibit a tight spatial register of their individual RFs. When examined with multisensory stimuli, these neurons show response

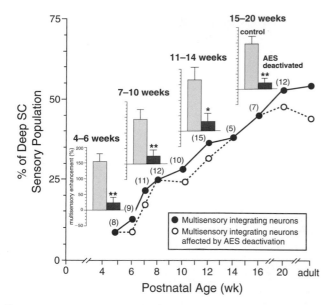

FIGURE 39.10 For the population of SC neurons, there is a strong correlation between the appearance of multisensory integration and the ability to compromise that integration via anterior ectosylvian sulcus (AES) deactivation in the cat. Line graphs chart the growth in the multisensory integrative population during postnatal development (solid symbols and line) and the parallel growth in neurons affected by AES deactivation (open symbols and dotted line). Bar graphs show the gain in the response during multisensory stimulation (i.e., multisensory enhancement) for those neurons capable of integration under control and AES deactivated conditions at four different age intervals. Although there was a substantial increase in the multisensory integrative population as development progressed, individual integrative neurons exhibited similar magnitudes of multisensory enhancement regardless of age. In all cases, this integration was severely compromised during AES deactivation. *P < 0.05; **P < 0.01. (From Wallace & Stein, 2001.)

interactions very much like those seen in the SC. In most instances, the presentation of stimuli together in space, and thus within their respective RFs, results in response enhancements, whereas spatially disparate pairings in which one of the stimuli is outside its RF result in no interaction or a response depression. Similar to SC neurons, AES multisensory neurons are also dependent on the temporal and physical features of the stimuli that are combined.

Preliminary recordings suggest that the development of multisensory neurons in AES bears many similarities to the development of their subcortical counterparts. Thus, multisensory neurons have yet to be found in AES at the earliest stages of postnatal development, stages in which modality-specific auditory and somatosensory neurons can be readily recorded. When first isolated, multisensory neurons in AES have very large RFs (Fig. 39.12). In addition, these early multisensory neurons appear to lack the ability to integrate their

multisensory inputs, again resembling the early multisensory population in the SC. Although provocative, these findings are preliminary and are derived from a limited sample. A more detailed examination of this population should shed light on both the similarities and the differences in the maturation of subcortical and cortical multisensory circuits.

Role of experience in multisensory development

The postnatal appearance and maturation of multisensory integration suggests that sensory experiences derived after birth play a critical role in these processes. In addition, the fundamental importance of cortex in these events further underscores the likely importance of sensory experience, since in the visual, somatosensory, and auditory systems, cortical development is strongly shaped by postnatal experience (Bavelier et al., 2001; Carvell & Simons, 1996; Daw, Reed, Wang, & Flavin, 1995; Diamond, Armstrong-Jones, & Ebner, 1993; Feldman, 2001; Finnerty, Roberts, & Connors, 1999; Kilgard et al., 2001; King, Parsons, & Moore, 2000; Simons & Land, 1987). Thus, by way of its impact on cortical maturational processes and the consequent development of a functional corticotectal pathway, sensory experience may ultimately control the maturation of SC multisensory integration.

In order to test the importance of sensory experience in multisensory development, we began with a straightforward manipulation, namely, eliminating experience in one sensory modality—vision. Animals were raised in complete darkness from birth until adulthood. When we examined animals that had been reared in this manner, we were surprised to see that substantial numbers of multisensory neurons, many with visual responses, were still present in the SC (Fig. 39.13). Nonetheless, despite their multisensory identity, these neurons were strikingly different from similar neurons in age-matched controls. Multisensory neurons in dark-reared animals had substantially larger RFs (Fig. 39.14). On average, these RFs were more than 50% larger than those measured in the control population. As in neonatal animals, this enlargement serves to degrade the spatial register of an individual neuron's RFs. Most important, multisensory neurons in dark-reared animals were found to lack the ability to integrate their multiple sensory cues as their adult counterparts did (Fig. 39.15). The similarities between multisensory neurons in these dark-reared animals and multisensory neurons in newborn, normally reared animals suggests that experiential deprivation delays or eliminates the maturation of the integrative capacity of these neurons. Experiments are ongoing to test whether this effect is reversible

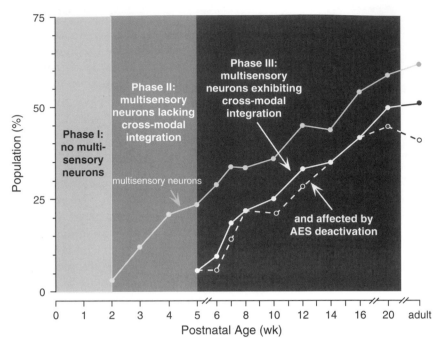

FIGURE 39.11   The SC passes through three developmental stages. Line graphs plot the developmental chronology of multisensory neurons, those exhibiting adultlike integration, and those affected by AES deactivation. Multisensory neurons are initially absent in the SC (phase 1; weeks 0–2), then appear but lack integrative characteristics (phase 2; weeks 2–5), and finally mature to achieve the adult proportion and characteristics (phase 3).

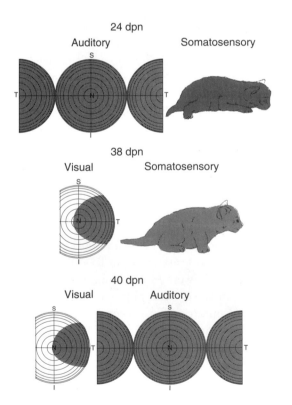

FIGURE 39.12   Receptive fields in multisensory AES neurons in neonatal animals are very large. Shown are the RFs (shaded areas) of three representative multisensory neurons near the earliest time points at which each could be recorded from AES (ages are shown above each panel). Conventions are as in Figure 39.4.

through subsequent adult experience, or whether the absence of visual-nonvisual experiences in early development permanently precludes the appearance of multisensory integration in the SC. In addition, we will test the hypothesis that the lack of multisensory integration in these neurons reflects the lack of a functional corticotectal pathway.

Future directions

The studies described in this chapter raise more questions than they answer. An important issue is that although the parallels between the physiology of multisensory neurons and behavior and perception in the adult provide strong suggestions as to the neural substrates for multisensory integration, little has been done to date to relate across these levels in a developing system. Although behavioral studies in humans, mammals, and birds have illustrated the sensitivity of the developing nervous system to multisensory cues, we have yet to glean substantial insight into the neural mechanisms driving these behaviors. In some circumstances, the neural and behavioral data sets acquired so far fail to map directly onto one another. For example, we have seen that for neurons in the cat SC, the temporal window for multisensory integration begins quite narrow and expands with age. However, in human infants, an opposite trend is seen (see Lewkowicz & Kraebel,

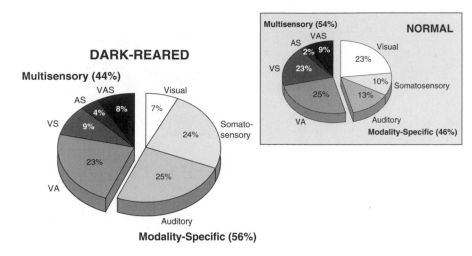

FIGURE 39.13 The relative incidence of sensory-responsive neuron types in the dark-reared and normal (inset) cat SC. Data from the dark-reared group were collected from adults that had been raised in complete darkness from birth. Note the slight decline in the multisensory population in dark-reared animals and the retention of a significant percentage of visually responsive neurons.

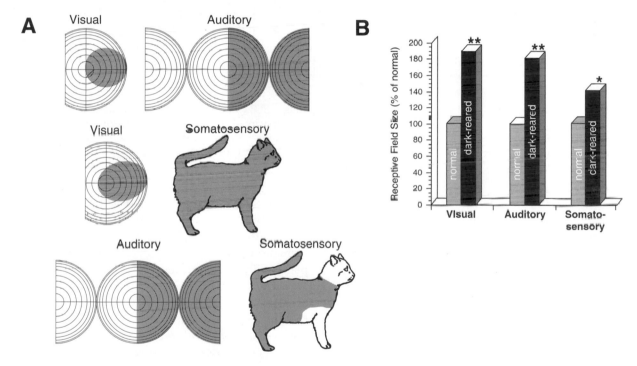

FIGURE 39.14 Receptive fields in the SC of dark-reared animals are significantly larger than in normally reared animals. (A) RFs (shaded areas) from representative visual-auditory (top), visual-somatosensory (middle), and auditory-somatosensory (bottom) neurons in the dark-reared population. (B) Bar graphs contrasting the proportionate difference in RF area between normal (gray bars; convention established at 100%) and dark-reared (black bars) animals for each represented modality. Comparisons are made between RFs at similar locations. *$P < 0.05$; **$P < 0.01$.

Chap. 41, this volume). Here, the temporal tolerance of this system appears to be greatest early in development and becomes increasingly refined with age. Although there are a number of possibilities for reconciling these seemingly disparate findings, here we simply highlight the need for studies in which neural and behavioral development can be examined in parallel. With such an

approach in hand, a number of straightforward questions spring immediately to mind. For example, does the appearance of the ability to use multisensory cues synergistically in order to enhance (or depress) behavior correspond to the appearance of a substantial complement of multisensory integrative neurons? Along similar lines, does the magnitude of the behavioral

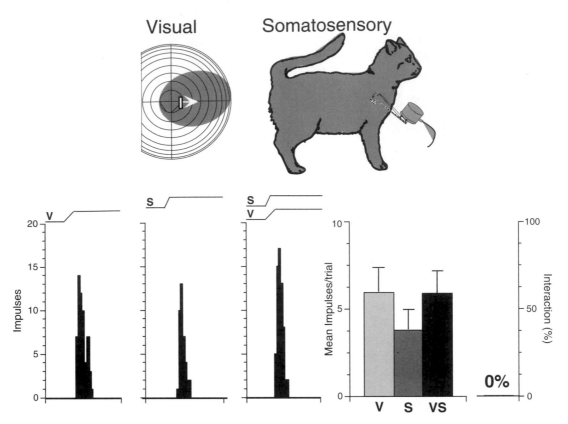

FIGURE 39.15 Multisensory integration is absent in dark-reared animals. Shown at the top are RFs (shaded area) and locations of sensory stimuli (icons) used to quantitatively test the multisensory capacity of this visual-somatosensory neuron. Histograms and summary bar graphs illustrate this neuron's response to the visual-alone, somatosensory-alone, and stimulus combination conditions. Note that the response to the stimulus combination is statistically indistinguishable from the response to either of the modality-specific components. Conventions are as in Figure 39.6.

changes exhibited at various ages relate to the magnitude of the activity changes seen in the multisensory population, the number of neurons exhibiting such changes, or some combination of these factors? Only by investigating and answering these questions will we come to understand the relationships between the maturation of multisensory networks and the behaviors that ultimately depend on them.

Concluding remarks

The development of cross-modal processes, like the development of each of the different sensory systems, is critically dependent on the experiences acquired during early postnatal life. Such experiences shape the manner in which stimuli from the different modalities are combined within the nervous system, as well as dictating the salience of these cross-modal combinations. Altering the normal associations between stimuli from the different senses compromises the ability of the nervous system to effectively utilize multiple sensory channels for behavioral and perceptual gain. Nonetheless, such changes appear to set in motion a cascade of

events that may enhance the processing capabilities of the remaining modality or modalities, compensating in part for the lost modality-specific and multisensory information. Although these data attest to the remarkably plastic nature of the developing brain, recent work in a variety of systems suggests that the adult brain may also have a significant capacity for such reorganization. Characterizing this adult plasticity in sensory and multisensory processes represents an exciting new realm in neuroscience research and one that has profound implications for the treatment of nervous system disorders and damage.

REFERENCES

Andreassi, J. L., & Greco, J. R. (1975). Effects of bisensory stimulation on reaction time and the evoked cortical potential. *Physiology and Psychology, 3,* 189–194.

Bavelier, D., Brozinsky, C., Tomann, A., Mitchell, T., Neville, H., & Liu, G. (2001). Impact of early deafness and early exposure to sign language on the cerebral organization for motion processing. *Journal of Neuroscience, 21,* 8931–8942.

Benedek, G., Mucke, L., Norita, M., Albowitz, B., & Creutzfeldt, O. D. (1988). Anterior ectosylvian visual area

(AEV) of the cat: Physiological properties. *Progress in Brain Research, 75,* 245–255.

Bernstein, I. H., Clark, M. H., & Edelstein, B. A. (1969). Effects of an auditory signal on visual reaction time. *Journal of Experimental Psychology, 80,* 567–569.

Berson, D. M. (1985). Cat lateral suprasylvian cortex: Y-cell inputs and corticotectal projection. *Journal of Neurophysiology, 53,* 544–556.

Berson, D. M., & McIlwain, J. T. (1982). Retinal Y-cell activation of deep-layer cells in superior colliculus of the cat. *Journal of Neurophysiology, 47,* 700–714.

Burton, H., Mitchell, G., & Brent, D. (1982). Second somatic sensory area in the cerebral cortex of cats: Somatotopic organization and cytoarchitecture. *Journal of Comparative Neurology, 210,* 109–135.

Carvell, G. E., & Simons, D. J. (1996). Abnormal tactile experience early in life disrupts active touch. *Journal of Neuroscience, 16,* 2750–2757.

Clarey, J. C., & Irvine, D. R. (1986). Auditory response properties of neurons in the anterior ectosylvian sulcus of the cat. *Brain Research, 386,* 12–19.

Clemo, H. R., & Stein, B. E. (1982). Somatosensory cortex: A "new" somatotopic representation. *Brain Research, 235,* 162–168.

Clemo, H. R., & Stein, B. E. (1983). Organization of a fourth somatosensory area of cortex in cat. *Journal of Neurophysiology, 50,* 910–925.

Clemo, H. R., & Stein, B. E. (1991). Receptive field properties of somatosensory neurons in the cat superior colliculus. *Journal of Comparative Neurology, 314,* 534–544.

Daw, N. W., Reid, S. N., Wang, X. F., & Flavin, H. J. (1995). Factors that are critical for plasticity in the visual cortex. *Ciba Foundation Symposium, 193,* 258–276.

Diamond, M. E., Armstrong-James, M., & Ebner, F. F. (1993). Experience-dependent plasticity in adult rat barrel cortex. *Proceedings of the National Academy of Sciences, USA, 90,* 2082–2086.

Edwards, S. B., Ginsburgh, C. L., Henkel, C. K., & Stein, B. E. (1979). Sources of subcortical projections to the superior colliculus in the cat. *Journal of Comparative Neurology, 184,* 309–329.

Feldman, D. E. (2001). A new critical period for sensory map plasticity. *Neuron, 31,* 171–173.

Finnerty, G. T., Roberts, L. S., & Connors, B. W. (1999). Sensory experience modifies the short-term dynamics of neocortical synapses. *Nature, 400,* 367–371.

Fox, M. W. (1970). Reflex development and behavioural organization. In W. A. Himwich (Ed.), *Developmental neurobiology* (pp. 553–580). Springfield, IL: Thomas.

Frens, M. A., Van Opstal, A. J., & Van der Willigen, R. F. (1995). Spatial and temporal factors determine auditory-visual interactions in human saccadic eye movements. *Perception & Psychophysics, 57,* 802–816.

Gielen, S. C., Schmidt, R. A., & Van den Heuvel, P. J. (1983). On the nature of intersensory facilitation of reaction time. *Perception & Psychophysics, 34,* 161–168.

Goldring, J. E., Dorris, M. C., Corneil, B. D., Ballantyne, P. A., & Munoz, D. P. (1996). Combined eye-head gaze shifts to visual and auditory targets in humans. *Experimental Brain Research, 111,* 68–78.

Harrington, L. K., & Peck, C. K. (1998). Spatial disparity affects visual-auditory interactions in human sensorimotor processing. *Experimental Brain Research, 122,* 247–252.

Hershenson, M. (1962). Reaction time as a measure of intersensory facilitation. *Journal of Experimental Psychology, 63,* 289–293.

Hoffmann, K. P. (1973). Conduction velocity in pathways from retina to superior colliculus in the cat: A correlation with receptive-field properties. *Journal of Neurophysiology, 36,* 409–424.

Huerta, M., & Harting, J. (1984). The mammalian superior colliculus: Studies of its morphology and connections. In H. Vanegas (Ed.), *Comparative neurology of the optic tectum* (pp. 687–773). New York: Plenum.

Hughes, H. C., Reuter-Lorenz, P. A., Nozawa, G., & Fendrich, R. (1994). Visual-auditory interactions in sensorimotor processing: Saccades versus manual responses. *Journal of Experimental Psychology: Human Perception and Performance, 20,* 131–153.

Jiang, H., Lepore, F., Ptito, M., & Guillemot, J. P. (1994a). Sensory interactions in the anterior ectosylvian cortex of cats. *Experimental Brain Research, 101,* 385–396.

Jiang, H., Lepore, F., Ptito, M., & Guillemot, J. P. (1994b). Sensory modality distribution in the anterior ectosylvian cortex (AEC) of cats. *Experimental Brain Research, 97,* 404–414.

Jiang, W., Wallace, M. T., Jiang, H., Vaughan, J. W., & Stein, B. E. (2001). Two cortical areas mediate multisensory integration in superior colliculus neurons. *Journal of Neurophysiology, 85,* 506–522.

Jiang, W., Jiang, H., & Stein, B. E. (2002). Two corticotectal areas facilitate multisensory orientation behavior. *Journal of Cognitive Neurosciences, 14,* 1240–1255.

Kadunce, D. C., Vaughan, J. W., Wallace, M. T., Benedek, G., & Stein, B. E. (1997). Mechanisms of within- and cross-modality suppression in the superior colliculus. *Journal of Neurophysiology, 78,* 2834–2847.

Kao, C. Q., McHaffie, J. G., Meredith, M. A., & Stein, B. E. (1994). Functional development of a central visual map in cat. *Journal of Neurophysiology, 72,* 266–272.

Kawamura, S., Hattori, S., Higo, S., & Matsuyama, T. (1982). The cerebellar projections to the superior colliculus and pretectum in the cat: An autoradiographic and horseradish peroxidase study. *Neuroscience, 7,* 1673–1689.

Kawamura, K., & Konno, T. (1979). Various types of corticotectal neurons of cats as demonstrated by means of retrograde axonal transport of horseradish peroxidase. *Experimental Brain Research, 35,* 161–175.

Kilgard, M. P., Pandya, P. K., Vazquez, J., Gehi, A., Schreiner, C. E., & Merzenich, M. M. (2001). Sensory input directs spatial and temporal plasticity in primary auditory cortex. *Journal of Neurophysiology, 86,* 326–338.

King, A. J., Parsons, C. H., & Moore, D. R. (2000). Plasticity in the neural coding of auditory space in the mammalian brain. *Proceedings of the National Academy of Sciences, USA, 97,* 11821–11828.

Levine, M. S., Hull, C. D., & Buchwald, N. A. (1980). Development of motor activity in kittens. *Developmental Psychobiology, 13,* 357–371.

McIlwain, J. T., & Buser, P. (1968). Receptive fields of single cells in the cat's superior colliculus. *Experimental Brain Research, 5,* 314–325.

Meredith, M. A., & Clemo, H. R. (1989). Auditory cortical projection from the anterior ectosylvian sulcus (Field AES) to the superior colliculus in the cat: An anatomical and electrophysiological study. *Journal of Comparative Neurology, 289,* 687–707.

Meredith, M. A., Clemo, H. R., & Stein, B. E. (1991). Somatotopic component of the multisensory map in the deep laminae of the cat superior colliculus. *Journal of Comparative Neurology, 312,* 353–370.

Meredith, M. A., & Stein, B. E. (1986a). Spatial factors determine the activity of multisensory neurons in cat superior colliculus. *Brain Research, 365,* 350–354.

Meredith, M. A., & Stein, B. E. (1986b). Visual, auditory, and somatosensory convergence on cells in superior colliculus results in multisensory integration. *Journal of Neurophysiology, 56,* 640–662.

Middlebrooks, J. C., & Knudsen, E. I. (1984). A neural code for auditory space in the cat's superior colliculus. *Journal of Neuroscience, 4,* 2621–2634.

Middlebrooks, J. C., Xu, L., Eddins, A. C., & Green, D. M. (1998). Codes for sound-source location in nontonotopic auditory cortex. *Journal of Neurophysiology, 80,* 863–881.

Mize, R. R. (1983). Patterns of convergence and divergence of retinal and cortical synaptic terminals in the cat superior colliculus. *Experimental Brain Research, 51,* 88–96.

Morrell, L. K. (1968). Temporal characteristics of sensory interaction in choice reaction times. *Journal of Experimental Psychology, 77,* 14–18.

Mucke, L., Norita, M., Benedek, G., & Creutzfeldt, O. (1982). Physiologic and anatomic investigation of a visual cortical area situated in the ventral bank of the anterior ectosylvian sulcus of the cat. *Experimental Brain Research, 46,* 1–11.

Norita, M., Mucke, L., Benedek, G., Albowitz, B., Katoh, Y., & Creutzfeldt, O. D. (1986). Connections of the anterior ectosylvian visual area (AEV). *Experimental Brain Research, 62,* 225–240.

Nozawa, G., Reuter-Lorenz, P. A., & Hughes, H. C. (1994). Parallel and serial processes in the human oculomotor system: Bimodal integration and express saccades. *Biological Cybernetics, 72,* 19–34.

Olson, C. R., & Graybiel, A. M. (1987). Ectosylvian visual area of the cat: Location, retinotopic organization, and connections. *Journal of Comparative Neurology, 261,* 277–294.

Perrott, D. R., Saberi, K., Brown, K., & Strybel, T. Z. (1990). Auditory psychomotor coordination and visual search performance. *Perception & Psychophysics, 48,* 214–226.

Scannell, J. W., Sengpiel, F., Tovee, M. J., Benson, P. J., Blakemore, C., & Young, M. P. (1996). Visual motion processing in the anterior ectosylvian sulcus of the cat. *Journal of Neurophysiology, 76,* 895–907.

Segal, R. L., & Beckstead, R. M. (1984). The lateral suprasylvian corticotectal projection in cats. *Journal of Comparative Neurology, 225,* 259–275.

Simons, D. J., & Land, P. W. (1987). Early experience of tactile stimulation influences organization of somatic sensory cortex. *Nature, 326,* 694–697.

Stein, B. E., & Arigbede, M. O. (1972). Unimodal and multimodal response properties of neurons in the cat superior colliculus. *Experimental Neurology, 36,* 179–196.

Stein, B. E., Huneycutt, W. S., & Meredith, M. A. (1988). Neurons and behavior: The same rules of multisensory integration apply. *Brain Research, 448,* 355–358.

Stein, B. E., Labos, E., & Kruger, L. (1973). Sequence of changes in properties of neurons of superior colliculus of the kitten during maturation. *Journal of Neurophysiology, 36,* 667–679.

Stein, B. E., Magalhaes-Castro, B., & Kruger, L. (1976). Relationship between visual and tactile representations in cat superior colliculus. *Journal of Neurophysiology, 39,* 401–419.

Stein, B. E., & Meredith, M. A. (1993). *The merging of the senses.* Cambridge, MA: MIT Press.

Stein, B., Meredith, M., Huneycutt, W., & McDade, L. (1989). Behavioral indices of multisensory integration: Orientation to visual cues is affected by auditory stimuli. *Journal of Cognitive Neuroscience, 1,* 12–24.

Stein, B. E., Spencer, R. F., & Edwards, S. B. (1983). Corticotectal and corticothalamic efferent projections of SIV somatosensory cortex in cat. *Journal of Neurophysiology, 50,* 896–909.

Stein, B. E., & Wallace, M. T. (1996). Comparisons of cross-modality integration in midbrain and cortex. *Progress in Brain Research, 112,* 289–299.

Sterling, P., & Wickelgren, B. G. (1969). Visual receptive fields in the superior colliculus of the cat. *Journal of Neurophysiology, 32,* 1–15.

Straschill, M., & Hoffmann, K. P. (1969). Functional aspects of localization in the cat's tectum opticum. *Brain Research, 13,* 274–283.

Tamai, Y., Miyashita, E., & Nakai, M. (1989). Eye movements following cortical stimulation in the ventral bank of the anterior ectosylvian sulcus of the cat. *Neuroscience Research, 7,* 159–163.

Tortelly, A., Reinoso-Suarez, F., & Llamas, A. (1980). Projections from non-visual cortical areas to the superior colliculus demonstrated by retrograde transport of HRP in the cat. *Brain Research, 188,* 543–549.

Villablanca, J. R., & Olmstead, C. E. (1979). Neurological development of kittens. *Developmental Psychobiology, 12,* 101–127.

Wallace, M. T., Meredith, M. A., & Stein, B. E. (1992). Integration of multiple sensory modalities in cat cortex. *Experimental Brain Research, 91,* 484–488.

Wallace, M. T., Meredith, M. A., & Stein, B. E. (1993). Converging influences from visual, auditory, and somatosensory cortices onto output neurons of the superior colliculus. *Journal of Neurophysiology, 69,* 1797–1809.

Wallace, M. T., & Stein, B. E. (1994). Cross-modal synthesis in the midbrain depends on input from cortex. *Journal of Neurophysiology, 71,* 429–432.

Wallace, M. T., & Stein, B. E. (1997). Development of multisensory neurons and multisensory integration in cat superior colliculus. *Journal of Neuroscience, 17,* 2429–2444.

Wallace, M. T., & Stein, B. E. (2000). Onset of cross-modal synthesis in the neonatal superior colliculus is gated by the development of cortical influences. *Journal of Neurophysiology, 83,* 3578–3582.

Wallace, M. T., & Stein, B. E. (2001). Sensory and multisensory responses in the newborn monkey superior colliculus. *Journal of Neuroscience, 21,* 8886–8894.

Welch, R. B., & Warren, D. H. (1986). Intersensory interactions. In K. R. Boff, L. Kaufman, & J. P. Thomas (Eds.), *Handbook of perception and human performance, Vol. 1: Sensory processes and perception* (pp. 25.21–25.36). New York: Wiley.

Wilkinson, L. K., Meredith, M. A., & Stein, B. E. (1996). The role of anterior ectosylvian cortex in cross-modality orientation and approach behavior. *Experimental Brain Research, 112,* 1–10.

Xu, L., Furukawa, S., & Middlebrooks, J. C. (1998). Sensitivity to sound-source elevation in nontonotopic auditory cortex. *Journal of Neurophysiology, 80,* 882–894.

40 Perceptual Development and the Origins of Multisensory Responsiveness

ROBERT LICKLITER AND LORRAINE E. BAHRICK

Introduction

Most objects and events present a mix of visual, auditory, tactile, and olfactory stimulation simultaneously. How do young infants come to perceive and derive meaning from this array of multimodal stimulation? How do young infants determine which sights and sounds constitute unitary objects and events and which patterns of stimulation are unrelated to one another?

Historically, two prevailing theoretical views, known as the integration view and the differentiation view, have dominated attempts to address these important questions regarding the development of intersensory perception (see Bahrick & Pickens, 1994; Gibson & Pick, 2000; Lewkowicz, 1994). Generally speaking, the *integration view* proposes that the different sensory modalities function as separate sensory systems during the initial stages of postnatal development and gradually become integrated during the course of development through the infant's activity and repeated experience with concurrent information provided to the different sensory modalities (Birch & Lefford, 1963; Friedes, 1974; Piaget, 1952). According to this view, young organisms must learn to coordinate and integrate the separate senses during early development. The *differentiation view* holds that the different senses form a primitive unity early in development, and as the infant develops, the sensory modalities differentiate from one another. In this view, the senses are initially unified, and infants differentiate finer and more complex multimodal relationships through their experience over the course of development (Bower, 1974; Gibson, 1969; Marks, 1978).

As a result of these opposing views, the most prominent question guiding behavioral research on early intersensory development over the past several decades has focused on whether intersensory development proceeds from initially separate senses that become increasingly integrated through the infant's ongoing experience, eventually resulting in coordinated multimodal perception, or whether the development of intersensory perception is a process of differentiation and increasing specificity (Kellman & Arterberry, 1998; Lewkowicz & Lickliter, 1994a; Rose & Ruff, 1987).

In recent years the discussion has become less polarized, due in large part to the adoption of a more systems-based approach to the development of perception, according to which any given perceptual skill or ability is generated by a network of multiple, cocontributing neural, physiological, and behavioral factors (Gottlieb, Wahlsten, & Lickliter, 1998; Lewkowicz, 2000; Lickliter & Bahrick, 2000; Thelen & Smith, 1994). Although some controversy remains as to whether perceptual development proceeds from a wholistic unity to differentiated sensory modalities or from separated senses to coordinated multimodal experience (i.e., Bushnell, 1994; Maurer, 1993), the dominant view at present argues against an all-or-none dichotomy between integration and differentiation views of perceptual development. The increasing research focus on the processes and mechanisms underlying human and animal infant intersensory perception over the past several decades has provided mounting evidence that the separate senses are not so separate, highlighting the importance of differentiation in early development. Moreover, both differentiation and integration processes appear to be involved in perceptual development and function in an intercoordinated manner. In this chapter, we briefly review converging evidence across species, developmental periods, and properties of objects and events suggesting a general developmental trajectory in which differentiation of amodal and modality-specific stimulus properties emerges in a coordinated and interdependent manner, with the detection of more global, amodal stimulus properties leading and constraining perceptual responsiveness to more specific properties of objects and events.

Infant perception of multimodal information

There is now compelling neural, electrophysiological, and behavioral evidence of strong intermodal linkages in newborns and young of a variety of avian and mammalian species, including humans (e.g., Carlsen & Lickliter, 1999; Frost, 1990; King & Carlile, 1993; Knudsen & Brainard, 1991, 1995; Lewkowicz & Turkewitz, 1981; Lickliter & Banker, 1994; Mellon, Kraemer, & Spear, 1991; Stein & Meredith, 1993; Withington-Wray, Binns, & Keating, 1990). For example, infant animals have been shown to be more sensitive to intersensory correspondences than older animals in a classical conditioning learning paradigm (Spear & McKinzie, 1994). Animal and human infants also demonstrate an array of intermodal perceptual skills in the weeks and months following birth, including the detection of temporal and spatial contiguity between auditory and visual stimulation, the detection of multimodal information specifying the self and body motion, and intersensory facilitation, in which stimulation in one modality enhances responsiveness to stimuli in other modalities (Lickliter & Stoumbos, 1991; Lyons-Ruth, 1977; Morrongiello, Fenwick, & Chance, 1998; Rochat, 1995; Spelke, 1979; Turkewitz & Mellon, 1989).

Of particular interest is the fact that human infants have been shown to be skilled perceivers of *amodal* stimulus properties in the first several months following birth (Bahrick, 1988, 1992; Bahrick, Flom, & Lickliter, 2002; Bahrick & Lickliter, 2000; Bahrick & Pickens, 1994; Lewkowicz, 2000; Walker-Andrews, 1986, 1997). Amodal stimulus properties are those that can be conveyed by more than one sensory modality, whereas modality-specific properties can only be conveyed by one particular sensory modality. Thus, temporal synchrony, spatial collocation, intensity, rate, duration, and rhythm are all examples of amodal stimulus properties that can be specified simultaneously by several sensory modalities. They stand in contrast to modality-specific stimulus properties, which can only be conveyed by one particular sensory modality, such as color, pitch, or sweetness. As a case in point, the sights and sounds of hands clapping share temporal synchrony, a common tempo of action, and a common rhythm. The amodal properties of synchrony, tempo, and rhythm are thus concurrently available both visually and acoustically. Detection of this information enables the infant to perceive sights and sounds that belong together. Given that the role of integration has often been seen to link together separate sensations to form a unified percept (Piaget, 1952; von Helmholtz, 1968), infants' ready detection of amodal stimulus properties makes the need for intersensory integration unnecessary and unlikely.

A large body of developmental research utilizing infant habituation techniques has demonstrated that infants are adept at perceiving and responding to a host of amodal relations uniting stimulation across visual, auditory, vestibular, tactile, and proprioceptive stimulation in the first months following birth (see Gibson & Pick, 2000; Lewkowicz & Lickliter, 1994a, for reviews). This early detection of amodal information provides support for the view that development proceeds from a global unity of the senses to increasing differentiation of finer levels of stimulation (see Bahrick, 2001; Lickliter & Bahrick, 2000, for further discussion).

On the other hand, infants can also detect perceptual information that is not amodal in the months following birth. Infants clearly become more skilled at detecting intersensory relations that are modality-specific or arbitrary in their co-occurrence over the course of the first year of life (Bahrick, 1994, 2001; Bushnell, 1994; Lewkowicz, 1994). Many relations between stimulus properties conveyed concurrently to different modalities are arbitrary in the sense that they are not united by redundant information common across the different sensory modalities and thus can vary as a function of context or stimulus domain. For example, the relation between the appearance of an object and the verbal label we give it, or that between a person's appearance and the specific sound of his or her voice, or that between the type of sound a particular toy produces and its color and shape are cases of arbitrary pairings of concurrent stimulation across two or more sensory modalities. Given that there is no common information that links the specific characteristics of stimulation presented to the two or more modalities, arbitrary relations must be learned by experiencing the information in the modalities together, and may thus be characterized as depending on some process of association or integration. Research findings indicate that this process is likely initially guided by the detection of amodal relations, including temporal synchrony, temporal microstructure, and spatial collocation (Bahrick, 2001; Gogate & Bahrick, 1998; Hernandez-Reif & Bahrick, 2001; Lewkowicz, 2002). For example, young infants can learn to relate specific sounds with objects of a particular appearance, but only when temporal synchrony unites the motion of the object and sound (Bahrick, 1994; Gogate & Bahrick, 1998). The detection of global, amodal information appears to guide and constrain the detection of more specific information, both ontogenetically and within a given episode of exploration, so that unitary multimodal objects and events are explored first and modality-specific details are perceived in the context of more general principles that organize these details.

In sum, it appears that both integration and differentiation processes are involved in the emergence and maintenance of various types of intersensory functioning. The recognition of the important role of these processes and their interaction has led several investigators, including Bahrick (1994), Botuck and Turkewitz (1990), Lewkowicz and Lickliter (1994b), Smith (1994), Thelen and Smith (1994), and Werner (1957), to suggest that integration and differentiation processes are best considered as complementary rather than competitive or mutually exclusive processes. Recent work in developmental psychology and psychobiology is providing a clearer picture of how differentiating amodal relations *and* integrating arbitrary or modality-specific information across the senses can interact with one another in the development of early percpetual and cognitive skills. A brief review of this body of work provides a forum for exploring its implications for a more fully realized understanding of the origins and development of intersensory perception.

The salience of amodal stimulus properties during early development

What causes some patterns of sensory stimulation to be salient, attended to, and remembered by young organisms, and other patterns of stimulation to be ignored? Although we are not yet able to conclusively answer this important question regarding selective attention, a growing body of evidence from developmental psychology and psychobiology suggests that infants' adept detection of amodal relations is a fundamental component of selective attention during early development (Bahrick, 1992, 1994, 2001; Lickliter, Bahrick, & Honeycutt, 2002; Slater, Guinn, Brown, & Hayes, 1999). In particular, the detection of amodal relations appears to specify the unity of multimodal stimulation, capture and direct infant attention, and facilitate the further differentiation of a coordinated multimodal object or event (Bahrick & Lickliter, 2000; Bahrick & Pickens, 1994; Lickliter & Bahrick, 2001). Such detection of amodal relations can guide and constrain the detection of other nested intersensory relations, including modality-specific and arbitrary stimulus relations.

As a case in point, 7-month-old infants have been shown to be capable of learning the arbitrary relation between an object and a speech sound, but only when the object is moved in temporal synchrony with the sound. When the object is still or moved asynchronously with the speech sound, 7-month-olds show no evidence of linking the speech sound and the object (Gogate & Bahrick, 1998). In this example, learning of arbitrary relations appeared to be (at least initially) guided and

facilitated by the detection of amodal relations present in multimodal stimulation. Hernandez-Reif and Bahrick (2001) have likewise shown that 6-month-old infants can detect the arbitrary relation between the tactually perceived shape of an object and a specific color or pattern, but only under conditions when amodal information for object shape unites their visual and tactile exploration. In other words, the relation between an object's color or pattern and its shape appears to be learned by young infants only in the presence of amodal shape information made concurrently available to vision and touch.

Related research has also found a developmental lag between the detection of amodal and arbitrary relations provided by a given event during early development. By 3 months of age, infants viewing objects striking a surface are capable of detecting the amodal audiovisual relations of temporal synchrony and the temporal microstructure specifying an object's composition. However, not until 7 months of age do infants detect the arbitrary relation between the pitch of the impact sound and the color and shape of the objects (Bahrick, 1992, 1994). Further, it was found that even when modality-specific properties (the pitch of a sound and the color of moving objects) were made more readily discriminable, amodal relations were nevertheless perceived developmentally prior to these modality-specific relations. Such findings suggest that the redundant, amodal properties of objects and events are typically more salient and perceived earlier than modality-specific or arbitrary multimodal relations.

This developmental sequence, whereby perceptual learning progresses from detection of amodal to arbitrary and modality-specific relations, promotes learning about consistencies and regularities across the senses during early development. For example, detection of amodal stimulus properties such as temporal synchrony and spatial collocation can foster appropriate, veridical generalizations on the part of the young organism and can minimize inappropriate generalizations about arbitrary stimulus relations that vary widely across contexts or are specific to only certain objects or events. In this scenario, detection of amodal relations are thought to guide and constrain perceptual learning about modality-specific relations such that general perceptual principles (e.g., voices go with faces, single objects make single impact sounds) are well established prior to learning more specific details of these events (e.g., Mary's face goes with a soft, high-pitched voice; the blue rattle makes a jingling sound when dropped). Bahrick's (1992, 1994) findings that 3-month-old infants were able to detect temporal synchrony and amodal information specifying object composition in single and multiple objects striking a surface, but not until 7 months of age could infants could detect the arbitrary, modality-specific relation between the pitch of the sound and the color and shape of the moving objects, provides support for the view that detection of amodal relations can guide and constrain early perceptual learning.

Although these results and those from other investigations of infants' capabilities for perceiving amodal relations (for reviews, see Lewkowicz, 2000; Walker-Andrews, 1997) indicate that young infants are remarkably skilled at perceiving coherent multimodal objects and events from the flow of sensory stimulation, the origins of this capacity and its implications for perceptual and cognitive development remain poorly understood. Recent evidence from comparative psychology and developmental psychobiology utilizing animal embryos and infants has, however, provided some insight into the emergence and maintenance of intersensory functioning (Lickliter, 2000a; Lickliter & Bahrick, 2000; Lewkowicz & Lickliter, 1994a). This body of work, along with parallel findings from the neural and electrophysiological literature, indicates a strong link between sensory systems and a functional distinction between unimodal and multimodal stimulation during early development (see Stein & Meredith, 1993; Stein, Meredith, & Wallace, 1994; Stein, Wallace, & Stanford, 2000). In particular, research with both animal and human infants indicates that different properties of stimuli are highlighted and attended to when concurrent multimodal stimuli rather than unimodal stimuli are made available to young organisms.

Differential effects of unimodal and multimodal stimulation

Functioning tactile, vestibular, chemical, and auditory modalities are likely interacting during the late stages of prenatal development in precocial animal species, and the onset of visual experience at birth or hatching significantly increases opportunities for multimodal stimulation during the postnatal period (Gottlieb, 1971a; Lickliter 2000b). Relatively little is known about the nature of perinatal intersensory interactions and the possible contributions of different types of sensory experience to newborns' perceptual preferences and abilities (but see Lickliter, 1995; Tees & Symons, 1987; Turkewitz, 1994; Turkewitz, Gilbert, & Birch, 1974). Converging research from both neural and behavioral levels of analyses has, however, consistently indicated differential effects of unimodal versus multimodal sensory stimulation on young and mature organisms' perceptual responsiveness.

For example, a number of neurophysiological studies of the adult cat have indicated that the temporal and spatial pairing of stimuli from different sensory modalities can elicit a neural response that is greater than the sum of the neural responses to the unimodal components of stimulation considered separately (Stein & Meredith, 1993; Stein et al., 1994). Spatially coordinated multimodal stimulus combinations produce significant increases over unimodal responses in an array of extracellular measures of neural activity in adult animals, including response reliability, number of impulses evoked, peak impulse frequency, and duration of the discharge train. This superadditive effect of bimodal stimulation, in which the magnitude of neural effects resulting from bimodal stimulation exceeds the level predicted by adding together responsiveness to each single-modality stimulus alone, has also been reported in behavioral investigations. Stein, Meredith, Honeycutt, and McDade (1989) have also demonstrated that the effectiveness of a visual stimulus in eliciting attentive and orientation behaviors in cats is dramatically affected by the presence of a temporally congruent and spatially collocated stimulus in the auditory modality. Responses made by cats to spatially coincident audiovisual stimuli were more accurate than those made to either form of unimodal stimulation.

In a similar vein, communicative displays like the threat expressions of macaque monkeys and the recruitment signals of ants have been shown to have different consequences on the behavior of conspecifics, depending on their unimodal or multimodal presentation (see Partan & Marler, 1999). Taken together, these various findings provide converging support for the notion that unimodal and multimodal stimulation elicit differential responsiveness across different species, different developmental stages, and different tasks.

Research with precocial avian embryos and hatchlings has consistently demonstrated the importance of multimodal sensory stimulation in the emergence and maintenance of normal or species-typical patterns of perceptual organization. Beginning with the pioneering work of Gottlieb (1971b) on the development of species identification in precocial birds, a large body of work has accumulated indicating that multimodal experience in the period following hatching is a key component in the development and maintenance of the early perceptual and social preferences underlying species identification (e.g., Gottlieb, 1993; Johnston & Gottlieb, 1981; Lickliter, Dyer, & McBride, 1993). More recently, studies of precocial bird embryos and hatchlings have demonstrated that subjects denied normal levels of multimodal stimulation during the early postnatal period show impaired perceptual responsiveness to both unimodal and multimodal maternal information

(Columbus & Lickliter, 1998; Columbus, Sleigh, Lickliter, & Lewkowicz, 1998; Gottlieb, 1993; Sleigh, Columbus, & Lickliter, 1998). As a case in point, quail chicks receiving enhanced exposure to unimodal (either auditory or visual) maternal stimulation following hatching showed altered patterns of responsiveness to both unimodal and bimodal maternal information. Regardless of whether their unimodal maternal experience was auditory or visual, chicks demonstrated enhanced unimodal and delayed bimodal responsiveness when compared with control chicks receiving typical levels of multimodal stimulation (Sleigh et al., 1998).

Related work with both quail chicks and ducklings on the effects of reducing available multimodal stimulation following hatching has also demonstrated altered patterns of auditory learning (Gottlieb, 1993; Lickliter & Hellewell, 1992) and attenuated intersensory functioning (Columbus & Lickliter, 1998), further highlighting the importance of multimodal stimulation to the normal emergence of intra- and intersensory functioning in early development. Similar findings from several other species of birds and mammals examined at the neural level of analysis also indicate that the uncoupling of multimodal experience can lead to significant changes in the young organism's normal developmental trajectory (King, Hutchings, Moore, & Blakemore, 1988; Knudsen & Brainard, 1991, 1995; Withington-Wray et al., 1990).

Recent evidence also indicates that experiential modifications of prenatal unimodal or bimodal sensory experience can alter neuroanatomical structure, physiological regulation, and perceptual learning during the period prior to birth or hatching. For example, Carlsen (1999) examined the effects of differing amounts of unusually early visual stimulation of quail embryos in the period prior to hatching on the dendritic morphology of neurons in the area of the telencephalon known as the visual Wulst, a structure similar to the mammalian visual cortex. The Wulst has a layered organization and response properties very similar to mammalian striate cortex (Pettigrew & Konishi, 1976). Quail embryos exposed to prenatal visual stimulation showed altered patterns of intersensory responsiveness to maternal auditory and visual cues and were also shown to have significant changes in the number of spines and degree of branching of dendrites in the Wulst when compared with control chicks not receiving prenatal visual stimulation. Embryos receiving relatively small amounts (10 min/h) of prenatal visual stimulation in the days prior to hatching showed enhanced audiovisual responsiveness to maternal cues and had significantly fewer dendritic spines than controls following hatching. In contrast, embryos receiving relatively large amounts

(40 min/h) of prenatal visual experience showed delayed intersensory responsiveness following hatching and had a significantly greater number of spines and more branching than control chicks. These results suggest that providing embryos with unusually early visual experience can modify emerging patterns of neural pruning and resulting architecture. How modifications in prenatal auditory experience would affect neuronal structure in the visual Wulst remains to be explored, but existing behavioral evidence demonstrating effects of prenatal auditory stimulation on subsequent visual responsiveness (Lickliter & Stoumbos, 1991; Sleigh & Lickliter, 1997) suggests that similar patterns of neuronal change in visual areas (in addition to the auditory region of the telencephalon) are plausible following augmented prenatal auditory stimulation.

Differential effects of unimodal versus bimodal stimulation during prenatal development have also been demonstrated at the physiological level of analysis. Reynolds and Lickliter (2002) found that quail embryos' heart rate is significantly affected by the type of prenatal sensory stimulation (unimodal vs. bimodal) provided during the period prior to hatching. Embryos exposed to concurrent but asynchronous bimodal (auditory/ visual) stimulation displayed significant increases in heart rate during stimulus exposure, whereas the heart rate of embryos exposed to concurrent intramodal (auditory/auditory) stimulation or unimodal (auditory or unimodal) visual stimulation remained near baseline during stimulus exposure. These results are consistent with behavioral evidence drawn from studies of prenatal perceptual learning in bird embryos. A number of studies have reported that when embryos are unimodally exposed to an individual maternal call in the days prior to hatching, they subsequently prefer this familiar maternal call over an unfamiliar maternal call in postnatal testing (Gottlieb, 1988; Gottlieb, Tomlinson, & Radell, 1989; Lickliter & Hellewell, 1992). However, when embryos are exposed to an individual maternal call concurrently with noncongruent stimulation to another sensory system (i.e., visual or vestibular), they fail to demonstrate a preference for the familiar call during postnatal testing (Honeycutt & Lickliter, 2001; Lickliter & Hellewell, 1992; Radell & Gottlieb, 1992). Concurrent (but asynchronous) bimodal stimulation appears to alter both physiological and behavioral arousal (Reynolds & Lickliter, 2002) and can interfere with prenatal perceptual learning. On the other hand, recent evidence indicates that *redundant*, synchronous bimodal stimulation can facilitate perceptual learning, suggesting that different types of multimodal stimulation have different effects on emerging physiological and behavioral organization during early development.

In summary, several related themes can be drawn from recent comparative research on the development of intersensory responsiveness in birds and mammals: (1) There appears to be enhanced behavioral responsiveness to coordinated multisensory stimulation as compared with unimodal stimulation. (2) Multimodal experience appears to lead to different developmental outcomes than unimodal experience. (3) The uncoupling of multimodal experience can lead to abnormal perceptual organization during early development. (4) Modifications in normal types and amounts of prenatal sensory stimulation can lead to altered neural development and increased physiological and behavioral arousal.

The role of intersensory redundancy in early perceptual development

We have proposed an *intersensory redundancy* hypothesis to describe how attention and perceptual processing of different stimulus properties are influenced by unimodal versus multimodal stimulation (Bahrick & Lickliter, 2000, 2002). In light of converging evidence drawn from physiological and behavioral studies highlighting the differential effects of unimodal and multimodal stimulation during early development, the intersensory redundancy hypothesis synthesizes knowledge gained from research on animal and human intersensory development and identifies some of the processes thought to underlie the emergence of intersensory perception. *Intersensory redundancy* refers to the spatially coordinated and concurrent presentation of the same information (e.g., rate, rhythm, intensity) across two or more sensory modalities. For the auditory and visual modalities, this also entails the temporally synchronous alignment of the bimodal information. In our view, intersensory redundancy is a particularly important and salient form of stimulation in early development. The intersensory redundancy hypothesis proposes that information presented redundantly across two or more sensory modalities selectively recruits young organisms' attention during early development, causing amodal (redundant) stimulus properties to become foreground and other stimulus properties to become background during exploration of an object or event. According to the intersensory redundancy hypothesis, selective attention on the part of the infant gives initial advantage to the perceptual processing, learning, and memory of stimulus properties that are redundantly specified over the processing, learning, or memory of nonredundant properties of sensory stimulation. In other words, information that is simultaneously presented across two or more modalities is thought to be highly salient to infants and can direct attentional selectivity at the expense of information that is not redundant (Bahrick & Lickliter, 2000; Bahrick & Pickens, 1994; Bahrick, Walker, & Neisser, 1981; Bahrick et al., 2002; Slater et al., 1999).

More than 20 years ago, Bahrick et al. (1981) demonstrated the salience of intersensory redundancy for directing selective attention during early development. Infants viewed films of two superimposed events (e.g., a toy Slinky moving and a hand-clapping game). For the adult viewer, when the two superimposed events were viewed silently, they appeared to be an amalgamation of ghostly images passing through one another. However, as soon as the sound track to one was turned on, the sound-specified event suddenly stood out from the other event, creating a strong impression of figure and ground. Infants also appeared to be affected this way by the addition of the sound track. By playing the synchronous soundtrack to one of the superimposed events, the investigators were able to direct infants' attentional selectivity to that event, causing them to ignore the silent one. However, once the sound track was turned off and the films were separated (appearing side by side) intersensory redundancy was no longer available, and infants preferred to view the novel, previously silent film. Control studies confirmed this interpretation, in that when infants were presented with only one centrally projected event with sound, followed by silent trials of the two events side by side (familiar vs. novel films), they preferred the previously absent (novel) film. Taken together, these results demonstrate that the intersensory redundancy provided by the natural, synchronous sound track to a visible event can guide infants' visual selectivity, even when another visual event occupies the same spatial location. This behavioral evidence is consistent with findings of heightened neural responsiveness to coordinated multimodal stimulation in adult animals (see Stein & Meredith, 1993).

More recently, intersensory redundancy has also been found to facilitate perceptual learning of amodal properties such as rhythm and tempo in early infancy (Bahrick & Lickliter, 2000; Bahrick et al., 2002). For example, in the Bahrick and Lickliter (2000) study, 5-month-old infants were habituated to films of a hammer tapping out one of two distinct irregular rhythms. The rhythms were presented visually (seeing the hammer) or acoustically (hearing the hammer tapping) or visually and acoustically (bimodal condition). Infants then received test trials depicting either a change in rhythm or no change in rhythm. Results indicated that infants were able to discriminate between the two irregular rhythms when they were presented bimodally (across both the auditory and visual modalities) and therefore redundantly, but not when the rhythms were

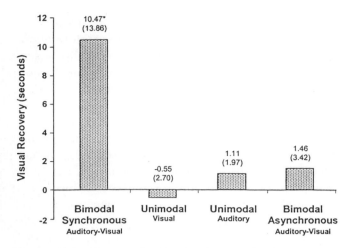

FIGURE 40.1 Five-month-old infants' mean visual recovery to a change in rhythm following bimodal (synchronous vs. asynchronous) or unimodal habituation. Visual recovery is the difference score between visual fixation during the test trials and visual fixation during posthabituation trials. Standard deviations appear in parentheses. *$p < 0.05$.

presented unimodally (only in the auditory or visual modality) or bimodally but out of temporal synchrony (Fig. 40.1). Concurrent and redundant stimulation of the auditory and visual modalities appeared to selectively guide infants' attention to the bimodally specified property of rhythm, fostering successful discrimination, whereas unimodal stimulation did not.

Parallel findings have been obtained demonstrating the importance of intersensory redundancy for detecting the amodal property of tempo in 3-month-old infants (Bahrick et al., 2002). In this study, infants were found to discriminate a change in tempo following bimodal but not unimodal familiarization (Fig. 40.2). Because most objects and events are multimodal,

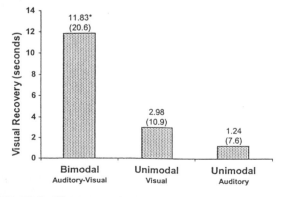

FIGURE 40.2 Three-month-old infants' mean visual recovery to a change in tempo following bimodal or unimodal habituation. Visual recovery is the difference score between visual fixation during test trials and visual fixation during posthabituation trials. Standard deviations appear in parentheses. *$p < 0.05$.

perceptual processing, learning, and memory for stimulus properties specified in more than one sensory modality will be promoted and develop earlier than processing of other properties. Conversely, when multimodal stimulation is not available, attention is likely to be more broadly focused on a variety of stimulus properties, including those that are specific to individual sensory modalities. It is important to note that the salience of redundant stimulation for directing attentional selectivity is expected to be most pronounced during early perceptual learning in a given domain, as infants are clearly capable of detecting amodal stimulus properties in unimodal stimulation within the first months of life (Lewkowicz & Lickliter, 1994a; Rose & Ruff, 1987).

In contrast to the facilitative effects of intersensory redundancy for perceptual learning about amodal stimulus properties, intersensory redundancy can also hinder or constrain learning about modality-specific stimulus properties. Because redundancy selectively focuses attention on the redundant aspects of stimulation and away from other aspects, detection and learning of properties such as pitch, color, or orientation would be attenuated in the presence of redundancy and enhanced in its absence. This attenuation effect was found for the perception of orientation of a moving object in 5-month-old infants (Bahrick, Lickliter, & Flom, 2000). In this study, infants exposed to a hammer tapping out a distinctive rhythm were able to perceive a change in the modality-specific property of orientation (movement upward vs. downward) when the event was experienced unimodally (visual presentation), but not when experienced bimodally (auditory-visual presentation). The addition of redundancy under the bimodal condition appeared to selectively recruit attention to redundantly specified stimulus properties (such as rhythm and tempo) at the expense of the unimodally specified property of orientation.

A focus on the nature of intersensory relationships and the role of intersensory redundancy in early perceptual and cognitive development has also been extended into the prenatal period with studies of animal embryos (see Lickliter, 1995). Given that the prenatal environment of both avian and mammalian species provides a rich array of tactile, vestibular, chemical, and auditory stimulation (Gottlieb, 1971a), it seems plausible that the developing embryo or fetus could be responsive to redundant multisensory information. In this light, we recently explored aspects of the intersensory redundancy hypothesis in precocial quail embryos and found that redundancy across modalities can also facilitate perceptual learning during the prenatal period (Lickliter et al., 2002). Quail embryos were exposed to an individual maternal call for 10 min/h across 6, 12, or 24 hours prior to hatching, under conditions of (1) unimodal auditory stimulation, (2) concurrent but asynchronous auditory and visual stimulation, or (3) redundant and synchronous auditory and visual stimulation. Subjects were then tested one day after hatching to determine if they preferred the familiar maternal call over an unfamiliar variant of the maternal call. Results indicated that for all exposure durations chicks that received the redundant audiovisual familiarization as embryos significantly preferred the familiar call, whereas those that received the nonredundant audiovisual familiarization failed to show a preference for the familiar call. Chicks that received the unimodal auditory familiarization showed eventual perceptual learning, preferring the familiar call following the longest period (24 hours) of prenatal exposure (Fig. 40.3). Thus, embryos receiving redundant information to the auditory and visual modalities about synchrony, tempo, rhythm, and duration required only one-quarter the exposure durations of embryos receiving unimodal information.

These results are the first to show enhanced prenatal perceptual learning when amodal information (tempo, rhythm, duration) is presented redundantly across two sensory modalities. Synchronous bimodal stimulation makes overlapping, temporally coordinated information available to the different senses and can facilitate perceptual learning and memory for redundant, amodal stimulus properties common across sensory modalities, even during the prenatal period (see also Honeycutt & Lickliter, 2002). In contrast, concurrent bimodal stimulation that is not redundant provides the young organism with competing sources of information, potentially interfering with the embryo's ability to successfully attend to either source of information (Lickliter & Hellewell, 1992; Radell & Gottlieb, 1992).

Additional support for this view has recently been provided by Reynolds and Lickliter (2001). Quail embryos exposed to concurrent but asynchronous auditory-visual stimulation had significantly higher baseline heart rates following stimulus exposure and significantly greater changes from baseline during stimulus exposure when compared with embryos that received synchronous (redundant) auditory-visual stimulation or unimodal auditory stimulation. The increased physiological arousal elicited by asynchronous bimodal stimulation may exceed some optimal range of arousal and interfere with perceptual learning, given that precocial avian embryos appear unable to demonstrate prenatal auditory learning of a maternal call when presentation is paired with concurrent but asynchronous patterned visual stimulation (Gottlieb et al., 1989; Lickliter & Hellewell, 1992). In contrast, redundant bimodal stimulation appears to regulate arousal levels in a range that supports and even facilitates prenatal perceptual learning (Lickliter et al., 2002).

Additional studies assessing physiological and behavioral arousal during and following specific types of sensory stimulation should provide further insight into the processes and mechanisms contributing to the origins and development of intersensory perception, learning, and memory. What seems clear at present

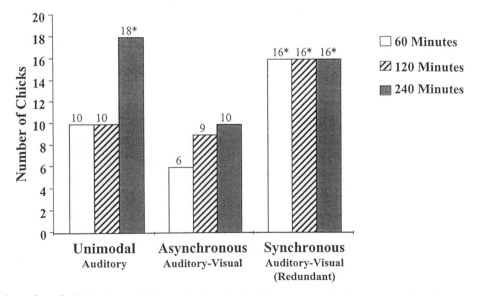

FIGURE 40.3 Number of quail chicks (out of 20) preferring the familiar maternal call over an unfamiliar maternal call following 60 minutes, 120 minutes, or 240 minutes of unimodal, concurrent but asynchronous, or redundant, synchronous prenatal exposure. *$p < 0.05$.

from converging evidence across different levels of analysis and from a variety of animal species is that temporally aligned multimodal stimulation (intersensory redundancy) is particularly salient during early development and is important for initially guiding and constraining selective attention and perceptual learning.

Conclusions

Converging evidence from both the neural (Calvert, 2001; Giard & Peronnet, 1999) and the behavioral sciences (Lewkowicz, 2000; Lickliter & Bahrick, 2000; Massaro, 1998) is providing a new framework for the study of multisensory perception. This framework acknowledges the multimodal nature of both the structure of the organism and the structure of its environment and recognizes that the separate senses interact and influence one another more than has been appreciated until very recently. In particular, we now know that intersensory interactions are present during both the prenatal period and the early postnatal period, raising the interesting question of how such interactions serve to influence subsequent perceptual organization. Although more research with both animal and human subjects is needed to further examine and clarify the role of intersensory responsiveness on perception, learning, and memory during early development, the evidence reviewed in this chapter suggests that overlapping or redundant sensory information can initially guide infants' selective attention and enhance perceptual discrimination and learning of amodal properties of stimulation. The consistent pattern of findings across different measures of responsiveness, different species, and different stages of development suggests that (1) redundant bimodal stimulation is attention getting, (2) redundant bimodal stimulation can lead to enhanced neural and behavioral responsiveness and facilitate adaptive levels of arousal, and (3) redundant bimodal stimulation promotes exploration and learning of global, amodal properties of objects and events. Intersensory redundancy appears to be an important cornerstone of early perceptual development (at least in precocial animal infants; see Wallace & Stein, 1997, for contrasting results with an altricial animal infant) and may be meaningfully investigated as a general principle, potentially applicable across a variety of avian and mammalian species. We propose that differentiation of amodal and modality-specific stimulus properties emerges in a coordinated manner, with the detection of more global, amodal properties leading and constraining perceptual responsiveness to more specific properties of objects and events. Thus, the detection of amodal relations promoted by redundancy across sensory modalites facilitates perceptual organization in young organisms in a manner that can provide an efficient and effective means of acquiring the skills and knowledge of adult perceivers.

REFERENCES

Bahrick, L. E. (1988). Intermodal learning in infancy: Learning on the basis of two kinds of invariant relations in audible and visible events. *Child Development, 59,* 197–209.

Bahrick, L. E. (1992). Infants' perceptual differentiation of amodal and modality specific audio-visual relations. *Journal of Experimental Child Psychology, 53,* 180–199.

Bahrick, L. E. (1994). The development of infants' sensitivity to arbitrary intermodal relations. *Ecological Psychology, 6,* 111–123.

Bahrick, L. E. (2001). Increasing specificity in perceptual development: Infants' detection of nested levels of multimodal stimulation. *Journal of Experimental Child Psychology, 79,* 253–270.

Bahrick, L. E., Flom, R., & Lickliter, R. (2002). Intersensory redundancy facilitates discrimination of tempo in 3-month-old infants. *Developmental Psychobiology, 41,* 352–363.

Bahrick, L. E., & Lickliter, R. (2000). Intersensory redundancy guides attentional selectivity and perceptual learning in infancy. *Developmental Psychology, 36,* 190–201.

Bahrick, L. E., & Lickliter, R. (2002). Intersensory redundancy guides early perceptual and cognitive development. *Advances in Child Development and Behavior, 30,* 153–187.

Bahrick, L. E., Lickliter, R., & Flom, R. (2000). *Intersensory redundancy: Infants' detection of unimodal properties of events.* Paper presented at a meeting of the International Society for Developmental Psychobiology, New Orleans, LA.

Bahrick, L. E., & Pickens, J. (1994). Amodal relations: The basis for intermodal perception and learning in infancy. In D. J. Lewkowicz & R. Lickliter (Eds.), *The development of intersensory perception: Comparative perspectives* (pp. 205–233). Hillsdale, NJ: Erlbaum.

Bahrick, L. E., Walker, A. S., & Neisser, U. (1981). Selective looking by infants. *Cognitive Psychology, 13,* 377–390.

Birch, H., & Lefford, A. (1963). *Intersensory development in children. Monographs of the Society for Research in Child Development, 28.*

Botuck, S., & Turkewitz, G. (1990). Intersensory functioning: Auditory-visual pattern equivalence in younger and older children. *Developmental Psychology, 26,* 115–120.

Bower, T. G. R. (1974). *Development in infancy.* San Francisco: Freeman.

Bushnell, E. W. (1994). A dual-processing approach to cross-modal matching: Implications for development. In D. J. Lewkowicz & R. Lickliter (Eds.), *The development of intersensory perception: Comparative perspectives* (pp. 19–38). Hillsdale, NJ: Erlbaum.

Calvert, G. A. (2001). Crossmodal processing in the human brain: Insights from functional neuroimaging studies. *Cerebral Cortex, 11,* 1110–1123.

Carlsen, R. M. (1999). *Neural plasticity and the development of intersensory functioning in bobwhite quail.* Unpublished doctoral dissertation, Virginia Polytechnic Institute and State University, Blacksburg, VA.

Carlsen, R. M., & Lickliter, R. (1999). Augmented prenatal tactile and vestibular stimulation alters postnatal auditory and visual responsiveness in bobwhite quail chicks. *Developmental Psychobiology, 35*, 215–225.

Columbus, R. F., & Lickliter, R. (1998). Modified sensory features of social stimulation alters the perceptual responsiveness of bobwhite quail chicks. *Journal of Comparative Psychology, 112*, 161–169.

Columbus, R. F., Sleigh, M. J., Lickliter, R., & Lewkowicz, D. J. (1998). Unimodal maternal experience interferes with responsiveness to the spatial contiguity of multimodal maternal cues in bobwhite quail chicks. *Infant Behavior and Development, 21*, 397–409.

Friedes, D. (1974). Human information processing and sensory modality: Cross-modal functions, information complexity, and deficit. *Psychological Bulletin, 81*, 242–310.

Frost, D. O. (1990). Sensory processing by novel, experimentally induced cross-modal circuits. *Annals of the New York Academy of Sciences, 608*, 92–112.

Giard, M. H., & Peronnet, F. (1999). Auditory-visual integration during multimodal object recognition in humans: A behavioral and electrophysiological study. *Journal of Cognitive Neuroscience, 11*, 473–490.

Gibson, E. J. (1969). *Principles of perceptual learning and development.* Englewood Cliffs, NJ: Prentice Hall.

Gibson, E. J., & Pick, A. D. (2000). *An ecological approach to perceptual learning and development.* New York: Oxford University Press.

Gogate, L. J., & Bahrick, L. E. (1998). Intersensory redundancy facilitates learning of arbitrary relations between vowel sounds and objects in seven-month-old infants. *Journal of Experimental Child Psychology, 69*, 133–149.

Gottlieb, G. (1971a). Ontogenesis of sensory function in birds and mammals. In E. Tobach, L. Aronson, & E. Shaw (Eds.), *The biopsychology of development* (pp. 66–128). New York: Academic Press.

Gottlieb, G. (1971b). *Development of species-identification in birds.* Chicago: University of Chicago Press.

Gottlieb, G. (1988). Development of species identification in ducklings: XV. Individual auditory recognition. *Developmental Psychobiology, 21*, 509–522.

Gottlieb, G. (1993). Social induction of malleability in ducklings: Sensory basis and psychological mechanism. *Animal Behavior, 45*, 707–719.

Gottlieb, G., Tomlinson, W. T., & Radell, P. L. (1989). Developmental intersensory interference: Premature visual experience suppresses auditory learning in ducklings. *Infant Behavior and Development, 12*, 1–12.

Gottlieb, G., Wahlsten, D., & Lickliter, R. (1998). The significance of biology for human development: A developmental psychobiological systems view. In R. Lerner (Ed.), *Handbook of child psychology, Vol. 1: Theoretical models of human development* (pp. 233–273). New York: Wiley.

Hernandez-Reif, M., & Bahrick, L. E. (2001). The development of visual-tactile perception of objects: Amodal relations provide the basis for learning arbitrary relations. *Infancy, 2*, 51–72.

Honeycutt, H., & Lickliter, R. (2001). Order-dependent timing of unimodal and multimodal stimulation affects prenatal auditory learning in bobwhite quail embryos. *Developmental Psychobiology, 38*, 1–10.

Honeycutt, H., & Lickliter, R. (2002). Prenatal experience and postnatal perceptual preferences: Evidence for attentional bias in bobwhite quail embryos. *Journal of Comparative Psychology, 116*, 270–276.

Johnston & Gottlieb (1981). Development of visual species identification in ducklings: What is the role of imprinting? *Animal Behaviour, 29*, 1082–1099.

Kellman, P. J., & Arterberry, M. E. (1998). *The cradle of knowledge: Development of perception in infancy.* Cambridge, MA: MIT Press.

King, A. J., & Carlile, S. (1993). Changes induced in the representation of auditory space in the superior colliculus by rearing ferrets with binocular lid suture. *Experimental Brain Research, 94*, 444–455.

King, A. J., Hutchings, M. E., Moore, D. R., & Blakemore, C. (1988). Developmental plasticity in visual and auditory representation in the mammalian superior colliculus. *Nature, 332*, 73–76.

Knudsen, E. I., & Brainard, M. S. (1991). Visual instruction of the neural map of auditory space in the developing optic tectum. *Science, 253*, 85–87.

Knudsen, E. I., & Brainard, M. S. (1995). Creating a unified representation of visual and auditory space in the brain. *Annual Review of Neuroscience, 18*, 19–43.

Lewkowicz, D. J. (1994). Development of intersensory perception in human infants. In D. J. Lewkowicz & R. Lickliter (Eds.), *The development of intersensory perception: Comparative perspectives* (pp. 165–204). Hillsdale, NJ: Erlbaum.

Lewkowicz, D. J. (2000). The development of intersensory temporal perception: An epigenetic systems/limitations view. *Psychological Bulletin, 126*, 281–308.

Lewkowicz, D. J. (2002). Heterogeneity and heterochrony in the development of Intersensory perception. *Cognitive Brain Research, 14*, 41–63.

Lewkowicz, D. J., & Lickliter, R. (1994a). *The development of intersensory perception: Comparative perspectives.* Hillsdale, NJ: Erlbaum.

Lewkowicz, D. J., & Lickliter, R. (1994b). Insights into mechanisms of intersensory development: The value of a comparative, convergent-operations approach. In D. J. Lewkowicz & R. Lickliter (Eds.), *The development of intersensory perception: Comparative perspectives* (pp. 403–413). Hillsdale, NJ: Erlbaum.

Lewkowicz, D. J., & Turkewitz, G. (1981). Intersensory interaction in newborns: Modification of visual preferences following exposure to sound. *Child Development, 52*, 827–832.

Lickliter, R. (1990). Premature visual stimulation accelerates intersensory functioning in bobwhite quail neonates. *Developmental Psychobiology, 23*, 15–27.

Lickliter, R. (1995). Embryonic sensory experience and intersensory development in precocial birds. In J. P. Lecanuet, W. P. Fifer, N. A. Krasnegor, & W. P. Smotherman (Eds.), *Fetal development: A psychobiological perspective* (pp. 281–294). Hillsdale, NJ: Erlbaum.

Lickliter, R. (2000a). An ecological approach to behavioral development: Insights from comparative psychology. *Ecological Psychology, 12*, 319–334.

Lickliter, R. (2000b). The role of sensory stimulation in perinatal development: Insights from comparative research for the care of the high-risk infant. *Journal of Developmental and Behavioral Pediatrics, 21,* 437–447.

Lickliter, R., & Bahrick, L. E. (2000). The development of infant intersensory perception: Advantages of a comparative convergent-operations approach. *Psychological Bulletin, 126,* 260–280.

Lickliter, R., & Bahrick, L. E. (2001). The salience of multimodal sensory stimulation in early development: Implications for the issue of ecological validity. *Infancy, 2,* 447–463.

Lickliter, R., Bahrick, L. E., & Honeycutt, H. (2002). Intersensory redundancy facilitates prenatal perceptual learning in bobwhite quail embryos. *Developmental Psychology, 38,* 15–23.

Lickliter, R., & Banker, H. (1994). Prenatal components of intersensory development in precocial birds. In D. J. Lewkowicz & R. Lickliter (Eds.), *The development of intersensory perception: Comparative perspectives* (pp. 59–80). Hillsdale, NJ: Erlbaum.

Lickliter, R., Dyer, A., & McBride, T. (1993). Perceptual consequences of early social experience in precocial birds. *Behavioural Processes, 30,* 185–200.

Lickliter, R., & Hellewell, T. B. (1992). Contextual determinants of auditory learning in bobwhite quail embryos and hatchlings. *Developmental Psychobiology, 25,* 17–24.

Lickliter, R., & Lewkowicz, D. J. (1995). Intersensory experience and early perceptual development: Attenuated prenatal sensory stimulation affects postnatal auditory and visual responsiveness in bobwhite quail chicks. *Developmental Psychology, 31,* 609–618.

Lickliter, R., & Stoumbos, J. (1991). Enhanced prenatal auditory experience facilitates postnatal visual responsiveness in bobwhite quail chicks. *Journal of Comparative Psychology, 105,* 89–94.

Lyons-Ruth, K. (1977). Bimodal perception in infancy: Response to auditory-visual incongruity. *Child Development, 48,* 820–827.

Marks, L. E. (1978). *The unity of the senses: Interrelations among the modalities.* New York: Academic Press.

Massaro, D. W. (1998). *Perceiving talking faces: From speech perception to a behavioral principle.* Cambridge, MA: MIT Press.

Maurer, D. (1993). Neonatal synesthesia: Implications for the processing of speech and faces. In B. de Boysson-Bardies, S. de Schonen, P. Jusczyk, P. McNeilage, & J. Morton (Eds.), *Speech and face processing in the first year of life* (pp. 109–124). Boston: Kluwer Academic.

Mellon, R. C., Kraemer, P. J., & Spear, N. E. (1991). Intersensory development and Pavlovian conditioning: Stimulus selection and encoding of lights and tones in the preweanling rat. *Journal of Experimental Psychology: Animal Behavior Processes, 17,* 448–464.

Morrongiello, B. A., Fenwick, K. D., & Chance, G. (1998). Cross-modal learning in newborn infants: Inferences about properties of auditory-visual events. *Infant Behavior and Development, 21,* 543–554.

Partan, S., & Marler, P. (1999). Communication goes multimodal. *Science, 283,* 1272–1273.

Pettigrew, J. D., & Konishi, M. (1976). Neurons selective for orientation and binocular disparity in the visual Wulst of the barn owl. *Science, 193,* 675–678.

Piaget, J. (1952). *The origins of intelligence.* New York: Norton.

Radell, P. L., & Gottlieb, G. (1992). Developmental intersensory interference: Augmented prenatal sensory experience interferes with auditory learning in duck embryos. *Developmental Psychology, 28,* 795–803.

Reynolds, G. D., & Lickliter, R. (2001). *Effects of intersensory redundancy on physiological arousal in bobwhite quail embryos.* Paper presented at the annual meeting of the International Society for Developmental Psychobiology, San Diego, CA.

Reynolds, G. D., & Lickliter, R. (2002). Effects of prenatal sensory stimulation on heart rate and behavioral measures of arousal in bobwhite quail embryos. *Developmental Psychobiology, 41,* 112–122.

Rochat, P. (1995). *The self in infancy: Theory and research.* Amsterdam: Elsevier.

Rose, S. A., & Ruff, H. A. (1987). Cross-modal abilities in human infants. In J. D. Osofsky (Ed.), *Handbook of infant development* (pp. 318–362). New York: Wiley.

Slater, A., Quinn, P. C., Brown, E., & Hayes, R. (1999). Intermodal perception at birth: Intersensory redundancy guides newborns' learning of arbitrary auditory-visual pairings. *Developmental Science, 2,* 333–338.

Sleigh, M. J., Columbus, R. F., & Lickliter, R. (1998). Intersensory experience and early perceptual development: Postnatal experience with multimodal maternal cues affects intersensory responsiveness in bobwhite quail chicks. *Developmental Psychology, 34,* 215–223.

Sleigh, M. J., & Lickliter, R. (1997). Augmented prenatal auditory stimulation alters postnatal perception, arousal, and survival in bobwhite quail chicks. *Developmental Psychobiology, 30,* 201–212.

Smith, L. B. (1994). Forward. In D. J. Lewkowicz & R. Lickliter (Eds.), *The development of intersensory perception: Comparative perspectives* (pp. ix–xix). Hillsdale, NJ: Erlbaum.

Spear, N. E., & McKinzie, D. L. (1994). Intersensory integration in the infant rat. In D. J. Lewkowicz & R. Lickliter (Eds.), *The development of intersensory perception: Comparative perspectives* (pp. 133–161). Hillsdale, NJ: Erlbaum.

Spelke, E. S. (1979). Perceiving bimodally specified events in infancy. *Developmental Psychology, 15,* 626–636.

Stein, B. E., & Meredith, M. A. (1993). *The merging of the senses.* Cambridge, MA: MIT Press.

Stein, B. E., Meredith, M. A., Huneycutt, W. S., & McDade, L. (1989). Behavioral indices of multisensory integration: Orientation to visual cues is affected by auditory stimuli. *Journal of Cognitive Neuroscience, 1,* 12–24.

Stein, B. E., Meredith, M. A., & Wallace, M. (1994). Development and neural basis of multisensory integration. In D. J. Lewkowicz & R. Lickliter (Eds.), *The development of intersensory perception: Comparative perspectives* (pp. 81–105). Hillsdale, NJ: Erlbaum.

Stein, B. E., Wallace, M., & Stanford, T. R. (2000). Merging sensory signals in the brain: The development of multisensory integration in the superior colliculus. In M. S. Gazzaniga (Ed.), *The new cognitive neurosciences* (pp. 55–71). Cambridge, MA: MIT Press.

Tees, R. C., & Symons, L. A. (1987). Intersensory coordination and the effect of early sensory deprivation. *Developmental Psychobiology, 23,* 497–507.

Thelen, E., & Smith, L. B. (1994). *A dynamic systems approach to the development of cognition and action.* Cambridge, MA: MIT Press.

Turkewitz, G. (1994). Sources of order for intersensory functioning. In D. J. Lewkowicz & R. Lickliter (Eds.), *The development of intersensory perception: Comparative perspectives* (pp. 3–17). Hillsdale, NJ: Erlbaum.

Turkewitz, G., Gilbert, M., & Birch, H. G. (1974). Early restriction of tactile stimulation and visual functioning in the kitten. *Developmental Psychobiology, 7,* 243–248.

Turkewitz, G., & Mellon, R. C. (1989). Dynamic organization of intersensory function. *Canadian Journal of Psychology, 43,* 286–301.

von Helmholtz, H. (1968). The origin of the correct interpretation of our sensory impressions. In R. M. Warren & R. P. Warren (Eds.), *Helmholtz on perception: Its physiology and development* (pp. 247–266). New York: Wiley.

Walker-Andrews, A. S. (1986). Intermodal perception of expressive behaviors: Relation of eye and voice? *Developmental Psychology, 22,* 373–377.

Walker-Andrews, A. S. (1997). Infants' perception of expressive behavior: Differentiation of multimodal information. *Psychological Bulletin, 121,* 437–456.

Wallace, M. T., & Stein, B. E. (1997). Development of multisensory neurons and multisensory integration in cat superior colliculus. *Journal of Neuroscience, 17,* 2429–2444.

Werner, H. (1957). The concept of development from a comparative and organismic point of view. In D. B. Harris (Ed.), *The concept of development* (pp. 125–148). Minneapolis: University of Minnesota Press.

Withington-Wray, D. J., Binns, K. E., & Keating, M. J. (1990). The maturation of the superior colliculus map of auditory space in the guinea pig is disrupted by developmental visual deprivation. *European Journal of Neuroscience, 2,* 682–692.

41 The Value of Multisensory Redundancy in the Development of Intersensory Perception

DAVID J. LEWKOWICZ AND KIMBERLY S. KRAEBEL

Introduction

Most species are endowed with multiple sensory systems that enable them to rely on a combination of multisensory signals for perception and action (Stein & Meredith, 1993). Moreover, as noted by Maier and Schneirla (1964), the reliance on multisensory inputs for control of behavior becomes the rule rather than the exception as one ascends the vertebrate phylogenetic scale from fish to human. Given these two facts, the obvious question is whether redundant, multisensory event and object specification is advantageous from the standpoint of perception and action. This question has figured more or less prominently in various recent discussions about the role of multisensory control pertaining to perception and information processing in general (Massaro, 1998), brain-behavior relations (Damasio, 1989; Edelman, 1992; Edelman & Tononi, 2000; Ettlinger & Wilson, 1990; Stein & Meredith, 1993), and neural and behavioral development (Edelman, 1992; Lewkowicz & Lickliter, 1994; Thelen & Smith, 1994).

In general, it is reasonable to conclude that the widespread evolutionary emergence of multisensory perception and action in the animal kingdom is likely to reflect the fact that multisensory input and the redundancy that input provides have adaptive value (J. J. Gibson, 1966, 1979; Maier & Schneirla, 1964; Marks, 1978; Piaget, 1952; Werner, 1973). For example, a predator that can spot a prey regardless of whether it can smell it, hear it, or see it is at an adaptive advantage over one that can only smell the prey. Likewise, a prey that can avoid a predator regardless of whether it can smell it, hear it, or see it is also at an adaptive advantage. As we will show, empirical evidence from studies of adult organisms indicates that multisensory redundancy provides a variety of advantages. This chapter reviews the available empirical evidence on the development of intersensory perception in human and animal infants to determine whether the same might be true in early development.

Theoretical foundations

Underlying a multisensory redundancy advantage is the implicit assumption that multiple sources of information can provide a perceiver with a more veridical picture of the world. The problem, however, of having access to multiple sources of sensory input via multiple and specialized sensory systems is that all this information must somehow be integrated into a meaningful whole. Various theoretical solutions to this problem have been proposed. J. J. Gibson (1966, 1979) proposed a highly parsimonious solution in his theory of direct perception. According to Gibson, sensory stimulation is registered by a set of perceptual systems that are directly responsive to the amodal invariants (i.e., stimulus properties that are equivalent across modalities) that normally specify objects and events. As a result, taking advantage of diverse sensory inputs meant that the observer simply needed to pick up the amodal invariants and in this way could perceive a world of unified objects and events. A key assumption made by Gibson was that the perceiver did not have to perform any active intersensory integration because the information specified in the external environment is already structured and integrated (i.e., in terms of amodal invariants). Unfortunately, Gibson did not offer any discussion of the underlying mechanisms making the pickup of amodal invariants possible except to say that perceivers somehow abstract these invariants from the perceptual array.

Other theoretical approaches to the problem of intersensory integration assume that some sort of active internal process is involved. For example, Massaro (1998) advocates an information processing view according to which intersensory perception is part of a general perceptual recognition process. For Massaro, perceptual recognition involves the operation of three sequentially dependent subprocesses: evaluation of input, its integration, and decision processes that compare the input to prototypes stored in long-term memory. Bertelson (1999), in his work on the intersensory integration of space, makes the assumption that the integration of audible and visible indices of spatial location occurs in an automatic fashion, but rather than occurring at the perceptual level, as in Gibson's theory, integration occurs at the sensory level. Welch (1999) takes issue with Bertelson's view and argues that top-down cognitive influences play an important role in intersensory integration of space. Finally, Stein and Meredith (1993) argue that the nervous system plays an active role in constructing a multisensory view of space.

Gibson's claim that amodal invariants are directly available to perceptual systems and that, as a result, no intervening neural integration processes are needed to achieve intersensory integration runs counter to empirical evidence. It is now clear that the brain is not a passive recipient of already synthesized multisensory arrays but that, at least in some cases, it actively synthesizes multisensory signals into coherent percepts. For example, Stein and colleagues (Stein, 1998) have shown that the deep layers of the adult mammalian superior colliculus (SC) contain mostly multisensory cells and that these cells exhibit a marked enhancement in activity when near-threshold auditory and visual stimuli are presented together in space and time. This enhancement is critically dependent on the association cortex, which sends down projections to the SC. When this cortex is inactivated, the multisensory cells stop integrating. Of particular interest from a developmental standpoint is the fact that these cells are not present at birth, and even when they begin to appear later, they do not exhibit mature functional properties. Moreover, when they first begin to integrate, their ability to integrate is directly dependent on influences from the association cortex. In other words, almost from the very beginning of life, the nervous system actively synthesizes heteromodal inputs, and, thus, studies of the role of multisensory redundancy in behavior should recognize the rich amodal structure available in the sensory array as well as the intimate role that the nervous system plays in its perception.

Evidence of a multisensory redundancy advantage

Findings that illustrate the benefits of multisensory redundancy in adults abound. Among these are findings showing that (1) adult humans and many adult nonhuman species perform more efficiently and accurately on various attentional, discriminative, and learning tasks when multiple sources of sensory information are available (Rowe, 1999), (2) many species rely on concurrent, multisensory cues in social communication (Partan & Marler, 1999), (3) adult humans perceive speech considerably better when it is jointly specified by audible and visible attributes (Summerfield, 1979), and (4) cats exhibit more vigorous behavioral and neural responsiveness on a spatial localization task when location is signaled by auditory and visual cues than when it is signaled by a unisensory cue (Stein & Meredith, 1993). In addition, some evidence suggests that infants respond in a more robust manner and show better discriminative responsiveness to bisensory events as opposed to unisensory ones (Bahrick & Lickliter, 2000; Lewkowicz, 1988a, 1988b, 1992c, 1996a, 1998, 2000b).

Evidence that even infants show greater responsiveness to multisensory inputs leads to the strong theoretical assumption that multisensory control of action and perception might be advantageous in early development as well. Although this may be a reasonable assumption, it has never actually been evaluated from an empirical point of view. To do so, it must first be established whether and how well young organisms can integrate multisensory information. To accomplish this task, in the following sections we will (1) discuss theoretical conceptions of intersensory perceptual development, (2) formulate the developmental question relating to intersensory perception, (3) discuss the unique contribution of developmental factors to the effects of multisensory redundancy, (4) argue that the neglected distinction between the perception of intersensory equivalence, on the one hand, and the perception of modality-specific relations, on the other, is key for determining whether a multisensory redundancy advantage is possible in early development, (5) consider the empirical evidence on infants' perception of intersensory equivalence, (6) consider several hypotheses that provide specific suggestions regarding infants' response to multisensory redundancy, and (7) end with a review of the empirical evidence that speaks most directly to the question of whether multisensory redundancy confers a sensory processing or perceptual advantage in early development.

Theoretical conceptions of intersensory perceptual development

Discussions of the developmental aspects of intersensory perception have long and deep historical roots going back to antiquity. Aristotle posited that the different senses, working in concert with one another, provide us with "common sensibles," and that these in turn provide us with basic and unique categories of experience (Marks, 1978). In the seventeenth and eighteenth centuries, the British empiricists Berkeley and Locke also recognized the value of multiple sense data, and in addition, asked how our ability to utilize such data comes about in development. Their answer was that our ability to take advantage of multisensory specification comes about through our everyday experiences with our world as we grow. This view foreshadowed Piaget's (1952) view that intersensory integration comes about gradually during early development and that it is intimately tied to the child's constant interaction with the world. Nativists such as Kant and Descartes took the opposite view and maintained that all knowledge was given at birth, and thus implied that experience-based integration of sense data was not necessary.

The empiricist versus nativist dichotomy has greatly influenced modern-day thinking, both about the value of multiple sense data for perception and action and about the developmental origins of intersensory integration. It has given rise to two modern, equally dichotomous theoretical views on the developmental origins of intersensory perception. One of them, known as the *developmental integration view,* is similar in concept to the experience-based view of Berkeley and Locke and proposes that the cooperative use of the different sensory modalities emerges in a gradual manner over many months or even years (Birch & Lefford, 1963, 1967; Piaget, 1952, 1954). The infant is presumed to come into the world with uncoordinated sensory modalities and only through active exploration and interaction with the world learns to associate separate sensations into coherent and meaningful experiences. In contrast, and similar to the nativist view of Kant and Descartes, variations on what has been dubbed the *developmental differentiation view* (Bower, 1974; E. J. Gibson, 1969; Werner, 1973) hold that infants come into the world with a relatively unified set of sensory modalities and that during development, the senses become gradually differentiated from one another. Eleanor Gibson's theory (1969), which is an extension of J. J. Gibson's theory of perception to development, is the prototypical example of this view. It holds that infants are born with perceptual systems that are ready to pick up amodal invariants, and that as development progresses, the ability to pick up more complex invariants improves. This in turn results in increasingly greater sophistication in the perception of intersensory relations. Unfortunately, this theory does not provide a developmental inventory of the particular invariants that become available to perceptual systems as infants develop, nor does it provide a priori criteria for making predictions regarding the types of invariants that infants should be sensitive to at a particular point in development, and the reasons why.

Defining the developmental question

Developing organisms face a unique problem because they are, by definition, immature, and thus, despite the clear advantage that multisensory input might confer on behavior, it is possible that they either may not be able to take advantage of it or may respond to it in a different way. It could be argued, for example, that the multisensory complexity introduced by the proliferation of multisensory sources of input during evolution actually created a problem of "intersensory confusion" for developing organisms.

Although intersensory confusion is a possibility, Turkewitz and Kenny (1982, 1985) have proposed an alternative and intriguing view based on Oppenheim's (1981) theory of ontogenetic adaptations. Oppenheim argued that development should not be viewed as a progressive change from an immature, maladapted state to a mature, adapted one. Instead, he suggested that development should be viewed as a series of stages during which the organism's structural and functional features and capacities evolve to be optimally adapted to their niche at their respective points in development. Turkewitz and Kenny applied this notion to intersensory functioning in early development and proposed that rather than thinking of structural and functional limitations of early development as imposing immature forms of intersensory organization, such limitations should be thought of as providing different but equally adapted and useful forms of intersensory organization. One example of this type of adaptation is the finding by Lewkowicz and Turkewitz (1980) that neonates can make low-level intersensory matches based on stimulus intensity and that, in contrast to adults, they do so spontaneously, without any prior training. These authors argued that this form of intersensory integration is unique to neonates because of their sensory and perceptual immaturity. Furthermore, based on Schneirla's (1965) view that young organisms are primarily responsive to intensity, they suggested that this form of integration actually offers a way of "bootstrapping" the perceptual system and getting it on its way to form new intersensory liaisons between the newly functional visual modality and other sensory modalities. Thus, consistent with Turkewitz and

Kenny's view, this initial immaturity is not an obstacle but a good starting point for solving the intersensory integration problem.

As Lewkowicz and Turkewitz's (1980) findings show, the theoretical scenario that infants enter the world with some basic capacity to integrate multisensory inputs but that this capacity is limited by the structural and functional limitations of early development is plausible. Given this fact, it is possible that the ever-present multisensory array of input leads to some confusion, but that this confusion is precisely what delivers a "push" to the infant's sensory-perceptual system to advance to higher forms of responsiveness. A recent study by Adolph (2000) on infants' depth avoidance behaviors provides a good example of how a push by external input can lead to sensorimotor reorganization. Adolph's work has shown that as infants pass from one motor milestone (e.g., sitting) to another (e.g., crawling), they must relearn to avoid depth. Adolph argues that this is because they must recalibrate the control variables determining balance control for a new posture. In the process of doing so, they form new perception-action couplings that are appropriate to the new posture. From the current perspective, as infants begin to crawl, they are able to venture out and explore beyond their immediate environment. This newfound ability affords new sensory experiences, but at a cost. If an infant sees some interesting toy, she can now crawl over and get it, but sometimes getting to that toy might involve traversing a gap. Being able to judge the size of the gap involves coordination among motor systems controlling balance and visual, kinesthetic, and vestibular input. This means that as infants reach new motor milestones, they must form new perception-action couplings to engage in adaptive behaviors. In other words, changing motor capacities provide new sensory opportunities, which in turn force reorganization.

Adolph's findings nicely illustrate a constructivist, epigenetic systems view of development. According to this view, the development of behavior consists of the constant interplay between the developing organism's structural and functional abilities at a given time in development and the exigencies of the world in which the organism develops (Piaget, 1952, 1954; Thelen & Smith, 1994). According to this view, simply positing innate abilities without specifying their developmental origins is not sufficient for understanding the development of intersensory integration and the effects of multisensory redundancy on behavior. What is ultimately needed is a description and explication of the process by which various systems, at various levels of organization, participate in the development of particular intersensory skills (Lewkowicz, 2000a).

From an epigenetic systems theoretical perspective, neither the developmental integration view nor the developmental differentiation view adequately captures the processes underlying the development of intersensory perception. According to the developmental integration view and its assumption that initially infants cannot perform intersensory integration, infants should not be able to take full advantage of multisensory redundancy. In contrast, according to the developmental differentiation view and its assumption that infants can perform integration, infants should be able to take advantage of it. It turns out, however, that when the extant findings on human infants' perception of intersensory relations are considered together, they suggest that neither of these predictions is an accurate depiction of the developmental process. The integration and differentiation views were proposed before sufficient empirical evidence regarding infant intersensory capacities was available, and represent the extreme ends of the theoretical spectrum. Over the past 25 years a sizable body of empirical evidence on the development of intersensory perceptual functions has been amassed, and it is now becoming clear that the developmental emergence of intersensory functions is likely the result of the joint action of developmental integration and differentiation processes (Lewkowicz, 1999).

Developmental factors and their unique importance

Although on logical grounds it might be expected that young, developing organisms may take advantage of multisensory redundancy, a priori this may not necessarily be the case because of uniquely developmental reasons. First, development is a dynamic process that consists of the continual reorganization of coacting systems (Gottlieb, 1991, 1997; Kuo, 1976; Schneirla, 1957; Thelen & Smith, 1994). In altricial vertebrate species (e.g., rats, cats, humans), the sensory systems are immature at birth and gradually become mature over time. In human infants in particular, such basic functions as visual acuity, binocularity, color perception, smooth pursuit, depth perception, motion perception, and edge detection are all immature at birth and change substantially during the first year of life (Hainline, 1998; Kellman & Arterberry, 1998). Likewise, basic auditory abilities such as frequency discrimination (Olsho, 1984), temporal discrimination (Trehub, Schneider, & Henderson, 1995), and basic speech-related abilities such as the detection of phonemic, prosodic, allophonic, and phonotactic cues all change during infancy (Jusczyk, Houston, & Goodman, 1998). Complicating the picture even more is the fact that the different sensory systems develop in sequence, with the tactile modality beginning to function first, followed by the vestibular, chemical, auditory, and finally the visual, with the first four beginning to function prior to birth (Gottlieb, 1971). This means that a given sensory modality might be functionally ahead of another and that this may lead to sensory processing hierarchies. (Lewkowicz, 1988a, 1988b).

Changes at the behavioral and neural level that specifically underlie intersensory integration are also known to occur. Knudsen and colleagues (Knudsen, 1985; Knudsen & Knudsen, 1985) have shown that the behavioral correction of auditory localization errors resulting from the insertion of an earplug into one ear of young barn owls is critically dependent on the visual spatial cues that are available to the owl at the same time. Moreover, these changes are reflected at the neural level in bisensory tectal units. Similarly, King and Carlile (1993) found that ferrets deprived of visual experience during early development showed abnormal topography and precision in the spatial tuning of individual acoustically tuned neurons in the SC, and that this resulted in the misalignment of the auditory and visual spatial maps. Finally, as noted earlier, Wallace and Stein (1997) found that the structures that ultimately become multisensory cells in the deep layers of the SC of the cat are initially not multisensory and only over time begin to exhibit multisensory response properties. Even more interesting is the finding that this is the case in primates as well (Wallace & Stein, 2001), even though primates are more developmentally precocial than cats and possess multisensory neurons in the deep layers of the SC at birth. Thus, the neural underpinnings of multisensory integration are not present even in a primate species that is more developmentally advanced at birth. According to Wallace and Stein (2001), these animals require substantial postnatal experience to develop normal integrative functions. In keeping with these kinds of findings, studies of intersensory integration in human infants also have shown that responsiveness to various types of intersensory relations changes in early development (Bushnell, 1994; Lewkowicz, 2000a; Lickliter & Bahrick, 2000; Walker-Andrews, 1997).

It is likely that the changing nature of intersensory functions observed in early development is partly due to a highly plastic neural substrate. Initially in development the brain is full of exuberant neural connections that link the various sensory-specific areas. As the organism develops, these connections are pruned and replaced by experience-dependent connections (Frost, 1990; Innocenti & Clarke, 1984). One rather dramatic

example of such plasticity comes from a study by von Melchner, Pallas, and Sur (2000) showing that it is possible to induce visual responsiveness in auditory thalamus and cortex by redirecting retinal projections to auditory thalamus in early development. In general, early neural plasticity enables sensorimotor experiences during infancy to leave lasting structural and functional traces that shape intersensory interactions for the rest of the organism's life. Interestingly, certain forms of plasticity continue even into adulthood, as evidenced by the fact that sensory-specific areas retain their capacity to respond to inputs that originate in other modalities (Kujala, Alho, & Näätänen, 2000).

The foregoing empirical findings suggest the following general conclusions. First, the neural substrate needed for responsiveness to multisensory information and its integration may not initially be available. Second, the neural substrate required for responsiveness to multisensory inputs changes in early development. Finally, experience contributes in important ways to the development of functional connectivity and ultimately to intersensory integration. These conclusions, and the empirical findings that support them, are consistent with a view expressed many years ago by Schneirla (1965) that the effective significance of a given set of sensory inputs may be quite different for infants and adults even when the inputs are objectively identical. Applied to intersensory functions, this principle suggests that a given constellation of multisensory redundant inputs may not have the same facilitating role in early development as it might have later in adulthood simply because some of those inputs either may not be registered or may be perceived differently than they are later. Despite these developmental limitations and the likelihood that infants experience a different "multisensory mix" than do children and adults, they still have the daunting task of constructing a unified and meaningful world out of the multisensory inputs that often redundantly specify objects and events. Indeed, as we will show later, a growing body of empirical evidence indicates that human infants do possess a variety of intersensory integration skills. At the same time, however, we will argue that we are far from understanding how these skills develop and change, and what role intersensory redundancy plays in the overall picture.

Important distinctions between different types of perceptual cues

To understand the effects of multisensory inputs on responsiveness, it is helpful to distinguish between self-generated inputs, on the one hand, and externally generated inputs on the other. Self-generated inputs are produced by an organism's own motion through the environment and can consist of kinesthetic and somatosensory sensations as well as self-induced transformations of the external array impinging on the visual, auditory, and perhaps olfactory modalities. Integration of these types of sensations is important for the perception of self and its intersensory unity. Externally generated inputs can consist of any combination of auditory, visual, olfactory, gustatory, tactile, and kinesthetic sensations that are produced by forces external to the organism. Under normal circumstances, self-generated and externally generated multisensory inputs are present at all times, and it is this constantly changing conglomeration of sensations that controls behavior in an ongoing fashion.

The internally and externally generated array of multisensory inputs can consist either of amodal or modality-specific perceptual attributes. Amodal attributes are those that can be specified equally well across the different modalities, provide the same information regardless of sensory modality, and thus provide the basis for the perception of intersensory equivalence. These are Aristotle's "common sensibles" and Gibson's amodal invariants and include, among others, intensity, shape, texture, spatial extent, spatial location, duration, temporal rate, and rhythm. Modality-specific attributes are those stimulus properties that uniquely specify perceptual experiences in one particular modality (to Aristotle these were the special objects of each sensory modality). They can include such sensory properties as color, temperature, timbre, pitch, taste, and olfactory quality.

Usually, a multisensory object or event is specified by a combination of amodal and modality-specific attributes. For example, when an infant interacts with an adult, he usually can see a moving face and lips and hear a voice modulating over time. Embedded in this audiovisual scene is a great deal of concurrent amodal and modality-specific information. The lips' motion and the modulations of the voice are temporally synchronized and spatially colocated, the visual and auditory attributes of each utterance have the same duration, and the visual and audible attributes of multiple utterances have the same tempo and overall rhythmic patterning over time. In addition, however, a variety of modality-specific attributes is available. The adult's face and hair have a certain color, the voice has a certain timbre, the hands have a certain temperature, and the adult might even give off a certain smell. This complex sensory-perceptual situation is actually commonplace and presents the researcher with the challenge of determining how infants select relevant and meaningful information from such a mélange of input.

Given that extraction of meaning from a multisensory event must involve intersensory integration, the traditional approach has been to ask whether infants can perceive the amodal invariance inherent in such prototypical situations. The interaction example shows, however, that infants must deal with a panoply of amodal and modality-specific attributes on a continuous basis. This means that the infant's perceptual task is more complicated than simply to abstract amodal invariance. Thus, the ultimate answer to how infants select and integrate the relevant information must recognize that the processes underlying the perception of amodal invariance are likely to be different from those underlying the perception of modality-specific attribute relations (Bahrick & Pickens, 1994; Lewkowicz, 2000a). That is, the perception of amodal information requires the extraction of similar features out of a sensory array of physically different inputs, whereas the perception of modality-specific intersensory relations requires the operation of associative processes. As a result, the key question is how these two types of processes interact in early development and how they make it possible for infants to perceive the integral nature of multisensory input.

Bahrick (1994) has addressed this question directly by proposing what she refers to as the increasing specificity view of intermodal development. Drawing on E. Gibson's (1969) theory of perceptual development, Bahrick proposed that initial attention to amodal invariants provides infants with the opportunity to subsequently perceptually differentiate arbitrary, modality-specific associations and that the detection of amodal invariant relations precedes the learning of modality-specific relations. Indeed, several studies have shown that the detection of modality-specific attribute relations emerges rather late in development. For example, in studies in which different types of objects made visible impacts while a sound corresponded to one of them, Bahrick (1992, 1994) found that 3½-month-old infants matched the visible and audible impacts on the basis of intersensory synchrony and temporal microstructure relations. In contrast, infants did not detect the association between the color or shape of an object and its pitch until 7 months of age. Consistent with the latter findings, Reardon and Bushnell (1988) reported that 7-month-old infants could associate the color of an object and its taste. Finally, Hernandez-Reif and Bahrick (2001) found that both 4- and 6-month-old infants could make visual-tactual matches, but that only 6-month-olds could associate color or pattern with shape.

It is interesting to note that aside from intensity (Lewkowicz & Turkewitz, 1980), the single most important perceptual attribute that infants seem to rely on in their developmentally earliest attempt to abstract the multisensory unity of the perceptual array is temporal synchrony (Lewkowicz, 2000a). For example, 3-month-old infants can make arbitrary matches of faces and voices on the basis of synchrony (Brookes et al., 2001), and 4-month-olds can match moving objects with their synchronous sounds (Lewkowicz, 1992b). Even newborn infants can make intersensory associations between a line of a particular orientation and a particular speech token (Slater, Quinn, Brown, & Hayes, 1999) and between an object and a sound (Morrongiello, Fenwick, & Chance, 1998). Strictly speaking, however, temporal synchrony is not an amodal invariant in the same sense that attributes such as intensity, shape, size, rhythm, or tempo are. Unlike true amodal invariant properties, temporal synchrony is an emergent property of two or more sensory inputs being available at the same time, and thus cannot be perceived independently in different sensory modalities. The fact that temporal synchrony does not qualify as an amodal invariant and the fact that even newborn infants are capable of making arbitrary intersensory associations on the basis of temporal synchrony leave many questions unanswered. In particular, it is still far from clear which true amodal invariants infants can perceive and when they can do so in development, and how responsiveness to these interacts with infants' responsiveness to modality-specific attributes during early development.

THE EFFECT OF MODALITY-SPECIFIC CUES ON PERCEPTION OF AN AMODAL INVARIANT   For purposes of the current discussion, we will define multisensory redundancy as the condition in which an object or event is specified by some combination of amodal and modality-specific attributes. This definition is broader than other definitions (Bahrick & Lickliter, 2000) in that it is more agnostic with respect to the contribution of concurrent modality-specific attributes to the redundancy of the multisensory array. Moreover, this definition recognizes that synchrony plays a key role in the integration of multisensory signals, regardless of whether they are amodal or modality-specific, and that synchrony-based integration is likely to be mediated by a different mechanism than the perception of amodal invariance. Our definition of redundancy is consistent with others' use of the term. For example, in her discussion of the kinds of multicomponent signals that characterize sexual, warning, and aggressive displays throughout the animal kingdom, Rowe (1999) refers to "the evolutionary scenario where a signaler sends redundant signals containing the same information." Given this definition, one might ask at what point in development infants become capable of selecting the salient and critical aspects of multisensory objects and events. Does multisensory redundancy make it easier to learn about objects and events, or do the multiple sources of information create confusion? How do developing infants deal with the onslaught of multisensory inputs against the backdrop of constantly changing sensory, motor, perceptual, and cognitive capacities?

The answers to these questions require an understanding of how infants respond to amodal and modality-specific intersensory relations, and how the perception of one might affect the perception of the other. For example, infants might be able to perceive the amodal character of some aspect of a talking person (e.g., the equal duration and rhythm of lip motion and voice modulation), but the visual information might play a greater role than the auditory information, and certain audible or visible modality-specific features (e.g., eye or hair color or the timbre of the voice) also might influence the way they perceive that person. Bahrick's increasing specificity view would suggest that modality-specific attributes should not affect the perception of amodal invariants because they tend to be in the background until amodal invariant relations are first differentiated. Is it possible, however, that modality-specific attributes can, under certain circumstances, influence the learning and perception of amodal invariant relations? This question has not been asked before, but it is critical if we are to have a more complete understanding of the interaction between amodal and modality-specific attributes.

As an initial attempt to address this question, we recently conducted two experiments (Lewkowicz & Schwartz, 2002). In the first experiment, we habituated 2-, 4-, 6-, 8-, and 10-month-old infants to a movie showing a woman's face with a large stationary blue or orange hat on her head. The woman could be seen and heard repeatedly uttering a single syllable /ba/ (300 ms in duration) in a rhythmic fashion (either in a 2-2 or a 3-1 repeating pattern). Once infants met a habituation criterion, they were given two test trials: a modality-specific test trial in which only the color of the hat was changed and an amodal test trial in which only the rhythmic pattern of the syllable was changed (the familiar hat was still present). As can be seen in Figure 41.1, regardless of age, infants discriminated the color change ($P < 0.05$) but did not discriminate the rhythm change. In the second experiment, we tested infants' discrimination of the two rhythmic patterns in the absence of the modality-specific information (i.e., the hat

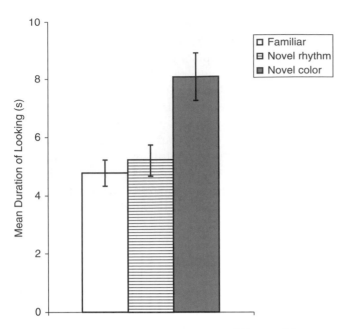

FIGURE 41.1 Response of infants to different bisensory rhythms in the presence of a salient modality-specific cue (a colored hat). Graphed are mean durations of looking to the familiar rhythm, novel rhythm, and novel color. Error bars indicate ± SEM.

was absent). As Figure 41.2 shows, this time infants easily discriminated between the two rhythms ($P < 0.001$). Together, these findings show that infants could perceive the amodal information but that they did not

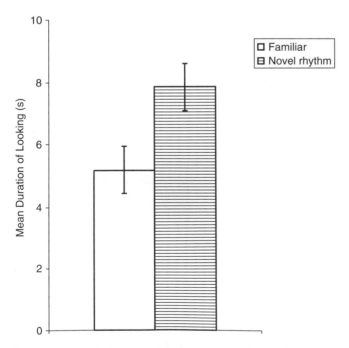

FIGURE 41.2 Response of infants to different bisensory rhythms in the absence of a modality-specific cue. Graphed are mean durations of looking to the familiar and novel rhythms. Error bars indicate ±SEM.

attend to it when a highly salient modality-specific attribute competed for attention. These findings show that, under some circumstances, modality-specific attributes may have processing priority over amodal cues. This observation raises the possibility that the Gibsonian view that infants are primarily attentive to amodal invariants may not fully capture the true complexity of the perceptual task.

OTHER TYPES OF INTERSENSORY INTERACTIONS   As already shown, intersensory interactions can produce integration and thus reduction of the overall amount of multisensory information through (1) the perception of invariance and (2) the perception of intersensory associations. In addition to these two major outcomes of intersensory integration, at least three other kinds of outcomes are possible: (1) sensory dominance or inhibition, (2) facilitation, or (3) induction of a novel perceptual experience (illusions). Although the perception of these types of effects has been studied far less in infants, there is a small literature on this topic. For example, Lewkowicz (1988a) found evidence of auditory dominance when infants' responsiveness to a flashing/beeping checkerboard was studied. In this study, infants did not respond to changes in the rate at which the checkerboard flashed when it was presented concurrently with the beeping sound but did respond to it when it was presented without the beeping sound. In addition, Lewkowicz found evidence of bisensory facilitation in a series of studies comparing infants' responses to unisensory versus bisensory changes in a compound auditory-visual (AV) stimulus. These studies are described in detail later in this chapter. Likewise, Bahrick and Lickliter (2000) have shown that infants learn about a rhythmical event more easily when it is specified concurrently by sensory inputs in more than one modality.

Two types of intersensory illusions previously reported in adults have now been reported in infants as well. A study by Rosenblum, Schmuckler, and Johnson (1997) investigated whether infants might be sensitive to the types of effects usually observed in the McGurk illusion (McGurk & MacDonald, 1976). They tested 5-month-old infants with AV pairs of conflicting syllables and found that infants exhibited responsiveness consistent with the induction of the McGurk effect. A more recent study by Scheier, Lewkowicz, and Shimojo (2003) found that infants' perception of an ambiguously moving visual object can be changed dramatically by the concurrent presentation of a brief and simple sound. This latter finding is based on an earlier study by Sekuler, Sekuler, and Lau (1997) showing that adults watching an ambiguous motion display reported perceptual reorganization of that display depending on the spatiotemporal relation of a simple sound to the motion of the two objects in the display. When subjects viewed two identical disks moving along the same path toward, through, and away from each other and heard a brief sound each time the objects coincided in the center, they reported seeing visual bouncing. When the sound did not correspond to the objects' spatial coincidence, they did not report bouncing. To determine when this AV illusion might emerge in development, Scheier et al. habituated 4-, 6-, and 8-month-old infants to such an ambiguous motion display while a sound occurred either at the point of the objects' coincidence (Experiment 1) or prior to or following coincidence (Experiment 2). During the test trials, the relation of the sound with respect to visual coincidence was changed (prior or following coincidence in Experiment 1 and during coincidence in Experiment 2). In both experiments, the 6- and 8-month-old infants detected the change in the spatiotemporal relation between the sound and the visual display, suggesting that they discriminated between the illusory and nonillusory displays. In a final experiment, infants were habituated to the ambiguous visual display together with a sound synchronized with the objects' coincidence and tested with disks that actually bounced against each other while the auditory stimulus was sounded. This time infants did not exhibit response recovery, as would have been expected if they had perceived the two events as bouncing.

Perception of amodal invariance in early development

As the preliminary findings from our "hat" study show, modality-specific cues can actually prevent infants from extracting what is otherwise a salient amodal invariant. This raises the obvious question of whether infants can perceive amodal invariance and when. Much of the research on this question has been reviewed elsewhere (Lewkowicz, 2000a; Lewkowicz & Lickliter, 1994; Lickliter & Bahrick, 2000; Rose & Ruff, 1987; Walker-Andrews, 1997), and therefore we will only highlight some of the major findings. For example, it has been shown that infants can perceive the following: (1) the amodal invariance of auditory and visual inputs on the basis of intensity shortly after birth (Kraebel, Vizvary, & Spear, 1998; Lewkowicz & Turkewitz, 1980), (2) the amodal invariance of audible and visible information specifying a syllable at 4 months of age (Kuhl & Meltzoff, 1982), (3) amodal invariance of multisensory emotional expressions by 7 months of age (Walker-Andrews, 1986), (4) AV synchrony and temporal microstructure relations in spatially dynamic events at 3½ months of age (Bahrick, 1988, 1992; Lewkowicz, 1992b, 1992c, 1996b) and

synchrony/duration-based AV relations in spatially static visual events by 6 months of age (Lewkowicz, 1986), (5) visual-proprioceptive relations specifying self-produced motion at 5 months of age (Bahrick & Watson, 1985; Schmuckler, 1996), and (6) visual-tactile shape relations by 6 months of age (Rose, 1994). Of greatest interest from the present standpoint is that when the available data are considered together, they indicate that the detection of specific types of intersensory equivalence relations emerges at different ages and that the specific age of emergence may depend on the particular nature of the information, sensory-perceptual maturity, experience, and so on.

In addition to the fact that skills for the detection of specific intersensory relations emerge at different ages, there are some findings in the literature showing that some of these skills either may not be fully developed at the ages tested or may not exist. For example, Spelke (1979) reported that 4-month-old infants performed AV matching on the basis of temporal rate, but a number of subsequent studies (Humphrey & Tees, 1980; Lewkowicz, 1985, 1992b, 1994a, 1994b) have been unable to obtain such matching. Likewise, Meltzoff and Borton (1979) reported that neonates can perform oral-visual transfer of shape information, but Maurer, Stager, and Mondloch (1999) failed to replicate this finding.

Perhaps of greatest interest has been the report by Meltzoff and Moore (1977) that newborn infants can imitate a variety of modeled actions. Because such an ability involves matching of visual and kinesthetic sensations, these findings would suggest that this form of intersensory integration is present at birth, and thus that extended experience with such relations is largely unnecessary for the perception of their multisensory unity. Unfortunately, subsequent studies (Anisfeld et al., 2001; McKenzie & Over, 1983) have not been able to replicate Meltzoff and Moore's initial findings. To some extent, the failure to obtain imitation is not surprising and is consistent with the fact that it is not until 5 months of age that infants exhibit statistically robust sensitivity to visual-proprioceptive relations (Bahrick and Watson [1985] did report a trend in this direction in some 3-month-olds, but overall, this was not a statistically significant finding). Finally, Lewkowicz has found in a number of studies that infants' response to the disruption of intersensory equivalence relations is not always consistent with what might be expected if they were perceiving amodal invariance. Specifically, Lewkowicz found that infants often failed to detect disruptions in amodal invariance, regardless of whether the invariance was specified by simple flashing checkerboards and pulsing tones (Lewkowicz, 1988a, 1988b, 1992c) or by human faces engaged in the act of speaking (Lewkowicz, 1996a, 1998, 2000b).

Solutions to the problem of multisensory inputs

We now return to the central question posed earlier: Do infants possess the requisite attentional and integrative mechanisms necessary to select the relevant and "correct" information from the panoply of multisensory information? By "correct" we mean the information that provides the most economical and unified snapshot of the world. Several hypotheses have been proposed that attempt to answer this question. The *intensity hypothesis,* proposed by Lewkowicz and Turkewitz (1980), is based on T. C. Schneirla's (1965) idea that initially in development, young organisms respond primarily to the quantitative aspects of stimulation. Applied to intersensory functioning in particular, the intensity hypothesis predicts that, unlike adults, young infants should engage in spontaneous, intensity-based, intersensory matching. As shown earlier, this is precisely what Lewkowicz and Turkewitz (1980) found. Based on this finding, they postulated that intensity provides an important and early basis for intersensory perception in infancy and a foundation for the construction of an intermodally unified perceptual world. In addition, Lewkowicz and Turkewitz proposed that as development progresses, intensity is replaced as a global intersensory integrator by higher-level, qualitative types of stimulus features.

At the time that Lewkowicz and Turkewitz proposed the intensity hypothesis, the literature on human infants' response to multisensory information was very sparse. Since that time, a sizable portion of the research on infant intersensory perception has been directed toward investigating the perception of temporally based intersensory relations, for the obvious reason that the temporal domain provides an entire class of stimulus features (e.g., synchrony, duration, rate, rhythm) that make the perception of intersensory relations possible. As noted earlier, one of the principal findings that has emerged from this research is that, like intensity, temporal synchrony plays a key and early role in intersensory integration in human infants (Bahrick, 1988; Lewkowicz, 1992a, 1996b). In fact, in a recent review of this research, Lewkowicz (2000a) proposed a model in which intersensory temporal synchrony is seen as providing an initial and foundational basis for the development and emergence of responsiveness to other, more complex types of temporal intersensory relations.

A third hypothesis, proposed by Walker-Andrews (1997), deals mainly with infants' perception of expressive behaviors but is notable in the current context because it emphasizes the importance of multisensory perception. Based on E. Gibson's (1969) amodal perception view, Walker-Andrews's hypothesis proposes that infants' presumed sensitivity to amodal invariants makes them selectively responsive to affect that is represented by multisensory attributes earlier in development than to affect that is represented by unisensory attributes. In other words, Walker-Andrews makes the claim that multisensory, redundant specification makes it possible for infants to perceptually differentiate and respond to affect earlier in development than they might respond to it if it is specified only by unisensory attributes.

A fourth and final hypothesis, proposed by Bahrick and Lickliter (2000), is conceptually similar to Walker-Andrews's hypothesis because it is also based on the Gibsonian assumption that infants are able to pick up amodal invariants. Bahrick and Lickliter dubbed it the *intersensory redundancy hypothesis* and proposed that intersensory redundancy directs and constrains infants' attention to bisensory information. Specifically, Bahrick and Lickliter suggest that when infants are first learning about a multisensory event, they attend selectively to its amodal properties precisely because the multisensory information is redundant. Attention to the event's amodal properties creates a developmental and episodic (i.e., during exploration) processing priority for amodal properties. Once the amodal properties are differentiated, modality-specific properties are then differentiated. If, however, multisensory stimulation is not available, Bahrick and Lickliter suggest that infants focus their attention more broadly on a variety of properties that are unique to individual modalities.

Bahrick and Lickliter (2000) put forth the intersensory redundancy hypothesis on the basis of studies in which they compared 5-month-old infants' ability to learn an audiovisual rhythmic pattern with their ability to learn a visual-only or an auditory-only rhythmic pattern. They showed that infants who were habituated to a specific audiovisual, intermodally synchronized rhythmic pattern detected a change in that pattern when tested with its visual representation. In contrast, infants who were habituated either to a specific rhythm specified by unisensory attributes or to a specific audiovisual rhythm whose auditory and visual attributes were desynchronized did not detect the pattern change. Thus, bisensory specification facilitated learning, but only if the audible and visible components of the rhythmic pattern were synchronized. The fact that synchrony drove the effect is of particular importance in the context of our earlier discussion of the operational definition of intersensory redundancy. Bahrick and Lickliter defined redundancy as "the spatially coordinated and concurrent presentation of the same information," where "concurrent" means intermodally synchronous. As noted earlier, however, intersensory temporal synchrony is not a true amodal invariant because, as in the case of cross-modal transfer, it is possible to perceive amodal invariance even when two or more heteromodal inputs are not temporally synchronous. Thus, responsiveness to an amodal invariant inherent in a multisensory, temporally synchronous event may be based on amodal invariance (e.g., rhythmic pattern), intersensory temporal synchrony, or on both properties working together. If it is based on synchrony, then it cannot be concluded that amodal redundancy drives the effect. To draw such a conclusion one must either investigate infants' ability to perceive intersensory equivalence per se or show that infants can learn the invariant rhythm even in the intermodally desynchronized case. The latter type of finding would be similar to Walker-Andrews's (1986) report showing that 7-month-old but not 5-month-old infants could match the affective tone of a voice with a face expressing the same affect despite the fact that the two were not synchronized. In sum, the interpretation of the underlying basis for what appears to be amodal redundancy effects must distinguish between the perception of temporal synchrony, on the one hand, and the perception of intersensory equivalence relations, on the other. This is key, because the underlying mechanisms for the perception of these two types of stimulus properties are different.

The four hypotheses discussed above build on the original and opposing theoretical propositions of Piaget, Birch, and Lefford, on the one hand, and E. Gibson, on the other. What makes them more useful is that they go beyond the broad and nonspecific principles of the classic views. They are more specific about the types of intersensory relations that infants are expected to perceive, specify more precisely the points in development when infants might be able to perceive these relations, and propose specific mechanisms that might underlie the emergence of such specific intersensory skills.

Human infants' responsiveness to multisensory compounds

Earlier we defined multisensory redundancy as the specification of an object or event by some combination of amodal and modality-specific attributes. In addition, we wondered at what point in development infants become capable of selecting the salient and critical aspects of multisensory objects and events, and whether multisensory redundancy makes it easier to do so. According to Bahrick and Lickliter's (2000) intersensory redundancy hypothesis, infants are selectively attentive to bisensory information, and their results showed that infants learned successfully only when rhythm was specified concurrently in the auditory and visual modalities.

In other words, it appeared that the learning of bisensory events (as long as their auditory and visual attributes are synchronous) is more effective than the learning of unisensory events.

Lewkowicz (1988a, 1988b, 1992c, 1996a, 1998, 2000b) has published a series of articles detailing the results of studies that shed further light on the role of redundant multisensory specification in infant perception and learning. In all of these studies, infants were first habituated to a compound AV stimulus and then were given several test trials in which various unisensory or bisensory attributes of the compound stimulus were changed. The basic feature of all of these studies was that responsiveness to the unisensory attributes was always studied in the context of the sensory input in the other modality. This was done explicitly to reflect the fact that infants normally have to deal with a multisensory world, and that responsiveness to input in one modality rarely, if ever, occurs in the absence of concurrent input in other modalities.

Three types of test trials were presented. Two of these were unisensory test trials and consisted of an auditory test trial (A), in which some attribute of the auditory component was changed while the visual component remained unchanged, and a visual (V) test trial, in which some attribute of the visual component was changed while the auditory component remained unchanged. The third test trial was the auditory-visual (AV) test trial in which a given auditory and visual attribute of the compound stimulus were changed simultaneously. The three different types of test trials made it possible to determine how auditory and visual inputs contributed separately as well as together to responsiveness. In addition, it was possible to determine whether infants perceived the relation between the auditory and visual information because the intersensory relation between these two components was disrupted in each of the unisensory test trials.

RESPONSE TO KINETICALLY STATIC AND DYNAMIC MULTISENSORY STIMULATION Responsiveness to a wide range of multisensory compounds was tested across the various experiments. In one series of experiments (Lewkowicz, 1988a, 1988b), responsiveness to kinetically static compounds was studied. Infants (6- and 10-month-olds) were first habituated to flashing checkerboards and beeping tones. Across the various experiments, the auditory and visual attributes of the compound stimulus were presented either in a temporally concordant fashion (e.g., the checkerboard flashed and a tone beeped synchronously at 2 or 4 Hz in some experiments and at 1 and 0.5 Hz in others) or in a temporally discordant fashion (e.g., the checkerboard flashed at 2 Hz and the tone beeped at 4 Hz, or vice versa). The ensuing test trials consisted of changes in the temporal properties of either the checkerboard, the beeping tone, or both. In some experiments, only rate changed, whereas in others, a constant duty cycle across different rates was used to control for the overall amount of stimulation, and thus rate and duration changed at the same time.

The design of these various experiments meant that in some of them, infants were habituated to a unitary multisensory event that provided a clear amodal invariant. In such a case, the auditory and visual attributes were presented in perfect one-to-one temporal synchrony and corresponded perfectly in terms of rate and duration. In other experiments, infants were habituated to a discordant multisensory event that, as a result, did not provide a clear amodal invariant. Two examples of the latter type of event can be seen in Figure 41.3. Panel *A* shows an event composed of auditory and visual components of equal "on" duration that differed in their temporal rate. Panel *B* shows an event composed of auditory and visual components that differed both in duration and in temporal rate. What makes these compound events particularly interesting is that even though they were not intermodally unified in terms of rate or duration, or by a one-to-one synchrony relation, they were still unified by higher-order synchrony relations. That is, the onset and offset of the slower component corresponded to the onset and offset of every other occurrence of the faster component (Fig. 41.3).

Table 41.1 shows the findings from the static compound experiments consisting of Experiments 1–7 from

TABLE 41.1

Results from Lewkowicz's studies of infants' responses to bisensory compounds

	A	V	AV
Lewkowicz (1988a)			
Experiment 1	−	−	√
Experiment 2	√	−	√
Experiment 3	Marg.	−	√
Experiment 4	−	−	√
Experiment 7	√	−	√
Lewkowicz (1988b)			
Experiment 1	√	−	√
Experiment 2	√	√	√
Experiment 3	√	√	√
Experiment 4	−	−	√
Experiment 5	√	√	√
Lewkowicz (1992c)			
Experiment 1	√	√	√
Experiment 2	√	√	√

Symbols: √ means positive result and − means negative result.

Lewkowicz (1988a) and Experiments 1–5 from Lewkowicz (1988b). Overall, two findings of particular interest emerged. First, infants responded consistently to the bisensory changes, confirming the theoretical expectation that bisensory changes should be highly salient. The consistency of the response to the bisensory changes is particularly notable from the standpoint of redundancy because infants responded to these changes regardless of whether the compound stimulus they first learned during habituation was amodally

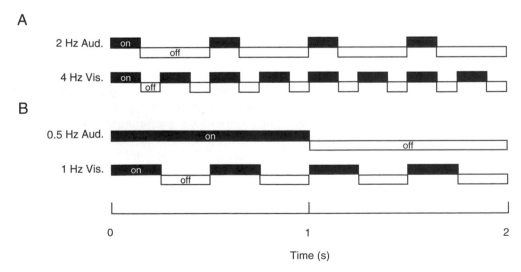

FIGURE 41.3 Schematic representation of the temporal distribution of stimulation in two kinds of intermodally discordant compounds stimulus events. (*A*) An event in which the stimulus "on" time was constant across different temporal rates of stimulus presentation in the different modalities. (*B*) An event in which the "on" time differed across rate to control the duty cycle.

invariant or not, and regardless of whether the components of the compound were synchronous. Based on Bahrick and Lickliter's (2000) findings and their intersensory redundancy hypothesis that amodal information has perceptual precedence and selectively facilitates perceptual learning, infants should not have learned the intermodally discordant compounds as well as the concordant ones. Thus, they should not have exhibited discrimination of the bisensory changes. This overall pattern of findings suggests that multisensory redundancy can indeed facilitate perceptual learning in early development, but that the facilitation is not based on (or at least does not require) the availability of a an amodal invariant. It seems that what is essential is some sort of intersensory temporal synchrony between the heteromodal components. What is key is that this synchrony does not have to be of a one-to-one nature but can be of a higher-order nature as well.

The second finding of interest from the experimental findings in Table 41.1 is that infants responded to the auditory and/or visual changes in a number of cases. For example, Figure 41.4 shows that when 10-month-old infants were habituated to a concordant compound stimulus, they responded not only to the bisensory change but also to the two unisensory ones. The finding that in some cases infants also responded to the unisensory changes suggests that redundant specification, even when it is in terms of a higher-order intersensory synchrony relation, can support the learning and differentiation of unisensory information and its relation to information in the other modality.

The static compound stimulus experiments suggested that the visual temporal information was less

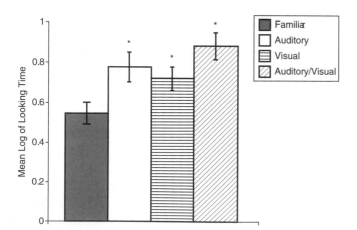

FIGURE 41.4   Mean log of looking duration at auditory, visual, and bisensory component changes in a flashing/beeping checkerboard. Asterisks indicate significant response recovery, and error bars indicate ± SEM.

discriminable than the auditory information. This observation raised the possibility that successful responsiveness to the auditory changes was due to the fact that auditory stimulation was more appropriate to the specialization of the auditory modality than was the visual stimulation to the specialization of the visual modality. Such an interpretation is consistent with a *modality appropriateness* hypothesis put forth by Welch and Warren (1986), which holds that audition is specialized for the processing of temporal information, whereas vision is specialized for the processing of motion. If that is the case, then it might not be surprising that the visual information was less discriminable and suggests that introducing motion in the visual modality might make the temporal information in vision more discriminable. This is likely given that motion is a powerful visual attribute and that infants are highly responsive to it from an early age (Kaufmann, Stucki, & Kaufmann-Hayoz, 1985; Volkmann & Dobson, 1976).

To test the possibility that visual motion might enable infants to respond to the visual information as well, Lewkowicz (1992c) habituated 2-, 4-, 6-, and 8-month-old infants to a bouncing object (a small disk) that could be seen moving up and down. A tone was sounded each time the object reversed its motion trajectory when it reached bottom. Following habituation, infants' perception of the unisensory and bisensory temporal attributes of this bouncing object were tested by changing the rate of visual and/or audible bouncing. Two such experiments were conducted, with the second one being essentially a replication of the first (the only difference was that two additional habituation trials were presented in Experiment 2 to test for spontaneous regression to the mean effects during habituation). Table 41.1 shows the results from both of these experiments and Figure 41.5 shows the mean amount of looking during the different test conditions in Experiment 1. As can be seen, the pattern of results is similar to that depicted in Figure 41.4. Infants responded not only to the bisensory change but also to both unisensory changes (Table 41.1 shows that this finding was replicated in Experiment 2). Together, the results from the static and dynamic compound experiments show that infants discriminated bisensory changes most easily, even after first learning a compound stimulus that was specified by discordant auditory and visual components, and often found the unisensory changes as easy to perceive as the bisensory ones. As before, these findings suggest that bisensory specification can facilitate perceptual learning and differentiation not only of bisensory information but of unisensory information and its relation to information in the other modality as well.

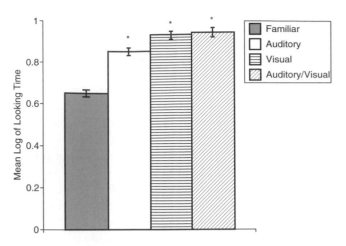

FIGURE 41.5   Mean log of looking duration at auditory, visual, and bisensory component changes of a bouncing/sounding disk. Asterisks indicate significant response recovery, and error bars indicate ± SEM.

RESPONSE TO AUDIOVISUAL SPEECH AND SINGING   It might be argued that the findings from the studies listed in Table 41.1 are not representative of infants' true perceptual skills because the stimulus materials used in these studies were artificial and impoverished from the point of view of infants' actual ecological experience (Lewkowicz, 2001). To determine whether this might be the case, a series of studies was conducted in which infants' response to ecologically meaningful events such as audiovisual speech and singing was studied.

In the first of this series of studies (Lewkowicz, 1996a), 4-, 6-, and 8-month-old infants were habituated to an audiovisual recording of a person speaking a continuous utterance in an adult-directed (AD) manner. The actor producing the utterance could be seen and heard speaking at a regular pace with minimal voice intonation variations and minimal head movements. Given the findings from Experiments 1 and 2 from Lewkowicz (1992c) showing that motion cues facilitate responsiveness to the visual attribute of an AV compound stimulus, it was expected that infants would find the visual changes easier to discriminate than the auditory ones, and/or that the detection of visual attribute changes might be found earlier in development. Table 41.2 shows the results of all of these studies. The overall pattern of findings is consistent with predictions. Except for the 4-month-olds in the first experiment, infants exhibited consistent detection of bisensory changes across all experiments and across all ages. In addition, infants exhibited responsiveness to visual changes more often than to auditory ones.

Figure 41.6 illustrates the findings from the first of these experiments (the AD→AD Experiment). In this case, infants were habituated to a person speaking a continuous script in the AD manner and then were tested for discrimination by hearing, seeing, or both hearing and seeing a different person speaking a different script. As can be seen, 4-month-old infants did not respond to any of the changes, whereas 6- and 8-month-old infants responded to the visual and bisensory changes. What is particularly interesting about these findings is that the 4-month-old infants did not even respond to the bisensory change, even though on this test trial they saw and heard a different person uttering a different script. In other words, they failed to detect the difference despite having access to two different, bisensory and amodally invariant events.

The subsequent experiments in this series were designed to further explore the role of various discriminative cues in infants' response to audiovisual speech. Thus, in the next two experiments gender and/or manner-of-speech differences were added to determine whether these cues might aid in discrimination. Specifically, in the second experiment (the AD→AD & Gender Experiment in Table 41.2), the actor seen and/or heard speaking during the test trials was of a different sex, whereas in the third experiment (the AD→ID & Gender Experiment in Table 41.2) this actor was not only of a different sex but also spoke in an infant-directed (ID) manner. This meant that the actor spoke in a prosodically exaggerated manner. As can be seen in Table 41.2, when gender alone was added, the 4-month-old infants also discriminated the visible and bisensory changes, but none of the age groups discriminated the audible changes. When ID speech was added as a discriminative cue, the 6- and 8-month-old infants responded to the audible changes as well, although the 4-month-olds still did not. When the results from the first three experiments are considered together, they show once again that the bisensory changes were the easiest to detect. In addition, these findings are consistent with the findings from the prior studies (Lewkowicz, 1992c) in showing that as long as objects moved, infants responded to the visual changes (the only exception were the 4-month-old infants in the first experiment).

Finally, because infants are highly responsive to exaggerated prosody (Fernald & Simon, 1984), two additional experiments were conducted in which discrimination of AD speech from singing was investigated (Lewkowicz, 1998). In one experiment the actor was of the same sex across habituation and test trials, whereas in the other experiment the actors were of different sexes. The additional prosody features were expected to make it possible for the infants to detect some of the unisensory and/or bisensory differences earlier in development. To test this possibility, a group of 3-month-old infants was added to

TABLE 41.2

Results from Lewkowicz's studies of infants' responses to bisensory continuous utterances, singing, and bisensory syllables

Continuous Utterance/Singing Studies (Lewkowicz, 1996a, 1998)				Syllable Studies (Lewkowicz, 2000b)			
Type of Change:	A	V	AV	Type of Change:	A	V	AV
AD→AD				*AD→AD*			
4 month	−	−	−	4 month	√	−	√
6 month	−	√	√	6 month	√	−	√
8 month	−	√	√	8 month	√	√	√
AD→AD & Gender				*AD→ID*			
4 month	−	√	√	4 month	√	√	√
6 month	−	√	√	6 month	√	√	√
8 month	−	√	√	8 month	√	√	√
AD→ID & Gender							
4 month	−	√	√				
6 month	√	√	√				
8 month	√	√	√				
AD→Song							
3 month	−	√	√				
4 month	√	√	√				
6 month	√	√	√				
8 month	√	√	√				
AD→Song & Gender							
3 month	√	√	√				
4 month	√	√	√				
6 month	√	√	√				
8 month	√	√	√				

Symbols: √ means positive result and − means negative result.

this study. Table 41.2 shows the results from these two experiments (the AD→Song and the AD→Song & Gender experiments). Except for the 3-month-old infants not

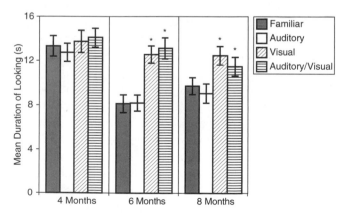

FIGURE 41.6 Mean duration of looking at auditory, visual, and bisensory component changes in 4-, 6-, and 8-month-old infants habituated to a female speaker uttering a script in an adult-directed (AD) manner and tested with components of a different female speaker also speaking in the AD manner. Asterisks indicate significant response recovery, and error bars indicate ± SEM.

responding to the audible change, infants between 3 and 8 months of age responded to all three types of changes. Thus, as expected, the differences in these experiments appeared to be easier to discriminate than in the three earlier experiments, and the ability to make these discriminations emerged earlier in development. Of greatest interest was the finding that unlike the earlier compound stimulus studies, which presented beeping checkerboards or bouncing objects, in these experiments infants responded to unisensory differences as easily as to the bisensory ones. This difference most likely reflects differences in the salience of the information, which in turn is probably due in part to differential experience effects with these types of stimuli.

The overall findings from the audiovisual speech/ singing studies suggest that the specific nature of the information making up a multisensory compound stimulus might play an important role in the overall pattern of responsiveness to the three types of test trials. In particular, ongoing speech is characterized by a variety of suprasegmental features, and so it is possible that these kinds of features might have contributed to the specific pattern of responsiveness. To determine if this was the case, infants' responsiveness to simpler audiovisual speech, consisting of isolated syllables, was investigated in the latest set of experiments (Lewkowicz, 2000b). Infants were habituated to a repeatedly presented syllable (either a /ba/ or a /sha/) and then tested to determine what aspects of the audible and/or visible attributes of the syllable they perceived. In this case the person the infants saw and heard was the same in the habituation and test phases. Results from two of these experiments are given in the Syllable Studies column of Table 41.2. As in all the previous studies, infants of all ages responded to the bisensory change in both experiments. It is particularly interesting to note, however, that infants in the first of the syllable experiments responded in a manner opposite that in the continuous speech studies. That is, infants at all three ages responded to the audible changes, but the 4- and 6-month-old infants did not respond to the visible changes. To test the possibility that it might have been difficult for infants to discriminate the syllables on the basis of lip movement alone, the difference between the habituation and test trial stimuli was increased in the second of these experiments by having the actor utter the test syllable in the ID manner. This meant that the syllable was uttered in a slower and more exaggerated manner. As can be seen in Table 41.2, this additional kinetic information enabled infants of all ages to now discriminate the visual change. Overall, and as before, the results from these two experiments showed that although infants responded most consistently to the bisensory changes, they also largely responded to the unisensory changes.

SUMMARY OF FINDINGS ON INFANTS' RESPONSE TO MULTISENSORY COMPOUNDS When the results from Lewkowicz's studies of infants' responsiveness to AV compounds are considered together, they yield the following findings of interest. First, infants exhibited the most reliable response to the bisensory changes. Second, responsiveness to the unisensory components of bisensory compounds appeared to depend on the nature of the information available. When presented with an AV compound composed of a flashing checkerboard and a beeping sound, infants responded more often to the audible than to the visible information. In contrast, when presented with a talking or singing face, infants responded more often to the visible than to the audible information. In addition, when infants were presented with a simple bouncing/sounding object, they responded to all three types of changes. Finally, and most important from the present standpoint, in many cases infants responded to unisensory changes as well as to the bisensory ones.

Interpretation of the findings from the compound stimulus studies hinges in part on the fact that the unisensory change trials involved not only changes in some attribute in that modality but also a concurrent change in the intersensory relation between the auditory and visual components of that compound as well. This makes it possible that the response in the unisensory change trials might have been due to a combination of the change in that particular modality as well as to a change in the intersensory relations inherent to that particular compound. It should be noted, however, that if infants were responding to the disruption of the intersensory relations in all the unisensory test trials, they should have exhibited a significant discriminative response on all these trials across all the experiments. The fact that they did not suggests that, at least in those experiments where they exhibited a discriminative response, they were responding only to the unisensory change. This conclusion is further supported by independent studies that addressed the question of intersensory matching directly. Specifically, in these studies, utilizing the identical stimulus materials as were used in the compound stimulus studies, Lewkowicz failed to find rate-based intersensory matching, both in studies presenting flashing checkerboards and beeping sounds (Lewkowicz, 1985) and moving objects and their synchronous and matching impact sounds (Lewkowicz, 1992b). Infants' failure to make intersensory matches in these two studies shows that it is unlikely that the overall response pattern in the unisensory change trials observed in Table 41.1 reflects infants' response to the disruption of intersensory relations. The more likely interpretation is that infants were treating the information in the two modalities as two separate streams of a compound stimulus, regardless of whether the components were synchronized in terms of a one-to-one or a higher-order temporal relation.

PERCEPTION OF INTERSENSORY EQUIVALENCE IN MULTISENSORY COMPOUNDS Infants' ability to perceive intersensory equivalence relations is important to the intersensory redundancy hypothesis because the advantage of multisensory redundancy derives in part from the fact that redundant multisensory inputs specify equivalent properties across different sensory modalities and thus facilitate unified perceptual experiences (Bahrick & Lickliter, 2000). By specifying a single, unitary perceptual experience, bisensory information is presumed to direct and constrain attention to bisensory information and thus make infants (particularly young ones who are learning to differentiate their world) attend selectively to amodal properties. We concluded earlier that the data from the compound stimulus experiments do not support the conclusion that amodal invariance per se is necessary for a redundancy advantage. In fact, the results from the compound stimulus studies also provide important clues regarding infants' response to amodal invariance.

If infants perceived and encoded the relation between the auditory and visual components of the compound stimulus during the habituation phase, then they should have responded to a disruption of that relation regardless of whether it was achieved by changing the auditory or the visual information. Therefore, instances in which infants failed to respond to both types of unisensory changes would provide the strongest evidence that they did not perceive the intersensory relation. Examination of Tables 41.1 and 41.2 reveals that there were a number of instances in which infants did not exhibit response recovery to both types of unisensory changes. The strictest criterion that can be used to examine this question is to consider only those experiments in which infants were habituated to a concordant AV compound stimulus. Considering just these experiments, results showed that there were cases in which infants failed to respond to an auditory and/or visual change in Experiments 1, 3, and 7 in Lewkowicz (1988a), in Experiment 1 in Lewkowicz (1988b), in all three experiments in Lewkowicz (1996a), in one experiment in Lewkowicz (1998), and in one of the two experiments in Lewkowicz (2000b). When these findings are considered together with the previously cited failures to obtain perception of intersensory equivalence, they suggest that the strong form of the Gibsonian view that infants are selectively tuned to amodal invariants may not be accurate.

The evidence that infants responded most easily to bisensory changes even after they were habituated to compounds that were composed of discordant auditory and visual components suggests that multisensory redundancy may provide its greatest benefit via the temporal synchrony route rather than the amodal invariance route. We recall here that even the discordant compounds were related in terms of higher-order synchrony relations. It should be emphasized, however, that concluding that intersensory temporal synchrony drives perception does not mean that responsiveness to amodal invariance does not play a role in perceptual learning and differentiation. It does, but in a theoretically unexpected way that runs counter to the Gibsonian amodal detection view. Specifically, in his model of the development of intersensory perception, Lewkowicz (2000a) suggested that intersensory temporal synchrony provides the initial basis for the perception of intersensory temporal relations. What our review of the extant data suggests, however, is that amodal invariants may play a role in intersensory integration not envisioned by Lewkowicz's (2000a) model.

The extant data suggest that amodal invariants do not drive perception early in development but rather that they provide support to the perception of intersensory temporal synchrony relations. This is best illustrated by considering the case of a bisensory compound stimulus whose auditory and visual streams are equivalent in terms of duration, tempo, or rhythm (e.g., a tapping hammer or a person uttering a nursery rhyme). The heteromodal elements making up the separate sensory streams of such events are, under normal conditions, in perfect synchrony. Thus, in the case of the talking person, the visible and audible attributes of each word making up the rhyme have synchronous onsets and offsets. As a result, the common rhythm across the two modalities actually helps to highlight the intersensory temporal synchrony relations by making them pop out perceptually. In this way, the overall event becomes more salient. There are two critical points that follow from this view. First, it is already clear that infants can perceive bisensory temporal patterns (Lewkowicz, in press) as well as unisensory ones (Lewkowicz, 1988a); this is really not the issue here. The real issue is whether infants are able to detect the specific temporal pattern as an independent perceptual feature regardless of modality (i.e., a true amodal invariant). If it can be shown that they can, then it can be argued that amodal invariants may provide a redundancy benefit. To date, however, the evidence is not clear on this possibility, and convincing proof will require a demonstration that infants can perceive intersensory equivalence of various amodal invariants *in the absence of intersensory temporal synchrony*. In the absence of such proof, the most parsimonious explanation of redundancy effects to date is that they are mediated by intersensory temporal synchrony relations.

Interestingly enough, the new interpretation can account for the developmentally later emergence of modality-specific associations. As noted earlier, infants do not make shape or color and pitch associations until the latter part of the first year of life (Bahrick, 1992, 1994). According to the interpretation offered here, it is not that the ability to perceive amodal invariants emerges earlier in development than the ability to perceive modality-specific associations. Rather, it is that the ability to perceive the temporal co-occurrence of the heteromodal components specifying bisensory events emerges before the ability to make arbitrary types of associations because the latter do not pop out in the same way that amodally related events do.

It should be emphasized that even though this developmental scenario may primarily reflect the perception of temporal intersensory relations in development, it may apply equally well to spatial intersensory relations (Lewkowicz, 1999). In addition, it should be noted that the developmental scenario may turn out to be even more complicated when the concurrent influence of modality-specific attributes is considered. The findings from the "hat" study showed that sometimes, even if a clearly detectable amodal invariant is available, infants may not attend to the invariant in the presence of a highly salient modality-specific attribute.

Responsiveness to multisensory compounds in other species

The results of the compound stimulus studies reviewed in the previous section showed that infants often responded to unisensory changes as easily as to the bisensory ones, suggesting that they might have perceived the differences on the basis of unisensory information. It should be emphasized, however, that the initial learning in Lewkowicz's studies was based on bisensory information, making it impossible to determine directly whether learning based on bisensory information is more effective than learning based on unisensory information. Bahrick and Lickliter (2000) did make that comparison directly and found that bisensory learning is more effective. Studies with animal infants have provided additional data with respect to these issues. In addition, they provide data on whether two different unisensory attributes can provide facilitation similar to that produced by a bisensory compound stimulus. In general, these studies have shown that sometimes multisensory signals may elicit greater responsiveness than unisensory signals, but sometimes they may not.

Kraebel and Spear (2000) found greater cardiac orienting to a compound stimulus composed of a moderate-intensity light and a moderate-intensity tone than to either the moderate-intensity light presented alone or the moderate-intensity tone presented alone. This same pattern of results was observed for low-intensity auditory and visual stimuli, suggesting that the enhanced orienting to the compound stimuli was due to responsiveness to the net intensity of the compound's elements. In some cases, however, combining single-element stimuli into a compound stimulus did not always produce greater orienting. For example, cardiac orienting to a compound stimulus composed of a moderate-intensity tone and a low-intensity light was not significantly greater than orienting to the moderate-intensity tone presented alone. The absence of greater orienting to the compound stimulus in this case was not due to an intermixing, and possible overshadowing, of intensity values, because greater orienting was observed to a compound composed of a moderate-intensity light and a low-intensity tone than to the moderate-intensity light presented alone.

Kraebel and Spear (2000) suggested that the differential effects of the compound stimuli used in their study were related to the developmental status of the infant's sensory systems. In rats, the auditory system becomes functional several days before the visual system does. As a result, by day 17—the age at which the animals were tested by Kraebel and Spear (2000)—an infant rat is more proficient at processing tones than lights. It is possible that overshadowing of a low-intensity stimulus may occur in a situation in which the compound is composed of mixed intensity levels (one moderate, one low) and in which the modality of the higher-intensity stimulus is dominant because of greater experience with that sensory modality. In this instance, at postnatal day 17, audition may be dominant over vision, given the earlier onset of auditory functioning.

The earlier development of audition may also partly account for the findings reported by Reynolds and Lickliter (2002) in a study of bobwhite quail embryos' response to multisensory (auditory/visual), intrasensory compound (two different auditory stimuli), and unisensory stimulation. The multisensory compound stimulus elicited greater behavioral arousal and cardiac responsiveness (acceleration) than did a unisensory stimulus, and the intramodal compound stimulus elicited greater cardiac responsiveness (but deceleration). Generally, deceleration is taken to be an index of the orienting response, whereas acceleration is taken to be an index of the defensive reflex. The former is considered to be the more mature form of the cardiac response because it is associated with information processing. These embryos already had fairly extensive auditory experience listening to their own and broodmates' vocalizations, and thus the two maternal bobwhite calls that made up the intramodal compound most likely had acoustic elements that were "interesting" to the birds. In contrast, the flashing strobe light that was the visual component of the bisensory compound might have been aversive to the less mature visual system.

Do multisensory signals confer a learning advantage?

The studies that provide the best evidence of facilitated learning with multisensory stimuli in infant rats are those that investigated a phenomenon known as *potentiation*. In these studies, Spear and his colleagues examined ontogenetic differences in learning and memory of multisensory versus unisensory stimuli in albino rats using associative learning procedures. The general design of these studies involved conditioning one group of animals to associate a neutral stimulus (A) with an unpleasant event, such as a foot shock, and conditioning another group to associate a compound stimulus (AB) with a foot shock. Both groups were then tested for fear to stimulus A presented alone. The compound stimulus was composed either of stimuli from two different sensory modalities or from the same modality. The question of interest was whether and how the addition of stimulus B influenced or "potentiated" learning of stimulus A. From the current perspective, the question of particular interest was whether stimulus B facilitated learning of stimulus A. In terms of the distinctions drawn earlier, this type of conditioning would represent a form of intersensory conjunction.

Mellon, Kraemer, and Spear (1991) demonstrated potentiation using auditory and visual stimuli. The AB compound stimulus consisted of a light and a tone, and the results showed that young rats exhibited greater behavioral suppression to a light if that light had previously been paired with a tone than if it had been presented alone. Likewise, Hinderliter and Misanin (1988) demonstrated potentiation in adolescent rats using a saccharin solution and maple odor. Potentiation can also be obtained when one of the elements of the compound stimulus is a nonpunctate stimulus. For example, Miller, Scherer, and Jagielo (1995) conditioned preweanling rats to an odor presented in a black chamber or to the black chamber alone and found that preweanlings showed greater behavioral suppression (freezing) in the black chamber if that black chamber had been previously paired with the odor. Together, these results show that redundant, multisensory signals that are not in any way amodally invariant do facilitate learning in infant rats.

Interestingly enough, and key from an intersensory redundancy point of view, potentiation can also be obtained with multiple cues from the same modality. For example, potentiation in young rats has been found when the compound stimulus consisted of solutions of sucrose and coffee (Kucharski & Spear, 1985), salt and saccharin, or sucrose and lemon (Spear & Kucharski, 1984a, 1984b). Potentiation also was found in infant rats when olfactory stimuli (lemon and orange odors) served as the elements of the compound stimulus (Spear & Kucharski, 1984a). Thus, concurrent presentation of two distinct cues enhances learning, and it does so regardless of whether the source of stimulation is the same

modality or in two different modalities. In other words, at least in the case of associative learning in infant rats, any form of redundancy is advantageous, and no special advantage accrues to multisensory redundancy.

As noted earlier, one of the solutions to the problem of "multisensory confusion" in early development is that the temporal synchrony of heteromodal inputs can serve as one initial basis for "clarifying" the intersensory relations and thus aiding in integration (Lewkowicz, 2000a). Lickliter, Bahrick, and Honeycutt (2002) have provided an example of this by showing that bobwhite embryos exposed to a pulsed maternal call and a synchronously flashing light preferred the familiar call in postnatal testing after less overall prenatal exposure than animals receiving nonsynchronous or unisensory prenatal stimulation. Studies of associative learning in infant rats have found similar results. For example, Kucharski and Spear (1985) gave infant rats oral infusions of a sucrose and coffee solution either concurrently or separated by three minutes, and then an injection of lithium chloride. Results showed that infants given the sucrose and coffee simultaneously ingested less sucrose at test than infants who were given sucrose and coffee sequentially. This enhancement of learning with simultaneous conditional stimulus (CS) presentation in comparison to sequential CS presentation has been observed using other associative procedures (sensory preconditioning, latent inhibition, and second-order conditioning) and has occurred when the conditional stimuli were either from the same modality (i.e., two odors) or from different modalities (i.e., a light and a tone; see Spear & McKinzle, 1994, for a review).

It appears that even though temporal synchrony is sufficient for learning conjunctions, it may not be essential, at least in the case of certain types of conditioning effects. In studies of what Spear and McKinzie (1994) and Spear, Kraemer, Molina, and Smoller (1988) have dubbed acquired equivalence, infant rats were given exposure to stimulus A paired with a neutral event C, then given exposure to stimulus B also paired with neutral event C, and then finally the value of stimulus A was modified by pairing it with an aversive unconditional stimulus (US). Results showed that when responsiveness to stimulus B was tested, infants responded to it as aversive, even though it had not been directly paired with the US. For infants, pairing a common event (C) with both A and B caused them to functionally respond to A and B equivalently. Thus, acquired equivalence studies demonstrate that temporal synchrony may be sufficient but not necessary for the acquisition of similarity between stimuli from separate modalities in infant rats. In addition, as with the potentiation studies, the elements can be from two different modalities or from the same modality.

Studies examining the role of context on conditioning also have shown that an enhanced context (i.e., a strong odor or a flashing light) aids in the acquisition of a response. For example, McKinzie and Spear (1995) and Brasser and Spear (1998) have examined trace learning in infant rats. In trace learning a short delay is introduced between the CS and US and the usual finding, and one consistent with the importance of temporal contiguity, is that learning is rather weak. McKinzie and Spear (1995) and Brasser and Spear (1998) showed that the strength of learning could be improved in this case by introducing extra sensory information (a strong odor and/or a flashing light) throughout the training and test sessions (in this case, the extra sensory information is presented both simultaneously and sequentially with regard to the CS). In addition, infant rats exhibit greater responsiveness to neutral stimuli and to aversive events (US) in enhanced contexts. For example, cardiac orienting to an auditory stimulus is greater in an enhanced context than in a plain context (Kraebel, Vizvary, Heron, & Spear, 1998), and infants exhibit greater ultrasonic vocalizations to foot shock in an enhanced context than in a plain context (Brasser & Spear, 1998). Because all of these studies used heteromodal stimuli (i.e., odor-tone, light-tone) it is not possible to assess the differential role of heteromodal versus homomodal stimulation. What is interesting about them, however, is that they suggest that these types of effects are mediated by generalized arousal that is induced by the contextual cues, and that this in turn makes the CS and US more salient to the animal.

In sum, associative learning in neonatal rats is facilitated when a stimulus is presented in combination with other sensory stimuli either as a discrete stimulus or as diffuse contextual stimulation. This learning is facilitated regardless of whether the "extra" stimulation is in the same or different modality. Finally, synchrony appears to facilitate learning, although it does not appear to be essential.

The uniqueness of infantile intersensory integration

One of the most fascinating findings that has emerged from the animal infant learning studies comes from studies of subthreshold conditioning (Molina, Hoffmann, Serwatka, & Spear, 1991; Spear et al., 1988). In this type of study, infant rats are first conditioned to an odor paired with foot shock, such that the odor produces an aversive response (phase 1). Then they are given subthreshold conditioning: a black chamber is paired with a foot shock, but the number of pairings given is not sufficient to produce conditioning (phase 2). One set of control subjects receives the odor and foot shock unpaired, and another set receives the black chamber and foot shock unpaired. All animals are then tested in a chamber of which one half was painted black and the other half painted white. Only those animals that received the foot shock paired with both the odor (phase 1) and the black chamber (phase 2) showed a strong aversion to the black side. These results suggest that the infant rats generalized between an olfactory CS and a visual CS when they had been paired with a common US. Further studies showed that when the association between the olfactory stimulus and foot shock was weakened via a standard extinction process, a concomitant decrease in aversion to the black side was found. In addition, other studies showed that the transfer of learning that was observed in the subthreshold conditioning procedure is critically dependent on the two CS's being associated with a common US. Of greatest interest from a developmental standpoint, however, is the finding that adult animals do not exhibit such subthreshold effects. In other words, the propensity to generalize across sensory modalities and to conjoin multisensory cues appears to be a uniquely infantile form of responsiveness.

Concluding remarks

We asked whether multisensory redundancy facilitates perception, attention, and learning in early development, and in general we have found that it does, but with some important caveats. We showed that the available findings from studies on human infants and birds suggest that multisensory redundancy is generally advantageous, but that findings from studies on infant rats show that multiple, unisensory signals can be advantageous as well. It is not possible at this time to determine whether multiple unisensory inputs might also facilitate perception in human infants because studies comparing infants' responsiveness to multiple unisensory inputs versus responsiveness to multisensory inputs have not been done.

We concluded that multisensory facilitation in human infants is based primarily on intersensory temporal synchrony relations rather than on amodal invariant relations (at this point, it could be argued that the same is true in birds). The same does not, however, appear to be the case for infant rats, because they exhibit facilitation effects even in the absence of intersensory temporal synchrony. At this point it is not clear whether the effects found in infant rats are confined to conditioning procedures or whether they reflect true differences in intersensory organization. One way to tell would be to conduct comparable conditioning studies in human infants, but this is a difficult task, given that such conditioning procedures involve extended testing that is very difficult to do in human infants. In lieu of that we can offer some speculations.

The apparently greater role for intersensory temporal synchrony in human infants may reflect a cross-species difference in developmental maturity. Even at birth, vision and audition in humans are more structurally and functionally advanced than they are in a newborn rat. This developmental difference is more exaggerated by the fact that most of the redundancy effects observed in human infants come from studies of infants 3 months of age and older. This means that human infants' performance reflects months of sensory-perceptual experience, further ensuring more sophisticated forms of responsiveness. In contrast, preweanlings rats' responsiveness is likely to consist primarily of changes in their state of arousal in response to overall amounts of stimulation (Lewkowicz, 1991; Turkewitz, Lewkowicz, & Gardner, 1983). These speculations provide a fertile new ground for future investigations of multisensory redundancy effects in early development. They also caution us to respect species differences, developmental differences, and general characteristics and principles of development when exploring such effects in future studies.

REFERENCES

Adolph, K. E. (2000). Specificity of learning: Why infants fall over a veritable cliff. *Psychological Science, 11*, 290–295.

Anisfeld, M., Turkewitz, G., Rose, S. A., Rosenberg, F. R., Shelber, F. J., Couturier Fagan, D. A., et al. (2001). No compelling evidence that newborns imitate oral gestures. *Infancy, 2*, 111–122.

Bahrick, L. E. (1988). Intermodal learning in infancy: Learning on the basis of two kinds of invariant relations in audible and visible events. *Child Development, 59*, 197–209.

Bahrick, L. E. (1992). Infants' perceptual differentiation of amodal and modality-specific audio-visual relations. *Journal of Experimental Child Psychology, 53*, 180–199.

Bahrick, L. E. (1994). The development of infants' sensitivity to arbitrary intermodal relations. *Ecological Psychology, 2*, 111–123.

Bahrick, L. E., & Lickliter, R. (2000). Intersensory redundancy guides attentional selectivity and perceptual learning in infancy. *Developmental Psychology, 36*, 190–201.

Bahrick, L. E., & Pickens, J. (1994). Amodal relations: The basis for intermodal perception and learning in infancy. In D. J. Lewkowicz & R. Lickliter (Eds.), *Development of intersensory perception: Comparative perspectives* (pp. 205–233). Hillsdale, NJ: Erlbaum.

Bahrick, L. E., & Watson, J. S. (1985). Detection of intermodal proprioceptive-visual contingency as a potential basis of self-perception in infancy. *Developmental Psychology, 21*, 963–973.

Bertelson, P. (1999). A case of crossmodal perceptual grouping. In G. Aschersleben, T. Bachman, & J. Musseler (Eds.),

Cognitive contributions to the perception of spatial and temporal events. Amsterdam: Elsevier.

Birch, H. G., & Lefford, A. (1963). *Intersensory development in children. Monographs of the Society for Research in Child Development,* 25.

Birch, H. G., & Lefford, A. (1967). *Visual differentiation, intersensory integration, and voluntary motor control. Monographs of the Society for Research in Child Development, 32*, 1–87.

Bower, T. G. R. (1974). *Development in infancy.* San Francisco: Freeman.

Brasser, S. M., & Spear, N. E. (1998). A sensory-enhanced context facilitates learning and multiple measures of unconditioned stimulus processing in the preweanling rat. *Behavioral Neuroscience, 112*, 126–140.

Brookes, H., Slater, A., Quinn, P. C., Lewkowicz, D. J., Hayes, R., & Brown, E. (2001). Three-month-old infants learn arbitrary auditory-visual pairings between voices and faces. *Infant and Child Development, 10*, 75–82.

Bushnell, E. W. (1994). A dual-processing approach to cross-modal matching: Implications for development. In D. J. Lewkowicz & R. Lickliter (Eds.), *The development of intersensory perception: Comparative perspectives* (pp. 19–38). Hillsdale, NJ: Erlbaum.

Damasio, A. R. (1989). Time-locked multiregional retroactivation: A systems-level proposal for the neural substrates of recall and recognition. *Cognition, 33*, 25–62.

Edelman, G. M. (1992). *Bright air, brilliant fire.* New York: Basic Books.

Edelman, G. M., & Tononi, G. (2000). *A universe of consciousness: How matter becomes imagination.* New York: Basic Books.

Ettlinger, G., & Wilson, W. A. (1990). Cross-modal performance: Behavioural processes, phylogenetic considerations and neural mechanisms. *Behavioural Brain Research, 40*, 169–192.

Fernald, A., & Simon, T. (1984). Expanded intonation contours in mothers' speech to newborns. *Developmental Psychology, 20*, 104–113.

Frost, D. O. (1990). Sensory processing by novel, experimentally induced cross-modal circuits. In A. Diamond (Ed.), *The development and neural bases of higher cognitive functions* (Vol. 608, pp. 92–112). New York: New York Academy of Sciences.

Gibson, E. J. (1969). *Principles of perceptual learning and development.* New York: Appleton.

Gibson, J. J. (1966). *The senses considered as perceptual systems.* Boston: Houghton-Mifflin.

Gibson, J. J. (1979). *An ecological approach to perception.* Boston: Houghton-Mifflin.

Gottlieb, G. (1971). Ontogenesis of sensory function in birds and mammals. In E. Tobach, L. R. Aronson, & E. Shaw (Eds.), *The biopsychology of development* (pp. 67–128). New York: Academic Press.

Gottlieb, G. (1991). Experiential canalization of behavioral development: Theory. *Developmental Psychology, 27*, 35–39.

Gottlieb, G. (1997). *Synthesizing nature-nurture: Prenatal roots of instinctive behavior.* Mahwah, NJ: Erlbaum.

Hainline, L. (1998). How the visual system develops: Normal and abnormal development. In A. Slater (Ed.), *Perceptual development: Visual, auditory, and speech perception in infancy* (pp. 5–50). Hove, England: Psychology Press.

Hernandez-Reif, M., & Bahrick, L. E. (2001). The development of visual-tactual perception of objects: Amodal relations provide the basis for learning arbitrary relations. *Infancy, 2,* 51–72.

Hinderliter, C. F., & Misanin, J. R. (1988). Weanling and senescent rats process simultaneously presented odor and taste differently than young adults. *Behavioral and Neural Biology, 49,* 112–117.

Humphrey, K., & Tees, R. C. (1980). Auditory-visual coordination in infancy: Some limitations of the preference methodology. *Bulletin of the Psychonomic Society, 16,* 213–216.

Innocenti, G. M., & Clarke, S. (1984). Bilateral transitory projection to visual areas from auditory cortex in kittens. *Developmental Brain Research, 14,* 143–148.

Jusczyk, P. W., Houston, D., & Goodman, M. (1998). Speech perception during the first year. In A. Slater (Ed.), *Perceptual development: Visual, auditory, and speech perception in infancy* (pp. 357–388). Hove, England: Psychology Press.

Kaufmann, F., Stucki, M., & Kaufmann-Hayoz, R. (1985). Development of infants' sensitivity for slow and rapid motions. *Infant Behavior and Development, 8,* 89–98.

Kellman, P. J., & Arterberry, M. E. (1998). *The cradle of knowledge: Development of perception in infancy.* Cambridge, MA: MIT Press.

King, A. J., & Carlile, S. (1993). Changes induced in the representation of auditory space in the superior colliculus by rearing ferrets with binocular eyelid suture. *Experimental Brain Research, 94,* 444–455.

Knudsen, E. I. (1985). Experience alters the spatial tuning of auditory units in the optic tectum during a sensitive period in the barn owl. *Journal of Neuroscience, 5,* 3094–3109.

Knudsen, E. I., & Knudsen, P. F. (1985). Vision guides the adjustment of auditory localization in young barn owls. *Science, 230,* 545–548.

Kraebel, K. S., & Spear, N. E. (2000). Infant rats are more likely than adolescents to orient differentially to amodal (intensity-based) features of single-element and compound stimuli. *Developmental Psychobiology, 36,* 49–66.

Kraebel, K. S., Vizvary, L. M., Heron, J. S., & Spear, N. E. (1998). Effect of context salience on heart rate orienting and habituation in preweanling and periadolescent rats. *Behavioral Neuroscience, 112,* 1080–1091.

Kraebel, K. S., Vizvary, L. M., & Spear, N. E. (1998). Stimulus intensity modulates associative and nonassociative responding in preweanling rats. *Developmental Psychobiology, 32,* 199–214.

Kucharski, D., & Spear, N. E. (1985). Potentiation and overshadowing in preweanling and adult rats. *Journal of Experimental Psychology: Animal Behavior Processes, 11,* 15–34.

Kuhl, P. K., & Meltzoff, A. N. (1982). The bimodal perception of speech in infancy. *Science, 218,* 1138–1141.

Kujala, T., Alho, K., & Näätänen, R. (2000). Cross-modal reorganization of human cortical functions. *Trends in Neurosciences, 23,* 115–120.

Kuo, Z. Y. (1976). *The dynamics of behavior development: An epigenetic view.* New York: Plenum Press.

Lewkowicz, D. J. (1985). Bisensory response to temporal frequency in 4-month-old infants. *Developmental Psychology, 21,* 306–317.

Lewkowicz, D. J. (1986). Developmental changes in infants' bisensory response to synchronous durations. *Infant Behavior and Development, 9,* 335–353.

Lewkowicz, D. J. (1988a). Sensory dominance in infants: I. Six-month-old infants' response to auditory-visual compounds. *Developmental Psychology, 24,* 155–171.

Lewkowicz, D. J. (1988b). Sensory dominance in infants: II. Ten-month-old infants' response to auditory-visual compounds. *Developmental Psychology, 24,* 172–182.

Lewkowicz, D. J. (1991). Development of intersensory functions in human infancy: Auditory/visual interactions. In M. J. S. Weiss & P. R. Zelazo (Eds.), *Newborn attention: Biological constraints and the influence of experience* (pp. 308–338). Norwood, NJ: Ablex.

Lewkowicz, D. J. (1992a). The development of temporally-based intersensory perception in human infants. In F. Macar, V. Pouthas & W. J. Friedman (Eds.), *Time, action and cognition: Towards bridging the gap* (pp. 33–43). Dordrecht, Netherlands: Kluwer Academic.

Lewkowicz, D. J. (1992b). Infants' response to temporally based intersensory equivalence: The effect of synchronous sounds on visual preferences for moving stimuli. *Infant Behavior and Development, 15,* 297–324.

Lewkowicz, D. J. (1992c). Infants' responsiveness to the auditory and visual attributes of a sounding/moving stimulus. *Perception & Psychophysics, 52,* 519–528.

Lewkowicz, D. J. (1994a). Limitations on infants' response to rate-based auditory-visual relations. *Developmental Psychology, 30,* 880–892.

Lewkowicz, D. J. (1994b). Reflections on infants' response to temporally based intersensory equivalence: Response to Spelke (1994). *Infant Behavior and Development, 17,* 289–292.

Lewkowicz, D. J. (1996a). Infants' response to the audible and visible properties of the human face: I. Role of lexical-syntactic content, temporal synchrony, gender, and manner of speech. *Developmental Psychology, 32,* 347–366.

Lewkowicz, D. J. (1996b). Perception of auditory-visual temporal synchrony in human infants. *Journal of Experimental Psychology: Human Perception and Performance, 22,* 1094–1106.

Lewkowicz, D. J. (1998). Infants' response to the audible and visible properties of the human face: II. Discrimination of differences between singing and adult-directed speech. *Developmental Psychobiology, 32,* 261–274.

Lewkowicz, D. J. (1999). The development of temporal and spatial intermodal perception. In G. Aschersleben, T. Bachman, & J. Müsseler (Eds.), *Cognitive contributions to the perception of spatial and temporal events* (pp. 395–420). Amsterdam: Elsevier.

Lewkowicz, D. J. (2000a). The development of intersensory temporal perception: An epigenetic systems/limitations view. *Psychological Bulletin, 126,* 281–308.

Lewkowicz, D. J. (2000b). Infants' perception of the audible, visible and bimodal attributes of multimodal syllables. *Child Development, 71,* 1241–1257.

Lewkowicz, D. J. (2001). The concept of ecological validity: What are its limitations and is it bad to be invalid? *Infancy, 2,* 437–450.

Lewkowicz, D. J. (2003). Learning and discrimination of audiovisual events in human infants: The hierarchical relation between intersensory temporal synchrony and rhythmic pattern cues. *Developmental Psychology, 39,* 795–804.

Lewkowicz, D. J., & Lickliter, R. (1994). *The development of intersensory perception: Comparative perspectives.* Hillsdale, NJ: Erlbaum.

Lewkowicz, D. J., & Schwartz, B. I. (2002). *Intersensory perception in infancy: Response to competing amodal and modality-specific attributes.* Paper presented at the International Conference on Infant Studies, Toronto, Canada.

Lewkowicz, D. J., & Turkewitz, G. (1980). Cross-modal equivalence in early infancy: Auditory-visual intensity matching. *Developmental Psychology, 16,* 597–607.

Lickliter, R., & Bahrick, L. E. (2000). The development of infant intersensory perception: Advantages of a comparative convergent-operations approach. *Psychological Bulletin, 126,* 260–280.

Lickliter, R., Bahrick, L. E., & Honeycutt, H. (2002). Intersensory redundancy facilitates prenatal perceptual learning in bobwhite quail (*Colinus virginianus*) embryos. *Developmental Psychology, 38,* 15–23.

Maier, N. R. F., & Schneirla, T. C. (1964). *Principles of animal psychology.* New York: Dover Publications.

Marks, L. (1978). *The unity of the senses.* New York: Academic Press.

Massaro, D. W. (1998). *Perceiving talking faces: From speech perception to a behavioral principle.* Cambridge, MA: MIT Press.

Maurer, D., Stager, C. L., & Mondloch, C. J. (1999). Cross-modal transfer of shape is difficult to demonstrate in one-month-olds. *Child Development, 70,* 1047–1057.

McGurk, H., & MacDonald, J. (1976). Hearing lips and seeing voices. *Nature, 264,* 229–239.

McKenzie, B. E., & Over, R. (1983). Young infants fail to imitate facial and manual gestures. *Infant Behavior and Development, 6,* 85–95.

McKinzie, D. L., & Spear, N. E. (1995). Ontogenetic differences in conditioning to context and CS as a function of context saliency and CS-US interval. *Animal Learning and Behavior, 23,* 304–313.

Mellon, R. C., Kraemer, P. J., & Spear, N. E. (1991). Development of intersensory function: Age-related differences in stimulus selection of multimodal compounds in rats as revealed by Pavlovian conditioning. *Journal of Experimental Psychology: Animal Behavior Processes, 17,* 448–464.

Meltzoff, A. N., & Borton, R. W. (1979). Intermodal matching by human neonates. *Nature, 282,* 403–404.

Meltzoff, A. N., & Moore, M. K. (1977). Imitation of facial and manual gestures by human neonates. *Science, 198,* 75–78.

Miller, J. S., Scherer, S. L., & Jagielo, J. A. (1995). Enhancement of conditioning by a nongustatory CS: Ontogenetic differences in the mechanisms underlying potentiation. *Learning and Motivation, 26,* 43–62.

Molina, J. C., Hoffmann, H., Serwatka, J., & Spear, N. E. (1991). Establishing intermodal equivalence in preweanling and adult rats. *Journal of Experimental Psychology: Animal Behavior Processes, 17,* 433–447.

Morrongiello, B. A., Fenwick, K. D., & Chance, G. (1998). Crossmodal learning in newborn infants: Inferences about properties of auditory-visual events. *Infant Behavior and Development, 21,* 543–554.

Olsho, L. W. (1984). Infant frequency discrimination. *Infant Behavior and Development, 7,* 27–35.

Oppenheim, R. W. (1981). Ontogenetic adaptations and retrogressive processes in the development of the nervous system and behavior: A neuroembryological perspective. In K. J. Connolly & H. F. R. Prechtl (Eds.), *Maturation and development: Biological and psychological perspectives* (pp. 73–109). Philadelphia: Lippincott.

Partan, S., & Marler, P. (1999). Communication goes multimodal. *Science, 283,* 1272–1273.

Piaget, J. (1952). *The origins of intelligence in children.* New York: International Universities Press.

Piaget, J. (1954). *The construction of reality in the child.* London: Routledge & Kegan.

Reardon, P., & Bushnell, E. W. (1988). Infants' sensitivity to arbitrary pairings of color and taste. *Infant Behavior and Development, 11,* 245–250.

Reynolds, G. D., & Lickliter, R. (2002). Effects of prenatal sensory stimulation on heart rate and behavioral measures of arousal in bobwhite quail embryos. *Developmental Psychobiology, 41,* 112–122.

Rose, S. A. (1994). From hand to eye: Findings and issues in infant cross-modal transfer. In D. J. Lewkowicz & R. Lickliter (Eds.), *The development of intersensory perception: Comparative perspectives* (pp. 265–284). Hillsdale: Erlbaum.

Rose, S. A., & Ruff, H. A. (1987). Cross-modal abilities in human infants. In J. Osofsky (Ed.), *Handbook of infant development* (2nd ed., pp. 318–362). New York: Wiley.

Rosenblum, L. D., Schmuckler, M. A., & Johnson, J. A. (1997). The McGurk effect in infants. *Perception & Psychophysics, 59,* 347–357.

Rowe, C. (1999). Receiver psychology and the evolution of multicomponent signals. *Animal Behaviour, 58,* 921–931.

Scheier, C., Lewkowicz, D. J., & Shimojo, S. (2003). Sound induces perceptual reorganization of an ambiguous motion display in human infants. *Developmental Science, 6,* 233–244.

Schmuckler, M. A. (1996). Visual-proprioceptive intermodal perception in infancy. *Infant Behavior and Development, 19,* 221–232.

Schneirla, T. C. (1957). The concept of development in comparative psychology. In D. B. Harris (Ed.), *The concept of development* (pp. 78–108). Minneapolis: University of Minnesota Press.

Schneirla, T. C. (1965). Aspects of stimulation and organization in approach/withdrawal processes underlying vertebrate behavioral development. In D. S. Lehrman, R. A. Hinde & E. Shaw (Eds.), *Advances in the study of behavior* (pp. 1–71). New York: Academic Press.

Sekuler, R., Sekuler, A. B., & Lau, R. (1997). Sound alters visual motion perception. *Nature, 385,* 308.

Slater, A., Quinn, P. C., Brown, E., & Hayes, R. (1999). Intermodal perception at birth: Intersensory redundancy guides newborn infants' learning of arbitrary auditory-visual pairings. *Developmental Science, 3,* 333–338.

Spear, N. E., Kraemer, P. J., Molina, J. C., & Smoller, D. E. (1988). Developmental change in learning and memory: Infantile disposition for "unitization." In J. Delacour & J. D. S. Levy (Eds.), *Systems with learning and memory abilities* (pp. 27–52). Amsterdam: Elsevier-North Holland.

Spear, N. E., & Kucharski, D. (1984a). Ontogenetic differences in stimulus selection during conditioning. In R. Kail & N. E. Spear (Eds.), *Comparative perspectives on the development of memory* (pp. 227–252). Hillsdale, NJ: Erlbaum.

Spear, N. E., & Kucharski, D. (1984b). Ontogenetic differences in the processing of multi-element stimuli. In H. Roitblatt, T. Bever & H. Terrace (Eds.), *Animal cognition* (pp. 545–567). Hillsdale, NJ: Erlbaum.

Spear, N. E., & McKinzie, D. L. (1994). Intersensory integration in the infant rat. In D. J. Lewkowicz & R. Lickliter (Eds.), *The development of intersensory perception: Comparative perspectives* (pp. 133–161). Hillsdale, NJ: Erlbaum.

Spelke, E. S. (1979). Perceiving bimodally specified events in infancy. *Developmental Psychology, 15,* 626–636.

Stein, B. E. (1998). Neural mechanisms for synthesizing sensory information and producing adaptive behaviors. *Experimental Brain Research, 123,* 124–135.

Stein, B. E., & Meredith, M. A. (1993). *The merging of the senses.* Cambridge, MA: MIT Press.

Summerfield, A. Q. (1979). Use of visual information in phonetic perception. *Phonetica, 36,* 314–331.

Thelen, E., & Smith, L. B. (1994). *A dynamic systems approach to the development of cognition and action.* Cambridge, MA: MIT Press.

Trehub, S. E., Schneider, B. A., & Henderson, J. L. (1995). Gap detection in infants, children, and adults. *Journal of the Acoustical Society of America, 98,* 2532–2541.

Turkewitz, G., & Kenny, P. A. (1982). Limitations on input as a basis for neural organization and perceptual development: A preliminary theoretical statement. *Developmental Psychobiology, 15,* 357–368.

Turkewitz, G., & Kenny, P. A. (1985). The role of developmental limitations of sensory input on sensory/perceptual organization. *Journal of Developmental and Behavioral Pediatrics, 6,* 302–306.

Turkewitz, G., Lewkowicz, D. J., & Gardner, J. (1983). Determinants of infant perception. In C. Rosenblatt, C. Beer, R. Hinde, & M. Busnel (Eds.), *Advances in the study of behavior* (pp. 39–62). New York: Academic Press.

Volkmann, F. C., & Dobson, M. V. (1976). Infant responses of ocular fixation to moving visual stimuli. *Journal of Experimental Child Psychology, 22,* 86–99.

von Melchner, L., Pallas, S. L., & Sur, M. (2000). Visual behaviour mediated by retinal projections directed to the auditory pathway. *Nature, 404,* 871–876.

Walker-Andrews, A. S. (1986). Intermodal perception of expressive behaviors: Relation of eye and voice? *Developmental Psychology, 22,* 373–377.

Walker-Andrews, A. S. (1997). Infants' perception of expressive behaviors: Differentiation of multimodal information. *Psychological Bulletin, 121,* 437–456.

Wallace, M. T., & Stein, B. E. (1997). Development of multisensory neurons and multisensory integration in cat superior colliculus. *Journal of Neuroscience, 17,* 2429–2444.

Wallace, M. T., & Stein, B. E. (2001). Sensory and multisensory responses in the newborn monkey superior colliculus. *Journal of Neuroscience, 21,* 8886–8894.

Welch, R. B. (1999). Meaning, attention, and the "unity assumption" in the intersensory bias of spatial and temporal perception. In G. Aschersleben, T. Bachman, & J. Musseler (Eds.), *Cognitive contributions to the perception of spatial and temporal events* (Vol. 129, pp. 371–387). Amsterdam: Elsevier.

Welch, R. B., & Warren, D. H. (1986). Intersensory interactions. In K. R. Boff, L. Kaufman, & J. P. Thomas (Eds.), *Handbook of perception and human performance: Sensory processes and perception* (Vol. 1, pp. 1–36). New York: Wiley.

Werner, H. (1973). *Comparative psychology of mental development.* New York: International Universities Press.

VII CROSS-MODAL PLASTICITY

42 Rewiring Cortex: Cross-Modal Plasticity and Its Implications for Cortical Development and Function

MRIGANKA SUR

Introduction

How do individual cortical areas come to process unique kinds of information and contribute to particular behaviors? This question lies at the heart of understanding how the cortex develops and acquires its functional capacities, yet there have been few direct approaches to answering it. In particular, it has proved difficult with the classical models of cortical development to separate intrinsic aspects of developmental programs from those that are influenced by extrinsic factors. A different paradigm for examining the question comes from cross-modal plasticity. Such plasticity, induced by rewiring the brain early in life, utilizes the inputs of one modality to drive cortical areas that normally process information from a different modality. These experiments provide important evidence that several aspects of cortical development and function are crucially influenced by the nature of input activity. This chapter reviews the logic of rewiring experiments in which visual inputs are induced to drive the auditory cortex, the physiological and behavioral consequences of rewiring, and the implications of these findings for mechanisms by which cortical areas acquire unique identities and processing functions or are able to carry out multisensory integration.

Development of cortical networks for vision

An area of cortex is characterized by specific inputs, processing networks, and outputs, all of which together enable the area to play a particular role in behavior. Traditional approaches to understanding the role of environmental influences on the development of cortical connections and networks have involved reductions in activity (Angelucci, Sharma, & Sur, 2000; Sur,

Angelucci, & Sharma, 1999). For example, the development and plasticity of ocular dominance columns in primary visual cortex (V1) have been an important proving ground for examining whether and how thalamocortical patterning and connections are regulated by visual inputs (Katz & Shatz, 1996). Ocular dominance columns in V1 arise by the segregation of inputs from the two eyes, relayed through eye-specific layers of the lateral geniculate nucleus (LGN). A vast body of evidence demonstrates that visual deprivation paradigms, such as suturing the lids of one eye during a critical period early in life, reduce the proportion of cells driven by the sutured eye (Wiesel & Hubel, 1965), and also reduce the size of ocular dominance columns related to the sutured eye (Antonini & Stryker, 1993; Shatz & Stryker, 1978). These experiments demonstrate ocular dominance plasticity whereby the open or untreated eye dominates the cortex both physiologically and anatomically, presumably by a dynamic mechanism of competition between axons from the two eyes for cortical territory and synaptic linkage with target cells. Activity in not only the presynaptic axons but also the target cells plays a role in regulating the outcome of the competition, because inhibiting cortical cells causes the less active axons to dominate cortex (Hata & Stryker, 1994; Reiter & Stryker, 1988). Whether or not the initial formation of ocular dominance columns entails the same mechanisms as those necessary for their maintenance remains an open question (Katz & Crowley, 2002; Sur & Leamey, 2001).

Until recently, the mechanisms of ocular dominance column formation and maintenance were thought to be similar. According to this view, axons from the two eyes initially overlap in cortex and subsequently segregate because of correlated activity in one eye and uncorrelated activity between the two eyes (Miller, Keller, &

Stryker, 1989). Indeed, the activity of adjacent retinal ganglion cells is correlated (Galli & Maffei, 1988), and waves of activity sweep across the retina during early life (Meister, Wong, Baylor, & Shatz, 1991), consistent with the hypothesis that correlated retinal activity has a role in the patterning of inputs from the two eyes in the LGN and subsequently in the cortex. Altering retinal waves reduces the degree of segregation of fibers from the two eyes in the LGN (Stellwagen & Shatz, 2002). Furthermore, the spontaneous activity of LGN cells appears to be correlated within one eye-specific layer but not across eye-specific layers (Weliky & Katz, 1999). Interestingly, however, the correlations depend on input from the cortex rather than from the retina, because ablating the cortex abolishes the correlations, whereas enucleation of the eyes does not. Thus, if correlations are important for setting up ocular dominance columns, these correlations must arise from a thalamocortical and corticothalamic loop (Sur & Leamey, 2001) rather than from retinal sources—a situation facilitated by the early development of pathways from the thalamus to the cortex (Johnson & Casagrande, 1993; Hermann, Antonini, & Shatz, 1994) and from the cortex back to the thalamus (Clasca, Angelucci, & Sur, 1995).

An alternative possibility is that the initial formation of ocular dominance columns is determined by matching molecular cues between LGN axons and target regions in V1. It turns out that ocular dominance columns can form very early in life, even when LGN axons first grow into layer 4 of V1, so that axons from each eye-specific layer project to nonoverlapping zones from the outset (Crowley & Katz, 2000; cf. Crair, Horton, Antonini, & Stryker, 2001). This is different from previous findings that the early innervation of cortex by LGN axons includes a significant overlap of terminations from the two eyes. It has been argued (Katz & Crowley, 2002) that the previously used technique of intraocular injection of tritiated proline for labeling the retinogeniculocortical projection (via transsynaptic transport of label from retinal axons through the LGN to geniculocortical axon terminals in V1) caused spillover in the LGN and in the cortex, and thus obscured the segregation. Consistent with the finding that the initial targeting of LGN axons is specific to ocular dominance zones, it has been shown that they develop even in the absence of retinal input, for removing the eyes does not immediately degrade the patchy geniculocortical termination zones (Crowley & Katz, 1999). Similarly, monocular deprivation very early in life has no effect on eye-specific driving in V1 for a time immediately after the deprivation, followed by a reduction in responses from the closed eye (Crair, Gillespie, &

Stryker, 1998). Thus, the initial development of ocular dominance projections appears to follow an intrinsic developmental program, and it would seem unlikely that activity instructs their formation. Although specific molecules related to left and right eye regions have not been discovered, the available evidence is consistent with the possibility that such molecules exist and have a role in setting up at least an initial scaffold of terminations. Yet activity can, in certain situations, play an instructive role in the formation of eye-specific domains in retinal targets: in frogs implanted with a third eye, axons from two retinas innervate a single tectum and form eye-specific stripes there (Constantine-Paton & Law, 1978). An instructive role for patterned activity in shaping the cortical columns is indicated by experiments that involve artificially induced strabismus, which causes V1 neurons to become almost exclusively monocular (Hubel & Wiesel, 1965; Van Sluyters & Levitt, 1980) and ocular dominance columns to sharpen and alter their spacing (Shatz, Lindstrom, & Wiesel, 1977; Lowel, 1994). Insofar as strabismus simply creates a spatial mismatch between the two eyes (thus reducing the spatial correlation between activity from the two eyes), these findings indicate that instruction by correlated input activity has a role at least in sculpting the final size and shape of ocular dominance columns.

A second system for examining the role of activity in the development of visual cortex connections involves orientation selectivity. Orientation-selective cells and orientation columns in V1 involve a more complex network than the termination of thalamocortical axons in eye-specific regions. Orientation selectivity arises in V1 cells by inputs from the LGN that are aligned along the axis of orientation (Ferster & Miller, 2000; Hubel & Wiesel, 1968), although considerable evidence indicates that thalamic inputs are amplified by local intracortical connections that sharpen orientation tuning and contribute to contrast gain control (Somers, Dragoi, & Sur, 2001; Somers, Nelson, & Sur, 1995). Orientation-selective cells in at least the superficial layers of V1 are organized into an orientation map (Bonhoeffer & Grinvald, 1991). Columns of cells that prefer a particular orientation are preferentially linked by long-range horizontal connections in V1 that are intrinsic to the superficial layers and are important for generating the orientation map (Gilbert & Wiesel, 1989).

Like ocular dominance, the development of orientation selectivity in V1 has been extensively studied and its plasticity examined with visual deprivation programs. Orientation selectivity is present in V1 of monkeys at birth (Wiesel & Hubel, 1974), and in cats and ferrets at eye opening, although selectivity sharpens a great deal with visual experience (Chapman & Stryker, 1993; Fregnac & Imbert, 1984; Sherman & Spear, 1982). Visual deprivation impairs but does not completely prevent the development of orientation-selective responses (Chapman & Stryker, 1993; Fregnac & Imbert, 1984; Sherman & Spear, 1982). Although long-range horizontal connections are present in cats and ferrets just before eye opening, the connections are refined after the onset of vision, and visual deprivation prevents the refinement (Callaway & Katz, 1990, 1991; Ruthazer & Stryker, 1996). The orientation map in V1 develops alongside the sharpening of horizontal connections, but the size and distribution of orientation domains remain stable while development proceeds (Chapman, Stryker, & Bonhoeffer, 1996). Visual deprivation does not alter the layout of the map, although it causes the map driven by a deprived eye to have weaker signals and less order (Crair et al., 1998). In cat V2, short-term monocular lid suture after the orientation map has formed causes the map driven by the closed eye to deteriorate, but a reverse suture (so that the formerly closed eye is now opened) restores the map (Kim & Bonhoeffer, 1994). Alternating suture, in which one eye or the other is sutured alternately so that the two eyes never have a common visual experience, nonetheless causes the maps from the two eyes to be in close register (Godecke & Bonhoeffer, 1996). Electric stimulation of an optic nerve in ferrets with patterned bursts for a few hours each day, starting close to the time of eye opening, broadens orientation selectivity of single neurons but does not change the layout of the orientation map (Weliky & Katz, 1997). These findings have been taken to indicate that orientation selectivity and orientation maps in V1 depend on an intrinsic scaffold of connections and depend little on visual influences.

The weight of evidence for a role for activity in the formation of ocular dominance columns—and hence for whether activity influences thalamocortical connectivity—indicates that the initial formation of the columns requires at most the presence of thalamocortical activity, although visually driven activity is required to sharpen the columns and to maintain them. The evidence in the case of orientation column formation—and hence for the role of activity in generating intracortical connectivity—is more complicated to interpret. Most of the experiments examining activity-dependent effects on orientation maps have suffered from two drawbacks. First, they commonly involved either lid suture to block visual inputs or infusion of tetrodotoxin into the eyes to block all retinal activity—both techniques that reduce afferent activity in visual pathways nonspecifically. The experiments hence largely addressed the effect on development of manipulating the *amount* rather than the *pattern* of activity, and thus were not suited for addressing an instructive role for activity. Second, it is now clear that in many instances the manipulations were initiated relatively late in development, after thalamocortical axons were already in place and even after much of the intracortical connections had started to organize (see Sur & Leamey, 2001). Thus, the experiments addressed the role of activity in the maintenance of columns rather than in their development. In general, classical paradigms such as lid suture starting near the time of eye opening are not adequate for examining whether or not the pattern of input activity instructs extrinsic aspects of cortical developmental programs.

Routing visual inputs to the auditory pathway: Why and how

A powerful way to address whether the pattern of input activity has a role in the development of cortical connections is to route axons that convey information about one sensory modality into central structures that normally process a different modality (Sur & Leamey, 2001; Sur et al., 1990). An early discovery by Schneider (1973; see also Frost, 1982) demonstrated that axons from the retina could be directed into the auditory thalamus in hamsters if the auditory thalamus was deafferented in newborn animals. We chose to work with ferrets, which have a well-developed visual pathway and are born at a very early stage in development, when axons from the retina are still developing projections to the thalamus and thalamic axons have not yet innervated the cortical plate. The goal of the experiments was to route retinal axons into the auditory thalamus in neonatal animals, thereby providing a pathway for visual inputs to drive the auditory thalamus and subsequently the auditory cortex (Fig. 42.1). We reasoned the following: (1) because the pattern of electric activity due to vision has a different spatial and temporal structure than that due to audition, auditory structures would develop with a very different pattern of input activity than normal; (2) such rerouting would leave intact the anatomical pathways leading away from the auditory thalamus, such as the thalamocortical projection from the auditory thalamus to primary auditory cortex, but cause them to convey a different pattern of activity; and (3) the change in input activity to the auditory cortex, without altering the anatomical identity of thalamocortical projections, would occur at a very early stage in development, and thus the experiment would address whether and how activity influences the initial formation of intracortical connections (rather than just their maintenance). If the auditory cortex in rewired

A Normal

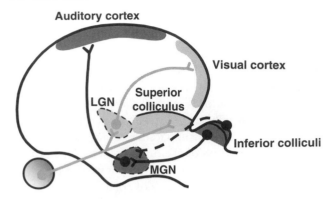

B Rewired

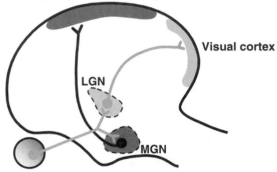

FIGURE 42.1 Visual and auditory pathways in normal animals, and the visual pathway to auditory cortex in rewired animals. (*A*) In normal ferrets, the major projections of the retina are to the lateral geniculate nucleus (LGN) and the superior colliculus; the LGN in turn projects to primary visual cortex and other cortical fields. The auditory pathway starts with the cochlea and consists of projections from the inferior colliculi in the two hemispheres to each medial geniculate nucleus (MGN), which projects to the primary auditory cortex and other cortical fields. (*B*) Deafferenting the MGN in neonatal ferrets by removing ascending auditory projections causes retinal fibers to innervate the MGN. The MGN still projects to the auditory cortex, but now relays visual information. Thus, the thalamocortical projections are anatomically the same in rewired animals as in normal animals, but in rewired animals they are driven by a very different spatiotemporal pattern of activity. This has a profound effect on the development of networks in auditory cortex and on the function of auditory cortex. (Adapted from Sur & Leamey, 2001.)

animals developed networks similar to those in visual cortex, it would provide powerful evidence that the formation of visual processing networks in cortex is influenced in instructive fashion by vision and is not simply due to the passive presence of activity or intrinsic developmental programs.

Retinal projections can be induced to innervate the medial geniculate nucleus (MGN) of the auditory thalamus following extensive surgical deafferentation of

the MGN in newborn ferrets (Sur, Garraghty, & Roe, 1988). The procedure involves sectioning the brachium of the inferior colliculus in order to remove ipsilaterally projecting ascending auditory fibers to the MGN, combined with ablating the superior colliculus (SC) down to the deep layers in order to remove contralaterally projecting ascending fibers (Angelucci, Clascà, & Sur, 1998). Molecular factors contribute to making the rerouting possible. One key molecule that has a role is the EphA system of receptor tyrosine kinases and their associated ephrin-A ligands, which have been implicated in topographic mapping of retinal projections to central targets (Feldheim et al., 2000). The ligands are expressed in a gradient in the MGN, with high expression along the border of the MGN and the optic tract, and they normally repel receptor-bearing retinal axons of the optic tract (Lyckman et al., 2001). Mutant mice in which genes for two of the ephrin-A ligands, ephrin-A2 and ephrin-A5, are deleted show a significant increase in the extent of retino-MGN projections compared with wild-type mice (Lyckman et al., 2001), primarily because of a major enhancement of projections from the ipsilateral retina (Ellsworth, Lyckman, & Sur, 2001). The likely reason for this result is that fibers from the temporal retina that give rise to the ipsilateral projection normally project to low-ephrin-A-expressing regions of the MGN. Removing the expression of the ligands by deleting the genes that make them expands the potential target space for axons from temporal retina (Ellsworth, Lyckman, & Sur, 2002). Thus, molecules that regulate topography can also regulate confinement of retinal projections to normal targets, and altering their expression can alter the specificity of retinothalamic projections. At the same time, other molecular systems are also likely to be involved in target specificity and plasticity: mice lacking ephrin-A ligands do not develop aberrant retinal projections to the MGN without deafferentation of the MGN, implying that other molecules, possibly including those upstream of the ephrins, have a role in confining retinothalamic projections.

The retinal projection to the MGN in ferrets arises from most of the major retinal ganglion cell types (Vitek, Schall, & Leventhal, 1985), prominently including W cells (Roe, Garraghty, Esguerra, & Sur, 1993), as well as other retinal ganglion cell classes (Angelucci et al., 1998). It is reasonable to propose that the key aspect of retinal ganglion cells that induces them to project to the MGN is the timing of axon outgrowth in the optic tract. Retinal ganglion cells that are generated around birth in ferrets, when the rewiring procedure is carried out, are likely to target novel locations; these include W cells from most of the retina as well as other cell classes from more peripheral regions of the retina (Angelucci et al., 1998).

Physiological and anatomical consequences of rewiring: Visual networks in auditory cortex

Rewired ferrets are a unique model for examining how the pattern of electric activity in space and time shapes processing networks and the role in behavior of a cortical area. The projection from the retina is chiefly to the ventral or principal division of the MGN and provides secure driving of MGN neurons (Fig. 42.2). MGN neurons in rewired ferrets have center-surround visual

A. Cortical cells

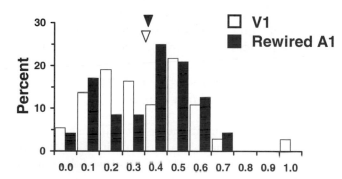

B. MGN cells

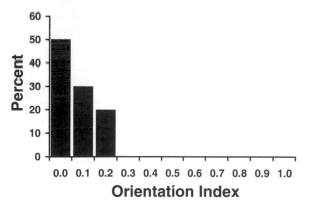

FIGURE 42.2   Orientation selectivity of cells in V1 of normal ferrets and in A1 of rewired ferrets, and a comparison with cells in the MGN of rewired ferrets. (*A*) Histogram of the orientation selectivity index of cells in V1 and rewired A1 demonstrates that cells are similarly tuned in the two areas. Orientation index = (Response at the preferred orientation − Response at the orthogonal orientation)/(Response at the preferred orientation + Response at the orthogonal orientation). (Adapted from Roe et al., 1992.) (*B*) Histogram of the orientation index for MGN cells shows that the cells are unselective or at most weakly selective for orientation. Thus, orientation selectivity arises in A1 of rewired ferrets, as it does in V1 of normal ferrets. (Adapted from Roe et al., 1993.)

receptive fields (RFs) (Roe et al., 1993). Retinal axons also map systematically to the ventral division of the MGN, with the central retina represented medially, the peripheral retina represented laterally, the ventral retina represented dorsally, and the dorsal retina represented ventrally within the MGN (Roe, Hahm, & Sur, 1991). Retinal axons have focal terminations within the MGN (Pallas, Hahm, & Sur, 1994), although the arbors are represented within MGN lamellae and are aligned along them (Pallas & Sur, 1994). Furthermore, retinal axons from each eye start out occupying overlapping territories but then segregate into eye-specific clusters within the MGN, although each cluster is smaller than the eye-specific layers that characterize the normal LGN (Angelucci, Clasca, Bricolo, Cramer, & Sur, 1997). These findings indicate that afferent axons have a significant effect on the structure of sensory pathways through the thalamus, but that the target also regulates key aspects of the projection.

The ventral division of the MGN projects heavily to primary auditory cortex (A1), and in rewired ferrets the thalamocortical projections convey visual drive to A1 rather than auditory drive. A map of visual space arises in rewired A1 (Roe, Pallas, Hahm, & Sur, 1990); the map provides important clues to how the pattern of input activity shapes the strength of thalamocortical synapses during development. In normal ferrets, A1 contains a one-dimensional map of sound frequency, with low frequencies represented laterally and high frequencies represented medially in cortex. The orthogonal (anteroposterior) axis is one of isofrequency, that is, the same frequency is remapped along it. Consistent with this mapping, the terminal arbors of single axons from the MGN to A1 are narrow along the variable-frequency axis but widespread along the isofrequency axis (Pallas, Roe, & Sur, 1990). The anatomical pattern of thalamocortical projections is not altered in rewired ferrets, and it predicts that visual RFs along the anteroposterior axis of rewired A1 would be highly overlapped and elongated in size and shape. Yet the physiological RFs, and the map itself, indicate otherwise: RFs are restricted in size, and there is a systematic progression along the anteroposterior dimension of A1. Thus, not all parts of thalamocortical axon arbors convey equal drive to postsynaptic neurons in rewired A1: either the weights of thalamocortical synapses are altered, or there is an increase in cortical inhibition, so as to cancel the widespread excitation supplied by the thalamus (Sur, Pallas, & Roe, 1990). Whereas altering the nature of input activity to A1 early in development does not seem to significantly alter the anatomical structure of thalamocortical arbors, the functional consequence of the projection is significantly changed, presumably due to correlated inputs from adjacent retinal and MGN loci that provide the substrate for focal functional connections within rewired A1.

Rewired A1 also develops visual orientation-selective cells and an orientation map. Single neurons within A1 are less responsive to visual stimuli compared to V1 neurons in normal animals (Roe, Pallas, Kwon, & Sur, 1992), but have orientation and direction tuning that is comparable in degree to that in V1 (Sharma, Angelucci, & Sur, 2000). In particular, the orientation selectivity arises in rewired A1 itself, just as it does within V1, because neurons in the rewired MGN exhibit significantly less selectivity (Fig. 42.2). Thus, it seems that the same mechanisms operate within rewired A1 as in normal V1 in order to generate orientation selectivity. These mechanisms include feed-forward excitation from the thalamus, combined with recurrent connections in the cortex to amplify the tuning (Somers et al., 1995, 2001). The intracortical connections may be a ubiquitous feature of A1 that is common to cortical areas, whereas the feed-forward projections are likely to be shaped by the nature of visual input: visual edges in natural scenes and other visual stimuli can provide correlated inputs to the MGN and to A1 in rewired animals that may be used by cortical neurons to generate orientation selectivity. The development of orientation selectivity in rewired A1 strongly implies that a similar mechanism could be used to generate orientation selectivity in V1 in normal animals, where the influence of activity has been difficult to resolve with other experimental models.

The strongest evidence that the pattern of input activity can shape intracortical networks is provided by the orientation map and the structure of long-range horizontal connections within rewired A1 (Sharma et al., 2000). Optical imaging of intrinsic signals demonstrates that domains of neurons in rewired A1 respond to the same preferred orientation; these domains are organized systematically around pinwheel centers to form a map of orientation-selective cells (Fig. 42.3). The pinwheel organization of the map is similar to that in V1 and indicates that the pinwheel structure is an important means by which the mapping of orientation selectivity relates to other maps and representations within V1. Long-range connections within rewired A1 connect domains that have the same orientation preference, and hence obey the same principle as do connections in V1. However, the orientation maps in rewired A1 and V1 also have differences: the orientation domains are larger in size in rewired A1 and seem to be less orderly in their spacing. Similar to the orientation map, horizontal connections in rewired A1 also seem to be less orderly than those in V1. Still, the pattern of horizontal connections in rewired A1 is significantly different from that in normal A1, and resembles in essential aspects the connections in V1 (Fig. 42.4). In V1, the connections are patchy and periodic, and often elongated along the orientation axis of the injection site. In A1, the connections are bandlike and extend along the isofrequency axis of the cortical sound frequency map. In rewired A1, the connections form patches that are much smaller than the bands in normal A1 (see Gao & Pallas, 1999), and the patches tend to extend along the orientation axis of the injection site. Thus, input activity has a significant role in shaping horizontal connections within the cortex. In rewired A1, input correlations driven by visual stimuli of the same orientation influence horizontal connections that come to interconnect cells responsive to the same visual orientation. In normal A1, the correlations are driven by auditory stimuli of the same frequency, and horizontal connections interconnect cells responsive to the same sound frequency (Read, Winer, & Schreiner, 2001).

The behavioral consequences of routing visual projections to the auditory pathway

The routing of retinal inputs to the auditory thalamus and the shaping of networks in the auditory cortex raise the question, what is the role in behavior of the rewired projection? In other words, is visual activation of the rewired projection interpreted by the ferrets as a visual stimulus or as an auditory one? If the behavioral role of a cortical area is set independent of its inputs, then activation of the auditory cortex by any stimulus (auditory or visual) would be interpreted as auditory. But if the nature of the inputs has a role in determining the function of a cortical area, rewired animals should interpret visual activation of the cortex as a visual stimulus.

Although this is a fundamental question about cortical function, there are few ways of answering it outside of a paradigm such as rewiring. Von Melchner, Pallas, and Sur (2000) used a selective training and stimulus presentation procedure in rewired ferrets to address the issue. Ferrets were rewired in the left hemisphere and were trained to discriminate between light and sound (Fig. 42.5). Sound stimuli (clicks or tone bursts) were presented at a range of locations, and animals received a juice reward for correct identification at one reward spout (the "auditory" spout). Light stimuli (red LEDs) were presented in the left monocular field, and hence were seen only by the right, or normal, hemisphere; animals received a juice reward for correct identification at a different reward spout (the "visual" reward spout). Thus, animals eventually learned to associate one reward location with sound and another

A. Normal V1   # B. Rewired A1

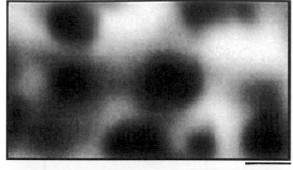

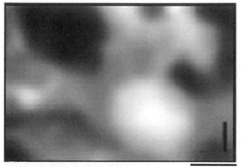

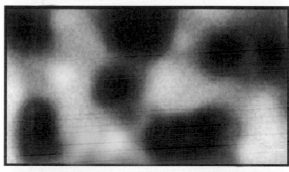

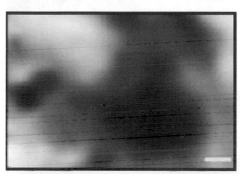

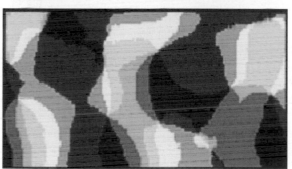

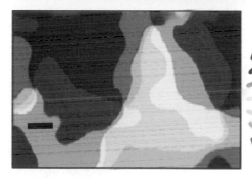

FIGURE 42.3   The orientation map in normal V1 and in rewired A1. (*A*) Optical imaging of an expanse of V1 (crosshatched on line drawing of ferret brain at top) shows domains of cortex (black blobs in middle images) that respond to vertically oriented gratings (upper image), and other domains that respond to horizontally oriented gratings (lower image). From a number of such images obtained in response to a stimulus of a single orientation, a composite orientation map is obtained by vector averaging the response at each pixel (bottom). Here, the angle of the average orientation vector is represented by the key at right. (*B*) Similar optical imaging data from an expanse of A1 in a rewired ferret (crosshatched on line drawing at top), including images obtained in response to vertical or horizontal gratings (middle) and a composite orientation map (bottom). Although the orientation map in rewired A1 has larger domains with variable spacing, an important similarity between the composite maps in rewired A1 and normal V1 is the presence of pinwheels around which cells preferring different orientations are systematically represented. Scale bars below upper images = 0.5 mm. (Adapted from Sharma et al., 2000.)

with light. After training was complete, the response of animals was tested with light stimuli presented in the right monocular field; these stimuli were projected into the left, or rewired, hemisphere. Reward was given indiscriminately at either reward spout for light or sound stimuli. (Visual stimuli were also presented at other locations for comparison; however, the critical part of the experiment involved the right monocular field.) In

the first stage of testing, animals responded overwhelmingly at the visual reward spout, indicating that the visual stimulus was seen. This was not surprising, because the rewired, or left, hemisphere contained two parallel pathways from eye to brain: the normal projection from the retina to the LGN and lateral-posterior nucleus (LP) to visual cortex, and the rewired projection from the retina to the MGN to auditory cortex. In

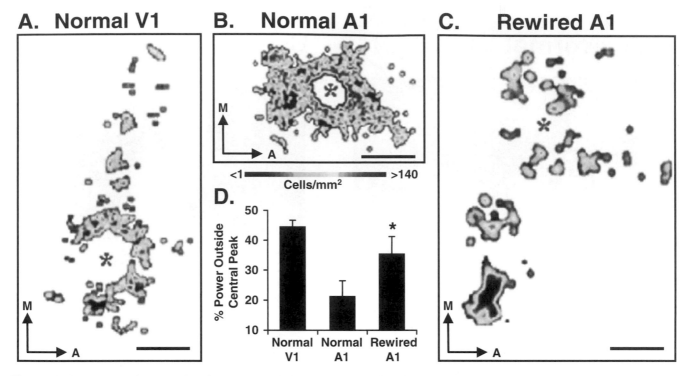

A. Normal V1   **B. Normal A1**   **C. Rewired A1**

D.

Figure 42.4   Horizontal connections in cortex and the effect of rewiring. (*A*) In V1 of a normal ferret, an injection of cholera toxin B (at the site marked by a star) retrogradely labeled cells that projected to the injection site. The cortex was sectioned parallel to the pia, and the density of horizontally projecting cells in layer 3 is depicted by the key in the middle. Horizontal connections of cells in the superficial layers of V1 are patchy and link cells with similar orientation preference. (*B*) In A1 of a normal ferret, horizontal connections spread along the isofrequency axis of cortex. (*C*) In A1 of a rewired ferret, horizontal connections are patchy and resemble connections in V1. (*D*) A power spectrum analysis of the spatial pattern of horizontal connections reveals the extent of periodicity of the connections: the more the power outside the central DC peak, the more periodic the connection pattern. Horizontal connections are highly periodic in V1, and are significantly more periodic in rewired A1 than in normal A1 (star denotes $P < 0.05$ comparing rewired and normal A1). Scale bars = 0.5 mm. (Adapted from Sharma et al., 2000.)

the second stage of testing, the LGN/LP in the rewired hemisphere was ablated with ibotenic acid and animals were tested after a period of recovery. In this instance, the only projection from the retina was that to the MGN; animals still responded overwhelmingly at the visual reward spout, indicating that the visual stimulus was again seen. In the third stage of testing, the auditory cortex was lesioned, and animals were tested after a period of recovery. In this instance, animals responded at chance levels at the visual reward spout, indicating that the animals were blind in the right visual field and the visual stimulus was not seen (Fig. 42.5).

Several kinds of control experiments demonstrated that rewired ferrets indeed perceived the visual stimuli with their rewired projection. In one control, normal animals were trained in the identical way to discriminate visual stimuli presented in the left monocular field and auditory stimuli. In the testing phase, they were presented with visual stimuli in the right monocular field, and they responded overwhelmingly at the visual reward spout, indicating that the stimuli were seen. In

the second phase of the control experiment, the LGN/LP and the SC in the left hemisphere were lesioned with ibotenic acid; animals were again tested with visual stimuli presented in the right monocular field and responded at chance levels at either reward spout, indicating that they were blind in the right visual field. In contrast to these animals, however, rewired ferrets had their left SC lesioned at birth (as part of the procedure to induce rewiring), and the left LGN/LP was lesioned prior to the second phase of testing. They were still able to perceive visual stimuli in the right visual field with the rewired projection in their left hemisphere, and were functionally blind only when their left auditory cortex was ablated. Thus, the rewired projection from the retina through the MGN to auditory cortex is able to mediate visual behavior.

What is the quality of visual sensation (*qualia*) evoked in the rewired projection, and does it resemble normal vision? To ascertain how different the perception of light was from sound in the rewired animals, another set of control ferrets were trained to respond to light stimuli

A.

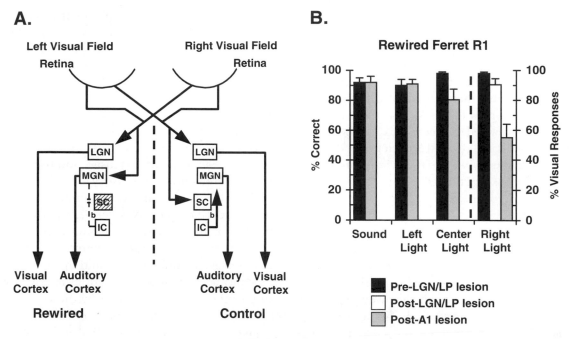

B.

Figure 42.5 The behavioral consequence of routing retinal projections to the auditory thalamus and of visual activation of auditory cortex. (*A*) Visual pathways in the normal hemisphere (right) and in the rewired hemisphere (left). The projection from the inferior colliculus (IC) to the medial geniculate nucleus (MGN) courses through the brachium (b) of the IC. In the rewired hemisphere, this projection was sectioned and the SC was ablated. Ferrets were trained to respond at one reward spout when visual stimuli were presented in the left visual field (which is seen by the right, or normal, hemisphere) and at a different reward spout when auditory stimuli were presented. After training was complete, ferrets were tested with visual stimuli presented in the center or in the right visual field, and responses were noted. (*B*) Ferrets learned to associate one reward spout with sound and another with light presented in the left visual field. When light was subsequently presented in the center or right visual field, they responded at the visual reward spout, indicating that the stimulus was seen (e.g., black bar in rightmost column). In the second phase of testing, the visual thalamus (LGN/LP) in the rewired hemisphere was lesioned, leaving the retina-MGN-A1 projection as the only pathway conveying visual information in the rewired hemisphere. Animals still responded at the visual reward spout to light in the right visual field (white bar in rightmost column). In the third phase of testing, A1 was lesioned. Now animals responded at chance levels to light in the right field (gray-shaded bar in rightmost column), indicating that they were blind in the right field. Of note, in the second phase, a visual stimulus in the right field was seen even when only the retina-MGN-A1 projection was intact and the key visual structures in the thalamus and midbrain were lesioned. Furthermore, visual percepts were blocked in these animals after ablation of A1 in the third phase (and not any visual area). Thus, the rewired projection is capable of mediating visual behavior. See text for details. (Adapted from von Melchner et al., 2000.)

alone or sound stimuli alone. That is, they were trained to associate one reward spout with their training stimulus and were then presented with the other stimulus. Animals trained on sound alone never responded at the sound reward spout when a light was presented to their rewired projection, indicating that the representation of the light was substantially different from sound (at least the training set of sounds). Animals trained on light alone always responded at the light reward spout when light was presented to the rewired projection, indicating that the representation of the light was similar in their normal and rewired projections. Furthermore, the representation of sound was generalized substantially by the rewired ferrets. Although they were trained with a restricted set of sounds, they routinely responded at the sound reward spout when they were tested with a broad range of sounds. Thus, it is

unlikely that the quality of representation of visual stimuli was simply another form of audition in rewired ferrets. Rather, the available evidence indicates that light stimuli were indeed perceived as visual, and as different from sound.

A final line of evidence that rewired ferrets can use their rewired projection for visual function comes from examining their ability to detect gratings of different contrasts and spatial frequencies. Animals with only the rewired projection from the retina to MGN to auditory cortex (that is, with the LGN/LP lesioned) were trained to respond at a reward spout only if a grating was visible in the right monocular field, but not otherwise (Von Melchner et al., 2000). Contrast-response functions were derived, and these demonstrated that the response of animals scaled with contrast: the higher the contrast, the greater the visibility of the grating via the rewired projection as measured by the accuracy of response. This was similar to the response of normal animals and of the normal hemisphere in rewired animals. Although the spatial acuity of the rewired pathway was lower than that of the normal visual pathway (likely due to the fact that retinal W cells form the primary source of inputs to the MGN), these findings indicate that the rewired projection is competent to mediate vision. Similarly, rewired hamsters can discriminate visual patterns with their rewired projection (Frost, Boire, Gingras, & Ptito, 2000).

One explanation for these results is that the capacity for visual or auditory function resides in some later, as yet unspecified location in the brain, and routing visual inputs to the auditory thalamus causes a switch in this location so that it interprets visual activation of auditory pathways as vision. For example, higher cortical areas in the ferret brain might be critically involved in perceptual specification, and rewiring might induce a change in the projection from the auditory cortex to such areas that then lead to the perception of vision. However, a more parsimonious explanation of these results, and one that invokes induction of function, is that vision is a distributed property of networks that receive inputs from the retina. Thus, visual inputs routed to the auditory thalamus induce visual function in subsequent "auditory" pathways and networks; pathways central to the MGN in rewired animals, including the pathways to auditory cortex, networks within auditory cortex, intracortical pathways between auditory areas, and descending projections from the auditory cortex, are all induced to be visual and thus to mediate vision. That is, brain pathways and networks derive function from their inputs.

Cross-modal plasticity in humans, and the lack of perceptual plasticity associated with phantom limbs

The conclusion that cortical areas derive function from their inputs is consistent with evidence from congenitally blind humans indicating involvement of visual cortex in nonvisual tasks. Visual cortex in such individuals shows activation in somatosensory tasks (Kujala et al., 1997; Sadato et al., 1996), as well as, under different conditions, in auditory tasks (Bavelier et al., 2001; Neville, Schmidt, & Kutas, 1983; Weeks et al., 2000). Conversely, auditory cortex in congenitally deaf individuals can be activated by visual tasks (Bavelier & Neville, 2002; Finney, Fine, & Dobkins, 2001; Neville et al., 1983). Of note, the quality of sensation associated with activating the visual cortex in congenitally blind individuals, or the auditory cortex in congenitally deaf

individuals, appears to derive from the nature of inputs. That is, visual inputs are perceived as visual even when auditory cortex is activated, just as auditory (or somatosensory) inputs are perceived as auditory (or somatosensory) in spite of activating visual cortex (at the least, the quality of the percept is not reported as different between situations that activate novel cortex and those that activate traditional sensory cortex). Furthermore, even in normal, nondeprived humans, there is evidence for extensive multisensory interactions whereby primary sensory areas of the cortex can be activated in a task-specific manner by stimuli of other modalities (Bavelier & Neville, 2002). Common to these findings is the principle that inputs recruit pathways, cortical areas, and networks within and between areas that process the information, and the sensoriperceptual modality associated with the input is driven by the nature of the input rather than by the cortical area activated per se. Of course, under normal conditions, the primary sensory areas are the first and most consistently activated cortical regions associated with the vast majority of modality-specific processing, and it is reasonable to conclude that their activity might intrinsically process a given modality. It is situations in which other modalities are adaptively processed by a cortical area without altering qualia that provide the strongest evidence for input-based functions of cortex.

One important instance in which the nature of the input does not adaptively change the perceptual role of a cortical area is the phantom limb percept. Here, sensory stimulation of a forelimb stump or the skin on the face leads to a percept of the missing limb being touched (Ramachandran & Rogers-Ramachandran, 2000). Removal of peripheral input causes a remapping of the cortical territory associated with the remaining skin, and this remapping is thought to underlie the phantom percept. Thus, removing the digits of the hand or deafferenting the arm causes an expansion of the cortical territory representing the face (Merzenich et al., 1984; Pons et al., 1991). The mechanism for this expansion is likely to be both an unmasking of divergent projections to cortex from peripheral receptors relayed through brainstem and thalamic somatosensory nuclei to primary somatosensory cortex, and the growth of new connections in subcortical and cortical areas (Florence, Taub, & Kaas, 1998; Jain, Florence, Qi, & Kaas, 2000; Jones & Pons, 1998). When the face is stimulated, its expanded cortical representation within the former hand and arm representation is activated, in addition to the extant face area. Activation of the former hand/arm cortex is considered to underlie the phantom percept, but the percept is a maladaptive one: sensory stimulation of one body region, the face, is associated with a wrong region of the body, a missing limb.

Why does the brain signal a wrong percept even though the primary somatosensory cortex has been remapped? One possibility is that the body image resides in some higher, fixed, cortical locus, and even though the primary somatosensory cortex is remapped, this later area continues to interpret activation from the face as arising from the limb. However, this possibility is unlikely. The remapping of primary somatosensory cortex ensures that later cortical areas would also be remapped, for they are all driven by the postcentral cortex and from the new face input. Furthermore, compared with primary somatosensory cortex, the capacity for plasticity is likely to be even more pronounced in the later areas. Interestingly, there is one pathway that likely remains unchanged even after deafferentation—the descending pathway from somatosensory cortex to the spinal cord. These projections from the hand/arm region are likely to continue targeting the appropriate spinal cord segments, even though the cortex is now receiving input from the face via subcortical or intracortical projections. The implication of this hypothesis is that a percept is due not only to the sensory input but also to the outflow, and the two have to be consistent in order to interpret an input as arising from a part of the body or from a modality. In this view, the phantom limb percept arises by a combination of sensory stimulation from the face (which activates remapped cortex) but an output referral to the spinal segments that still relate to the missing limb.

In rewired ferrets, then, it is important that not only the inputs to auditory cortex be visual but also that the output projections of auditory cortex be consistent with the input, that is, be able to mediate visual responses. One possibility is that the outflow of the auditory cortex should now target existing visual structures. But our data to date indicate that this is unlikely: the inputs to primary auditory cortex in rewired ferrets arise from essentially the same cortical areas that provide input to auditory cortex in normal ferrets (Pallas & Sur, 1993), and it is likely that the connections are reciprocal. Furthermore, rewired auditory cortex projects downstream to auditory thalamic nuclei and not to visual thalamic nuclei. More likely is that due to deafferentation of the MGN, auditory input is absent in ascending pathways in the rewired hemisphere, so that all of the "auditory" structures have simply been turned visual. This complete takeover of pathways and networks is in fact essential for respecifying the perceptual role of the auditory cortex as visual.

Similarly, it is reasonable to propose that in congenitally deprived humans, there exists a consistent set of pathways to and from cortex that allows the cortex to process information from a new modality. In normal, undeprived humans, we propose that the recruitment of cortical areas of one modality for tasks of another that nonetheless preserve a modality-specific percept would involve rules that match the output to the input. Specifically, the activation of a novel area by a particular sensory modality should not involve the output cells of the area, and the processed output should preserve the specificity of the input modality.

Conclusions

Cross-modal plasticity provides an important means by which natural stimuli, rather than deprivation paradigms, can be used to examine a central issue in brain development: to what extent are the connectivity and function of a cortical area influenced by its inputs during development? Routing retinal inputs to the MGN causes the auditory cortex to be driven by spatial and temporal patterns of electric activity due to vision, without altering the thalamocortical pathways from the MGN to auditory cortex. Several features of auditory cortex are subsequently altered, including thalamocortical connections and intracortical networks that map visual space and process visual orientation selectivity. The perceptual role of auditory cortex is also altered, so that rewired ferrets interpret activation of the auditory cortex by visual stimuli as vision. Thus, the nature of input activity has a profound role in the construction of cortical networks that process the input. In normal development, mechanisms of plasticity provide a means by which processing networks are matched to the input without explicit specification of network connectivity—this is a means of self-organization of cortical processing networks. The behavioral findings underscore the importance of output as well as input projections in perception and indicate that the role in behavior of an area of the cortex arises from a consistent set of inputs, processing networks, and outputs.

ACKNOWLEDGMENTS   The research described in this chapter was supported by grants from the National Institutes of Health and the March of Dimes.

REFERENCES

Angelucci, A., Clasca, F., Bricolo, E., Cramer, K. S., & Sur, M. (1997). Experimentally induced retinal projections to the ferret auditory thalamus: Development of clustered eye-specific patterns in a novel target. *Journal of Neuroscience, 17,* 2040–2055.

Angelucci, A., Clasca, F., & Sur, M. (1998). Brainstem inputs to the ferret medial geniculate nucleus and the effect of early deafferentation on novel retinal projections to the auditory thalamus. *Journal of Comparative Neurology, 400,* 417–439.

Angelucci, A., Sharma, J., & Sur, M. (2000). The modifiability of neocortical connections and function during development. In J. H. Kaas (Ed.), *The mutable brain* (pp. 351–392). Amsterdam: Harwood Academic.

Antonini, A., & Stryker, M. P. (1993). Rapid remodeling of axonal arbors in the visual cortex. *Science, 260,* 1819–1821.

Bavelier, D., & Neville, H. J. (2002). Cross-modal plasticity: Where and how? *Nature Reviews: Neuroscience, 3,* 443–452.

Bavelier, D., Brozinsky, C., Tomann, A., Mitchell, T., Neville, H., & Lin, G. (2001). Impact of early deafness and early exposure to sign language on the cerebral organization for motion processing. *Journal of Neuroscience, 21,* 8931–8942.

Bonhoeffer, T., & Grinvald, A. (1991). Iso-orientation domains in cat visual cortex are arranged in pinwheel-like patterns. *Nature, 353,* 429–431.

Callaway, E. M., & Katz, L. C. (1990). Emergence and refinement of clustered horizontal connections in cat striate cortex. *Journal of Neuroscience, 10,* 1134–1153.

Callaway, E. M., & Katz, L. C. (1991). Effects of binocular deprivation on the development of clustered horizontal connections in cat striate cortex. *Proceedings of the National Academy of Sciences, USA, 88,* 745–749.

Chapman, B., & Stryker, M. P. (1993). Development of orientation selectivity in ferret visual cortex and effects of deprivation. *Journal of Neuroscience, 13,* 5251–5262.

Chapman, B., Stryker, M. P., & Bonhoeffer, T. (1996). Development of orientation preference maps in ferret primary visual cortex. *Journal of Neuroscience, 16,* 6443–6453.

Clasca, F., Angelucci, A., & Sur, M. (1995). Layer-specific programs of development in neocortical projection neurons. *Proceedings of the National Academy of Sciences, USA, 92,* 11145–11149.

Constantine-Paton, M., & Law, M. I. (1978). Eye-specific termination bands in tecta of three-eyed frogs. *Science, 202,* 639–641.

Crair, M. C., Gillespie, D. C., & Stryker, M. P. (1998). The role of visual experience in the development of columns in cat visual cortex. *Science, 279,* 566–570.

Crair, M. C., Horton, J. C., Antonini, A., & Stryker, M. P. (2001). Emergence of ocular dominance columns in cat visual cortex by 2 weeks of age. *Journal of Comparative Neurology, 430,* 235–249.

Crowley, J. C., & Katz, L. C. (1999). Development of ocular dominance columns in the absence of retinal input. *Nature Neuroscience, 2,* 1125–1130.

Crowley, J. C., & Katz, L. C. (2000). Early development of ocular dominance columns. *Science, 290,* 1321–1324.

Ellsworth, C. A., Lyckman, A. W., & Sur, M. (2001). Eye-specific patterning of retinogeniculate terminations in the medial geniculate nucleus of rewired mice. *Society of Neuroscience Abstracts, 27,* 27.13.

Ellsworth, C. A., Lyckman, A. W., & Sur, M. (2002). Ephrin-a mediates eye-specific patterning of retinogeniculate projections in rewired mice. *Society of Neuroscience Abstracts, 28,* 820.823.

Feldheim, D. A., Kim, Y. I., Bergemann, A. D., Frisen, J., Barbacid, M., & Flanagan, J. G. (2000). Genetic analysis of ephrin-A2 and ephrin-A5 shows their requirement in multiple aspects of retinocollicular mapping. *Neuron, 25,* 563–574.

Ferster, D., & Miller, K. D. (2000). Neural mechanisms of orientation selectivity in the visual cortex. *Annual Review of Neuroscience, 23,* 441–471.

Finney, E. M., Fine, I., & Dobkins, K. R. (2001). Visual stimuli activate auditory cortex in the deaf. *Nature Neuroscience, 4,* 1171–1173.

Florence, S. L., Taub, H. B., & Kaas, J. H. (1998). Large-scale sprouting of cortical connections after peripheral injury in adult macaque monkeys. *Science, 282,* 1062–1063.

Fregnac, Y., & Imbert, M. (1984). Development of neuronal selectivity in primary visual cortex of cat. *Physiological Review, 64,* 325–434.

Frost, D. O. (1982). Anomalous visual connections to somatosensory and auditory systems following brain lesions in early life. *Brain Research, 255,* 627–635.

Frost, D. O., Boire, D., Gingras, G., & Ptito, M. (2000). Surgically created neural pathways mediate visual pattern discrimination. *Proceedings of the National Academy of Sciences, USA, 97,* 11068–11073.

Galli, L., & Maffei, L. (1988). Spontaneous impulse activity of rat retinal ganglion cells in prenatal life. *Science, 242,* 90–91.

Gao, W., & Pallas, S. L. (1999). Cross-modal reorganization of horizontal connectivity in auditory cortex without altering thalamocortical projections. *Journal of Neuroscience, 19,* 7940–7950.

Gilbert, C. D., & Wiesel, T. N. (1989). Columnar specificity of intrinsic horizontal and corticocortical connections in cat visual cortex. *Journal of Neuroscience, 9,* 2432–2442.

Godecke, I., & Bonhoeffer, T. (1996). Development of identical orientation maps for two eyes without common visual experience. *Nature, 379,* 251–254.

Hata, Y., & Stryker, M. P. (1994). Control of thalamocortical afferent rearrangement by postsynaptic activity in developing visual cortex. *Science, 265,* 1732–1735.

Herrmann, K., Antonini, A., & Shatz, C. J. (1994). Ultrastructural evidence for synaptic interactions between thalamocortical axons and subplate neurons. *European Journal of Neuroscience, 6,* 1729–1742.

Hubel, D. H., & Wiesel, T. N. (1965). Binocular interaction in striate cortex of kittens reared with artificial squint. *Journal of Neurophysiology, 28,* 1041–1059.

Hubel, D. H., & Wiesel, T. N. (1968). Receptive fields and functional architecture of monkey striate cortex. *Journal of Physiology, 195,* 215–243.

Jain, N., Florence, S. L., Qi, H. X., & Kaas, J. H. (2000). Growth of new brainstem connections in adult monkeys with massive sensory loss. *Proceedings of the National Academy of Sciences, USA, 97,* 5546–5550.

Johnson, J. K., & Casagrande, V. A. (1993). Prenatal development of axon outgrowth and connectivity in the ferret visual system. *Vision and Neuroscience, 10,* 117–130.

Jones, E. G., & Pons, T. P. (1998). Thalamic and brainstem contributions to large-scale plasticity of primate somatosensory cortex. *Science, 282,* 1121–1125.

Katz, L. C., & Crowley, J. C. (2002). Development of cortical circuits: Lessons from ocular dominance columns. *Nature Reviews: Neuroscience, 3,* 34–42.

Katz, L. C., & Shatz, C. J. (1996). Synaptic activity and the construction of cortical circuits. *Science, 274,* 1133–1138.

Kim, D. S., & Bonhoeffer, T. (1994). Reverse occlusion leads to a precise restoration of orientation preference maps in visual cortex. *Nature, 370,* 370–372.

Kujala, T., Alho, K., Huotilainen, M., Ilmoniemi, R. J., Lehtokoski, A., Leinonen, A., et al. (1997). Electrophysiological evidence for cross-modal plasticity in humans with early- and late-onset blindness. *Psychophysiology, 34,* 213–216.

Lowel, S. (1994). Ocular dominance column development: Strabismus changes the spacing of adjacent columns in cat visual cortex. *Journal of Neuroscience, 14,* 7451–7468.

Lowel, S., & Singer, W. (1992). Selection of intrinsic horizontal connections in the visual cortex by correlated neuronal activity. *Science, 255,* 209–212.

Lyckman, A. W., Jhaveri, S., Feldheim, D. A., Vanderhaeghen, P., Flanagan, J. G., & Sur, M. (2001). Enhanced plasticity of retinothalamic projections in an ephrin-A2/A5 double mutant. *Journal of Neuroscience, 21,* 7684–7690.

Meister, M., Wong, R. O., Baylor, D. A., & Shatz, C. J. (1991). Synchronous bursts of action potentials in ganglion cells of the developing mammalian retina. *Science, 252,* 939–943.

Merzenich, M. M., Nelson, R. J., Stryker, M. P., Cynader, M. S., Schoppmann, A., & Zook, J. M. (1984). Somatosensory cortical map changes following digit amputation in adult monkeys. *Journal of Comparative Neurology, 224,* 591–605.

Miller, K. D., Keller, J. B., & Stryker, M. P. (1989). Ocular dominance column development: Analysis and simulation. *Science, 245,* 605–615.

Neville, H. J., Schmidt, A., & Kutas, M. (1983). Altered visual-evoked potentials in congenitally deaf adults. *Brain Research, 266,* 127–132.

Pallas, S. L., Hahm, J., & Sur, M. (1994). Morphology of retinal axons induced to arborize in a novel target, the medial geniculate nucleus: I. Comparison with arbors in normal targets. *Journal of Comparative Neurology, 349,* 343–362.

Pallas, S. L., Roe, A. W., & Sur, M. (1990). Visual projections induced into the auditory pathway of ferrets: I. Novel inputs to primary auditory cortex (AI) from the LP/pulvinar complex and the topography of the MGN-AI projection. *Journal of Comparative Neurology, 298,* 50–68.

Pallas, S. L., & Sur, M. (1993). Visual projections induced into the auditory pathway of ferrets: II. Corticocortical connections of primary auditory cortex. *Journal of Comparative Neurology, 337,* 317–333.

Pallas, S. L., & Sur, M. (1994). Morphology of retinal axon arbors induced to arborize in a novel target, the medial geniculate nucleus: II. Comparison with axons from the inferior colliculus. *Journal of Comparative Neurology, 349,* 363–376.

Pons, T. P., Garraghty, P. E., Ommaya, A. K., Kaas, J. H., Taub, E., & Mishkin, M. (1991). Massive cortical reorganization after sensory deafferentation in adult macaques. *Science, 252,* 1857–1860.

Ramachandran, V. S., & Rogers-Ramachandran, D. (2000). Phantom limbs and neural plasticity. *Archives of Neurology, 57,* 317–320.

Read, H. L., Winer, J. A., & Schreiner, C. E. (2001). Modular organization of intrinsic connections associated with spectral tuning in cat auditory cortex. *Proceedings of the National Academy of Sciences, USA, 98,* 8042–8047.

Reiter, H. O., & Stryker, M. P. (1988). Neural plasticity without postsynaptic action potentials: Less-active inputs become dominant when kitten visual cortical cells are pharmacologically inhibited. *Proceedings of the National Academy of Sciences, USA, 85,* 3623–3627.

Roe, A. W., Garraghty, P. E., Esguerra, M., & Sur, M. (1993). Experimentally induced visual projections to the auditory thalamus in ferrets: Evidence for a W cell pathway. *Journal of Comparative Neurology, 334,* 263–280.

Roe, A. W., Hahm, J.-O., & Sur, M. (1991). Experimentally induced establishment of visual topography in auditory thalamus. *Society of Neuroscience Abstracts, 17,* 898.

Roe, A. W., Pallas, S. L., Hahm, J. O., & Sur, M. (1990). A map of visual space induced in primary auditory cortex. *Science, 250,* 818–820.

Roe, A. W., Pallas, S. L., Kwon, Y. H., & Sur, M. (1992). Visual projections routed to the auditory pathway in ferrets: Receptive fields of visual neurons in primary auditory cortex. *Journal of Neuroscience, 12,* 3651–3664.

Ruthazer, E. S., & Stryker, M. P. (1996). The role of activity in the development of long-range horizontal connections in area 17 of the ferret. *Journal of Neuroscience, 16,* 7253–7269.

Sadato, N., Pascual-Leone, A., Grafman, J., Ibanez, V., Deiber, M. P., Dold, G., et al. (1996). Activation of the primary visual cortex by Braille reading in blind subjects. *Nature, 380,* 526–528.

Schneider, G. E. (1973). Early lesions of superior colliculus: Factors affecting the formation of abnormal retinal projections. *Brain, Behavior and Evolution, 8,* 73–109.

Sharma, J., Angelucci, A., & Sur, M. (2000). Induction of visual orientation modules in auditory cortex. *Nature, 404,* 841–847.

Shatz, C. J., Lindstrom, S., & Wiesel, T. N. (1977). The distribution of afferents representing the right and left eyes in the cat's visual cortex. *Brain Research, 131,* 103–116.

Shatz, C. J., & Stryker, M. P. (1978). Ocular dominance in layer IV of the cat's visual cortex and the effects of monocular deprivation. *Journal of Physiology* (London), *281,* 267–283.

Sherman, S. M., & Spear, P. D. (1982). Organization of visual pathways in normal and visually deprived cats. *Physiological Review, 62,* 738–855.

Somers, D. C., Dragoi, V., & Sur, M. (2001). Orientation selectivity and its modulation by local and long-range connections in visual cortex. In A. Peters & B. Payne (Eds.), *Cerebral cortex: The cat primary visual cortex* (pp. 471–520). San Diego, CA: Academic Press.

Somers, D. C., Nelson, S. B., & Sur, M. (1995). An emergent model of orientation selectivity in cat visual cortical simple cells. *Journal of Neuroscience, 15,* 5448–5465.

Stellwagen, D., & Shatz, C. J. (2002). An instructive role for retinal waves in the development of retinogeniculate connectivity. *Neuron, 3,* 357–367.

Sur, M., Angelucci, A., & Sharma, J. (1999). Rewiring cortex: The role of patterned activity in development and plasticity of neocortical circuits. *Journal of Neurobiology, 41,* 33–43.

Sur, M., Garraghty, P. E., & Roe, A. W. (1988). Experimentally induced visual projections into auditory thalamus and cortex. *Science, 242,* 1437–1441.

Sur, M., & Leamey, C. A. (2001). Development and plasticity of cortical areas and networks. *Nature Reviews, Neuroscience, 2,* 251–262.

Sur, M., Pallas, S. L., & Roe, A. W. (1990). Cross-modal plasticity in cortical development: Differentiation and specification of sensory neocortex. *Trends in Neurosciences, 13,* 227–233.

Swindale, N. V., Shoham, D., Grinvald, A., Bonhoeffer, T., & Hubener, M. (2000). Visual cortex maps are optimized for uniform coverage. *Nature Neuroscience, 3,* 822–826.

Van Sluyters, R. C., & Levitt, F. B. (1980). Experimental strabismus in the kitten. *Journal of Neurophysiology, 43,* 686–699.

Vitek, D. J., Schall, J. D., & Leventhal, A. G. (1985). Morphology, central projections, and dendritic field orientation of retinal ganglion cells in the ferret. *Journal of Comparative Neurology, 241,* 1–11.

Von Melchner, L., Pallas, S. L., & Sur, M. (2000). Visual behaviour mediated by retinal projections directed to the auditory pathway. *Nature, 404,* 871–876.

Weeks, R., Horwitz, B., Aziz-Sultan, A., Tian, B., Wessinger, C. M., Cohen, L. G., et al. (2000). A positron emission tomographic study of auditory localization in the congenitally blind. *Journal of Neuroscience, 20,* 2664–2672.

Weliky, M., Bosking, W. H., & Fitzpatrick, D. (1996). A systematic map of direction preference in primary visual cortex. *Nature, 379,* 725–728.

Weliky, M., & Katz, L. C. (1997). Disruption of orientation tuning in visual cortex by artificially correlated neuronal activity. *Nature, 386,* 680–685.

Weliky, M., & Katz, L. C. (1999). Correlational structure of spontaneous neuronal activity in the developing lateral geniculate nucleus in vivo. *Science, 285,* 599–604.

White, L. E., Coppola, D. M., & Fitzpatrick, D. (2001). The contribution of sensory experience to the maturation of orientation selectivity in ferret visual cortex. *Nature, 411,* 1049–1052.

Wiesel, T. N., & Hubel, D. H. (1965). Comparison of the effects of unilateral and bilateral eye closure on cortical unit responses in kittens. *Journal of Neurophysiology, 28,* 1029–1040.

Wiesel, T. N., & Hubel, D. H. (1974). Ordered arrangement of orientation columns in monkeys lacking visual experience. *Journal of Comparative Neurology, 158,* 307–318.

43 Cross-Modal Consequences of Visual Deprivation in Animals

JOSEF P. RAUSCHECKER

Introduction

Anecdotal evidence abounds that blind people develop better capacities in their nondeprived sensory modalities than sighted individuals do. There are many examples of blind musicians. Louis Braille became blind at an early age and developed a tactile system for reading and writing that was later adopted the world over. Perhaps most famous is Helen Keller, who overcame deficits in both vision and hearing. As these examples suggest, the human brain seems to have the capacity to compensate for the loss of some sensory information by invoking other input channels.

However, the concept of cross-modal compensatory plasticity has not gone unchallenged. Early reports often claimed that individuals with blindness or deafness were generally impaired and had lower intelligence. Although such claims can in retrospect be dismissed as uncontrolled observations and most likely reflected additional neurological insults or birth defects that went undetected in prescientific medicine, another challenge to compensatory plasticity in the blind is more serious. A philosophical argument can be made that the concept of space in hearing (or perhaps any concept of space) depends largely on visual input (Fisher, 1964; Worchel, 1951). Supporters of such theories have often claimed an "innate dominance of vision over audition in the development and maintenance of sound localization" (Knudsen & Knudsen, 1989). Individuals who are blind from birth, therefore, should show impairments in sound localization, because the visual reference frame is missing.

Thus, we are left with two diametrically opposed viewpoints whose resolution requires empirical studies. In fact, the viewpoints seem almost mutually exclusive, so that a resolution one way or another should be straightforward. If the compensatory plasticity hypothesis holds, blind humans or animals should be just as good as sighted individuals (or even better) on any complex auditory task, and particularly on sound localization. If the general degradation hypothesis holds, blind individuals should show marked impairment in these capacities. An auxiliary argument can be made on the basis of comparisons between individuals who became blind early or late in life. Although early-blind individuals would be expected to have better-developed audition according to the compensatory plasticity hypothesis, late-blind individuals should have better audition according to the general degradation hypothesis, because they at least had a chance to build up an auditory space concept using vision while they were able to see early in their lives.

Auditory behavior in visually deprived mammals and blind humans

Qualitative observations in cats that were binocularly lid-sutured from birth for several months do not yield evidence of overt impairments in behavior, as they would be predicted as a consequence of the general degradation hypothesis. Quantitative measurements of sound localization behavior confirm this impression. Sound localization error was measured in a task that required cats to walk toward a sound source that varied randomly in azimuth location in order to get a food reward. The error was consistently smaller in visually deprived cats than in sighted controls (Rauschecker & Kniepert, 1994). The improvement was largest for lateral and rear positions of space, but even in straight-ahead positions, where the localization error is already small in normal controls, no deterioration by any means was found.

Identical results have been found in visually deprived ferrets (King & Parsons, 1999; King & Semple, 1996), thus confirming the results of the earlier studies in cats. Similar findings have also been reported for blind humans (Lessard, Pare, Leporé, & Lassonde, 1998; Muchnik, Efrati, Nemeth, Malin, & Hildesheimer, 1991; Röder et al., 1999). The study by Röder et al. confirmed the results of the animal studies in specific detail, in that it found the improvements to be most significant in lateral azimuth positions and no evidence of deterioration in straight-ahead positions. These recent studies also accord extremely well with the classic findings by Rice and colleagues, who analyzed the echolocation abilities of blind humans and found them to be improved, particularly in lateral positions of space (Rice, 1970; Rice, Feinstein, & Schusterman, 1965).

Lessard et al. (1998) add an interesting twist in that they demonstrate individuals who are partially blind to be worst on sound localization. The authors' interpretation was that a conflict of information is created by two different frames of reference in these individuals.

Behavioral observations in blind owls

In contrast to visually deprived cats, ferrets, and humans, barn owls that were visually deprived after hatching do not show the same kind of cross-modal compensation. On the contrary, "[s]ound localization behavior was significantly less precise in blind-reared owls than in normal owls" (Knudsen, Esterly, & du Lac, 1991). Thus, the results from this species seem to support the general degradation hypothesis, in which vision is indispensable for normal development of auditory spatial behavior and acts as the master, while audition is the slave.

Physiological and structural changes in the midbrain tectum

Neurophysiological and neuroanatomical studies in visually deprived barn owls have revealed severe structural changes in the midbrain tectum (superior colliculus, or SC)(Knudsen et al., 1991). Thus, the auditory behavioral deterioration of visually deprived owls seems to be a direct consequence of degradations in the circuitry of these midbrain nuclei, which are thought to govern sound localization behavior in amphibians, birds, and, to some extent, mammals. Indeed, topographic maps of auditory space have been found in the SC of owls (Knudsen & Konishi, 1978), ferrets, and guinea pigs (Palmer & King, 1982).

Similar structural degradations in the tectal auditory space map as in visually deprived owls have been found in visually deprived ferrets and guinea pigs (King & Carlile, 1993; Withington, 1992). Thus, we are now left with an interesting paradox in the latter two species: although the changes in the space map of the midbrain seem to support a general degradation hypothesis, the behavioral data from blind ferrets mentioned earlier (King & Parsons, 1999; King & Semple, 1996) clearly support the compensatory plasticity theory. Could it be that other, "higher" parts of the brain determine the sound localization behavior of ferrets (and mammals in general) to a greater extent than the midbrain SC?

Role of auditory cortex in sound localization

Lesions of auditory cortex in a number of mammalian species, including humans, result in severe deficits of sound localization behavior (Beitel & Kaas, 1993; Heffner & Heffner, 1990; Jenkins & Merzenich, 1984). While older studies assumed that primary auditory cortex (A1) itself was the locus of auditory space processing, more recent studies point to an involvement of nonprimary areas (Korte & Rauschecker, 1993; Middlebrooks, Clock, Xu, & Green, 1994). Analysis of the functional specialization of auditory cortical areas in the rhesus monkey suggests the existence of a processing stream for auditory space that originates in A1 and projects posteriorly (Rauschecker, 1998a, 1998b; Rauschecker & Tian, 2000; Recanzone, 2000; Tian, Reser, Durham, Kustov, & Rauschecker, 2001) and dorsally up to posterior parietal (PP) cortex and on to dorsolateral prefrontal (DLPF) cortex (Romanski et al., 1999). Both PP and DLPF have long been known to participate in spatial processing within the visual domain, but their involvement in auditory space processing is a more recent proposition (Rauschecker, 1998a, 1998b). These findings from animal studies are now supported by a growing body of evidence from functional neuroimaging work in humans as well (Alain, Arnot, Hevenor, Graham, & Grady, 2001; Bushara et al., 1999; Griffiths et al., 1998; Maeder et al., 2001; Warren, Zielinski, Green, Rauschecker, & Griffiths, 2002; Weeks et al., 1999; Zatorre, Bouffard, Ahad, & Belin, 2002).

Anterior ectosylvian cortex in normal and visually deprived cats

A possible functional homologue of primate PP cortex in cats is the anterior ectosylvian (AE) cortex in the anterior ectosylvian sulcus (AES). This conclusion can be drawn on the basis of both anatomical and physiological arguments. Anatomically, AES is the strongest source of auditory input to the SC (Meredith & Clemo, 1989). Physiologically, representations of the three main sensory modalities are found in close proximity to each other, with some overlap between them (Benedek, Mucke, Norita, Albowitz, & Creutzfeldt, 1988; Clarey & Irvine, 1990; Clemo & Stein, 1983; Jiang, Leporé, Ptito, & Guillemot, 1994; Mucke, Norita, Benedek, & Creutzfeldt, 1983; Olson & Graybiel, 1987).

In cats that were visually deprived from birth by means of binocular lid suture (and lids reopened for testing), the visual area (AEV) in the fundus of the AES had all but vanished. However, neurons in this region did not simply become unresponsive to sensory stimulation altogether. Instead, they were found to be briskly responsive to auditory and (to some extent) tactile stimulation. In other words, the neighboring auditory and somatosensory fields had expanded into the formerly visual territory, at the expense of area AEV (Rauschecker & Korte, 1993).

The response properties of the expanded anterior ectosylvian auditory area (AEA) in the AES of blind cats were similar to those of neighboring auditory fields. In particular, auditory spatial tuning (tuning for the location of a sound source in free field) was significantly sharper in the whole AE region than in sighted control animals (Korte & Rauschecker, 1993). Whereas the control group comprised roughly 50% spatially tuned cells (with a spatial tuning ratio of better than 2:1), the blind animals had close to 90% spatially specific auditory neurons in the AE region. In addition, neurons with spatial tuning ratios of 10:1 or better were much more common in blind cats.

The increased number of auditory neurons, together with their sharpened spatial filtering characteristics, is likely to improve the sampling density of auditory space and is thought to underlie the improved spatial abilities of early blind animals (Rauschecker, 1995). Sharper tuning does increase the efficiency of a population code, in the sense that fewer neurons are required to achieve a given acuity (Fitzpatrick, Batra, Stanford, & Kuwada, 1997). If the number of neurons increases, the resulting acuity increases, too. Related theoretical considerations lead to the conclusion that a tuning optimum for best performance can be found (Baldi & Heiligenberg, 1988), and it appears that the tuning values found in blind cats come closer to this optimum. The reason why this optimum is not reached in sighted cats lies in the limit on the number of auditory-responsive neurons imposed by the competing visual input.

Controversy between mammals and owls resolved?

The results in visually deprived cats, ferrets, and owls, taken together, permit only one conclusion. Sound localization behavior in blind owls seems to correlate with the state of the tectal space map. Although in visually deprived ferrets the auditory map of space in the midbrain tectum is perturbed as badly as in blind owls, sound localization behavior in visually deprived ferrets is normal or even improved, as it is in visually deprived cats. Thus, the degradation of the midbrain space map does not have a significant influence on the ferrets' behavior, which instead appears to be governed by cortical mechanisms, as demonstrated by the physiological data

from visually deprived cats. In other words, auditory spatial behavior is more "corticalized" in mammals than it is in birds, with their more limited forebrain volume. Although some influence of forebrain structures on auditory space processing can also be demonstrated in barn owls (Cohen, Miller, & Knudsen, 1998; Miller & Knudsen, 1999), their behavior seems more dominated by the evolutionarily older midbrain.

It is conceivable that different effects could be demonstrated with different behavioral tasks. More reflexive, automatic behaviors that inevitably depend more on midbrain structures might reveal detrimental effects of visual deprivation on spatial hearing also in mammals. Conversely, auditory behavior that involves memory or higher perceptual learning may eventually uncover compensatory mechanisms in owls. Generally speaking, the type of compensatory cross-modal reorganization described in this chapter is a domain of neocortex, with its highly plastic synaptic connections, possibly based on an abundance of NMDA receptors (Rauschecker, 1991). In fact, neocortex is so powerful in its effects on mammalian behavior that it is capable, in most overtly visible cases, of overruling and amending changes in subordinate structures. Clear corticofugal influences can even be demonstrated at the single-neuron level (Suga, Gao, Zhang, Ma, & Olsen, 2000).

Calibration signals for auditory space processing

The results in blind mammals, including humans, demonstrate unequivocally that vision is not necessary to establish precise spatial hearing. This is not to say that vision plays no role in cross-modal development, if it is available. Various lines of evidence, including the effects of prism rearing (Hyde & Knudsen, 2002; Knudsen & Knudsen, 1989; Kohler, 1964), do point to the powerful influence of vision on multisensory coordination and sensorimotor learning. However, vision is only one of several calibration signals that shape and fine-tune auditory spatial perception, and the absence of vision, therefore, does not jeopardize this process. Again, we may be dealing with a fundamental difference between the SC and the cerebral cortex. The former harbors a map of auditory space in its deeper layers that is in close communication with an overlying retinotopic visual map in its superficial layers. By contrast, space coding in the mammalian neocortex, especially the parietal areas, is achieved in body-centered coordinates, regardless of sensory modality (Andersen, 1997; Colby, 1998; Colby & Goldberg, 1999).

Several layers of calibration signals for auditory space processing in the cerebral cortex are available in the absence of vision (Lewald, 2002; Lewald, Foltys, & Topper, 2002; Lewald & Karnath, 2000). One of these signals is provided by proprioceptive feedback from muscle and joint receptors, which inform the auditory system about head and body position in space. Auditory motion also plays a role in spatial perception, as it does in the visual domain, by producing a shift or parallax signal. Cats that are visually deprived from birth develop new patterns of head and pinna movements (Rauschecker & Henning, 2001), which may help in generating both proprioceptive feedback and auditory motion parallax.

The fact that the scanning movements in blind cats are found exclusively along a vertical axis points to the possibility that different calibration signals may be used in azimuth and elevation, and the two dimensions could therefore be affected differently by loss of vision (Lewald & Ehrenstein, 2001). Sound localization in the vertical domain, which is largely accomplished by evaluating spectral cues originating from the head and pinnae (head-related transfer functions, HRTF), may depend more on calibration by vision than does sound localization in the horizontal domain, as it has been tested in most pertinent studies. Indeed, recent observations in blind humans indicate a somewhat lesser degree of compensation in elevation than in azimuth (Zwiers, Van Opstal, & Cruysberg, 2001).

Attentional modulation or structural reorganization?

Although the existence of compensatory plasticity in the blind has been disputed by some because of a postulated need for vision to calibrate auditory space perception, others have belittled it as an almost trivial phenomenon. Just as closing one's eyes or operating in the dark makes it easier to "concentrate" on the auditory modality, it has been argued, blindness improves certain aspects of hearing by focusing attention (more or less temporarily) on that modality. According to this view, cross-modal reassignment is nothing more than a task-dependent modulation of cortical circuitry, similar to a shift of attention.

There is no question that attention plays a role during the process of cross-modal reorganization, and short-term changes during blindfolding periods of a few days may indeed be related to task-dependent attentional modulation (Pascual-Leone & Hamilton, 2001). However, as deprivation persists, the neural circuitry is changed on a more permanent basis, as the above results from anesthetized animals show. Cortical reorganization is thought of as an activity-dependent process, and attention can certainly increase firing rates of participating neurons. Therefore, attentional

modulation may hasten cross-modal modifications and trigger the cascade of biochemical events that eventually lead to structural changes.

Unimodal training effects or cross-modal reassignment?

Another and related argument in these attempts to trivialize cross-modal compensatory plasticity has been to say that it "merely" reflects training effects in the nondeprived modalities, which of course must come to bear with the extended training periods that blind individuals spend on auditory and tactile tasks. Sighted individuals, if given the opportunity to practice as much as blind ones, would inevitably show the same amount of reorganization and improvement in performance. It is difficult to refute this logic, because studies in which a normal control group is forced to practice Braille, for instance, as much (and with the same motivation or attention!) as a blind group are difficult to perform.

It is indisputable that exercising one channel (in the case of blindness, audition or touch) helps with the refinement and expansion of that channel and its underlying neural machinery. The real question is whether silencing a competing channel, in this case vision, through deprivation helps even more. The available evidence suggests an unequivocal yes. Neonatal enucleation of mice or rats, for instance, leads to an expansion of somatosensory barrel cortex by up to 30% (Rauschecker, Tian, Korte, & Egert, 1992; Toldi, Farkas, & Volgyi, 1994). One might argue that the same effect could be achieved by unimodal activation of the whisker-barrel pathway in a tactile training paradigm. However, what this argument overlooks is that improvement of cognitive functions goes hand in hand with recruitment of additional neural resources, presumably an expansion of cortical tissue devoted to these functions (Merzenich, Recanzone, Jenkins, Allard, & Nudo, 1988; Merzenich & Sameshima, 1993). If one cortical area expands, then another must shrink and accordingly lose functionality, because the overall size of the cortex is fixed. Such a "zero-sum game" assumption may not be strictly true, but there can be no doubt that removing patterned input of one sort from a cortical system provides a competitive advantage to other potential sources of input.

Neural mechanisms of compensatory plasticity

The concept of competition between afferent input fibers for synaptic space on common target neurons is a central one in various types of plasticity, including studies of neuromuscular junction (Lichtman & Balice-Gordon,

1990), cerebellum (Sotelo, 1990), but above all developing visual cortex. The idea is that activating one input channel while silencing another hastens the increases in synaptic efficacy of the first one and helps drive down the other. Classical studies of ocular dominance plasticity (Wiesel & Hubel, 1963) are usually explained in those terms (Blakemore, Van Sluyters, & Movshon, 1976; Guillery & Stelzner, 1970).

Concretely, afferent fibers coming from different layers of the lateral geniculate nucleus (LGN), which carry activity from the left or right eye, respectively, are thought to compete for space on the postsynaptic membranes of cortical target neurons or for neurotrophic factors from the targets. At birth, the axonal arbors of the afferents are still diffuse and overlapping. During postnatal development, neuronal activity in the two pathways will lead to consolidation of synapses driven successfully by afferent activity. Lack of activity in the competing afferent pathway, while the postsynaptic neuron is being activated by other inputs, will lead not only to a lack of consolidation but also to an active elimination of the corresponding synapses from the target neurons.

Synaptic efficacy is based on both pre- and postsynaptic mechanisms, and both have been postulated to be modifiable as a result of neural activity. Particular consideration has classically been given to the conjunction of pre- and postsynaptic activation (Rauschecker, 1991; Singer, 1995), as proposed by Hebb (1949). Hebb's rules can be modified to accommodate the concept of competition between different neural input systems, resulting in what is sometimes referred to as an "anti-Hebb" rule.

The concept of competition has later been extended to accommodate cross-modal plasticity as well (Rauschecker, 1996, 1997). Competing pathways now consist of afferents from different sensory systems converging on target neurons in multimodal regions of cerebral cortex, such as the cat's anterior ectosylvian cortex (AEC). By analogy, much overlap exists at birth between representations of, e.g., visual and auditory inputs in AEC (Rauschecker, 1995). This overlap is reduced during normal development; with early blindness, however, competition leads to an overrepresentation of auditory compared to visual input, as described earlier in this chapter.

This massive expansion of nonvisual domains into formerly visual territory suggests an actual reassignment of visual cortical resources to the auditory (and somatosensory) modalities (Rauschecker & Korte, 1993; Hyvärinen et al., 1981). Because the long-term results of this cross-modal reassignment can be measured in anesthetized animals, which are not prone to shifts of attention, it must be based on changes in the "hard-ware" of these cortical areas rather than on temporary, task-dependent modulations of cortical circuitry. This is not to say that short-term changes of the kind described recently by Pascual-Leone and colleagues (Kauffman, Theoret, & Pascual-Leone, 2002; Pascual-Leone & Hamilton, 2001) cannot take place as temporary alterations of cortical circuitry. Short-term changes may be converted into long-term changes by cascades of molecular and biochemical processes.

Despite decades of research the actual nature of any of these circuitry changes is presently still unclear. Short-term changes could simply consist of modulations of synaptic transmission by various neuromodulatory agents, such as actylcholine and noradrenaline (Edeline, 2003). This would require that circuitry underlying both sets of connectivity is pre-existing and is only shifted between different states. In other words, many more connections would have to exist than are overtly visible with recording of suprathreshold activity, and brain regions classically assumed to be unimodal would in fact have to be multi- or metamodal according to this concept (Pascual-Leone & Hamilton, 2001). Recent anatomical studies with more sensitive tracers in nonhuman primates have indeed revealed previously undocumented projections from auditory to visual cortex (Falchier et al., 2002; Rockland & Ojima, 2003). These projections may only be the tip of the iceberg in a metamodal brain. Backprojections from multimodal brain regions, e.g., frontal or parietal cortex, by definition also carry a multimodal signal, which would render "unimodal" areas in fact multimodal.

Unmasking of existing connections has also been postulated for some time as a possible substrate in other cases of cortical plasticity because of their apparent speed with which they happen. Long-term changes in the actual hardware may include not only synaptic weight changes or unmasking of preexisting connections but also sprouting of new connections, permanent pruning of axonal and dendritic arbors, synapse creation and elimination, or all of the above (Florence & Kaas, 1995; Gilbert et al., 1996; Jones, 2000; Raineteau & Schwab, 2001). A view of the brain's circuitry as undergoing constant remodeling and restructuring is probably not far off the mark. Although the basic layout with its macroscopic design in terms of lobes, areas, and even columnar organization may be genetically determined, the fine structure in terms of synaptic connections is highly plastic and in permanent flux, even in adult brains, as long as they still respond to experience and learning.

ACKNOWLEDGMENTS Substantial portions of the text appeared in slightly different form in Rauschecker (2002, 2003) and are reproduced here by permission of the publishers.

REFERENCES

Alain, C., Arnott, S. R., Hevenor, S., Graham, S., & Grady, C. L. (2001). "What" and "where" in the human auditory system. *Proceedings of the National Academy of Sciences, USA, 98,* 12301–12306.

Andersen, R. A. (1997). Multimodal integration for the representation of space in the posterior parietal cortex. *Philosophical Transactions of the Royal Society of London, Series B: Biological Sciences, 352,* 1421–1428.

Baldi, P., & Heiligenberg, W. (1988). How sensory maps could enhance resolution through ordered arrangements of broadly tuned receivers. *Biology and Cybernetics, 59,* 313–318.

Beitel, R. E., & Kaas, J. H. (1993). Effects of bilateral and unilateral ablation of auditory cortex in cats on the unconditioned head orienting response to acoustic stimuli. *Journal of Neurophysiology, 70,* 351–369.

Benedek, G., Mucke, L., Norita, M., Albowitz, B., & Creutzfeldt, O. D. (1988). Anterior ectosylvian visual area (AEV) of the cat: Physiological properties. *Progress in Brain Research, 75,* 245–255.

Blakemore, C., Van Sluyters, C. V., & Movshon, J. A. (1976). Synaptic competition in the kitten's visual cortex. *Cold Spring Harbor Symposia on Quantitative Biology, 40,* 601–609.

Bushara, K. O., Weeks, R. A., Ishii, K., Catalan, M.-J., Tian, B., Rauschecker, J. P., et al. (1999). Modality-specific frontal and parietal areas for auditory and visual spatial localization in humans. *Nature Neuroscience, 2,* 759–766.

Clarey, J. C., & Irvine, D. R. F. (1990). The anterior ectosylvian sulcal auditory field in the cat: I. An electrophysiological study of its relationship to surrounding auditory cortical fields. *Journal of Comparative Neurology, 301,* 289–303.

Clemo, H. R., & Stein, B. E. (1983). Organization of a fourth somatosensory area of cortex in cat. *Journal of Neurophysiology, 50,* 910–923.

Cohen, Y. E., Miller, G. L., & Knudsen, E. I. (1998). Forebrain pathway for auditory space processing in the barn owl. *Journal of Neurophysiology, 79,* 891–902.

Colby, C. L. (1998). Action-oriented spatial reference frames in cortex. *Neuron, 20,* 15–24.

Colby, C. L., & Goldberg, M. E. (1999). Space and attention in parietal cortex. *Annual Review of Neuroscience, 22,* 319–349.

Edeline, J. M. (2003). The thalamo-cortical auditory receptive fields: Regulation by the states of vigilance, learning and the neuromodulatory systems. *Experimental Brain Research, 153,* 554–572.

Falchier, A., Clavagnier, S., Barone, P., and Kennedy, H. (2002). Anatomical evidence of multimodal integration in primate striate cortex. *Journal of Neuroscience, 22,* 5749–5759.

Fisher, G. H. (1964). Spatial localization by the blind. *American Journal of Psychology, 77,* 2–133.

Fitzpatrick, D. C., Batra, R., Stanford, T. R., & Kuwada, S. (1997). A neuronal population code for sound localization. *Nature, 388,* 871–874.

Florence, S. L., & Kaas, J. H. (1995). Large-scale reorganization at multiple levels of the somatosensory pathway follows therapeutic amputation of the hand in monkeys. *Journal of Neuroscience, 15,* 8083–8095.

Gilbert, C. D., Das, A., Ito, M., Kapadia, M., & Westheimer, G. (1996). Spatial integration and cortical dynamics. *Proceedings of the National Academy of Sciences, USA, 93,* 615–622.

Griffiths, T. D., Rees, G., Rees, A., Green, G. G., Witton, C., Rowe, D., et al. (1998). Right parietal cortex is involved in the perception of sound movement in humans. *Nature Neuroscience, 1,* 74–79.

Guillery, R. W., & Stelzner, D. J. (1970). The differential effects of unilateral lid closure upon the monocular and binocular segments of the dorsal lateral geniculate nucleus in the cat. *Journal of Comparative Neurology, 139,* 413–421.

Hebb, D. O. (1949). *The organization of behavior.* New York: Wiley.

Heffner, H. E., & Heffner, R. S. (1990). Effect of bilateral auditory cortex lesions on sound localization in Japanese macaques. *Journal of Neurophysiology, 64,* 915–931.

Hyde, P. S., & Knudsen, E. I. (2002). The optic tectum controls visually guided adaptive plasticity in the owl's auditory space map. *Nature, 415,* 73–76.

Hyvärinen, J., Carlson, S., & Hyvärinen, L. (1981). Early visual deprivation alters modality of neuronal responses in area 19 of monkey cortex. *Neuroscience Letters, 4,* 239–243.

Jenkins, W. M., & Merzenich, M. M. (1984). Role of cat primary auditory cortex for sound-localization behavior. *Journal of Neurophysiology, 52,* 819–847.

Jiang, H., Leporé, F., Ptito, M., & Guillemot, J. P. (1994). Sensory modality distribution in the anterior ectosylvian cortex (AEC) of cats. *Experimental Brain Research, 97,* 404–414.

Jones, E. G. (2000). Cortical and subcortical contributions to activity-dependent plasticity in primate somatosensory cortex. *Annual Review of Neuroscience, 23,* 1–37, 2000.

Kauffman, T., Theoret, H., & Pascual-Leone, A. (2002). Braille character, discrimination in blindfolded human subjects. *Neuroreport, 13,* 571–574.

King, A. J., & Carlile, S. (1993). Changes induced in the representation of auditory space in the superior colliculus by rearing ferrets with binocular eyelid suture. *Experimental Brain Research, 94,* 444–455.

King, A. J., & Parsons, C. (1999). Improved auditory spatial acuity in visually deprived ferrets. *European Journal of Neuroscience, 11,* 3945–3956.

King, A. J., & Semple, D. J. (1996). Improvement in auditory spatial acuity following early visual deprivation in ferrets. *Society for Neuroscience Abstracts.*

Knudsen, E. I., Esterly, S. D., & du Lac, S. (1991). Stretched and upside-down maps of auditory space in the optic tectum of blind-reared owls: Acoustic basis and behavioral correlates. *Journal of Neuroscience, 11,* 1727–1747.

Knudsen, E. I., & Knudsen, P. F. (1989). Vision calibrates sound localization in developing barn owls. *Journal of Neuroscience, 9,* 3306–3313.

Knudsen, E. I., & Konishi, M. (1978). A neural map of auditory space in the owl. *Science, 200,* 795–797.

Kohler, I. (1964). *The formation and transformation of the perceptual world* [*Über Aufbau und Wandlungen der Wahrnehmungswelt,* R. M. Rohrer, Vienna, 1951]. Vienna: International Universities Press.

Korte, M., & Rauschecker, J. P. (1993). Auditory spatial tuning of cortical neurons is sharpened in cats with early blindness. *Journal of Neurophysiology, 70,* 1717–1721.

Lessard, N., Pare, M., Leporé, F., & Lassonde, M. (1998). Early-blind human subjects localize sound sources better than sighted subjects. *Nature, 395,* 278–280.

Lewald, J. (2002). Opposing effects of head position on sound localization in blind and sighted human subjects. *European Journal of Neuroscience, 15,* 1219–1224.

Lewald, J., & Ehrenstein, W. H. (2001). Effect of gaze direction on sound localization in rear space. *Neuroscience Research, 39,* 253–257.

Lewald, J., Foltys, H., & Topper, R. (2002). Role of the posterior parietal cortex in spatial hearing. *Journal of Neuroscience, 22,* RC207.

Lewald, J., & Karnath, H. O. (2000). Vestibular influence on human auditory space perception. *Journal of Neurophysiology, 84,* 1107–1111.

Lichtman, J. W., & Balice-Gordon, R. J. (1990). Understanding synaptic competition in theory and in practice. *Journal of Neurobiology, 21,* 99–106.

Maeder, P. P., Meuli, R. A., Adriani, M., Bellmann, A., Fornari, E., Thiran, J. P., et al. (2001). Distinct pathways involved in sound recognition and localization: A human fMRI study. *NeuroImage, 14,* 802–816.

Meredith, M. A., & Clemo, H. R. (1989). Auditory cortical projection from the anterior ectosylvian sulcus (Field AES) to the superior colliculus in the cat: An anatomical and electrophysiological study. *Journal of Comparative Neurology, 289,* 687–707.

Merzenich, M. M., Recanzone, G., Jenkins, W. M., Allard, T. T., & Nudo, R. J. (1988). Cortical representational plasticity. In P. Rakic & W. Singer (Eds.), *Neurobiology of neocortex,* (pp. 41–67). New York: Wiley.

Merzenich, M. M., & Sameshima, K. (1993). Cortical plasticity and memory. *Current Opinion in Neurobiology, 3,* 187–196.

Middlebrooks, J. C., Clock, A. E., Xu, L., & Green, D. M. (1994). A panoramic code for sound location by cortical neurons. *Science, 264,* 842–844.

Miller, G. L., & Knudsen, E. I. (1999). Early visual experience shapes the representation of auditory space in the forebrain gaze fields of the barn owl. *Journal of Neuroscience, 19,* 2326–2336.

Muchnik, C., Efrati, M., Nemeth, E., Malin, M., & Hildesheimer, M. (1991). Central auditory skills in blind and sighted subjects. *Scandinavian Audiology, 20,* 19–23.

Mucke, L., Norita, M., Benedek, G., & Creutzfeldt, O. D. (1983). Physiologic and anatomic investigation of visual cortical area situated in the ventral bank of the anterior ectosylvian sulcus of the cat. *Experimental Brain Research, 46,* 1–11.

Olson, C. R., & Graybiel, A. M. (1987). Ectosylvian visual area of the cat: Location, retinotopic organization, and connections. *Journal of Comparative Neurology, 261,* 277–294.

Palmer, A. R., & King, A. J. (1982). The representation of auditory space in the mammalian superior colliculus. *Nature, 299,* 248–249.

Pascual-Leone, A., & Hamilton, R. (2001). The metamodal organization of the brain. *Progress in Brain Research, 134,* 427–445.

Raineteau, O., & Schwab, M. E. (2001). Plasticity of motor systems after incomplete spinal cord injury. *Nature Reviews Neuroscience, 2,* 263–273.

Rauschecker, J. P. (1991). Mechanisms of visual plasticity: Hebb synapses, NMDA receptors and beyond. *Physiological Review, 71,* 587–615.

Rauschecker, J. P. (1995). Compensatory plasticity and sensory substitution in the cerebral cortex. *Trends in Neurosciences, 18,* 36–43.

Rauschecker, J. P. (1996). Substitution of visual by auditory inputs in the cat's anterior ectosylvian cortex. *Progress in Brain Research, 112,* 313–323.

Rauschecker, J. P. (1997). Mechanisms of compensatory plasticity in the cerebral cortex. In H.-J. Freund, B. A. Sabel, & O. W. Witte (Eds.), *Brain plasticity. Advances in Neurology, 73,* 137–146.

Rauschecker, J. P. (1998a). Cortical processing of complex sounds. *Current Opinion in Neurobiology, 8,* 516–521.

Rauschecker, J. P. (1998b). Parallel processing in the auditory cortex of primates. *Audiology & Neuro-otology, 3,* 86–103.

Rauschecker, J. P. (2002). Cortical map plasticity in animals and humans. *Progress in Brain Research, 138,* 73–88.

Rauschecker, J. P. (2003). Auditory reassignment. In *Handbook of neuropsychology* (2nd ed.), *Vol. 9: Plasticity and rehabilitation.* (F. Boller & J. Grafman, vol. eds.) (pp. 167–176). Amsterdam: Elsevier.

Rauschecker, J. P., & Henning, P. (2001). Crossmodal expansion of cortical maps in early blindness. In J. Kaas (Ed.), *The mutable brain* (pp. 243–259). Singapore: Harwood Academic Publishers.

Rauschecker, J. P., & Kniepert, U. (1994). Enhanced precision of auditory localization behavior in visually deprived cats. *European Journal of Neuroscience, 6,* 149–160.

Rauschecker, J. P., & Korte, M. (1993). Auditory compensation for early blindness in cat cerebral cortex. *Journal of Neuroscience, 13,* 4538–4548.

Rauschecker, J. P., & Tian, B. (2000). Mechanisms and streams for processing of "what" and "where" in auditory cortex. *Proceedings of the National Academy of Sciences, USA, 97,* 11800–11806.

Rauschecker, J. P., Tian, B., Korte, M., & Egert, U. (1992). Crossmodal changes in the somatosensory vibrissa/barrel system of visually deprived animals. *Proceedings of the National Academy of Sciences, USA, 89,* 5063–5067.

Recanzone, G. H. (2000). Spatial processing in the auditory cortex of the macaque monkey. *Proceedings of the National Academy of Sciences, USA, 97,* 11829–11835.

Rice, C. E. (1970). Early blindness, early experience, and perceptual enhancement. *Research Bulletin of the American Foundation for the Blind, 22,* 1–22.

Rice, C. E., Feinstein, S. H., & Schusterman, R. J. (1965). Echo-detection ability of the blind: Size and distance factor. *Journal of Experimental Psychology, 70,* 246–251.

Rockland, K. S., & Ojima, H. (2003). Multisensory convergence in calcarine visual areas in macaque monkey. *International Journal of Psychophysiology, 50,* 19–26.

Röder, B., Teder-Sälejärvi, W., Sterr, A., Rösler, F., Hillyard, S. A., & Neville, H. J. (1999). Improved auditory spatial tuning in blind humans. *Nature, 400,* 162–166.

Romanski, L. M., Tian, B., Fritz, J., Mishkin, M., Goldman-Rakic, P. S., & Rauschecker, J. P. (1999). Dual streams of auditory afferents target multiple domains in the primate prefrontal cortex. *Nature Neuroscience, 2,* 1131–1136.

Singer, W. (1995). Development and plasticity of cortical processing architectures. *Science, 270,* 758–764.

Sotelo, C. (1990). Cerebellar synaptogenesis: What we can learn from mutant mice. *Journal of Experimental Biology, 153,* 225–249.

Suga, N., Gao, E., Zhang, Y., Ma, X., & Olsen, J. F. (2000). The corticofugal system for hearing: Recent progress. *Proceedings of the National Academy of Sciences, USA, 97,* 11807–11814.

Tian, B., Reser, D., Durham, A., Kustov, A., & Rauschecker, J. P. (2001). Functional specialization in rhesus monkey auditory cortex. *Science, 292,* 290–293.

Toldi, J., Farkas, T., & Volgyi, B. (1994). Neonatal enucleation induces cross-modal changes in the barrel cortex of rat: A behavioural and electrophysiological study. *Neuroscience Letters, 167,* 1–4.

Warren, J. D., Zielinski, B. A., Green, G. G. R., Rauschecker, J. P., & Griffiths, T. D. (2002). Analysis of sound source motion by the human brain. *Neuron, 34,* 1–20.

Weeks, R., Horwitz, B., Aziz-Sultan, A., Tian, B., Wessinger, C. M., Cohen, L., et al. (2000). A positron emission tomographic study of auditory localisation in the congenitally blind. *Journal of Neuroscience, 20,* 2664–2672.

Weeks, R. A., Aziz-Sultan, A., Bushara, K. O., Tian, B., Wessinger, C. M., Dang, N., et al. (1999). A PET study of human auditory spatial processing. *Neuroscience Letters, 262,* 155–158.

Wiesel, T. N., Hubel, D. H. (1963). Single-cell responses in striate cortex of kittens deprived of vision in one eye. *Journal of Neurophysiology, 26,* 1003–1017.

Withington, D. J. (1992). The effect of binocular lid suture on auditory responses in the guinea-pig superior colliculus. *Neuroscience Letters, 136,* 153–156.

Worchel, P. (1951). Space perception and orientation in the blind. *Psychological Monographs, 65,* 1–28.

Zatorre, R. J., Bouffard, M., Ahad, P., & Belin, P. (2002). Where is "where" in the human auditory cortex? *Nature Neuroscience, 5,* 905–909.

Zwiers, M. P., Van Opstal, A. J., & Cruysberg, J. R. (2001). Two-dimensional sound-localization behavior of early-blind humans. *Experimental Brain Research, 140,* 206–222.

44 Visual Cortical Involvement in Normal Tactile Perception

K. SATHIAN, S. C. PRATHER, AND M. ZHANG

Introduction

Over the past few years, increasing evidence has been accumulating that visual cortical areas are closely involved in certain aspects of normal tactile perception. Such findings of cross-modal cortical recruitment challenge the notion that the senses are rigidly distinct from one another, emphasizing instead their close-knit nature. In this chapter we review the empirical evidence for visual cortical involvement in tactile perception in normally sighted humans. This evidence stems from functional neuroimaging studies in humans, which have shown that visual cortical regions are recruited during a number of tactile tasks and in a manner that is highly task-specific. Studies of the sighted and of individuals with visual deprivation of long (see Fridman, Celnik, & Cohen, Chap. 45, this volume) or short term are mutually complementary.

Visual cortical involvement in tactile discrimination of grating orientation

In a task that is frequently used to study tactile spatial acuity (Sathian & Zangaladze, 1996; van Boven & Johnson, 1994a, 1994b), plastic gratings consisting of alternating ridges and grooves of equal width are applied to the fingerpad and subjects are asked to discriminate whether the gratings are oriented along or across the finger. We employed this task in a positron emission tomographic (PET) study in normally sighted humans (Sathian, Zangaladze, Hoffman, & Grafton, 1997). The hand-held gratings, oriented either along or across the long axis of the finger, were applied to the immobilized right index fingerpad. There were two main tasks. In the experimental task, subjects reported grating orientation and ignored grating dimensions. In a control task, they ignored grating orientation and reported whether the grooves were wide or narrow (spacing task). By using identical stimuli in both tasks, we controlled for basic somatosensory processing. A subtraction approach (orientation minus spacing) was adopted to reveal brain regions more active in the grating orientation task than in the spacing task. Subtraction images revealed activation at a single focus, located in a region of left extrastriate visual cortex, close to the parieto-occipital fissure (Fig. 44.1). This study was the first to report activity in a visual cortical area during a tactile task in the sighted.

The parieto-occipital locus had previously been shown to be active during visual discrimination of grating orientation (Sergent, Ohta, & MacDonald, 1992) and other tasks requiring spatial mental imagery (Mellet et al., 1996). Hence, we suggested (Sathian et al., 1997) that it is involved in visuospatial processes common to tactile and visual orientation discrimination. Although it remains uncertain which area of macaque cerebral cortex is homologous to this human cortical region, its location in the vicinity of the parieto-occipital fissure suggests that it may be the counterpart of an area in the macaque parieto-occipital fissure known as V6 or PO, in which a high proportion of neurons are orientation-selective (Galletti, Battaglini, & Fattori, 1991).

To rule out the possibility that visual cortical activation in our task was merely an epiphenomenon, we proceeded to use transcranial magnetic stimulation (TMS) to test whether blocking visual cortical processing disrupts tactile perception. Earlier studies had shown that focal TMS over occipital cortex could transiently interfere with visual perception (Amassian et al., 1989; Epstein, Verson, & Zangaladze, 1996; Epstein & Zangaladze, 1996). In our TMS study (Zangaladze, Epstein, Grafton, & Sathian, 1999), an electromechanical device was used to apply gratings to the immobilized right index fingerpad of subjects with normal vision. As in the PET study, the gratings were oriented either along or across the long axis of the finger, and subjects were required to discriminate grating orientation in the experimental task. The control task involved discrimination of grating spacing. Single-pulse TMS was applied over a number of scalp locations using a magnetic stimulator with a high-efficiency iron-core coil. A variable delay circuit was used to deliver TMS at particular delays following the onset of the tactile stimulus. TMS applied at certain occipital sites significantly disrupted

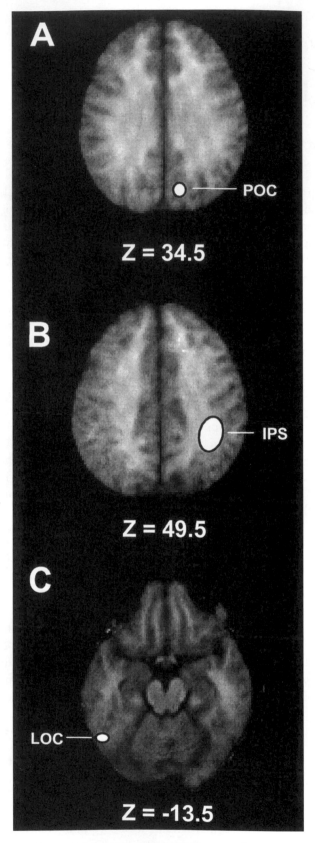

performance on the orientation task, with a peak effect at a delay of 180 ms. The effect of TMS was spatially restricted over the scalp. It was present directly over the locus of PET activation in the left hemisphere and at sites close to it, but not at more distant sites. Computation of the presumptive boundaries of the physiological effects of TMS in the cerebral cortex (the isopotential lines, corresponding to 90% of the motor threshold, of the calculated electric field induced in the brain by TMS) indicated that the PET activation locus was within these boundaries for TMS at effective sites but not ineffective sites. This observation is consistent with the idea that the left hemisphere locus identified in our PET study (Sathian et al., 1997) is critical for tactile discrimination of orientation. Crucially, the effect was specific for the orientation task, because TMS at any of the occipital sites tested had no effect on discrimination of grating spacing.

When TMS was delivered over primary somatosensory cortex at a 30 ms delay, its effect was nonspecific, impairing both orientation and spacing discrimination. This observation is not surprising, because interfering with somatosensory cortical function should disrupt processing of all tactile input. In contrast, occipital TMS specifically interfered with orientation and not spacing discrimination. Subjective reports were consistent with the effects of TMS on performance. During occipital TMS, subjects reported feeling the grating but being unsure about its orientation (but not spacing). However, during TMS over primary somatosensory cortex, they had difficulty even feeling the grating. This study (Zangaladze et al., 1999) was the first to indicate that the activity of extrastriate visual cortex during tactile perception is not just an epiphenomenon but is essential for optimal tactile performance.

Visual cortical activation during perception and mental rotation of two-dimensional tactile forms

We were interested in whether recruitment of visual cortical processing during tactile perception generalizes to other tasks. To address this question, we performed

FIGURE 44.1   Sites in extrastriate visual cortex that were active during tactile tasks in PET studies from our laboratory, displayed on horizontal anatomic MR slices of an image derived by averaging across a number of normal brains. Radiologic convention is used, so that the right hemisphere is on the left, and vice versa. Talairach z values (Talairach & Tournoux, 1988) are shown below each slice. Only approximate regions of activation are illustrated here. Full details can be found in the original reports. (A) Left parieto-occipital cortical (POC) activation for discrimination of grating orientation versus spacing. (B) Left intraparietal sulcus (IPS) activation for mental rotation versus mirror-image discrimination. (C) Right lateral occipital complex (LOC) activation for discrimination of global two-dimensional form versus bar orientation.

another PET study (Prather, Votaw, & Sathian, 2002) using a variety of two-dimensional form stimuli presented again to the immobilized fingerpad of subjects with normal vision while the subjects were engaged in perceptual tasks. So as not to bias processing toward the visual domain, we took care that subjects never saw the stimuli used in these studies. (In the PET study of grating orientation discrimination, subjects had seen the stimuli prior to tactile stimulation.) One task of particular interest was discrimination between mirror-image stimuli. It is well known that, when subjects perform this task with visually presented stimuli, their response times increase as a function of the angular disparity between the pair of stimuli presented (Shepard & Metzler, 1971). This phenomenon is considered to indicate that subjects mentally rotate the image of one member of the pair to bring it into congruence with the other before making a perceptual decision. Thus, it is a task calling for mental imagery. Similar findings have been obtained with tactually presented stimuli (Marmor & Zaback, 1976; Prather & Sathian, 2002).

In the PET study, the stimulus used was the upside-down letter J. The stimulus angle with respect to the long axis of the finger was either 0 degrees (pure mirror-image discrimination condition) or quite large (135–180 degrees, mental rotation condition). Mirror-image discrimination was required by asking subjects to report which of two mirror-image configurations they perceived. In the mental rotation condition, subjects were explicitly asked to mentally rotate the stimulus into the canonical orientation (0 degrees) before reporting their decision. Subjects reported that they did, in fact, mentally rotate in this condition. This subjective report was confirmed psychophysically by finding longer response times for the mental rotation condition compared to the mirror-image condition. Additional conditions in this PET study included a global form condition, in which subjects were asked to distinguish between the upside-down letters T and V; a condition requiring detection of microspatial detail, in which subjects reported whether or not a bar, oriented along the finger, contained a gap (measuring 3 or 4 mm); and an orientation condition, in which subjects reported whether a bar was oriented along the long axis of the fingerpad or at a 45-degree angle to it.

In this study, the mental rotation condition consistently yielded an active region in the left superior parietal cortex near the intraparietal sulcus (Fig. 44.1), when contrasted with any of the other conditions. This focus in the *dorsal* visual pathway is also active during mental rotation of visual stimuli (Alivisatos & Petrides, 1997), consistent with the notion that multisensory parietal regions support the complex spatial transformations involved in

mental rotation and mirror-image discrimination and in agreement with earlier electrophysiological findings for tactile stimuli (Röder, Rösler, & Hennighausen, 1997). Relative to the orientation condition, the form condition recruited a focus in the right occipitotemporal region (Fig. 44.1) within the lateral occipital complex (LOC), a visual object-selective region in the *ventral* visual pathway (Malach et al., 1995) that appears to be homologous with macaque inferotemporal cortex (Grill-Spector et al., 1998). Thus, the findings of this PET study (Prather et al., 2004) indicate that recruitment of extrastriate visual cortex during tactile perception parallels the general organization of visual information flow into a dorsal cortical pathway for spatial processing and into a ventral cortical pathway for form processing (Mishkin, Ungerleider, & Macko, 1983; Ungerleider & Haxby, 1994), and the specific segregation of mental rotation and object recognition of visual stimuli in dorsal versus ventral visual areas, respectively (Gauthier et al., 2002).

Next, we asked whether the presence or extent of visual cortical recruitment during tactile perception depends on spatial scale. Tactile features can be categorized (Grant, Thiagarajah, & Sathian, 2000; Roland & Mortensen, 1987) as macrospatial (e.g., shape, size, orientation) or microspatial (e.g., surface texture, irregularities). Vision is superior to touch in analyzing macrospatial features, whereas the reverse is true for microspatial features (Heller, 1989). Further, as reviewed earlier in this chapter, tactile discrimination of grating orientation, a macrospatial task, recruits visual cortical activity that is functionally relevant to performance, but tactile discrimination of grating spacing, a microspatial task, does not (Sathian et al., 1997; Zangaladze et al., 1999). Hence, macrospatial tactile tasks might be preferentially associated with visual processing, as suggested by others (Klatzky, Lederman, & Reed, 1987). To further test this idea, we used the global form discrimination and gap detection tasks described above in a study (Stoesz et al., 2003) using functional magnetic resonance imaging (fMRI). Compared with a baseline rest condition, activity was present bilaterally in the LOC during the (macrospatial) form discrimination task but not in the (microspatial) gap detection task. A direct contrast between the tasks confirmed that LOC activity was greater during the former task than during the latter task (Fig. 44.2). LOC activity was greater on the right side than on the left, even though stimuli were presented to the right hand. Thus, this fMRI study (Stoesz et al., 2003), together with our first PET study (Sathian et al., 1997), indicates that macrospatial tactile tasks are indeed more effective at recruiting extrastriate visual cortex than microspatial tasks.

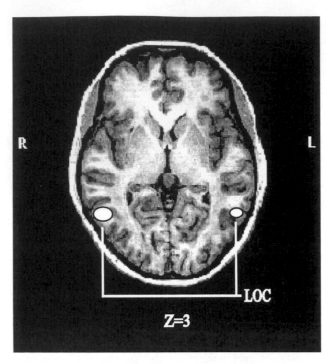

FIGURE 44. 2   Bilateral activations in the lateral occipital complex (LOC) during global two-dimensional form discrimination contrasted with gap detection in an fMRI study from our laboratory. Activations are displayed on a horizontal slice through an anatomic MR image from a single subject. Other details as in Figure 44.1.

Visual cortical activation during tactile perception of three-dimensional forms

A number of fMRI studies have revealed that visual cortical areas are also active when normal subjects engage in active haptic exploration of objects in three dimensions, with the goal of object identification. In the first of these studies (Deibert, Kraut, Kremen, & Hart, 1999), haptic object recognition was contrasted with haptic texture discrimination. This study found activity in occipital cortex, including both striate and extrastriate areas. Activation was bilateral although only the right hand was used for haptic exploration. Another group reported that selectivity in the LOC for objects compared to textures, originally described for visual stimuli (Malach et al., 1995), also extended to haptic stimuli, with a subregion of the LOC being active during both visual and haptic presentations (Amedi, Jacobson, Hendler, Malach, & Zohary, 2001). Such multisensory activity tended to be associated with a preference for graspable visual objects over other visual stimuli (Amedi, Malach, Hendler, Peled, & Zohary, 2002). LOC activity was again bilateral even though only the right hand was used in the haptic conditions (Amedi et al., 2001, 2002). The LOC appears to be specifically concerned with object shape,

since it was not activated by object-specific sounds (Amedi et al., 2002), although object identification from auditory cues was not explicitly called for in this study.

The overlap of activity in the LOC during visual and haptic exploration of objects was confirmed by another group (James et al., 2002). In this study, haptic exploration was bimanual and, not surprisingly, LOC activity was bilateral. Further, both visual and haptic exploration appear to engage a common neural representation, since cross-modal priming effects have been described in two fMRI studies. Amedi et al. (2001) reported that haptic object exploration evoked a smaller fMRI signal in the LOC for previously seen objects, compared to previously unseen ones. This is analogous to priming effects in the LOC within the visual modality (Grill-Spector et al., 1999). James et al. (2002) reported fMRI priming effects in the opposite direction, with *greater* LOC activity during vision of previously explored objects: the magnitude of such neural priming was similar for prior visual and haptic exposure. The reason for the unusual direction of the priming effect in the latter study is not clear; the authors attributed it to their use of novel objects. Regardless, these two studies indicate the presence of cross-modal neural priming effects. These neural effects may be related to psychophysical observations that cross-modal visuohaptic priming can be as effective as within-modality priming (Easton, Greene, & Srinivas, 1997; Easton, Srinivas, & Greene, 1997; Reales & Ballesteros, 1999). Converging evidence that visual and haptic inputs share a common neural representation is offered by the case report of a patient with both visual and tactile agnosia (a specific inability to recognize objects), despite otherwise intact somatic sensation, following a lesion of the left occipitotemporal cortex that presumably damaged the LOC (Feinberg, Gonzalez Rothi, & Heilman, 1986).

Visual cortical activation during tactile perception of motion

A PET study (Hagen et al., 2002) used radial visual motion to define the motion-sensitive area that is thought to be the human homologue of the middle temporal visual area (MT/V5) in macaque monkeys. This area was found to be active bilaterally when subjects attended to the motion of a brush stroked along the right forearm. Overlapping activity during the tactile and visual motion conditions was also found bilaterally near the intraparietal sulcus. Although there was no task in either the visual or tactile modality in this study, the colocalization of activity during the tactile and visual motion conditions again suggests a common, multisensory neural substrate.

Why is visual cortex involved in normal tactile perception?

The studies reviewed to this point permit the general conclusion that visual cortical processing is common during tactile perception, especially during macrospatial tasks. This processing appears to be task-specific, such that the specific areas of extrastriate visual cortex that mediate particular visual tasks are recruited in the corresponding tactile tasks. Moreover, our TMS study (Zangaladze et al., 1999) showed that extrastriate visual cortical activity is actually necessary for optimal tactile perception of certain object properties. These conclusions, and the observations on which they are based, fly in the face of common belief that separate neural systems process input from each sense, with the information being later combined in higher-order areas to provide unified object percepts. Rather, it appears that neural systems may not be exclusively devoted to processing a single kind of sensory input. Specifically, visual cortical regions are intimately involved in processing at least certain kinds of tactile information. Why might this be?

One possibility is that visual cortical recruitment during tactile tasks reflects visual imagery. Unfamiliarity with the stimuli or tasks in the tactile domain might trigger translation into a more familiar visual format for more efficient processing. Such cross-modal recoding may in fact be quite general, especially when complex information is involved (Freides, 1974). In support of a visual imagery explanation is that subjects across multiple studies in our laboratory consistently reported mentally visualizing tactile stimuli, even when they had not encountered them visually and even when the task itself did not explicitly call for mental imagery. Of note, in all these studies from our laboratory, stimulus variations occurred in no more than two spatial dimensions. Our results thus accord with psychophysical findings suggesting that visual mediation of haptic recognition is especially prominent for two-dimensional object representations (Lederman, Klatzky, Chataway, & Summers, 1990). In contrast, haptic recognition of three-dimensional forms might not require visual recoding (Lederman et al., 1990).

In our fMRI study (Stoesz et al., 2003), we found greater activation of the LOC during the macrospatial global form task than the microspatial gap detection task. Correspondingly, most subjects in this study reported using visual imagery during the macrospatial but not the microspatial task. This observation suggests that visual imagery is associated with effective recruitment of the LOC. On the other hand, Amedi et al. (2001) reported that active visual imagery evoked only one-fifth the activity in the LOC that haptic object identification did, and hence argued that LOC activity during haptic perception is not due to visual imagery. However, another group found clear recruitment of the left LOC during mental imagery of object shape (De Volder et al., 2001). In this PET study, mental imagery was triggered by auditory cues that had previously been associated with the objects during an initial phase of exploration that was visual in a group of sighted subjects and haptic in a group of blind subjects. Thus, activity in the LOC can be generated during perception as well as imagery, whether visual or haptic.

Another piece of evidence favoring a visual imagery explanation stems from the time course of TMS (and corresponding event-related potential) effects over occipital cortex during tactile grating orientation discrimination (Zangaladze et al., 1999). Both effects peak at about 180 ms following the onset of a (62.5-ms-duration) tactile stimulus presentation, compared to a 30–50 ms latency for somatosensory cortical effects. This delay between somatosensory and visual cortical effects seems unduly long for a purely feed-forward mechanism based on direct somatosensory inputs to visual cortical areas, but is certainly consistent with a scenario where a visual representation is activated in a top-down manner for comparison with the bottom-up somatosensory input. The top-down activation might represent processes involved in visual imagery. Further study of the time course of visual cortical activation during tactile tasks would be fruitful.

There are certainly other possible explanations for visual cortical recruitment during tactile perception. The simplest possibility is that there are direct, feed-forward somatosensory inputs to the visual cortical areas implicated in tactile perception. At present there is no evidence for this. Investigation of this issue using functional neuroimaging methods to probe functional connectivity, or better yet, direct neuroanatomical studies in nonhuman primates, would be helpful. Another possibility is that these areas are part of a multisensory network that can be activated through more than one sensory modality, perhaps via feedback connections from higher-order regions that receive multisensory input. In this context, a neurophysiological study in behaving monkeys found that some neurons in area V4 (in the ventral visual pathway) demonstrated selectivity for the orientation of either a tactile or a visual grating when it served as a cue to be matched to a subsequently presented visual stimulus (Haenny, Maunsell, & Schiller, 1988). The response to the tactile cue was not sensory, because it disappeared when the sensory information was irrelevant to the task. These potential explanations are not mutually exclusive; indeed, there may be multiple reasons underlying visual cortical involvement in touch. It has even been proposed (Pascual-Leone & Hamilton, 2001) that functional specificity in cerebral cortex is dependent on task rather than modality. In this view, occipital cortex is specialized for high-acuity spatial processing and may become devoted primarily (but not exclusively) to vision as a result of competition between sensory inputs during development.

Conclusions

A number of visual cortical areas are intimately involved in tactile perception. A variety of tactile tasks recruit visual cortical processing, and in a manner that appears to be quite task-specific. The mechanisms underlying visual cortical recruitment for tactile perception are still uncertain. Possibilities include involvement of visual imagery and/or multisensory processing, either directly via ascending somatosensory projections or indirectly via descending connections from higher-order multisensory areas. However, the work reviewed in this chapter, together with the other chapters in this volume, makes it clear that multisensory interactions are commonplace rather than exceptional. The challenge is to achieve a synthesis that defines the nature of normal cross-modal interactions and their alteration by sensory deprivation.

ACKNOWLEDGMENTS The research reviewed in this chapter was supported by grants from the NEI and NINDS.

REFERENCES

Alivisatos, B., & Petrides, M. (1997). Functional activation of the human brain during mental rotation. *Neuropsychologia, 36*, 111–118.

Amassian, V. E., Cracco, R. Q., Maccabee, P. J., Cracco, J. B., Rudell, A., & Eberle, L. (1989). Suppression of visual perception by magnetic coil stimulation of human occipital cortex. *EEG Clin Neurophysiology, 74*, 458–462.

Amedi, A., Jacobson, G., Hendler, T., Malach, R., & Zohary, E. (2002). Convergence of visual and tactile shape processing in the human lateral occipital complex. *Cerebral Cortex, 12*, 1202–1212.

Amedi, A., Malach, R., Hendler, T., Peled, S., & Zohary, E. (2001). Visuo-haptic object-related activation in the ventral visual pathway. *Nature Neuroscience, 4*, 324–330.

De Volder, A. G., Toyama, H., Kimura, Y., Kiyosawa, M., Nakano, H., Vanlierde, A., et al. (2001). Auditory triggered mental imagery of shape involves visual association areas in early blind humans. *NeuroImage, 14*, 129–139.

Deibert, E., Kraut, M., Kremen, S., & Hart, J. (1999). Neural pathways in tactile object recognition. *Neurology, 52*, 1413–1417.

Easton, R. D., Greene, A. J., & Srinivas, K. (1997). Transfer between vision and haptics: Memory for 2-D patterns and 3-D objects. *Psychonomic Bulletin and Review, 4*, 403–410.

Easton, R. D., Srinivas, K., & Greene, A. J. (1997). Do vision and haptics share common representations? Implicit and explicit memory within and between modalities. *Journal of Experimental Psychology: Learning, Memory, and Cognition, 23*, 153–163.

Epstein, C. M., Verson, R., & Zangaladze, A. (1996). Magnetic coil suppression of visual perception at an extracalcarine site. *Journal of Clinical Neurophysiology, 13*, 247–252.

Epstein, C. M., & Zangaladze, A. (1996). Magnetic coil suppression of extrafoveal visual perception using disappearance targets. *Journal of Clinical Neurophysiology, 13*, 242–246.

Feinberg, T. E., Gonzalez Rothi, L. J., & Heilman, K. M. (1986). Multimodal agnosia after unilateral left hemisphere lesion. *Neurology, 36*, 864–867.

Freides, D. (1974). Human information processing and sensory modality: Cross-modal functions, information complexity and deficit. *Psychological Bulletin, 81*, 284–310.

Galletti, C., Battaglini, P. P., & Fattori, P. (1991). Functional properties of neurons in the anterior bank of the parietooccipital sulcus of the macaque monkey. *European Journal of Neuroscience, 3*, 452–461.

Gauthier, I., Hayward, W. G., Tarr, M. J., Anderson, A. W., Skudlarski, P., & Gore, J. C. (2002). BOLD activity during mental rotation and viewpoint-dependent object recognition. *Neuron, 34*, 161–171.

Grant, A. C., Thiagarajah, M. C., & Sathian, K. (2000). Tactile perception in blind Braille readers: A psychophysical study of acuity and hyperacuity using gratings and dot patterns. *Perception & Psychophysics, 62*, 301–312.

Grill-Spector, K., Kushnir, T., Edelman, S., Avidan, G., Itzchak, Y., & Malach, R. (1999). Differential processing of objects under various viewing conditions in the human lateral occipital complex. *Neuron, 24*, 187–203.

Grill-Spector, K., Kushnir, T., Hendler, T., Edelman, S., Itzchak, Y., & Malach, R. (1998). A sequence of object-processing stages revealed by fMRI in the human occipital lobe. *Human Brain Mapping, 6*, 316–328.

Haenny, P. E., Maunsell, J. H. R., & Schiller, P. H. (1988). State dependent activity in monkey visual cortex: II. Retinal and extraretinal factors in V4. *Experimental Brain Research, 69*, 245–259.

Hagen, M. C., Franzen, O., McGlone, F., Essick, G., Dancer, C., & Pardo, J. V. (2002). Tactile motion activates the human middle temporal/V5 (MT/V5) complex. *European Journal of Neuroscience, 16*, 957–964.

Heller, M. A. (1989). Texture perception in sighted and blind observers. *Perception & Psychophysics, 45*, 49–54.

James, T. W., Humphrey, G. K., Gati, J. S., Servos, P., Menon, R. S., & Goodale, M. A. (2002). Haptic study of three-dimensional objects activates extrastriate visual areas. *Neuropsychologia, 40*, 1706–1714.

Klatzky, R. L., Lederman, S. J., & Reed, C. (1987). There's more to touch than meets the eye: The salience of object attributes for haptics with and without vision. *Journal of Experimental Psychology: General, 116*, 356–369.

Lederman, S. J., Klatzky, R. L., Chataway, C., & Summers, C. D. (1990). Visual mediation and the haptic recognition of two-dimensional pictures of common objects. *Perception & Psychophysics, 47*, 54–64.

Malach, R., Reppas, J. B., Benson, R. R., Kwong, K. K., Jiang, H., Kennedy, W. A., et al. (1995). Object-related activity revealed by functional magnetic resonance imaging in human occipital cortex. *Proceedings of the National Academy of Sciences, USA, 92,* 8135–8139.

Marmor, G. S., & Zaback, L. A. (1976). Mental rotation by the blind: Does mental rotation depend on visual imagery? *Journal of Experimental Psychology: Human Perception and Performance, 2,* 515–521.

Mellet, E., Tzourio, N., Crivello, F., Joliot, M., Denis, M., & Mazoyer, B. (1996). Functional anatomy of spatial mental imagery generated from verbal instructions. *Journal of Neuroscience, 16,* 6504–6512.

Mishkin, M., Ungerleider, L., & Macko, K. (1983). Object vision and spatial vision: Two cortical pathways. *Trends in the Neurosciences, 6,* 414–417.

Pascual-Leone, A., & Hamilton, R. (2001). The metamodal organization of the brain. *Progress in Brain Research, 134,* 427–445.

Prather, S. C., & Sathian, K. (2002). Mental rotation of tactile stimuli. *Cognitive Brain Research, 14,* 91–98.

Prather, S. C., Votaw, J. R., & Sathian, K. (2004). Task-specific recruitment of dorsal and ventral visual areas during tactile perception. *Neuropsychologia,* in press.

Reales, J. M., & Ballesteros, S. (1999). Implicit and explicit memory for visual and haptic objects: Cross-modal priming depends on structural descriptions. *Journal of Experimental Psychology: Learning, Memory and Cognition, 25,* 644–663.

Roland, P. E., & Mortensen, E. (1987). Somatosensory detection of microgeometry, macrogeometry and kinesthesia in man. *Brain Research Review, 12,* 1–42.

Röder, B., Rösler, F., & Hennighausen, E. (1997). Different cortical activation patterns in blind and sighted humans during encoding and transformation of haptic images. *Psychophysiology, 34,* 292–307.

Sathian, K., & Zangaladze, A. (1996). Tactile spatial acuity at the human fingertip and lip: Bilateral symmetry and inter-digit variability. *Neurology, 46,* 1464–1466.

Sathian, K., Zangaladze, A., Hoffman, J. M., & Grafton, S. T. (1997). Feeling with the mind's eye. *NeuroReport, 8,* 3877–3881.

Sergent, J., Ohta, S., & MacDonald, B. (1992). Functional neuroanatomy of face and object processing: A positron emission tomography study. *Brain, 115,* 15–36.

Shepard, R. N., & Metzler, J. (1971). Mental rotation of three-dimensional objects. *Science, 171,* 701–703.

Stoesz, M., Zhang, M., Weisser, V. D., Prather, S. C., Mao, H., & Sathian, K. (2003). Neural networks active during tactile form perception: Common and differential activity during macrospatial and microspatial tasks. *International Journal of Psychophysiology, 50,* 41–49.

Talairach, J., & Tournoux, P. (1988). Co-planar stereotaxic atlas of the brain. New York: Thieme.

Ungerleider, L. G., & Haxby, J. V. (1994). "What" and "where" in the human brain. *Current Opinion in Neurobiology, 4,* 157–165.

van Boven, R. W., & Johnson, K. O. (1994a). A psychophysical study of the mechanisms of sensory recovery following nerve injury in humans. *Brain, 117,* 149–167.

van Boven, R. W., & Johnson, K. O. (1994b). The limit of tactile spatial resolution in humans: grating orientation discrimination at the lip, tongue and finger. *Neurology, 44,* 2361–2366.

Zangaladze, A., Epstein, C. M., Grafton, S. T., & Sathian, K. (1999). Involvement of visual cortex in tactile discrimination of orientation. *Nature, 401,* 587–590.

45 Visual Cortex Engagement in Tactile Function in the Presence of Blindness

ESTEBAN A. FRIDMAN, PABLO CELNIK, AND LEONARDO G. COHEN

Introduction

The primary visual cortex (V1) represents the first cortical relay of visual input. Basic aspects of an object are initially analyzed at this level. Similarly, somatosensory information is initially processed in the primary somatosensory areas. The central nervous system (CNS) integrates information originating in different modalities. Such integration is thought to occur in association areas of the cerebral cortex (Hadjikhani & Roland, 1998; Mesulam, 1998). However, recently acquired evidence challenges this assumption. For example, the perception of colors is possible even after damage to V1. It has been proposed that a pathway connecting the pulvinar with V4 could mediate such transfer, bypassing V1 (for a review, see Zeki, 2001). It is likely, therefore, that integration of multisensory information could take place at different levels of the nervous system.

Plasticity within and across sensory modalities

Reorganization in the human CNS occurs in specific sensory or motor modalities in association with chronic (Cohen, Bandinelli, Findley, & Hallett, 1991; Cohen, Bandinelli, Topka, et al., 1991; Elbert et al., 1994; Flor et al., 1995; Fuhr et al., 1992; Hall, Flament, Fraser, & Lemon, 1990; Kew et al., 1994, 1997; Knecht et al., 1996; Pascual-Leone, Peris, Tormos, Pascual, & Catala, 1996; Ridding & Rothwell, 1995) and acute deafferentation (Birbaumer et al., 1997; Brasil-Neto et al., 1992, 1993; Ridding & Rothwell, 1995; Ziemann, Corwell, & Cohen, 1998; Ziemann, Hallett, & Cohen, 1998); during skill acquisition (Pascual-Leone, Grafman, & Hallett, 1994; Pascual-Leone, Wassermann, Sadato, & Hallett, 1995); and after short-term motor practice (Classen, Liepert, Hallett, & Cohen, 1996; Classen, Liepert, Wise, Hallett, & Cohen, 1998). Additionally, cortical reorganization occurs across sensory modalities, a phenomenon called *cross-modal plasticity*. In this case, a modality-specific brain area that is deprived of its normal sensory input may become responsive to input originating in different sensory modalities.

Cross-modal plasticity between visual and somatosensory cortical representations

Cross-modal plasticity has been described after loss of visual input in blind individuals. In subjects who became blind at a very early age (early blind), the occipital cortex is activated in association with the performance of tactile discrimination tasks, such as Braille reading. Sadato and co-workers used positron emission tomography (PET) to measure activation during Braille reading and tactile discrimination tasks in patients who became blind early in life and in healthy controls (Sadato et al., 1996). Blind subjects showed activation of primary and secondary visual cortical areas during Braille reading, with lesser activation during performance of other tactile discriminative tasks. Performance of the same tasks in sighted controls was associated with deactivation of visual cortical areas. Occipital areas remained inactive in both groups when a simple tactile task that did not involve discriminative efforts was presented. Therefore, in blind subjects, cortical areas that normally process visual input are active during the performance of tactile discriminative tasks, a conclusion consistent with previous studies (Uhl, Franzen, Lindinger, Lang, & Deecke, 1991; Wanet-Defalque et al., 1988). In a follow-up study, Sadato et al. (1998) showed that, in sighted subjects, non-Braille tactile discrimination tasks activated the secondary somatosensory area and suppressed activity in the occipital regions. Conversely, in blind individuals, the occipital region, including V1, was activated during the task. This finding suggests that, in the blind, the neural network usually reserved for visual shape discrimination processing (including BA 7, BA 17 and 18) is used for the evaluation of spatial information.

Although this experiment and others showed that patterns of brain activation during tactile discrimination tasks clearly differ in normal subjects and in blind Braille readers, the functional role of this activation remained unclear. Cohen and co-workers later studied whether these areas contributed to performance of the tactile task or were activated incidentally. Using repetitive transcranial magnetic stimulation (rTMS), they studied the effect of disrupting the activity of different cortical regions on reading performance of Braille and embossed roman letters (Cohen et al., 1997). rTMS was applied to induce a focal transient disruption of activity in underlying cortical sites. This form of stimulation causes a "virtual lesion" that is reversible after the end of the stimulation train. Trains of rTMS with a frequency of 10 Hz were applied to occipital regions while early-blind subjects read Braille and while blind subjects and sighted volunteers performed a tactile discrimination task (consisting of reading embossed roman letters). A figure-8-shaped, water-cooled coil (7 cm outer diameter of each coil; Cadwell Laboratories, Kennewick, WA) was used. The stimulus intensity was 10% above the resting motor threshold of the first dorsal interosseus (FDI) muscle. TMS was delivered randomly to several locations (OZ, O1, O2, P3, P4, and Fz of the international 10–20 system of electrode placement, and to the contralateral sensorimotor area). As a sham stimulation control, rTMS was delivered into the air to simulate the sound of the stimulator. Subjects were asked to identify letters and read them aloud one by one as quickly and accurately as possible. In the blind subjects, disruption of occipital activity with rTMS while reading Braille resulted in more accuracy errors than sham stimulation (Fig. 45.1). The application of rTMS to occipital sites elicited distorted somatosensory perceptions only in the blind group: blind subjects reported negative ("missing dots"), positive ("phantom dots"), and confusing sensations ("dots don't make sense") associated with occipital stimulation. These results indicate that disruption of occipital activity substantially affected performance on tactile discrimination tasks in early-blind individuals but not in the control group.

Consistent with the hypothesis of a substantial engagement of the visual cortex in tactile discrimination in blind persons, a case was recently reported of a blind woman, a skilled Braille reader, who lost her reading skills after an occipital ischemic stroke (Hamilton, Keenan, Catala, & Pascual-Leone, 2000). This case demonstrates the involvement and relevance of the striate and peristriate cortex for Braille reading in subjects who lose their vision.

Period of susceptibility to experience cross-modal plasticity

These and other studies firmly determined the existence of cross-modal plasticity after long-term visual deprivation in humans. A further question arose concerning whether a critical time window exists for visual deprivation to lead to such cross-modal plasticity. Information from animals studies is consistent with the idea that such a time window in cats and monkeys is limited to the first weeks or months of life (Crair, 1998; Hubel & Wiesel, 1970; Regal, Boothe, Teller, & Sackett, 1976; von Noorden, 1972), but in humans it may last substantially longer. For example, the ability of the visual cortex to reorganize during the second decade of life has been demonstrated in the setting of amblyopia (Epelbaum, Milleret, Buisseret, & Dufier, 1993; Keech & Kutschke, 1995; Vaegan, 1979).

The existence of differences in processing between human subjects who are blind from early life versus those who become blind later in life has been demonstrated by Buchel et al. The authors demonstrated different task-specific activation of visual areas during Braille reading compared with auditory word processing (Buchel, Price, Frackowiak, & Friston, 1998). Blind subjects who lost their sight after puberty showed activation in V1 and extrastriate visual areas, whereas early-blind subjects had activation only in the extrastriate regions on the same tasks. The authors suggested that visual imagery present in the population of blind subjects who lost their sight after puberty might be responsible for the striate cortex activation. In a study using a different tactile discriminative task, Cohen et al. also found differences in task-related activation of the visual cortex between early- and late-blind subjects (Fig. 45.2; Color Plate 22.) (Cohen et al., 1999). Consistent with these PET findings, rTMS delivered to the occipital cortex of late-blind individuals failed to disrupt performance on the tactile discriminative task (Fig. 45.3).

These results were interpreted to indicate that the window of opportunity for cross-modal plasticity in blind humans is limited to childhood and that reorganizational processes might play a compensatory role when the visual loss occurs within a window of opportunity before age 14 years (Cohen et al., 1999).

Performance on tactile discriminative tasks by blind subjects

When Louis Braille, blinded at the age of 3, created the special system that allows blind people to read, he speculated that the blind may have better tactile perceptual

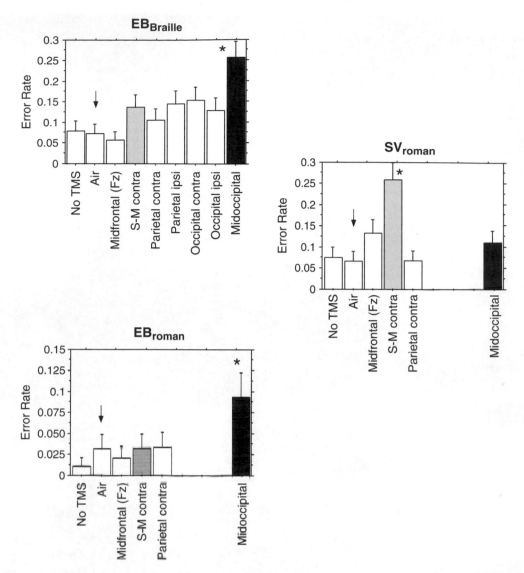

FIGURE 45.1   Error rates (mean ± SE) for stimulation of different positions in the three groups studied (early-blind subjects reading Braille, early-blind subjects reading roman letters, and sighted volunteers reading roman letters). Missing bars indicate that stimulation at that position was not performed in that specific group. Black bars indicate error rates induced by stimulation of the midoccipital position, and gray bars indicate error rates induced by stimulation of the contralateral sensorimotor cortex. In both groups of early-blind subjects, stimulation of the midoccipital position induced more errors in reading Braille characters and roman letters than stimulation of any other position, whereas in the sighted volunteers, stimulation of the contralateral primary sensorimotor region induced more errors than stimulation of any other position. Asterisks indicate scalp positions where significantly more errors occurred than control (air, marked with arrows). S-M, sensorimotor cortex; contra, contralateral; ipsi, ipsilateral; EB$_{Braille}$, early-blind subjects reading Braille; EB$_{roman}$, early-blind subjects reading roman letters; SV$_{roman}$, sighted volunteers reading roman letters. *$P < 0.001$. (Modified from Cohen et al., 1997.)

skills than sighted subjects. Although several studies have evaluated the tactile capacities of blind individuals compared with sighted controls, most were unable to show significant differences. Evaluation of light-touch threshold detection using von Frey-type nylon monofilaments did not reveal such differences between blind subjects and sighted persons (Heinrichs & Moorhouse, 1969; Pascual-Leone & Torres, 1993; Sterr et al., 1998).

Likewise, vibratory detection thresholds (Heinrichs & Moorhouse, 1969) and threshold detection of electric pulses (Pascual-Leone & Torres, 1993) did not differ significantly between blind and sighted subjects.

More recently, evaluation of tactile discriminative skills in different fingers showed that blind subjects who read Braille with multiple fingers had lower tactile thresholds at two of their three reading fingers and at a

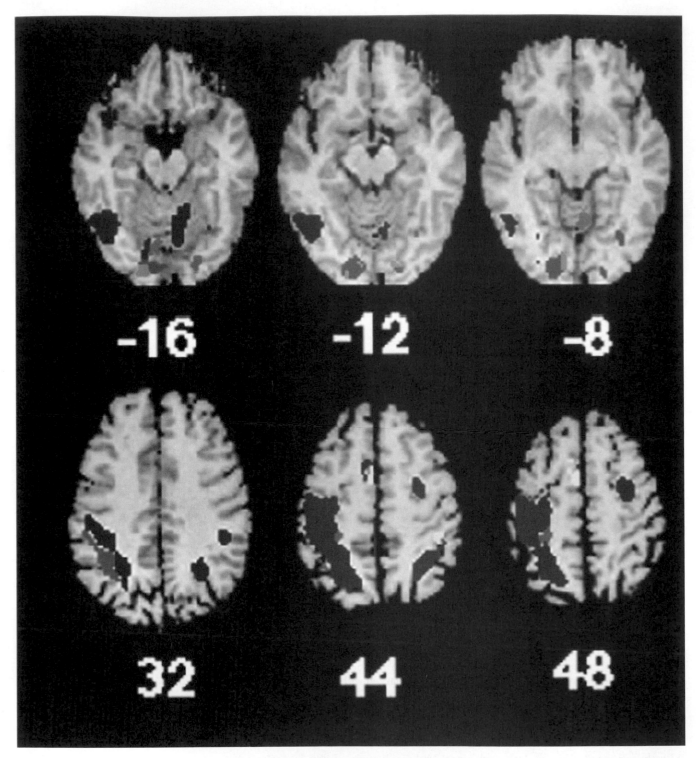

FIGURE 45.2 Conjunction analysis of activation by Braille discrimination task by congenitally blind ($n = 4$), early-blind ($n = 4$), and late-blind ($n = 4$) groups, superimposed on typical MR images unrelated to the study's subjects. Transaxial images 4–16 mm below and 32–52 mm above the anteroposterior commissural line are shown. The pixels show levels of statistical significance above $P < 0.05$ with correction for multiple comparisons at voxel level. Areas commonly activated in congenitally blind, early-blind, and late-blind subjects (violet), congenitally blind and early-blind but not late-blind individuals (red), congenitally blind and late-blind but not early-blind individuals (yellow), early-blind and late-blind but not congenitally blind individuals (green), early-blind individuals only (light blue), and late-blind individuals only (pink) are shown. The primary visual cortex is commonly activated in congenitally blind and early-blind individuals but not in late-blind individuals. (Modified from Cohen et al., 1999.) (See Color Plate 22.)

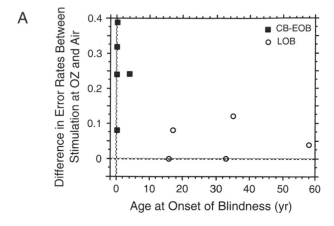

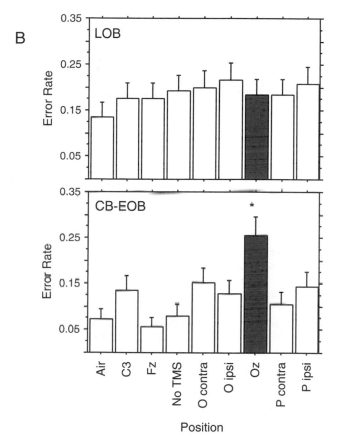

FIGURE 45.3 (*A*) Difference in error rates with stimulation over the midoccipital region (OZ) and control (Air) as a function of age at onset of blindness. (*B*) Error rates (mean ± SE) for stimulation of different scalp positions in the late-onset blind (LOB) group (top) and in the congenitally blind (CB) + early-onset blind (EOB) group (shown for comparison) (bottom). Solid columns indicate error rates induced by stimulation of the midoccipital position. Note that in the CB + EOB group, stimulation of midoccipital positions elicited the largest error rate. In the LOB group, there are no differences in error rates by stimulation position. *Scalp positions where significantly more errors occurred than control (air). TMS, transcranial magnetic stimulation; Air, no

brain stimulation (control); C3, sensorimotor cortex; contra, contralateral; ipsi, ipsilateral. (Modified from Cohen et al., 1999.)

single nonreading finger (Sterr et al., 1998). Similarly, blind subjects who read Braille with only a single finger had lower thresholds in that finger compared to sighted subjects at their reading finger, as well as at a nonreading finger (Sterr et al., 1998). Studies that evaluated conventional two-point discrimination tasks (Heinrichs & Moorhouse, 1969; Pascual-Leone & Torres, 1993) have not found blind persons to have superior abilities. Therefore, the issue is not completely settled.

The design and varied methods of two-point discrimination tests provide a variety of nonspatial neural cues for performance. For example, nonsimultaneous skin contact of two points provides a temporal cue for discrimination from a single point. Furthermore, it has recently been shown (Vega-Bermudez & Johnson, 1999) that a single tactile stimulus evokes higher firing rates in primary afferents than two tactile stimuli presented simultaneously. Positional cues are also important. It has been reported that blind subjects can better identify a pair of narrowly separated points pressed onto the finger when placed orthogonal but not longitudinal to the long axis of the finger (Stevens, Foulke, & Patterson, 1996). The same study also reported that blind subjects are better able to detect a change in orientation from longitudinally positioned points when presentations are paired with orthogonally positioned points. The neural basis for these differences remains to be determined.

In a study of tactile letter recognition and gap detection tasks at the fingertip using the Optacon stimulator (a device in which the stimuli are an array of pins activated by way of piezoelectrically driven pulse taps; Tele Sensory Co., Mountainview, CA), naive blind Braille readers performed better than naive sighted subjects on both tasks. Van Boven and co-workers recently utilized a grating orientation discrimination task for the middle and index fingers of blind Braille readers compared to sighted control subjects (Van Boven, Hamilton, Kauffman, Keenan, & Pascual-Leone, 2000). They found superior tactile spatial acuity in blind individuals, measured as significantly lower grating orientation thresholds.

The intensive practice associated with Braille reading in individuals who are blind from an early age may lead to maladaptive phenomena. For example, blind subjects who read Braille using multiple fingers mislocalize tactile stimuli more than sighted subjects when touched with von Frey-type nylon filaments (Sterr et al., 1998).

Interestingly, although individuals with early-onset (before 5 years) blindness can detect a significantly finer offset in the alignment of a row of three embossed dots than sighted subjects at initial (task-naive) testing, no difference in performance is noted by the third test session a few days later (Grant, Thiagarajah, & Sathian, 2000).

This information points to a greater involvement of the occipital cortex in performance on nonvisual (tactile) tasks in blind individuals than in sighted controls. However, some level of tactile processing is known to take place even in sighted individuals. Zangaladze and associates (see also Sathian, Prather, & Zhang, Chap. 44, this volume) instructed sighted subjects to discriminate the orientation of a grating applied to the right index finger with their eyes closed (Zangaladze, Epstein, Grafton, & Sathian, 1999). TMS applied to occipital sites at a 180-ms delay markedly impaired task performance. In contrast, TMS applied ipsilateral to the hand undergoing the discriminative task had no deleterious effects on performance. In addition, TMS applied during a control task to test whether the disruption of tactile performance by occipital TMS was specific to discrimination of orientation or texture did not affect performance. However, when TMS was applied over the contralateral somatosensory cortex, it blocked discrimination of both grating texture and orientation. Taken together, the findings of these studies suggest that the visual cortex may participate in processing of some tactile tasks even in sighted individuals.

Summary

Long-term deafferentation in the visual domain leads to the involvement of the occipital cortex in performance on tactile discriminative tasks. The magnitude of such capacity appears limited to a window of opportunity that is maximal before puberty. The finding that some aspects of tactile processing may take place in the occipital cortex of sighted volunteers raises the possibility of relatively hidden cross-modal capacities in the intact occipital cortex that are unmasked and enhanced by long-term deafferentation and prolonged practice of the tactile task.

REFERENCES

Birbaumer, N., Lutzenberger, W., Montoya, P., Larbig, W., Unertl, K., Topfner, S., et al. (1997). Effects of regional anesthesia on phantom limb pain are mirrored in changes in cortical reorganization. *Journal of Neuroscience, 17,* 5503–5508.

Brasil-Neto, J. P., Cohen, L. G., Pascual-Leone, A., Jabir, F. K., Wall, R. T., & Hallett, M. (1992). Rapid reversible modulation of human motor outputs after transient deafferentation of the forearm: A study with transcranial magnetic stimulation. *Neurology, 42,* 1302–1306.

Brasil-Neto, J. P., Valls-Sole, J., Pascual-Leone, A., Cammarota, A., Amassian, V. E., Cracco, R., et al. (1993). Rapid modulation of human cortical motor outputs following ischaemic nerve block. *Brain, 116,* 511–525.

Buchel, C., Price, C., Frackowiak, R. S., & Friston, K. (1998). Different activation patterns in the visual cortex of late and congenitally blind subjects. *Brain, 121,* 409–419.

Classen, J., Liepert, A., Hallett, M., & Cohen, L. G. (1996). Use-dependent modulation of movement representation in the human motor cortex. *Society of Neuroscience Abstracts, 22,* 1452.

Classen, J., Liepert, A., Wise, S. P., Hallett, M., & Cohen, L. G. (1998). Rapid plasticity of human cortical movement representation induced by practice. *Journal of Neurophysiology, 79,* 1117–1123.

Cohen, L. G., Bandinelli, S., Findley, T. W., & Hallett, M. (1991). Motor reorganization after upper limb amputation in man: A study with focal magnetic stimulation. *Brain, 114,* 615–627.

Cohen, L. G., Bandinelli, S., Topka, H. R., Fuhr, P., Roth, B. J., & Hallett, M. (1991). Topographic maps of human motor cortex in normal and pathological conditions: Mirror movements, amputations and spinal cord injuries. *Electroencephalography and Clinical Neurophysiology, Supplement, 43,* 36–50.

Cohen, L. G., Celnik, P., Pascual-Leone, A., Corwell, B., Falz, L., Dambrosia, J., et al. (1997). Functional relevance of cross-modal plasticity in blind humans. *Nature, 389,* 180–183.

Cohen, L. G., Weeks, R. A., Sadato, N., Celnik, P., Ishii, K., & Hallett, M. (1999). Period of susceptibility for cross-modal plasticity in the blind. *Annals of Neurology, 45,* 451–460.

Craig, J. C. (1988). The role of experience in tactual pattern perception: A preliminary report. *International Journal of Rehabilitation Research, 11,* 167–183.

Crair, M. C. (1998). The role of visual experience in the development of columns in cat visual cortex. *Science, 279,* 566–570.

Elbert, T., Flor, H., Birbaumer, N., Knecht, S., Hampson, S., Larbig, W., et al. (1994). Extensive reorganization of the somatosensory cortex in adult humans after nervous system injury. *Neuroreport, 5,* 2593–2597.

Epelbaum, M., Milleret, C., Buisseret, P., & Dufier, J. L. (1993). The sensitive period for strabismic amblyopia in humans. *Ophthalmology, 100,* 323–327.

Flor, H., Elbert, T., Knecht, S., Wienbruch, C., Pantev, C., Birbaumer, N., et al. (1995). Phantom-limb pain as a perceptual correlate of cortical reorganization following arm amputation. *Nature, 375,* 482–484.

Fuhr, P., Cohen, L. G., Dang, N., Findley, T. W., Haghighi, S., Oro, J., et al. (1992). Physiological analysis of motor reorganization following lower limb amputation. *Electroencephalography and Clinical Neurophysiology, 85,* 53–60.

Grafman, J. (2000). Conceptualizing functional plasticity. *Journal of Communication Disorders, 33,* 345–356.

Grant, A. C., Thiagarajah, M. C., & Sathian, K. (2000). Tactile perception in blind Braille readers: A psychophysical study of acuity and hyperacuity using gratings and dot patterns. *Perception & Psychophysics, 62,* 301–312.

Hadjikhani, N., & Roland, P. (1998). Cross-modal transfer of information between the tactile and the visual representation in the human brain: A positron emission tomographic study. *Journal of Neuroscience, 18,* 1072–1084.

Hall, E. J., Flament, D., Fraser, C., & Lemon, R. N. (1990). Non-invasive brain stimulation reveals reorganized cortical outputs in amputees. *Neuroscience Letters, 116,* 379–386.

Hamilton, R., Keenan, J., Catala, M., & Pascual-Leone, A. (2000). Alexia for Braille following bilateral occipital stroke in an early blind woman. *Neuroreport, 11,* 237–240.

Heinrichs, R. W., & Moorhouse, J. A. (1969). Touch-perception thresholds in blind diabetic subjects in relation to the reading of Braille type. *New England Journal of Medicine, 280,* 72–75.

Hubel, D. H., & Wiesel, T. N. (1970). The period of susceptibility to the physiological effects of unilateral-eye closure in kittens. *Journal of Physiology (London), 206,* 419–436.

Keech, R. V., & Kutschke, P. J. (1995). Upper age limit for the development of amblyopia. *Journal of Pediatric Ophthalmology and Strabismus, 32,* 89–93.

Kew, J. J., Halligan, P. W., Marshall, J. C., Passingham, R. E., Rothwell, J. C., Ridding, M. C., et al. (1997). Abnormal access of axial vibrotactile input to deafferented somatosensory cortex in human upper limb amputees. *Journal of Neurophysiology, 77,* 2753–2764.

Kew, J. J., Ridding, M. C., Rothwell, J. C., Passingham, R. E., Leigh, P. N., Sooriakumaran, S., et al. (1994). Reorganization of cortical blood flow and transcranial magnetic stimulation maps in human subjects after upper limb amputation. *Journal of Neurophysiology, 72,* 2517–2524.

Knecht, S., Henningsen, H., Elbert, T., Flor, H., Hohling, C., Pantev, C., et al. (1996). Reorganization and perceptual changes after amputation. *Brain, 119,* 1213–1219.

Mesulam, M. (1998). From sensation to cognition. *Brain, 121,* 1013–1052.

Pascual-Leone, A., Grafman, J., & Hallett, M. (1994). Modulation of cortical motor output maps during development of implicit and explicit knowledge. *Science, 263,* 1287–1289.

Pascual-Leone, A., Peris, M., Tormos, J. M., Pascual, A. P., & Catala, M. D. (1996). Reorganization of human cortical motor output maps following traumatic forearm amputation. *Neuroreport, 7,* 2068–2070.

Pascual-Leone, A., & Torres, F. (1993). Plasticity of the sensorimotor cortex representation of the reading finger in Braille readers. *Brain, 116,* 39–52.

Pascual-Leone, A., Wassermann, E. M., Sadato, N., & Hallett, M. (1995). The role of reading activity on the modulation of motor cortical outputs to the reading hand in Braille readers. *Annals of Neurology, 38,* 910–915.

Rauschecker, J. P. (1995). Compensatory plasticity and sensory substitution in the cerebral cortex. *Trends in the Neurosciences, 18,* 36–43.

Rauschecker, J. P., & Kniepert, U. (1994). Auditory localization behaviour in visually deprived cats. *European Journal of Neuroscience, 6,* 149–160.

Regal, D. M., Boothe, R., Teller, D. Y., & Sackett, G. P. (1976). Visual acuity and visual responsiveness in dark-reared monkeys (*Maccaca nemesterina*). *Vision Research, 16,* 523–530.

Ridding, M. C., & Rothwell, J. C. (1995). Reorganisation in human motor cortex. *Canadian Journal of Physiology and Pharmacology, 73,* 218–222.

Sadato, N., Pascual-Leone, A., Grafman, J., Ibanez, V., Deiber, M. P., Dold, G., et al. (1996). Activation of the primary visual cortex by Braille reading in blind subjects. *Nature, 380,* 526–528.

Sadato, N., Pascual-Leone, A., Grafman, J., Deiber, M. P., Ibanez, V., & Hallett, M. (1998). Neural networks for Braille reading by the blind. *Brain, 121,* 1213–1229.

Sathian, K., Zangaladze, A., Hoffman, J. M., & Grafton, S. T. (1997). Feeling with the mind's eye. *Neuroreport, 8,* 3877–3881.

Sterr, A., Muller, M. M., Elbert, T., Rockstroh, B., Pantev, C., & Taub, E. (1998). Perceptual correlates of changes in cortical representation of fingers in blind multifinger Braille readers. *Journal of Neuroscience, 18,* 4417–4423.

Stevens, J. C., Foulke, E., & Patterson, M. Q. (1996). Tactile acuity, aging and Braille reading in long-term blindness. *Journal of Experimental Psychology: Applications, 2,* 91–106.

Uhl, F., Franzen, P., Lindinger, G., Lang, W., & Deecke, L. (1991). On the functionality of the visually deprived occipital cortex in early blind persons. *Neuroscience Letters, 124,* 256–259.

Vaegan, T. D. (1979). Critical period for deprivation amblyopia in children. *Transactions of the Ophthalmological Society, UK, 99,* 432–439.

Van Boven, R. W., Hamilton, R. H., Kauffman, T., Keenan, J. P., & Pascual-Leone, A. (2000). Tactile spatial resolution in blind Braille readers. *Neurology, 54,* 2230–2236.

Vega-Bermudez, F., & Johnson, K. O. (1999). Surround suppression in the responses of primate SA1 and RA mechanoreceptive afferents mapped with a probe array. *Journal of Neurophysiology, 81,* 2711–2719.

Von Noorden, G. K. (1972). Experimental amblyopia. *Irish Journal of Medical Science, 8,* 1496–1499.

Wanet-Defalque, M-C., Veraart, C., De Volder, A., Metz, R., Michel, C., Dooms, G., et al. (1988). High metabolic activity in the visual cortex of early blind subjects. *Brain Research, 446,* 369–373.

Zangaladze, A., Epstein, C. M., Grafton, S. T., & Sathian, K. (1999). Involvement of visual cortex in tactile discrimination of orientation. *Nature, 401,* 587–590.

Zeki, S. (2001). Localization and globalization in conscious vision. *Annual Review of Neuroscience, 24,* 57–86.

Ziemann, U., Corwell, B., & Cohen, L. G. (1998). Modulation of plasticity in human motor cortex after forearm ischemic nerve block. *Journal of Neuroscience, 18,* 1115–1123.

Ziemann, U., Hallett, M., & Cohen, L. G. (1998). Mechanisms of deafferentation-induced plasticity in human motor cortex. *Journal of Neuroscience, 18,* 7000–7007.

46 Compensatory Plasticity as a Consequence of Sensory Loss

BRIGITTE RÖDER AND FRANK RÖSLER

Introduction

The concept of *sensory compensation* was proposed by the philosopher Diderot, in "Lettre sure les Aveugles," published in 1749. *Sensory compensation* refers to improvement in the remaining senses after the loss of one sensory system in order to counteract the lost capabilities. Along these lines, William James in 1890 proposed that loss of vision should promote the learning of extraordinary perceptual skills in the intact modalities. However, the empirical literature on this issue is inconclusive; both superior and inferior performance have been reported for blind individuals in comparison with sighted individuals and for deaf persons in comparison with normal-hearing individuals (for reviews, see Röder & Neville, 2003; Röder & Rösler, 2001). Reasons for the contradictory results on testing most likely originate in the characteristics of the participants recruited for the studies (e.g., etiology, degree, duration and age at onset of sensory impairment, age at testing) and the tasks used (e.g., different tasks were used for the experimental group and the control group, instructions were not always adequate for blind or deaf participants) (for detailed discussions of these issues, see Millar, 1982; Röder & Neville, 2003; Thinus-Blanc & Gaunet, 1997).

This chapter reviews findings in blind and deaf individuals for different functional domains, including perceptual, language, and spatial functions. To understand what the underlying neural mechanisms of cross-modal compensation are, some relevant findings from animal research are reported and the meaning of the term *neuroplasiticity* is discussed. The focus is on the visual deprivation model, but some parallel findings in the deaf are reported as well.

The sensory deprivation model for investigating compensatory plasticity

The term *compensation* needs to be clarified. Different outcomes are possible in behavioral studies that compare the performance of blind and sighted or deaf and hearing individuals. The following possible outcomes pertain to the visual deprivation model, but analogous outcomes are conceivable for the auditory deprivation model:

1. *Congenitally blind individuals show worse performance than sighted controls.* This result would point toward a dependency of the development of the investigated skill on visual input. Either lack of mutual interactions between the visual and the other sensory systems (auditory, tactile, etc.) or missing guidance by the visual modality could result in worse performance of blind individuals within their intact sensory systems. Inferior performance by blind individuals compared with sighted individuals would suggest incomplete or missing compensation.

2. *Congenitally blind individuals perform at the same level as sighted controls.* This result would indicate either that the function under consideration develops independently from the visual system or that the possibly facilitating visual input is counteracted by the other sensory systems. Therefore, no performance differences between sighted and blind individuals can be taken as evidence for compensation.

3. *Congenitally blind individuals show superior performance compared with a sighted control group.* This outcome would clearly indicate compensatory changes, including a possible release from functional inhibition, in the blind and has been called *hypercompensation* by Zwiers, Van Opstal, and Cruysberg (2001b). It could then be asked whether these improvements are sufficient to substitute for the visual input. It is well known that congruent simultaneous input from two or more modalities can enhance performance (e.g., result in lower thresholds or faster response times; e.g., Calvert, Brammer, & Iversen, 1998; Welch & Warren, 1986). Therefore, the question arises of whether the enhancements within the blind persons' intact sensory systems result in a performance level as high as the multisensory performance level of sighted individuals. If so, this result would suggest a replacement of visual input by the intact modalities, and this pattern of results would provide evidence for *sensory substitution*. However, from an evolutionary point of view, the substitution of one sensory system by another seems less likely; different sensory systems most likely developed because

they provide not only convergent but also complementary sources of information (Millar, 1994). Therefore, an enhancement of performance by the intact system may allow a performance level in the blind that settles somewhere between the unimodal and multisensory performance of sighted individuals.

4. If congenitally blind and late-blind individuals show similar performance, and that performance is either superior to or not different from the performance of sighted individuals, it is justified to concluded that the mechanisms underlying compensation are not linked to early developmental stages (so-called critical periods). If the late blind show less compensation than the congenitally blind but still exhibit higher performance than the sighted, it is plausible to infer that there are *sensitive periods* during early childhood in which the underlying compensatory mechanisms are most plastic, but that adaptations, although to a lower degree, are still possible later in life. The same performance level for late-blind and sighted individuals, but inferior performance compared with that of the congenitally blind, would suggest the existence of critical periods for compensatory behavior to emerge. A fundamental problem in comparing early- and late-blind individuals is that age at onset and the duration of blindness are confounded.

5. Superior performance of a late-blind group compared with a congenitally blind group, with both congenitally and late-blind individuals outperforming sighted control individuals would indicate that prior visual experience supports compensatory improvements in the intact senses. This result could be due to a double advantage of the late blind: they have experienced an intense training of their intact sensory systems but may still be able to activate (supplementory) visual concepts.

In recent years, researchers have wondered which, if any, changes of the central nervous system (CNS) underlie behavioral adaptations after sensory loss; that is, if the intact sensory systems increase their processing efficiency, possibly by expanding associated neural representations (*compensatory plasticity*). Some authors (e.g., Miller, 1992) have contrasted compensatory behavior based on neural reorganization and behavioral improvements based on changes in processing strategies. However, the use of different processing strategies causes a shift in the degree to which a particular system is used, and thus in turn may elicit use-dependent neural reorganization. Therefore, this distinction will not be made here.

The development and increased availability of functional neuroimaging techniques, including electrophysiological recordings, in recent years have made it possible to study neuroplasticity in humans (Poldrack, 2000). Studies using event-related potentials (ERPs), positron emission tomography (PET), functional magnetic resonance imaging (fMRI), and transcranial magnetic stimulation (TMS) have shown evidence of neural reorganization in blind and deaf humans and are discussed in the context of compensatory performance. Furthermore, the data in humans supplement data obtained in animals using invasive techniques. The latter have demonstrated reorganization that ranges from very local changes within the innervation zones of thalamic afferents up to cross-modal changes, i.e., an innervation of the deprived (cortical and subcortical) brain structures by the intact sensory systems (for reviews, see Kujala, Alho, & Näätänen, 2000; Rauschecker, 2001; Röder & Neville, 2003; Sur & Leamey, 2001).

In this chapter, different functional areas ranging from elementary perceptual processes to higher cognitive functions such as language are reviewed in blind and deaf people compared with sighted and hearing people, respectively. The use of less complex perceptual tasks allows a direct comparison with results from the animal literature, that is, with data obtained from investigations at the single-cell and molecular level that are not accessible in human studies. In contrast, possible alterations of higher cognitive functions can only be explored in humans, and therefore these studies extend the knowledge about the plasticity capabilities of the CNS derived from animal investigations. In many studies ERP methods have been used because the high temporal resolution of electrophysiological recordings allows researchers to differentiate the processing stages that are capable of change in order to adapt to altered requirements. Supplementary PET and fMRI studies have been used to more precisely localize the brain areas in which change due to sensory deprivation emerge. Data from these three sources—behavioral studies, ERP, and PET/fMRI studies—will be reviewed in order to draw conclusions about the extent and neural basis of cross-modal compensation.

What is neural plasticity?

"[The brain's] capacity for adaptation to change [. . . is] commonly referred to as neural plasticity" (Rauschecker, 1997, p. 137). In general, such changes occur at different organizational levels of the CNS, ranging from gene transcription through molecular, synaptic, neural, and systems levels up to the CNS as a whole, and to behavior (see Sejnowski & Churchland, 1989; Shaw & McEachern, 2001). Plastic changes at different levels of neural organization are most likely interdependent (Shaw & McEachern, 2001).

Neural plasticity has been classified according to different aspects. For example, *physiological plasticity* has been contrasted to *anatomical plasticity* (Birbaumer & Schmidt, 1991). Whereas physiological plasticity reflects changes in the response properties of neurons and neuronal assemblies (e.g., firing thresholds, long-term potentiation, long-term depression; see Cain, 2001; Teyler, 2001), anatomical plasticity involves changes in the structure of the neuron and neuropil (e.g., number and form of synapses, size of cell somata and dendritic trees). It is important to note that anatomical and physiological changes are not independent but interact. For example, during an initial learning phase, the firing rates of neurons change, possibly due to the disinhibition of silent synapses or to changes in the transmitter release of the presynaptic contact. The consecutive consolidation phase is characterized by structural changes that strengthen the initial physiological changes (see, e.g., Kolb & Whishaw, 1990). This points toward a classification of neural changes with respect to the elapsed time since the eliciting event, with a distinction made between rapid changes (those occurring within seconds to hours) and slow changes (those occurring over days and months). Although rapid changes most likely build on the unmasking, disinhibition, or potentiation of previously existing connections (the concept of "silent synapses," or physiological plasticity), slow changes most likely involve additional anatomical changes, including collateral sprouting and changes of the neuron's structure itself, contributing to the consolidation of rapid changes.

Anatomical and physiological changes have been observed in both the developing and the mature CNS. For example, the development of binocular response properties of visual cortex neurons depends on input from both eyes (Hubel & Wiesel, 1977). If input from one eye is missing (monocular deprivation) during early development (i.e., during "critical" or "sensitive" periods), neurons in visual cortex will still respond to input received through the intact eye only, even if the deprivation has been removed. Knudsen (1988) defines sensitive periods as the period in life during which "experience (including sensory deprivation) can cause abnormal development," and critical periods as "a period in life when experience enables normal development" (p. 305). Similar to the findings of Hubel and Wiesel (1977) in cats and primates, it has been shown in human infants that incongruent input through both eyes, for example because of a monocular cataract or strabismus, results in a dimness of vision in one eye, even though no defects of this eye are detectable (this phenomenon is known as amblyopia) (Keech & Kutschke, 1995; Kiorpes, Kiper, O'Keefe, Cavanaugh, &

Movshon, 1998). Moreover, it has been shown that congenital, dense binocular or monocular cataracts lead to impaired binocular depth perception in humans (Maurer, Lewis, & Brent, 1989), along with deficits in other visual tasks. In particular, the more complex visual functions that develop during the first months of life, including visual orienting (Goldberg, Maurer, Lewis, & Brent, 2001) and face perception (Le Grand, Maurer, & Brent, 2001), are affected (for a review, see Maurer & Lewis, 2001).

In adult animals it has been reported that neurons that originally had receptive fields (RFs) at a retinal location that was subsequently damaged develop new RFs at the border of the retinal lesion (Kaas et al., 1990). Therefore, the adult visual system is also capable of change. This holds for the other sensory systems as well: perceptual learning and local peripheral damage in adult individuals elicit reorganization of sensory maps of the somatosensory, auditory, and motor system as well (for reviews, see Fahle & Poggio, 2002; Kaas, 2000, 2001). Competition and cooperation have been proposed as the guiding principles of brain plasticity (Hebb, 1949). This is demonstrated by the fact that a reorganization in visual cortex after restricted retinal lesions are created in adult animals is induced only if a matching lesion is placed in the second eye (otherwise deprived neurons keep their RFs through the intact retina). It is interesting to note, however, that after a similar local lesion of the retina during the critical period, neurons develop two RFs, one for each eye, possibly contributing to local double images and/or blur (Chino, Smith, Mori, & Kaas, 2001). This demonstrates that although developmental and adult plasticity share many common characteristics they are not identical.

Studies on the effects of enriched versus impoverished environments on brain development have focused on anatomical plasticity. Animals raised in enriched environments have thicker and heavier cortices, a richer branching of dendrites, more dendritic spines, and a higher glia cell density (Rosenzweig & Leiman, 1982, cited in Birbaumer & Schmidt, 1991; Black, Jones, Nelson, & Greenough, 1998; Turner & Greenough, 1985). Importantly, enriched environments elicit similar, although smaller (Black et al., 1998) and qualitatively not entirely identical, anatomical changes (Kolb & Gibb, 2001) in adult animals (Green, Greenough, & Schlumpf, 1983). Moreover, animals raised in complex environments show faster learning, and the difference between them and their siblings raised in impoverished environments is the larger, the more complex the task is (see Black et al., 1998). These results have been related to findings demonstrating that new neurons are generated (in hippocampus and cortex) even in adult individuals

(Gould, Reeves, Graziano, & Gross, 1999; Gross, 2000; Ormerod & Galea, 2001; Shors et al., 2001; van Praag, Kempermann, & Gage, 2000), including humans (Eriksson et al., 1998). Neurogenesis in the hippocampus has been demonstrated to contribute functionally to learning (Shors et al., 2001).

A classification of neuroplasticity according to the eliciting factor was suggested by Sheedlo and Turner (1992, p. 8): "Neuroplasticity, broadly defined, involves the ability of the nervous system to adapt its structural organization to altered circumstances arising from either developmental, environmental, or traumatic phenomena." Development and aging are accompanied by changes in the organization of the CNS. Moreover, extraordinary (e.g., intense practice) or everyday requirements elicit changes in the CNS that mediate learning and memory. Traumatic events that cause damage either to the CNS tissue proper or an indirect injury to the CNS are associated with sensory deprivation or deafferentation. Again, these three conditions eliciting plastic changes are not necessarily independent. For example, sensory deprivation is accompanied by a higher reliance on other sensory systems, causing use-dependent changes, and the extent of the latter may interact with the time in life at which the deprivation started.

Recently, Grafman (2000) proposed four major types of neuroplasticity, mainly guided by the CNS structures involved:

1. *Homologue area adaptation:* Cognitive processes are taken over by the corresponding regions of the opposite hemisphere. For example, patients who had suffered right parietal lesions in childhood showed relatively normal visual-spatial skills as adolescents but were impaired on arithmetic tasks, which are mediated in most healthy people by left parietal regions. It was assumed that the latter was due to a "crowding" of the left parietal areas by spatial processes, resulting in less synaptic space for arithmetic functions. Grafman proposed that this form of plasticity is restricted and most active during early developmental stages. However, it is worth noting that patients who sustain a left hemisphere lesion as adults and consecutively become aphasic show language-related activity in homologous regions of the right hemisphere (Thompson, 2000). Nevertheless, the functional significance of homologous brain activation for recovery of language functions is not yet clear. For example, those patients who had some remaining activity in the left hemisphere during language tasks were those who recovered best, while the degree of right hemispheric activity did not correlate with language skills (Rosen et al., 2000).

2. *Cross-modal reassignment:* Brain structures previously devoted to the processing of a particular kind of sensory input now accept input from a different modality. It is assumed that such input substitution takes place when there is similarity between the information normally processed in this area and the new information now invading it. For example, Grafman assumes that Braille reading is accompanied by an activation of the "visual" cortex in blind readers, because Braille and printed letters share some common abstract features. In fact, both Braille and printed words activate left basal, posterior temporal brain regions, which have been associated with reading (Büchel, Price, & Friston, 1998). More generally, it has been argued that primary sensory areas share several characteristics: they all consist of six layers and contain a layer with small cells known as the granular layer (layer IV). Moreover, sensory areas possess widespread horizontal connections that link cortical columns of similar functionality. Columns in turn are characterized by typical interlaminar connection patterns. Universal functional characteristics are, for example, some kind of topographic organization and lateral inhibition (i.e., contrast enhancement) and neurons selective for such features as orientation. Sur and co-workers (Sur & Leamey, 2001; Sur, Pallas, & Roe, 1990) hypothesized that common features are genetically predetermined, whereas differences between sensory areas (e.g., cytoarchitectonic features: corticocortical and subcortical connectivity, topography, and response properties of neurons) are specified by extrinsic input during development. Given the universal features of cortical tissue, it could be proposed that a sensory area is also capable of processing input from a different modality. In line with this view, neural transplant studies have shown that visual cortex tissue that is transplanted into somatosensory cortex acquires the functional properties of somatosensory rather than visual cortex (Schlaggar & O'Leary, 1991). Furthermore, rewiring experiments have shown that visual input that is rerouted to the auditory cortex (by ablating the visual targets and deafferenting auditory afferents) induces the development of a retinotopically organized map in auditory cortex, and animals rewired in such a manner seem to react differently to visual and auditory stimuli (reviewed in Pallas, 2001; Sur & Leamey, 2001).

3. *Map expansion:* According to Grafman, functional brain regions enlarge as a result of functional requirements. For example, the intense use of some fingers, such as by Braille readers (Hamilton & Pascual-Leone, 1998) or by stringed instrument players (Elbert, Pantev, Wienbruch, Rockstroh, & Taub, 1995), has been found to be accompanied by an expansion of the associated neural representations in sensory cortex. However, it should be noted that sensory map expansions are seen, sometimes to a larger degree, after deafferentation as

well. For example, after amputation of one finger, neurons in somatosensory cortex that were formally associated with the deafferented finger develop RFs at the adjacent fingers. The functional significance of the latter changes is unclear, and there is even evidence that deafferentation-induced reorganizations of sensory maps are maladaptive (Flor et al., 1995; Irvine, 2000; Mühlnickel, Elbert, Taub, & Flor, 1998), possibly being associated with phantom pain and tinnitus. On the other hand, perceptual learning does not always cause sensory map expansion (Gilbert, Sigman, & Crist, 2001; Ohl, Scheich, & Freeman, 2001; Recanzone, Merzenich, & Schreiner, 1992).

4. *Compensatory masquerade* denotes a novel allocation of particular neurocognitive processes to perform a task formerly mediated by the damaged system. The proposal of this fourth type of plasticity is reminiscent of the older "structural" versus "strategic" distinction (e.g., Miller, 1992). The underlying idea here is that no physiological or anatomical changes are involved if the system, as a result of peripheral or central damage, performs particular tasks via a different route. One example would be to remember routes by verbally mediated route memory after parietal cortex damage.

In the context of neuroplasticity elicited by sensory deprivation, a distinction between *intramodal* and *intermodal* (or *cross-modal*) changes has been suggested (Röder & Neville, 2003). Sensory-specific systems associated with the intact modalities may reorganize after deprivation of one sensory system as a result of the greater reliance (use dependence) of the individual on that system (intramodal changes). Moreover, if parts of one sensory system are deafferented, the rest of the system may change. On the other hand, brain areas normally associated with a totally deprived modality may be innervated by the intact sensory systems (intermodal/cross-modal changes or functional reallocation), resulting in an expansion of the intact sensory systems across modality borders. Again, these different types of plasticity are distinguished based on the presumed locus of neural changes. The intra-/intermodal classification may be extended to a system level: *intrasystem changes* would refer to neural changes (both physiological and anatomical) within a functional system that is linked to specific brain regions (i.e., an increase in processing efficiency), while *intersystem changes* would refer to changes of the neuroanatomical correlates of a functional system (e.g., activation of homologous brain areas of the right hemisphere for language after left hemisphere damage, or recruitment of visual brain areas for nonvisual tasks in blind individuals).

In this discussion, the term *reorganization* is used to describe changes with respect to the normal (i.e., evolutionarily determined) specialization of different parts of the brain, and can therefore also be used in discussing neuroplasticity studies in congenitally blind or deaf individuals.

Perceptual functions

After the deafferentation of parts of one sensory system, the associated sensory maps change (Buonomano & Merzenich, 1998; Cruikshank & Weinberger, 1996; Kaas, 1991, 2000). For example, if a finger is amputated, neurons with an RF on that finger develop RFs on adjacent fingers (Merzenich & Jenkins, 1993). Corresponding changes have been reported after lesions of the retina (Chino, Kaas, Smith, Langston, & Cheng, 1992; Eysel et al., 1999; Kaas et al., 1990) and the cochlea (Irvine, 2000), and similar sensory map changes are observed after perceptual training (Buonomano & Merzenich, 1998; Cruikshank & Weinberger, 1996; Gilbert, 1995; Gilbert et al., 2001; Kaas, 1991, 2000; Sathian, 1998). In the latter case, the "disruption" of the normal functional specialization of sensory cortex is not as large as after peripheral injury (Pons et al., 1991), and the reorganization is not as extensive. Sensory map changes have been demonstrated in humans after partial deafferentation, such as in amputees (Elbert et al., 1994; Flor et al., 1995; Grüsser et al., 2001) and in tinnitus patients (Hoke, Feldmann, Pantev, Lütkenhäner, & Lehnertz, 1989; Mühlnickel et al., 1998), and have also been demonstrated during the course of perceptual learning (Braun, Schweizer, Elbert, Birbaumer, & Taub, 2000; Braun, Wilms, et al., 2000; Elbert et al., 1995; Menning, Roberts, & Pantev, 2000; Pantev & Lütkenhäner, 2000; Pantev et al., 1998).

If visual input is missing, then the perceptual system relies more heavily on input from the intact sensory systems. Thus, it is plausible to expect similar use-dependent neural changes in blind people as those observed in healthy people after periods of intense perceptual training.

Anatomical studies in visually deprived animals reported an increase of the neuropil (dendrites, synapses) in auditory areas in mice (Gyllensten, Malmfors, & Norrlin, 1966) and rats (Ryugo, Ryugo, Globus, & Killackey, 1975), as well as an enlargement of the barrel fields in mice, which was most likely due to an increased use of the facial vibrissae for tactile orienting (Rauschecker, Tian, Korte, & Egert, 1992).

For auditory discrimination thresholds (e.g., for frequency, interaural time differences, and amplitude modulations), no differences have been detected between blind and sighted people (Bross & Borenstein, 1982; Niemeyer & Starlinger, 1981; Starlinger &

Niemeyer, 1981). However, the time resolution within the auditory system has been found to be superior in the blind (Muchnik, Efrati, Nemeth, Malin, & Hildesheimer, 1991; Rammsayer, 1992). As for the auditory modality, absolute tactile sensitivity does not seem to differ between the sighted and the blind (Axelrod, 1959; Pascual-Leone & Torres, 1993; Röder & Neville, 2003). On some tactile discrimination tasks, such as two-point discrimination (Röder & Neville, 2003), tactile hyperacuity tasks (Grant, Thiagarajah, & Sathian, 2000), and grating orientation tasks (Van Boven, Hamilton, Kauffman, Keenan, & Pascual-Leone, 2000), superior performance has been obtained by blind Braille readers (also see Sathian, 2000). Superior tactile resolution was related to an increased cortical sensory and motor representation of the Braille reading hand (Pascual-Leone & Torres, 1993; Pascual-Leone et al., 1993).

Moreover, early electrophysiological studies demonstrated shorter latencies for auditory (Niemeyer & Starlinger, 1981) and somatosensory (Feinsod, Bach-y-Rita, & Madey, 1973) brain ERPs in blind individuals compared with sighted humans. These findings have been replicated for both the auditory and the somatosensory system (Röder, Rösler, Hennighausen, & Näcker, 1996) and extended by demonstrating shorter discrimination times in the same blind individuals (Fig. 46.1). Moreover, no difference in the scalp distribution of this early potential shift (N1) was observed between blind groups and sighted groups. Therefore, Röder et al. (1996) concluded that the perceptual processing step indicated by N1 is mediated in the blind by the same neural systems as in the sighted, but that blind individuals may have increased their processing efficiency (intramodal plasticity). The N1 latency differences between the sighted group and the blind group do not explain the total reaction time advantage of the blind. However, there is no one-to-one matching between ERP latencies and reaction times (Hillyard & Picton, 1987). The importance of the N1 latency differences for the behavioral outcome is, however, suggested by the fact that the group differences were larger both for the N1 latencies and for reaction times for somatosensory than auditory stimuli.

Another possibility for investigating the excitability of neural networks is to study the refractoriness of ERPs. Stimulus repetition usually results in an amplitude reduction of several potential deflections, and the degree of this attenuation is a function of the interstimulus interval (ISI) between the consecutive events. The refractory periods depend on the ERP component; for example, P3 recovers within 1 s, while it takes 10–15 s for the N1–P2 complex (vertex potential) to recover completely (Näätänen, 1992). The relative refractory period has been regarded as an index of the excitability of cortical cell assemblies under stimulation conditions and has been related to processing rate and efficiency (Neville, Schmidt, & Kutas, 1983).

Röder, Rösler, and Neville (1999) presented frequent standard tones and rare target tones (differing in frequency) with varying ISIs (500, 1000, and 2000 ms) to a group of 11 congenitally blind and 11 age-, sex-, and handedness-matched sighted adults. The participants' task was to detect the target stimuli and to press a button as fast as possible. It was found that the auditory N1 and P2 potentials varied as a function of ISI in both groups (Fig. 46.2). However, in blind participants, N1 recovered earlier over temporal recording sites and P2 recovered earlier over frontal cortex than in sighted participants (Fig. 46.2). In contrast, no group differences in the scalp distribution of N1 and P1 (including the refractory effect for both potential shifts) were observed. Therefore, the shorter recovery cycle for the vertex potential suggests an enhanced excitability of the auditory system proper in blind individuals. It might be speculated that this change originates in a hypertrophy within auditory areas, as has been observed previously in visually deprived animals (Gyllensten et al., 1966; Ryugo et al., 1975). Therefore, intramodal changes may have contributed to an increased auditory processing efficiency contributing to shorter target detection times in the same blind individuals. It is interesting that similar results have been reported for musicians (Pantev et al., 1998): on magnetoencephalographic (MEG) recordings, a higher amplitude of the magnetic equivalent of N1 to tones was found in musicians than in control participants. Therefore, perceptual learning rather than blindness per se may be crucial for the shorter refractoriness of the vertex potential in the blind.

Group differences in scalp topography were observed for a later ERP wave: N2, elicited by targets, had a larger amplitude over centroposterior brain areas in the blind than in the sighted (Fig. 46.3). Data from patients with focal brain damage (Knight, 1990) and intracranial recordings in humans (Halgren et al., 1995) suggest that the parietal lobe, as well as multisensory areas of the temporoparietal junction, contributes to the generation of N2. It was speculated that visual parts or multisensory neurons of these polymodal fields are occupied by the intact modalities in the blind participants, similar to what has been observed in visually deprived animals (Hyvärinen, Hyvärinen, & Linnankoski, 1981; Rauschecker, 1995). This may have resulted in stronger and more posteriorly oriented N2 generators in blind than in sighted humans. Because N2 has been associated with early semiautomatic classification processes (Näätänen & Picton, 1986; Ritter, Simon, &

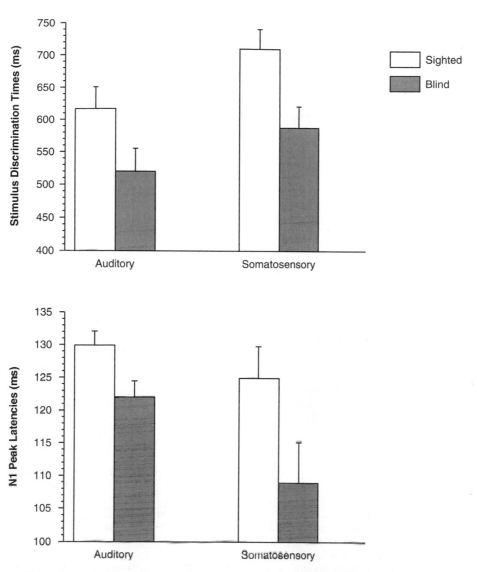

FIGURE 46.1   Perceptual functions. *Top:* Auditory and somatosensory discrimination times (with SE bars) for blind and sighted adults. *Bottom:* Auditory and somatosensory N1 latencies (with SE bars) for the same participants. Blind individuals showed shorter target discrimination times for both auditory and somatosensory stimuli and had shorter latencies for the N1 potential. (Adapted from Röder et al., 1996. © 1996 Elsevier Science Ireland Ltd.)

Vaughan, 1983), a reorganization or expansion of this system may have contributed to the superior discrimination speed of the blind as well. It should be noted that the posteriorly shifted N2 topography of the blind is one of the most reliable findings to emerge from ERP investigations in blind humans and has been reported both for the auditory system and the somatosensory system by several laboratories (Kujala et al., 1995; Liotti, Ryder, & Woldorff, 1998; Röder et al., 1996; Röder, Teder-Sälejärvi, et al., 1997).

In deaf people, basic visual functions such as brightness discrimination (Bross, 1979), flicker fusion threshold (Bross & Sauerwein, 1980), contrast sensitivity (Finney, Fine, & Dobkins, 2001), and preattentive texture segregation (Rettenbach, Diller, & Sireteanu, 1999) do not differ from those of hearing controls. As in the blind, superior performance by deaf seems to arise on more attention-demanding tasks (Rettenbach et al., 1999). For example, deaf people have shown superior performance when rare movement changes in the peripheral part of one hemifield had to be detected while the same changes in any other location had to be ignored (Bavelier et al., 2001; Neville & Lawson, 1987). A greater recruitment of visual motion areas (MT/MST) in the deaf was also observed with fMRI in a peripheral but not central motion detection task (Bavelier et al., 2000). Neville et al. (1983) investigated the functionality of the visual system in deaf people by measuring

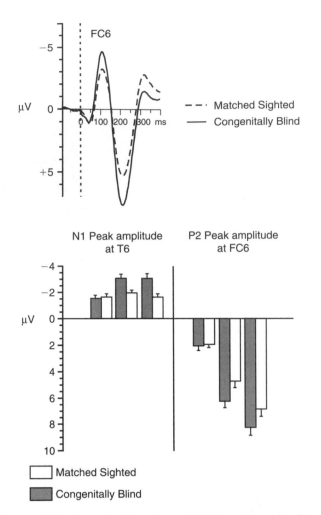

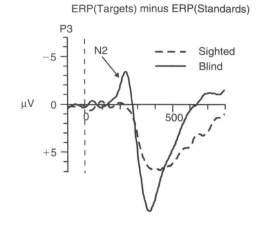

FIGURE 46.2 Perceptual functions. *Top:* Grand average of the auditory ERPs elicited by tones presented after a 2000 ms ISI. *Bottom:* Mean peak amplitude (with SE bars) of N1 at a temporal site (left) and P2 at a frontal site (right) as a function of ISI. The congenitally blind showed shorter refractory periods than the sighted. (Adapted from Röder, Rösler, et al., 1999. © 1999 Elsevier Science Ireland Ltd.)

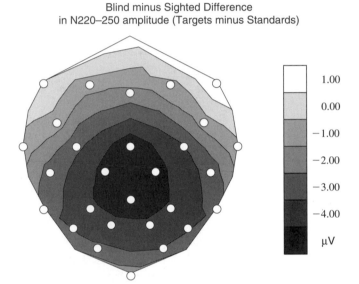

FIGURE 46.3 Perceptual functions. *Top:* The ERP(Targets) minus ERP(Standards) difference wave at the parietal site P3 averaged across sighted and blind participants, respectively. N2 was seen only at frontocentral sites in the sighted. *Bottom:* Topographic map showing the group difference in the scalp distribution of the N2 wave (average amplitude, 220–250 ms). The darker the gray shading, the more negative the N2 of the blind compared with the sighted. The group difference is largest at centroparietal recording sites located above multimodal brain structures. (Adapted from Röder, Rösler, et al., 1999. © 1999 Elsevier Science Ireland Ltd.).

refractory periods of visual ERPs (N150 and P230); they found that they recover faster in auditorily deprived adults than in hearing adults. These data, together with the corresponding results in the blind (Röder, Rösler, & Neville, 1999), suggest that an increase in the excitability of sensory areas associated with the intact modalities reflects a general adaptation of the CNS to sensory loss. Finally, tactile deviant detection was found to be superior in deaf people, whereas tactile frequency discrimination thresholds were not (Levänen & Hamdorf, 2001).

Studies in deaf individuals suggest that changes at the perceptual level can occur together with, or may contribute to, changes in more complex perceptual-cognitive functions (Neville & Bavelier, 2000). Similarly, researchers have argued that some impairments in higher cognitive functions (e.g., specific language im-

pairments) originate in deficits of elementary perceptual skills (Tallal et al., 1996). Moreover, it has been proposed that the degree of potential reorganization increases with each processing step and is larger for sensory association cortex than for primary sensory cortex or the thalamus (Kaas, 1991). Thus, sensory deprivation should result in changes in higher cognitive functions, such as language and spatial reasoning, both at the behavioral level and at the neural level.

Language function

Studies on language in the blind have mainly focused on language acquisition. Researchers have wondered if there is a unique or specific contribution of the visual system to language learning that might lead to deviations and delays in the language acquisition of blind children. On the other hand, it has been argued that blind people, including blind children, need language much more extensively in order to acquire knowledge about the world. Therefore, Chomsky (cited in Andersen, Dunlea, & Kekelis, 1993) hypothesized that blind children should pick up language more rapidly than their sighted counterparts. Empirical studies have supported the first hypothesis; delays and deviations in the acquisition of different aspects of language, including semantics, syntax, and phonology, have been observed in blind children (Dunlea, 1989; Mills, 1983, 1988; Pèrez-Pereira, & Conti-Ramsden, 1999). For example, the lack of overgeneralization and the reduced number of word inventions in blind children's language have been interpreted as indicating impaired category formations, reflecting a general cognitive deficit that is mirrored in language (Andersen, Dunlea, & Kekelis, 1984, 1993). Most prominently, the term *verbalism* has repeatedly been associated with the language of blind people. The term encapsulates the assumption that blind people use words—for example, visual terms—without being aware of the underlying meaning. However, there is now convincing evidence that blind people use visual words such as "look" or "see" with the meaning of, for example, "explore haptically" and "meet," respectively (Landau & Gleitman, 1985). Landau and Gleitman (1985) proposed that a word's meaning can be learned without direct sensory experience, based on the word's position within a sentence, an idea called "bootstrapping." Although there is evidence that concept formation is delayed in the blind child, these initial disadvantages seem to dissipate with age and are negligible after the age of 10 (Pèrez-Pereira & Conti-Ramsden, 1999). Moreover, the reduced number of overgeneralizations observed in blind children most likely arises from the smaller number of visual features of their concepts rather than from a general cognitive deficit, because blind children do overgeneralize on the basis of auditory or tactile features (Mills, 1988).

As for the acquisition of semantic aspects of language, the initial development of syntax in the blind is characterized by delays and deviations from the normal time course. For example, blind children use functional words later than their sighted counterparts, and their early speech contains an unusually high number of imperatives. However, these and other differences vanish with age too, and have been mainly attributed to altered child-parent interactions as a secondary consequence of blindness. For example, a common attentional space is created between a sighted child and a parent when the two look at the same object, a communication tool not available to blind children. As a result, blind children's parents use more imperatives, and this speech pattern in turn is mirrored by their children.

Additionally, the general developmental delay of blind children has to be taken into account when discussing language skills in blind compared with sighted children. Its origins have been seen in an impoverished input or less active environmental stimulation for the blind child. Nevertheless, blind children do finally master language acquisition, and it seems that from then on, they use language as their main tool to acquire knowledge about the world (Pèrez-Pereira & Conti-Ramsden, 1999). For example, spatial skills improve faster once language and abstract verbal reasoning have been mastered (Pèrez-Pereira & Conti-Ramsden, 1999).

Other studies on language in the blind have focused on the use of Braille (the writing and reading system of the blind), and on the effects of Braille acquisition on language perception in general. For example, it has been hypothesized that reading Braille (similar to other tactile tasks; Summers & Lederman, 1990) entails spatial components that are not part of reading print. It has been suggested that, as a consequence, Braille reading involves right hemisphere functions to a larger degree, which in turn may result in a higher importance of right hemisphere structures in the processing of spoken language as well (Hermelin & O'Connor, 1971; Karavatos, Kapromos, & Tzavaras, 1984). It has been reported that blind pupils did not show the typical right ear/left hemisphere advantage for the perception of dichotically presented consonant-vowel-consonant strings (Larsen & Hakonsen, 1983). Moreover, it has been observed that with increasing proficiency in Braille reading, the left hemisphere advantage for spoken language perception vanishes (Karavatos et al., 1984). These reports, however, contrast with the results of Bertelson, Morais, Mousty, and Hublet (1987) demonstrating an even larger right side/left hemisphere advantage for the perception of auditorily presented consonant-vowel strings in blind adults. Therefore, the effects of using Braille instead of print on the cerebral organization of language are not yet clear. Moreover, all studies on language lateralization in the blind have used only indirect measures to determine cerebral processing asymmetries, and most studies have been conducted in children or adolescents. There are only a few studies on speech perception skills in blind adults, and those studies primarily focused on the perceptual aspects of speech comprehension rather than on language functions proper. These studies found superior performance on single word identification for the blind, particularly under conditions of a low signal-to-noise ratio (S/N) (Muchnik et al., 1991; Niemeyer & Starlinger, 1981).

This section discusses studies that focused on semantic and syntactic aspects of language and their cerebral organization in congenitally blind versus sighted adults. The studies used spoken language because this is the language modality both sighted and blind people are most familiar with from early in life.

In the first study to be discussed, Röder, Rösler, and Neville (2000) recorded ERPs while congenitally blind adults and sighted controls matched for age, handedness, sex, and education listened to short sentences. A paradigm was used that is well regarded in the ERP literature for the investigation of semantic aspects of language and that provides information about syntactic processing functions as well. The sentences terminated either with a highly expected, congruous word or a nonexpected, incongruous word. The participant's task was to decide whether or not the sentence was meaningful. FRPs were measured for both words in the middle and words at the end of sentences. Because a delayed response mode was used, only accuracy data could be obtained. Error rates were low (<2%) and did not differ between groups. In agreement with the results of other studies (Brown, Hagoort, & Kutas, 2000), incongruous final sentence words elicited a negativity (N400) with a left frontocentrotemporal distribution (Hagoort & Brown, 2000; Holcomb & Neville, 1991). The same effect was detected in the blind participants but with an earlier onset, indicating that they had detected the incongruency earlier (Fig. 46.4). Moreover, the N400 in the blind had a symmetrical and posteriorly extended scalp topography, suggesting that the cerebral organization of language in blind individuals may differ from that of sighted persons. The N400 scalp topography of blind participants resembled that of children before they learn to read and write (Holcomb, Coffey, & Neville, 1992). It was hypothesized that owing to the lack of visual input, less competition between areas and hemispheres in blind individuals results in a representation of language that is extended bilaterally and posteriorly. This hypothesis has been supported by fMRI studies (Röder, Stock, Bien, Neville, & Rösler, 2002). Whereas in right-handed, sighted young adults, mainly the left hemisphere perisylvian cortex (including Broca's and Wernicke's area) was activated during speech processing (Röder, Stock, Neville, Bien, & Rösler, 2002), congenitally blind adults of the same age, sex, and handedness had additional activations in homologous regions in the right hemisphere. Moreover, activation of visual

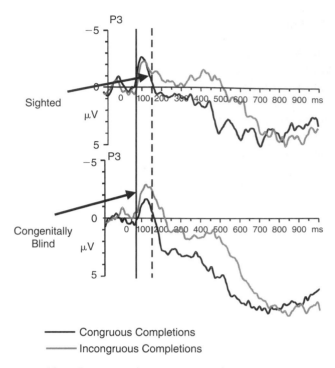

FIGURE 46.4 Language functions. Grand average of ERPs for congruous (black line) and incongruous completions (gray line) for sighted (top) and congenitally blind (bottom) participants. Blind participants detected nonmatching sentence final words faster than sighted participants. (Adapted from Röder et al., 2000. © 2000 Elsevier Science Ireland Ltd.)

cortex areas was found in the blind participants but not in the sighted participants (Fig. 46.5).

The ERP study focused on the incongruity effect for words at the end of the sentence, that is, words that were or were not semantically and syntactically primed. Therefore, it is not clear from which aspect of processing the advantage of the blind participants arose. Röder et al. (2000) reported evidence for enhanced processing of syntactic language elements as well; functional words as compared with content words elicited a pronounced negativity in the blind participants that was not seen in the sighted participants. Therefore, the hypothesis was put forward that in blind people, the processing of functional words is particularly enhanced. This enhanced processing may have two, nonexclusive causes. On the one hand, building an expectancy on the basis of the syntactic context (e.g., by using functional words) speeds up the comprehension of the next content word. On the other hand, in the context of a noisy background, the understanding of function words suffers relatively more than the intelligibility of content words, because function words are more acoustically degraded (Herron & Bates, 1997). In these situations, with a low S/N, sighted people make additional use of facial cues not available to the blind in order to enhance

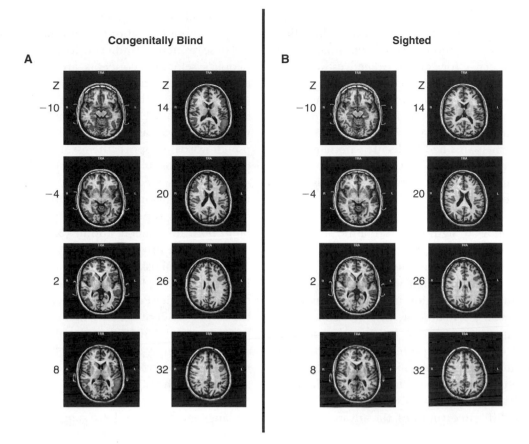

Congenitally Blind

A

Sighted

B

FIGURE 46.5   Language functions. Brain activation pattern during speech processing in sighted (left) and congenitally blind (right) adults as revealed with fMRI. The activations are projected on a series of horizontal sections of the brain of one participant. Neuroradiological convention is used; that is, the left side of the brain is shown at right, and visa versa. Although sighted participants activated nearly exclusively left hemispheric perisylvian brain regions, the congenitally blind showed activations in the homologous right hemispheric areas as well as in visual cortex (From Röder, Stock, et al., 2002. © Federation of the European Neuroscience Societies.)

speech intelligibility (Calvert et al., 1998). As a matter of fact, the N1 to function words was larger in amplitude than the N1 to content words in blind but not in sighted participants. Insofar as N1 amplitude is a function of attention allocated to a stimulus, this result indicates an enhanced processing of function words by the blind participants (Hillyard, Hink, Schwent, & Picton, 1973).

However, it could be hypothesized that in the experiment of Röder et al. (2000), blind participants finished the perceptual analysis of the words earlier than sighted participants rather than using the semantic or syntactic context more efficiently.

To find out which processing stages differ in the blind, a semantic and morphosyntactic priming experiment was conducted (Röder, Demuth, Streb, & Rösler, 2002). It is well known that words embedded in a semantic-associative or syntactic context are processed faster than words presented in a neutral or incongruent context, or else in isolation (e.g., Balota, 1994). A comparison of semantic and morphosyntactic priming effects between

blind and sighted people would be expected to reveal those subsystems of speech comprehension that contribute to, or cause, faster speech understanding in the blind: (1) If blind people have less elaborated semantic-conceptual networks, as has been argued for blind children (Pring, Freistone, & Katan, 1990), smaller semantic priming effects would be expected for them than for sighted controls (see earlier discussion of the language acquisition literature). (2) If blind people make more efficient use of the syntactical context, they should show larger syntactic priming effects than sighted controls. (3) If blind people have superior performance on perceptual processing steps, they should show shorter reaction times in all conditions and for pseudowords as well.

A lexical decision task was used in which adjectives were presented as primes and nouns or pseudowords as targets. There were 91 stimulus sets, each consisting of one adjective, four legitimate German nouns, and four pronounceable pseudowords. One of the four legitimate nouns was semantically and syntactically, one only semantically, one only syntactically, and one neither semantically nor syntactically associated with the adjective. The syntactic relation was operationalized by inflecting the adjective for gender. Adjectives were spoken by a male voice and nouns by a female voice. Neither mean word frequencies nor stimulus length differed significantly between the four conditions with legitimate nouns. Stimuli were presented via headphones, and participants had to decide whether or not the target noun was a legitimate German word. Twelve congenitally blind adults and 14 sighted controls of the same mean age, sex distribution, and education took part.

The results showed significant semantic and morphosyntactic priming effects, both of about equal size (Fig. 46.6). Moreover, the combined semantic/syntactic priming effect was larger than would have been expected by summing the reaction time advantage of the conditions with only semantically or only syntactically congruent context information. Neither the size nor the pattern of these priming effects differed between sighted and blind groups (Fig. 46.6). However, overall lexical decision times for the blind participants were shorter, particularly for pseudowords. Because the groups did not differ in error rates, the advantage of the

blind could not be explained by a hypothesis that blind people do not care about committing errors.

These results contradict both the hypothesis that blind people's semantic concepts are impoverished (Pring et al., 1990) and the hypothesis put forward by Röder et al. (2000) that the blind make more extended use of syntactic context. However, the finding of a general reaction time advantage for the blind (most clearly for pseudowords) supports the assumption that perceptual processing aspects rather than specific language functions are enhanced in the blind. This observation fits with other behavioral and/or neurophysiological studies demonstrating superior auditory perceptual skills in the blind both for speech stimuli (Niemeyer & Starlinger, 1981; Röder, Rösler, et al., 1999) and for simple tones (Kujala, Lehtokoski, Alho, Kekoni, & Näätänen, 1997; Röder et al., 1996; Röder, Rösler, et al., 1999) (see earlier discussion under Perceptual Functions). With respect to the earlier onset of the ERP incongruity effect reported by Röder et al. (2000), the results of Röder, Demuth, et al. (2002) imply that it very likely stems from a perceptual rather than from a semantic or syntactic processing advantage of the blind.

Finally, it should be pointed out that the experiments on language discussed here suggest that blind adults do

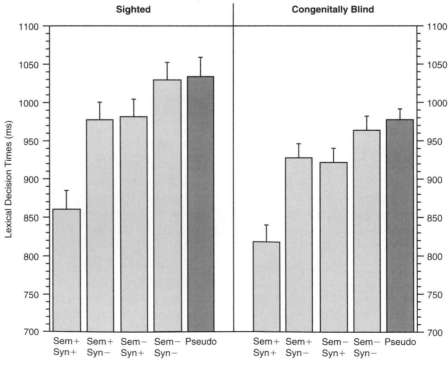

FIGURE 46.6   Language functions. Mean lexical decision times as a function of semantic and syntactic priming. Sem+, semantically primed; Syn+, morphosyntactically primed; Sem−, not semantically primed; Syn−, not morphosyntactically primed; Pseudo, pronounceable nonword. Priming effects were similar in the blind and sighted group but the blind had overall shorter lexical decision times. (Adapted from Röder, Demuth, et al., 2002. © Psychology Press.)

not show impaired language abilities, as was suggested by the language acquisition literature. In contrast, speech comprehension seems to be enhanced, or faster, in the congenitally blind. The present evidence supports the idea that this can be attributed to more enhanced perceptual processing skills rather than more efficient semantic or syntactic processing in the blind. A corresponding mutual dependence of basic perceptual functions and language-related processes was reported for children with specific language impairments (Tallal et al., 1996).

Differences in the cerebral organization of language as a result of altered language input due to auditory deprivation have been observed in deaf signers as well (Neville & Bavelier, 2000). Native deaf signers display a pronounced right hemispheric activation both during processing American Sign Language (ASL) and English (Neville & Bavelier, 2000; Neville et al., 1998). Since a similar brain activation pattern as in the deaf was seen in healthy individuals who learned ASL as their first language, it was concluded that the acquisition of a sign language rather than auditory deprivation proper contributes to the stronger right hemispheric involvement in language processing. Moreover, the latter was found to be only partial if ASL was acquired late (Newman, Pancheva, Ozawa, Neville, & Ullman, 2001), suggesting a more pronounced plasticity of the language system during development. For processing written English, a larger effect of late acquisition due to auditory deprivation is seen for syntactic than semantic processing aspects (Neville, Mills, & Lawson, 1992).

It is interesting to note that both in the blind and in the deaf, there seems to be a mutual interdependence between changes in perceptual functions and alterations in some aspects of language processing. In sum, these studies demonstrate that different subcomponents of complex functions have to be analyzed in order to conclude which subsystem is capable of change and may contribute to behavioral changes such as faster speech comprehension.

Spatial functions

Animal studies have clearly demonstrated that there are interdependencies between the senses in spatial processes associated with the localization of an event. For example, the spatial position of an audiovisual stimulus is determined more accurately than that of the auditory or the visual part alone. In cats and monkeys, polymodal brain areas (including the superior colliculus [SC] and the anterior ectosylvian area) have been found to contain neurons that are responsive to stimuli of more than one modality, many of them having spatially over-lapping RFs (for reviews, see B. A. Stein, Wallace, & Stanford, 2000; B. E. Stein, 1998; B. E. Stein & Meredith, 1993). If, for example, both the auditory and the visual part of an object fall within the overlapping part of a neuron's RFs (Kadunce, Vaughan, Wallace, & Stein, 2001), the neuron fires more vigorously than would have been expected by the maximum response to either single modality. Similar interactions between the different modalities at the neural level exist in humans as well (Driver & Spence, 1998), and moreover, it has been found that spatial attention, e.g., to visual stimuli, affects the processing of auditory stimuli at the attended location as early as 100 ms after stimulus onset (e.g., Eimer, Cockurn, Smedley, & Driver, 2001; Hillyard, Simpson, Woods, VanVoorhis, & Münte, 1984). Given these interdependencies between sensory systems, it has been proposed that the visual system, which has the highest spatial resolution, possesses an instructive role in the generation of spatial maps assessed by the other modalities. Visual maps are a simple retinotopic projection onto brain structures such as the SC and visual cortex. By contrast, auditory space maps have to be computed from several nontopographic cues (interaural time and level differences, spectral cues) and have to be adjusted through development, especially because of the growth of the head and ears. Therefore, auditory maps are more adaptable.

To test the role of visual cues in the generation and adaption of auditory spatial representations, visually deprived animals, as well as blind humans, have been tested on auditory localization tasks. Studies in owls rearing with prisms displacing their angle of view showed that auditory space maps in the optical tectum shifted with the visual displacement, suggesting a visual dominance of auditory space representations (e.g., DeBello & Knudsen, 2001). Moreover, binocularly deprived owls displayed less precisely tuned auditory space maps than sighted owls (Knudsen, Esterly, & du Lac, 1991). These results have been interpreted as evidence that the visual system guides the setup of auditory space maps. However, studies in other species, including humans, have not always confirmed the findings in owls. It is important to note, though, that the auditory system of owls differs in may respects from that of cats and primates (including humans). The ears of owls are arranged asymmetrically, and they are hardly able to move their eyes. The latter may favor a very tight relationship between auditory and visual spatial representations because a continuous recalculation of auditory and visual input into a common reference frame (eye- vs. head-centered) is not necessary. Moreover, the spatial tuning of tectal neurons is, possibly as a consequence, much more precise, and their RFs are smaller than those in the SC of cats or primates (see DeBello & Knudsen, 2001). Nevertheless, results from studies in blind humans are far from being consistent either. On the behavioral level, auditory localization skills have been reported to be worse (Zwiers, Van Opstal, & Cruysberg, 2001a), equal (Ashmead et al., 1998; Wanet & Veraart, 1985; Zwiers et al., 2001b), and better (Lessard, Paré, Leporé, & Lassonde, 1998; Muchnik et al., 1991; Rice, 1970).

In a series of experiments with visually deprived cats, Rauschecker and co-workers (reviewed in Rauschecker, 1995, 2001) found that neurons of visual subareas of the polymodal anterior ectosylvian cortex became responsive to auditory and somatosensory stimuli. Most important, the number and sharpness of spatially tuned auditory neurons were increased (Korte & Rauschecker, 1993; Rauschecker & Korte, 1993). On the behavioral level, visually deprived cats showed better auditory localization, particularly at lateral and rear positions (Rauschecker & Kniepert, 1994).

Since the research series of Rauschecker and co-workers established an animal model both at the neural and at the behavioral level, it was used to design a corresponding study in humans (Röder, Teder-Sälejärvi, et al., 1999). The goal of the study on auditory localization in humans was to investigate both the localization accuracy at the behavioral level and spatial tuning at the neural level. Because a direct measurement of the spatial tuning of neurons (i.e., the assessment of the RF of a neuron) is not possible in humans, ERPs were used to assess the width of the spatial attention focus, which is limited by the spatial resolution of auditory networks. It is well established that several components of the ERPs are modulated by spatial attention (e.g., Hillyard, Mangun, Woldorff, & Luck, 1995; Mangun & Hillyard, 1995; Näätänen, 1992). The N1 of auditory ERPs displays the largest increase in amplitude for stimuli presented exactly at the attended location and a smaller amplitude modulation for tones from adjacent positions (Teder-Sälejärvi & Hillyard, 1998). The steepness of the N1 amplitude gradients can be used to assess the sharpness of auditory spatial tuning in humans. Picking up on this idea, Röder, Teder-Sälejärvi, et al. (1999) presented short noise bursts at a high rate from eight speakers, four located in front of the participants (central array) and four on the right side (peripheral array) (Fig. 46.7, top). In alternating blocks, participants had to attend to the central speaker at zero degrees and to the rightmost speaker at 90 degrees azimuth in order to detect a rare deviant sound there. Both frequent ($P = 0.84$, standards) and rare noise bursts ($P = 0.16$, deviants) were presented with the same probability from all eight speakers. This paradigm allows for the assessment of localization accuracy by calculating the response rates to deviants (hit responses and false alarms). Additionally, spatial tuning of auditory processes can be estimated by analyzing the gradients of N1 amplitude modulation around the attended sound source. Eight congenitally blind adults and eight sighted controls matched for age, handedness, and sex took part. In agreement with the results of psychophysical research (Mills, 1972), a less precise localization of sounds from peripheral than from central sources was found at the behavioral level in both sighted and blind participants (Fig. 46.7, left). However, response gradients were steeper for the blind than for the sighted participants when the most peripheral speaker had to be attended to, indicating that they had a specific advantage in localizing lateral sound sources. Corresponding results were found for the N1 amplitude gradients (Fig. 46.7, right). For centrally presented sounds, the N1 modulation due to attention decreased as a function of the distance of the sound from the attended loudspeaker proper. Although the steepness of the central N1 amplitude gradients was similar in both groups, it was greater in the blind for sounds from the periphery. These results suggest that early spatial filtering mechanisms are more sharply tuned in the blind than in the sighted, resulting in a more precise preselection of sound sources. That this was true only for peripheral sound sources indicates that the superior performance of the blind is very specific and cannot be explained by nonspecific factors such as greater vigilance or motivation. The findings match well those of Rauschecker and co-workers in visually deprived cats and those of King and Parsons (1999) in visually deprived ferrets.

The processing advantage of peripheral sounds in the blind is further substantiated by the shorter latencies of the N1, N2, and P3 potentials, particularly for peripheral targets. In addition to the sharper tuning of the N1 amplitude gradients, a posteriorly shifted scalp topography of the spatial attention effect was observed in the blind, that is, they showed a more central rather than frontal maximum than did the sighted. It was speculated that this shift might originate in a reorganization of multisensory brain areas similar to that reported previously for visually deprived cats (Korte & Rauschecker, 1993; Rauschecker & Korte, 1993) and monkeys (Hyvärinen, Hyvärinen, et al., 1981). Evidence from a PET experiment with human participants also points toward this idea: Weeks et al. (2000) found a larger PET activation of parietal brain areas in a group of early-blind humans compared with a sighted control group while they were performing an auditory localization task. Moreover, this activation extended to parieto-occipital association

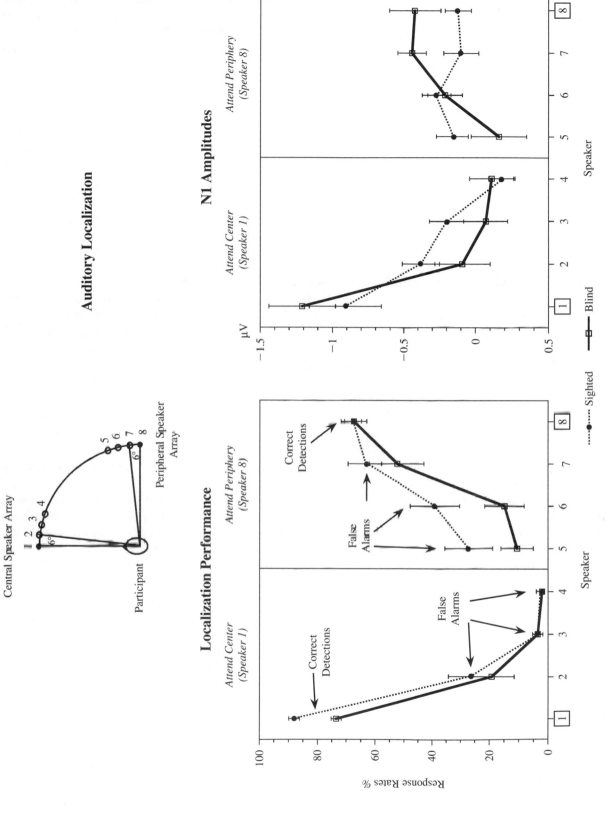

Auditory Localization

Central Speaker Array

Peripheral Speaker Array

Participant

N1 Amplitudes

Attend Center (Speaker 1)

Attend Periphery (Speaker 8)

μV

Speaker

Localization Performance

Attend Center (Speaker 1)

Attend Periphery (Speaker 8)

Correct Detections

False Alarms

Correct Detections

False Alarms

Response Rates %

Speaker

····· Sighted

—— Blind

FIGURE 46.7 Spatial functions. A schematic drawing of the speaker array is shown on top. Localization performance when speaker 1 was attended ("attend center") and when speaker 8 was attended ("attend periphery") is shown in the lower left panel. At right, the amplitude of the auditory N1 is shown for standards from speakers 1–4 for the "attend center" condition and speakers 5–8 for the "attend periphery" condition. The data on the blind and sighted subjects are superimposed. The congenitally blind showed more precise localization of sound from the periphery, which was accompanied by a sharper spatial tuning of the N1. (Adapted from Röder, Teder-Sälejärvi, et al., 1999. © 1999 Macmillian Magazines, Ltd.)

733

areas. A correlation analysis of the activation levels of different brain areas revealed a positive relationship between right posterior parietal and right occipital areas in the blind but a negative relation in the sighted, which was interpreted as further evidence for a functional connection between the two areas in the blind.

A recent study, however, observed disadvantages for congenitally blind compared with sighted participants on an auditory elevation judgment task in which spectral cues became the essential feature for localization (Zwiers et al., 2001a). However, in the same year and in the same blind sample, the same authors reported equal performance on a series of experiments that required localizing sounds at different azimuths and elevations (Zwiers et al., 2001b). Missing advantages for the blind may have been due to the fact that Zwiers et al. (2001a, 2001b) tested only sound positions covering central space, for which neither Rauschecker (1995) nor Röder, Teder-Sälejärvi, et al. (1999) had found advantages for blind individuals.

Finally, the question arises of how the improved auditory localization performance develops in the congenitally blind. Developmental studies have observed an earlier onset of auditory than visual orienting in both animals (Philipps & Brugge, 1985) and humans (Morrongiello, 1994). Therefore, auditory spatial representations may initially evolve by the activity of sensorimotor feedback loops (auditory, tactile proprioceptive interactions) without visual guidance. In sighted individuals theses first spatial maps may reorganize as soon as visual input becomes available (DeBello & Knudsen, 2001; Turkewitz & Kenny, 1982), while they refine in their absence. This idea is supported by the differential advantage for blind people found by Röder, Teder-Sälejärvi, et al. (1999) and Rauschecker (1995), that is, their performance was superior only at peripheral (90 degrees) and rear locations, where sight does not provide any useful information (field of view: ±80 degrees). For central space, there might be a recalibration or refinement of auditory maps by visual input that possibly reduces the variability of elevation judgments in the sighted (Zwiers et al., 2001a). Both in cats (Wallace & Stein, 1997) and in monkeys (Wallace & Stein, 2001), multisensory enhancement emerges during the first month of life. Furthermore, patients with macular degeneration show worse localization in frontal but not in peripheral space (Lessard et al., 1998). In these patients, the distorted information for the central field of view might have caused a distorted auditory map as well (similar to that seen in owls reared wearing prisms). The higher reliance on audition for monitoring the environment may have led to a refinement of auditory peripheral space representations in the blind, possibly by an expansion of these representations in multisensory brain areas where peripheral space is dominant (Hikosaka, Iwai, Hide-Aki, & Tanaka, 1988).

These reports on auditory spatial attention in blind individuals correspond to findings in the deaf. Enhanced processing of visual events in peripheral but not in central space has been found repeatedly in deaf adults (Bavelier et al., 2000; Neville & Lawson, 1987; Neville et al., 1983). It is worth noting that the brain responses of the blind and the deaf differed from those of the sighted and hearing, respectively, as early as 100 ms after stimulus onset—that is, in the same time range that has been found to be sensitive to cross-modal spatial attention (Eimer et al., 2001; Hillyard et al., 1984).

Recent fMRI studies in the deaf have confirmed and extended the electrophysiological findings by demonstrating a more extended activation of the motion-selective area MT-MST in the deaf than in hearing controls for peripheral but not central attention (Bavelier et al., 2000). Moreover, a recruitment of the polymodal posterior superior temporal sulcus and a stronger activation of posterior parietal cortex during a luminance and velocity detection task has been reported for the same deaf signers (Bavelier et al., 2001). Therefore, data from electrophysiological and imaging studies give rise to the possibility that a reorganization of multimodal brain areas contributes to compensatory behavior changes—in other words, to improved auditory localization in the early blind and enhanced visual attention in the deaf.

Although auditory localization involves distal space, other studies on space perception in the blind have focused on near space, that is, spatial positions that can be explored with the hands (reviewed in Röder & Neville, 2003; Thinus-Blanc & Gaunet, 1997). For example, spatial imagery tasks in congenitally and late-blind adults were used (Röder & Rösler, 1998; Röder, Rösler, Heil, & Hennighausen, 1993; Röder, Rösler, & Hennighausen, 1997). Hardly any performance difference between blind and sighted groups has been obtained. Moreover, electrophysiological data (see also the PET data of Weeks et al., 2000) suggested an involvement of parietal regions, which have often been recognized to be important for spatial processes (Andersen, Snyder, Bradley, & Xong, 1997) not only in sighted but also in blind people. The latter finding questions the proposal that blind individuals succeed on spatial tasks because they activate alternative verbal strategies (Dodds 1983).

For deaf signers, it has been hypothesized that they may possess superior visuospatial imagery abilities (Emmorey, Kosslyn, & Bellugi, 1993). In sign language space, mediates grammatical functions. For example, what is subject and what is object is expressed by pointing to particular locations, and verb signs move between these locations. The generation of complex images was indeed found to be enhanced in deaf native signers (Emmorey et al., 1993). The fact that hearing native signers showed a similar advantage suggests that the early exposure to sign language rather than deafness resulted in the superior performance of the signers. No group differences were found for other spatial tasks, including mental rotation speed and spatial memory (Emmorey et al., 1993).

Mechanisms

The central issue now is what can be learned about the compensatory plasticity capabilities of the CNS from studies in the blind and the deaf. First, for studies reported in the blind, it is important that they show superior performance on auditory tasks of different complexities on which they rely heavily in everyday life (auditory discrimination, auditory localization, speech comprehension, short- and long-term memory [not reviewed here]). According to the listing of possible outcomes of studies comparing congenitally blind and sighted controls (discussed earlier under Sensory Deprivation Model), these findings indicate a "hypercompensation" in the blind, that is, an improvement above and beyond the performance level of sighted individuals. This raises the question of whether the improvements within the intact sensory systems are able to substitute for the lost visual input. This question was explicitly tested in a voice recognition experiment (in Röder & Neville, 2003), and no evidence for such a substitution was demonstrated: sighted participants recognized persons on the basis of faces with a higher probability of being correct than congenitally blind participants did on the basis of voices, although the blind had superior voice recognition abilities. Other results that are inconsistent with the substitution assumption come from the auditory localization study (Röder, Teder-Sälejärvi, et al., 1999): although the localization skills of the blind participants were superior to those of the sighted, they did not match the visual or combined auditory-visual localization accuracy of sighted individuals.

Other studies, in particular those investigating spatial skills in near space, did not obtain performance differences between sighted and blind groups (for details, see Röder & Neville, 2003). This means either that these functions are independent of visual input or that the blind are able to compensate for the lack of additional visual information. Given the repeatedly demonstrated interactions between the representations of space of different modalities, the former assumption seems implausible for the case of spatial tasks. Therefore, equal performance here most likely indicates compensation. The spatial representations generated on the basis of haptic and auditory input by the blind seem to have the same properties as those generated on the basis of visual input in the sighted. When tested directly (Röder & Rösler, 1998), no additional advantage (with respect to mental scanning speed) arose from additional visual input. This result favors a substitution account. Unfortunately, however, the time participants took to learn the spatial layout was not systematically recorded. However, post hoc we realized that both sighted and blind haptically learning participants needed more time than visually or visually and haptically learning sighted participants. This observation suggests that although the properties of visually and haptically acquired spatial representations were similar, it was more effortful for the blind (and for the sighted) to generate this representation haptically than it was for the sighted to build it visually, a finding that questions an unrestricted substitution account.

Millar (1994) argued that the different sensory modalities provide both convergent and complementary information about the environment. If information provided by the different sensory systems were totally redundant, it would not make much sense to have different sensory channels at all. It can be assumed that the performance of the blind is partially based on redundancies across modalities, resulting in a performance level on some tasks at least equal to the performance of sighted individuals. The adaptive capacities of the intact senses seem to counteract to some degree the detrimental effects of the missing visual input. This may lead to higher performance levels on tasks for which no additional visual input is available for sighted controls. Nevertheless, blind persons are not able to fully replace visual input by the other modalities (see also Rauschecker, 1997): sighted individuals perform still better than blind individuals when they have access to visual input.

What are the neural correlates of compensation and hypercompensation? Three nonexclusive mechanisms have been proposed by Röder and Neville (2003): (1) Sensory-specific systems associated with the intact modalities reorganize to increase their processing efficiency (intramodal changes). (2) In polymodal brain structures, the subareas normally associated with the deprived modality may respond to stimuli of the intact senses, and multisensory cells may retain responsiveness to stimuli of the nondeprived modalities only. (3) Brain areas normally primarily associated with the deprived modality may be occupied by input of the intact sensory systems (inter-/cross-modal plasticity, also called functional reallocation).

This classification schema focuses on the brain systems that change rather than on the eliciting factors. Others have distinguished *use-dependent* and *lesion-induced plasticity;* in other words, intense practice and peripheral or central lesions trigger reorganizations of the CNS. The loss of input from one sensory system (as a total peripheral lesion) is commonly followed by a more intense use of the remaining senses. The intensity of the "perceptual training" that accompanies visual loss can hardly be matched in a perceptual training experiment with sighted participants. Therefore, it is difficult to determine which changes in the blind are use-dependent and which are primarily deafferentation (lesion)-induced; in fact, both causes may interact. Nevertheless, several comparisons can be made to distinguish between primarily lesion-induced and primarily use-dependent neural changes after sensory deprivation: (1) Blind people can be compared with sighted people who have engaged in intense perceptual trainings (e.g., Braille readers; Sterr et al., 1998) and with sighted people who have been exposed to long-duration tactile stimulation (Braun, Schweizer, et al., 2000; Schweizer et al., 2001). (2) Early blind adults (Röder et al., 1996; Röder, Rösler, et al., 1999) can be compared with people who are forced to use their haptic (Elbert et al., 1995) or auditory sensory systems intensely (Pantev et al., 1998; Pantev, Roberts, Schulz, Engelien, & Ross, 2001). (3) Training-induced changes in healthy people (Braun, Schweizer, et al., 2000; Menning et al., 2000) can be compared with deafferentation-induced plasticity, such as occurs in amputees (Flor et al., 1995; Grüsser et al., 2001) or in patients with tinnitus (Mühlnickel et al., 1998).

The following discussion considers the possible contribution of the three neural mechanisms—intramodal plasticity, reorganization of polymodal brain structures, and cross-/intermodal changes—to behavioral changes after sensory deprivation, with a focus on the blind. Where possible, findings from animal studies and from other studies in humans on neural plasticity are taken into account.

1. INTRAMODAL/INTRASYSTEM PLASTICITY Extended use or deafferentation of a subregion of the sensory epithelium leads to both physiological and morphological changes at the synapses within the sensory representational zone (intramodal changes; e.g., changes of synaptical weights, as associated with long-term potentiation and depression [e.g., Teyler, 2001]; changes in the number of spines, the morphology of postsynaptic endings, growth of horizontal connections, dendritic trees, and cell somata [reviewed in Kolb & Whishaw, 1998]). In the case of perceptual learning, this may result in an

enlargement of or more efficient processing algorithms within associated neural networks (Gilbert et al., 2001). In the case of peripheral lesions, an invasion of adjacent sensory areas into the deafferented brain zone has been observed; that is, neighboring representations enlarge (for recent reviews, see Buonomano & Merzenich, 1998; Elbert, Heim, & Rockstroh, 2001; Gilbert et al., 2001; Kaas, 2000). Accordingly, this type of plasticity has been called "map expansion" by Grafman (2000). Intramodal reorganization has been well documented both at the cortical and subcortical level, and the changes seen at different neural levels most likely interact (Ergenzinger, Glasier, Hahm, & Pons, 1998; Jones & Pons, 1998; Kaas, 1999).

The shorter refractory periods for ERPs in the blind (Röder, Rösler, et al., 1999) are very similar to the larger dipole moments for somatosensory and auditory magnetic activity found in musicians (Elbert et al., 1995; Pantev et al., 1998). This similarity may point toward primarily use-dependent intramodal changes in the representational maps of blind persons associated with their intact modalities (Elbert et al., 2002). This hypothesis is further supported by the repeatedly observed shorter latencies of both the auditory and somatosensory N1 reported in blind participants (Röder et al., 1996) and the simultaneous lack of a difference between sighted and blind groups in the scalp topography of the N1 to targets. Shorter reaction times in the blind suggest that an increased efficiency (e.g., timing of processing steps) contributes to compensatory behavior in the blind. Parallel findings have been reported for the deaf: shorter refractory periods for visual ERPs (Neville et al., 1983) and enhanced activity of visual motion areas (MT-MST) (Bavelier et al., 2000) point toward a use-dependent reorganization of visual brain systems after loss of hearing.

2. REORGANIZATION OF POLYMODAL BRAIN AREAS Deprivation is a more extreme form of imbalance induced to sensory maps than intense practice. Instead of a disequilibrium between different parts of one sensory system, a total deprivation of input to one sensory modality results in ill-balanced relations across the neural representations of the different sensory systems, particularly within the polymodal brain areas where afferents of the different sensory systems converge. Therefore, no new mechanisms in addition to competition and cooperation (e.g., the Hebbian rule) have to be proposed to explain reorganization of multimodal brain structures: the higher activity level of the intact sensory afferents very likely causes an expansion of the representation associated with the intact modalities (Rauschecker, 1997). Neurons with multisensory

responsiveness already exist at birth (Wallace & Stein, 2001). The integrative effects—that is, cross-modal facilitation or inhibition—however, emerge postnatally (B. A. Stein et al., 2000). Therefore, it is easy to imagine that the congenital lack of input from one modality may result in the replacement or suppression of the deprived afferents.

In visually deprived animals, reorganization of poly-modal brain structures, for example, the SC as a subcortical brain structure (Rauschecker & Harris, 1983; Vidyasagar, 1978) and cortical areas of the temporal, parietal, and parieto-occipital lobes (Hyvärinen, Carlson, & Hyvärinen, 1981; Hyvärinen & Hyvärinen, 1979; Hyvärinen, Hyvärinen, et al., 1981; Yaka, Yinon, & Wollberg, 1999), has been reported. Corresponding to these observations in animals, enhanced blood flow changes in parieto-occipital areas were observed in blind humans (e.g., De Volder et al., 1997; Weeks et al., 2000). Electrophysiological recordings in humans have repeatedly revealed an enhancement and a posterior shift of the N2 potential in the blind (Alho et al., 1993; Liotti et al., 1998; Röder et al., 1996; Röder, Rösler, et al., 1999; Röder, Teder-Sälejärvi, et al., 1997) (see Fig. 46.3). The N2 is believed to be generated in multisensory cortex, including the parietal lobe (Knight, 1990; Woods, Knight, & Scabini, 1993). Therefore, it could be hypothesized that a reorganization of multimodal brain regions contributes to compensatory performance in the blind. Moreover, the observation that latencies of N2 elicited by sounds from peripheral locations (for which enhanced performance was found in the blind) were shorter in the blind than in the sighted suggests that the reorganization of multimodal brain areas is functionally adaptive. It is unknown if a deprivation-induced reorganization of multimodal structures can take place in adults as well. Moreover, it may be hypothesized that a massive disequilibrium, such as the total loss of input to one sensory system, is a prerequisite for cross-modal changes in polymodal brain structures to occur. By contrast, intense practice may not be sufficient to elicit such changes. Preliminary evidence for these hypotheses comes from an auditory localization study in conductors (Münte, Kohlmetz, Nager, & Altenmüller, 2001). Like the blind, conductors showed more precise auditory spatial selection at a processing stage around 100 ms after stimulus presentation. However, the ERP effect was posteriorly shifted in the blind only and not in the conductors, indicating the involvement of different neural mechanisms. However, the specific training of the conductors did not begin before adulthood. Therefore, the lack of a topographic difference either may be due to the existence of a critical period for cross-modal reorganization in early development or may originate in the weaker imbalance between the input of different modalities induced by practice within one sensory system alone. A comparison of late-blind and congenitally blind adults could shed additional light on this issue. In fact, Kujala et al. (1997) found a similar posterior shift of the auditory N2 in late-blind adults, suggesting that total deprivation rather than age at onset of the deprivation determines the occurrence of reorganizations in multimodal brain areas. Röder and Neville (2003) proposed that an irreversible reorganization of these multimodal brain areas (Carlson, Pertovaara, & Tanila, 1987) in early-blind individuals whose cataracts were removed in adulthood was responsible for the lack of recovery of higher visual functions such as depth perception (Ackroyd, Humphrey, & Warrington, 1974), spatial attention (Goldberg et al., 2001), or face recognition (Le Grand et al., 2001) (for a review, see Sacks, 1995)—in other words, visual functions that rely on sensory association areas.

Evidence for a reorganization of polymodal brain areas in the deaf (e.g., of the posterior superior temporal sulcus) has recently been reported as well (Bavelier et al., 2001). A stronger visual-processing-related activation of the latter was only seen in deaf, not in hearing signers, indicating that a reorganization of multimodal brain areas may be a common consequence of sensory deprivation. In agreement with this hypothesis is the finding that sign language activated classical language areas (i.e., auditory association areas) but not primary auditory cortex (Nishimura et al., 1999). Conversely, stimulation though a cochlear implant activated primary auditory cortex but not auditory association areas in prelingually deaf people. By contrast, in postlingually deaf persons, both primary and secondary auditory areas are activated by stimulation through a cochlear implant (Hirano et al., 1996). These findings are in agreement with neurophysiological and anatomical studies in deaf cats (Klinke, Kral, Heid, Tillein, & Hartman, 1999), and it may be that, as in visually deprived monkeys, a reorganization of multisensory association cortex during a critical period is irreversible, preventing a successful functional recovery after a late cochlear implementation in the prelingually deaf (Lehnhardt & Achendorff, 1993; Shepard, Hartmann, Heid, Hardie, & Klinke, 1997).

A reorganizations that crosses modality borders in polymodal brain structures is, according to the classification schema introduced in earlier in this chapter, a type of cross-modal or intermodal plasticity, or "cross-modal reassignment," according to Grafman (2000). From a neuroanatomical point of view, however, a categorization as *intrasystem* rather than *intersystem change* would be appropriate.

3. Intermodal/Intersystem Plasticity A proper intersystem change would mean that brain areas not involved in a particular task in healthy individuals are now involved in this function. An example is brain structures primarily associated with the visual system that are activated by nonvisual input after the loss of sight.

An aberrant innervation of thalamic modality-specific relay nuclei has been reported in rewiring experiments (for recent reviews, see Pallas, 2001; Sur & Leamey, 2001). Because these nuclei continue to project to their normal targets, activation from a different modality is transmitted to sensory cortex. For example, a simultaneous ablation of auditory afferents and visual target structures in ferrets results in an innervation of the medial geniculate body by visual afferents and in turn in a retinotopically organized map in what is normally auditory cortex. A similar rerouting of visual input can be induced in somatosensory cortex (Frost, 1992) and seems to occur in blind mole rats even without surgical interventions. Moreover, in the latter, both somatosensory (Necker et al., 1992) and auditory (Bronchti et al., 2002) input have been found to activate visual cortex. In addition, in binocularly deprived ferrets, cells in extrastriate cortex have been observed to respond to auditory stimuli both in dark-reared and in enucleated animals (animals whose eyes had been removed). Moreover, a small number of striate cortex cells gained auditory responsiveness in enucleated animals (Yaka, Yinon, Rosner, & Wollberg, 2000; Yaka et al., 1999). A stabilization or failure to inhibit thalamocortical or corticocortical connections present (Falchier, Calvagier, Baron, & Kennedy, 2002; Innocenti & Clarke, 1984) or a growth of new connections could also contribute to nonvisual information flow to the occipital cortex after early visual deprivation.

As mentioned earlier, activation of "visual" brain regions in blind humans has been reported for a number of tasks, including Braille reading and tactile discrimination (Büchel, Price, Frackowiak, & Friston, 1998; Röder et al., 1996; Sadato et al., 1998; Uhl, Franzen, Podreka, Steiner, & Deecke, 1993), auditory discrimination (Röder et al., 1996), auditory localization (De Volder et al., 1999; Weeks et al., 2000), auditory object recognition (Arno et al., 2001), haptic-spatial imagery (Röder, Rösler, et al., 1997), auditory imagery (De Volder et al., 2001), and speech processing (Röder, Rösler, et al., 2000; Röder, Stock, Bien, et al., 2002). It remains to be clarified whether "visual" cortex activation is essential or at least contributes to compensatory behavior in the blind. A disruption of tactile discrimination ability by TMS at occipital sites in blind but not in sighted adults (Cohen et al., 1997) suggests a behavioral relevance of "visual" cortex areas in the blind.

However, the great variety of tasks eliciting occipital cortex activation in the blind opens the possibility that these brain regions may be coactivated whenever other cortical areas are put into a higher excitation level in attentionally demanding tasks, and that a reduced efficiency of inhibitory circuits (Rozas et al., 2001; Singer & Tretter, 1976) facilitates such coactivation (for a detailed discussion, see Röder & Neville, 2003). A recent fMRI study found a deactivation of auditory areas during visual stimulus presentation, and vice versa (Laurienti et al., 2002). This study and other brain imaging studies (e.g., Calvert & Lewis, Chap. 30, Macaluso & Driver, Chap. 33, this volume) and electrophysiological studies on multisensory perception (e.g., Eimer, Chap. 34, this volume) have demonstrated that the stimuli of one sense can cause changes in sensory-specific areas of another sensory system. It could be speculated that if the circuits that cause the reported deactivation of visual brain areas during auditory processing do not work in the blind (and vice versa in the deaf) visual (auditory) brain areas are relatively more activated in the blind (deaf) during auditory (visual) processing. It has to be noted that in the blind, an activation of, for example, auditory or somatosensory areas was observed during auditory and tactile processing, respectively, as was observed in the sighted, but in addition, visual cortex activity was found. Such a reduced inhibition or deactivation of visual cortex in nonvisual tasks could also explain the similar activation patterns in late- and early-blind individuals that are sometimes observed, and also the recent results from blindfolding studies (Pascual-Leone & Hamilton, 2001). Wearing a blindfold elicited visual hallucinations that quickly disappeared after removal of the blindfold. Moreover, fMRI showed increasing visual cortex activity during tactile and auditory tasks in the blindfolded participants. This activity disappeared after the blindfold was removed as well. These results suggest that physiological rather than structural changes contribute to visual cortex activation after visual deprivation.

Another possible explanation for the great variety of tasks accompanied by an activation of the occipital cortex in the blind is that for different tasks, different striate or extrastriate areas are activated, but that the spatial resolution of brain imaging techniques, particularly electrophysiological recordings, is not adequate to detect such local specificity. In addition, it could be that this local functional specialization of occipital brain tissue varies across blind individuals and is masked by group average data (a related idea was expressed in a discussion by J. Rauschecker, 1999).

Regardless of its functional role, it is still unknown if an activation of cortex predominantly associated with the deprived modality is linked to a critical period during early development or if it can be induced, possibly to a lesser degree, in the mature CNS as well. Some authors have not found different activation patterns in congenitally and late-blind adults (while both of these groups differed from the sighted controls) (Kujala et al., 1997; Rösler, Röder, Heil, & Hennighausen, 1993). In contrast, other authors have not found activation differences between late-blind and sighted groups (while both differed from a congenitally blind group) (Cohen et al., 1999; Veraart et al., 1990). Furthermore, Büchel, Price, Frackowiak, et al. (1998) reported striate cortex activation in late-blind but not in congenitally blind adults. Late-blind adults are a very heterogeneous group, differing in age at onset, duration, and cause of the blindness, the degree of visual impairments prior to the onset of total blindness, and the extent of rehabilitation training. It is very likely that this heterogeneity may have contributed to the discrepancies between studies with late-blind individuals.

There is now a lot of evidence that neural changes can be elicited both in the developing and adult CNS. At least for some systems, the extent of possible plastic changes is larger during early development than during adulthood. For example, the amount of change in representational maps of musicians or amputees is larger the earlier the musical training started or the deafferentation happened (Elbert et al., 1995; Pantev et al., 1998, 2001; for a review, see Elbert et al., 2001). Similarly, owls reared wearing prisms for a short time epoch during early development retained the enhanced adaptation capacities of auditory maps into adulthood, long after removal of the prisms (Knudsen, 1998). The early deviant experience of these owls was obviously able to expand the normal adult adaptive capabilities of their neural systems. The existence of critical and sensitive periods in life is now well accepted, and most likely there are multiple sensitive periods for different functions (Gilbert et al., 2001; Le Grand et al., 2001; Maurer & Lewis, 1993; Neville et al., 1992; Stiles & Thal, 1993). Berardi, Pizzorusso, and Maffei (2000) proposed that the length of the critical periods is a function of total life span and brain complexity (operationalized by brain weight). It is assumed that experience elicits the development of inhibitory circuits that in turn terminates critical periods. Moreover, Berardi et al. (2000) suggested that the delayed development of inhibitory circuits results in a time window during which excitation dominates what in turn results in an enhanced susceptibility to sensory experience. A critical period ends with the emergence of a particular function. Accordingly, those subfunctions that develop late are most susceptible to environmental factors (Maurer & Lewis,

1993). Although there seems to be an overlap between the neural mechanisms underlying learning in childhood and adulthood (Kandel & O'Dell, 1992; Neville & Bavelier, 2001), the existence of critical periods and the higher plasticity capacities of the developing CNS suggest differences as well (Neville & Bavelier, 2001).

Finally, recent findings indicate that neurogenesis continues into adulthood and exists even in cortex (Gould, Reeves, Graziano, et al., 1999; for a review, see Ormerod & Galea, 2001; van Praag et al., 2000). This raises the possibility that even in adulthood, a much more extended rewiring of the CNS may be possible than originally thought. It has been shown that newly generated neurons in the hippocampus are important for learning (Shors et al., 2001), but it remains to be demonstrated whether neurogenesis plays a role in cross-modal plasticity. Nevertheless, it is interesting to note that newly produced neurons were detected in association cortex (prefrontal, inferior temporal, and parietal cortex), but not in sensory areas (occipital cortex), and moreover, the new neurons built short rather than long extending axons. Therefore, it may be hypothesized that neurogenesis contributes to adaptive changes within multisensory brain areas rather than primary sensory areas.

Outlook and summary

Although the term neuroplasticity commonly has a positive connotation, reorganization can have maladaptive consequences as well; examples include phantom pain (Flor et al., 1995), tinnitus (Mühlnickel et al., 1998), and problems with motor control (Candia et al., 1999). The increasing knowledge of how extended neural reorganization can be elicited has recently been used to develop new treatment programs to reverse maladaptive reorganizations caused by direct or indirect injuries to the CNS. For example, Flor, Denke, Schaefer, and Grüsser (2001) trained upper arm amputees to discriminate tactile stimuli at the stump. Based on the findings that intensive behavior-relevant stimulation of parts of the sensory epithelium results in an enlargement of the associated neural representations (Buonomano & Merzenich, 1998; Elbert et al., 1995), they hypothesized that the deafferentation-induced expansion of facial representations into the hand area in somatosensory cortex, which they had shown to correlate with phantom pain in upper arm amputees, should be opposed by an intense use of the stump. The maladaptive neural reorganizations were indeed reversed through tactile discrimination training and phantom pain decreased, while two-point threshold at the stump declined. Similar neural mechanisms may contribute to the lower occurrence of phantom pain in artificial-limb-wearing amputees (Lotze et al., 1999; Weiss, Miltner, Adler, Brücker, & Taub, 1999). Similarly, constraining the mobility of a healthy limb in stroke patients (constraint-induced movement therapy; Liepert et al., 1998; Taub et al., 1993) resulted in improved motor functions of the former paretic upper arm (e.g., Miltner, Bauder, Sommer, Dettmer, & Taub, 1998). The functional recovery was accompanied by a regaining of the excitability of the associated motor cortex (Liepert et al., 1998). Forcing musicians who suffer from dystonia of their intensely and monotonously used fingers to move the latter in isolation by constraining some fingers of the affected hand (Candia et al., 1999) or temporarily medically paralyzing involved muscles (Chen & Hallett, 1998; Cole, Hallett, & Cohen, 1995) effectively reduces the motor impairments. The concept underlying all these treatment programs is that training or constraining counteracts the use-dependent, ill-balanced neural representational changes caused by injury or intense practice.

Reminiscent of the findings of Knudsen (1998) are observations in people born deaf who learned ASL either as their first native language or as their first language, but late in life (after the age of 9) (Mayberry, Lock, & Kazmir, 2002). Those who had learned ASL on schedule outperformed the late learners, even though both groups were matched for the duration they had used ASL. However, more interesting is the comparison of the ASL proficiency of the congenitally deaf late learners with that of late-deaf late learners. The latter group (although slightly worse than the native learners) showed a higher proficiency in ASL than the first group, although both groups were matched for chronological age and years of ASL experience (Mayberry et al., 2002). This observation means that adult late-deaf signers who had learned a language (although an oral language) on schedule outperformed congenitally deaf signers who started learning ASL at the same late age (and used it for the same time period) but had learned neither a sign language nor an oral language in childhood. Therefore, similar to what was found in prism-reared owls (Knudsen, 1998), the late-deaf late learners showed enlarged adaptive capacities: the exposure to a language from early on facilitated or made possible the acquisition of another language as adults (just as everyone is able to learn a second language to some degree), but the lack of early language exposure prevented congenitally deaf late learners from gaining proficiency in sign language. This finding supports earlier single case reports showing that children deprived of speech in early childhood are not able to acquire any language (e.g., Curtiss, 1977). If there is no adequate input in early childhood during periods of enhanced plasticity, if neural systems are not set up for a particular function, some capabilities (e.g., language) are irrevocably lost. These findings have direct consequences for the setup and timing of educational programs. In particular, they suggest that for individuals who have lost sight or hearing, interventions should start as early as possible. Initial delays in language acquisition in the blind were attributed to a less rich language environment (Andersen et al., 1993). However, since language is the most important communication medium for the blind child, the child is nevertheless continuously exposed to speech, and finally succeeds. Less favorable are findings on motor development, which is also delayed in blind children (Tröster, Hecker, & Brambring, 1994). The reduced mobility of blind children has been related to stereotyped motor behavior, which shows a high persistence (Brambring & Tröster, 1992) through adulthood. Moreover, although language seems to develop and reorganize continuously up to about the age of 8 years (Friederici, 1992), critical periods for spatial functions seem to terminate earlier (Stiles, 2001; Stiles & Thal, 1993). Therefore, it could be hypothesized that reduced possibilities for safely exploring the environment and a late onset of mobility training favor deficits in spatial skills in blind persons (Ungar, 2000).

The research discussed in this chapter concerning blind individuals indicates that they show better or equal performance when compared with sighted controls on several perceptual-cognitive tasks. Improvements observed in the blind and in the deaf, however, are not able to substitute visual or auditory input, respectively. Changes at the behavioral level are accompanied by both intramodal and cross-modal neural reorganizations. Finally, not all compensatory changes seem to be linked to critical periods.

REFERENCES

Ackroyd, C., Humphrey, N. K., & Warrington, E. K. (1974). Lasting effects of early blindness: A case study. *Quarterly Journal of Experimental Psychology, 26,* 114–124.

Alho, K., Kujala, T., Paavilainen, P., Summala, H., & Näätänen, R. (1993). Auditory processing in visual brain areas of the early blind: Evidence from event-related potentials. *Electroencephalography and Clinical Neurophysiology, 86,* 418–427.

Andersen, E. S., Dunlea, A., & Kekelis, L. (1984). Blind children's language: Resolving some differences. *Journal of Child Language, 11,* 645–664.

Andersen, E. S., Dunlea, A., & Kekelis, L. (1993). The impact of input: Language acquisition in the visually impaired. *First Language, 13,* 23–49.

Andersen, R. A., Snyder, L. H., Bradley, D. C., & Xong, J. (1997). Multimodal representation of space in the posterior cortex and its use in planning movements. *Annual Review of Neuroscience, 20,* 303–330.

Arno, P., De Volder, A., Vanlierde, A., Wanet-Defalque, M.-C., Streel, E., Robert, A., et al. (2001). Occipital activation by pattern recognition in the early blind using auditory substitution for vision. *NeuroImage, 13,* 632–645.

Ashmead, D. H., Wall, R. S., Ebinger, K. A., Eaton, S. B., Snook-Hill, M.-M., & Yang, X. (1998). Spatial hearing in children with visual disabilities. *Perception, 27,* 105–122.

Axelrod, S. (1959). *Effects of early blindness: Performance of blind and sighted children on tactile and auditory tasks* (pp. 1–83). New York: American Foundation for the Blind.

Balota, D. A. (1994). Visual word recognition. In M. A. Gernsbacher (Ed.), *Handbook of psycholinguistics* (pp. 334–357). New York: Academic Press.

Bavelier, D., Brozinsky, C., Tomann, A., Mitchell, T., Neville, H. J., & Liu, G. (2001). Impact of early deafness and early exposure to sign language on the cerebral organization for motion processing. *Journal of Neuroscience, 21,* 8931–8942.

Bavelier, D., Tomann, A., Hutton, C., Mitchell, T., Corina, D., Liu, G., & Neville, H. J. (2000). Visual attention to the periphery is enhanced in congenitally deaf individuals. *Journal of Neuroscience, 20*(RC93), 1–6.

Berardi, N., Pizzorusso, T., & Maffei, L. (2000). Critical periods during sensory development. *Current Opinion in Neurobiology, 10,* 138–145.

Bertelson, P., Morais, J., Mousty, P., & Hublet, C. (1987). Spatial constraint on attention to speech in the blind. *Brain and Language, 32,* 68–75.

Birbaumer, N., & Schmidt, R. F. (1991). *Biologische Psychologie.* Berlin: Springer.

Black, J. E., Jones, T. A., Nelson, C. A., & Greenough, W. T. (1998). Neuroplasticity and the developing brain. In N. Alessi, J. T. Coyle, S. I. Harrison, & S. Eth (Eds.), *The handbook of child and adolescent psychiatry* (pp. 31–53). New York: Wiley.

Brambring, M., & Tröster, H. (1992). On the stability of stereotyped behaviors in blind infants and preschoolers. *Journal of Visual Impairment and Blindness, 86,* 105–110.

Braun, C., Schweizer, R., Elbert, T., Birbaumer, N., & Taub, E. (2000). Differential activation in somatosensory cortex for different discrimination tasks. *Journal of Neuroscience, 20,* 446–450.

Braun, C., Wilms, A., Schweizer, R., Godde, B., Preissl, H., & Birbaumer, N. (2000). Activity patterns of human somatosensory cortex adapt dynamically to stimulus properties. *Neuroreport, 11,* 2977–2980.

Bronchti, G., Heil, P., Sadka, R., Hess, A., Scheich, H., & Wollberg, Z. (2002). Auditory activation of "visual" cortical areas in the blind mole rat (*Spalax ehrenbergi*). *European Journal of Neuroscience, 16,* 311–329.

Bross, M. (1979). Residual sensory capacities of the deaf: A signal detection analysis of visual discrimination task. *Perceptual and Motor Skills, 48,* 187–194.

Bross, M., & Borenstein, M. (1982). Temporal auditory acuity in blind and sighted subjects: A signal detection analysis. *Perceptual and Motor Skills, 55,* 963–966.

Bross, M., & Sauerwein, H. (1980). Signal detection analysis of visual flicker in deaf and hearing individuals. *Perceptual and Motor Skills, 51,* 839–843.

Brown, C. M., Hagoort, P., & Kutas, M. (2000). Postlexical integration processes in language comprehension: Evidence from brain-imaging research. In M. S. Gazzaniga (Ed.), *The new cognitive neurosciences* (pp. 881–895). Cambridge, MA: MIT Press.

Büchel, C., Price, C. J., Frackowiak, R. S. J., & Friston, K. J. (1998). Different activation patterns in the visual cortex of late and congenitally blind subjects. *Brain, 121,* 409–419.

Büchel, C., Price, C. J., & Friston, K. J. (1998). A multimodal language region in the ventral visual pathway. *Nature, 394,* 274–277.

Buonomano, D. V., & Merzenich, M. M. (1998). Cortical plasticity: From synapses to map. *Annual Review of Neuroscience, 21,* 149–186.

Cain, D. P. (2001). Synaptic models of neuroplasticity: What is LTP? In C. A. Shaw & J. C. McEachern (Eds.), *Toward a theory of neuroplasticity* (pp. 118–129). Hove, England: Psychology Press.

Calvert, G. A., Brammer, M. J., & Iversen, S. D. (1998). Cross modal identification. *Trends in Cognitive Sciences, 2,* 247–253.

Candia, V., Elbert, T., Altenmüller, E., Rau, H., Schäfer, T., & Taub, E. (1999). Constraint-induced movement therapy for focal hand dystonia in musicians. *Lancet, 353,* 1273–1274.

Carlson, S., Pertovaara, A., & Tanila, H. (1987). Late effects of early binocular visual deprivation on the function of Brodmann's area 7 of monkeys (*Macaca arctoides*). *Developmental Brain Research, 33,* 101–111.

Chen, R., & Hallett, M. (1998). Focal dystonia and repetitive motion disorders. *Clinical Orthopedics, 351,* 102–106.

Chino, Y., Smith, E. M. K., Mori, T. Z. B., & Kaas, J. H. (2001). Recovery of binocular responses by cortical neurons after early monocular lesions. *Nature Neuroscience, 4,* 689–690.

Chino, Y. M., Kaas, J. H., Smith, E. L., Langston, A. L., & Cheng, H. (1992). Rapid reorganization of cortical maps in adult cats following restricted deafferentation in retina. *Vision Research, 32,* 789–796.

Cohen, L. G., Celnik, P., Pascual-Leone, A., Corwell, B., Faiz, L., Dambrosia, J., et al. (1997). Functional relevance of cross-modal plasticity in blind humans. *Nature, 389,* 180–183.

Cole, R., Hallett, M., & Cohen, L. G. (1995). Double-blind trail of botulinum toxin for treatment of focal hand dystonia. *Movement Disorders, 10,* 466–471.

Cruikshank, S. J., & Weinberger, N. M. (1996). Evidence for the Hebbian hypothesis in experience-dependent physiological plasticity of neocortex: A critical review. *Brain Research Review, 22,* 191–228.

Curtiss, S. (1977). *Genie: A psycholinguistic study of a modern-day "wild child."* New York: Academic Press.

De Volder, A. G., Bol, A., Blin, J., Robert, A., Arno, P., Grandin, C., et al. (1997). Brain energy metabolism in early blind subjects: Neural activity in the visual cortex. *Brain Research, 750,* 235–244.

De Volder, A. G., Catalán-Ahumada, M., Robert, A., Bol, A., Labar, D., Copperns, A., et al. (1999). Changes in occipital cortex activity in early blind humans using a sensory substitution device. *Brain Research, 826,* 128–134.

De Volder, A. G., Toyama, H., Kimura, Y., Kiyosawa, M., Nakano, H., Vanlierde, A., et al. (2001). Auditory triggered mental imagery of shape involved visual association areas in early blind humans. *NeuroImage, 14,* 129–139.

DeBello, W. M., & Knudsen, E. I. (2001). Adaptive plasticity of the auditory space map. In C. A. Shaw & J. C. McEachern (Eds.), *Toward a theory of neuroplasticity* (pp. 13–30). Hove, England: Taylor & Francis/Psychology Press.

Dodds, A. G. (1983). Mental rotation and visual imagery. *Journal of Visual Impairment and Blindness, 77,* 16–18.

Driver, J., & Spence, C. (1998). Crossmodal links in spatial attention. *Philosophical Transactions of the Royal Society of London, 353,* 1319–1331.

Dunlea, A. (1989). *Vision and the emergence of meaning.* Cambridge, England: Cambridge University Press.

Eimer, M., Cockurn, D., Smedley, B., & Driver, J. (2001). Cross-modal links in endogenous spatial attention are mediated by common external locations: Evidence from event-related brain potentials. *Experimental Brain Research, 139,* 398–411.

Elbert, T., Flor, H., Birbaumer, N., Knecht, S., Hampson, S., Larbig, W., et al. (1994). Extensive reorganization of the somatosensory cortex in adult humans after nervous system injury. *Neuroreport, 5,* 2593–2597.

Elbert, T., Heim, S., & Rockstroh, B. (2001). Neural plasticity and development. In C. Nelson & M. Luciana (Eds.), *Handbook of developmental cognitive neuroscience* (pp. 191–202). Cambridge, MA: MIT Press.

Elbert, T., Pantev, C., Wienbruch, C., Rockstroh, B., & Taub, E. (1995). Increased cortical representation of the fingers of the left hand in string players. *Science, 270,* 305–307.

Elbert, T., Sterr, A., Rockstroh, B., Pantev, C., Müller, M. M., & Taub, E. (2002). Expansion of the tonotopic area in the auditory cortex of the blind. *Neuroscience, 22,* 9941–9944.

Emmorey, K., Kosslyn, S. M., & Bellugi, U. (1993). Visual imagery and visual-spatial language: Enhanced imagery abilities in deaf and hearing ASL signers. *Cognition, 46,* 139–181.

Ergenzinger, E. R., Glasier, M. M., Hahm, J. O., & Pons, T. P. (1998). Cortically induced thalamic plasticity in the primate somatosensory system. *Nature Neuroscience, 1,* 226–229.

Eriksson, P. W. W. S., Perfilieva, E., Björk-Eriksson, T., Alborn, A.-M., Nordborg, C., Peterson, D. A., et al. (1998). Neurogenesis in the adult human hippocampus. *Nature and Medicine, 4,* 1313–1317.

Eysel, U. T., Schweigart, G., Mittmann, T., Eyding, D., Qu, Y., Vandesande, F., et al. (1999). Reorganization in the visual cortex after retinal and cortical damage. *Restorative Neurology and Neuroscience, 15,* 153–164.

Fahle, M., & Poggio, T. (2002). *Perceptual learning.* Cambridge, MA: MIT Press.

Falchier, A., Clavagnier, S., Barone, P., & Kennedy, H. (2002). Anatomical evidence of multimodal integration in primate striate cortex. *Journal of Neuroscience, 22,* 5749–5759.

Feinsod, M., Bach-y-Rita, P., & Madey, J. M. (1973). Somatosensory evoked responses: Differences in blind and sighted persons. *Brain Research, 60,* 219–223.

Finney, E. M., Fine, I., & Dobkins, K. R. (2001). Visual stimuli activate auditory cortex in the deaf. *Nature Neuroscience, 4,* 1171–1173.

Flor, H., Denke, C., Schaefer, M., & Grüsser, S. (2001). Effect of sensory discrimination training on cortical reorganisation and phantom limb pain. *Lancet, 357,* 1763–1764.

Flor, H., Elbert, T., Knecht, S., Wienbruch, C., Pantev, C., Birbaumer, N., et al. (1995). Phantom-limb pain as a perceptual correlate of cortical reorganization following arm amputation. *Nature, 375,* 482–484.

Friederici, A. D. (1992). Development of language relevant processing systems: The emergence of a cognitive module. In B. Boysson-Bardies, S. de Schonen, P. Jusczyk, P. McNeilage, & J. Morton (Eds.), *Developmental neurocogni-*

tion: Speech and face processing in the first year of life (pp. 451–459). Dordrecht: Kluwer Academic.

Frost, D. O. (1992). Visual processing by novel, surgically created neural circuits. In D. M. K. Lam & G. M. Bray (Eds.), *Regeneration and plasticity in the mammalian visual system* (pp. 197–219). London: Bradford Books.

Gilbert, C. D. (1995). Dynamic properties of adult visual cortex. In M. S. Gazzaniga (Ed.), *The cognitive neurosciences* (pp. 73–90). Cambridge, MA: MIT Press.

Gilbert, C. D., Sigman, M., & Crist, R. E. (2001). The neural basis of perceptual learning. *Neuron, 31,* 681–697.

Goldberg, M., Maurer, D., Lewis, T. L., & Brent, P. (2001). The influence of binocular visual deprivation on the development of visual-spatial attention. *Developmental Neuropsychology, 19,* 53–81.

Gould, E., Reeves, A. J., Fallah, M., Tanapat, P., Gross, C., & Fuchs, E. (1999). Hippocampal neurogenesis in adult old world primates. *Proceedings of the National Academy of Sciences, USA, 96,* 5263–5267.

Gould, E., Reeves, A. J., Graziano, M. S. A., & Gross, C. G. (1999). Neurogenesis in the neocortex of adult primates. *Science, 286,* 548–552.

Grafman, J. (2000). Conceptualizing functional neuroplasticity. *Journal of Communication Disorders, 33,* 345–356.

Grant, A. C., Thiagarajah, M. C., & Sathian, K. (2000). Tactile perception in blind Braille readers: A psychophysical study of acuity and hyperacuity using gating and dot patterns. *Perceptions in Psychophysics, 62,* 301–312.

Green, E. J., Greenough, W. T., & Schlumpf, B. E. (1983). Effects of complex or isolated environments on cortical dendrites of middle-aged rats. *Brain Research, 264,* 233–240.

Gross, C. G. (2000). Neurogenesis in the adult brain: Death of a dogma. *Nature Reviews: Neuroscience, 1,* 67–73.

Grüsser, S. M., Winter, C., Mühlnickel, W., Denke, C., Karl, A., Villringer, K., et al. (2001). The relationship of perceptual phenomena and cortical reorganization in upper extremity amputees. *Neuroscience, 102,* 263–272.

Gyllensten, L., Malmfors, T., & Norrlin, M.-L. (1966). Growth alteration in the auditory cortex of visually deprived mice. *Journal of Comparative Neurology, 126,* 463–470.

Hagoort, P., & Brown, C. (2000). ERP effects of listening to speech: Semantic ERP effects. *Neuropsychologia, 38,* 1518–1530.

Halgren, E., Baudena, P., Clark, J. M., Heit, G., Liégeois, C., Chauvel, P., et al. (1995). Intracerebral potentials to rare target and distractor auditory and visual stimuli: I. Superior temporal plane and parietal lobe. *Electroencephalography and Clinical Neurophysiology, 94,* 191–220.

Hamilton, R. H., & Pascual-Leone, A. (1998). Cortical plasticity associated with Braille learning. *Trends in Cognitive Sciences, 2,* 168–169.

Hebb, D. O. (1949). *The organization of behavior: A neurophysiological theory.* New York: Wiley.

Hermelin, B., & O'Connor, N. (1971). Right and left handed reading of Braille. *Nature, 231,* 470.

Herron, D. T., & Bates, E. A. (1997). Sentential and acoustic factors in the recognition of open- and closed-class words. *Journal of Memory and Language, 37,* 217–239.

Hikosaka, K., Iwai, E., Hide-Aki, S., & Tanaka, K. (1988). Polysensory properties of neurons in the anterior bank of the caudal superior temporal sulcus of the macaque monkey. *Journal of Neurophysiology, 60,* 1615–1637.

Hillyard, S. A., Hink, R. F., Schwent, V. L., & Picton, T. W. (1973). Electrical signs of selective attention in the human brain. *Science, 182,* 177–188.

Hillyard, S. A., Mangun, G. R., Woldorff, M. C., & Luck, S. J. (1995). Neural systems mediating selective attention. In M. S. Gazzaniga (Ed.), *The cognitive neurosciences* (pp. 665–681). Cambridge, MA: MIT Press.

Hillyard, S. A., & Picton, T. W. (1987). Electrophysiology of cognition. In *Handbook of physiology: Section 1. The nervous system. V. Higher functions of the brain: Part 2* (E. Plum, Ed.) (pp. 519–584). Bethesda, MD: American Physiology Society.

Hillyard, S. A., Simpson, G. V., Woods, D. L., VanVoorhis, S., & Münte, T. F. (1984). Event-related brain potentials in selective attention to different modalities. In F. Reinoso-Suárez & C. Ajmone-Marsan (Eds.), *Cortical integration* (pp. 395–414). New York: Raven Press.

Hirano, S., Kojima, H., Naito, Y., Honjo, I., Kamoto, Y., Okazawa, H., et al. (1996). Cortical speech processing mechanisms while vocalizing visually presented speech. *Neuroreport, 8,* 363–367.

Hoke, M., Feldmann, H., Pantev, M., Lütkenhäner, B., & Lehnertz, K. (1989). Objective evidence of tinnitus in auditory evoked magnetic fields. *Hearing Research, 37,* 281–286.

Holcomb, P. J., Coffey, S. A., & Neville, H. J. (1992). Visual and auditory sentence processing: A developmental analysis using event-related brain potentials. *Developmental Neuropsychology, 8,* 203–241.

Holcomb, P. J., & Neville, H. J. (1991). Nature speech processing: An analysis using event-related brain potentials. *Psychobiology, 19,* 286–300.

Hubel, D. H., & Wiesel, T. N. (1977). Functional architecture of macaque monkey visual cortex. *Proceedings of the Royal Society of London, Series B: Biological Sciences, 198,* 1–59.

Hyvärinen, J., Carlson, S., & Hyvärinen, L. (1981). Early visual deprivation alters modality of neuronal responses in area 19 of monkey cortex. *Neuroscience Letters, 26,* 239–243.

Hyvärinen, J., & Hyvärinen, L. (1979). Blindness and modification of association cortex by early binocular deprivation in monkeys. *Child: Care, Health and Development, 5,* 385–387.

Hyvärinen, J., Hyvärinen, L., & Linnankoski, I. (1981). Modification of parietal association cortex and functional blindness after binocular deprivation in young monkeys. *Experimental Brain Research, 42,* 1–8.

Innocenti, C. M., & Clarke, S. (1984). Bilateral transitory projection to visual areas from auditory cortex in kittens. *Developmental Brain Research, 14,* 143–148.

Irvine, D. R. F. (2000). Injury- and use-related plasticity in the adult auditory system. *Journal of Communication Disorders, 33,* 293–312.

Jones, E. G., & Pons, T. P. (1998). Thalamic and brainstem contributions to large-scale plasticity of primate somatosensory cortex. *Science, 282,* 1121–1125.

Kaas, J. H. (1991). Plasticity of sensory and motor maps in adult mammals. *Annual Review of Neuroscience, 14,* 137–167.

Kaas, J. H. (2000). The reorganization of sensory and motor maps after injury in adult mammals. In M. S. Gazzaniga (Ed.), *The new cognitive neurosciences* (pp. 223–236). Cambridge, MA: MIT Press.

Kaas, J. H. (2001). The mutability of sensory representations after injury in adult mammals. In C. A. Shaw & J. C. McEachern (Eds.), *Toward a theory of neuroplasticity* (pp. 323–334). Hove, England: Taylor & Francis/Psychology Press.

Kaas, J. H., Krubitzer, L. H., Chino, Y. M., Langston, A. L., Polley, E. H., & Blair, N. (1990). Reorganization of retinotopic cortical maps in adult mammals after lesion of the retina. *Science, 248,* 229–231.

Kadunce, D. C., Vaughan, W., Wallace, M. T., & Stein, B. E. (2001). The influence of visual and auditory receptive field organization on multisensory integration in the superior colliculus. *Experimental Brain Research, 139,* 303–310.

Kandel, E. R., & O'Dell, T. J. (1992). Are adult learning mechanisms also used for development? *Science, 258,* 243–245.

Karavatos, A., Kapromos, G., & Tzavaras, A. (1984). Hemispheric specialization for language in the congenitally blind: The influence of the Braille system. *Neuropsychologia, 22,* 521–525.

Keech, R. V., & Kutschke, P. J. (1995). Upper age limit for the development of amblyopia. *Journal of Pediatric Ophthalmology and Strabismus, 32,* 89–93.

King, A. J., & Parsons, C. H. (1999). Improved auditory spatial acuity in visually deprived ferrets. *European Journal of Neuroscience, 11,* 3945–3956.

Kiorpes, L., Kiper, D. C., O'Keefe, L. P., Cavanaugh, J. R., & Movshon, A. J. (1998). Neuronal correlates of ambyopia in the visual cortex of macaque monkeys with experimental strabismus and anismetropia. *Journal of Neuroscience, 18,* 6411–6424.

Klinke, R., Kral, A., Heid, S., Tillein, J., & Hartmann, R. (1999). Recruitment of the auditory cortex in congenitally deaf cats by long-term cochlear electrostimulation. *Science, 285,* 1729–1733.

Knight, R. T. (1990). Neuronal mechanisms of event-related potentials: Evidence from human lesion studies. In J. W. Rohrbauch, R. Parasuraman, & R. J. Johnson (Eds.), *Event-related brain potentials: Basic issues and applications* (pp. 3–18). New York: Oxford University Press.

Knudsen, E. I. (1998). Capacity for plasticity in the adult owl auditory system expanded by juvenile experience. *Science, 279,* 1531–1533.

Knudsen, E. I., Esterly, S. D., & du Lac, S. (1991). Stretched and upside-down maps of auditory space in the optic tectum of blind-reared owls: Acoustic basis and behavioral correlates. *Journal of Neuroscience, 11,* 1727–1747.

Kolb, B., & Gibb, R. (2001). Early brain injury, plasticity and behavior. In C. Nelson & M. Luciana (Eds.), *Handbook of developmental cognitive neuroscience* (pp. 175–190). Cambridge, MA: MIT Press.

Kolb, B., & Whishaw, I. Q. (1998). Brain plasticity and behavior. *Annual Review of Psychology, 49,* 43–64.

Kolb, B., & Whishaw, I. Q. (1990). *Fundamentals of human neuropsychology.* New York: Freeman.

Korte, M., & Rauschecker, J. P. (1993). Auditory spatial tuning of cortical neurons is sharpened in cats with early blindness. *Journal of Neurophysiology, 70,* 1717–1721.

Kujala, T., Alho, K., Huotilainen, M., Ilmoniemi, R. J., Lehtokoski, A., Leinonen, A., Rinne, T., Salonen, O., Sinkkonen, J., Standertskjald-Nordenstam, & Näätänen, R. (1997). Electrophysiological evidence for cross-modal plasticity in humans with early- and late-onset of blindness. *Psychophysiology, 34*(2), 213–216.

Kujala, T., Alho, K., Kekoni, J., Hämäläinen, H., Reinikainen, K., Salonen, O., et al. (1995). Auditory and somatosensory event-related brain potentials in early blind humans. *Experimental Brain Research, 104,* 519–526.

Kujala, T., Alho, K., & Näätänen, R. (2000). Cross-modal reorganization of human cortical functions. *Trends in Neurosciences, 23,* 115–120.

Kujala, T., Lehtokoski, A., Alho, K., Kekoni, J., & Näätänen, R. (1997). Faster reaction times in the blind than sighted during bimodal divided attention. *Acta Psychologica, 96,* 75–82.

Landau, B., & Gleitman, L. R. (1985). *Language and experience: Evidence from the blind child.* Cambridge, MA: Harvard University Press.

Larsen, S., & Hakonsen, K. (1983). Absence of ear asymmetry in blind children in a dichotic listening task compared to sighted controls. *Brain and Language, 18,* 192–198.

Laurienti, P. J., Burdette, J. H., Wallace, M. T., Yen, Y.-F. Y., Field, A. S., & Stein, B. E. (2002). Deactivation of sensory-specific cortex by cross-modal stimuli. *Journal of Cognitive Neuroscience, 14,* 420–429.

Le Grand, R., Maurer, D., & Brent, H. P. (2001). Early visual experience and face processing. *Nature, 410,* 890.

Lehnhardt, E., & Achendorff, A. (1993). Prognostic factors in 187 adults provided with the Nucleus Cochlear Mini-System 22. In B. Fraysse & O. Deguine (Eds.), *Cochlear implants: New perspectives* (pp. 146–152). Basel: Karger.

Lessard, N., Paré, M., Leporé, F., & Lassonde, M. (1998). Early-blind human subjects localize sound sources better than sighted subjects. *Nature, 395,* 278–280.

Levänen, S., & Hamdorf, D. (2001). Feeling vibrations: Enhanced tactile sensitivity in congenitally deaf humans. *Neuroscience Letters, 301,* 75–77.

Liepert, J., Miltner, W. H. R., Bauder, H., Sommer, M., Dettmers, C., Taub, E., et al. (1998). Motor cortex plasticity during constraint-induced movement therapy in stroke patients. *Neuroscience Letters, 250,* 5–8.

Liotti, M., Ryder, K., & Woldorff, M. G. (1998). Auditory attention in congenitally blind: Where, when and what gets reorganized. *Neuroreport, 9,* 1007–1012.

Lotze, M., Grodd, W., Birbaumer, N., Erb, M., Huse, E., & Flor, H. (1999). Does use of a myoelectric prosthesis prevent cortical reorganization and phantom pain. *Nature Neuroscience, 2,* 501–502.

Mangun, G. R., & Hillyard, S. A. (1995). Mechanisms and models of selective attention. In M. D. Rugg & M. G. H. Coles (Eds.), *Electrophysiology of mind: Event-related potentials and cognition* (pp. 40–85). Oxford, England: Oxford University Press.

Maurer, D., & Lewis, T. L. (2001). Visual acuity and spatial contrast sensitivity: Normal development and underlying mechanisms. In C. A. Nelson & M. Luciana (Eds.), *Handbook of developmental cognitive neuroscience* (pp. 237–251). Cambridge, MA: MIT Press.

Maurer, D., Lewis, T. L., & Brent, H. (1989). The effects of deprivation on human visual development. Studies in children treated with cataracts. In F. J. Morrison, C. Lord, & D. P. Keating (Eds.), *Applied developmental psychology* (pp. 139–227). San Diego: Academic Press.

Mayberry, R. I., Lock, E., & Kazmi, H. (2002). Linguistic ability and early language exposure. *Nature, 417,* 38.

Menning, H., Roberts, L. E., & Pantev, C. (2000). Plastic changes in the auditory cortex induced by intensive frequency discrimination training. *Neuroreport, 11,* 817–822.

Merzenich, M. M., & Jenkins, W. M. (1993). Reorganization of cortical representations of the hand following alterations of skin input induced by nerve injury, skin island transfer, and experience. *Journal of Hand Therapy, 6,* 89–104.

Millar, S. (1982). Studies of the deaf and the blind. In A. Burton, (Ed.), *The pathology and psychology of cognition* (pp. 135–168). London: Methuen.

Millar, S. (1994). *Understanding and representing space: Theory and evidence from studies with blind and sighted children.* Oxford, England: Clarendon Press.

Miller, L. (1992). Diderot reconsidered: Visual impairment and auditory compensation. *Journal of Visual Impairment and Blindness, 86,* 206–210.

Mills, A. (1972). Auditory localization. In J. V. Fobias (Ed.), *Foundations of modern auditory theory* (pp. 303–348). New York: Academic Press.

Mills, A. E. (1983). *Language acquisition in the blind child.* London & Canberra: Croom Helm.

Mills, A. E. (1988). Visual handicap. In D. Bishop & K. Mogford (Eds.), *Language development in exceptional circumstances* (pp. 150–163). Edinburgh, Scotland: Churchill Livingstone.

Miltner, W. H. R., Bauder, H., Sommer, M., Dettmer, C., & Taub, E. (1998). Effects of constraint-induced movement therapy on patients with chronic motor deficits after stroke: A replication. *Stroke, 30,* 586–592.

Morrongiello, B. A. (1994). Effects of colocation on auditory-visual integrations and crossmodal perception in infants. In D. J. Lewkowicz & R. Lickliter (Eds.), *The development of intersensory perception* (pp. 235–263). Hillsdale, NJ: Lawrence Erlbaum Associates.

Muchnik, C., Efrati, M., Nemeth, E., Malin, M., & Hildesheimer, M. (1991). Central auditory skills in blind and sighted subjects. *Scandinavian Audiology, 20,* 19–23.

Mühlnickel, W., Elbert, T., Taub, E., & Flor, H. (1998). Reorganization of auditory cortex in tinnitus. *Proceedings of the National Academy of Sciences, USA, 95,* 10340–10343.

Münte, T. F., Kohlmetz, C., Nager, W., & Altenmüller, E. (2001). Superior auditory spatial tuning in conductors. *Nature, 409,* 580.

Näätänen, R. (1992). *Attention and brain function.* Hillsdale, NJ: Erlbaum.

Näätänen, R., & Picton, T. W. (1986). N2 and automatic versus controlled processes. In W. C. McCallum, R. Zappolini, & F. Denoth (Eds.), *Cerebral psychophysiology: Studies in event-related potentials (EEG Suppl. 38)* (pp. 169–186). Amsterdam: Elsevier.

Necker, R., Rehkämper, G., & Nevo, E. (1992). Electrophysiological mapping of body representation in the blind mole rat. *Neuroreport, 3,* 505–508.

Neville, H., & Bavelier, D. (2000). Specificity and plasticity in neurocognitive development in humans. In M. S. Gazzaniga (Ed.), *The cognitive neurosciences* (pp. 83–98). Cambridge, MA: MIT Press.

Neville, H. J., & Bavelier, D. (2001). Specificity of developmental neuroplasticity in humans: Evidence from sensory deprivation and altered language experience. In C. A. Shaw & J. C. McEachern (Eds.), *Toward a theory of neuroplasticity* (pp. 261–274). Hove: Taylor & Francis, Psychology Press.

Neville, H. J., Bavelier, D., Corina, D., Rauschecker, J., Karni, A., Lalwani, A., et al. (1998). Cerebral organization for language in deaf and hearing subjects: Biological constraints and effects of experience. *Proceedings of the National Academy of Sciences, USA, 95,* 922–928.

Neville, H. J., & Lawson, D. (1987). Attention to central and peripheral visual space in a movement detection task: An event-related potential and behavioral study. II. Congenitally deaf adults. *Brain Research, 405,* 268–283.

Neville, H. J., Mills, D. L., & Lawson, D. L. (1992). Fractionating language: Different neuronal subsystems with different sensitive periods. *Cerebral Cortex, 2,* 244–258.

Neville, H. J., Schmidt, A., & Kutas, M. (1983). Altered visual-evoked potentials in congenitally deaf adults. *Brain Research, 266,* 127–132.

Newman, A. J., Pancheva, R., Ozawa, K., Neville, H. J., & Ullman, M. T. (2001). An event-related fMRI study of syntactic and semantic violations. *Journal of Psycholinguist Research, 30,* 339–364.

Niemeyer, W., & Starlinger, I. (1981). Do blind hear better? Investigations on auditory processing in congenital early acquired blindness. II. Central functions. *Audiology, 20,* 510–515.

Nishimura, H., Hashikawa, K., Doi, K., Iwaki, T., Watanabe, Y., Kusuoka, H., et al. (1999). Sign language 'heard' in the auditory cortex. *Nature, 397,* 116.

Ohl, F. W., Scheich, H., & Freeman, W. J. (2001). Change in pattern of ongoing cortical activity with auditory category learning. *Nature, 412,* 733–736.

Ormerod, B. K., & Galea, L. A. M. (2001). Mechanism and function of adult neurogenesis. In C. A. Shaw & J. C. McEachern (Eds.), *Toward a theory of neuroplasticity* (pp. 223–243). Hove, England: Taylor & Francis/ Psychology Press.

Pallas, S. L. (2001). Intrinsic and extrinsic factors that shape neocortical specification. *Trends in Neurosciences, 24,* 417–423.

Pantev, C., & Lütkenhäner, B. (2000). Magnetoencephalographic studies of functional organization and plasticity of the human auditory system. *Clinical Neurophysiology, 17,* 130–142.

Pantev, C., Oostenveld, R., Engelien, A., Ross, B., Roberts, L. E., & Hike, M. (1998). Increased auditory cortical representation in musicians. *Nature, 393,* 811–814.

Pantev, C., Roberts, L. E., Schulz, M., Engelien, A., & Ross, B. (2001). Timbre-specific enhancement of auditory cortical representations in musicians. *Neuroreport, 12,* 169–174.

Pascual-Leone, A., Cammarota, A., Wassermann, E. M., Brasil-Neto, J. P., Cohen, L. G., & Hallett, M. (1993). Modulation of motor cortical outputs of the reading hand of Braille readers. *Annals of Neurology, 34,* 33–37.

Pascual-Leone, A., & Hamilton, R. (2001). The metamodal organization of the brain. *Progress in Brain Research,* 428–445.

Pascual-Leone, A., & Torres, F. (1993). Plasticity of the sensorimotor cortex representation of the reading finger in braille readers. *Brain, 116,* 39–52.

Pèrez-Pereira, M., & Conti-Ramsden, G. (1999). *Language development and social interaction in blind children* (pp. 1–197). Hove, England: Psychology Press.

Philipps, D. P., & Brugge, J. F. (1985). Progress in the neurophysiology of sound localization. *Annual Review of Psychology, 36,* 245–274.

Poldrack, R. A. (2000). Imaging brain plasticity: Conceptual and methodological issues. A theoretical review. *NeuroImage, 12,* 1–13.

Pons, T. P., Garraghty, P. E., Ommaya, A. K., Kaas, J. H., Taub, E., & Mishkin, M. (1991). Massive cortical reorganization after sensory deafferentation in adult macaques. *Science, 252,* 1857–1860.

Pring, L., Freistone, S. E., & Katan, S. A. (1990). Recalling pictures and words: Reversing the generation effect. *Current Psychology Research, 9,* 35–45.

Rammsayer, T. (1992). Zeitdauerdiskriminationsleistung bei Blinden und Nicht-Blinden: Evidenz für biologischen Zeitmechanismus. *Kognitionswissenschaft, 2,* 180–188.

Rauschecker, J. P. (1995). Compensatory plasticity and sensory substitution in the cerebral cortex. *Trends in Neurosciences, 18,* 36–43.

Rauschecker, J. P. (1997). Mechanisms of compensatory plasticity in the cerebral cortex. In H.-J. Freund, B. A. Sabel, & O. W. Witte (Eds.), *Brain plasticity, advances in neurology* (pp. 137–146). Philadelphia: Lippinott-Raven.

Rauschecker, J. P. (2001). Developmental neuroplasticity within and across sensory modalities. In C. A. Shaw & J. C. McEachern (Eds.), *Toward a theory of neuroplasticity* (pp. 244–260). Hove, England: Taylor & Francis/ Psychology Press.

Rauschecker, J. P., & Harris, L. R. (1983). Auditory compensation of the effect of visual deprivation in cats' superior colliculus. *Experimental Brain Research, 50,* 63–83.

Rauschecker, J. P., & Kniepert, U. (1994). Auditory localization behavior in visually deprived cats. *European Journal of Neuroscience, 6,* 149–160.

Rauschecker, J. P., & Korte, M. (1993). Auditory compensation for early blindness in cat cerebral cortex. *Journal of Neuroscience, 13,* 4538–4548.

Rauschecker, J. P., Tian, B., Korte, M., & Egert, U. (1992). Crossmodal changes in the somatosensory vibrissa/barrel system of visually deprived animals. *Proceedings of the National Academy of Sciences, USA, 89,* 5063–5067.

Recanzone, G. H., Merzenich, M. M., & Schreiner, C. E. (1992). Changes in the distributed temporal response properties of SI cortical neurons reflect improvements in performance on a temporally based tactile discrimination task. *Journal of Neurophysiology, 67,* 1071–1091.

Rettenbach, R., Diller, G., & Sireteanu, R. (1999). Do deaf people see better? Texture segmentation and visual search compensate in adult but not in juvenile subjects. *Journal of Cognitive Neuroscience, 11,* 560–583.

Rice, C. E. (1970). Early experience and perceptual enhancement. *Research Bulletin, American Foundation for the Blind, 22,* 1–22.

Ritter, W., Simon, R., & Vaughan, H. G. J. (1983). Event-related potential correlates of two stages of information processing in physical and semantic discrimination task. *Psychophysiology, 20,* 168–179.

Röder, B., Demuth, L., Streb, J., & Rösler, F. (2003). Semantic and syntactic priming in auditory word recognition in congenitally blind adults. *Language and Cognitive Processes, 18,* 1–20.

Röder, B., & Neville, H. (2003). Developmental functional plasticity. In J. Grafman & I. Robertson (Eds.), *Handbook of Neuropsychology.* New York: Elsevier.

Röder, B., & Rösler, F. (1998). Visual input does not facilitate the scanning of spatial images. *Journal of Mental Imagery, 22,* 165–182.

Röder, B., & Rösler, F. (2001). Ein Vergleich haptischer Wahrnehmungsleistungen zwischen blinden und sehenden Personen. In M. Grunwald & L. Beyer (Eds.), *Der bewegte Sinn: Grundlagen und Anwendungen zur haptischen Wahrnehmung* (pp. 89–98). Basel: Birkhäuser Verlag.

Röder, B., Rösler, F., Heil, M., & Hennighausen, E. (1993). DC-Correlates of haptic mental rotation in blind and sighted subjects. *Psychophysiology, 30*(Suppl. 1), 55.

Röder, B., Rösler, F., & Hennighausen, E. (1997). Different cortical activation patterns in blind and sighted humans during encoding and transformation of haptic images. *Psychophysiology, 34,* 292–307.

Röder, B., Rösler, F., Hennighausen, E., & Näcker, F. (1996). Event-related potentials during auditory and somatosensory discrimination in sighted and blind human subjects. *Cognitive Brain Research, 4,* 77–93.

Röder, B., Rösler, F., & Neville, H. J. (1999). Effects of interstimulus interval on auditory event-related potentials in congenitally blind and normally sighted humans. *Neuroscience Letters, 264,* 53–56.

Röder, B., Rösler, F., & Neville, H. J. (2000). Event-related potentials during language processing in congenitally blind and sighted people. *Neuropsychologia, 38,* 1482–1502.

Röder, B., Stock, O., Bien, S., Neville, H., & Rösler, F. (2002). Speech processing activates visual cortex in congenitally blind adults. *European Journal of Neuroscience, 16,* 930–936.

Röder, B., Stock, O., Neville, H., Bien, S., & Rösler, F. (2002). Brain activation modulated by the comprehension of normal and pseudo-word sentences of different processing demands: A functional magnetic resonance imaging study. *NeuroImage, 15,* 1003–1014.

Röder, B., Teder-Sälejärvi, W., Sterr, A., Rösler, F., Hillyard, S. A., & Neville, H. J. (1997). *Auditory-spatial tuning in sighted and blind adults: Behavioral and electrophysiological evidence* (abstract). 27th Annual Meeting of the Society for Neuroscience, New Orleans, October 25–30.

Röder, B., Teder-Sälejärvi, W., Sterr, A., Rösler, F., Hillyard, S. A., & Neville, H. J. (1999). Improved auditory spatial tuning in blind humans. *Nature, 400,* 162–166.

Rosen, H. J., Petersen, S. E., Linenweber, M. R., Snyder, A. Z., White, D. A., Chapman, L., et al. (2000). Neural correlates of recovery from aphasia after damage to left inferior frontal cortex. *Neurology, 55,* 1883–1894.

Rösler, F., Röder, B., Heil, M., & Hennighausen, E. (1993). Topographic differences of slow event-related brain potentials in blind and sighted adult human subjects during haptic mental rotation. *Cognitive Brain Research, 1,* 145–159.

Rozas, C., Frank, H., Heynen, A. J., Morales, B., Bear, M. F., & Kirkwood, A. (2001). Developmental inhibitory gate controls the relay of activity to the superficial layers of the visual cortex. *Journal of Neuroscience, 21,* 6791–6801.

Ryugo, D. K., Ryugo, R., Globus, A., & Killackey, H. P. (1975). Increased spine density in auditory cortex following visual or somatosensoric deafferentation. *Brain Research, 90,* 143–146.

Sacks, O. (1995). To see and not to see. In O. Sacks (Ed.), *An anthropologist on Mars* (pp. 108–152). New York: Vintage Books.

Sadato, N., Pascual-Leone, A., Grafman, J., Deiber, M.-P., Ibanez, V., & Hallett, M. (1998). Neural networks for Braille reading by the blind include visual cortex. *Brain, 121,* 1213–1229.

Sathian, K. (1998). Perceptual learning. *Current Science, 75,* 451–457.

Sathian, K. (2000). Practice makes perfect: Sharper tactile perception in the blind. *Neurology, 54,* 2203–2204.

Schlaggar, B. L., & O'Leary, D. D. M. (1991). Potential of visual cortex to develop an array of functional units unique to somatosensory cortex. *Science, 252,* 1556–1560.

Schweizer, R., Braun, C., Fromm, C., Wilms, A., & Birbaumer, N. (2001). The distribution of mislocalizations across fingers demonstrates training-induced neuroplastic changes in somatosensory cortex. *Experimental Brain Research, 139,* 435–442.

Sejnowski, T. J., & Churchland, P. S. (1989). Brain and cognition. In M. Posner (Ed.), *Foundations of cognitive science* (pp. 301–356). Cambridge, MA: MIT Press.

Shaw, C. A., & McEachern, J. C. (2000). *Toward a theory of neuroplasticity.* Hove, England: Psychology Press.

Sheedlo, H. J., & Turner, J. E. (1992). Historical perspective on regeneration and plasticity in the visual system. In D. M. K. Lam & G. M. Bray (Eds.), *Regeneration and plasticity in the mammalian visual system* (pp. 3–13). London: MIT Press.

Shepard, R. K., Hartmann, R., Heid, S., Hardie, N., & Klinke, R. (1997). The central auditory system and auditory deprivation: Experience with cochlear implants in the congenitally deaf. *Acta Otolaryngology* (Suppl. 532), 28–33.

Shors, R. J., Miesegaes, G., Beylin, A., Zhao, M., Rydel, T., & Gould, E. (2001). Neurogenesis in the adult involved in the formation of trace memories. *Nature, 410,* 372–376.

Singer, W., & Tretter, F. (1976). Receptive-field properties and neuronal connectivity in striate and parastriate cortex of contour-deprived cats. *Journal of Neurophysiology, 39,* 613–629.

Starlinger, J., & Niemeyer, W. (1981). Do the blind hear betterü Investigation in congenital or early blindness. *Audiology, 20,* 503–509.

Stein, B. A., Wallace, M. T., & Stanford, T. R. (2000). Merging sensory signals in the brain: The development of multisensory integration in the superior colliculus. In M. S. Gazzaniga (Ed.), *The new cognitive neurosciences* (pp. 55–71). Cambridge, MA: MIT Press.

Stein, B. E. (1998). Neural mechanisms of synthesizing sensory information and production adaptive behaviors. *Experimental Brain Research, 123,* 124–135.

Stein, B. E., & Meredith, M. A. (1993). *The merging of the senses.* Cambridge, MA: MIT Press.

Sterr, A., Müller, M., Elbert, T., Rockstroh, B., Pantev, B., & Taub, E. (1998). Perceptual correlates of changes in cortical representation of fingers in blind multifinger readers. *Journal of Neuroscience, 18,* 4417–4423.

Stiles, J. (2001). Neural plasticity and cognitive development. *Developmental Neuropsychology, 18,* 237–272.

Stiles, J., & Thal, D. (1993). Linguistic and spatial cognitive development following early focal brain injury: Patterns of deficit recovery. In M. H. Johnson (Ed.), *Brain development and cognition* (pp. 643–664). Oxford, England: Blackwell.

Summers, D. C., & Lederman, S. J. (1990). Perceptual asymmetries in the somatosensory system: A dichhaptic experiment and critical review of the literature from 1929 to 1986. *Cortex, 26,* 201–226.

Sur, M., & Leamey, A. (2001). Development and plasticity of cortical areas and networks. *Nature Reviews: Neuroscience, 2,* 251–262.

Sur, M., Pallas, S. L., & Roe, A. W. (1990). Cross-modal plasticity in cortical development: Differentiation and specification of sensory neocortex. *Trends in Neurosciences, 13,* 227–233.

Tallal, P., Miller, S. L., Bedi, G., Byma, G., Wang, X., Nagaraja, S. S., et al. (1996). Language comprehension in language-learning impaired children improve with acoustically modified speech. *Science, 271,* 81–84.

Taub, E., Miller, N. E., Novack, T. A., Cook, E. W., Fleming, W. C., Nepomuiceno, C. S., et al. (1993). Technique to improve chronic motor deficit after stroke. *Archives of Physical Medicine and Rehabilitation, 74,* 347–354.

Teder-Sälejärvi, W., & Hillyard, S. A. (1998). The gradient of spatial auditory attention in free field: An event-related potential study. *Perception & Psychophysics, 60,* 1228–1242.

Teyler, T. J. (2001). LTP and the superfamiliy of synaptic plasticities. In C. A. Shaw & J. C. McEachern (Eds.), *Toward a theory of neuroplasticity* (pp. 101–117). Hove, England: Psychology Press/Taylor & Francis.

Thinus-Blanc, C., & Gaunet, F. (1997). Representation of space in blind persons: Vision as a spatial sense? *Psychological Bulletin, 121,* 20–42.

Thompson, C. K. (2000). Neuroplasticity: Evidence from aphasia. *Journal of Communication Disorders, 33,* 357–366.

Tröster, H., Hecker, W., & Brambring, M. (1994). Longitudinal study of cross-motor development in blind infants and preschoolers. *Early Child Development and Care, 104,* 61–78.

Turkewitz, G., & Kenny, P. A. (1982). Limitations on input as a basis for neural organization and perceptual development: A preliminary theoretical statement. *Developmental Psychobiology, 15,* 357–368.

Turner, A. M., & Greenough, W. Z. (1985). Differential rearing effects on rat visual cortex synapses. I Synaptic and neuronal density and synapses per neuron. *Brain Research, 329,* 195–203.

Uhl, F., Franzen, P., Podreka, I., Steiner, M., & Deecke, L. (1993). Increased regional cerebral blood flow in inferior occipital cortex and cerebellum of early blind humans. *Neuroscience Letters, 150,* 162–164.

Ungar, S. (2000). Cognitive mapping without visual experience. In R. Kitchin & S. Freundschuh (Eds.), *Cognitive mapping: Past, present and future.* London: Routledge.

Van Boven, R. W., Hamilton, R. H., Kauffman, T., Keenan, J. P., & Pascual-Leone, A. (2000). Tactile spatial resolution in blind Braille readers. *Neurology, 54,* 2230–2236.

van Praag, H., Kempermann, G., & Gage, F. H. (2000). Neural consequences of environmental enrichment. *Nature Reviews: Neuroscience, 1,* 191–198.

Veraart, C., De Volder, A. G., Wanet-Defalque, M. C., Bol, A., Michel, C., & Goffinet, A. M. (1990). Glucose utilization in human visual cortex is abnormally elevated in blindness of early onset but decreases in blindness of late onset. *Brain Research, 510,* 115–121.

Vidyasagar, T. R. (1978). Possible plasticity in the superior colliculus. *Nature, 275,* 140–141.

Wallace, M. T., & Stein, B. E. (1997). Development of multisensory neurons and multisensory integration in cat superior colliculus. *Journal of Neuroscience, 17,* 2429–2444.

Wallace, M. T., & Stein, B. E. (2001). Sensory and multisensory responses in the newborn monkey superior colliculus. *Journal of Neuroscience, 21,* 8886–8894.

Wanet, M. C., & Veraart, C. (1985). Processing of auditory information by the blind in spatial localization task. *Perception & Psychophysics, 38,* 91–96.

Weeks, R., Horwitz, B., Aziz-Sultan, A., Tian, B., Wessinger, C. M., Cohen, L. G., et al. (2000). A positron emission tomographic study of auditory localization in the congenitally blind. *Journal of Neuroscience, 20,* 2664–2672.

Weiss, T., Miltner, W. H. R., Adler, T., Brücker, L., & Taub, E. (1999). Decrease in phantom limb pain associated with prosthesis induced increased use of an amputation stump in humans. *Neuroscience Letters, 272,* 131–134.

Welch, R. B., & Warren, D. H. (1986). Intersensory interaction. In K. R. Boff, L. Kaufman, & J. P. Thomas (Eds.), *Handbook of perception and human performance* (pp. 25-1–25-36). New York: Wiley.

Woods, D. L., Knight, R. T., & Scabini, D. (1993). Anatomical substrates of auditory selective attention: Behavioral and electrophysiological effects of posterior association cortex lesion. *Cognitive Brain Research, 1,* 227–240.

Yaka, R., Yinon, U., Rosner, M., & Wollberg, Z. (2000). Pathological and experimentally induced blindness induces auditory activity in the cat primary visual cortex. *Experimental Brain Research, 131,* 144–148.

Yaka, R., Yinon, U., & Wollberg, Z. (1999). Auditory activation of cortical visual areas in cats after early visual deprivation. *European Journal of Neuroscience, 11,* 1301–1312.

Zwiers, M. P., Van Opstal, A. J., & Cruysberg, J. R. M. (2001a). A spatial hearing deficit in early-blind humans. *Journal of Neuroscience, 21*(RC142), 1–5.

Zwiers, M. P., Van Opstal, A. J., & Cruysberg, J. R. M. (2001b). Two-dimensional sound-localization behavior of early-blind humans. *Experimental Brain Research, 140,* 206–222.

47 Audiovisual Speech Perception in Deaf Adults and Children Following Cochlear Implantation

TONYA R. BERGESON AND DAVID B. PISONI

Introduction

Cochlear implants (CIs) are electronic auditory prostheses developed to enable individuals with severe to profound hearing impairment to perceive speech and understand spoken language. A CI consists of an external microphone and speech processor, which convert sound into an electrical signal, and an external transmitter, which transmits the electrical signal to an internal receiver, which then sends the electrical signal to an array of electrodes (located in the cochlea) that stimulate the auditory nerve. Although CIs work well in many patients, the benefits to individual users vary substantially. Auditory-alone (A-alone) performance measures have demonstrated that some users of CIs are able to communicate successfully using speech over a telephone even when lipreading cues are unavailable (e.g., Dorman, Dankowski, McCandless, Parkin, & Smith, 1991). Other users show little benefit in open-set speech perception tests under A-alone listening conditions but report that the CI helps them understand speech when visual information is also available in face-to-face conversation.

One source of these individual differences is undoubtedly the way in which the surviving neural elements in the cochlea are stimulated with electrical currents provided by the speech processor (Fryauf-Bertschy, Tyler, Kelsay, Gantz, & Woodworth, 1997). Other sources of individual differences, however, result from the way in which these initial sensory inputs are coded and processed by higher cortical centers in the auditory system (Pisoni, 2000; Pisoni, Cleary, Geers, & Tobey, 2000). In this chapter, we present a review and theoretical interpretation of new findings on the central cognitive factors related to audiovisual (AV) speech perception that contribute to the individual differences in outcome and benefit with CIs in profoundly deaf adults and children.

Although there are many important clinical reasons for investigating the basis for the variation and variability in outcome measures of speech and language among deaf adults and children who have received CIs, there are also several theoretical reasons, having to do with issues in neural and behavioral development, for carrying out research in this unique population. Deaf adults and children who receive CIs afford an unusual opportunity to study the effects of auditory deprivation on sensory, perceptual, and cognitive development, specifically the cognitive mechanisms that underlie the development of speech and language processing skills after the introduction of novel auditory input to the nervous system. For ethical reasons, it is not possible to carry out sensory deprivation experiments with adults and children, and it is impossible to delay or withhold medical treatment for an illness or disability that has been identified and diagnosed. Thus, for studies of this kind in humans, it becomes necessary to rely on clinical populations that are receiving medical interventions of various kinds and hope that appropriate experimental designs can be developed that will yield new scientific knowledge and understanding about the basic underlying neural mechanisms and processes.

Fortunately, in everyday experience, speech communication is not limited to input from the auditory sensory modality alone. Visual information about speech articulation and spoken language obtained from lipreading has been shown to improve speech understanding in listeners with normal hearing (Erber, 1969; Sumby & Pollack, 1954), listeners with hearing loss (Erber, 1972, 1975), and hearing-impaired listeners with CIs (Tyler, Parkinson, Woodworth, Lowder, & Gantz, 1997). Although lipreading cues have been shown to enhance speech perception, the sensory, perceptual, and cognitive processes underlying the multisensory gain in performance are not well understood, especially in special clinical populations, such as adults and children who are hearing-impaired and subsequently acquire or reacquire hearing via CIs.

In one of the first studies to investigate AV speech perception, Sumby and Pollack (1954) demonstrated that visual cues to speech greatly enhance speech intelligibility for normal hearing (NH) listeners, especially when the acoustic signal is masked by noise. They found that performance on several closed-set word recognition tasks increased substantially under AV presentation compared to A-alone presentation. This increase in performance was comparable to the gain observed when the auditory signal was increased by about 15 dB SPL under A-alone perception conditions (Summerfield, 1987). Since this research was reported almost 50 years ago, numerous other studies have demonstrated that visual information from lipreading improves speech perception performance over A-alone conditions in NH adults (Massaro & Cohen, 1995) as well as in adults and children with varying degrees of hearing impairment (Erber, 1975, 1979; Geers, 1994; Geers & Brenner, 1994; Geers, Brenner, & Davidson, 2003; Grant, Walden, & Seitz, 1998; Massaro & Cohen, 1999).

Cross-modal speech perception and the cognitive processes by which individuals combine and integrate auditory and visual speech information with lexical and syntactic knowledge have become major areas of research in the field of speech perception (e.g., Massaro, 1998; Massaro & Cohen, 1995). AV speech perception appears to be much more complicated than just the simple addition of auditory and visual cues to speech (e.g., Massaro & Cohen, 1999). That is, the gain in performance obtained from combined AV information is superadditive. For example, Sumby and Pollack (1954) and Erber (1969) observed that although speech intelligibility decreased in A-alone conditions when the signal-to-noise ratio (S/N) decreased, word recognition dramatically increased under AV conditions, with the visual contribution increasing in importance when the speech signal was less audible.

A well-known example of visual bias in AV speech perception is the McGurk effect (McGurk & MacDonald, 1976). When presented with an auditory /ba/ stimulus and a visual /ga/ stimulus simultaneously, many listeners report hearing an entirely new stimulus, a perceptual /da/. Thus, information from separate sensory modalities is combined to produce percepts that differ predictably from either the auditory or the visual signal alone. However, these findings are not observed in all individuals (see Massaro & Cohen, 2000). Grant and Seitz (1998) suggested that listeners who are more susceptible to the McGurk effect also are better at integrating auditory and visual speech cues. Grant et al. (1998) proposed that some listeners could improve consonant perception skills by as much as 26% by sharpening their integration abilities. Their findings on AV speech perception may have important clinical implications for intervention and aural rehabilitation strategies with deaf and hearing-impaired listeners because consonant perception accounted for approximately half of the variance of word and sentence recognition in their study.

In an important theoretical paper on AV speech perception, Summerfield (1987) identified two major reasons to study AV integration in speech perception. First, studies of AV integration allow researchers to investigate the independent and collaborative contribution of individual auditory and visual modalities. Second, AV integration occurs to varying degrees in all perceivers. Even NH listeners benefit from lipreading cues when they are required to recognize speech in background noise or under other degraded listening conditions. Moreover, many hearing-impaired listeners depend heavily on lipreading cues for everyday communication purposes without the availability of reliable auditory information to support speech perception. Thus, the study of cross-modal speech perception and AV integration may provide speech researchers with new insights into the fundamental cognitive processes used in spoken language processing.

Summerfield (1987) proposed five mechanisms that could account for AV speech perception. These mechanisms ranged from the "vision:place, audition:manner" or VPAM hypothesis, in which place evidence is categorized by the visual modality and manner evidence is categorized by the auditory modality before the information is integrated, to a modality-free dynamical representation of AV speech perception. At the present time, the debate concerning the underlying neural and perceptual mechanisms of AV integration is unresolved, with some researchers supporting modality-neutral, early-integration theories of AV speech perception (e.g., Fowler, 1986; Rosenblum, in press; Rosenblum & Gordon, 2001) and others arguing for modality-specific, late-integration theories (e.g., Bernstein, Auer, & Moore, Chap. 13, this volume) of AV speech perception. Our recent findings, reported later in this chapter, on deaf adults and children who received CIs add new knowledge and may inform this debate by determining the relative contributions of visual and severely compromised auditory modalities when the auditory modality is restored with a CI.

Because postlingually deaf adults have to readjust their perceptual strategies to compensate for the loss of hearing or degraded auditory input, and may have to rely more heavily on visual cues to spoken language than

NH adults, it seems reasonable to suppose that hearing loss alone would naturally lead to increased lipreading abilities. However, research investigating this hypothesis has led to inconclusive results. Some investigators have found no lipreading advantage for hearing-impaired adults (e.g., Massaro, 1987; Mogford, 1987; Rönnberg, 1995), whereas other researchers have found better lipreading performance in some deaf adults than in NH adults (Bernstein, Demorest, & Tucker, 2000). In a recent study, Bernstein, Auer, and Tucker (2001) reported that NH adults who were self-selected as "good lipreaders" could actually lipread words in sentences just as well as deaf adults. However, the deaf adults' lipreading accuracy was superior to that of NH adults only when the sentences were scored in terms of phonemes correct, which reflects the use of partial stimulus information.

One reason for the equivocal results on this issue is that there is enormous variability in the lipreading skills of the deaf adult population. Such variability in deaf adults' lipreading skills may be explained by the age at onset of the hearing loss: adults who experienced a hearing loss earlier in life may be better lipreaders than adults who acquired a hearing loss later in life, simply because they have had more exposure and experience with the visual properties of speech articulation and were forced to actively code and process visual speech cues to engage in meaningful speech communication activities on a daily basis. In fact, it has been reported that many deaf adults with early-onset deafness are better lipreaders than NH adults (see Bernstein et al., 2000). However, there has been very little research conducted on this problem or the underlying factors that are responsible for these individual differences in lipreading skills.

In a study on the effects of age at onset of deafness, Tillberg, Rönnberg, Svärd, and Ahlner (1996) measured speech perception in A-alone, visual-alone (V-alone), and AV modalities in adults with early-onset versus late-onset deafness and found no differences in performance between the two groups in A-alone and AV conditions. However, they did find better performance for adults with early-onset deafness than for adults with late-onset deafness in the V-alone condition. The differences in lipreading performance between the early-onset and late-onset groups most likely were due to experience and activities with visual speech cues. That is, adults with an early-onset hearing loss spend a greater proportion of their lives using visual rather than auditory cues to perceive speech, whereas adults with a late-onset hearing loss depend primarily on auditory cues to speech for a longer time and thus have much less lipreading experience overall.

Among audiologists and speech and hearing scientists who work with the deaf, it is generally assumed that the primary modality for speech perception is different for hearing-impaired and NH populations (e.g., Erber, 1969; Gagné, 1994; Seewald, Ross, Giolas, & Yonovitz, 1985). The primary modality for speech perception is audition for NH people, but it is vision for hearing-impaired people. In fact, CIs were historically thought of as sensory aids to lipreading, with vision considered to be the primary modality for speech perception and spoken language in this population (Gantz et al., 1988; Tyler et al., 1985; Tyler, Tye-Murray, & Lansing, 1988). Early single-channel CIs provided minimal auditory information about speech and spoken language and coded only duration and amplitude, with little if any of the fine spectral detail needed for phonetic perception and spoken word recognition (Gantz, Tye-Murray, & Tyler, 1989). However, even the addition of subthreshold auditory signals or gross acoustic cues such as duration, amplitude, and fundamental frequency significantly improves speech recognition scores over lipreading alone (e.g., Boothroyd, Hnath-Chisolm, Hanin, & Kishon-Rabin, 1988; Breeuwer & Plomp, 1986; Erber, 1969, 1979).

As CI technology has advanced over the years, so have the speech perception abilities of hearing-impaired listeners who have received CIs (Fryauf-Bertschy, Tyler, Kelsay, & Gantz, 1992; Fryauf-Bertschy et al., 1997; Miyamoto, Kirk, et al., 1997; Miyamoto, Svirsky, & Robbins, 1997; Waltzman et al., 1997). If deaf adults who depend primarily on the visual sensory channel for speech perception are better lipreaders than NH adults, what happens to their lipreading abilities once the auditory channel is restored via a CI after a period of deafness? Does reliance on the primary sensory channel change and reorganize following implantation? It could be that adult CI recipients still depend primarily on visual speech cues and merely supplement this information with the auditory input from the implant. It is also conceivable that postlingually deaf adults have the opportunity to revert back to the auditory channel as their primary input for speech perception, but whether this occurs or not will depend on the nature of the sensory information provided by the CI.

Studies of postlingually deaf adults have assumed that AV integration ability is intact prior to onset of deafness. How did adults acquire this ability in the first place? Are hearing and vision both initially necessary to be able to integrate A and V information? It has been commonly thought that postlingually deaf children and adults without an auditory communication channel must use lipreading as their primary communication channel, but relatively little is actually known about the lipreading skills of prelingually, profoundly deaf children who have never experienced sound or had any exposure to speech or spoken language via the auditory sensory modality prior to receiving a CI.

A number of years ago, Seewald et al. (1985) reported that differential reliance on either audition or vision as the primary modality for speech perception was related to level of hearing impairment in prelingually deaf children. When faced with conflicting auditory and visual information in a speech perception test, children who had higher hearing thresholds were biased toward the visual input, whereas children with lower hearing thresholds were biased toward auditory input. More recent research on prelingually deaf children with CIs has shown that combined AV information in tests of spoken language recognition improves performance over A-alone and V-alone conditions (Geers, 1994; Geers & Brenner, 1994; Geers et al., 2003; Staller, Dowell, Beiter, & Brimacombe, 1991; Tyler, Fryauf-Bertschy, et al., 1997; Tyler, Opie, Fryauf-Bertschy, & Gantz, 1992). But how do profoundly deaf children acquire lipreading skills in the first place when they have received little if any auditory input during the critical period for language development? How do congenitally deaf children recover the articulatory gestures of the talker and use that source of information to recognize words and understand spoken language?

In this chapter, we review recent findings on the AV speech perception skills of deaf adults and children who have received CIs, and provide an interpretation of the results in terms of perceptual learning and the effects of experience on perceptual and linguistic development. Our findings from studies of both postlingually deaf adults and prelingually deaf children offer some new insights into the development of multimodal speech perception after hearing has been restored via a CI. These results also contribute to the current theoretical debate about the nature of the processes underlying AV speech perception.

Audiovisual integration in postlingually deaf adults following cochlear implantation

AV speech perception often provides large benefits to individuals with some degree of hearing impairment, including CI recipients (Erber, 1972, 1975; Tyler, Parkinson, et al., 1997). In everyday activities, listeners with CIs perceive speech in a wide variety of contexts, including television, face-to-face conversation, and over the telephone. Success in recognizing spoken words and understanding the talker's intended message differs substantially under these diverse listening conditions.

To investigate the ability of postlingually deaf adult CI users to integrate the limited auditory information they receive from their implant with visual speech cues during spoken word recognition, Kaiser, Kirk, Lachs, and Pisoni (2003) examined the spoken word recognition skills of two groups of listeners who were tested under three presentation conditions: A-alone, V-alone, and AV. NH adults (mean age, 42 years) and postlingually deaf adult users of CIs (mean age, 50 years) were presented with digitally recorded monosyllabic English words produced by several different male and female talkers. The word lists were balanced across presentation formats (A-alone, V-alone, AV) in terms of lexical competition (lexically easy vs. lexically hard words) and talker variability (single talker vs. multiple talkers). The speech signals were presented via a loudspeaker at 70 dB SPL (C weighted) for participants using CIs. To prevent the NH participants from attaining ceiling performance on the task, they were tested using a -5 dB S/N in speech spectrum noise. All participants were asked to verbally repeat aloud the words that they heard.

Because of the differences in testing procedures for the NH listeners (i.e., speech presented in noise) and CI patients (i.e., speech presented in quiet via a CI) in A-alone and AV presentation formats, it was not appropriate to compare absolute A-alone scores between these two groups of listeners. The nature of the signal degradation resulting from the presentation of speech in noise to NH listeners was not equivalent to the transformation of speech by a CI and then presented as an electrical signal to a hearing-impaired listener's auditory system. Thus, only patterns of performance within each group could be compared.

In both groups of listeners, performance in the AV condition was better than in the A-alone condition, followed by performance in the V-alone condition (Fig. 47.1). When tested under identical presentation conditions for V-alone stimuli, CI users obtained higher scores than their NH counterparts. This finding was not surprising, because the adults with hearing impairment had much more extensive experience than the NH listeners in utilizing visual speech cues to supplement information received through a degraded auditory channel. NH and CI listeners achieved roughly the same level of performance in the AV condition.

CI users made somewhat better use of visual information in more difficult listening conditions compared to NH listeners, such as when there was ambiguity about the talker or when they were forced to make fine phonetic discriminations among acoustically confusable or lexically hard words. Thus, the deaf adults with CIs combined visual information with the available auditory information conveyed by their CI to support open-set word recognition, but they did so in somewhat different ways than the NH listeners, perhaps relying more on visual cues than auditory cues to speech. Taken together, the

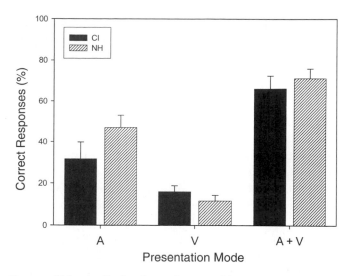

FIGURE 47.1 Audiovisual word recognition: mean percent correct word recognition under auditory-alone (A), visual-alone (V), and audiovisual (AV) presentation conditions in normal-hearing (NH) adults and adults with a cochlear implant (CI). (Data from Kaiser, Kirk, Lachs, & Pisoni, 2003.)

results suggested that reliable information in either sensory modality could compensate for impoverished sensory information in the other modality. Nevertheless, the overall pattern of results across the three presentation conditions was strikingly similar for NH adults and postlingually deaf adults with CIs. This is not surprising, because the adults with CIs in the study of Kaiser et al. (2003) were all postlingually deafened individuals who had acquired language normally prior to the onset of their hearing loss.

The CI users in the study by Kaiser et al. (2003) also varied greatly in terms of age at onset of profound deafness, ranging from 3 years to 65 years. Tillberg et al. (1996) found that hearing-impaired adults with an early onset of deafness were better lipreaders than hearing-impaired adults with a late onset of deafness. To investigate the effects of age at onset of deafness on the word recognition abilities of postlingually deaf adults whose hearing has been restored via a CI, we reanalyzed the data of Kaiser et al. We found a significant negative correlation between age at onset of deafness and V-alone word recognition scores ($r = -0.60$, $p < 0.01$), but no significant correlations between age at onset of deafness and A-alone ($r = -0.30$, Ns) or AV ($r = -0.40$, Ns) word recognition scores. Thus, similar to the results of Tillberg et al. (1996), we found that adults with early-onset deafness and CIs are better lipreaders than adults with late-onset deafness and CIs, whereas age at onset of deafness has no effect on A-alone and AV word recognition abilities.

The adult CI users in the study of Kaiser et al. (2003) were all progressively deafened postlingually. It is possible that, while hearing declines over time, gradual reliance on lipreading eventually leads to greater use of the visual correlates of speech when the auditory information in the speech signal is no longer sufficient to support reliable word recognition. On the other hand, it may be the case that people who sustain the sudden onset of hearing impairment simply do not have as much experience as people with a progressive hearing loss in extracting visual speech cues to compensate for compromised hearing. To investigate the effects of the time course of hearing loss on AV speech perception in postlingually deaf adults following CI, we carried out a retrospective analysis of patient data from the clinical records of the Department of Otolaryngology–Head and Neck Surgery at Indiana University (Bergeson, Pisoni, Reese, & Kirk, 2003).

Adult CI users who were analyzed in this study experienced either a sudden hearing loss ($n = 13$), defined as the onset of a profound hearing loss within 1 month, or a progressive hearing loss ($n = 32$), defined as the gradual onset of a profound hearing loss over a period of time greater than 1 month (mean, 25.0 years; range, 1–45 years). As part of routine clinical testing, these patients were given the City University of New York (CUNY) sentence recognition test (Boothroyd, Hanin, & Hnath, 1985). In this test, the patient is asked to repeat aloud meaningful English sentences presented under three conditions: A-alone, V-alone, and combined AV. The listeners' responses are scored in terms of correctly identified key words in each sentence.

Our analyses revealed that both groups of postlingually deaf adult CI users performed best in the AV condition, followed by the A-alone condition, and worst in the V-alone condition. These findings are similar to the results obtained in postlingually deaf adult CI users by Kaiser et al. (2003). There were no significant differences in performance across the two groups of patients in A-alone and AV conditions. However, adult CI users with progressive hearing loss performed better than those with sudden hearing loss in the V-alone condition. Thus, CI users with a progressive hearing loss appear to be somewhat better lipreaders than those who experienced a sudden hearing loss. These results are most likely due to the fact that adults who lose their hearing over a long period of time are able to gain more experience at extracting visual articulation cues from talkers while their hearing is slowly declining over time. Lipreading appears to be a perceptual skill that is difficult to learn easily in a short period of time in the laboratory (e.g., Berger, 1972; Gesi, Massaro, & Cohen, 1992). Perhaps it is the implicit nature of learning from the gradual reliance on visual speech cues when auditory speech cues are degraded that leads to better lipreading performance in progressively deafened adults. Nevertheless, it is clear from our recent findings that experience and activities with the visual correlates of speech over an extended period of time affect the development of lipreading skills in this population of hearing-impaired listeners (Bernstein et al., 2001).

In summary, postlingually deaf adults with CIs exhibit similar AV speech perception as NH adults. Word recognition performance is best when combined auditory and visual information is available, followed by A-alone information, and then V-alone information. These results are not surprising, given that both NH adults and postlingually deaf adults with CIs have had a period of normal linguistic experience. Moreover, neither group had any central brain damage, so there is no reason to believe that the fundamental AV integration skills are substantially different across groups. Our new retrospective studies also showed that age at onset of deafness and rate of hearing loss influence lipreading abilities, with better lipreading performance in CI adults with early onset of deafness and progressive hearing loss than in adults with a late onset of deafness and sudden hearing loss (Bergeson, Pisoni, Reese, et al., 2003; Kaiser et al., 2003). Thus, experience with language matters for A-alone and AV speech perception, whereas experience of hearing loss over a longer period of time matters for V-alone speech perception, or lipreading.

Audiovisual integration in prelingually deaf children following cochlear implantation

The studies described in the preceding section show that postlingually deaf adults benefit from AV speech information over and above A-alone and V-alone speech cues. That is, they show cross-modal enhancement effects under AV conditions. Is AV integration possible only for those perceivers who have had experience with both auditory and visual cues to speech from birth? Many studies over the years have shown that NH children and even young infants are capable of cross-modal perception (Desjardins, Rogers, & Werker, 1997; Kuhl & Meltzoff, 1982; Lewkowicz, 1992, 2000; Lewkowicz & Kraebel, Chap. 41, this volume; MacKain, Studdert-Kennedy, Spieker, & Stern, 1983; Spelke, 1979, 1981). Moreover, early experience with cross-modal stimuli may be a necessary prerequisite for the development of auditory and visual sensory systems and the integration of common information from each modality (Lewkowicz & Kraebel, Chap. 41, this volume).

It is possible, then, that children who have been deprived of auditory sensory input since birth may not be able to acquire language through normal sensory means, that is, AV speech cues. However, with the con-tinued broadening of candidacy criteria and the numerous technological advances in CI signal processing, more children than ever before have the potential to develop spoken language processing skills using electrical signals provided by CIs. Are prelingually deaf children who receive CIs capable of AV integration? More specifically, after their hearing is restored via a CI, will these children show evidence of AV benefit? How is AV integration influenced by auditory deprivation and early experience?

Previous research investigating auditory skills in deaf children who have received CIs has shown that there are enormous individual differences in pediatric CI outcome measures of speech and language (e.g., Fryauf-Bertschy et al., 1997; Miyamoto et al., 1989; Tyler, Fryauf-Bertschy, et al., 1997). Some children can learn to communicate extremely well using the auditory/oral modality and acquire age-appropriate language skills, whereas other children may display only minimal spoken word recognition skills or show very delayed language abilities (e.g., Robbins, Svirsky, & Kirk, 1997; Tomblin, Spencer, Flock, Tyler, & Gantz, 1999). At the present time, these differences in speech and language outcomes after implantation cannot be predicted very well from measures obtained. before implantation. Instead, they appear to emerge only after electrical stimulation has commenced (see Pisoni, 2000; Pisoni et al., 2000).

Previous research has demonstrated that several key demographic and audiological factors contribute to success with a CI. Numerous studies have shown that children with superior spoken word recognition scores after implantation typically received implants at a very young age (Fryauf-Bertschy et al., 1997; Kirk, Pisoni, & Miyamoto, 2000; Osberger, Todd, Berry, Robbins, & Miyamoto, 1991; Waltzman & Cohen, 1988; Waltzman et al., 1994, 1997). Thus, children with a shorter duration of deafness before implantation are better at recognizing spoken words and understanding spoken language than children with a longer duration of deafness.

It is very likely that duration of deafness also affects AV speech perception skills in children, too. Such effects are inversely related to the length of deafness in postlingually deaf adults. As noted earlier, Tillberg et al. (1996) found that adults with early-onset deafness were better lipreaders than adults with late-onset deafness. It is possible that prelingually deaf children who receive implants at an older age (i.e., experience a longer period of deafness) are better lipreaders than those children who receive implants earlier (i.e., experience a shorter period of deafness). This might be the case because children who receive implants at a later age and who therefore have less experience with auditory sensory input than children who receive implants at an earlier age presumably must rely primarily on visual rather than auditory cues to speech to communicate.

Another source of variability that has been shown to contribute to success and benefit with a CI is the nature of the early sensory and linguistic environment deaf children are immersed in after receiving a CI. Although deaf children with CIs may experience a range of language, from signed to oral-aural, clinicians typically divide deaf children according to one of two predominant communication modes: oral communication (OC), in which children utilize auditory-oral skills and are educated using that approach, and total communication (TC), in which children utilize simultaneous signed and spoken English. Oral communication methods can range from auditory-verbal therapy, in which auditory information is heavily emphasized and lipreading is discouraged (Ling, 1993; Rhoades, 1982), to cued speech, in which specific hand cues are used to supplement lip-read information (Cornett & Daisey, 2000). Similarly, total or simultaneous communication can range from an emphasis on spoken English, to equal emphasis on signed and spoken English (e.g., Signing Exact English; Gustason & Zawolkow, 1993), and finally to an emphasis on manual signs (Geers et al., 1999). Note that even the latter extreme, which places emphasis on manual signs, is still not a completely unimodal manual sign language, such as American Sign Language (ASL).

Previous studies have demonstrated that OC children have significantly better spoken word recognition abilities, on average, than TC children (e.g., Kirk et al., 2000; Miyamoto, Kirk, Svirsky, & Sehgal, 1999; Tobey et al., 2000). Other research has also documented that OC children have better expressive language and speech intelligibility skills than TC children (Cullington, Hodges, Butts, Dolan-Ash, & Balkany, 2000; Hodges, Dolan-Ash, Balkany, Schloffman, & Butts, 1999; Kirk et al., 2000; Svirsky, Robbins, Kirk, Pisoni, & Miyamoto, 2000). Interestingly, TC children who rely more on speech than sign also have better speech perception and speech intelligibility skills than TC children who rely more on sign than speech (Geers, Spehar, & Sedey, 2002). Finally, a recent study has reported longer digit spans and faster speaking rates in OC children (Pisoni & Cleary, 2003). These results suggest that OC children may have larger working memory capacities and more efficient verbal rehearsal processes than TC children (Burkholder & Pisoni, 2003; Pisoni & Cleary, 2003, in press). To date, however, little is known about the extent to which early experience and activity affect the development of AV speech perception skills in young deaf children who receive CIs. In the remainder of this chapter, we report some new findings on these issues and then discuss their theoretical implications.

Early investigations of the AV speech perception skills of children showed that visual lipreading information improved speech perception performance over A-alone conditions in deaf and NH children (Erber, 1972, 1975). How do prelingually deaf children with CIs use both auditory and visual sources of information about speech? Some preliminary findings have shown that children with CIs do experience a gain in performance and display enhancement effects from the combined AV inputs relative to A-alone or V-alone input (Bergeson, Pisoni, & Davis, 2003a; Geers, 1994; Geers & Brenner, 1994; Geers et al., 2003; Geers & Moog, 1992; Tyler, Fryauf-Bertschy, et al., 1997; Tyler et al., 1992). Tyler, Fryauf-Bertschy, et al. (1997) also reported that children with implants showed improvement in lipreading ability over time. As the children accumulated experience with the implant, their lipreading skills in perceiving speech via vision alone also improved. Finally, Geers and Moog (1992) found that 16- to 17-year-old OC students had better V-alone and AV sentence comprehension scores than TC students. These results suggest that, aside from providing access to the auditory sensory modality, a CI also allows the child to develop more fully specified phonetic and phonological representations of the articulatory form of speech, especially if that child is in an OC environment. Moreover, access to sound and the auditory sense provided by a CI could affect general information processing skills, such as attention, perceptual learning, and memory, needed for coding speech and creating permanent phonological and lexical representations of words in long-term memory (Pisoni & Cleary, in press).

In a recent study, Lachs, Pisoni, and Kirk (2001) directly examined the relationship between A-alone measures of spoken language processing and the use of AV information in prelingually deafened hearing-impaired children who had used their CIs for a period of two years. The Common Phrases (CP) test (Robbins, Renshaw, & Osberger, 1995) was administered to 27 prelingually deaf children with CIs under three presentation conditions: A-alone, V-alone, and AV. The CP test is an open-set clinical measure of sentence comprehension that is used frequently with deaf children to assess their ability to understand phrases used in everyday situations. To minimize the visual differences between mouthed-only sentences and spoken sentences in the V condition, the children were often asked to turn off their CIs while the clinician presented the sentences aloud. Examples of sentences included in the CP test and typical responses are shown in Table 47.1. The CP test is routinely administered live-voice with ten trials in each condition, chosen from a total of six different

TABLE 47.1
Examples of phrases and correct responses in the Common Phrases Test

Phrase	Correct Responses
1. When is your birthday?	"When is your birthday?" "July."
2. What color are your eyes?	"What color are your eyes?" "Brown."
3. Clap your hands.	"Clap your hands." Child follows direction by clapping hands.
4. What time is it?	"What time is it?" "It's three o'clock."

sentence lists. Performance in each condition was scored as the percentage of phrases correctly repeated in their entirety, questions correctly answered, or directions correctly followed by the child.

As shown in Figure 47.2, Lachs et al. (2001) found that prelingually deaf children with CIs performed better on AV than on either the A-alone or V-alone conditions of the CP test. This pattern is quite similar to previous results observed with postlingually deaf adults with CIs (Dowell et al., 1982; Kaiser et al., 2003). However, there was no difference between performance in the A-alone and V-alone conditions. This pattern is different from the results observed with postlingually deaf adult CI users, who performed better in A-alone than V-alone conditions (Bergeson, Pisoni, Reese, et al., 2003; Kaiser et al., 2003). Thus, there was no overall tendency for these children to rely more on

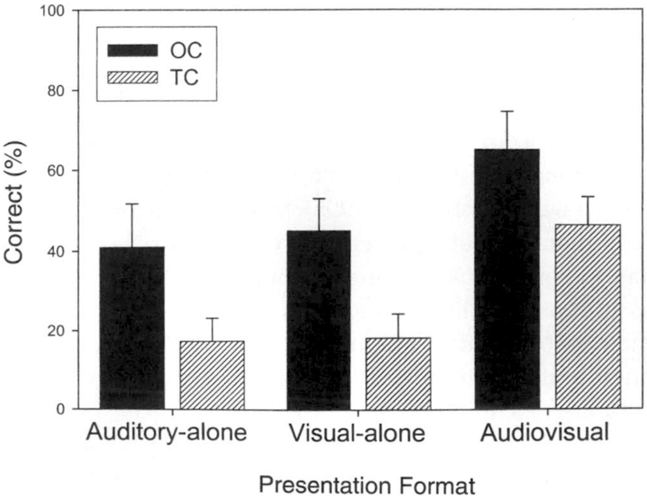

FIGURE 47.2 Common phrase recognition: mean percent of phrases correctly repeated or answered as a function of presentation condition and communication mode 2 years after implantation of a cochlear device. (Adapted from Lachs, Pisoni, & Kirk, 2001.)

one input modality than the other. However, when Lachs et al. examined the scores for individual children, it became clear that some children tended to rely on one sensory modality more often than the other. In addition, the children in the study of Lachs et al. exhibited a wide range of variability in combining multisensory inputs, which is a typical result frequently reported in the CI literature.

Overall, the Lachs et al. (2001) results show that prelingually deaf children who use CIs also show enhancement and benefit when speech is presented in an AV format compared to A-alone and V-alone formats. Interestingly, for most of the children, AV performance did not exceed the scores predicted by the simple sum of performance in the unimodal conditions. That is, there did not appear to be a superadditive effect of AV integration in perceiving highly familiar test sentences in these children. This pattern of results with CI children differs from what would be expected based on the published literature for NH adults, in which AV performance routinely exceeded the sum of A-alone and V-alone performance (Grant et al., 1998; Massaro & Cohen, 1999; Sumby & Pollack, 1954).

More interestingly, however, Lachs et al. (2001) carried out a series of other analyses and found that the skills in deriving benefit from AV sensory input were not isolated or independent but were closely related to A-alone spoken word recognition and speech production abilities, which make use of a common set of underlying phonological processing abilities. These processing abilities involve decomposition of the sensory input into a structural description consisting of sequences of phonemes and then the reassembly of these segments into a highly organized sequence of gestures for use in speech production and articulation.

Lachs et al. (2001) examined the relative gains in AV speech perception that result from the additional visual information to the A-alone condition (visual gain = $(AV - A)/(100 - A)$) and the additional auditory

TABLE 47.2
Characteristics of participants

Communication Mode	Age at Implantation (mo)	Unaided PTA (dB HL)	Aided PTA (CI) (dB HL)	Number of Electrodes
Oral communication (n = 39)	51 (17–106)	112 (98–121) (n = 32)	33 (22–40) (n = 37)	19.53 (8–22)
Total communication (n = 41)	59 (22–106)	115 (106–122) (n = 35)	35 (21–58) (n = 38)	20.53 (8–22)

Note: Values in table are means (range).

information compared to the V-alone condition (auditory gain = $(AV - V)/(100 - V)$). The children who derived more gain from the combined sensory inputs were also better performers on the Lexical Neighborhood Test (Kirk, Eisenberg, Martinez, & Hay-McCutcheon, 1999; Kirk, Pisoni, & Osberger, 1995), an A-alone measure of open-set spoken word recognition (visual gain $r = +0.90$; auditory gain $r = +0.78$). Moreover, the children who derived more AV benefit also produced more intelligible speech on an independent test that assessed speech production skills of these children (visual gain $r = +0.42$; auditory gain $r = +0.54$). Finally, Lachs et al. (2001) also found that visual gain was a better predictor of speech intelligibility for OC children ($r = +0.46$) than TC children ($r = -0.19$). These correlations demonstrate a relation between early sensory experience and language processing activities and the ability to integrate auditory and visual sources of information about speech.

The recent study by Lachs et al. (2001) showed two important findings in this clinical population: first, strong relations between AV integration and speech and spoken language outcomes, and second, large effects of communication mode on AV integration. We believe these results are theoretically important because they show that AV speech perception skills are not just isolated or autonomous perceptual skills but are correlated with other components of speech and language. The cross-sectional results reported by Lachs et al. (2001) are informative, but it is also important to look at change over time to investigate the development of AV integration skills in this clinical population. It is here that we can begin to see the effects of early experience and study the time course of perceptual learning and development both before and after cochlear implantation, when hearing is introduced for the first time. To do this, we investigated the speech perception skills of 80 prelingually deaf children with CIs longitudinally, from before implantation to 5 years after implantation

(see Bergeson, Pisoni, & Davis, 2003). Children were tested once every 6 months for the first 3 years of CI use, and then once every year thereafter; not all children were tested at each test interval over the 5-year period. Table 47.2 provides a summary of the demographics of these children. The CP test was administered live-voice under three presentation conditions: A-alone, V-alone, and combined AV.

A summary of the results obtained by Bergeson, Pisoni, and Davis (2003b) is shown in Figure 47.3. Table 47.3 shows the number of participants tested at each interval. Overall, the results of the longitudinal analysis revealed that prelingually deaf children with CIs performed better in the AV condition than in the A-alone and V-alone conditions. As expected, performance improved over time after cochlear implantation, regardless of communication mode and presentation format. Nevertheless, children's performance increased at a greater rate over time following cochlear implantation in A-alone and AV conditions than in the V-alone condition.

Bergeson, Pisoni, and Davis (2003b) also found a strong effect of early experience and communication mode on children's comprehension performance. OC children performed consistently better than TC children under all presentation conditions both prior to implantation and across the 5 years following implantation. It is interesting that the difference between OC and TC children's test scores is quite large before implantation in the V-alone condition. Moreover, OC children's test scores gradually increased over time, whereas TC children's scores were initially much lower before implantation and then increased sharply across time. After 5 years of implant experience, the TC children tended to catch up to the performance levels of the OC children.

We believe these new AV speech perception results are theoretically and clinically important. Our findings demonstrate selective effects of early experience and processing activities on performance in all three

TABLE 47.3

TABLE 47.3
Number of participants at each testing interval

Condition, Modality	Implant Use (yr)					
	0	1	2	3	4	5
Auditory-alone						
OC	9	16	19	24	19	11
TC	14	17	24	27	25	14
Visual-alone						
OC	6	14	16	22	17	10
TC	14	19	25	26	24	11
Audiovisual						
OC	8	17	16	22	17	10
TC	14	19	25	26	24	11

Note: Modality: OC, oral communication; TC, total communication.

presentation formats of the CP test. The results of the Bergeson, Pisoni, and Davis (2003b) study reveal that the visual input about speech and speech articulation that OC children receive even prior to cochlear implantation actually improves their sensitivity and attention to both auditory and visual cues to speech. The coupled and complementary cross-modal inputs about speech from both vision and sound may serve to focus attention on the distinctive properties of language, such as the linguistically significant gestures and differences between words. OC children may have more experience focusing attention on combined auditory and visual articulation information even before they receive CIs than do TC children, who must share and divide their limited visual attention between the talker's face and hands (Pisoni & Cleary, 2003, in press).

It has been suggested that prelingually deaf children with CIs follow the same biologically based language development schedule as NH children once their hearing is restored (e.g., Lenneberg, 1967; Pinker, 1994; Pisoni et al., 2000). However, the results of the Bergeson, Pisoni, and Davis (2003b) study demonstrate that novel sensory interactions and perceptual learning begin to emerge even prior to implantation in OC children. That is, the time course of spoken language development may be more delayed for TC children than OC children, especially when compared with NH children who display typical cross-modal speech perception skills. Our results are also important because of the clinical implications for achieving optimal benefit or outcome in prelingually deaf children with CIs. OC children receive more robust sensory information specifying the linguistically significant contrasts between words and also produce more intelligible speech contrasts than TC children (e.g., Tobey et al., 2000), who may develop underspecified phonological representations of spoken words.

Another important factor that emerged from our analysis of the CP test was the effect of duration of deafness before receiving a CI. When scores on the CP test were averaged over all 5 years, we found that children who received CIs at a younger age (i.e., those who had a shorter period of deafness) performed much better than children who received implants later in life (i.e., had a longer period of deafness; Fig. 47.4). We expected this finding, insofar as large effects of age at implantation are consistently reported in the literature (Fryauf-Bertschy et al., 1997; Kirk et al., 2000; Osberger et al., 1991; Waltzman et al., 1994, 1997). However, although children who received implants at an earlier age performed better than children who received implants at a later age in both the A-alone and AV presentation conditions, we also found that children who received implants at an earlier age performed worse than children who received implants at a later age in the V-alone presentation condition. Thus, children who were profoundly deaf for longer periods of time before implantation actually turned out to be better lipreaders than children who were profoundly deaf for shorter periods of time. This is a novel finding with prelingually deaf children that replicates the earlier research findings reported by Tillberg et al. (1996), who found that adults with early-onset deafness performed more accurately on V-alone word and sentence recognition tests than adults with late-onset deafness.

CORRELATIONS OF COMMON PHRASES WITH OUTCOME MEASURES OF SPEECH AND LANGUAGE   The findings obtained in the recent study by Bergeson, Pisoni, and Davis (2003b) on cross-modal speech perception in prelingually deaf children following cochlear implantation can stand on their own as an independent contribution of new knowledge demonstrating the effects of early

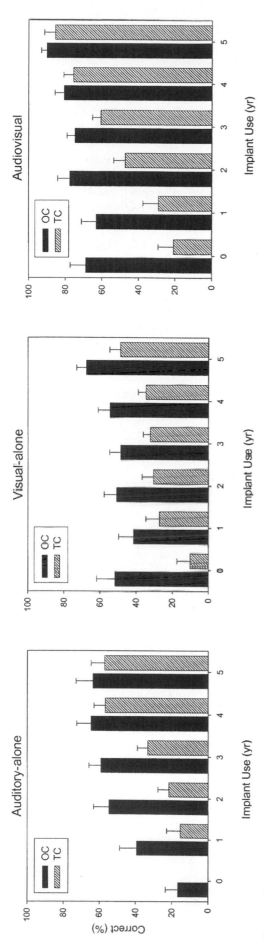

FIGURE 47.3   Mean percent correct sentence comprehension over time on the Common Phrases Test under auditory-alone, visual-alone, and audiovisual conditions for oral communication (OC) and total communication (TC) children. Error bars represent SE. (From Bergeson, Pisoni, & Davis, 2003.)

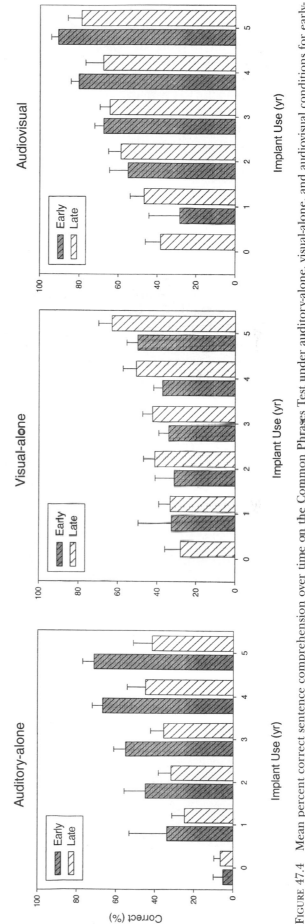

FIGURE 47.4   Mean percent correct sentence comprehension over time on the Common Phrases Test under auditory-alone, visual-alone, and audiovisual conditions for early-implanted (Early) and late-implanted (Late) children. Error bars represent SE. (From Bergeson, Pisoni, & Davis, 2003b.)

sensory experience on speech perception and spoken language processing. However, because the CP data used in this study were collected as part of a larger longitudinal project at the Indiana University School of Medicine dealing with the speech and language skills of deaf children who use CIs, we had a unique opportunity to look beyond the AV scores from this particular study to explore the relations between cross-modal speech perception measures and several other aspects of speech and language development in these children.

What do the AV speech perception scores tell us about the development of speech and spoken language processing skills in this unique population? Are the measures of cross-modal speech perception obtained from the CP test related to other outcome measures of speech perception, speech production, and language processing? Two different sets of correlations were carried out to gain some broader perspective on the clinical significance of these results.

First, we looked at the intercorrelations between scores on the CP test and a small, representative set of outcome measures of speech and language obtained 3 years after implantation to assess the validity of cross-modal speech perception measures. The *Phonetically Balanced–Kindergarten Test* (PBK; Haskins, 1949) is a live-voice, open-set test used to assess A-alone speech perception. The *Peabody Picture Vocabulary Test* (PPVT; Dunn & Dunn, 1997) is a closed-set test used to assess

receptive vocabulary knowledge. The *Reynell Developmental Language Scales 3rd Edition* (RDLS-III; Edwards et al., 1997; Reynell & Huntley, 1985) is a test used to assess children's receptive and expressive language skills. The PPVT and RDLS-III are administered using the child's preferred mode of communication, either spoken English or Signing Exact English, which is simultaneously signed and spoken English. Finally, the *Beginner's Intelligibility Test* (BIT; Osberger, Robbins, Todd, Riley & Miyamoto, 1994) is a test used to assess the intelligibility of children's speech productions.

We found strong and positive correlations of the CP scores with independent measures of spoken word recognition, receptive vocabulary development, expressive and receptive language, and speech intelligibility (Table 47.4). The strongest correlations observed with these outcome measures, with the exception of the PPVT test, were found with the A-alone and AV scores on the CP test. Also, the correlations of the CP test with these five outcome measures were consistently much stronger for the OC children than the TC children, although both groups showed similar overall patterns.

The strong intercorrelations observed 3 years after implantation suggest that the measures of cross-modal speech perception obtained using the CP test share a common source of variance with other behavioral tests that are routinely used to measure speech and language skills in this clinical population. The pattern of

TABLE 47.4

Correlations for Common Phrases and outcome measures 3 years after implantation

Test, Correlation	Oral Communication			Total Communication		
	A	V	AV	A	V	AV
PBK—words						
r	0.635**	0.313	0.559**	0.561**	−0.234	0.388
N	24	21	22	25	25	24
PBK—phonemes						
r	0.657**	−0.062	0.471*	0.705**	−0.250	0.197
N	24	21	22	25	25	24
PPVT						
r	0.422*	0.628**	0.577**	−0.009	0.484*	0.310
N	23	20	21	25	25	24
RDLS-III Expressive						
r	0.704**	0.572*	0.789**	0.214	0.454*	0.500*
N	13	14	13	20	20	20
RDLS-III Receptive						
r	0.688**	0.385	0.815**	0.018	0.332	0.406
N	14	14	12	20	21	20
BIT						
r	0.734**	0.557*	0.734**	0.611**	0.038	0.526*
N	16	15	16	17	18	17

*$P < 0.05$, **$P < 0.01$.

correlations is revealing because it indicates that the basic underlying sensory, cognitive, and linguistic processes used to carry out cross-modal speech perception are also accessed and used in other behavioral speech perception and language tests that are used to measure open-set word recognition, receptive vocabulary development, expressive and receptive language, and speech production. Thus, the three scores on the CP test are not measuring some isolated and independent set of perceptual skills that are highly task-specific and do not generalize beyond the specific experimental paradigm. The behavioral tests included in Bergeson, Pisoni, and Davis (2003b) to measure audiological outcomes, such as open-set word recognition, sentence comprehension, and speech production, all involve rapid phonological encoding of sequential patterns and then reproduction or imitation of presented items. Thus, higher-level cognitive processes such as perception, attention, learning, and memory, as well as phonological and lexical coding and language, play an important role in these outcome measures (see Pisoni et al., 2000).

In addition to the intercorrelations with these outcome measures after 3 years of implant use, we also carried out a set of correlations between the preimplantation CP V-alone and AV scores and the same set of speech and language outcome measures after 3 years of implant use. This analysis was done to determine whether we could identify early predictors of speech and language outcome from behavioral measures of cross-modal speech perception obtained before the time of implantation. In order to obtain an adequate sample size for this analysis, the correlations were carried out by combining the scores for both OC and TC children. As shown in Table 47.5, all of the correlations were strong, positive, and significant. Interestingly, in all cases the V-alone CP pre-implantation measure was the strongest predictor of speech and language outcomes after 3 years of CI use.

These findings suggest that preimplantation lipreading and cross-modal speech perception scores can be used to predict open-set word recognition and speech intelligibility after several years of implant use. Measures of cross-modal speech perception may provide reliable behavioral markers that can be used to predict and identify the children who will obtain the most benefit from their CIs at an early point following implantation. Although the preimplantation correlations are based on small samples, the results of Bergeson, Pisoni, and Davis (2003b) suggest that measures of AV speech perception obtained before implantation may reveal fundamental perceptual and cognitive processes that are used to recover the linguistically significant gestures of the speaker that encode and represent distinc-

TABLE 47.5

Correlations for preimplant Common Phrases and 3 years postimplant outcome measures

Test, Correlation	V	AV
PBK—words		
r	0.906**	0.724**
N	10	17
PBK—phonemes		
r	0.814**	0.760**
N	10	17
PPVT		
r	0.704*	0.679**
N	9	16
BIT		
r	0.883*	0.839**
N	6	11

$*P < 0.05, **P < 0.01.$
Note: V, visual-alone; AV, audiovisual.

tive phonological contrasts in the sound system of the target language in the child's environment.

We know of only two previous studies that have attempted to identify preimplantation predictors of success with CIs. Knutson et al. (1991) presented a series of digits at a rate of one every 2 s and asked postlingually deaf adults to respond when the digits reflected a pattern of even-odd-even numbers. They found that preimplantation performance on the visual monitoring task predicted audiological outcome after 18 months of implant use. Knutson et al. (1991) concluded that the cognitive processing operations and skills needed to rapidly extract information from sequentially arrayed visual stimuli may also be used in processing complex auditory signals, and may underlie the successful use of a CI. In a more recent study of prelingually deaf children with CIs, Tait, Lutman, and Robinson (2000) found that preverbal communicative or autonomy behaviors (i.e., turn-taking behaviors that cannot be predicted from a conversational partner's preceding turn) that are present before implantation are associated with speech perception and language comprehension 3 years after implantation. Given the relative lack of reliable preimplantation predictors of success with a CI, the present findings are important, because AV integration may be the type of outcome measure that should be used to assess performance in prelingually deaf children who receive CIs. Such underlying preverbal communication skills may function as the "prerequisites" for speech and language and may reflect cross-modal interactions between perception and action that are not tied to a specific sensory modality.

Discussion

The studies reviewed in this chapter have shown that postlingually deaf adults who use CIs process AV speech in ways that are fundamentally quite similar to NH adults (Kaiser et al., 2003). Performance is best in the AV condition, followed by the A-alone condition and then the V-alone condition. Moreover, postlingually deaf adults with CIs who experienced an early onset of deafness or a progressive hearing loss were found to be better lipreaders than adults who experienced a late onset of deafness or a sudden hearing loss (Bergeson, Pisoni, Reese, et al., 2003; Kaiser et al., 2003).

Lachs et al. (2001) also documented a similar pattern of results in a cross-sectional study of prelingually deaf children 2 years after cochlear implantation. They found that these children comprehended common sentences better when the sentences were presented in an AV format than when the sentences were presented in an A-alone or V-alone format. Furthermore, OC children tended to score higher on the CP test, as well as on other outcome measures of spoken word recognition and speech intelligibility, than TC children did. Finally, the results of Lachs et al. (2001) showed that children who received more AV benefit in the CP test also produced more intelligible speech, suggesting a common underlying linguistic basis for speech perception and speech production that involves the construction of a discrete phonological representation from cues encoded from the initial acoustic signal. It is assumed that phonological representations such as these are used in both speech perception and production (Abler, 1989; Studdert-Kennedy, 1998).

Finally, several consistent patterns of performance emerged from the recent analysis of the longitudinal data carried out by Bergeson, Pisoni, and Davis (2003b) on a large group of prelingually deaf children with the CP test over a period of 5 years following cochlear implantation. We found that these children performed better under AV conditions compared to A-alone and V-alone conditions. Moreover, performance in the A-alone and AV conditions improved more rapidly over time following cochlear implantation compared to performance in the V-alone condition. OC children displayed consistently higher scores in the CP test than TC children in all three presentation conditions, even prior to implantation. Also, children who received implants at an earlier age performed much better than children who received implants at a later age in the A-alone and AV conditions, whereas children who received implants at a later age performed better than those who received implants at an earlier age in the V-alone condition. Finally, Bergeson, Pisoni, and Davis (2003b) found that AV sen-

tence comprehension skills in the CP test were strongly correlated with several clinical outcome measures of speech perception, speech intelligibility, and language skills. Preimplantation performance on the CP test was also strongly correlated with 3-year postimplantation performance on clinical outcome measures of speech perception, speech intelligibility, and language skills.

SOME EFFECTS OF DURATION OF DEAFNESS ON AUDIOVISUAL SPEECH PERCEPTION Our reanalysis of the data of Kaiser et al. (2003) revealed an interesting dissociation in postlingually deaf adult CI users' reliance on auditory and visual information on a word recognition task. Adults with early-onset deafness and CIs were better lipreaders than adults with late-onset deafness and CIs, whereas duration of deafness had no effect on A-alone and AV word recognition abilities. These results replicate the earlier findings of Tillberg et al. (1996), who found more accurate lipreading performance for adults with early-onset deafness than late-onset deafness, but no differences in performance between the two groups in A-alone and AV conditions. It is likely that adults with early-onset hearing loss have much more lipreading expe- rience than adults with late-onset hearing loss and thus depend more on visual than on auditory cues to speech.

In addition to documenting changes in performance on the three versions of the CP test after implantation, Bergeson, Pisoni, and Davis (2003b) also uncovered several other developmental findings that were related to the duration of deafness before implantation. As noted earlier, age at implantation is related to duration of deafness prior to implantation. Thus, the children who received their implants at older ages were deprived of sound for longer periods of time than the children who received their implants at younger ages. Two closely related findings emerged from our analyses of the effects of age at implantation, suggesting a close coupling and complementary relationship of the auditory and visual sensory inputs used in speech perception. First, we found that as age at implantation increased, performance on the A and AV conditions declined. This result is not surprising, and it replicates earlier findings reported consistently in the literature on pediatric cochlear implantation (Fryauf-Bertschy et al., 1997; Kirk et al., 2000; Osberger et al., 1991; Waltzman et al., 1994, 1997). As the duration of deafness before implantation increases, performance on a wide range of auditory-based outcome measures declines. These results are part of the motivation to provide deaf children with CIs as early as possible before the neural populations decline from lack of auditory input and stimulation (e.g., Neville & Bruer, 2001; Teoh, Pisoni, & Miyamoto, in press a, in press b).

Second, we found a reversal of this pattern when we examined the lipreading skills in the V condition. As age at implantation increased, scores on the V-alone presentation conditions improved, demonstrating a double dissociation between auditory and visual inputs as a function of early sensory experience. Thus, early experience and processing activities with spoken language before implantation affects auditory and visual modalities selectively in different ways. The consequences of early visual sensory experiences in the absence of sound and hearing can been seen over time after hearing is introduced with a CI. The lipreading results observed in this population of children are consistent with other reports in the literature on the lipreading and visual speech perception skills of congenitally deaf individuals who use oral language as their primary means of communication (e.g., Bernstein et al., 2000). Individuals with congenital deafness who acquire and use oral language at an early age often have excellent lipreading skills that they have slowly acquired over a very long period of time from visual input about speech articulation that they are exposed to in their language-learning environment.

The earlier studies of the lipreading skills of deaf children with CIs never investigated the changes in performance over time after implantation or assessed the effects of age at implantation on performance (Geers, 1994; Geers & Brenner, 1994; Geers & Moog, 1992; Geers et al., 2003; Staller et al, 1991; Tyler, Fryauf-Bertschy, et al., 1997; Tyler et al., 1992). The developmental findings of Bergeson, Pisoni, and Davis (2003b) demonstrate a trade-off between auditory and visual cues to speech as a function of early experience and activities both before and after implantation. These results suggest that the differential reliance on auditory and visual cues to speech may not be rigidly fixed and may change significantly over time as hearing either declines due to the onset of deafness or improves after the restoration of hearing with a hearing aid or CI.

Duration of deafness prior to cochlear implantation is an extremely important demographic factor because a period of auditory deprivation at an early age may result in significant cortical reorganization in the central auditory system. Early cochlear implantation in children may lead to restoration of auditory abilities due to neural plasticity. However, neural plasticity and the potential for neural reorganization after implantation may occur only during critical or sensitive periods of development (e.g., up to 6 years of age) (Beggs & Foreman, 1980; Bruer, 2001; Moore, 2002; Neville & Bruer, 2001; Robinson, 1998; Shepherd & Hardie, 2001; Shepherd et al., 1997; Teoh et al., 2003; Wolff & Thatcher, 1990). Ponton and colleagues have found very different patterns of cortical auditory evoked potentials in NH

children and early-implanted, prelingually deaf children with CIs compared to prelingually deaf CI users who received implants much later in life, and they concluded that the underlying cortical plasticity ends at 12 years of age (Eggermont, Ponton, Don, Waring, & Kwong, 1997; Ponton, Don, Eggermont, Waring, & Masuda, 1996; Ponton & Eggermont, 2001). In a recent study of cortical response latencies to speech in congenitally deaf children and adults with CIs, Sharma, Dorman, & Spahr (2002) found maximal plasticity in a sensitive period lasting up to $3\frac{1}{2}$ years of age, with plasticity remaining in some children even up to 7 years of age (see also Gordon, Papsin, & Harrison, 2003).

EFFECTS OF EARLY EXPERIENCE AFTER IMPLANTATION
How does the early sensory and linguistic experience in the language-learning environment affect a deaf child's information processing skills after receiving a CI? This is an important fundamental question about perceptual learning, memory, and the effects of early experience that can be addressed directly by several of the findings obtained in our research on AV speech perception in deaf children with CIs. Although it has been well documented that a child's communication mode plays an important role in the development of speech and oral language skills following implantation, there has been little if any discussion of the underlying sensory and cognitive mechanisms that are responsible for these differences in performance. Numerous studies have reported that deaf children immersed in OC programs do much better on a range of oral language tasks than deaf children who are in TC programs. Tests assessing speech feature discrimination, comprehension, spoken word recognition, receptive and expressive language, and speech intelligibility all consistently show that deaf children in OC programs do much better than deaf children in TC programs. Why does this difference occur and what factors are responsible for the better performance of OC children?

We found a similar pattern of results in our own AV speech perception studies. Prelingually deaf children who received CIs performed better on the CP test regardless of presentation format if they were immersed in OC programs compared to deaf children who were enrolled in TC programs (Bergeson, Pisoni, & Davis, 2003b; Lachs et al., 2001) (see Figs. 47.2 and 47.3). Moreover, Bergeson, Pisoni, and Davis (2003b) found that the advantage for OC children was present even prior to implantation, which demonstrates the importance of early experience on sentence comprehension performance. Finally, deaf children who received implants at younger ages exhibited better sentence comprehension skills when the sentences were presented in

A-alone and AV formats, whereas children who received implants at a later age displayed better performance when the sentences were presented in the V-alone format (Bergeson, Pisoni, & Davis, 2003b), again revealing the differential effects of early experience and processing activities on AV speech perception capacities.

Why do the children who are placed in TC environments do worse on a wide range of outcome measures than children in OC environments? Several factors may be responsible for the differences in performance between these two groups of children. Understanding these differences may provide some important new insights into how the child's early sensory experience and processing activities affect the development of phonological coding skills that are used on a range of behavioral tasks. It is important to note here that deaf children are not randomly assigned to OC and TC education methods. Parents enroll their deaf children into one of these two educational approaches when they first discover their children's deafness, prior to cochlear implantation (Yoshinaga-Itano, 2000). Moreover, the CI children we studied generally did not change education methods over time, so it cannot be argued that OC children perform better than TC children because all children who are less successful with CIs switch to a TC education method and vice versa.

The most striking difference between children in OC and TC environments is that children in TC environments typically use simultaneous communication methods. Speech is routinely combined with some form of manual communication such as Signing Exact English. One consequence of using simultaneous communication is that the rate of articulation and information transfer may be much slower than using speech alone without the production of any manual signs. Slower presentation rates of speech and spoken language may affect the speed and efficiency of verbal rehearsal processes of working memory and may reduce processing capacity in language comprehension and production tasks (Carpenter, Miyake, & Just, 1994).

Another reason for the poorer performance of TC children may be due to the competition between speech and manual communication for controlled attention and limited processing resources in working memory, both of which are assumed to play major roles in language comprehension and spoken word recognition (Baddeley, Gathercole, & Papagno, 1998). Under simultaneous communication methods, speech and sign do not specify the same gestures and common underlying articulatory events of the talker. Information from the two sensory channels cannot be integrated quickly in the same way as it is when a listener simultaneously sees the talker's lips and hears speech under cross-modal, AV presentation conditions. Moreover, because the child is looking at the talker's hands rather than his or her face, reliable lipreading cues may not be readily available to provide additional complementary phonetic information about the speech signal that is coded in the visual display of the talker's face. Thus, little facilitation or enhancement can be gained from the manual visual input; if anything, substantial competition and even inhibition effects resulting from two divergent input signals may occur (see Doherty-Sneddon, Bonner, & Bruce, 2001).

It is also important to emphasize strongly here that almost all deaf children who receive CIs have hearing parents who often do not have a good working knowledge of sign language and manual communication methods. One consequence of this is that the language samples that deaf children in TC environments are exposed to are very likely to reflect an incomplete or impoverished model of language (Moeller & Luetke-Stahlman, 1990; Swisher & Thompson, 1985). Thus, the child not only gets exposed to poor instances of manual signs, but at the same time he or she receives degraded and impoverished auditory signals via the CI. Thus, input from neither sensory modality is sufficient for optimal language acquisition.

Finally, it is also possible, and perhaps very likely, that these differences in early linguistic experience after implantation between the TC and OC children may produce different effects on the initial encoding of speech signals into phonetic representations and subsequent verbal rehearsal processes used to maintain phonological representations in short-term memory. Because TC children have less extensive exposure to speech and spoken language than OC children in their language-learning environment after implantation and are not explicitly forced to engage frequently in linguistically meaningful activities such as talking and answering questions on the fly, they may actually have two separate problems in processing phonological information. The first problem concerns the initial encoding and perception of linguistically significant patterns. The competing auditory and visual (i.e., manual) input may limit TC children's exposure to speech, which in turn may affect the development of automatic attention strategies and the speed with which spoken language can be rapidly identified and recoded into stable and robust phonological representations in working memory. Thus, as a result of early differences in perception, TC children may have difficulty in scanning and retrieving verbal information rapidly in short-term memory (e.g., Burkholder & Pisoni, 2003).

The second problem deals with verbal rehearsal processes used to maintain phonological representations in working memory for use on a wide range of behavioral tasks, such as open-set word recognition, vocabulary and language comprehension, and speech intelligibility. In addition to problems with scanning and retrieving information in short-term memory, TC children may also have slower and less efficient verbal rehearsal processes once phonological and lexical information actually gets into working memory simply because they have had less experience and processing activities in producing in spoken language (Pisoni & Cleary, 2003).

Passive exposure to spoken language without explicit analysis and conscious manipulation of the auditory patterns and internal phonological structure may not be sufficient to develop stable and robust lexical representations of spoken words and high levels of verbal fluency needed to control speech production. Like NH children, deaf children who receive CIs may need to be actively engaged in processing spoken language in order to develop automaticity and automatic attention strategies that can be carried out rapidly without conscious effort or increased demands on their limited processing resources. This may be one important direct benefit of oral-only educational programs. The excellent expressive language skills displayed by deaf children in aural-oral programs may simply reflect the development of highly automatized phonological analysis skills which permit the child to engage in active processing strategies in perception that initially involve decomposition of a novel speech pattern into a sequence of discrete phonological units and then the reassembly of those individual components into a highly organized and precise coordinated sequence of gestures for use in speech production and articulation. These types of phonological analysis skills are all used in word recognition, sentence comprehension, speech intelligibility, and nonword repetition tasks that require imitation and reproduction of sound patterns.

Highly automatized phonological coding skills of this kind involving perceptually guided action patterns in speech production may result in increases in the speed and efficiency of rapidly constructing phonological representations of spoken words in working memory. Recovering the internal structure of a sensory pattern in speech perception tasks and then rapidly reconstructing the same motor pattern in speech production tasks may function to establish permanent links between speech perception and production and may lead to further development of highly efficient sensorimotor articulatory programs that are routinely used for verbal rehearsal and maintenance of detailed phonological patterns in working memory. Thus, highly automatized phonological processing skills may simply be a byproduct of the primary focus on speech and oral language

activities that are strongly emphasized in oral-only educational environments. These differences in the early experiences and activities of OC children may account for why OC children consistently display better scores on a wide range of outcome measures of speech and language, especially outcome measures that require repetition of phonological patterns in open-set tasks, such as tests of word recognition (PBK), sentence comprehension (CP test), and speech intelligibility (BIT).

AUDIOVISUAL PROPERTIES OF SPEECH AND SPOKEN LANGUAGE Taken together, the results of the studies presented in this chapter on deaf adults and children suggest that although traditional end-point behavioral measures of AV speech perception appear to reflect the use of equivalent sources of sensory information in speech obtained from separate auditory and visual domains, such behavioral equivalence does not necessarily preclude modality specificity at the neural level. This appears to be the case for both postlingually deaf adults and prelingually deaf children who receive CIs to restore their hearing after a period of profound deafness. Because normal intersensory integration follows a developmental sequence (e.g., Gogate, Walker-Andrews, & Bahrick, 2001; Lewkowicz, 2002) involving experience- and activity-dependent neural processes, it is remarkable that even children who were congenitally deaf, and therefore deprived of auditory sensory input since birth, are capable of learning to integrate the auditory and visual attributes of speech in such a way that leads to AV enhancement effects similar to those observed in NH adults, NH children, and postlingually deaf adults with CIs. In general, although the results of the present studies reveal large differences in outcome after cochlear implantation, many adults and children can and do make optimal use of AV information in speech to understand spoken language.

In a recent paper, Grant et al. (1998) proposed that AV enhancement in hearing-impaired adults may depend on one's lipreading skills, with highly successful lipreaders exhibiting larger AV benefit than poor lipreaders. It is possible that these exceptionally good lipreaders are more sensitive to the underlying kinematics common to both auditory and visual speech patterns. In fact, several studies have shown that NH adults display benefits under highly degraded A-alone conditions when auditory input (e.g., words, sentences) is paired with point light displays (PLDs) of speech, which isolate the kinematic properties of a speaker's face (Lachs, 2002; Rosenblum, Johnson, & Saldaña, 1996; Rosenblum & Saldaña, 1996). More recently, we have investigated AV word recognition using PLDs of speech in a small group of postlingually deaf adults with CIs and found similar AV enhancement effects (Bergeson, Pisoni, Lachs, & Reese, 2003). The adult CI users in our study displayed sensitivity to the kinematic properties in speech represented by the dynamic changes in PLDs of speech, and they were able to use kinematics to improve their AV word recognition performance compared to A-alone performance.

However, the strong association between lipreading skill and AV enhancement may exist only for hearing-impaired or deaf adults and children who have compromised auditory systems. It has generally been assumed that the primary modality for speech perception is audition for NH people but vision for hearing-impaired people (e.g., Erber, 1969; Gagné, 1994; Seewald et al., 1985). As mentioned earlier, Seewald et al. (1985) found that hearing-impaired children who had higher hearing thresholds were biased toward visual input, whereas children with lower hearing thresholds were biased toward auditory input. A more recent study investigating hearing-impaired adults showed that adults with early-onset deafness were better lipreaders than adults with late-onset deafness (Tillberg, 1996). Moreover, we found that postlingually deaf adult CI users who experienced progressive hearing loss were better lipreaders than adults who experienced sudden hearing loss (Bergeson, Pisoni, Reese, et al., 2003). Does primary reliance on the visual sensory channel change following cochlear implantation? What is the best way to determine which modality is the "primary" sensory system for speech?

Although we did not attempt to directly assess the primary sensory modality for speech in the studies presented in this chapter, an examination of the findings on AV speech perception in prelingually deaf children with CIs can begin to answer these questions. We found differences, prior to implantation, in perception of visual speech information on the CP test depending on children's early experience or communication mode (OC vs. TC) (Bergeson, Pisoni, & Davis, 2003). Also, we found that children's performance did not improve across time in the V-alone condition after implantation, whereas their performance did improve across time in the A-alone and AV conditions. Finally, deaf children who received implants later in life (i.e., after longer periods of deafness) had better lipreading scores and worse A and AV scores than deaf children who received implants earlier in life (i.e., after shorter periods of deafness). Taken together, these three results suggest that prelingually deaf children rely primarily on the visual sensory channel prior to cochlear implantation, particularly those children who receive implants later in life, but that over time, after sound and audition are introduced, they gradually learn to rely on information provided by the auditory sensory channel in similar ways as NH children and adults.

It is important to note that, although the studies reported in this chapter did not obtain any direct assessments of the underlying neural mechanisms involved in AV integration, the present findings contribute valuable new information about the way questions concerning such mechanisms are formulated and assessed based on this unique clinical population. AV perception researchers generally support either "modality-neutral," early-integration theories (e.g., Fowler, 1986; Rosenblum, in press; Rosenblum & Gordon, 2001) or "modality-specific," late-integration theories (e.g., Bernstein, Auer, & Moore, Chap. 13, this volume) of AV speech perception. However, these two accounts of AV integration assume that both auditory and visual sensory systems are intact and have developed normally. As we have shown in the present chapter, AV speech perception can be dramatically influenced by hearing impairment and restoration of the auditory modality with a CI.

The studies reviewed in this chapter raise a number of new theoretical issues that any theory of AV speech perception should be able to explain: the effects of early experience (OC vs. TC), the effects of duration of deafness prior to implantation (early implantation versus late implantation in prelingually deaf children; early-onset deafness versus late-onset deafness in postlingually deaf adults), the differential effects of presentation method (A-alone, V-alone, AV), and the effects of perceptual learning (development of AV speech perception over time following cochlear implantation in prelingually deaf children). For example, Bergeson, Pisoni, and Davis (2003) found that lipreading skills did not improve as much as A-alone and AV skills over time following cochlear implantation. If AV speech perception was simply an amodal process reflecting a common event structure, one might expect that lipreading skills would improve over time at the same rate as auditory skills.

Similarly, the effects of early implantation on A-alone and V-alone speech perception are not consistent with an amodal or modality-neutral view of speech perception and spoken language processing. The Bergeson, Pisoni, and Davis (2003b) findings of better auditory perception skills in children who received implants early and better lipreading skills in children who received implants at a later age are more consistent with a modality-specific model in which the auditory and visual systems are independent. Although performance for both the early-implanted and late-implanted groups of children was similar in the AV presentation condition, the mechanisms and processes used by these two groups of children most likely differ, with the group receiving implants at an earlier age primarily using the auditory modality and the group receiving implants at a later age primarily using the visual modality. Our recent findings are not only consistent with a modality-specific model of AV speech perception, they are also compatible with recent studies on the neural basis of auditory deprivation and cortical plasticity (Armstrong, Neville, Hillyard, & Mitchell, 2002; Eggermont et al., 1997; Ponton et al., 1996; Ponton & Eggermont, 2001; Sharma et al., 2002) and AV integration or multisensory convergence (Fort, Delpuech, Pernier, & Giard, 2002; Meredith, 2002; Olson, Gatenby, & Gore, 2002; Patton, Belkacem-Boussaid, & Anastasio, 2002; Teder-Sälejärvi, McDonald, Di Russo, & Hillyard, 2002).

Future studies examining AV speech perception in both postlingually deaf adults and prelingually deaf children who receive CIs should be invaluable in terms of informing this current theoretical debate, because these unique clinical populations afford a way to study differences in early experience and developmental history before and after cochlear implantation using traditional behavioral techniques.

Conclusions

The AV speech perception results from our studies of profoundly deaf children with CIs demonstrate clearly that the processes employed in integrating cross-modal sensory information from auditory and visual modalities reflect a number of fundamental information processing operations associated with phonetic coding and the construction of phonological and lexical representations of spoken language. The basic information processing operations measured by the AV tests used in these studies are not task-specific but are more general in nature because they are also deployed in a range of other speech and language processing tasks that are routinely used to measure audiological outcome and assess benefit following cochlear implantation.

Measures of AV integration skills may therefore reflect important milestones in neural development related to the sensory, cognitive, and linguistic processes that underlie speech and language development in this unique clinical population. Moreover, measures of AV speech perception in this population may provide new behavioral markers of how information about the phonetic events is combined and integrated across sensory domains before implantation and then after hearing is introduced for the first time following a period of auditory deprivation.

Our findings from the longitudinal study of deaf children before and after cochlear implantation revealed that measures of AV speech perception and the

enhancement obtained under cross-modal presentation conditions were strongly correlated with both receptive and expressive outcome measures of speech and language. These correlations have both theoretical and clinical significance. Theoretically, the findings suggest close links and tight coupling between speech perception and production and a common source of shared variance among all these tasks that reflects the use of abstract phonological knowledge of the sound structure and sound patterns of the target language in the ambient environment. Knowledge of phonology, phonological constraints, and the use of phonological processing skills involving decomposition and reassembly processes emerge as important contributors to success and benefit with a CI. This is particularly true for children who were immersed in OC educational environments. They consistently showed large differences in performance in a range of language processing tasks compared to children in TC environments.

The differences in performance observed between OC and TC environments demonstrate the substantial contribution of early sensory and linguistic experience and phonological processing activities to the development of speech perception skills and the underlying cognitive processes that are used in these behavioral tasks. What the child does with the limited sensory information received through the CI is shaped and modulated by the routine and highly practiced linguistic activities and processes that operate on these early sensory representations in both speech perception and production. Not only does extensive practice speaking and listening in OC environments serve to create permanent phonological memory codes for speech and language but these particular kinds of linguistic activities also encourage and promote the development of highly automatized processing and attentional strategies that contribute to the speed and fluency of spoken language processing, one of the primary hallmarks of linguistic competence observed in typically developing NH children.

Clinically, the preimplantation correlations provide some additional new insights into the important role of cross-modal speech perception in this unique population. These correlations suggest that even before a deaf child receives a CI, it is possible to obtain some reliable behavioral measures based on V-alone speech perception that will predict outcome and benefit after implantation. We believe this is an important new finding from our research on AV speech perception. Although lipreading scores do not reflect direct sensory input from the peripheral auditory system, measures of lipreading skills in a deaf child prior to implantation may provide an initial index of the coupling and interactions between auditory and visual systems and the potential for unity and convergence of processing common phonetic events between these two different sensory systems even in the absence of sound and hearing. Thus, the development of cross-modal speech perception skills may serve as a valuable window on the underlying neural information processing operations used in speech and language perception and provide both clinicians and researchers with new measures of how a deaf child somehow manages to recover the vocal gestures and linguistically significant articulatory events of the talker to comprehend the intended message.

ACKNOWLEDGMENTS This work was supported by NIH-NIDCD Training Grant T32DC00012 and NIH-NIDCD Research Grant R01DC00111 to Indiana University, and NIH-NIDCD Research Grant R01DC00064 to the Indiana University School of Medicine. We thank Amy Teoh, Elizabeth Collison, Cindy Hiltgen, and Lindsey Reese for their help in testing the children and adults.

REFERENCES

Abler, W. L. (1989). On the particulate principle of self-diversifying systems. *Journal of Social and Biological Structures, 12,* 1–13.

Armstrong, B. A., Neville, H. J., Hillyard, S. A., & Mitchell, T. V. (2002). Auditory deprivation affects processing of motion, but not color. *Cognitive Brain Research, 14,* 422–434.

Baddeley, A., Gathercole, S. E., & Papagno, C. (1998). The phonological loop as a language learning device. *Psychological Review, 105,* 158–173.

Beggs, W. D. A., & Foreman, D. L. (1980). Sound localization and early inaural experience in the deaf. *British Journal of Audiology, 14,* 41–48.

Berger, K. W. (1972). *Speechreading: Principles and methods.* Baltimore: National Educational Press.

Bergeson, T. R., Pisoni, D. B., & Davis, R. A. O. (2003a). A longitudinal study of audiovisual speech perception by children with hearing loss who use cochlear implants. *The Volta Review, 163,* monograph, 347–370.

Bergeson, T. R., Pisoni, D. B., & Davis, R. A. O. (2003b). *Development of audiovisual comprehension skills in prelingually deaf children with cochlear implants.* Manuscript submitted for publication.

Bergeson, T. R., Pisoni, D. B., Lachs, L., & Reese, L. (2003, August). *Audiovisual integration of point light displays of speech by deaf adults following cochlear implantation.* Poster presented at the 15th International Congress of Phonetic Sciences, Barcelona, Spain.

Bergeson, T. R., Pisoni, D. B., Reese, L., & Kirk, K. I. (2003, February). *Audiovisual speech perception in adult cochlear implant users: Effects of sudden vs. progressive hearing loss.* Poster presented at the annual midwinter research meeting of the Association for Research in Otolaryngology, Daytona Beach, Florida.

Bernstein, L. E., Auer, E. T., Jr., & Tucker, P. E. (2001). Enhanced speechreading in deaf adults: Can short-term training/practice close the gap for hearing adults? *Journal of the Acoustical Society of America, 90,* 2971–2984.

Bernstein, L. E., Demorest, M. E., & Tucker, P. E. (2000). Speech perception without hearing. *Perception & Psychophysics, 62,* 233–252.

Boothroyd, A., Hanin, L., & Hnath, T. (1985). *A sentence test of speech perception: Reliability, set equivalence, and short term learning* (Internal Report RCI 10). New York: City University of New York.

Boothroyd, A., Hnath-Chisolm, T., Hanin, L., & Kishon-Rabin, L. (1988). Voice fundamental frequency as an auditory supplement to the speechreading of sentences. *Ear and Hearing, 9,* 306–312.

Breeuwer, M., & Plomp, R. (1986). Speechreading supplemented with auditorily presented speech parameters. *Journal of the Acoustical Society of America, 79,* 481–499.

Bruer, J. T. (2001). A critical and sensitive period primer. In D. B. Bailey, J. T. Bruer, F. J. Symons, & J. W. Lichtman (Eds.), *Critical thinking about critical periods* (pp. 3–26). Baltimore: Paul H. Brookes.

Burkholder, R. A., & Pisoni, D. B. (2003). Speech timing and working memory in profoundly deaf children after cochlear implantation. *Journal of Experimental Child Psychology, 85,* 63–88.

Carpenter, P. A., Miyake, A., & Just, M. A. (1994). Working memory constraints in comprehension: Evidence from individual differences, aphasia, and aging. In M. A. Gernsbacher (Ed.), *Handbook of psycholinguistics* (pp. 1075–1122). San Diego, CA: Academic Press.

Cornett, R. O., & Daisey, M. E. (2000). *The cued speech resource book for parents of deaf children.* Cleveland, OH: The National Cued Speech Association.

Cullington, H., Hodges, A. V., Butts, S. L., Dolan-Ash, S., & Balkany, T. J. (2000). Comparison of language ability in children with cochlear implants placed in oral and total communication education settings. *Annals of Otology, Rhinology, and Laryngology, 185,* 121–123.

Desjardins, R. N., Rogers, J., & Werker, J. F. (1997). An exploration of why preschoolers perform differently than do adults in audiovisual speech perception tasks. *Journal of Experimental Child Psychology, 66,* 85–110.

Doherty-Sneddon, G., Bonner, L., & Bruce, V. (2001). Cognitive demands of face monitoring: Evidence for visuospatial overload. *Memory & Cognition, 29,* 909–919.

Dorman, M. F., Dankowski, K., McCandless, G., Parkin, J. L., & Smith, L. B. (1991). Vowel and consonant recognition with the aid of a multichannel cochlear implant. *Quarterly Journal of Experimental Psychology, 43,* 585–601.

Dowell, R. C., Martin, L. F., Tong, Y. C., Clark, G. M., Seligman, P. M., & Patrick, J. E. (1982). A 12-consonant confusion study on a multiple-channel cochlear implant patient. *Journal of Speech and Hearing Research, 25,* 509–516.

Dunn, L., & Dunn, L. (1997). *Peabody Picture Vocabulary Test—Third Edition.* Circle Pines, MN: American Guidance Service.

Edwards, S., Fletcher, P., Garman, M., Hughes, A., & Letts, C., & Sinka, I. (1997). *Reynell Developmental Language Scales—Third Edition.* Windsor, England: NFER-Nelson Publishing Company.

Eggermont, J. J., Ponton, C. W., Don, M., Waring, M. D., & Kwong, B. (1997). Maturational delays in cortical evoked potentials in cochlear implant users. *Acta Oto-laryngologica, 17,* 161–163.

Erber, N. P. (1969). Interaction of audition and vision in the recognition of oral speech stimuli. *Journal of Speech and Hearing Research, 12,* 423–425.

Erber, N. P. (1972). Auditory, visual, and auditory-visual recognition of consonants by children with normal and impaired hearing. *Journal of Speech and Hearing Research, 15,* 413–422.

Erber, N. P. (1975). Auditory-visual perception of speech. *Journal of Speech and Hearing Disorders, 40,* 481–492.

Erber, N. P. (1979). Speech perception by profoundly hearing-impaired children. *Journal of Speech and Hearing Disorders, 44,* 255–270.

Fort, A., Delpuech, C., Pernier, J., & Giard, M.-H. (2002). Early auditory-visual interactions in human cortex during nonredundant target identification. *Cognitive Brain Research, 14,* 20–30.

Fowler, C. A. (1986). An event approach to the study of speech perception from a direct-realist perspective. *Journal of Phonetics, 14,* 3–28.

Fryauf-Bertschy, H., Tyler, R. S., Kelsay, D., & Gantz, B. (1992). Performance over time of congenitally deaf and postlingually deafened children using a multichannel cochlear implant. *Journal of Speech and Hearing Research, 35,* 913–920.

Fryauf-Bertschy, H., Tyler, R. S., Kelsay, D., Gantz, B., & Woodworth, G. (1997). Cochlear implant use by prelingually deafened children: The influences of age at implant and length of device use. *Journal of Speech, Language, and Hearing Research, 40,* 183–199.

Gagné, J.-P. (1994). Visual and audiovisual speech perception training: Basic and applied research needs. In J.-P. Gagné & N. Tye-Murray (Eds.), *Research in audiological rehabilitation: Current trends and future directions* [Monograph]. *Journal of the Academy of Rehabilitative Audiology, 27,* 133–159.

Gantz, B. J., Tye-Murray, N., & Tyler, R. S. (1989). Word recognition performance with single-channel and multichannel cochlear implants. *American Journal of Otology, 10,* 91–94.

Gantz, B. J., Tyler, R. S., Knutson, J. F., Woodworth, G., Abbas, P., McCabe, B. F., et al. (1988). Evaluation of five different cochlear implant designs: Audiologic assessment and predictors of performance. *Laryngoscope, 98,* 1100–1106.

Geers, A. (1994). Techniques for assessing auditory speech perception and lipreading enhancement in young deaf children [Monograph]. *Volta Review, 96,* 85–96.

Geers, A., & Brenner, C. (1994). Speech perception results: Audition and lipreading enhancement. *Volta Review, 96,* 97–108.

Geers, A., Brenner, C., & Davidson, L. (2003). Factors associated with development of speech perception skills in children implanted by age five. *Ear and Hearing, 24,* 24S–35S.

Geers, A. E., & Moog, J. S. (1992). Speech perception and production skills of students with impaired hearing from oral and total communication education settings. *Journal of Speech and Hearing Research, 35,* 1384–1393.

Geers, A., Nicholas, J., Tye-Murray, N., Uchanski, R., Brenner, C., Crosson, J., et al. (1999). Cochlear implants and education of the deaf child: Second-year results. Periodic Progress Report No. 35, Central Institute for the Deaf (pp. 5–16).

Geers, A., Spehar, B., & Sedey, A. (2002). Use of speech by children from total communication programs who wear cochlear implants. *American Journal of Speech-Language Pathology, 11,* 50–58.

Gesi, A. T., Massaro, D. W., & Cohen, M. M. (1992). Discovery and expository methods in teaching visual consonant and word identification. *Journal of Speech and Hearing Research, 35,* 1180–1188.

Gogate, L. J., Walker-Andrews, A. S., & Bahrick, L. E. (2001). The intersensory origins of word comprehension: An ecological–dynamic systems view. *Developmental Science, 4,* 1–37.

Gordon, K. A., Papsin, B. C., & Harrison, R. V. (2003). Activity-dependent developmental plasticity of the auditory brain stem in children who use cochlear implants. *Ear and Hearing, 24,* 485–500.

Grant, K. W., & Seitz, P. F. (1998). Measures of auditory-visual integration in nonsense syllables and sentences. *Journal of the Acoustical Society of America, 104,* 2438–2450.

Grant, K. W., Walden, B. E., & Seitz, P. F. (1998). Auditory-visual speech recognition by hearing-impaired subjects: Consonant recognition, sentence recognition, and auditory-visual integration. *Journal of the Acoustical Society of America, 103,* 2677–2690.

Gustason, G., & Zawolkow, E. (1993). *Signing Exact English.* Los Alamitos, CA: Modern Signs Press.

Haskins, H. A. (1949). *A phonetically balanced test of speech discrimination for children.* Unpublished master's thesis, Northwestern University, Evanston, IL.

Hodges, A. V., Dolan-Ash, M., Balkany, T. J., Schloffman, J. J., & Butts, S. L. (1999). Speech perception results in children with cochlear implants: Contributing factors. *Otolaryngology–Head and Neck Surgery, 12,* 31–34.

Kaiser, A. R., Kirk, K. I., Lachs, L., & Pisoni, D. B. (2003). Talker and lexical effects on audiovisual word recognition by adults with cochlear implants. *Journal of Speech, Language, and Hearing Research, 46,* 390–404.

Kirk, K. I., Eisenberg, L. S., Martinez, A. S., & Hay-McCutcheon, M. (1999). The Lexical Neighborhood Tests: Test-retest reliability and interlist equivalency. *Journal of the American Academy of Audiology, 10,* 113–123.

Kirk, K. I., Pisoni, D. B., & Miyamoto, R. T. (2000). Lexical discrimination by children with cochlear implants: Effects of age at implantation and communication mode. In S. Waltzman & N. Cohen (Eds.), *Proceedings of the Vth International Cochlear Implant Conference* (pp. 252–253). New York: Thieme.

Kirk, K. I., Pisoni, D. B., & Osberger, M. J. (1995). Lexical effects on spoken word recognition by pediatric cochlear implant users. *Ear and Hearing, 16,* 470–481.

Knutson, J. F., Hinrichs, J. V., Tyler, R. S., Gantz, B. J., Schartz, H. A., & Woodworth, G. (1991). Psychological predictors of audiological outcomes of multichannel cochlear implants: Preliminary findings. *Annals of Otology, Rhinology, and Laryngology, 100,* 817–822.

Kuhl, P. K., & Meltzoff, A. N. (1982). The bimodal perception of speech in infancy. *Science, 218,* 1138–1141.

Lachs, L. (2002). Vocal tract kinematics and crossmodal speech information. *Research on Spoken Language Processing* (Technical Report No. 10). Bloomington, IN: Speech Research Laboratory.

Lachs, L., Pisoni, D. B., & Kirk, K. I. (2001). Use of audiovisual information in speech perception by prelingually deaf children with cochlear implants: A first report. *Ear and Hearing, 22,* 236–251.

Lenneberg, E. H. (1967). *The biological foundations of language.* New York: Wiley.

Lewkowicz, D. J. (1992). Infants' responsiveness to the auditory and visual attributes of a sounding/moving stimulus. *Perception & Psychophysics, 52,* 519–528.

Lewkowicz, D. J. (2000). Infants' perception of the audible, visible, and bimodal attributes of multimodal syllables. *Child Development, 71,* 1241–1257.

Lewkowicz, D. J. (2002). Heterogeneity and heterochrony in the development of intersensory perception. *Cognitive Brain Research, 14,* 41–63.

Ling, D. (1993). Auditory-verbal options for children with hearing impairment: Helping to pioneer an applied science. *Volta Review, 95,* 187–196.

MacKain, K., Studdert-Kennedy, M., Spieker, S., & Stern, D. (1983). Infant intermodal speech perception is a left-hemisphere function. *Science, 219,* 1347–1349.

Massaro, D. W. (1987). Speech perception by ear and eye. In B. Dodd & R. Campbell (Eds.), *Hearing by eye: The psychology of lip-reading* (pp. 53–83). Hillsdale, NJ: Erlbaum.

Massaro, D. W. (1998). *Perceiving talking faces: From speech perception to a behavioral principle.* Cambridge, MA: MIT Press.

Massaro, D. W., & Cohen, M. M. (1995). Perceiving talking faces. *Current Directions in Psychological Science, 4,* 104–109.

Massaro, D. W., & Cohen, M. M. (1999). Speech perception in perceivers with hearing loss: Synergy of multiple modalities. *Journal of Speech, Language, and Hearing Research, 42,* 21–41.

Massaro, D. W., & Cohen, M. M. (2000). Tests of auditory-visual integration efficiency within the framework of the fuzzy logical model of perception. *Journal of the Acoustical Society of America, 108,* 784–789.

McGurk, H., & MacDonald, J. W. (1976). Hearing lips and seeing voices. *Nature, 264,* 746–748.

Meredith, M. A. (2002). On the neuronal basis for multisensory convergence: A brief overview. *Cognitive Brain Research, 14,* 31–40.

Miyamoto, R. T., Kirk, K. I., Robbins, A. M., Todd, S., Riley, A., & Pisoni, D. B. (1997). Speech perception and speech intelligibility in children with multichannel cochlear implants. In I. Honjo & H. Takahashi (Eds.), *Cochlear implant and related sciences update. Advances in otorhinolaryngology* (pp. 198–203). Basel, Switzerland: Karger.

Miyamoto, R., Kirk, K., Svirsky, M., & Sehgal, S. (1999). Communication skills in pediatric cochlear implant recipients. *Acta Oto-laryngologica, 119,* 219–224.

Miyamoto, R. T., Osberger, M. J., Robbins, A. M., Renshaw, J. J., Myres, W. A., Kessler, K., et al. (1989). Comparison of sensory aids in deaf children. *Annals of Otology, Rhinology, and Laryngology, 98,* 2–7.

Miyamoto, R. T., Svirsky, M. A., & Robbins, A. M. (1997). Enhancement of expressive language in prelingually deaf children with cochlear implants. *Acta Oto-laryngologica, 117,* 154–157.

Moeller, M. P., & Luetke-Stahlman, B. (1990). Parents' use of Signing Exact English: A descriptive analysis. *Journal of Speech and Hearing Disorders, 55,* 327–338.

Mogford, K. (1987). Lip-reading in the prelingually deaf. In B. Dodd & R. Campbell (Eds.), *Hearing by eye: The psychology of lip-reading* (pp. 191–211). Hillsdale, NJ: Erlbaum.

Moore, J. K. (2002). Maturation of human auditory cortex: Implications for speech perception. *Annals of Otology, Rhinology, and Laryngology, 111,* 7–10.

Neville, H. J., & Bruer, J. T. (2001). Language processing: How experience affects brain organization. In D. B. Bailey, J. T. Bruer, F. J. Symons, & J. W. Lichtman (Eds.), *Critical thinking about critical periods* (pp. 151–172). Baltimore: Paul H. Brookes.

Olson, I. R., Gatenby, J. C., & Gore, J. C. (2002). A comparison of bound and unbound audio-visual information processing in the human cerebral cortex. *Cognitive Brain Research, 14,* 129–138.

Osberger, M. J., Robbins, A. M., Todd, S. L., Riley, A. I., & Miyamoto, R. T. (1994). Speech intelligibility of children with cochlear implants. *Volta Review, 96,* 169–180.

Osberger, M. J., Todd, S. L., Berry, S. W., Robbins, A. M., & Miyamoto, R. T. (1991). Effect of age of onset of deafness on children's speech perception abilities with a cochlear implant. *Annals of Otology, Rhinology, and Laryngology, 100,* 883–888.

Patton, P., Belkacem-Boussaid, K., & Anastasio, T. J. (2002). Multimodality in the superior colliculus: An information theoretic analysis. *Cognitive Brain Research, 14,* 10–19.

Pinker, S. (1994). *The Language Instinct.* New York: William Morrow.

Pisoni, D. B. (2000). Cognitive factors and cochlear implants: Some thoughts on perception, learning, and memory in speech perception. *Ear and Hearing, 21,* 70–78.

Pisoni, D. B., & Cleary, M. (in press). Some new findings on learning, memory and cognitive processes in deaf children following cochlear implantation. In F. G. Zeng, A. N. Popper, & R. R. Fay (Eds.), S*pringer handbook of auditory research: Auditory prosthesis* (SHAR Volume X). Geneva: Springer-Verlag.

Pisoni, D. B., & Cleary, M. (2003). Measures of working memory span and verbal rehearsal speed in deaf children after cochlear implantation. *Ear and Hearing, 24,* 106S–120S.

Pisoni, D. B., Cleary, M., Geers, A. E., & Tobey, E. A. (2000). Individual differences in effectiveness of cochlear implants in children who are prelingually deaf: New process measures of performance. *Volta Review, 101,* 111–164.

Ponton, C. W., Don, M., Eggermont, J. J., Waring, M. D., & Masuda, A. (1996). Maturation of human cortical auditory function: Differences between normal-hearing children and children with cochlear implants. *Ear and Hearing, 17,* 430–437.

Ponton, C. W., & Eggermont, J. J. (2001). Of kittens and kids: Altered cortical maturation following profound deafness and cochlear implant use. *Audiology & Neuro-Otology, 6,* 363–380.

Reynell, J. K., & Huntley, M. (1985). *Reynell Developmental Language Scales—Revised, Edition 2.* Windsor, England: NFER-Nelson Publishing Company.

Rhoades, E. A. (1982). Early intervention and development of communication skills for deaf children using an auditory-verbal approach. *Topics in Language Disorders, 2,* 8–16.

Robbins, A. M., Renshaw, J. J., & Osberger, M. J. (1995). *Common Phrases Test.* Indianapolis: Indiana University School of Medicine.

Robbins, A. M., Svirsky, M. A., & Kirk, K. I. (1997). Children with implants can speak, but can they communicate? *Otolaryngology–Head and Neck Surgery, 117,* 155–160.

Robinson, K. (1998). Implications of developmental plasticity for the language acquisition of deaf children with cochlear implants. *International Journal of Pediatric Otorhinolaryngology, 46,* 71–80.

Rönnberg, J. (1995). Perceptual compensation in the deaf and blind: Myth or reality? In R. A. Dixon & L. Bäckman

(Eds.), *Compensating for psychological deficits and declines* (pp. 251–274). Mahwah, NJ: Erlbaum.

Rosenblum, L. D. (in press). The primacy of multimodal speech perception. In D. B. Pisoni & R. E. Remez (Eds.), *Handbook of speech perception*. Oxford, England: Blackwell.

Rosenblum, L. D., & Gordon, M. S. (2001). The generality of specificity: Some lessons from audiovisual speech. *Behavioral and Brain Sciences, 24*, 239–240.

Rosenblum, L. D., Johnson, J. A., & Saldaña, H. M. (1996). Point-light facial displays enhance comprehension of speech in noise. *Journal of Speech, Language, and Hearing Research, 39*, 1159–1170.

Rosenblum, L. D., & Saldaña, H. M. (1996). An audiovisual test of kinematic primitives for visual speech perception. *Journal of Experimental Psychology: Human Perception and Performance, 22*, 318–331.

Seewald, R. C., Ross, M., Giolas, T. G., & Yonovitz, A. (1985). Primary modality for speech perception in children with normal and impaired hearing. *Journal of Speech and Hearing Research, 28*, 36–46.

Sharma, A., Dorman, M. F., & Spahr, A. J. (2002). A sensitive period for the development of the central auditory system in children with cochlear implants: Implications for age of implantation. *Ear and Hearing, 23*, 532–539.

Shepherd, R. K., & Hardie, N. A. (2001). Deafness-induced changes in the auditory pathway: Implications for cochlear implants. *Audiology & Neuro-otology, 6*, 305–318.

Shepherd, R. K., Hartmann, R., Heid, S., Hardie, N., & Klinke, R. (1997). The central auditory system and auditory deprivation: Experience with cochlear implants in the congenitally deaf. *Acta Oto-laryngology, S532*, 28–33.

Spelke, E. S. (1979). Perceiving bimodally specified events in infancy. *Developmental Psychology, 15*, 626–636.

Spelke, E. S. (1981). The infant's acquisition of knowledge of bimodally specified events. *Journal of Experimental Child Psychology, 31*, 279–299.

Staller, S. J., Dowell, R. C., Beiter, A. L., & Brimacombe, J. A. (1991). Perceptual abilities of children with the Nucleus 22-Channel cochlear implant. *Ear and Hearing, 12*, 34S–47S.

Studdert-Kennedy, M. (1998). The particulate origins of language generativity: From syllable to gesture. In J. R. Hurford, M. Studdert-Kennedy, & C. Knight (Eds.), *Approaches to the evolution of language* (pp. 202–221). Cambridge, England: Cambridge University Press.

Sumby, W. H., & Pollack, I. (1954). Visual contribution to speech intelligibility in noise. *Journal of the Acoustical Society of America, 26*, 212–215.

Summerfield, Q. (1987). Some preliminaries to a comprehensive account of audio-visual speech perception. In B. Dodd & R. Campbell (Eds.), *Hearing by eye: The psychology of lipreading* (pp. 3–51). Hillsdale, NJ: Erlbaum.

Svirsky, M. A., Robbins, A. M., Kirk, K. I., Pisoni, D. B., & Miyamoto, R. T. (2000). Language development in profoundly deaf children with cochlear implants. *Psychological Science, 11*, 153–158.

Swisher, V., & Thompson, M. (1985). Mother's learning simultaneous communication: The dimensions of the task. *American Annals of the Deaf, 130*, 212–218.

Tait, M., Lutman, M. E., & Robinson, K. (2000). Preimplant measures of preverbal communicative behavior as predictors of cochlear implant outcomes in children. *Ear and Hearing, 21*, 18–24.

Teder-Sälejärvi, W. A., McDonald, J. J., Di Russo, F., & Hillyard, S. A. (2002). An analysis of audio-visual cross-modal integration by means of event-related potential (ERP) recordings. *Cognitive Brain Research, 14*, 106–114.

Teoh, S. W., Pisoni, D. B., & Miyamoto, R. T. (in press a). Cochlear implantation in adults with prelingual deafness: I. Clinical results. *Laryngoscope.*

Teoh, S. W., Pisoni, D. B., & Miyamoto, R. T. (in press b). Cochlear implantation in adults with prelingual deafness: II. Underlying constraints that affect audiological outcomes. *Laryngoscope.*

Tillberg, I., Rönnberg, J., Svärd, I., & Ahlner, B. (1996). Audio-visual speechreading in a group of hearing aid users: The effects of onset age, handicap age, and degree of hearing loss. *Scandinavian Audiology, 25*, 267–272.

Tobey, E., Geers, A., Douek, B., Perrin, J., Skellett, R., Brenner, C., & Torretta, G. (2000). Factors associated with speech intelligibility in children with cochlear implants. *Annals of Otology, Rhinology, and Laryngology, Supplement 185*, 28–30.

Tomblin, J. B., Spencer, L., Flock, S., Tyler, R., & Gantz, B. (1999). A comparison of language achievement in children with cochlear implants and children using hearing aids. *Journal of Speech, Language, and Hearing Research, 42*, 497–511.

Tyler, R. F., Fryauf-Bertschy, H., Kelsay, D. M., Gantz, B., Woodworth, G., & Parkinson, A. (1997). Speech perception by prelingually deaf children using cochlear implants. *Otolaryngology–Head and Neck Surgery, 117*, 180–187.

Tyler, R. S., Gantz, B. J., McCabe, B. F., Lowder, M. W., Otto, S. R., & Preece, J. P. (1985). Audiological results with two single channel cochlear implants. *Annals of Otology, Rhinology, and Laryngology, 94*, 133–139.

Tyler, R. F., Opie, J. M., Fryauf-Bertschy, H., & Gantz, B. J. (1992). Future directions for cochlear implants. *Journal of Speech-Language Pathology and Audiology, 16*, 151–163.

Tyler, R. F., Parkinson, A. J., Woodworth, G. G., Lowder, M. W., & Gantz, B. J. (1997). Performance over time of adult patients using the Ineraid or Nucleus cochlear implant. *Journal of the Acoustical Society of America, 102*, 508–522.

Tyler, R. S., Tye-Murray, N., & Lansing, C. R. (1988). Electrical stimulation as an aid to lipreading. In *New reflections on speechreading* [Special issue]. *Volta Review, 90*, 119–148.

Waltzman, S., & Cohen, N. L. (1988). Effects of cochlear implantation on the young deaf child. *American Journal of Otology, 19*, 158–162.

Waltzman, S. B., Cohen, N. L., Gomolin, R. H., Green, J. E., Shapiro, W. H., Hoffman, R. A., et al. (1997). Open set speech perception in congenitally deaf children using cochlear implants. *American Journal of Otology, 15*, 9–13.

Waltzman, S. B., Cohen, N. L., Gomolin, R. H., Shapiro, W. H., Ozdaman, S. R., & Hoffman, R. A. (1994). Long-term results of early cochlear implantation in congenitally and prelingually deafened children. *American Journal of Otology, 15*, 9–13.

Wolff, A. B., & Thatcher, R. W. (1990). Cortical reorganization in deaf children. *Journal of Clinical and Experimental Neuropsychology, 12*, 209–221.

Yoshinaga-Itano, C. (2000). Development of audition and speech: Implications for early intervention with infants who are deaf or hard of hearing. *Volta Review, 100*, 213–234.

48 Neuroimaging Studies of Cross-Modal Plasticity and Language Processing in Deaf People

RUTH CAMPBELL AND MAIRÉAD MACSWEENEY

Introduction

In this short chapter we focus on just two questions in the domain of cortical imaging of language and sensory processing. First, to what extent do cortical circuits that subserve spoken language in hearing people also support spoken language processing, in the form of speech-reading, in people born profoundly deaf? Second, do the cortical circuits for processing a visible language such as sign language involve auditory processing regions, and do these networks differ between deaf and hearing signers?

Before these questions can be answered, it is important to realize just how variable the world of the deaf child can be, compared with that of a hearing child. The child born deaf may be deprived of not one but two human faculties. Because most human languages are spoken, the loss of hearing can have major consequences for successful language acquisition. Sensitivity to heard speech has been demonstrated as early as the second trimester of fetal development (Mehler & Christophe, 1994), and spoken language development is heavily dependent on adequate auditory function throughout childhood. If hearing is lost, for example, by infectious disease such as meningitis within the first 5 years, its impact on spoken language development can be immense (Bedford et al., 2001). Furthermore, the great majority of deaf children are born to hearing parents and may therefore be deprived of a critical feature of the ecology of language development, a salient informative communicative context shared by child and caregivers (Vygotsky, 1962, 1978). However, approximately 5%–10% of the deaf population are born to deaf parents, the majority of whom use a signed language within the home. Thus, these deaf children are raised with exposure to a visuospatial language that has all the cognitive, linguistic, and communicative requirements of a spoken human language (Klima & Bellugi, 1979; Sutton-Spence & Woll, 2000). Moreover, this language is not related in any significant way to the spoken language of the host community. The signed language development of Deaf children of Deaf parents (DoD*) follows the characteristic course, both in timing and in structure, of spoken language acquisition by hearing children (e.g., Bellugi & Fischer, 1972; Klima & Bellugi, 1979; Liddell, 1980; Petitto et al., 2001; Sacks, 1989).

Before considering the neural systems supporting processing of signed languages in native users, we will explore an aspect of language processing in deaf people from a hearing home (DoH) that, until recently, was somewhat neglected in studies of the cognitive neuroscience of language: speech-reading. Hearing people make use of visible speech actions; in fact, they cannot avoid it (McGurk & MacDonald, 1976). Deaf people are exposed to speech and its visible effects. Nevertheless, skill in speech-reading varies enormously from one deaf child to another. The origin of this variability lies in the reduced input specificity of seen compared with heard speech. This difference can be demonstrated in terms of phonological structure. Speech that is seen but not heard can deliver only a small subset of the phonological categories available to the hearing perceiver of speech (see, e.g., Summerfield, 1987). But for a profoundly deaf child born into a hearing family, speech-reading may be the only means of access to the language that surrounds her. Although earlier tests suggested

---

*Deaf (upper case) denotes a person who self identifies with deaf culture. While such a person typically has a hearing loss, the degree of hearing loss may not itself predict this classification.

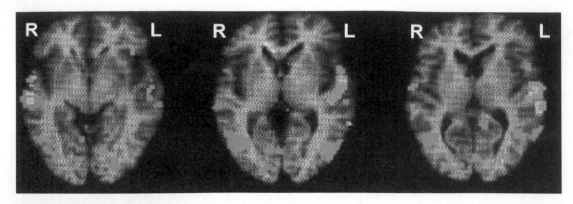

FIGURE 48.1   Speech-reading and listening to speech. Shown are group median activation maps for hearing subjects in three contiguous transaxial scans (n = 7). Blue indicates regions activated by hearing speech; pink indicates regions activated by watching silent speech. Yellow regions are activated both by heard and seen speech. The overlap areas are in auditory cortex on the superior surface of the temporal lobe (From Calvert et al., 1997.) (See Color Plate 23.)

otherwise (e.g., Mogford, 1987), careful recent tests of lipreading show that a proportion of people born deaf can become adept at spoken language processing and may be more skilled than the best hearing individuals at following silent, lip-read speech (Bernstein, Demorest, & Tucker, 2000). Our work has explored how cortical circuits for speech-reading become organized in people born profoundly deaf—people for whom a spoken, not a signed, language was the first language available in the home.

Seeing speech: Cortical correlates of silent speech-reading in hearing and deaf individuals

Calvert et al. (1997) were the first group to explore the cortical substrates for the processing of seen silent speech in a hearing population using functional magnetic resonance imaging (fMRI). Participants were given a simple speech-reading task: "Watch the face speaking random numbers between 1 and 9, and rehearse them silently to yourself." Silent speech-reading activated extensive visual cortical regions, including V5/MT and occipitotemporal regions. In addition, parts of the auditory speech processing system within the lateral temporal lobe were activated bilaterally at the group level. In particular, activation was observed in posterior parts of the superior temporal gyrus (STG), extending both ventrally into the superior temporal sulcus (STS) and superiorly onto the superior temporal plane, incorporating the tip of Heschl's gyrus (Brodmann's area 42; Fig. 48.1, Color Plate 23).

The most striking aspect of the study was that it demonstrated that parts of auditory cortex, defined functionally as those regions of superior temporal cortex that were activated by heard speech, could also be activated by watching the silent speaker. This result was

unexpected, because these areas had been considered to be specific to acoustic processing; they were in the regions that have been labeled primary (A1) and secondary (A2) auditory cortex (see Luria, 1973). Activation was not extensive within A1, and, given the spatial resolution of fMRI, appeared to be confined to the parabelt rather than to core regions of auditory cortex (Hackett, Preuss, & Kaas, 2001). These are the cytoarchitectonic Brodmann's areas 41 and 42. Activation was robust, and replicable (Campbell et al., 2001; MacSweeney et al., 2000, 2001; MacSweeney, Calvert, et al., 2002). Figure 48.2 illustrates the relative locations of these superior temporal regions. Two questions arose

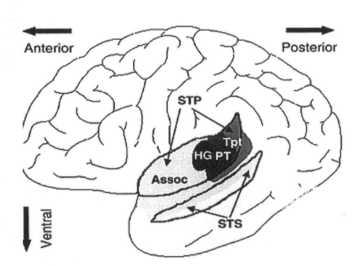

FIGURE 48.2   Schematic of the superior temporal plane (STP) of the human left hemisphere, unfolded to show relative positions of primary auditory cortex (black), including Heschl's gyrus (HG), and secondary auditory cortex (PT, Tpt; medium shading), on the superior surface of the posterior part of the superior temporal gyrus. The positions of the superior temporal sulcus (STS) and other associative auditory regions (light shading) are also shown. (From Wise et al., 2001.)

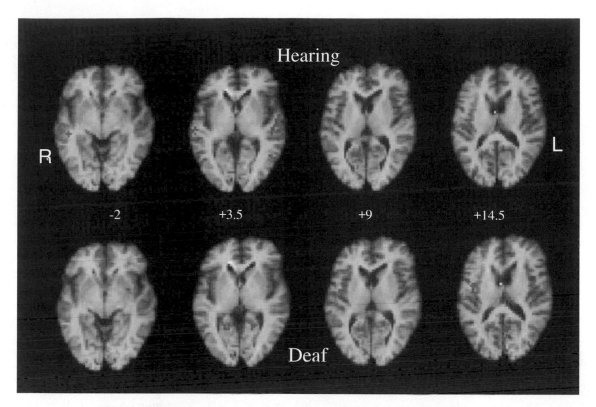

Hearing

R L

-2   +3.5   +9   +14.5

Deaf

FIGURE 48.3   Activation by speech-reading in hearing and deaf subjects. *Top:* Four contiguous axial images showing median activation by silent speech-reading in hearing subjects (n = 6). Superior temporal gyri were activated bilaterally, extending into auditory cortex. *Bottom:* Corresponding sections for deaf subjects (n = 6). Activation in the deaf subjects is in the right insular/frontal regions, the parahippocampal gyri bilaterally, and the posterior cingulate. There is no activation in auditory cortex-analogous regions. (Adapted from MacSweeney et al., 2001.) (See Color Plate 24.)

from these findings. First, was activation in auditory cortex specific to seen (silent) speech, or did it extend to nonlinguistic lip movement? Second, would the pattern be replicated in people born profoundly deaf?

To address the first of these questions, we compared speech-reading with the perception of mouth movements that could not be construed as speech—facial actions such as chewing. Many of the same regions were activated by both types of facial movement, including STS and posterior parts of STG (Calvert et al., 1997; Campbell et al., 2001). However, speech-reading activated superior lateral temporal regions (i.e., auditory cortex) to a greater extent than watching facial gurns. This activation was bilateral, whereas activation by facial gurns in these areas was right-lateralized. Do deaf people show a similar pattern when they watch speech? Does activation occur in regions corresponding to those activated by heard speech in hearing individuals? We tested six deaf adults using the same tasks. All were profoundly deaf from birth, had hearing parents, and their main mode of communication with hearing people was spoken English. All had attended schools where spoken English was the medium of instruction. They

were as good as the hearing group at identifying lip-spoken vocabulary items. However, their pattern of cortical activation differed significantly from that of the hearing group (MacSweeney et al., 2001; MacSweeney, Calvert, et al., 2002; Fig. 48.3, Color Plate 24). Specifically, there was no suggestion that left superior lateral temporal regions were activated consistently across this group during the speech-reading perception task. Deaf individuals showed activation in different regions of the left lateral temporal cortex; however, the focal location of these activations was inconsistent across individuals, and no lateral superior temporal activation was detected at the group level. Our interpretation of this lack of consistency in location of temporal activation was that it directly reflected the deaf participants' lack of experience with auditory correlates of visible speech. In hearing individuals, associations between vision and audition in speech are consistent throughout development. Functional imaging studies suggest that the STS may support audiovisual speech binding for normally occurring heard and seen speech, and can then modulate back-projections to sensory cortex. In hearing people, activation of STS is time-linked to activation in both sensory cortices when individuals are presented with coherent audiovisual speech. We have suggested that this is the mechanism that is responsible for activation in auditory processing regions when hearing people watch silent speech (Calvert, Campbell, & Brammer, 2000; Calvert et al., 1999).

In deaf people, even when behavioral measures suggest equivalent or superior skills to those of hearing controls, long-term absence of hearing has led to a change in the cortical associations that develop when speech is identified by eye. Instead of recruiting regions that support acoustic processing, regions that were consistently activated across participants included the posterior cingulate and parahippocampal gyrus (MacSweeney et al., 2001; MacSweeney, Calvert, et al., 2002; Fig. 48.3). This network of regions may be involved in integrating remembered events with on-line processing. The posterior cingulate in particular may perform a binding function, similar to that of the STS in hearing people, but in this case between visual analysis of seen speech and memories of previous encounters of that item. In the deaf group there was also activation of visual processing regions within the left lingual gyrus (V2/VP regions of visual cortex). Such activation can be observed during reading of written words (e.g., Kuriki, Takeuchi, & Hirata, 1998) and may also exhibit variable lateralization as a function of the attentional requirement to detect local (left-sided) or global (right-sided) visual target structure (Fink et al., 1997). Involvement of this region in speech-reading in deaf people, however, was a new finding, and it suggests that this area is indeed modifiable by language associations. In support of this hypothesis, Giraud, Price, Graham, Truy, and Frackowiak (2001), using positron emission tomography (PET), reported that adults with deafness of different kinds who had received a cochlear implant showed activation in visual cortex when they tried to *hear* lexical speech contrasts without any visual input whatsoever. The investigators speculated that this activation, which was most marked in visual region V2, may reflect associations established in deaf people, prior to prosthesis implantation and the restoration of acoustic function, between watching speech movements and the lexical correlates of seeing speech.

Thus, our studies and data from others' studies suggest that visual cortical regions might reorganize following early hearing loss. It has been suggested that posterior cortical regions may become relatively more active in the brains of deaf compared to hearing people, driven by the functional needs of the deaf person to "make vision work in place of hearing" (see Emmorey, 2001, for further discussion). The extent to which such reorganization may reflect structural changes in the visual system or differences in the allocation of attentional resource is a topic of intense study. Although it has not been possible to demonstrate advantages for low-level contrast sensitivity in deaf people (Finney & Dobkins, 2001), attention to motion in the visual periphery can sometimes be detected more readily by deaf signers than by hearing nonsigners and is accompanied by specific electrophysiological signatures (e.g., Neville & Lawson, 1987; see also Röder & Rösler, Chap. 46, this volume). In addition, a left hemisphere advantage for visual movement detection in deaf signers, which is absent or reversed in hearing populations, is reliably reported (Neville & Lawson, 1987, Bosworth & Dobkins, 1999). Bavelier et al. (2001) have shown that moving flow-field patterns requiring attention to spatial or featural aspects of the display generated relatively greater activity in the left MT/MST visual processing regions in deaf than in hearing people. Moreover, activation was enhanced when attention was required to detect peripheral visual movement. As originally suggested by Neville and Lawson (1987), these effects may reflect early exposure to sign language, leading to enhanced attentional processing of visual movement (Bavelier et al., 2000, 2001; Bosworth & Dobkins, 2002).

Although some reorganization of parts of visual cortex and their projections to and from (visual) association cortex may be predicted as a compensatory or learned aspect of cognition in deafness, the fate of auditory cortex in the absence of hearing is less clear. When measured prior to the implantation of a cochlear hearing aid, auditory cortex in deaf people is generally hypometabolic (Lee et al., 2001; Okazawa et al., 1996). Lee et al. (2001) reported a correlation between degree of hypometabolism in auditory cortex and effectiveness of speech processing after prosthesis implantation in prelingually deaf people. The less active the resting metabolism of the auditory cortical regions tested prior to implantation, the better the postimplantation hearing (of speech) appeared to be. They suggest that speech processing following implantation of an acoustic prosthesis must therefore depend on resistance to colonization from other modalities (such as visual input) in auditory cortex. We will return to this inference in our closing remarks. But is there direct evidence that auditory cortical regions in deaf people are modifiable, so that they become sensitive to inputs other than sound? Neurophysiological and behavioral studies of congenitally deaf cats suggest not. Studies by Klinke and colleagues (see Klinke, Krai, Heid, Tillein, & Hartmann, 1999) suggest that reafferentation of auditory inputs (from cochlear excitation) is the only means by which responsivity in auditory cortex can be attained. Without this, "afferent input . . . remains rudimentary."

Vibrotactile activation of auditory cortex? "Feeling" speech

A magnetoencephalographic (MEG) study by Levänen, Jousmaki, and Hari (1998) reported frequency-specific activation in auditory cortex in an elderly deaf man when he received vibrotactile stimulation on the fingers and palm of the hand. Activation was observed first in somatosensory cortex and somewhat later in auditory cortex. Auditory cortex activation was not observed in hearing controls. In the Tadoma method of speech-reading, which was originally developed for deaf-blind people, the perceiver senses as well as sees speech by resting his hand on the mouth, shoulder, and clavicle of the speaker. In this way the resonant body vibrations resulting from vocal cord vibration can be picked up. For the sighted deaf speech-reader, mouth movements are visible, but information about voicing patterns, which cannot be reliably gleaned from lip patterns, can still be usefully picked up by feeling clavicle vibrations. Moreover, this type of vibrotactile information appears to combine naturally with seen speech, so that "tactovisual" speech illusions, similar to the McGurk audiovisual speech illusion for hearing listeners, can be generated (Fowler & Dekle, 1991). It is unclear from the report of Levänen et al. whether their deaf participant, from a family that included deaf members, was a practiced Tadoma user, or whether he ever had usable hearing—for example, in the first year or two of life. Had that been the case, then activation in auditory processing regions could have occurred through established associations of vibrotactile processing with seen and heard speech. Levänen and Hamdorf (2001) also reported greater behavioral sensitivity to vibrotactile stimulation in deaf than in hearing individuals, but there are no further reports of deaf individuals showing vibrotactile-related activation in auditory cortex. It should be noted further that the resolution of MEG is not yet sufficient to confirm that *primary* auditory cortex was activated by vibrotactile perception, given the proximity of primary somatosensory cortex to Heschl's gyrus (see Fig. 48.2).

Conclusions: Silent speech-reading by deaf adults

Speech-reading (lipreading) is a window into the world of speech for the person born deaf. The highly skilled, deaf lipreader may closely resemble the hearing person in his or her reliance on verbal strategies for memory rehearsal and in perceptual sensitivity to phonetic structure in a range of language processing tasks, including reading (e.g., Leybaert, 2000; Leybaert, Alegria, Hage, & Charlier, 1998, for such behavioral evidence in deaf speech-readers who are also exposed to

phonetic manual cues). Nevertheless, there are clear indications that deaf and hearing speech-readers use different cortical resources. Hearing people show activation in superior temporal cortex, including primary and secondary auditory regions and the STS, when speech-reading. In contrast, only one deaf participant showed speech-reading-related activation in the region that would be classified as secondary auditory cortex in hearing people (MacSweeney et al., 2001). As a group, the deaf participants did not reliably activate these regions, but did make relatively greater use of visual processing systems, especially within the left lingual gyrus, that may be modulated by posterior cingulate activity. Reports of nonacoustic activation of primary auditory cortex by vibrotactile stimulation in deaf people require more detailed localization studies and replication. To date, it seems that speech-related activation within regions corresponding to primary auditory cortex can only be reliably observed when seen and heard speech have been experienced by the perceiver. Whether the same is true of a signed language input is discussed in the next section.

Signed language processing systems

Very few cases of sign language aphasia in deaf adults have been reported (see, e.g., Corina, 1998; Poizner, Klima, & Bellugi, 1987). These case studies suggest that the organization of processing systems supporting signed language is strikingly similar to that for spoken language (e.g., Hickok, Bellugi, & Klima, 1996). Lesions of the left hemisphere, in Broca's area within the left inferior frontal lobe, and in Wernicke's area (left posterior superior and middle temporal gyri, incorporating the supramarginal gyrus) have similar effects on signed language processing as they would on speech processing in hearing people. Neuroimaging studies provide supporting evidence that sign production implicates Broca's area, just as speech production does in hearing people (Corina & McBurney, 2001; McGuire et al., 1996), and, in a complementary way, Wernicke's area is activated when meaningful sign language is perceived (Neville et al., 1998; Nishimura et al., 1999; Petitto et al., 2000; Söderfeldt, Rönnberg, & Risberg, 1994; Söderfeldt et al., 1997). There is currently debate about the degree of lateralization of sign language perception in relation to speech lateralization (see Corina & McBurney, 2001; Hickok, Bellugi, & Klima, 1998; MacSweeney, Woll, Campbell, McGuire, et al., 2002; Neville et al., 1998; Paulesu & Mehler, 1998; Rönnberg, Söderfeldt, & Risberg, 2000), which will not be elaborated here. There is agreement, however, not only that the processing of signed languages activate regions involved in spoken language processing, including Wernicke's and Broca's areas, but also that there may be cortical regions recruited to sign language processing that are unlikely to be recruited to process speech. For example, the parietal lobes may be specifically involved in processing signed sentences that are spatially demanding (MacSweeney, Woll, Campbell, Calvert, et al., 2002). In contrast, these regions were not differentially activated in hearing people perceiving audiovisual spoken English versions of the same sentences. Thus, there are likely to be subtle differences in processing systems used for signed and spoken languages. However, for the purposes of this chapter, we will focus on the issue of whether signed languages may recruit auditory processing regions.

Auditory cortex: When can it be activated by visual stimuli?

Pioneering cortical imaging studies of sign language processing have all showed activation in superior temporal regions (Levänen, Uutela, Salenius, & Haari, 2001; Neville et al., 1998; Söderfeldt et al., 1994, 1997). None of these studies made explicit claims concerning activation, in people born profoundly deaf, of brain regions analogous to auditory cortex in hearing people. However, some recently published reports have done so.

Nishimura et al. (1999), using PET, reported that sign language stimuli could activate superior temporal regions, corresponding to auditory cortex in hearing people, in a man born profoundly deaf. This work explicitly distinguished between regions corresponding to primary (A1) and secondary (A2) auditory cortex. The authors found reliable activation by sign language only in A2-analogue regions and not within Heschl's gyrus (A1). Also using PET, Petitto et al. (2000) furthered this finding, reporting activation of secondary auditory cortex in deaf native signers but not in hearing nonsigners during perception of ASL signs. Furthermore, they reported the same pattern of activation for phonologically structured nonsense signs. On the basis of these data, the authors made the strong claim that superior temporal regions, including secondary auditory cortex, were *specifically* activated by phonologically structured input, regardless of whether the input was delivered auditorily through speech or visually through a signed language. Activation in this region was suggested to reflect the segmental structure—the phonology—of the language. Our own findings partly support Petitto's claims, but they also suggest further patterns.

When compared with viewing a still image of a person, our studies suggest that observing British Sign Language (BSL) sentences generated activation in the same region reported by Petitto et al., extending to the posterior STG bilaterally, in Deaf native signers (MacSweeney, Woll, Campbell, McGuire, et al., 2002). In a further study, we also observed activation in these regions when deaf participants watched meaningless arm and hand movements, based on the tic-tac signaling system used by bookmakers and their assistants to signal betting odds on the racetrack (MacSweeney et al., 2003). These displays do not form sequences that can be interpreted as signed language. Superior temporal regions that support heard speech analysis in hearing people have indeed become sensitive to sign language input, but this sensitivity may extend to *all* potentially meaningful arm and hand gestures.

A recent fMRI study by Finney, Fine, and Dobkins (2001) suggests that such activation may even extend beyond biological motion such as that of the hands and arms. They reported activation in cortical regions corresponding to primary auditory cortex when a group of prelingually deaf people viewed a simple moving-dot pattern. Activation of auditory cortex by such abstract visual input cannot be explained by possible early acquired associations between sight, sound, and touch for speech, as in the case of vibrotactile activation reported by Levänen et al. (1998).

Animal data suggest acoustic specificity for primary auditory cortex (Klinke et al., 1999). Thus the findings of Finney et al. (2001) of visual activation in primary auditory cortex in people born deaf raise important questions regarding the degree of cross-modal plasticity of A1 and its functional role. As Figure 48.2 indicates, primary auditory cortex is a difficult region to localize— whatever the means of neuroimaging. The transverse temporal gyrus (Heschl's gyrus) is located within the superior plane of the temporal lobe. This region is adjacent to a number of nonacoustic regions in the superior and inferior plane. Individuals vary in the extent, inclination, number of duplications, and gyral architecture of Heschl's gyrus (see Leonard, Puranik, Kuldau, & Lombardino, 1998). Therefore, mapping activation across different brains into a standardized space (as in Finney et al., 2001) may not be satisfactory when attempting to localize primary auditory cortex as a functional region at the group level. A further consideration is that the anatomy of this region in congenitally deaf people is only now being explored. Although early findings are negative (see Emmorey et al., 2003), there may be structural differences in this region between congenitally deaf and hearing populations of which we are not yet aware.

In our study (MacSweeney et al., 2003) we examined the claim that activation from a moving visual display (BSL and TicTac) might extend into primary auditory cortex. Using each individual's high-resolution structural image, we were able to locate Heschl's gyrus in each participant and look for corresponding activation within this region. There were no participants in whom the main focus of activation fell within Heschl's gyrus. Rather, in the majority of participants, the main focus of activation within this region was posterior to Heschl's gyrus, in the planum temporale. However, in one participant out of nine, this posterior activation did incorporate a medial posterior portion of Heschl's gyrus, the analogue of primary auditory cortex in hearing people. A more robust finding from this analysis, however, was that in half of the participants, this activation included the tip of Heschl's gyrus at its junction with STG, the analogue region of secondary auditory cortex. Thus, our studies to date suggest that in deaf people, secondary auditory cortex-analogue region is sensitive to varieties of visual movement and not, as hypothesized by Petitto et al. (2001), just to sign-structured input. However, with regard to activation within the medial portion of Heschl's gyrus, the pattern is still unclear. We have observed limited activation in this region in one of our deaf participants. Interestingly, there are also preliminary reports of activation of this region in hearing people during observation of moving-dot patterns (Bavelier & Neville, 2002). Therefore, the degree of cross-modal plasticity of this assumed unimodal area is far from fully understood.

Native signers: The role of hearing status

One remaining question is whether the visual activation observed in auditory regions in deaf native signers is related to early sign language knowledge or hearing status. In all our studies of BSL perception, a consistent finding has been that, compared with deaf people of similar sign background, hearing offspring of deaf parents show reduced activation in superior temporal regions, including auditory cortex. Whereas auditory regions in deaf people can become specialized for visual processing, in people with intact auditory function these regions remain dedicated to speech, even when it is not the first language to be acquired (MacSweeney, Woll, Campbell, McGuire, et al., 2002). Under these circumstances, sign language struggles to compete, within auditory cortex, with heard and spoken language, despite its early acquisition. Thus, congenital deafness rather than sign language knowledge appears to account for the recruitment of auditory cortices to visual motion processing. To test this hypothesis further it would be necessary to explore conditions under which auditory cortices are activated in congenitally profoundly deaf late learners of a signed language, a group not yet explored in neuroimaging studies of sign language processing.

Cortical plasticity of auditory speech processing regions in profound prelingual deafness: Conclusion

Lee et al. (2001) conclude their study of auditory cortex metabolism in deaf patients before and after cochlear implantation with a strong claim:

> If cross-modal plasticity [e.g., for sign language] restores metabolism in the auditory cortex before implantation, prelingually deaf patients will show no improvement in hearing function. . . . The resting cortical metabolism of untreated prelingually deaf patients represents a usurping by cross-modal plasticity, which deters the improvement of hearing capability and the restoration of normal function in the auditory temporal cortices after cochlear implantation. (p. 150)

In this statement Lee et al. appear to be advocating early cochlear implantation or restricting the exposure of a deaf child to a signed language in order to preserve the auditory function of auditory cortex. In our opinion, this contentious issue requires much more extensive research, especially in relation to age at which implantation is performed and language mastery prior to implantation. Our work does find evidence that auditory processing regions are reserved for spoken language processing in hearing people, even when a signed language was the first to be acquired. Hearing and deaf groups could be readily distinguished by activation in these regions. However, evidence for the "usurping" of primary auditory cortex by other modalities in people born deaf is far from clear. Animal studies do not conform with the suggestions of Lee et al. Klinke et al. (1999) have failed to find activation in primary auditory cortex in the congenitally deaf cat in response to visual or tactile input. In our own studies, in the absence of perceived acoustic structure, auditory-analogue regions do not develop a consistent specialization for speech-reading of a spoken language. Furthermore, although we have observed partial activation of Heschl's gyrus in some deaf participants, we have not yet observed focused and robust activation by visual stimulation in the medial portion of Heschl's gyrus—the region which, in hearing people, would be delineated as A1. Future studies with more deaf participants and with greater imaging resolution should enable us to obtain more authoritative information.

More generally, just as in hearing people superior temporal regions support not only speech but a range of complex acoustic analyses contributing, for example, to voice timbre and musical analysis (e.g., Belin, Zatorre, Lafaille, Ahad, & Pike, 2000; Griffiths, Büchel, Frackowiak, & Patterson, 1998), so in deaf people these regions may support a range of nonsign but complex patterns of visual movement processing. These patterns may include moving checkerboard and flow patterns (Bavelier et al., 2001; Finney et al., 2001), and also a range of biological movement patterns, including gestural patterns. The role of the STS in the analysis of communicative gesture in hearing people is well established (see Allison, Puce, & McCarthy, 2000, for a review). But our speculation here goes beyond this both functionally and anatomically: it is possible that the disposition of the brain for mastering signed language in a person born deaf may be associated with a reconfiguring of language cortex in the superior-posterior parts of the lateral temporal cortex to subserve the analysis of many varieties of nonlinguistic visual movement.

The close correspondence in patterns of cortical activation for speech in hearing people and for sign in deaf people strongly supports the view that language makes use of cortical substrates involved in processing communicative gesture. Such gesture patterns, whether vocal or manual, may have characteristics suited to the processing specialization of the superior-posterior temporal regions, especially in the left hemisphere. The elaboration of those characteristics in humans and in other primates may ultimately clarify how and why language evolves in all sentient human populations, irrespective of their hearing status.

REFERENCES

Allison, T., Puce, A., & McCarthy, G. (2000). Social perception from visual cues: Role of STS region. *Trends in Cognitive Sciences, 4,* 267–278.

Bavelier, D., Brozinsky, C., Tomann, A., Mitchell, T., Neville, H. J., & Liu, G. (2001). Impact of early deafness and early exposure to sign language on the cerebral organization for motion processing. *Journal of Neuroscience, 21,* 8931–8942.

Bavelier, D., & Neville, H. (2002). Cross-modal plasticity: Where and how? *Nature Reviews: Neuroscience, 3,* 443–452.

Bavelier, D., Tomann, A., Hutton, C., Mitchell, T., Corina, D., Liu, G., et al. (2000). Visual attention to the periphery is enhanced in congenitally deaf individuals. *Journal of Neuroscience, 20,* RC 93, 1–6.

Bedford, H., de Louvois, J., Halket, S., Peckham, C., Hurley, R., & Harvey, D. (2001). Meningitis in infancy in England and Wales: Follow up at age 5 years. *British Medical Journal, 323,* 533–536.

Belin, P., Zatorre, R. J., Lafaille, P., Ahad, P., & Pike, B. (2000). Voice selective areas in human auditory cortex. *Nature, 403,* 309–312.

Bellugi, U., & Fischer, S. (1972). A comparison of sign language and spoken language. *Cognition, 1,* 173–200.

Bernstein, L. E., Demorest, M. E., & Tucker, P. E. (2000). Speech perception without hearing. *Perception & Psychophysics, 62,* 233–252.

Bosworth, R. G., & Dobkins, K. R. (1999). Left hemisphere dominance for motion processing in deaf signers. *Psychological Science, 10,* 256–262.

Bosworth, R. G., & Dobkins, K. R. (2002). The effects of spatial attention on motion processing in deaf signers, hearing signers, and hearing nonsigners. *Brain and Cognition, 49,* 152–169.

Calvert, G. A., Brammer, M. J., Bullmore, E. T., Campbell, R., Iversen, S. D., & David, A. S. (1999). Response amplification in sensory-specific cortices during cross-modal binding. *Neuroreport, 10,* 2619–2623.

Calvert, G. A., Bullmore, E. T., Brammer, M. J., Campbell, R., Williams, S. C., McGuire, P. K., et al. (1997). Activation of auditory cortex during silent lipreading. *Science, 276,* 593–596.

Calvert, G. A., Campbell, R., & Brammer, M. J. (2000). Evidence from functional magnetic resonance imaging of crossmodal binding in the human heteromodal cortex. *Current Biology, 10,* 649–657.

Campbell, R., & Dodd, B. (1980). Hearing by eye. *Quarterly Journal of Experimental Psychology, 32,* 85–99.

Campbell, R., MacSweeney, M., Surguladze, S., Calvert, G., McGuire, P. K., Suckling, J., et al. (2001). Cortical substrates for the perception of face actions: An fMRI study of the specificity of activation for seen speech and for meaningless lower face acts. *Cognitive Brain Research, 12,* 233–243.

Corina, D. P. (1998). The processing of sign language: Evidence from aphasia. In B. Stemmer & H. Whitaker (Eds.), *Handbook of neurolinguistics* (pp. 313–329). New York: Academic Press.

Corina, D. P., & McBurney, S. L. (2001). The neural representation of language in users of American Sign Language. *Journal of Communication Disorders, 34,* 455–471.

Emmorey, K. (2001). *Language, cognition, and the brain: Insights from sign language research.* Mahwah, NJ: Erlbaum.

Emmorey, K., Allen, J. S., Bruss, J., Schenker, D., & Damasio, H. (2003). A morphometric analysis of auditory brain regions in congenitally deaf adults. *Proceedings of the National Academy of Sciences, USA, 100,* 10049–10054.

Fink, G. R., Halligan, P. W., Marshall, J. C., Frith, C. D., Frackowiak, R. S., & Dolan, R. J. (1997). Neural mechanisms involved in the processing of global and local aspects of hierarchically organized visual stimuli. *Brain, 120,* 1779–1791.

Finney, E. M., & Dobkins, K. R. (2001). Visual contrast sensitivity in deaf versus hearing populations: Exploring the perceptual consequences of auditory deprivation and experience with a visual language. *Cognitive Brain Research, 11,* 171–183.

Finney, E. M., Fine, I., & Dobkins, K. R. (2001). Visual stimuli activate auditory cortex in the deaf. *Nature Neuroscience, 4,* 1171–1173.

Fowler, C. A., & Dekle, D. J. (1991). Listening with eye and hand: Cross-modal contributions to speech perception. *Journal of Experimental Psychology: Human Perception and Performance, 17,* 816–828.

Giraud, A. L., Price, C. J., Graham, J. M., Truy, E., & Frackowiak, R. S. J. (2001). Cross-modal plasticity underpins language recovery after cochlear implantation. *Neuron, 30,* 657–663.

Griffiths, T. D., Büchel, C., Frackowiak, R. S. J., & Patterson, R. D. (1998). Analysis of temporal structure in sound by the human brain. *Nature Neuroscience, 1,* 422–427.

Hackett, T. A., Preuss, T. M., & Kaas, J. H. (2001). Architectonic identification of the core region in auditory cortex of macaques, chimpanzees, and humans. *Journal of Comparative Neurology, 441,* 197–222.

Hickok, G., Bellugi, U., & Klima, E. S. (1996). The neurobiology of sign language and its implications for the neural basis of language. *Nature, 381,* 699–702.

Hickok, G., Bellugi, U., & Klima, E. (1998). What's right about the neural organisation of sign language? A perspective on recent neuroimaging results. *Trends in Cognitive Sciences, 2,* 465–468.

Klima, E., & Bellugi, U. (1979). *The signs of language.* Cambridge, MA: Harvard University Press.

Klinke, R., Krai, A., Heid, S., Tillein, J., & Hartmann, R. (1999). Recruitment of the auditory cortex in congenitally deaf cats by longterm cochlear electrostimulation. *Science, 285,* 1729–1733.

Kuriki, S., Takeuchi, F., & Hirata, Y. (1998). Neural processing of words in the human extrastriate visual cortex. *Brain Research: Cognitive Brain Research, 63,* 193–203.

Lee, D. S., Lee, J. S., Oh, S. H., Kim, S. K., Kim, J. W., Chung, J. K., et al. (2001). Deafness: Cross-modal plasticity and cochlear implants. *Nature, 409,* 149–150.

Leonard, C. M., Puranik, C., Kuldau, J. M., & Lombardino, L. J. (1998). Normal variation in the frequency and location of human auditory cortex landmarks. Heschl's gyrus: Where is it? *Cerebral Cortex, 8,* 397–406.

Levänen, S., & Hamdorf, D. (2001). Feeling vibrations: Enhanced tactile sensitivity in congenitally deaf humans. *Neuroscience Letters, 301,* 75–77.

Levänen, S., Jousmaki, R., & Hari, R. (1998). Vibration-induced auditory-cortex activation in a congenitally deaf adult. *Current Biology, 8,* 869–872.

Levänen, S., Uutela, K., Salenius, S., & Haari, R. (2001). Cortical representation of sign language: Comparisons of deaf signers and hearing non-signers. *Cerebral Cortex, 11,* 506–512.

Leybaert, J. (2000). Phonology acquired through the eyes and spelling in deaf children. *Journal of Experiment Child Psychology, 75,* 291–318.

Leybaert, J., Alegria, J., Hage, C., & Charlier, B. (1998). The effect of exposure to phonetically augmented speech in the prelingually deaf. In R. Campbell, B. Dodd, & D. Burnham (Eds.), *Hearing by eye II* (pp. 283–302). Hove, England: Psychology Press.

Liddell, S. K. (1980). *American Sign Language syntax.* The Hague: Mouton.

Luria, A. R. (1973). *The working brain.* London: Penguin Books.

MacSweeney, M., Amaro, E., Calvert, G. A., Campbell, R., David, A. S., McGuire, P. K., et al. (2000). Activation of auditory cortex by silent speechreading in the absence of scanner noise: An event-related fMRI study. *Neuroreport, 11,* 1729–1734.

MacSweeney, M., Calvert, G. A., Campbell, R., McGuire, P. K., David, A. S., Williams, S. C. R., et al. (2002). Speechreading circuits in people born deaf. *Neuropsychologia, 40,* 801–807.

MacSweeney, M., Campbell, R., Calvert, G. A., McGuire, P. K., David, A. S., Suckling, J., et al. (2001). Activation of audi-

tory cortex by speechreading in congenitally deaf people. *Proceedings of the Royal Society of London, Series B: Biological Sciences, 26,* 451–457.

MacSweeney, M., Campbell, R., Woll, B., Amaro, E., McGuire, P. K., Calvert, G. A., et al. (2003). *Auditory cortex in deaf people can be activated by biological non-linguistic movement: An fMRI study of BSL and gesture perception.* Unpublished manuscript.

MacSweeney, M., Woll, B., Campbell, R., Calvert, G. A., McGuire, P. K., David, A. S., et al. (2002). Neural correlates of British Sign Language processing: Specific regions for topographic language? *Journal of Cognitive Neuroscience, 14,* 1064–1075.

MacSweeney, M., Woll, B., Campbell, R., McGuire, P. K., David, A. S., Williams, S. C. R., et al. (2002). Neural systems underlying British Sign Language and audiovisual English processing in native users. *Brain, 125,* 1583–1593.

McGurk, H., & MacDonald, J. (1976). Hearing lips and seeing voices. *Nature, 264,* 746–748.

McGuire, P. K., Robertson, D., Thacker, A., David, A. S., Kitson, N., Frackowiak, R. S. J., et al. (1996). Neural correlates of thinking in sign language. *Neuroreport, 8,* 695–698.

Mehler, J., & Christophe, A. (1994). Language in the infant's mind. *Philosophical Transactions of the Royal Society of London, Series B: Biological Sciences, 346,* 13–20.

Mogford, K. (1987). Lip-reading in the prelingually deaf. In B. Dodd & R. Campbell (Eds.), *Hearing by eye: The psychology of lip-reading* (pp. 191–211). Hillsdale, NJ: Erlbaum.

Neville, H. J., Bavelier, D., Corina, D. P., Rauschecker, R., Karni, J. P., Karni, A., et al. (1998). Cerebral organization for language in deaf and hearing subjects: Biological constraints and effects of experience. *Proceedings of the National Academy of Sciences, USA, 90,* 922–929.

Neville, H., & Lawson, D. (1987). Attention to central and peripheral visual space in a movement detection task: An event-related potential and behavioral study. II. Congenitally deaf adults. *Brain Research, 405,* 268–283.

Nishimura, H., Hashikawa, K., Doi, K., Iwaki, T., Watanabe, Y., Kusuoka, H., et al. (1999). Sign language "heard" in the auditory cortex. *Nature, 397,* 116.

Okazawa, H., Naito, Y., Yonekura, Y., Sadato, N., Hirano, S., Nishizawa, S., et al. (1996). Cochlear implant efficiency in pre- and post-lingually deaf subjects: A study with H2 (15)0 and PET. *Brain, 119,* 1297–1306.

Paulesu, E., & Mehler, J. (1998). Right on in sign language. *Nature, 392,* 233–234.

Petitto, L., Katerelos, M., Levy, B. G., Gauna, K., Tetreault, K., & Ferraro, V. (2001). Bilingual signed and spoken language acquisition from birth: Implications for the mechanisms underlying early bilingual language acquisition. *Journal of Child Language, 28,* 453–459.

Petitto, L., Zatorre, R. J., Gauna, K., Nikelski, E. J., Dostie, D., & Evans, A. C. (2000). Speechlike cerebral activity in profoundly deaf people processing signed languages: Implications for the neural basis of human language. *Proceedings of the National Academy of Sciences, USA, 97,* 13961–13966.

Poizner, H., Klima, E., & Bellugi, U. (1987). *What the hands reveal about the brain.* Cambridge, Mass.: MIT Press.

Rönnberg, J., Söderfeldt, B., & Risberg, J. (2000). The cognitive neuroscience of sign language. *Acta Psychologica, 105,* 237–254.

Sacks, O. (1989). *Seeing voices: A journey into the world of the deaf.* Berkeley: University of California Press.

Söderfeldt, B., Rönnberg, J., & Risberg, J. (1994). Regional cerebral blood flow in sign language users. *Brain and Language, 46,* 59–68.

Söderfeldt, B., Ingvar, M., Rönnberg, J., Eriksson, L., Serrander, M., & Stone-Elander, S. (1997). Signed and spoken language perception studied by positron emission tomography. *Neurology, 49,* 82–87.

Summerfield, A. Q. (1987). Some preliminaries to a comprehensive account of audio-visual speech perception. In B. Dodd & R. Campbell (Eds.), *Hearing by eye: The psychology of lip-reading.* Hillsdale, NJ: Erlbaum.

Sutton-Spence, R., & Woll, B. (1999). *The linguistics of BSL: An introduction.* Cambridge, UK: Cambridge University Press.

Vygotsky, L. S. (1962). *Thought and language.* Cambridge, MA: MIT Press.

Vygotsky, L. S. (1978). *Mind in society.* Cambridge, MA: Harvard University Press.

Wise, R. J. S., Scott, S. K., Blank, S. C., Mummery, C. J., Murphy, K., & Warburton, E. A. (2001). Separate neural subsystems within "Wernicke's" area. *Brain, 124,* 83–95.

VIII PERSPECTIVES DERIVED FROM CLINICAL STUDIES

49 Multisensory Integration: Resolving Ambiguities for Human Postural Control

LESLIE ALLISON AND JOHN J. JEKA

Introduction

Upright bipedal stance in humans may appear to be primarily an issue of musculoskeletal control; however, information from multiple sensory sources is crucial for normal balance function. Deficits in sensory integration processes are often suspected as an underlying source of balance disorders in individuals who have sustained brain changes due to disease, trauma, or aging. Rather than merely enhancing the resolution of a percept, sensory information from multiple modalities is essential to resolve ambiguities inherent to controlling the upright, multilinked, unstable human body. The focus of this chapter is a particularly important aspect of sensory integration for postural control: multisensory reweighting. Balance maintenance involves constant updating and prioritization of the sensory information generated by the surrounding environment (e.g., visual flow) and by self-motion (e.g., vestibular, proprioceptive). This updating and prioritizing process, which we refer to as *multisensory reweighting*, remains poorly understood. The first part of the discussion, then, reviews recently developed techniques that allow precise quantification of multisensory reweighting in the context of human postural control.

Postural control is achieved through a complex process involving the reception and integration of sensory inputs, motor planning, and muscular execution. To prevent balance loss, sensory systems must determine and monitor the position of the center of mass (COM) in relation to the body's base of support so that motor systems can control the COM and prevent it from exceeding its limits of stability. Correct estimation of COM position is reliant on multisensory integration, for two reasons. First, the COM is a calculated point in space that cannot be directly detected by any single sense. COM position must be derived from information gathered from three separate sensory modalities, the visual, vestibular, and somatosensory systems. Second,

each of these individual sensory modalities provides information that is often ambiguous; information from other senses is required to resolve these ambiguities. Despite the critical dependence of postural control on multisensory integration for COM estimation, the mechanisms underlying multisensory integration for postural control are essentially unknown.

The three primary peripheral sensory inputs contributing to postural control are the bilateral receptors of the somatosensory, visual, and vestibular systems. Each of the three sensory systems provides both unique and redundant information for postural control. Somatosensory receptors located in the joints, ligaments, muscles, and skin provide information about muscle length, stretch, tension, and contraction; pain, temperature, and pressure; and joint position. Central (or focal) vision allows environmental orientation, contributing to the perception of verticality and object motion. Peripheral (or ambient) vision detects the motion of the self in relation to the environment, including head movements and postural sway. Central visual inputs tend to receive more conscious recognition, but both are normally used for postural control. The vestibular system provides information about the motion of the head and its position in relation to gravity and other inertial forces.

Yet ambiguities exist within each sense (intrasensory conflict). Figure 49.1 illustrates inherent ambiguities associated with sensory systems that are important for postural control. The somatosensory system alone cannot distinguish between a change in surface tilt and changes in body inclination. The visual system alone cannot necessarily discriminate motion in the environment from self-motion. The vestibular system alone cannot determine whether head motion signaled by the semicircular canals is caused by flexion at the neck or flexion at the hips, or whether head motion signaled by the otoliths is due to head tilt or to linear acceleration or deceleration.

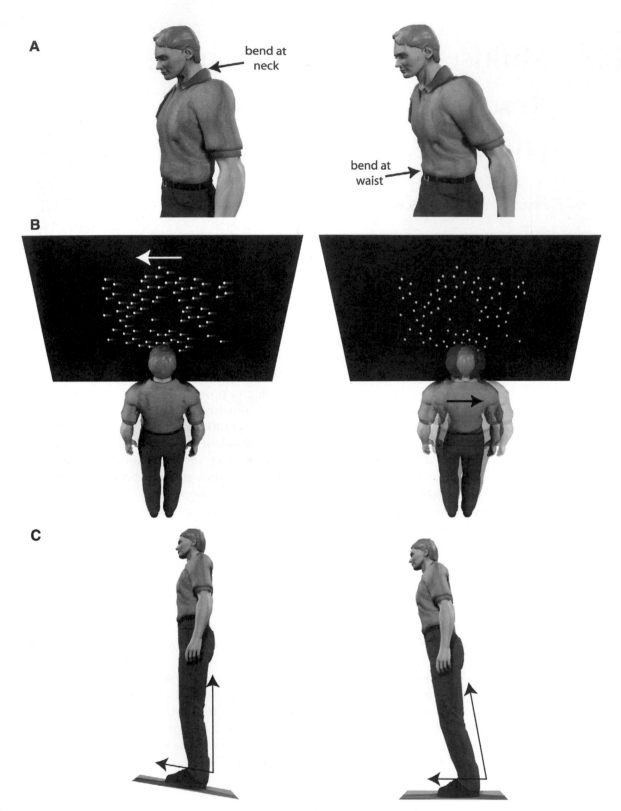

FIGURE 49.1 Each sensory system alone provides ambiguous information about body dynamics. (*A*) The vestibular system provides similar information when the head is tilted and when the trunk tilts at the waist. Somatosensory information from the neck or trunk is needed to resolve the ambiguity. (*B*) The visual system alone cannot resolve visual field motion generated from extrinsic movements in the surround versus intrinsic self-motion. Somatosensory and vestibular information about self-movement may resolve this ambiguity. (*C*) A change in ankle inclination due to forward body sway cannot be distinguished from the same ankle angle produced by support surface tilt without visual flow or vestibular information.

Multisensory integration permits resolution of these ambiguities by using information received simultaneously through other senses that may or may not be consistent with the information gained from a single modality. For example, somatosensation from neck and trunk muscles can resolve the problem of whether head motion is caused by neck versus hip flexion, and vision can resolve the problem of whether head motion is caused by head tilt versus linear acceleration or deceleration. Typically, body movements in space produce consistent information from all three senses. When one leans forward, the sensations experienced include pressure on the toes and stretch of the calf muscles (somatosensation), posterior peripheral visual flow and retinal image enlargement (vision), and forward head acceleration/deceleration. These sensations are collectively perceived as a forward body lean. Thus, accurate estimates of the COM are based on information from all three sensory systems involved in postural control.

Sensory ambiguities can also arise when information between systems is not synchronous (intersensory conflict). Multisensory integration must then function to resolve the ambiguity by recognizing any discrepancies and selecting the most useful inputs on which to base motor commands. For example, a driver stopped still at a red light suddenly hits the brake when an adjacent vehicle begins to roll: movement of the other car detected by the peripheral visual system is momentarily misperceived as self-motion. In this situation, the vestibular and somatosensory systems do not detect motion, but the forward visual flow is interpreted as backward motion. Because the brain failed to suppress the (mismatched) visual inputs, the braking response was generated. To resolve conflicts between two inconsistent sensory inputs, information from a third source may be necessary.

Sensory reweighting

A generally held view of the postural control system is that multiple sensory inputs are dynamically reweighted to maintain upright stance as sensory conditions change (Horak & Macpherson, 1996). Precise estimation of self-orientation is particularly important when an individual is confronted with new environmental conditions that require an immediate updating of the relative importance of different sources of sensory information. Environmental changes such as moving from a light to a dark room or from a smooth to an uneven support surface (e.g., from a paved road to a rocky surface) require an updating of sensory weights to current conditions so that muscular commands are based on the most precise and reliable sensory information

available. The ability to select and reweight alternative orientation references adaptively is considered one of the most critical factors in postural control in patient and elderly populations (Horak, Shupert, & Mirka, 1989).

The effects of sensory reweighting on postural control are difficult to characterize because postural control involves both sensory and motor processes. The most common research measure of postural control is the mean amplitude of postural sway, a behavioral "end-product" influenced by closely entwined sensory and motor mechanisms. Any interpretation of changes in postural sway behavior arising from sensory reweighting must eliminate the possibility that such changes are due to alterations in the motor components of the control system. Much of the current evidence for sensory reweighting is heavily reliant on a clinical protocol that selectively alters sensory information from either vision or somatosensation, or both. The Sensory Organization Test (SOT) uses a hydraulically controlled support platform and visual surround, pictured in Figure 49.2, both of which may be servo-linked to a person's body sway (NeuroCom International, Clackamas, OR; see Jacobson, Newman, & Kartush, 1997, for a description). The support surface is a force plate that detects body sway precisely. With such a device, changes in ankle angle that typically accompany forward and backward movements of the body can be attenuated by rotating the support surface around the axis of the ankle. Similarly, the visual surround can also be moved forward and backward with anterior-posterior body sway, negating any visual flow that typically accompanies such body movements. The movements of the support surface or visual surround are "sway-referenced" to the movements of the body. The SOT consists of a series of six different conditions, schematically shown in Figure 49.2, that allow postural performance to be compared under various combinations of visual, vestibular, and somatosensory information. For example, when the support surface is sway-referenced and the eyes are closed (SOT condition 5) or when both the support surface and the visual surround are sway-referenced (SOT condition 6), the individual is left with primarily vestibular information to maintain upright stance. Many patient populations and elderly individuals with balance problems fall immediately in SOT conditions 5 and 6, while young, healthy individuals are able to maintain upright stance (Woollacott, Shumway-Cook, & Nashner, 1986), although with significantly greater postural sway. Poor performance under these altered sensory conditions is widely interpreted as evidence of sensory reweighting deficits. This conclusion is intuitively appealing, because the motor demands of the standing

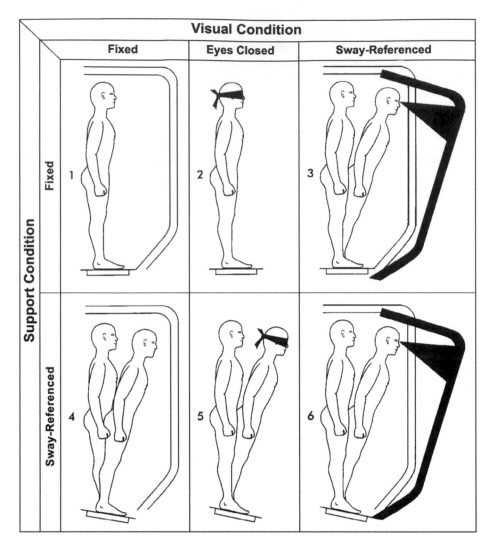

FIGURE 49.2   The Sensory Organization Test measures postural sway during quiet stance in six sensory conditions. Visual and somatosensory inputs are systematically manipulated to create environments in which one or both senses are rendered unusable for estimation of body position in space. *Condition 1:* Eyes open, on a fixed surface, all senses available and accurate. *Condition 2:* Eyes closed, on a fixed surface, vision absent. *Condition 3:* Visual surround sway-referenced, vision inaccurate. Both conditions 2 and 3 force reliance on somatosensory and vestibular inputs. *Condition 4:* Support surface sway-referenced, somatosensation inaccurate to induce reliance on vision and vestibular inputs. *Condition 5:* Eyes closed, on a sway-referenced surface, vision absent, and somatosensation inaccurate. *Condition 6:* Visual surround and support surface sway-referenced, vision and somatosensation inaccurate. Both conditions 5 and 6 induce sole reliance on vestibular inputs.

task are not changing but the sensory conditions under which balance must be maintained are changing. In our view, however, such evidence does not necessarily support sensory reweighting as the sole mechanism underlying changes in body sway, because measures of sway cannot by themselves distinguish whether the changes are dependent upon adaptations in sensory processes, motor processes, or some combination of the two.

For the past several years, we have been developing a quantitative model of how the nervous system might integrate sensory information for postural control (for modeling details, see Kiemel, Oie, & Jeka, in press; Oie, Kiemel, & Jeka, in press). The model contains parameters that characterize the stability of the postural control system (e.g., damping, stiffness) controlled by motor processes, as well as parameters that reflect how strongly the postural system is coupled to sensory information. The important point is that a change in virtually any parameter in the model can lead to changes in body sway similar to those observed in studies claiming reweighting of sensory inputs. For example, the increased loss of balance observed in elderly individuals when compared with younger adults on the SOT could be due to a change in stability parameters, a change in sensory weights, or both. Without directly testing experimental data relative to a quantitative model, it is impossible to identify the source of change within the nervous system. This limitation is important, because the source of change in balance control may vary from one population to the next, even though the effect on measures such as mean sway amplitude may be relatively similar.

The concept of reweighting as discussed above makes the prediction that changes in postural response in different sensory conditions should be due to changes in sensory weights. However, it is also possible that postural system parameters that are more related to musculoskeletal control may change instead of or in addition to changes in sensory weights. In the next section we illustrate a new technique that clearly attributes changes in postural sway to changes in sensory weights rather than to changes in the control strategy. Furthermore, we present preliminary data from an elderly population identified as at risk for falling. Even though standard measures from the SOT would suggest a sensory reweighting deficit in this population, the techniques we have developed provide clear evidence of multisensory reweighting in these fall-prone older adults.

Multisensory integration: The light-touch/vision paradigm

One of the primary methods to investigate sensorimotor integration in postural control evolved from linear systems analysis. An individual is typically "driven" by an oscillating pattern of sensory information. The resulting postural or orientation responses of the body are measured to determine "system" control properties. For example, the sinusoidal vertical axis rotation (SVAR) technique rotates seated subjects at a range of frequencies to measure the gain and phase of eye movements in the dark as an assessment of vestibular function (Howard, 1982; Krebs, Gill-Body, Riley, & Parker, 1993). Similarly, an oscillating visual "moving room" has been used to demonstrate the coupling of visual information with whole-body posture (Berthoz, Lacour, & Soechting, 1979; Dijkstra, Schöner, & Gielen, 1994; Dijkstra, Schöner, Giese, & Gielen, 1994; Lee & Lishman, 1975; Peterka & Benolken, 1995; Soechting & Berthoz, 1979; Talbott & Brookhart, 1980; van Asten, Gielen, & Denier van der Gon, 1988). These techniques have established that rate information is derived from sensory stimuli; that is, the vestibular system provides information about the angular acceleration of the head and the linear acceleration of the body (Benson, 1982), while the visual system is sensitive to the velocity of a stimulus (Dijkstra, Schöner, Giese, et al., 1994; Schöner, 1991).

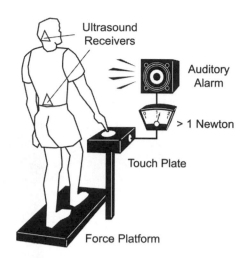

FIGURE 49.3   A subject standing on the force platform with his right index fingertip on the touch plate positioned at waist level. For the sake of illustration, the alarm is shown sounding due to an applied force on the touch plate of >1 N. This typically occurs on less than 2% of all experimental trials.

We have developed similar techniques to study the properties of somatosensory coupling to posture. In a series of studies, we have demonstrated that somatosensory cues derived from light-touch fingertip contact to a stationary surface provide orientation information for improved control of upright stance (Holden, Ventura, & Lackner, 1994; Jeka, Easton, Bentzen, & Lackner, 1996; Jeka & Lackner, 1994, 1995). Figure 49.3 illustrates the light-touch paradigm. Subjects stand in a tandem stance while maintaining fingertip contact with a stationary plate that measures the applied forces. Ultrasound receivers measure head and approximate COM kinematics. An auditory alarm sounds if above-threshold fingertip forces are applied, signaling the subject to reduce the applied force without losing contact with the plate. In general, the task is easy for healthy young subjects to execute. After one practice trial, participants rarely set off the alarm. The results have consistently shown that light-touch contact (<1 N) with the fingertip to a rigid surface attenuates postural sway just as well as mechanical contact of 10–20 N. Furthermore, the influence of fingertip contact with a moving surface on whole-body posture is as dramatic as with full-field visual displays (Jeka, Oie, Schöner, Dijkstra, & Henson, 1998; Jeka, Schöner, Dijkstra, Ribeiro, & Lackner, 1997). When the contact surface moves sinusoidally, postural sway adopts the frequency of contact surface motion. The predictions of a second-order, linear model support the hypothesis that body sway is coupled to the contact surface through the velocity of the somatosensory stimulus at the fingertip. More recent studies have replicated and extended these light-touch findings to other task

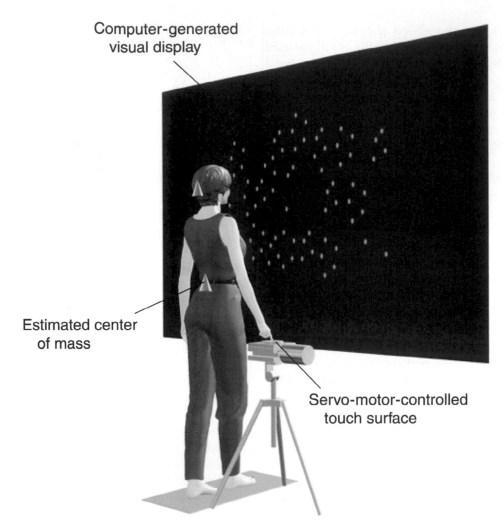

Computer-generated
visual display

Estimated center
of mass

Servo-motor-controlled
touch surface

FIGURE 49.4   Vision and light touch experimental setup. The participant is shown in a modified tandem stance standing in front of the visual display while contacting the touch surface with her right fingertip. The visual display and the touch plate can be stationary or computer-controlled to move at any frequency and amplitude.

situations (Clapp & Wing, 1999; Dickstein, Shupert, & Horak, 2001; Reginella, Redfern, & Furman, 1999; Riley, Wong, Mitra, & Turvey, 1997).

We have developed a new multisensory experimental paradigm using light-touch contact in combination with vision as sources of sensory information for postural control. Figure 49.4 shows the experimental setup. An advantage of using light-touch contact as a sensory source is that, like vision, it is easily manipulated (i.e., it is easy to add, remove, or vary its movement frequency and amplitude), making it possible to precisely vary vision and touch relative to one another and to investigate multisensory integration with regard to postural control.

In a recent study using the light-touch/vision paradigm, Oie et al. (in press) tested whether changes in postural sway could be attributed to multisensory reweighting of light touch and vision. Healthy young subjects were presented with sinusoidal 0.20 Hz visual display motion and sinusoidal 0.28 Hz fingertip touch surface motion. These frequencies were chosen at a ratio of approximately $\sqrt{2}$ to avoid overlapping harmonics in the stimuli. The peak amplitudes of the visual and somatosensory stimuli motion were manipulated in five conditions (vision:touch amplitude [mm]: 2:8, 2:4, 2:2, 4:2, 8:2). Figure 49.5 shows the stimuli and center of mass response from a 2:4 vision-touch trial. Figure 49.6 shows the frequency spectra of the visual, touch, and COM signals. Peaks in the COM signal at the frequencies corresponding to the visual and touch stimuli illustrate that body sway is responding to both stimuli simultaneously. Separating the response of the body to vision from the response of the body to touch in the frequency spectrum enables precise quantification of how vision and touch interact.

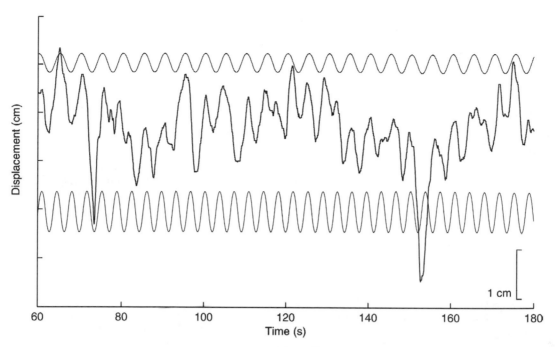

FIGURE 49.5 Exemplar time series. A 180 s segment of data showing the time series of visual display motion at 0.2 Hz with amplitude of 2 mm (upper trace), center of mass displacement (middle trace), and touch surface motion at 0.28 Hz with amplitude of 4 mm (lower trace).

Three different reweighting scenarios are possible in this situation: (1) no reweighting, (2) intramodality reweighting, and (3) intermodality reweighting (Fig. 49.7). No reweighting would be indicated by constant gain for both vision and touch across conditions, depicted in Figure 49.7A. Constant gain implies that no matter what amplitudes of sensory motion are provided from vision and touch, the same relative response amplitude is observed. Even though previous evidence makes a constant gain response unlikely (e.g., Peterka & Benolken, 1995), constant gain may be observed if stimulus parameters were chosen incorrectly. For example, if the stimulus amplitude was large enough to be easily discernible from self-motion, a weak postural response would be predicted, with a potential "basement" effect across conditions.

Intramodality reweighting would be evident if changes in stimulus amplitude were followed by corresponding changes in gain, but only within a particular modality. Figure 49.7B illustrates the intramodality scenario. Note that visual gain changes only in response to changes in visual stimulus amplitude (e.g., from condition 8:2 to 4:2) and touch gain changes only in response to changes in touch stimulus amplitude (e.g., from condition 2:8 to condition 2:4). Such results would indicate that the modalities operate in a relatively independent manner. Finally, Figure 49.7C illustrates results indica-

tive of both intramodality and intermodality reweighting. Note that changes in visual gain are observed not only when visual stimulus amplitude changes (e.g., from condition 8:2 to 4:2—intramodality reweighting), but also when touch stimulus amplitude changes (e.g., from condition 2:4 to 2:8—intermodality reweighting). Similar effects would be predicted for the influence of vision on touch gain (i.e., black squares in Figure 49.7C). The fact that changes in gain to vision and touch are dependent on both vision and touch would argue for both an intramodality and intermodality dependence. While intramodality reweighting is commonly observed (e.g., Peterka & Benolken, 1995), until recently there was no rigorous evidence for intermodality reweighting in the posture literature (Oie et al., 2002).

The results from Oie et al. (2002) clearly showed both an intra- and intermodality dependence on stimulus amplitude. For example, Figure 49.8 shows results from two exemplar subjects who showed both intramodality and intermodality reweighting. COM gain relative to touch (i.e., touch gain) increases from the 2:8 to the 2:4 condition. This increase in touch gain in response to a decrease in touch stimulus amplitude, interpreted as intramodality reweighting, is expected because previous results have shown that an increase in stimulus amplitude typically leads to a smaller response in body sway (e.g., Peterka & Benolken, 1995), most

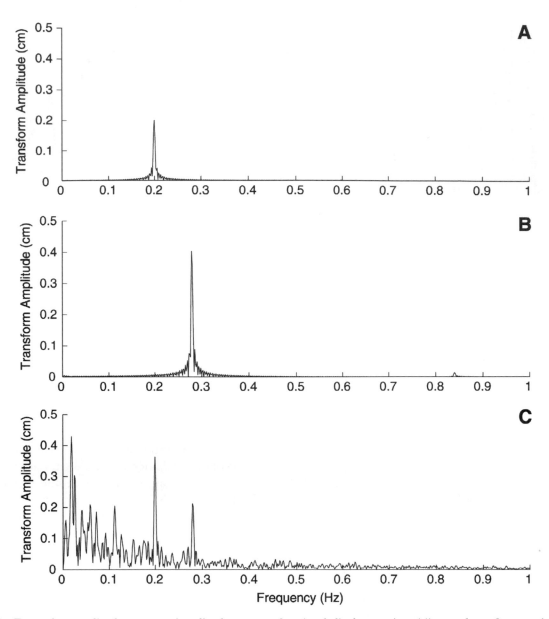

FIGURE 49.6   Exemplar amplitude spectra. Amplitude spectra for visual display motion (*A*), touch surface motion (*B*), and center of mass (COM) displacement (*C*) shown in Figure 49.5. Note the peaks in the COM spectrum corresponding to the visual and touch frequencies, indicating that body sway is responding to both stimuli simultaneously.

likely because a larger stimulus amplitude is more easily discernible from self-motion. The accompanying decrease of vision gain from the 2:8 to the 2:4 condition, however, cannot be due to visual stimulus amplitude, which is constant between these two conditions. The visual gain decrease is attributable to the decrease in touch stimulus amplitude, a clear instance of intermodality reweighting. Similar instances of intermodality reweighting can be observed across other conditions. We refer to this effect as *inverse gain reweighting*. To our knowledge, such intermodality reweighting has never been shown.

Fitting a third-order time series model to the sway trajectories provided additional evidence that changes in gain were due to sensory reweighting (for modeling details, see Oie et al., 2002). In terms of our theoretical framework, the fact that the two gains changed in opposite directions implies that the changes in gain are due to changes in estimation dynamics (i.e., sensory reweighting), not to changes in control dynamics. For example, if increasing the touch plate amplitude increased the stiffness and eigenfrequency associated with the control parameters of the model, then both gains would be expected to decrease. These fits showed

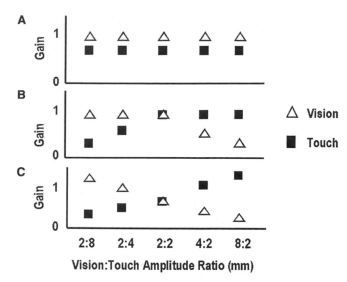

FIGURE 49.7 Hypothetical multisensory reweighting scenarios. (*A*) No reweighting: vision and touch gains are constant across conditions. (*B*) Intramodality reweighting: vision gain changes only when visual stimuli amplitudes change, and touch gain changes only when touch stimuli amplitudes change. (*C*) Intermodality and intramodality reweighting: vision gain changes in response to changes in touch stimulus amplitude (intermodality) and visual stimulus amplitude (intramodality); touch gain changes in response to changes in visual stimulus amplitude (intermodality) and touch stimulus amplitude (intramodality).

no significance dependence of the control parameters on the stimulus amplitudes (see Oie et al., 2002).

The techniques summarized in this section have allowed intermodality reweighting to be identified rigorously, to our knowledge, for the first time. A crucial aspect of the design was to present stimuli from different modalities at different frequencies so that the

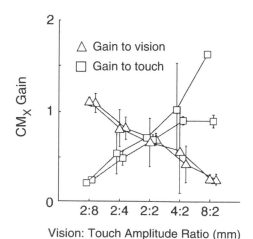

FIGURE 49.8 Inverse gain reweighting. Vision and touch gains from two healthy young subjects demonstrate both intra- and intermodality reweighting (see text for details).

response to each stimulus could be quantified separately, thus revealing their inherent interdependence. Moreover, fitting the data to model parameters ruled out any contribution from other aspects of the postural control system (e.g., nonlinear stiffness). These same techniques can now be applied to populations that have been previously hypothesized to have deficits in sensory reweighting, namely, the unstable elderly.

Sensory reweighting in the fall-prone elderly population

Central sensory selection and reweighting processes are thought to degrade with increasing age and are hypothesized to be particularly deficient in fall-prone versus healthy older adults (Alexander, 1994; Horak et al., 1989; Woollacott, 2000). Previous studies using the SOT paradigm described earlier found that postural sway in healthy older adults is very similar to that in young adults under conditions in which only one sense is altered (vision *or* somatosensory), but is significantly greater in conditions where both vision and somatosensory cues were disrupted (SOT conditions 5 and 6) (Baloh, Corona, Jacobson, & Enrietto, 1998; Baloh, Fife, & Zwerling, 1994; Shepard, Schultz, Alexander, Gu, Boisemier, 1993; Whipple, Wolfson, Derby, Singh, & Tobin, 1993). Young adults very rarely actually lost their balance during the SOT trials, while 20% of healthy older adults lost their balance *on the first trial* of conditions in which one input was sway-referenced, and 40% fell on the first trial of conditions in which both inputs were sway-referenced. These healthy older adults showed far fewer losses of balance on subsequent trials of the same conditions, indicating rapid adaptation to the altered environmental demands (Horak et al., 1989; Wolfson, Whipple, Derby, et al., 1992; Woollacott et al., 1986). One study found that healthy older adults standing on a sway-referenced surface had fewer losses of balance with no visual input (eyes closed, SOT condition 5) than with conflicting visual inputs (sway-referenced visual surround, SOT condition 6), reflecting a deficit in central suppression of inaccurate visual cues (Whipple et al., 1993).

Older adults with a history of falls or a high risk of falling were found to differ from healthy, age-matched counterparts on these tests of sensory integration. They failed to adapt to altered sensory conditions, often losing balance repeatedly despite continued exposure to the sensory condition (Horak et al., 1989; Whipple & Wolfson, 1989). Fallers demonstrated greater instability in conditions where only one sensory input was altered compared to their healthy counterparts (Anacker & DiFabio, 1992; Baloh, Spain, Socotch, Jacobson, & Bell,

1995; Shumway-Cook & Woollacott, 2000). They are hypothesized to be more visually dependent, failing to use reliable somatosensory cues in environments where visual inputs are unstable (Simoneau et al., 1999; Sundermier, Woollacott, Jensen, & Moore, 1996).

Age-related peripheral sensory loss is well documented and is hypothesized by some to be the primary reason why older adults lose their orientation sense (Whipple & Wolfson, 1989; Woollacott, 1993; Woollacott et al., 1986). Naturally, central sensory integration processes cannot successfully produce accurate estimations of spatial position if incoming information is inadequate. Substantial support exists, however, for the notion that central processing deficits play a major role in age-related balance decline (Stelmach, Teasdale, DiFabio, & Phillips, 1989; Teasdale, Bard, LaRue, & Fleury, 1993; Teasdale, Stelmach, & Breunig, 1991; Teasdale, Stelmach, Breunig, & Meeuwsen, 1991). Older adults who perform balance exercises designed to challenge the sensory systems demonstrate improved balance (Hu & Woollacott, 1994; Ledin et al., 1991; Rose & Clark, 2000). Obviously, such improvements cannot be attributed to a reversal of peripheral sensory loss, and instead are thought to reflect improved sensory integration processing.

Are central sensory reweighting deficits responsible, at least in part, for the postural control problems seen in healthy and fall-prone older adults? Conclusions from previous research seem to indicate so. Earlier studies, however, typically used postural sway measures such as mean sway amplitude that by themselves cannot determine whether changes in sway are due to changes in control parameters (motor processes), coupling parameters (sensory processes), or some combination of both (e.g., Anacker & DiFabio, 1992; Horak et al., 1989; Whipple & Wolfson, 1989; see also College et al., 1994). Many earlier studies also did not use careful controls for peripheral sensory loss, which if present may have confounded their results (e.g., Sundermier et al., 1996; Teasdale et al., 1991). Using the two-frequency light-touch/vision paradigm described above we are investigating hypothesized sensory reweighting deficits in fall-prone older adults (average age 83 years). Elderly subjects are excluded from the study if they have any medical diagnoses known to produce sensory deficits (e.g., diabetes, macular degeneration, vestibulopathy) or if they are found to have sensory loss on a clinical neurological screening. Subjects perform both the SOT and the two-frequency light-touch/vision tests. Preliminary results (first seven subjects out of 20 planned), shown in Figure 49.9, indicate that the subjects' performance on the SOT is consistent with prior research, that is, they have great difficulty remaining stable under conditions in which vision and somatosensory

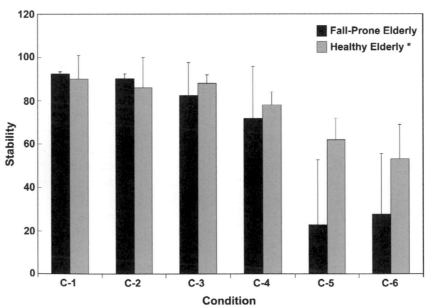

FIGURE 49.9 Sensory Organization Test results: mean stability scores for the fall-prone older adults (n = 7) and healthy older adults (*normative data from the manufacturer). High stability reflects little postural sway; low stability reflects excessive postural sway. Performance under conditions in which only one sense was altered at a time was not significantly different between the two groups, but fall-prone subjects were much less stable than their healthy counterparts when both vision and somatosensation were altered (conditions 5 and 6).

inputs are altered simultaneously (SOT conditions 5 and 6). Because subjects with vestibular deficits have been excluded from the study, poor performance on SOT conditions 5 and 6 implies that they have difficulty with sensory reweighting.

In contrast to the SOT results, the same group of subjects displayed clear evidence of multisensory reweighting on the two-frequency light-touch/vision experiment. Vision and touch gains for the fall-prone older adults versus a group of healthy young adults are shown in Figure 49.10. For the fall-prone older adults, intramodality reweighting is apparent for both modalities. Of note is the sharp decline in vision gain as the vision stimulus amplitude increased from 2:2 to 8:2, and the rise in touch gains as the touch stimulus amplitude decreased from 2:8 to 2:2. Intermodality reweighting is evident for vision, as there was a significant decrease in

the vision gain when the vision stimulus amplitude was constant while the touch stimulus amplitude was decreasing. Mean touch gains also rose (not significantly in these preliminary results) in conditions in which constant touch stimulus amplitudes were paired with increasing vision stimulus amplitudes. Thus, fall-prone elderly subjects showed a very similar pattern of gain change across conditions when compared with healthy young adults. Differences between the elderly and young groups are observed only in the absolute levels of gain, as the elderly showed larger gains in response to both vision and touch stimuli.

These data do not support the assumption that multisensory reweighting is deficient in fall-prone older adults. Rather, these unstable elderly subjects appear more coupled to and influenced by sensory stimuli than are healthy younger subjects. This is particularly so for the visual stimuli, potentially lending further support for "visual dependence" in this fall-prone population (Simoneau et al., 1999; Sundermier et al., 1996).

Summary

Sensory information from multiple modalities does not merely enhance balance control. Control of a multi-linked upright body with varying sensor locations would be impossible without multisensory information to resolve inherent ambiguities about body dynamics associated with any single modality. Moreover, as we have emphasized in this chapter, flexible adaptation to changing environmental conditions is a crucial component of everyday activity. Early studies of multisensory integration and postural control suggested a reweighting process in response to dramatic changes in the environment or nervous system (e.g., Nashner, 1982; Woollacott et al., 1989). More recent studies have shown that the nervous system is sensitive to extremely small changes in sensory conditions; sensory reweighting was observed in response to amplitude changes as small as 2 mm (e.g., Oie et al., 2002). The implication of such sensitivity is that the nervous system reweights multisensory information continually during normal everyday behavior in order to generate new estimates of the COM for upright stance control.

An important component of the new techniques reviewed here is the use of models to rule out aspects other than reweighting that could account for changes in the response to sensory stimulation. By fitting model parameters to the trajectories of postural sway, changes in gain to a sensory driving signal were attributed to sensory reweighting rather than to changes in control parameters such as stiffness (Oie et al., 2002). The ability to precisely identify the underlying source of change

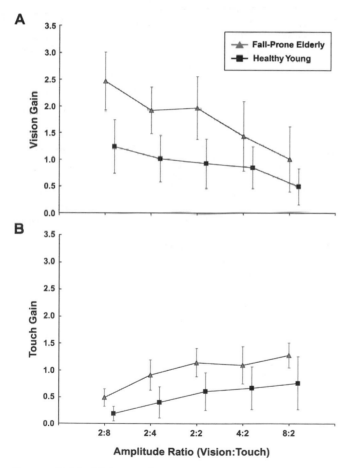

FIGURE 49.10 Vision and touch gains in fall-prone elderly versus young subjects. (A) Vision gains in both elderly and young subjects reflect both intramodality and intermodality reweighting. (B) Touch gains in both groups reflect intramodality but not intermodality reweighting. Vision and touch gains were significantly higher in the elderly than in the young across all amplitude ratio conditions.

is particularly important as different populations with balance problems are studied. Preliminary findings suggest, for example, that the underlying cause of balance problems in a group of elderly at-risk fallers is not a deficit in reweighting, as results from studies using the SOT suggest. In combination with the higher levels of sway amplitude observed in the elderly in both our two-frequency light-touch/vision protocol and the SOT, control parameters (e.g., damping, stiffness) for the elderly are expected to differ from young adults. Because fitting model parameters reliably requires a relatively large data set, confirmation of this prediction awaits the full set of 20 elderly fallers.

Many studies have cited "sensory selection" problems whenever abnormal levels of sway are observed in experimental conditions with an inaccurate sensory orientation reference. Such problems have been reported in stroke patients (DiFabio & Badke, 1990), traumatic brain injury patients (Shumway-Cook & Olmscheid, 1990), symptomatic elderly fallers (Black, Shupert, Horak, & Nashner, 1988; Horak et al., 1989) and children with developmental disorders (e.g., Nashner, Shumway-Cook, & Matin, 1983). We emphasize that such results are potentially related to multisensory reweighting deficits, but definitive evidence must be rigorously tested with a quantitative model to (1) show intra- and intermodality reweighting deficits, and (2) distinguish sensory reweighting deficits from changes in control parameters. The latter point is particularly important. Significant changes in the control strategy are probable with injured and aging nervous systems, and attributing differences in balance control to multisensory reweighting alone is in hindsight speculative.

ACKNOWLEDGMENTS Work was supported by National Institutes of Health grant R29 NS35070 and the Erickson Foundation (J. J. P.).

REFERENCES

Alexander, N. B. (1994). Postural control in older adults. *Journal of the American Geriatrics Society, 42,* 93–108.

Anacker, S. L., & DiFabio, R. P. (1992). Influence of sensory inputs on standing balance in community dwelling elders with a recent history of falling. *Physical Therapy, 72,* 575–584.

Baloh, R. W., Corona, S., Jacobson, K. M., Enrietto, J. A., & Bell, T. (1998). A prospective study of posturography in normal older people. *Journal of the American Geriatrics Society, 46,* 438–443.

Baloh, R. W., Fife, T. D., Zwerling, L., et al. (1994). Comparison of static and dynamic posturography in young and older normal people. *Journal of the American Geriatrics Society, 42,* 405–412.

Baloh, R. W., Spain, S., Socotch, T. M., Jacobson, K. M., & Bell, T. (1995). Posturography and balance problems in older people. *Journal of the American Geriatrics Society, 43,* 638–644.

Benson, A. J. (1982). The vestibular sensory system. In H. B. Barlow & J. D. Mollon (Eds.), *The senses* (pp. 333–368). New York: Cambridge University Press.

Berthoz, A., Lacour, M., Soechting, J. F., & Vidal, P. P. (1979). The role of vision in the control of posture during linear motion. *Progress in Brain Research, 50,* 197–209.

Black, F. O., Shupert, C., Horak, F. B., & Nashner, L. M. (1988). Abnormal postural control associated with peripheral vestibular disorders. In O. Pompeiano & J. Allum (Eds.), *Vestibulo-spinal control of posture and movement. Progress in Brain Research, 76,* 263–275.

Clapp, S., & Wing, A. M. (1999). Light touch contribution to balance in normal bipedal stance. *Experimental Brain Research, 125,* 521–524.

College, N. R., Cantley, P., Peaston, I., Brash, H., Lewis, S., & Wilson, J. A. (1994). Ageing and balance: The measurement of spontaneous sway by posturography. *Gerontology, 40,* 273–278.

Dickstein, R., Shupert, C. L., & Horak, F. B. (2001). Fingertip touch improves stability in patients with peripheral neuropathy. *Gait and Posture, 14,* 238–247.

DiFabio, R., & Badke, M. B. (1990). Relationship of sensory organization to balance function in patients with hemiplegia. *Physical Therapy, 70,* 543–552.

Dijkstra, T. M. H., Schöner, G., & Gielen, C. C. A. M. (1994). Temporal stability of the action-perception cycle for postural control in a moving visual environment. *Experimental Brain Research, 97,* 477–486.

Dijkstra, T. M. H., Schöner, G., Giese, M. A., & Gielen, C. C. A. M. (1994). Frequency dependence of the action-perception cycle for postural control in a moving visual environment: Relative phase dynamics. *Biology and Cybernetics, 71,* 489–501.

Holden, M., Ventura, J., & Lackner, J. R. (1994). Stabilization of posture by precision contact of the index finger. *Journal of Vestibular Research, 4,* 285–301.

Horak, F. B., & Macpherson, J. M. (1996). Postural orientation and equilibrium. In J. Shepard & L. Rowell (Eds.), *Handbook of physiology* (pp. 255–292). New York: Oxford University Press.

Horak, F. B., Shupert, C. L., & Mirka, A. (1989). Components of postural dyscontrol in the elderly: A review. *Neurobiology of Aging, 10,* 727–738.

Howard, I. P. (1982). *Human visual orientation.* New York: Wiley.

Hu, M. H., & Woollacott, M. H. (1994). Multisensory training of standing balance in older adults: Postural stability and one-leg stance balance. *Journal of Gerontology, 49,* M52–M61.

Jacobson, G. P., Newman, C. W., & Kartush, J. M. (1997). *Handbook of balance function testing.* Florence, KY: Delmar.

Jeka, J. J., Easton, R. D., Bentzen, B. L., & Lackner, J. R. (1996). Haptic cues for orientation and postural control in sighted and blind individuals. *Perception & Psychophysics, 58,* 409–423.

Jeka, J. J., & Lackner, J. R. (1994). Fingertip contact influences human postural control. *Experimental Brain Research, 100,* 495–502.

Jeka, J. J., & Lackner, J. R. (1995). The role of haptic cues from rough and slippery surfaces in human postural control. *Experimental Brain Research, 103,* 267–276.

Jeka, J. J., Oie, K. S., Schöner, G. S., Dijkstra, T. M. H., & Henson, E. M. (1998). Position and velocity coupling of postural sway to somatosensory drive. *Journal of Neurophysiology, 79,* 1661–1674.

Jeka, J. J., Schöner, G., Dijkstra, T. M. H., Ribeiro, P., & Lackner, J. R. (1997). Coupling of fingertip somatosensory information to head and body sway. *Experimental Brain Research, 113,* 475–483.

Kiemel, T., Oie, K. S., & Jeka, J. J. (in press). Multisensory fusion and the stochastic structure of postural sway. *Biology and Cybernetics.*

Krebs, D. E., Gill-Body, K. M., Riley, P. O., & Parker, S. W. (1993). Double-blind, placebo-controlled trial of rehabilitation for bilateral vestibular hypofunction: Preliminary report. *Otolaryngology—Head and Neck Surgery, 109,* 735–741.

Ledin, T., Kronhed, A. C., Moller, C., Moller, M., Odkvist, L. M., & Olsson, B. (1991). Effects of balance training in elderly evaluated by clinical tests and dynamic posturography. *Journal of Vestibular Research, 1,* 129–138.

Lee, D. N., & Lishman, J. R. (1975). Visual proprioceptive control of stance. *Journal of Human Movement Studies, 1,* 87–95.

Nashner, L. M. (1982). Adaptation of human movement to altered environments. *Trends in Neuroscience, 5,* 358–361.

Nashner, L. M., Shumway-Cook, A., & Marin, O. (1983). Stance posture control in select groups of children with cerebral palsy: Deficits in sensory organization and muscular coordination. *Experimental Brain Research, 49,* 393–409.

Oie, K. S., Kiemel, T. S., & Jeka, J. J. (2002). Multisensory fusion: Simultaneous reweighting of vision and touch for the control of human posture. *Cognitive Brain Research, 14,* 164–176.

Peterka, R. J., & Benolken, M. S. (1995). Role of somatosensory and vestibular cues in attenuating visually induced human postural sway. *Experimental Brain Research, 105,* 101–110.

Reginella, R. L., Redfern, M. S., & Furman, J. M. (1999). Postural sway with earth-fixed and body referenced finger contact in young and older adults. *Journal of Vestibular Research, 9,* 103–109.

Riley, M. A., Wong, S., Mitra, S., & Turvey, M. T. (1997). Common effects of touch and vision on postural parameters. *Experimental Brain Research, 117,* 165–170.

Rose, D. J., & Clark, S. (2000). Can the control of bodily orientation be significantly improved in a group of older adults with a history of falls? *Journal of the American Geriatrics Society, 48,* 275–282.

Schöner, G. (1991). Dynamic theory of action-perception patterns: The "moving room" paradigm. *Biology and Cybernetics, 64,* 455–462.

Shepard, N. T., Schultz, A., Alexander, N. B., Gu, M. J., & Boisemier, T. (1993). Postural control in young and elderly adults when stance is challenged: Clinical versus laboratory measurements. *Annals of Otology Rhinodogy Laryngology, 102*(7), 508–517.

Shumway-Cook, A., & Olmscheid, R. (1990). A systems analysis of postural dyscontrol in traumatically brain-injured patients. *Journal of Head Trauma and Rehabilitation, 5,* 51–62.

Shumway-Cook, A., & Woollacott, M. H. (2000). Attentional demands and postural control: The effect of sensory

context. *Journals of Gerontology, Series A: Biological Sciences and Medical Sciences, 55A,* M10–M16.

Simoneau, M., Teasdale, N., Bourdin, C., Bard, C., Fleury, M., & Nougier, V. (1999). Aging and postural control: Postural perturbations caused by changing the visual anchor. *Journal of the American Geriatrics Society, 47,* 235–240.

Soechting, J., & Berthoz, A. (1979). Dynamic role of vision in the control of posture in man. *Experimental Brain Research, 36,* 551–561.

Stelmach, G. E., Teasdale, N., DiFabio, R. P., & Phillips, J. (1989). Age-related decline in postural control mechanisms. *International Journal of Aging and Human Development, 29,* 205–223.

Sundermier, L., Woollacott, M. H., Jensen, J. L., & Moore, S. (1996). Postural sensitivity to visual flow in aging adults with and without balance problems. *Journals of Gerontology, Series A: Biological Sciences and Medical Sciences, 51A,* M45–M52.

Talbott, R. E., & Brookhart, J. M. (1980). A predictive model study of the visual contribution to canine postural control. *American Journal of Physiology, 239,* R80–R92.

Teasdale, N., Bard, C., LaRue, J., & Fleury, M. (1993). On the cognitive penetrability of postural control. *Experimental Aging Research, 19,* 1–13.

Teasdale, N., Stelmach, G. E., & Breunig, A. (1991). Postural sway characteristics of the elderly under normal and altered visual and support surface conditions. *Journals of Gerontology, Series A: Biological Sciences and Medical Sciences, 46,* B238–B244.

Teasdale, N., Stelmach, G. E., Breunig, A., & Meeuwsen, H. J. (1991). Age differences in visual sensory integration. *Experimental Brain Research, 85,* 691–696.

van Asten, N. J. C., Gielen, C. C. A. M., & Denier van der Gon, J. J. (1988). Postural adjustments induced by simulated motion of differently structured environments. *Experimental Brain Research, 73,* 371–383.

Whipple, R., & Wolfson, L. I. (1989). Abnormalities of balance, gait and sensorimotor function in the elderly population. In P. Duncan (Ed.), *Balance: Proceedings of the APTA Forum* (pp. 61–68). Alexandria, VA: American Physical Therapy Association.

Whipple, R., Wolfson, L., Derby, C., Singh, D., & Tobin, J. (1993). Altered sensory function and balance in older persons. *Journal of Gerontology, 48,* 71–76.

Wolfson, L., Whipple, R., Derby, C. A., et al. (1992). A dynamic posturography study of balance in the healthy elderly. *Neurology, 42,* 2069–2075.

Woollacott, M. H. (1993). Age-related changes in posture and movement. *Journal of Gerontology, 48,* 56–60.

Woollacott, M. H. (2000). Systems contributing to balance disorders in older adults. *Journals of Gerontology, Series A: Biological Sciences and Medical Sciences, 55A,* M424–M428.

Woollacott, M. H., Shumway-Cook, A., & Nashner, L. M. (1986). Aging and posture control: Changes in sensory organization and muscular coordination. *International Journal of Aging and Human Development, 23,* 97–114.

50 Neuropsychological Evidence of Integrated Multisensory Representation of Space in Humans

ELISABETTA LÀDAVAS AND ALESSANDRO FARNÈ

Introduction

This chapter focuses on multisensory behavioral phenomena that can be seen in humans affected by extinction or neglect, two neuropsychological signs related to altered functions of spatial perception. Through the study of pathologic behavioral phenomena that become manifest following damage to the central nervous system (CNS), neuropsychological studies have substantially contributed to our understanding of the normal organization of brain cognitive functions, and represent the natural interface among several diverse disciplines. In this chapter we describe a series of neuropsychological investigations of multimodal spatial phenomena that are tightly linked to other fields of neuroscience, such as neurophysiology and cognitive psychology, allowing for a direct comparison with the behavioral characteristics of the cross-modal construction of space in healthy subjects and the neural bases of cross-modal spatial behavior in both animals and humans.

We review several highly convergent behavioral findings that provide strong evidence in favor of the existence, in humans, of multimodal integration systems representing space through the multisensory coding of tactile-visual and tactile-auditory events, as well as visual-auditory events. In addition, these findings show that multimodal integration systems may differ with respect to some of their functional characteristics, such as the portion of space in which the multisensory integration occurs. For example, some types of integrated processing (e.g., those that involve the tactile modality) may take place in a privileged manner within a limited sector of space closely surrounding the body surface, that is, in near peripersonal space. Alternatively, the integrated processing of auditory and visual events may occur within a larger sector of space, in far peripersonal space. These findings are entirely consistent with the functional properties of multisensory neuronal structures coding (near and far) peripersonal space in animals, as well as with behavioral, electrophysiological, and neuroimaging evidence for the cross-modal coding of space in normal subjects. This high level of convergence ultimately favors the idea that multisensory space coding is achieved through similar multimodal structures in both humans and nonhuman primates.

Research in neuropsychology, as in many other psychological domains, has historically focused on a single sensory modality at a time. Because we typically receive a simultaneous flow of information from each of our different senses in real-world situations, however, our perception of objects in the world is also the product of integrated, multisensory processing. Providing animals with many sources of input that can operate simultaneously or substitute for one another when necessary frees them from many constraints. The integration of multiple sensory cues also provides animals with enormous flexibility, so that their reaction to the presence of one stimulus can be altered by the presence of another. The combination of, for example, visual and tactile cues or visual and auditory cues can enhance the result produced by the processing of a cue provided in a single modality and can also eliminate any ambiguity that might occur when a stimulus from one modality is not fully detected.

Some of the systems responsible for such integrative sensory processing have now been documented physiologically and their relevance for space coding has been shown. However, despite a long tradition of single-cell studies on multimodal neurons in animals, the existence of these integrated systems has only recently been investigated in humans. Such a relatively small (but rapidly increasing) number of studies is surprising, given that these multisensory systems offer a unique opportunity for recovery from cognitive impairment following brain lesions. For instance, altered performance in a unimodal sensory system can be influenced—enhanced or degraded—by the activation of another modality. Impairments in spatial representation, such as extinction or neglect, may be caused by a loss of neurons representing particular locations in space in one single modality (Pouget & Sejnowski, 1997). Stimuli presented in that portion of space are neglected or extinguished (Làdavas, Berti, & Farnè, 2000), whereas stimuli presented in the intact portion of space are detected. Whenever perceptual problems due to extinction or neglect are limited to the impairment of unimodal space representations, then detection in these patients can be obtained by the activation of an integrated system coding stimuli presented in the affected space in different modalities.

The neurophysiological bases that would be necessary for producing such a perceptual enhancement through multisensory integrative processing have been revealed in nonhuman primates. For example, neurons have been reported in the putamen and in the parietal and frontal cortices that are multimodal: they respond to both tactile and visual stimuli. Other multimodal neurons respond to tactile, visual, and auditory stimuli. Besides showing multisensory responses, these neurons are strongly activated only when visual or auditory stimuli are located in spatial proximity to a particular body part (e.g., to the face and hand) where the tactile receptive field (RF) of a given neuron is located. That is, multimodal responses are evoked most effectively by presenting visual and auditory stimuli within the visual and auditory RFs extending outward from their tactile RF. Therefore, these brain areas are specialized for the coding of visual-auditory space immediately surrounding the body (i.e., near peripersonal space).

Such a multisensory integration system would be very useful in recovery from tactile extinction, and in the first part of this chapter, we review evidence of the existence in humans of an integrated visuotactile system and an auditory-tactile system responsible for coding near peripersonal space, as well as their relevance for the modulation of tactile extinction.

In addition, neurophysiological studies in the cat and monkey have also revealed the existence of multimodal neurons in the superior colliculus (SC) that synthesize visual, auditory, and/or somatosensory inputs and are relevant for behavioral responses such as attending and orienting to sensory stimuli presented in far peripersonal space. Again, the activation of this integrated visual-auditory system could be very useful for recovery from visuospatial impairments such as visual neglect. In this respect, the integration of visual and auditory information can potentially enable patients with visual neglect to detect "bimodal" stimuli for which the visual unimodal component is below the behavioral threshold. Thus, in the second part of this chapter, we provide evidence of the existence in humans of an integrated visuo-auditory system responsible for the coding of far peripersonal space and its relevance for the temporary recovery from visual neglect.

Extinction and neglect as probes to investigate spatial multisensory interactions

The neuropsychological conditions called extinction and neglect represent two models that provide considerable insight into the behavioral characteristics of multimodal spatial representation in humans. Extinction (Loeb, 1885; Oppenheim, 1885) is a pathological sign that follows brain damage. In extinction, some patients fail to report a stimulus, presented to the contralesional affected side, only when a concurrent stimulus is presented on the ipsilesional side of the body, that is, under conditions of double simultaneous stimulation (Bender, 1952). Otherwise, when the same stimulus is delivered singly to the contralesional affected side, patients with extinction are able to detect its presence most of the time, indicating that extinction is not merely a consequence of a disorder of primary sensory processing, even if some sensory deficit is present (Làdavas, 1990). The phenomenon is most frequently associated with unilateral brain lesions on the right side (Barbieri & De Renzi, 1989), and so manifests as left-sided extinction. Extinction is easily uncovered by means of confrontation techniques. A confrontation technique in the visual modality, for example, might entail the examiner standing in front of the patient and wiggling the left, right, or both index fingers simultaneously while the patient is asked to verbally report which side has been stimulated. In this way, the patient's right or left visual field respectively is alternately or simultaneously stimulated by a brief visual stimulus, and the presence and severity of extinction can be detected and quantified. Impaired reporting of left-sided stimuli under conditions of double simultaneous stimulation as compared with left unilateral stimulation is the hallmark of visual extinction. The confrontation technique is also used to detect and quantify the presence of extinction in the tactile and auditory modalities.

The competitive nature of this phenomenon is clearly evident in the fact that patients no longer report the presence of the same contralesional stimulus when an identical stimulus is presented simultaneously on the ipsilesional side (di Pellegrino & De Renzi, 1995; Ward, Goodrich, & Driver, 1994). Among several interpretations of extinction phenomena (e.g., Posner, Walker, Friedrich, & Rafal, 1984; Robertson & Rafal, 2000), it has been suggested that extinction emerges as a consequence of an unbalanced competition between spared and affected representations of space, whereby ipsilesional and contralesional stimuli are associated with competitive weights of different strength for accessing limited attentional resources (Berti et al., 1999; di Pellegrino & De Renzi, 1995; Driver, 1998; Driver, Mattingley, Rorden, & Davis, 1997; Duncan, 1980, 1996). When two opposite stimuli compete in patients with extinction, the ipsilesional stimulus benefits from a higher weight with respect to the contralesional stimulus, whose competitive strength has been reduced by a lesion of a brain area representing a portion of contralateral space. As a result of this uneven competition, the contralesional stimulus loses, owing to a weaker activation of the representation of that portion of space, and is seemingly extinguished by the stronger ipsilesional stimulus (di Pellegrino, Basso, & Frassinetti, 1997; Ward et al., 1994).

Hemispatial neglect is another spatial disorder that is most frequently associated with right brain damage. In contradistinction to extinction, of which neglect has long been considered a major form, patients with neglect do not report left contralesional stimuli even when the stimuli are presented alone (Robertson & Marshall, 1993), that is, under conditions of left unilateral stimulation. However, hemispatial neglect seems to represent a distinct deficit rather than an exaggerated form of extinction, from which it differs in some respects. In particular, the fact that patients with right-sided brain damage can be selectively affected by neglect or extinction and the occurrence of double dissociations between these deficits (Bisiach, 1991; Cocchini, Cubelli, Della Sala, & Beschin, 1999; Goodrich & Ward, 1997; Liu, Bolton, Price, & Weintraub, 1992; Ro & Farnè, 2001) clearly illustrate that neglect and extinction are specific impairments associated with different underlying neural mechanisms. Hemispatial neglect is most often associated with lesions involving the inferior parietal lobule (Vallar & Perani, 1986; Mort et al., 2003), whereas lesions correlated with extinction often also involve subcortical structures such as the thalamus and basal ganglia (Vallar, Rusconi, Bignamini, Geminiani, & Perani, 1994).

In this chapter, we present a series of studies from our laboratory that illustrate that extinction can also occur between different sensory modalities, as well as the

characteristics that crucially contribute to exacerbate or, most interestingly, reduce the manifestations of cross-modal extinction (for a review, see, Làdavas, 2002) and neglect. Before describing the methods, the main results, and theoretical implications of these studies on cross-modal modulation, we will introduce some basic neurophysiological findings on multisensory processing in nonhuman primates. On the basis of this animal evidence, we propose that in humans as well, visual and tactile (or auditory) information is coded by an integrated multisensory system representing near peripersonal space.

Neuronal bases for multisensory processing of near peripersonal space

The last two decades of neurophysiological research have yielded a large body of evidence supporting the suggestion that multisensory integration at the single-neuron level is a frequent feature of spatial representation, especially in the coding of near peripersonal space (Duhamel, Colby, & Goldberg, 1991, 1998; Graziano & Gross, 1995, 1998a, 1998b; Hyvärinen & Poranen, 1974; Rizzolatti, Luppino, & Matelli, 1998; Rizzolatti, Scandolara, Matelli, & Gentilucci, 1981). It is now widely accepted that a number of structures and cortical areas of the monkey brain, such as the putamen, parietal areas 7b and VIP, and premotor areas (F2 and F4, following the nomenclature proposed by Rizzolatti and colleagues), play some special role in representing the space that closely surrounds the animal's body. These areas contain a high proportion of multimodal neurons that have a tactile and visual and/or auditory RF and exhibit good spatial registration among these different RFs. For example, visual and auditory RFs match the location of the somatosensory RF, extending only a few centimeters outward from the skin. These neurons respond to both tactile and visual (or auditory) stimuli, provided that the visual (or auditory) stimuli are presented immediately adjacent to a particular body part (e.g., the head or hand).

Although the different properties of multimodal neurons, as well as their possible functional role, are described elsewhere in this book, it is worth remembering some of their basic characteristics. For example, visual and auditory RFs of these neurons have a limited extension in depth, which is confined to the space immediately surrounding the monkey's body. Their visually and auditorily evoked activity shows gradients of response, such that the neuronal discharge decreases as the distance between visual or auditory stimuli and the cutaneous RF increases. In addition, vision-related activity seems to operate in coordinates that are centered on body parts; that is, visual RFs move in space according to the position of the associated tactile RF, located on a given body part, when this is moved. Similarly, the position of the visual RFs of multimodal neurons does not change when the monkey gazes in different directions. Finally, since the somatosensory RFs are somatotopically organized, the associated visual or auditory RFs form a multimodal map of the space immediately adjacent to the animal's body.

On the basis of these functional characteristics, several authors have suggested that the parieto-premotor areas and the putamen are part of a complex sensorimotor network, interfacing multisensory coding of near peripersonal space centered on body parts with the appropriate motor responses (Colby, Duhamel, & Goldberg, 1993; Duhamel et al., 1998; Fogassi et al., 1996, 1999; Graziano, Hu, & Gross, 1997). Indeed, multimodal neurons often discharge during both sensory stimulation and the voluntary execution of movements toward specific spatial locations. Because of these properties, the activation of multisensory neurons evoked, for example, by a visual stimulus presented near the hand or the face would activate the somatosensory representation of the hand or face. In this way, movements of the animal's body may be controlled by either somatosensory or visual information about an object's location, or by both inputs at the level of the same neuron. Indeed, recent evidence clearly supports the idea that defensive, reflexive movements might be almost directly coded by these multi-sensorimotor interfaces. Electric stimulation of precentral multimodal areas has been show to evoke complex avoidance or defensive actions "against an object in the bimodal RF" (Graziano, Taylor, & Moore, 2001).

Besides animal evidence, recent functional brain imaging studies have provided the first evidence of the existence of similar multimodal structures in human subjects (Bremmer, Schlack, Shah, et al., 2001). The following section addresses the behavioral relevance of sensory integration mechanisms in humans for space representation.

Visual modulation of tactile perception

Starting from the animal studies mentioned in the previous section, we propose that a similar multisensory system may operate in the human brain. To verify this possibility, we initially investigated whether competition between the right and left representations of space could lead to extinction across the visual and tactile modalities. Indeed, contralesional extinction has long been known to occur within different modalities (unimodal extinction), for example, when bilateral stimuli are both visual

(Làdavas, 1990; di Pellegrino & De Renzi, 1995; Ward et al., 1994) and auditory (De Renzi, 1982; De Renzi, Gentilini, & Pattaccini, 1984), olfactory (Bellas, Novelly, Eskenazi, & Wasserstein, 1988), or tactile (Bender, 1952; Gainotti, De Bonis, Daniele, & Caltagirone, 1989; Moscovitch & Behrmann, 1994; Vallar et al., 1994). However, the phenomenon of cross-modal extinction—that is, extinction between modalities—has been experimentally documented only in recent years in studies on patients with right-sided brain lesions and left unimodal tactile extinction. In particular, we have recently shown that the presentation of a visual stimulus in the right ipsilesional field can extinguish a tactile stimulus presented on the contralesional hand that is otherwise well detected by patients when presented alone (Bender, 1952; di Pellegrino, Làdavas, & Farnè, 1997; see also Mattingley, Driver, Beschin, & Robertson, 1997). Most relevant to this discussion, we asked whether the perception of contralesional tactile stimuli could be not only reduced but also increased by the simultaneous presentation of a visual stimulus, depending on the spatial arrangement, congruent or not, of visual and tactile stimuli with respect to the contralesional affected side of the body. Specifically, we predicted that visuotactile presentations (i.e., ipsilesional visual stimulus and contralesional tactile stimulus) would exacerbate the pathological phenomenon, that is, presenting a visual stimulus in the opposite side relative to the left hand (affected by tactile extinction) should result in a reduced perception of tactile events on that hand. On the contrary, visuotactile presentation would reduce this symptom: that is, presenting a visual stimulus to the same contralesional side should result in enhanced perception of tactile events on that hand. In addition, we predicted that if a multisensory (visuotactile) system processing tactile and visual stimuli near the body was responsible for coding left and right spatial representations, then the presentation of visual stimuli in the near as compared to the far peripersonal space would be much more effective in modulating cross-modal visuotactile extinction. Therefore, both the reduction and the enhancement of left tactile perception should be obtained most effectively following nearby visual stimulation.

These hypotheses were investigated in a group of ten patients with right-sided brain damage and left unimodal tactile extinction by means of a cross-modal stimulation paradigm (for details, see Làdavas, di Pellegrino, Farnè, & Zeloni, 1998). Some of the experimental conditions were aimed at investigating the cross-modal reduction of contralesional tactile perception; others were devised to verify the possibility of its cross-modal enhancement and will therefore be described separately.

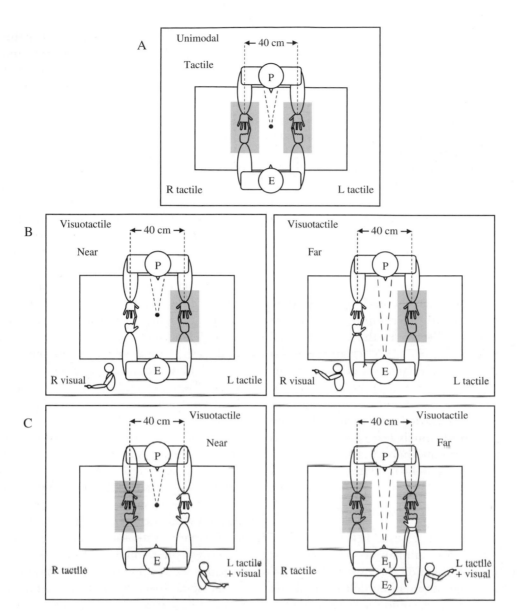

FIGURE 50.1 Schematic drawing of the experimental conditions used for assessing unimodal tactile extinction (*A*) and cross-modal reduction (*B*) or enhancement (*C*) of tactile perception on the contralesional hand. Depending on the condition, tactile and/or visual stimuli were presented by the experimenter (E) to the right (R), left (L), or both hands of a patient (P). Vision of tactile stimuli could be prevented by using cardboard shields (gray rectangles). In the cross-modal conditions (*B* and *C*), the visual stimulus was presented either near (left panels) or far (right panels) from the patients' hands. The location of near and far visual stimuli presented by the experimenter is also shown from the side at the bottom of each panel. The black dot represents a fixation point that patients were required to look at during stimulation. The experimenter's nose served as fixation point in the cross-modal far conditions (right panels). (Modified from Làdavas, E. [2002]. Functional and dynamic properties of visual peripersonal space. *Trends in Cognitive Sciences, 6,* 17–22. © 2002, Elsevier Science Publishing. Used by permission.)

REDUCING CONTRALESIONAL TACTILE PERCEPTION For this part of the investigation, patients sat at a table in front of the experimenter with their hands positioned palm down on the table surface, and had to maintain visual fixation on a central dot (Fig. 50.1). Visual stimuli (brief flexion-extension movement of the examiner's index finger) and tactile stimuli (unseen brief touches of the dorsal aspect of patients' index finger) were presented singly or simultaneously. Direct vision of tactile

stimuli was impeded (Fig. 50.1*B*). In separate blocks of trials, the visual stimulus was presented either near (about 5 cm) or far (about 30 cm) from the patient's hand. Patients were required to report verbally what they had felt or seen with the words "left," "right," "both," or "none," regardless of the stimulus modality.

The results confirmed that patients' tactile perception on the contralesional hand was relatively spared by the lesion, since they were highly accurate in reporting single left tactile stimulation (94% correct responses). They also manifested a severe unimodal tactile extinction, since they were able to report only a minority of left touches (less than 40% of trials) when both hands were simultaneously touched. Crucially, presenting a visual stimulus in the ipsilesional field also had a largely negative impact on the perceptual awareness of contralesional single touches. That is, perception of a single stimulus delivered in the tactile modality to the left hand, which would have been otherwise accurate, was instead substantially reduced by the simultaneous presentation of a single stimulus delivered ipsilesionally in the visual modality (incongruent visuotactile stimulation). This phenomenon of cross-modal visuotactile extinction was also clearly influenced by the distance of the ipsilesional visual stimulus with respect to the patient's right hand. A visual stimulus presented near the ipsilesional hand interfered so profoundly with perception of the tactile stimulus concurrently delivered to the contralesional hand (Fig. 50.1*B*, left) that patients were able to feel it on only 25% of the trials. In quantitative terms, left tactile perception was reduced by almost the same amount whether a visual stimulus was presented near the right hand or a tactile stimulus was delivered to the same hand (Fig. 50.1*A*). In contrast, much less interference was exerted on tactile perception when the same visual stimulus was presented away from the right hand (Fig. 50.1*B*, right), such that patients were able to feel most left tactile stimuli (75% of trials).

ENHANCING CONTRALESIONAL TACTILE PERCEPTION The experimental setting was similar to the one just described, but visual stimulation was now spatially congruent with the tactile stimulation delivered to the contralesional hand. Patients could receive a single tactile stimulation on the ipsilesional or contralesional hand, or both tactile stimulations simultaneously. In addition, a visual stimulus could be concurrently delivered in the contralesional field, in separate blocks, either near the patient's visible hand (about 5 cm) or far from the patient's hand (about 30 cm), which was screened from view to avoid tactile stimuli acting as visual cues (see Fig. 50.1). Visual stimuli were irrelevant to the task, and patients were required to respond verbally only to what they had felt, by saying "left," "right," "both," or "none."

The results showed that tactile extinction was dramatically reduced by the presentation of a contralesional visual stimulus close to the patients' left hand. In particular, the patients' ability to perceive a left touch under conditions of double tactile stimulation was very poor when only tactile stimuli were presented (mean accuracy of 39.5%). However, the simultaneous

presentation of a visual stimulus near the left contralesional hand (congruent visuotactile stimulation) substantially enhanced the perception of tactile stimuli delivered to that hand, which increased to an accuracy of 85.5%. Similar to the cross-modal extinction phenomenon described above, this cross-modal visuotactile enhancement was also clearly influenced by the distance from the patient's left hand at which the visual stimulus was presented. A visual stimulus presented near the left contralesional hand (see Fig. 50.1*C*, left) increased patients' tactile perception so much that their performance was almost comparable to that found under left unilateral stimulation (93.5% accuracy), when only a single tactile stimulus was presented. In stark contrast, patients' performance was not ameliorated significantly when the same visual stimulus was presented far from their contralesional hand (see Fig. 50.1*C*, right). In this latter case, patients reported having felt a touch on the left hand on only 48% of trials, thus showing that visual stimulation of the contralesional field is not sufficient per se to transiently improve tactile extinction and that a close spatial proximity of visual and tactile events is necessary for cross-modal enhancement of tactile perception to occur.

In summary, both parts of this study showed strong effects of the cross-modal modulation of tactile perception, which appeared to be (1) dependent on the spatial congruence of visuotactile inputs relative to the affected side and (2) most consistently manifest when visuotactile interaction occurred in the near peripersonal space. In agreement with the predictions of our hypothesis, both these phenomena constitute strong neuropsychological evidence that the human brain represents near peripersonal space through an integrated multisensory visuotactile system. Due to its activity, visual stimulation near the ipsilesional hand would strongly activate the somatosensory representation of that hand, as if it were a tactile stimulus. In patients with left tactile extinction, in whom spatial competition is biased ipsilesionally, the somatosensory representation of the left and right hands, activated by spatially incongruent tactile and visual stimuli, would largely extinguish contralesional tactile stimuli. This is because the processing of the somatosensory stimulation of the contralesional hand is disadvantaged in terms of competitive weights, and gives rise to a comparatively weaker representation. A similar line of reasoning indicates that the somatosensory representation of the left hand, once activated by spatially congruent visual and tactile stimuli, would be less extinguished by the concurrently activated somatosensory representation of the right hand. This is because the weaker contralesional representation can be enhanced by the simultaneous activation operated by a visual stimulus presented close to the same hand. This, in turn, would result in cross-modal boosting of the otherwise extinguished left tactile stimuli into perceptual awareness.

In the cases of both the reduction and enhancement of tactile perception, however, the presentation of the same visual stimulus in the far peripersonal space of the hands activated their somatosensory representations only weakly. As a consequence, the unbalanced competition cannot be effectively exaggerated and reduced, and cross-modal modulation of tactile perception is much decreased or absent.

Visual dominance over proprioception in cross-modal modulation

Although the spatial congruence of visual and tactile events (relative to the affected hand) clearly determines the worsening or improving nature of cross-modal modulation of tactile perception, the spatial distance of visual events from the patients' body is crucial for its occurrence. But how does the multisensory system estimate the distance between the hands and nearby visual objects? In humans, one possibility is by combining proprioception and vision (Haggard, Newman, Blundell, & Andrew, 2000; Rossetti, Desmurget, & Prablanc, 1995; van Beers, Sittig, & Gon, 1999). In monkeys, these inputs can be merged at the level of single, multimodal neurons that respond to near peripersonal visual stimuli even when proprioception is the only available source of information to reconstruct arm position, that is, when direct vision of the arm by the monkey is prevented. However, this proprioception-alone-based response is much weaker than that evoked when vision of the arm is also allowed (Graziano, 1999; MacKay & Crammond, 1987; Obayashi, Tanaka, & Iriki, 2000). Therefore, one may ask whether visual information regarding hand posture is more relevant than proprioceptive information for the cross-modal representation of near peripersonal space in humans.

Accordingly, we investigated whether the cross-modal modulation of tactile perception on the hand can still be obtained when the patient's hand is not visible (Làdavas, Farnè, Zeloni, & di Pellegrino, 2000). To verify this hypothesis, two different experiments were performed with another group of patients with right brain damage and left tactile extinction, one in which patients could see their hands and one in which they could not. The rationale and methods of these experiments were analogous to those adopted in the previous investigation: both the effects of cross-modal reduction and enhancement of contralesional tactile perception were investigated.

CROSS-MODAL REDUCTION OF TACTILE PERCEPTION In the case of spatially incongruent visuotactile stimulation, the reduction of contralesional tactile perception was much stronger when the visual stimulus was presented near the visible hand (35% accuracy) compared to the condition in which vision of the hand was prevented (58% accuracy). In fact, the amount of cross-modal extinction obtained when vision was prevented was comparable regardless of whether the visual stimulus was presented near or far from the patients' ipsilesional hand (58% and 61% accuracy, respectively). That is, cross-modal extinction was not prevalent in the near peripersonal space when only proprioceptive cues about hand position were available. This result indicates that proprioception only weakly mediates the representation of hand-centered visual peripersonal space.

CROSS-MODAL ENHANCEMENT OF TACTILE PERCEPTION In the case of spatially congruent visuotactile stimulation, the enhancement of contralesional tactile perception was much stronger when the visual stimulus was presented near the visible hand (91% accuracy) compared to the condition in which vision of the hand was prevented (65% accuracy). Actually, the improvement of the otherwise extinguished tactile stimuli was so marked that, under conditions of bilateral tactile stimulation, patients reported almost the same proportion of left touches as they perceived when tactile stimuli were delivered singly to their left, affected hand (93% accuracy). In other words, congruent visuotactile stimulation was able to "extinguish" the pathological signs of tactile extinction, but only when vision of the contralesional hand was allowed. Therefore, vision of hand position in space may have a major impact in coding the distance of visual stimuli from someone's hands, in agreement with the notion that visual information usually overwhelms low spatial resolution senses such as proprioception (Dassonville, 1995; Hay, Pick, & Ikeda, 1965; Mon-Williams, Wann, Jenkinson, & Rushton, 1997; Rock & Victor, 1964; Warren & Cleaves, 1971). Further studies are needed to clarify the possible interaction between the proximity of the visual input and the vision of the stimulated hand in producing spatially segregated cross-modal facilitatory effects.

Cross-modal interaction in the near peripersonal space of a fake hand

In case of illusory sensory conflict, normal subjects report feeling their hand where they see it (Mon-Williams et al., 1997), even if they are actually looking at a fake hand slightly displaced with respect to their own hand (Botvinick & Cohen, 1998; Pavani, Spence, & Driver,

2000). These illusory effects vanish when the rubber hands that the subjects are looking at are implausibly oriented in space with respect to their body, such as when fake hands are not aligned with subjects' shoulders.

We hypothesized that vision of a fake hand might be able to activate the corresponding visual peripersonal space representation. This hypothesis was investigated in a group of RBD patients, with right brain damage and reliable left tactile extinction, which was tested using synthetic probes analogous to Semmes-Weinstein monofilaments (for details, see Farnè, Pavani, Meneghello, & Làdavas, 2000). Visual stimuli were presented near a prosthetic right hand but far from the patient's ipsilesional hand, which was placed behind his or her back. Tactile stimuli were delivered to the left hand. In separate blocks of trials, the rubber hand was either visually aligned or misaligned with respect to the ipsilesional shoulder. Patients were simply required to verbally report the side(s) of stimulation, irrespective of the sensory modality.

In agreement with our prediction, the results showed that under conditions of spatially incongruent visuotactile stimulation, tactile perception on the contralesional hand was substantially reduced by a concurrent visual stimulus delivered near the rubber hand. Indeed, the patients' ability to perceive single touches on the left hand was well preserved (91% accuracy), but appeared to be strongly affected when the perihand space was visually stimulated (49% accuracy). Moreover, this cross-modal interference was more effective when the rubber hand appeared in a plausible orientation than in an implausible orientation. In the visually plausible condition (i.e., rubber hand spatially aligned with the shoulder), patients consistently failed to report a tactile stimulus delivered on the contralesional hand when a visual stimulus was simultaneously presented near the rubber hand (49% accuracy). In this case, the amount of cross-modal extinction was comparable to that obtained when a visual stimulus was presented near the patient's (real) right hand (41% accuracy). In contrast, the cross-modal interference exerted by incongruent cross-modal stimulation was much reduced when the rubber hand appeared in an implausible orientation (71% accuracy). In this visually incompatible condition (i.e., rubber hand not aligned with the shoulder), cross-modal extinction substantially decreased, the magnitude being comparable to that obtained by presenting a visual stimulus far from the patient's (real) ipsilesional hand (74% accuracy).

These findings clearly show that the integrated processing of visuotactile input in near peripersonal space can also be uniquely activated on the basis of visual information regarding hand position, whereas proprio-

ception per se does not seem to be crucial for the distinction between near and far space. The results also provide the first neuropsychological evidence that the human brain can form visual representations of the near peripersonal space of a nonowned body part, such as a rubber hand, as if it were a real hand. Indeed, the multisensory system coding hand-centered peripersonal space in humans uses mainly visual information to compute the spatial relation between the positions of hands and visual stimuli (see also Maravita, Spence, Clarke, Husain, & Driver, 2000). Thus, vision of a fake hand can dominate over conflicting information provided by proprioception, such that a visual stimulus presented far from a patient's real hand is processed as if it were in near peripersonal space. However, this phenomenon can take place only if the fake hand looks plausible with respect to the patient's body, showing that visual dominance is not complete and probably not necessary, because in normal situations, vision and proprioception convey congruent information. When extremely conflicting information is provided by the different senses, the seen rubber hand may no longer be processed as a personal belonging and thus does not capture the felt hand position. It is important to underline that this result is again fully consistent with neurophysiological evidence. When a fake realistic arm is visible instead of the arm of the animal, the activity of many visuotactile neurons in the ventral premotor and parietal areas is modulated by the congruent or incongruent location of a seen fake arm (Graziano, 1999; Graziano, Cooke, & Taylor, 2000).

On the other hand, vision of a body part not only can reduce tactile sensation, it can also help to enhance tactile sensitivity in both neurological patients (Halligan, Hunt, Marshall, & Wade, 1996; Halligan, Marshall, Hunt, & Wade, 1997) and normal subjects (Tipper, et al., 1998, 2001). Seeing the corporeal origin of a tactile sensation can ameliorate impaired somatosensory perception in brain-damaged patients with hemisensory loss of the upper limb (Halligan et al., 1996, 1997; Newport, Hindle, & Jackson, 2001). Similar to what was described earlier in patients, this has also been shown when the seen body part is a fake, rubber replica of a hand. Rorden and colleagues, for example, have shown that a patient with hemisensory loss could recover lost tactile sensitivity if a visual stimulus, presented in spatial congruence with the unseen tactile stimulation of the affected hand, was attached to a rubber hand mimicking the real one (Rorden, Heutink, Greenfield, & Robertson, 1999). By taking advantage of the rubber hand illusion, a patient's tactile sensitivity deficit could be dramatically ameliorated. Once again, the occurrence of cross-modal enhancement of tactile sensation strictly depended on the rubber hand's orientation with respect to the patient's shoulder. Indeed, the improvement was present only when the seen position of the rubber hand was visually compatible with the patient's body, that is, when the rubber hand was superimposed and aligned with the subject's hidden hand. Moreover, Kennett, Taylor-Clarke, and Haggard (2001) have recently shown in normal subjects that not only tactile detection but also two-point discrimination can be improved by viewing the tactually stimulated body part through a visual magnifying glass, even without the tactile stimulation being seen.

Visuotactile interactions near the face: Reduction and enhancement of tactile perception

Overall, the observed pattern of results is highly consistent with the functional properties of monkeys' multimodal neurons described earlier, and they also suggest that human and nonhuman primates are likely to share similar cerebral mechanisms for the representation of near space. If this is true, one would expect that humans represent near peripersonal space not only in relation to their hands but also in relation to other body parts, similar to what has been found in monkeys. Indeed, the RFs of multisensory neurons are distributed in a somatotopic manner over the hand and arm, trunk, and face. The face, for example, is widely represented in the ventral intraparietal area (VIP) of the parietal lobe (Colby et al., 1993; Duhamel et al., 1991, 1998). It is therefore possible that, similar to the hand, the space closely surrounding the human face could also be coded through the activity of a multisensory mechanism.

Therefore, analogous to the previous studies, we investigated whether presentation of visual stimuli, congruent or incongruent with tactile stimuli delivered to the affected side of the face, could modulate the phenomenon of tactile extinction. Opposite results (i.e., enhancement and reduction) were again expected in patients with extinction as a function of the spatial position from which the visual stimulus was presented. We also expected that the cross-modal modulation of extinction would be stronger for visual stimuli near the patient's face than for visual stimuli far from it.

This hypothesis was assessed in a group of patients with right brain damage and left unimodal tactile extinction (Fig. 50.2). In this study, tactile extinction was examined on the face by applying unilateral and bilateral touches to patients' cheeks. Patients were submitted to a cross-modal paradigm similar to that used for testing cross-modal modulation of tactile perception relative to the hand (see Làdavas, Zeloni, & Farnè, 1998). In the part of the investigation that was aimed at assessing the cross-modal reduction of contralesional tactile perception (Fig. 50.2B), patients were presented with tactile stimuli on their left affected cheek. Visual stimuli were concurrently presented in the right ipsilesional field (incongruent) and, in separate blocks, were presented near or far from the patient's right cheek. Patients were required to verbally report the side(s) of stimulation, irrespective of the sensory modality.

To assess the cross-modal enhancement of contralesional tactile perception (Fig. 50.2C), patients were presented with unilateral or bilateral tactile stimuli and, in addition, visual stimuli were concurrently presented in the contralesional affected cheek (congruent). In separate blocks of trials, visual stimuli (irrelevant for the task) were presented near or far from the left side of the patient's face. Patients were required to verbally report the side(s) of tactile stimulation.

The results clearly supported our predictions. As for the hand, spatially incongruent visual stimuli presented to the ipsilesional side produced a decrease in the detection of contralesional tactile stimuli, particularly when visual stimuli were presented near the ipsilesional cheek (Fig. 50.2B, left). In this condition, patients reported only 38% of touches to the left cheek, which were otherwise well perceived when delivered alone (94% accuracy). Again, the cross-modal reduction produced by nearby visual stimulation of the right cheek was so strong that the number of contralesional touches that patients were able to report was comparable to that obtained following bilateral tactile stimulation (33% accuracy). This phenomenon was much less severe when visual stimuli were delivered far from the face (Fig. 50.2B, right); in this case patients were still able to report 69% of contralesional touches.

As expected, opposite results were obtained when the visual stimuli were presented in spatial congruence with the tactile stimuli delivered to the left affected cheek. Under conditions of double tactile stimulation, patients' severe tactile extinction (only 33% accuracy) was substantially reduced by the presentation of a contralesional visual stimulus (congruent visuotactile stimulation). In particular, the presentation of a visual stimulus near the left contralesional cheek (Fig. 50.2C, left) substantially enhanced the perception of tactile stimuli delivered to that cheek, which increased to 79% accuracy. This cross-modal visuotactile enhancement of tactile perception was much reduced when the same visual stimulus was presented far from the patients' contralesional cheek (Fig. 50.2C, right). In this latter case, the amelioration of patients' perception resulted in an accuracy of 59%. This confirms that close spatial proximity of visual and tactile events is necessary for obtaining the strongest cross-modal enhancement of tactile

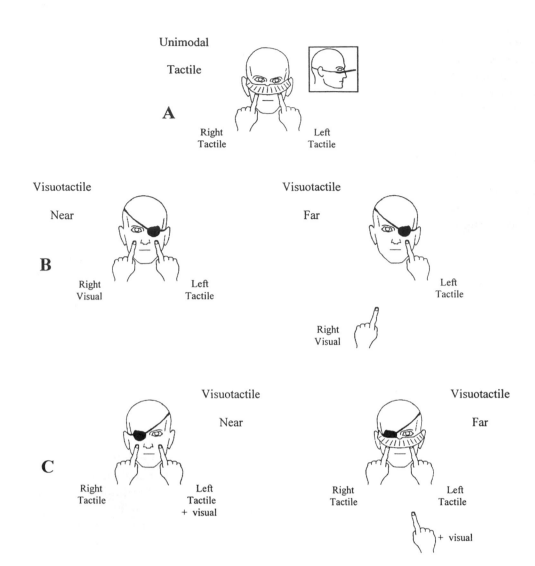

Unimodal

Tactile

A

Right
Tactile

Left
Tactile

Visuotactile

Near

B

Right
Visual

Left
Tactile

Visuotactile

Far

Left
Tactile

Right
Visual

Visuotactile

Near

C

Right
Tactile

Left
Tactile
+ visual

Visuotactile

Far

Right
Tactile

Left
Tactile

+ visual

FIGURE 50.2   Schematic drawing of the experimental conditions used for assessing unimodal tactile extinction (*A*) and cross-modal reduction (*B*) or enhancement (*C*) of tactile perception on the contralesional cheek. Depending on the condition, tactile and/or visual stimuli were presented by the experimenter (not shown) to the right, left, or both cheeks of a patient. Vision of tactile stimuli could be prevented by using monocular blindfolding or a wearable cardboard shield (depicted in the inset). In the cross-modal conditions (*B* and *C*), the visual stimulus was presented either near (left column) or far (right column) from the patients' cheeks. (Modified from Làdavas, E., et al. [1998]. Visual peripersonal space centered on the face in humans. *Brain, 121,* 2317–2326. Used by permission of Oxford University Press.)

perception. In close functional analogy with neurophysiological findings reported in the monkey literature, these findings further support the existence of an integrated system that controls both visual and tactile inputs within near peripersonal space around the face and the hand in humans (di Pellegrino, Làdavas, et al., 1997; Làdavas, di Pellegrino, et al., 1998; Làdavas, Zeloni, et al., 1998; Làdavas et al., 2000).

REFERENCE SYSTEM IN VISUOTACTILE PROCESSING   Besides the enhanced sensitivity to nearby visuotactile stimulation, another functional similarity between human and monkey multisensory integration systems consists of the reference system in which the near peripersonal space

seems to be coded. When the hands are crossed, for example, what is seen on the "right" could be felt as "left," and vice versa. We exploited this crossed-hand arrangement to investigate whether multisensory integration near the hand operates in a hand-centered coordinate system, as one might expect from several neurophysiological findings (Fogassi et al., 1996; Obayashi et al., 2000). Visuotactile extinction was investigated in one patient with right brain damage using the same paradigm described earlier, with the exception that the patient crossed his hands in front of himself, thus having the left hand in right hemispace and the right hand in left hemispace (di Pellegrino, Làdavas, et al., 1997). A strong reduction in contralesional tactile perception was observed when a visual stimulus was presented near the right hand, comparable to the reduction obtained in the canonical uncrossed posture. That is, the cross-modal extinction was not influenced by changing the hands' position, provided that the (incongruent) spatial arrangement of visual and tactile stimuli was kept constant.

This finding shows that the multisensory integration system represents visual peripersonal space in hand-centered coordinates and is in agreement with behavioral studies on normal subjects (Pavani et al., 2000; Spence, Pavani, & Driver, 1998, 2000), showing that cross-modal congruency effects are strongest near the body and do not change whether the hands are located in a crossed or uncrossed posture. Therefore, psychophysical, neuropsychological, and neurophysiological studies provide converging evidence to support the construct that multisensory coding of nearby space is body part centered, and the visuotactile spatial register can be remapped in accordance with changes in body posture. The recently discovered existence of bimodal areas in the human brain similar to those found in non-human primates provides likely candidates to account for all these different forms of cross-modal phenomena (Bremmer, Schlack, Shah, et al., 2001; Macaluso & Driver, 2001; Macaluso, Frith, & Driver, 2000a, 2000b). It would be interesting to determine whether the visual peripersonal space of the face can also be coded in face-centered coordinates, for example by investigating the amount of cross-modal extinction produced by visual stimuli approaching different portions of the face from different starting positions. In respect to the face, neurophysiological evidence supports the idea that proprioception can mediate multisensory coding together with visual and tactile information, because face-related bimodal neurons respond selectively to the projected point of impact of a visual stimulus approaching the face (Duhamel et al., 1998).

Auditory-tactile interactions in near auditory space

In the monkey, the multisensory integration involved in representing near peripersonal space combines both visual-tactile inputs and auditory-tactile inputs (Graziano, Reiss, & Gross, 1999). Similar to visuotactile neurons, some multisensory cells respond to both audition and touch, provided that the source of auditory input is located close to the animal's head. In addition, strong responses are evoked only by complex sounds (e.g., white noise bursts), and not by pure tones. Therefore, these neurons may represent the neural basis for building a spatial representation of the auditory peripersonal space surrounding the head.

In keeping with the idea that similar multimodal structures for the representation of near space are shared by human and nonhuman primates, one might ask whether spatially incongruent auditory tactile stimulation in patients with tactile extinction would reduce contralesional tactile perception, and thus lead to an exacerbation of unimodal tactile extinction. This result is exactly what would be expected if an integrated auditory-tactile system were responsible for processing perihead space representation in humans. It is indeed possible that, similar to what we have shown for visual stimuli, the somatosensory representation of a part of our body can be activated by an auditory stimulus presented in the space immediately surrounding that body part. The finding of an exaggerated cross-modal extinction, mainly at small distances of the auditory stimulus from the head, would further support the possibility that the human brain processes tactile and auditory inputs in a multisensory auditory-tactile system (Làdavas, Pavani, & Farnè, 2001).

We recently tested this hypothesis by investigating cross-modal extinction between a sound and a touch in a group of patients with right brain damage left tactile extinction. In this study, extinction was assessed by presenting bilateral touches at the level of the neck (Farnè & Làdavas, 2002). We predicted that an ipsilesional auditory stimulus would extinguish a spatially incongruent contralesional tactile stimulus (cross-modal auditory-tactile extinction). In addition, this phenomenon was expected to be sensitive to stimulus distance, and to be stronger when auditory stimuli originated near the ipsilesional side of the patients' head (at 20 cm from the right ear), than at a greater distance (70 cm from the right ear). Owing to integrative auditory-tactile processing, indeed, a sound presented near the right ear would effectively activate the somatosensory representation of the right side of the head. Therefore, the simultaneous activation of the somatosensory representations of the left and right sides of the head (evoked by touch and sound, respectively) would reduce the perception of the tactile stimulus delivered to the contralesional side of the neck. In contrast, a sound presented far from the right ear would weakly activate the somatosensory representation of the right side of the patient's head, and a weak reduction of contralesional touch perception would be produced. Finally, we predicted that cross-modal extinction would also be modulated by the type of sound, being stronger in response to complex sounds (white noise bursts) rather than simple frequencies (pure tones).

Patients' tactile sensitivity was well preserved for single stimulus detection on the left side of the neck (91% accuracy). In contrast, they reported only a small proportion of left stimuli with bilateral tactile stimulation

(36% accuracy). In agreement with a previous single-case study (Làdavas et al., 2001), the results of the cross-modal stimulation condition showed that strong contralesional extinction was obtained following the presentation of a sound near the right ear (43.5% accuracy). As expected, cross-modal interference with contralesional tactile perception was markedly reduced when the same sound originated from a farther location (66% accuracy), thus showing that auditory-tactile extinction was clearly modulated by the distance of the sound.

In addition, the spatial selectivity of this phenomenon for the perihead space was more consistent following the presentation of complex sounds than following the presentation of simple frequencies. Indeed, only in the case of peripersonal complex sounds was the amount of auditory-tactile extinction comparable to that induced by a tactile stimulus. In contrast, the amount of extinction produced by pure tones was significantly smaller than that induced by a touch, even when pure tones were presented close to the head.

In summary, these findings show the existence of a multisensory system that integrates auditory and tactile inputs within near peripersonal space around the head in humans, and are in agreement with the idea that this spatial representation might be functionally distinct from that which codes auditory information in far space (Brungart, Durlach, & Rabinowitz, 1999; Moore & King, 1999). In close analogy with the monkey data, these neuropsychological findings show that the human brain forms integrated auditory-tactile representations of the peripersonal space surrounding the head (Làdavas et al., 2001).

Taken together, the results of the studies reported here provide a remarkably convergent body of behavioral evidence demonstrating that multisensory systems coding near peripersonal space in humans are functionally very similar to those described in monkeys, and do not concern only the combination of visual and tactile modalities but also auditory and tactile modalities. Additionally, when multimodal integration involves the sense of touch, the behavioral consequences of the sensory interaction are likely to be limited to the space immediately surrounding the cutaneous surface of the body.

However, other kinds of multisensory interactions, not involving somatosensation, can be revealed in humans. Audiovisual interactions, for example, can give rise to important behavioral cross-modal effects that can take place in far peripersonal space. The following sections describe these cross-modal interactions, their functional characteristics, and their relevance for temporarily ameliorating spatial deficits such as visual neglect.

Visual neglect as a probe for investigating auditory-visual interactions

Patients with cerebral lesions involving the posterior-inferior parietal and the premotor cortex, most often in the right hemisphere, sometimes fail to explore the extrapersonal and personal sectors of space contralateral to the side of the lesion or to report stimuli presented in that portion of space. These patients have a bias to orient toward objects or events located to their right while neglecting those to the left, often being unaware of the latter. When asked to search for visual targets among distracters on cancellation tasks, right-hemisphere-damaged patients with neglect typically mark targets on the right, missing targets toward the left. In addition to the visual spatial deficit, they may also show an impairment of auditory space perception (Pavani, Làdavas, & Driver, 2002; Pavani, Meneghello, & Làdavas, 2001), as revealed by their inability to discriminate the relative spatial positions of sounds presented in contralesional space. In contrast, their performance is comparable to that of healthy controls when the acoustic stimuli are presented in ipsilesional space. The sound localization deficit in neglect has also been documented by Deouell and co-workers (Deouell, Bentin, & Soroker, 2000). They found that the typical event-related brain potentials elicited in response to a change in sound spatial position were reduced in neglect patients when the sound was presented in the left hemispace. This result can be interpreted as the consequence of the inability of these patients to perceive a change in sound position in contralesional space, owing to the auditory location deficit. Therefore, patients with visual neglect may be affected by spatial deficits in the auditory modality as well. Because of their auditory and visual spatial deficit, neglect patients are the best neuropsychological candidates in whom to verify whether the principles of multisensory integration that have been found in animals are also valid for humans. These principles and the neural substrate responsible for multisensory processing in far peripersonal space are described in the following section.

Neuronal bases for multisensory processing of far peripersonal space

Whenever different sensory information converges onto individual neurons in the CNS, there is the potential for multisensory integration. There are many sites in the brain where such convergence takes place. One of the densest concentrations of multisensory neurons is found in the deep layers of the SC (Gordon, 1973;

King & Palmer, 1985; Meredith & Stein, 1983, 1986a; Stein, 1984; Stein & Arigbede, 1972; Stein, Magalhaes-Castro, & Kruger, 1976). The SC receives visual, auditory and somatosensory inputs (Stein, 1984) and plays an important role in attending and orienting to these sensory stimuli (Sparks, 1990).

Although multisensory integration has been extensively investigated in the SC, the rules that govern the integration of multisensory information in this subcortical structure apply to other brain regions as well. These areas include the superior temporal polysensory (STP) area and the hippocampus of primates, the anterior ectosylvian sulcus (AES), the lateral suprasylvian cortex, and the visual cortex in cats (Clemo, Meredith, Wallace, & Stein, 1991; Stein & Meredith, 1993; Stein, Meredith, & Wallace, 1993; Wallace, Meredith, & Stein, 1992). The principles underlying this integration have been outlined by single-unit studies in cats, guinea pigs, and monkeys (King & Palmer, 1985; Meredith, Nemitz, & Stein, 1987; Meredith & Stein, 1983, 1986a, 1986b; Wallace & Stein, 2001; Wallace, Wilkinson, & Stein, 1996) and have largely been investigated with regard to the interaction between visual and auditory stimuli.

Multisensory enhancement in far space is determined by the spatial and temporal characteristics of the stimuli. By manipulating these parameters, the same combination of stimuli (e.g., visual and auditory) can produce response enhancement or depression in the same neurons. According to the spatial principle governing this type of multisensory integration (the so-called *spatial rule*), visual and auditory stimuli originating from the same position in space will fall within the excitatory RFs of a visual-auditory multisensory neuron. The physiological result of this pairing is an enhancement of the bimodal neuron's response.

The angular distance that can separate visual and auditory stimuli and still result in a facilitatory effect depends on the size of the visual and auditory RFs. Auditory RFs are larger than visual RFs (Jay & Sparks, 1987; King & Hutchings, 1987; King & Palmer, 1983; Knudsen, 1982; Middlebrooks & Knudsen, 1984) and, as a consequence, the auditory stimulus will excite neurons over a large region, including the region excited by the visual stimulus. In contrast, when a sound appears in a spatial position outside the excitatory RF of the bimodal neuron, the neural response to the visual stimulus is no longer enhanced. Alternatively, when a visual stimulus falls within an inhibitory region of the auditory RF, it will depress neuronal responses to the visual stimulus.

A second crucial aspect of multisensory integration concerns the relative timing of the two sensory events (the so-called *temporal rule*). Maximal multisensory interactions are achieved when periods of peak activity of the unimodal discharge train overlap. This situation is usually achieved when stimuli are presented simultaneously, although a temporal window for multisensory interactions overcomes small temporal discrepancies between the stimuli. A further principle of multisensory integration concerns the nature of the multimodal response. A simple inverse relationship exists between the effectiveness of the stimuli and the response evoked: combinations of weak unimodal stimuli produce the greatest enhancement. For example, even when the individual visual and auditory stimuli evoke no response, their combination becomes effective and produces a surprisingly vigorous response (Meredith & Stein, 1986a). This third principle, known as *inverse effectiveness,* provides an explanation for a greater enhancement when two weak rather than two potent stimuli are combined.

Auditory-visual modulation of neglect: Enhancement of contralesional unimodal visual perception through bimodal stimulation

In the neuropsychological domain there is no evidence that similar principles of multisensory visual-auditory integration apply in humans. However, such integrated systems, if they are shown to exist, could be useful in improving the performance of patients with visual neglect (i.e., patients with spatial representational deficits). The integration of visual and auditory information could improve patients' detection of bimodal stimuli of which the visual unimodal component goes undetected.

In this respect, it is worth noting that two unimodal visual stimuli, although presented in the same spatial position, do not produce an amelioration of visual detection deficits (Làdavas, Carletti, & Gori, 1994). When a left exogenous noninformative visual cue was presented immediately before the visual target, no amelioration of performance in left visual field target detection was found. At variance with unimodal visual presentation, and consistent with the expectation based on the neurophysiological studies, it was found that the bimodal presentation of auditory and visual stimuli improves visual stimulus detection in patients with visual neglect. In a recent study by Frassinetti and colleagues (Frassinetti, Pavani, & Làdavas, 2002), neglect patients were required to fixate a central stimulus and to detect visual stimuli horizontally displayed at 8, 24, and 40 degrees in the left visual field as well as in the right visual field. The task was performed either in a unimodal condition (i.e., only visual stimuli were presented) or in cross-modal

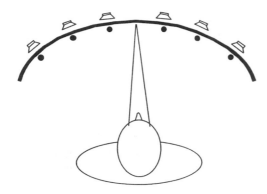

🔔 Auditory stimulus

• Visual stimulus

FIGURE 50.3 Schematic drawing (seen from above) of the experimental setup used to assess variations in visual detection following visual + auditory stimulation. The patient faced a semicircular black display. The apparatus consisted of six LEDs and six loudspeakers located at an eccentricity of 8, 24, and 40 degrees on either side of the central fixation point. A strip of black fabric concealed the loudspeakers from patient's view.

conditions (i.e., a sound was presented simultaneously with the visual target). In the cross-modal conditions, sounds were presented either at the same spatial position as the visual target or at one of the remaining five spatial positions (Fig. 50.3).

The results of this study show that a cue from one modality (audition) substantially modified stimulus detection in another modality (vision). In neglect patients, a sound presented at the same position (or at a small disparity) as a visual stimulus influenced detection of previously neglected visual targets. Moreover, by varying the positions of different sensory stimuli and evaluating their effect on visual detection, the authors found that the improvement was evident only when the two stimuli followed a rather clear-cut spatial rule. Indeed, auditory stimuli produced a great increase of visual responses either when the two stimuli were spatially coincident or when they were located near one another in space at a distance of 16 degrees. In contrast, when the spatial disparity between the two sensory stimuli was larger than 16 degrees, the patients' visual performance was unaffected by a concomitant sound.

The finding that an amelioration of neglect is observable only when the two stimuli are presented at the same position or at a small disparity cannot be explained as a result of an arousal phenomenon; that is, the presence of two stimuli, instead of one, might have produced

greater activity throughout the brain by generally increasing neural sensitivity to all stimuli. Recently, Robertson and colleagues (Robertson, Mattingley, Rorden, & Driver, 1998) have suggested that nonspatial phasic alerting events (for example, warning tones) can overcome a neglect patient's spatial bias in visual perceptual awareness. In that study, however, at variance with our results, the beneficial effect of sound on visual perception was not spatially specific. The relative acceleration of perceptual events on the contralesional side was found when the warning sound was presented on the left or the right side of the space. However, such an arousal effect cannot alone explain the pattern of results found in our study (Frassinetti et al., 2002). By varying the positions of different sensory stimuli and evaluating their effects on visual detection, we found that the improvement was evident only when stimuli followed a rather clear-cut spatial rule. Rather, our results are in keeping with the functional properties of multisensory neurons described in animal studies (Stein & Meredith, 1993). A functional property of bimodal neurons is that their response is enhanced only when both auditory and visual stimuli are located within their respective excitatory RFs. Because auditory RFs are larger than visual RFs, the auditory stimulus will excite neurons over a larger region. This explains why, in the study by Frassinetti et al., the influence of the auditory stimulus extended to visual stimuli located not only in the same position but also in a near position, at a disparity of 16 degrees (see also Spence, 2001).

Moreover, the cross-modal effects were more evident for the most peripheral stimuli in the left visual field, where neglect was more severe, and they were not found when the stimuli were presented in more medial positions, where neglect was very mild. This finding too, is consistent with neurophysiological findings (the inverse effectiveness rule), which showed a greater enhancement when two weak stimuli rather than two potent sensory stimuli were combined. In animal work (Meredith & Stein, 1986a), the enhancement of correct responses with combined stimuli was observed when single-modality stimuli evoked poor performance. Visually responsive multisensory neurons show proportionately greater response enhancement with subthreshold (undetected) stimuli. Overall, because the behavioral effects of cross-modal modulation revealed in humans parallel the functional properties of multisensory integration processes revealed in animals, the findings reviewed in this chapter might reflect the activity of mechanisms responsible for the facilitatory effects that have been reported in normal subjects on cross-modal cuing paradigms (for a discussion of this issue, see McDonald et al., 2001).

The omnipresent nature of multisensory representation of space in humans

The unitary perception of space actually reflects the outcome of a multimodular and multisensory computation that requires a considerable amount of fusion among the senses. Our everyday perceptual experience is the result of integrated multisensory processes that probably rely on the activity of different but interconnected sensory integration systems. The functional properties of these systems have been studied physiologically in nonhuman primates and their contribution to the coding of near or far peripersonal space through the integration of visual, tactile, proprioceptive, and auditory inputs has been documented.

In this chapter we reviewed the neuropsychological findings that shed light on brain mechanisms responsible for coding space through multisensory processing in humans. In a series of experiments, we took advantage of the spatial ipsilesional bias caused by right unilateral lesions to assess the functional organization of these multisensory processes. For our approach to work, the lesion responsible for the bias should not completely impair the circuit of multimodal brain areas, because any cross-modal spatial arrangement (congruent or not) would otherwise be ineffective. It would be interesting to relate the selectivity of cross-modal extinction for near peripersonal space with the location of brain damage. In agreement with the above prediction, a retrospective analysis (unpublished) of patient populations studied in previous work from our laboratory indicated that patients showing strong spatial selectivity tended to be affected by more restricted frontoparietal lesions than patients showing less or nonspecific effects. However, these data are only preliminary. Because of the large size and variable extent of the lesions in our groups of patients, it is difficult to relate precisely their cross-modal behavioral phenomena with a defined cerebral location, and more detailed analyses of the extent and precise locus of damage are needed.

Recent event-related potential (ERP) studies have shown that multisensory interactions can occur early in the cortical processing hierarchy, in putatively unimodal brain regions (Foxe et al., 2000). By specifically manipulating spatial attention, several behavioral and ERP studies have shown that cross-modal links between vision, audition, and touch can affect sensory perceptual processes within modality-specific cortical regions (for a review, see Eimer & Driver, 2001). These findings point to the possible (nonmutually exclusive) existence of bottom-up, feed-forward integration in early sensory processing, and top-down modulation of unimodal sensory areas through backward propagation of activity from multimodal areas. Whether the competition is more likely to occur directly in these structures or through backward modulation of primary areas (Driver & Spence, 2000; Eimer, 2001; Kennett, Eimer, Spence, & Driver, 2001; Macaluso et al., 2000a; Shimojo & Shams, 2001), it is noteworthy that cross-modal effects between opposite body parts appear to require intact interhemispheric connections (Spence, Kingstone, Shore, & Gazzaniga, 2001; Spence, Shore, Gazzaniga, Soto-Faraco, & Kingstone, 2001; see also Marzi, Girelli, Natale, & Miniussi, 2001).

In addition, it is important to establish whether other factors may affect the presence and strength of spatially selective cross-modal effects. In this respect, our retrospective study suggested that the presence of visual neglect in addition to tactile extinction, and the fact that patients were tested in a relatively acute stage, may negatively influence the emergence of selective cross-modal effects in near peripersonal space. These findings suggest that the severity of patients' clinical conditions (in terms of presence of neglect and testing during the acute or chronic phase) might obscure the differential spatial distribution of cross-modal extinction. Further studies are needed to clarify whether these factors may interact.

In aggregate, our studies show that the expression of cross-modal interaction seems to be a rather frequent occurrence that can be selectively modulated by several parameters relative to the relationship between the stimulus and the body, such as distance, spatial location, visual or proprioceptive information, visual plausibility of fake body parts, auditory complexity, and spatial and temporal coincidence. Therefore, our findings are in good agreement with a modular organization of space in which several neuronal structures are devoted to the processing of different space sectors, in different coordinates, and across different modalities, most probably for different behavioral purposes (Rizzolatti et al., 1998). Among these structures, the representation of near and far peripersonal space in humans parallels the functioning of the circuit of multisensory areas that has been well documented in monkeys, which is similarly sensitive to the same parameters as were just listed. This strongly supports our claim that human and nonhuman primate brains have similar multisensory integrated circuits (Làdavas, di Pellegrino, et al., 1998; Farnè & Làdavas, 2000). This idea received even more direct support from functional MRI studies showing that multimodal processing in both species displays a high degree of commonality, both anatomically and functionally (Bremmer, Schlack, Duhamel, et al., 2001; Bremmer, Schlack, Shah, et al., 2001; Macaluso et al., 2000a, 2000b).

REFERENCES

Barbieri, C., & De Renzi, E. (1989). Patterns of neglect dissociations. *Behavioral Neurology, 2,* 13–24.

Bellas, D. N., Novelly, R. A., Eskenazi, B., & Wasserstein, J. (1988). The nature of unilateral neglect in the olfactory sensory system. *Neuropsychologia, 26,* 45–52.

Bender, M. B. (1952). *Disorders in perception.* Springfield, IL: Thomas.

Berti, A., Oxbury, S., Oxbury, J., Affanni, P., Umiltà, C., & Orlandi, L. (1999). Somatosensory extinction for meaningful objects in a patient with right hemispheric stroke. *Neuropsychologia, 37,* 333–343.

Bisiach, E. (1991). Extinction and neglect: Same or different? In J. Paillard (Ed.), *Brain and space* (pp. 251–257). New York: Oxford University Press.

Botvinick, M., & Cohen, J. (1998). Rubber hands "feel" touch that eyes see. *Nature, 391,* 756.

Bremmer, F., Schlack, A., Duhamel, J. R., Graf, W., & Fink, G. R. (2001). Space coding in primate posterior parietal cortex. *NeuroImage, 14,* S46–S51.

Bremmer, F., Schlack, A., Shah, N. J., Zafiris, O., Kubischik, M., Hoffmann, K., et al. (2001). Polymodal motion processing in posterior parietal and premotor cortex: A human fMRI study strongly implies equivalencies between humans and monkeys. *Neuron, 29,* 287–296.

Brungart, D. S., Durlach, N. J., & Rabinowitz, W. M. (1999). Auditory localization of nearby sources: II. Localization of a broadband source. *Journal of the Acoustical Society of America, 106,* 1956–1968.

Clemo, H. R., Meredith, M. A., Wallace, M. T., & Stein, B. E. (1991). Is the cortex of cat anterior ectosylvian sulcus a polysensory area? *Society of Neuroscience Abstracts, 17,* 1585.

Cocchini, G., Cubelli, R., Della Sala, S., & Beschin, N. (1999). Neglect without extinction. *Cortex, 35,* 285–313.

Colby, C. L., Duhamel, J. R., & Goldberg, M. E. (1993). Ventral intraparietal area of the macaque: Anatomic location and visual response properties. *Journal of Neurophysiology, 69,* 902–914.

Dassonville, P. (1995). Haptic localization and the internal representation of the hand in space. *Experimental Brain Research, 106,* 434–448.

Deouell, L. Y., Bentin, S., & Soroker, N. (2000). Electrophysiological evidence for an early (preattentive) information processing deficit in patients with right hemisphere damage and unilateral neglect. *Brain, 123,* 353–365.

De Renzi, E. (1982). *Disorders of space exploration and cognition.* New York: Wiley.

De Renzi, E., Gentilini, M., & Pattaccini, F. (1984). Auditory extinction following hemisphere damage. *Neuropsychologia, 22,* 1231–1240.

di Pellegrino, G., & De Renzi, E. (1995). An experimental investigation on the nature of extinction. *Neuropsychologia, 33,* 153–170.

di Pellegrino, G., Basso, G., & Frassinetti, F. (1997). Spatial extinction to double asynchronous stimulation. *Neuropsychologia, 35,* 1215–1223.

di Pellegrino, G., Làdavas, E., & Farnè, A. (1997). Seeing where your hands are. *Nature, 338,* 730.

Driver, J. (1998). The neuropsychology of spatial attention. In H. Pashler (Ed.), *Attention* (pp. 297–340). Hove, England: Psychology Press.

Driver, J., Mattingley, J. B., Rorden, C., & Davis, G. (1997). Extinction as a paradigm measure of attentional bias and restricted capacity following brain injury. In P. Thier & H. O. Karnath (Eds.), *Parietal lobe contribution to orientation in 3D space* (pp. 401–429). Heidelberg: Springer Verlag.

Driver, J., & Spence, C. (2000). Multisensory perception: Beyond modularity and convergence. *Current Biology, 10,* R731–R735.

Duhamel, J. R., Colby, C. L., & Goldberg, M. E. (1991). Congruent representation of visual and somatosensory space in single neurons of monkey ventral intra-parietal area (VIP). In J. Paillard (Ed.), *Brain and space* (pp. 223–236). New York: Oxford University Press.

Duhamel, J. R., Colby, C. L., & Goldberg, M. E. (1998). Ventral intraparietal area of the macaque: Congruent visual and somatic response properties. *Journal of Neurophysiology, 79,* 126–136.

Duncan, J. (1980). The locus of interference in the perception of simultaneous stimuli. *Psychological Review, 87,* 272–300.

Duncan, J. (1996). Coordinated brain systems in selective perception and action. In T. Inui & J. L. McClelland (Eds.), *Attention and performance* (pp. 549–578). Cambridge, MA: MIT Press.

Eimer, M. (2001). Crossmodal links in spatial attention between vision, audition, and touch: Evidence from event-related brain potentials. *Neuropsychologia, 39,* 1292–1303.

Eimer, M., & Driver, J. (2001). Crossmodal links in endogenous and exogenous spatial attention: Evidence from event-related brain potential studies. *Neuroscience and Biobehavioral Review, 25,* 497–511.

Farnè, A., & Làdavas, E. (2000). Dynamic size-change of hand peripersonal space following tool use. *Neuroreport, 85,* 1645–1649.

Farnè, A., & Làdavas, E. (2002). Auditory peripersonal space in humans. *Journal of Cognitive Neuroscience, 14,* 1030–1043.

Farnè, A., Pavani, F., Meneghello, F., & Làdavas, E. (2000). Left tactile extinction following visual stimulation of a rubber hand. *Brain, 123,* 2350–2360.

Fogassi, L., Gallese, V., Fadiga, L., Luppino, G., Matelli, M., & Rizzolatti, G. (1996). Coding of peripersonal space in inferior premotor cortex (area F4). *Journal of Neurophysiology, 76,* 141–157.

Fogassi, L., Raos, V., Franchi, G., Gallese, V., Luppino, G., & Matelli, M. (1999). Visual responses in the dorsal premotor area F2 of the macaque monkey. *Experimental Brain Research, 128,* 194–199.

Foxe, J., Morocz, I. A., Murray, M. M., Higgins, B. A., Javitt, D. C., & Schroeder, C. E. (2000). Multisensory auditory-somatosensory interactions in early cortical processing revealed by high-density electrical mapping. *Cognitive Brain Research, 10,* 77–83.

Frassinetti, F., Pavani, F., & Làdavas, E. (2002). Acoustical vision of neglected stimuli! Interaction among spatially converging audio-visual inputs in neglect patients. *Journal of Cognitive Neuroscience, 14,* 62–69.

Gainotti, G., De Bonis, C., Daniele, A., & Caltagirone, C. (1989). Contralateral and ipsilateral tactile extinction in patients with right and left focal brain damage. *International Journal of Neuroscience, 45,* 81–89.

Goodrich, S., & Ward, R. (1997). Anti-extinction following unilateral parietal damage. *Cognitive Neuropsychology, 14,* 595–612.

Gordon, B. G. (1973). Receptive fields in the deep layers of the cat superior colliculus. *Journal of Neurophysiology, 36,* 157–178.

Graziano, M. S. A. (1999). Where is my arm? The relative role of vision and proprioception in the neuronal representation of limb position. *Proceedings of the National Academy of Sciences, USA, 96,* 10418–10421.

Graziano, M. S. A., Cooke, D. F., & Taylor, S. R. (2000). Coding the location of the arm by sight. *Science, 290,* 1782–1786.

Graziano, M. S. A., & Gross, C. G. (1995). The representation of extrapersonal space: A possible role for bimodal, visuo-tactile neurons. In M. S. Gazzaniga (Ed.), *The cognitive Neuroscience* (pp. 1021–1034). Cambridge, MA: MIT Press.

Graziano, M. S. A., & Gross, C. G. (1998a). Visual responses with and without fixation: Neurons in premotor cortex encode spatial locations independently of eye position. *Experimental Brain Research, 118,* 373–380.

Graziano, M. S. A., & Gross, C. G. (1998b). Spatial maps for the control of movement. *Current Opinion in Neurobiology, 8,* 195–201.

Graziano, M. S. A., Hu, X. T., & Gross, C. G. (1997). Visuospatial properties of ventral premotor cortex. *Journal of Neurophysiology, 77,* 2268–2292.

Graziano, M. S. A., Reiss, L. A. J., & Gross, C. G. (1999). A neuronal representation of the location of nearby sounds. *Nature, 397,* 428–430.

Graziano, M. S. A., Taylor, C. S. R., & Moore, T. (2001). Electrical stimulation of the bimodal, visual-tactile zone in the precentral gyrus evokes defensive movements. *Society for Neuroscience Abstracts, 129,* 8.

Haggard, P., Newman, C., Blundell, J., & Andrew, H. (2000). The perceived position of the hand in space. *Perception & Psychophysics, 62,* 363–377.

Halligan, P. W., Hunt, M., Marshall, J. C., & Wade, D. T. (1996). When seeing is feeling: Acquired synaesthesia or phantom touch? *Neurocase, 2,* 21–29.

Halligan, P. W., Marshall, J. C., Hunt, M., & Wade, D. T. (1997). Somatosensory assessment: Can seeing produce feeling? *Journal of Neurology, 244,* 199–203.

Hay, J. C., Pick, H. L., & Ikeda, K. (1965). Visual capture produced by prism spectacles. *Psychonomic Sciences, 2,* 215–216.

Hyvärinen, J., & Poranen, A. (1974). Function of the parietal associative area 7 as revealed from cellular discharges in alert monkeys. *Brain, 97,* 673–692.

Jay, M. F., & Sparks, D. L. (1987). Sensorimotor integration in the primate superior colliculus: II. Coordinates of auditory signals. *Journal of Neurophysiology, 57,* 35–55.

Kennett, S., Eimer, M., Spence, C., & Driver, J. (2001). Tactile-visual links in exogenous spatial attention under different postures: Convergent evidence from psychophysics and ERPs. *Journal of Cognitive Neuroscience, 13,* 462–478.

Kennett, S., Taylor-Clarke, M., & Haggard, P. (2001). Noninformative vision improves the spatial resolution of touch in humans. *Current Biology, 11,* 1188–1191.

King, A. J., & Hutchings, M. E. (1987). Spatial response property of acoustically responsive neurons in the superior colliculus of the ferret: A map of auditory space. *Journal of Neurophysiology, 57,* 596–624.

King, A. J., & Palmer, A. R. (1983). Cells responsive to free-field auditory stimuli in guinea-pig superior colliculus: Distribution and response properties. *Journal of Physiology, 342,* 361–381.

King, A. J., & Palmer, A. R. (1985). Integration of visual and auditory information in bimodal neurons in the guinea pig superior colliculus. *Experimental Brain Research, 60,* 492–500.

Knudsen, E. I. (1982). Auditory and visual maps of space in the optic tectum of the owl. *Journal of Neuroscience, 2,* 1177–1194.

Làdavas, E. (1990). Selective spatial attention in patients with visual extinction. *Brain, 113,* 1527–1538.

Làdavas, E. (2002). Functional and dynamic properties of visual peripersonal space in humans. *Trends in Cognitive Sciences, 6,* 17–22.

Làdavas, E., Berti, A., & Farnè, A. (2000). Dissociation between conscious and non-conscious processing in neglect. In Y. Rossetti & A. Revounsuo (Eds.), *Beyond dissociation: Interaction between dissociated implicit and explicit processing. Advances in Consciousness Research* (Vol. 22, pp. 175–193). Philadelphia: John Benjamins.

Làdavas, E., Carletti, M., & Gori, G. (1994). Automatic and voluntary orienting of attention in patients with visual neglect: Horizontal and vertical dimensions. *Neuropsychologia, 32,* 1195–1208.

Làdavas, E., di Pellegrino, G., Farnè, A., & Zeloni, G. (1998). Neuropsychological evidence of an integrated visuo-tactile representation of peripersonal space in humans. *Journal of Cognitive Neuroscience, 10,* 581–589.

Làdavas, E., Farnè, A., Zeloni, G., & di Pellegrino, G. (2000). Seeing or not seeing where your hands are. *Experimental Brain Research, 131,* 458–467.

Làdavas, E., Pavani, F., & Farnè, A. (2001). Feel the noise! A case of auditory-tactile extinction. *Neurocase, 7,* 97–103.

Làdavas, E., Zeloni, G., & Farnè, A. (1998). Visual peripersonal space centred on the face in humans. *Brain, 121,* 2317–2326.

Liu, G., Bolton, A. K., Price, B. H., & Weintraub, S. (1992). Dissociated perceptual-sensory and exploratory-motor neglect. *Journal of Neurology, Neurosurgery, and Psychiatry, 55,* 701–706.

Loeb, J. (1885). Die elementaren Störungen einfacher Funktionen nach ober-flächlicher, umschriebener Verletzung des Großhirns. *Pflugers Archivs, 37,* 51–56.

Macaluso, E., & Driver, J. (2001). Spatial attention and cross-modal interactions between vision and touch. *Neuropsychologia, 39,* 1304–1316.

Macaluso, E., Frith, C. D., & Driver, J. (2000a). Modulation of human visual cortex by crossmodal spatial attention. *Science, 289,* 1206–1208.

Macaluso, E., Frith, C. D., & Driver, J. (2000b). Selective spatial attention in vision and touch: Unimodal and multimodal mechanisms revealed by PET. *Journal of Neurophysiology, 63,* 3062–3085.

MacKay, W. A., & Crammond, D. J. (1987). Neuronal correlates in posterior parietal lobe of the expectation of events. *Behavioural Brain Research, 24,* 167–179.

Maravita, A., Spence, C., Clarke, K., Husain, M., & Driver, J. (2000). Vision and touch through the looking glass in a case of crossmodal extinction. *Neuroreport, 169*, 3521–3526.

Marzi, C. A., Girelli, M., Natale, E., & Miniussi, C. (2001). What exactly is extinguished in unilateral visual extinction? Neurophysiological evidence. *Neuropsychologia, 39*, 1354–1366.

Mattingley, J. B., Driver, J., Beschin, N., & Robertson, I. H. (1997). Attentional competition between modalities: Extinction between touch and vision after right hemisphere damage. *Neuropsychologia, 35*, 867–880.

McDonald, J. J., Teder-Salejarvi, W. A., & Ward, L. M. (2001). Multisensory integration and crossmodal attention effects in the human brain. *Science, 292*, 1791a.

Meredith, M. A., Nemitz, J. M., & Stein, B. E. (1987). Determinants of multisensory integration in superior colliculus neurons: I. Temporal factors. *Journal of Neuroscience, 7*, 3215–3229.

Meredith, M. A., & Stein, B. E. (1983). Interactions among converging sensory inputs in the superior colliculus. *Science, 221*, 389–391.

Meredith, M. A., & Stein, B. E. (1986a). Spatial factors determine the activity of multisensory neurons in cat superior colliculus. *Brain Research, 369*, 350–354.

Meredith, M. A., & Stein, B. E. (1986b). Visual, auditory and somatosensory convergence on cells in superior colliculus results in multisensory integration. *Journal of Neurophysiology, 56*, 640–662.

Middlebrooks, J. C., & Knudsen, E. I. (1984). A neural code for auditory space in the cat's superior colliculus. *Journal of Neuroscience, 4*, 2621–2634.

Mon-Williams, M., Wann, J. P., Jenkinson, M., & Rushton, K. (1997). Synaesthesia in the normal limb. *Proceedings of the Royal Society of London, 264*, 1007–1010.

Moore, D. R., & King, A. J. (1999). Auditory perception: The near and far of sound localization. *Current Biology, 9*, R361–R363.

Mort, D. J., Malhotra, P., Mannan, S. K., Rorden, C., Pambakian, A., Kennard, C., Husain, M. (2003). The anatomy of visual neglect. *Brain, 126*, 1986–1997.

Moscovitch, M., & Behrmann, M. (1994). Coding of spatial information in the somatosensory system: Evidence from patients with neglect following parietal lobe damage. *Journal of Cognitive Neuroscience, 6*, 151–155.

Newport, R., Hindle, J. V., & Jackson, S. R. (2001). Vision can improve the felt position of the unseen hand: Neurological evidence for links between vision and somatosensation in humans. *Current Biology, 11*, 1–20.

Obayashi, S., Tanaka, M., & Iriki, A. (2000). Subjective image of invisible hand coded by monkey intraparietal neurons. *Neuroreport, 11*, 3499–3505.

Oppenheim, H. (1885). Über eine durch eine klinisch bisher nicht verwetete Untersuchungsmethode ermittelte Sensibilitätsstörung bei einseitigen Erkrankungen des Großhirns. *Neurologische Centralblatt, 37*, 51–56.

Pavani, F., Làdavas, E., & Driver, J. (2002). Selective deficit of auditory localisation in patients with visuospatial neglect. *Neuropsychologia, 40*, 291–301.

Pavani, F., Meneghello, F., & Làdavas, E. (2001). Deficit of auditory space perception in patients with visuospatial neglect. *Neuropsychologia, 39*, 1401–1409.

Pavani, F., Spence, C., & Driver, J. (2000). Visual capture of touch: Out of the body experiences with rubber gloves. *Psychological Science, 11*, 353–359.

Posner, M. I., Walker, J. A., Friedrich, J., & Rafal, R. D. (1984). Effects of parietal injury on covert orienting of attention. *Journal of Neuroscience, 4*, 1863–1874.

Pouget, A., & Sejnowski, T. J. (1997). Lesion in a basis function model of parietal cortex: Comparison with hemineglect. In P. Thier & H. O. Karnath (Eds.), *Parietal lobe contribution to orientation in 3-D space* (pp. 521–538). Berlin: Springer-Verlag.

Rizzolatti, G., Luppino, G., & Matelli, M. (1998). The organization of the cortical motor system: New concepts. *Electroencephalography and Clinical Neurophysiology, 106*, 283–296.

Rizzolatti, G., Scandolara, C., Matelli, M., & Gentilucci, M. (1981). Afferent properties of periarcuate neurons in macaque monkeys: II Visual responses. *Behavioural Brain Research, 2*, 147–163.

Ro, T., & Farnè, A. (2001). Within-modal anti-extinction in multimodal "neglect." *Cognitive Neuroscience Society Abstracts, 103E*, 139.

Robertson, I. H., & Marshall, J. C. (1993). *Unilateral neglect: Clinical and experimental studies*. Hillsdale, NJ: Erlbaum.

Robertson, I. H., Mattingley, J. B., Rorden, C., & Driver, J. (1998). Phasic alerting of neglect patients overcomes their spatial deficit in visual awareness. *Nature, 395*, 169–172.

Robertson, I. H., & Rafal, R. D. (2000). Disorders of visual attention. In M. S. Gazzaniga (Ed.), *The new cognitive neuroscience* (pp. 633–649). Cambridge, MA: MIT Press.

Rock, I., & Victor, J. (1964). Vision and touch: An experimentally created conflict between the two senses. *Science, 143*, 594–596.

Rorden, C., Heutink, J., Greenfield, E., & Robertson, I. H. (1999). When a rubber hand "feels" what the real hand cannot. *Neuroreport, 10*, 135–138.

Rossetti, Y., Desmurget, M., & Prablanc, C. (1995). Vectorial coding of movement: Vision, proprioception or both? *Journal of Neurophysiology, 74*, 457–463.

Shimojo, S., & Shams, L. (2001). Sensory modalities are not separate modalities: Plasticity and interactions. *Current Opinion in Neurobiology, 11*, 505–509.

Sparks, D. L. (1990). Signal transformations required for the generation of saccadic eye movements. *Annual Review of Neuroscience, 13*, 309–336.

Spence, C. (2001). Crossmodal attentional capture: A controversy resolved? In C. Folk & B. Gibson (Eds.), *Attraction, distraction, and action: Multiple perspectives on attentional capture* (pp. 231–262). Amsterdam: Elsevier.

Spence, C., Kingstone, A., Shore, D., & Gazzaniga, M. S. (2001). Representation of visuotactile space in the split brain. *Psychological Science, 12*, 90–93.

Spence, C., Pavani, F., & Driver, J. (1998). What crossing the hands can reveal about crossmodal links in spatial attention. *Psychonomic Society Abstracts, 3*, 13.

Spence, C., Pavani, F., & Driver, J. (2000). Crossmodal links between vision and touch in covert endogenous spatial attention. *Journal of Experimental Psychology: Human Perception and Performance, 26*, 1298–1319.

Spence, C., Shore, D. I., Gazzaniga, M. S., Soto-Faraco, S., & Kingstone, A. (2001). Failure to remap visuotactile space across the midline in the split-brain. *Canadian Journal of Experimental Psychology, 55,* 133–140.

Stein, B. E. (1984). Multimodal representation in the superior colliculus and optic tectum. In H. Vanegas (Ed.), *Comparative neurology of the optic tectum* (pp. 819–841). New York: Plenum Press.

Stein, B. E., & Arigbede, M. O. (1972). Unimodal and multimodal response properties of neurons in the cat's superior colliculus. *Experimental Neurology, 36,* 179–196.

Stein, B. E., Huneycutt, W. S., & Meredith, M. A. (1988). Neurons and behaviour: The same rule of multisensory integration apply. *Brain Research, 448,* 355–358.

Stein, B. E., London, N., Wilkinson, L. K., & Price, D. D. (1996). Enhancement of perceived visual intensity by auditory stimuli: A psychophysical analysis. *Journal of Cognitive Neuroscience, 8,* 497–506.

Stein, B. E., Magalhaes-Castro, B., & Kruger, L. (1976). Relationship between visual and tactile representation in cat superior colliculus. *Journal of Neurophysiology, 39,* 401–419.

Stein, B. E., & Meredith, M. A. (1993). *The merging of the senses.* Cambridge, MA: MIT Press.

Stein, B. E., Meredith, M. A., Huneycutt, W. S., & McDade, L. W. (1989). Behavioural indices of multisensory integration: Orientation to visual cues is affected by auditory stimuli. *Journal of Cognitive Neuroscience, 1,* 12–24.

Stein, B. E., Meredith, M. A., & Wallace, M. T. (1993). Nonvisual responses of visually responsive neurons. *Progress in Brain Research, 95,* 79–90.

Tipper, S. P., Lloyd, D., Shorland, B., Dancer, C., Howard, L. A., & McGlone, F. (1998). Vision influences tactile perception without proprioceptive orienting. *Neuroreport, 9,* 1741–1744.

Tipper, S. P., Phillips, N., Dancer, C., Lloyd, D., Howard, L. A., & McGlone, F. (2001). Vision influences tactile perception at body sites that cannot be viewed directly. *Experimental Brain Research, 139,* 160–167.

Vallar, G., & Perani, D. (1986). The anatomy of unilateral neglect after right hemisphere stroke lesions: A clinical CT/scan correlation study in man. *Neuropsychologia, 24,* 609–622.

Vallar, G., Rusconi, M. L., Bignamini, L., Geminiani, G., & Perani, D. (1994). Anatomical correlates of visual and tactile extinction in humans: A clinical CT scan study. *Journal of Neurology, Neurosurgery, and Psychiatry, 57,* 464–470.

van Beers, R. J., Sittig, A. C., & Gon, J. J. (1999). Integration of proprioceptive and visual position-information: An experimentally supported model. *Journal of Neurophysiology, 81,* 1355–1364.

Wallace, M. T., Meredith, M. A., & Stein, B. E. (1992). Integration of multiple sensory modalities in cat cortex. *Experimental Brain Research, 91,* 484–488.

Wallace, M. T., & Stein, B. E. (2001). Sensory and multisensory responses in the newborn monkey superior colliculus. *Journal of Neuroscience, 21,* 8886–8894.

Wallace, M. T., Wilkinson, L. K., & Stein, B. E. (1996). Representation and integration of multiple sensory inputs in primate superior colliculus. *Journal of Neurophysiology, 76,* 1246–1266.

Ward, R., Goodrich, S., & Driver, J. (1994). Grouping reduces visual extinction: Neuropsychological evidence for weight-linkage in visual selection. *Vision and Cognition, 1,* 101–129.

Warren, D. H., & Cleaves, W. T. (1971). Visual-proprioceptive interaction under large amounts of conflict. *Journal of Experimental Psychology, 90,* 206–214.

51 Cross-Modal Integration and Spatial Attention in Relation to Tool Use and Mirror Use: Representing and Extending Multisensory Space Near the Hand

ANGELO MARAVITA AND JON DRIVER

Introduction

This chapter focuses on spatial cross-modal integration between visual and tactile stimuli, which is often thought to arise primarily in the peripersonal space near the body or hands within which objects can be touched and manipulated (see, e.g., Duhamel, Colby, & Goldberg, 1998; Fogassi et al., 1996; Gentilucci et al., 1988; Graziano & Gross, 1995; Rizzolatti, Scandolara, Matelli, & Gentilucci, 1981). We examine how such integration can be extended into more distant space, either when a person wields a tool that brings distant visual stimuli within touchable or manipulable reach or when the hands are seen in a mirror, so that their distant visual reflections can relate to touch at the hands' true location. Data from studies in normal and brain-damaged adult humans are tentatively related to the growing body of neurophysiological data on multisensory representations of space near the body at the single-cell level (see, e.g., Colby, Duhamel, & Goldberg, 1993; Gentilucci et al., 1988; Graziano & Gross, 1995; Graziano, Yap, & Gross, 1994; Leinonen, Hyvärinen, Nyman, & Linnankoski, 1979; Rizzolatti et al., 1981). The work reviewed shows how classical notions of the "body schema" (Head & Holmes, 1911; see also Ishibashi, Obayashi, & Iriki, Chap. 28, this volume, for a detailed discussion of this construct) may now be subjected to psychological and neuroscientific scrutiny (cf. Aglioti, Smania, Manfredi, & Berlucchi, 1996; Berlucchi & Aglioti, 1997; Frederiks, 1985), leading to more mechanistic formulations of how the space near

our body parts may be represented and how these spatial representations can be dynamically altered by wielding tools or viewing mirror reflections.

In the first section of the chapter, we discuss recent evidence that visual-tactile spatial integration can be modulated by the use of long tools. Wielding long tools not only extends reaching abilities into far space but also may modulate the integration between distant visual stimuli at the end of the tool (which become reachable by it) and tactile stimuli on the hands wielding the tool. Far visual events that can be reached by the tool start to influence tactile stimulation in a similar fashion to visual stimuli that are located nearer to the stimulated hand. In effect, the distant visual stimuli become "peripersonal" when a tool allows them to be reached.

In the second part of the chapter, we consider situations in which the hands are seen reflected in a mirror, so that their distant visual images reflect information that is actually located near (or at) the hands in external space. Intriguingly, in this situation, visual input from the mirror is seen as far away ("through the looking glass"), projecting the same optical images as those that would be produced by distant sources. We show that distant visual stimuli (now reflections in the mirror) can interfere with tactile stimuli in an analogous manner to visual stimuli that are directly seen as close to the hand, provided the mirror reflections are represented as having a peripersonal source, as when the true location of the source of the mirror image can be encoded. These results can be seen as analogous to the effects of tool use in some respects, with mirrors serving as a more abstract kind of tool that can also allow distant visual information to be related to touch on the body or hands. Finally, we discuss the possible roles of learning, or of top-down knowledge, in producing these various extensions of tactile-visual interactions into distant visual space.

Cross-modal integration modulated by wielding long tools

One of the characteristic features of human behavior is the ability to use a wide range of tools to increase motor interaction with external space. This feature is evident in many routine tasks of daily life. The evolutionary separation of the hands from human locomotion may have led to increased specialization in using them for many sensorimotor interactions with external objects, including tool manufacture and use (Paillard, 1993). Moreover, when using tools manually, we typically rely on a combination of visual, tactile, and proprioceptive information to guide our spatial actions with the tools, with such multisensory guidance prompting the question of how these different sources of information are integrated.

Although highly skilled tool use is characteristic of humans, other species, and in particular other primates, may also exhibit some degree of tool use. Chimpanzees may manipulate some tools in a seemingly insightful way, such as to reach a desired object that would otherwise be too far away (Kohler, 1927). Moreover, fascinating recent data have shown that even "lower" primates, such as the macaque, can be trained to use tools manually to perform elementary tasks, even though they may not do so spontaneously (Ishibashi, Hihara, & Iriki, 2000). These monkeys can be trained via shaping to use a long rake to retrieve pieces of food that would otherwise be out of reach. This learning usually requires a number of days or weeks, but thereafter the animals are able to use the rake efficiently whenever the situation requires it.

In a series of pioneering studies, Iriki and colleagues (Iriki, Tanaka, & Iwamura, 1996; Iriki et al., 2001; see also Ishibashi et al., Chap. 28, this volume) have observed that such tool use can plastically modulate the coding of multisensory space by cells in the anterior bank of the intraparietal sulcus (IPS). Multisensory cells in this region usually have a tactile receptive field (RF) on a specific body part (e.g., the hand) and a visual RF for the corresponding sector of space (see also Graziano & Gross, 1995; Rizzolatti, Fadiga, Fogassi, & Gallese, 1997). Critically, once the monkey has become skillful in using the rake as a tool to extend reachable space, just a few minutes of using the rake in this way can induce an expansion of the visual RF of such IPS

neurons into more distant space, so that they now start to respond to stimuli near the far end of the tool (Iriki et al., 1996). It has been proposed that this response may be a neural correlate of a change in the body schema representation of the hand to include the full length of the tool, with a corresponding expansion of the visual RFs for bimodal neurons responding to stimuli in the hand's peripersonal (reachable) space. Previous authors (e.g., Critchley, 1979; Head & Holmes, 1911; Paillard, 1971) had speculated, often based solely on human introspection, that external objects, including tools, might become incorporated into the body schema. The groundbreaking findings of Iriki et al. seem to demonstrate the neurobiological reality of these claims.

In the next section we introduce evidence from behavioral studies in normal and brain-damaged humans that wielding a long tool can have effects on human behavior that are somewhat analogous to the cellular effects found by Iriki and colleagues. Wielding a long tool can extend cross-modal integration between vision and touch that involves multisensory spatial representations such that more distant visual stimuli near the end of a wielded tool come to have similar effects as those lying close to the hand.

EFFECTS OF WIELDING A LONG TOOL ON THE SPATIAL NATURE OF CROSS-MODAL EXTINCTION   We sought to test in humans whether wielding a long tool could enhance the effect of a far visual stimulus (at the end of the tool) on responses to a tactile stimulus on one hand. Our first study examined a patient affected by unilateral left extinction after right hemisphere damage. This clinical sign is fairly common after various forms of right-sided brain lesion following stroke (Vallar, Rusconi, Bignamini, Geminiani, & Perani, 1994). Patients with extinction can typically detect isolated stimuli on either side but become unaware of stimulation on the contralesional (left) side if it is presented concurrently with ipsilesional (right) stimulation, so that the latter is said to extinguish awareness of the former. Various explanations have been proposed for why this might arise. In keeping with the competitive models of spatial attention (e.g., Bundesen, 1990; Desimone & Duncan, 1995), a common suggestion is that the lesion confers an advantage to right-sided stimuli whenever multiple concurrent stimuli compete for spatial attention (e.g., Driver, Mattingley, Rorden, & Davis, 1997).

The important point for our purposes is that left-sided extinction after right brain injury can arise even between stimuli presented in different modalities (Bender, 1970), as when a right visual event extinguishes awareness of a touch on the left hand that would otherwise have been felt (Mattingley, Driver, Beschin, & Robertson, 1997). Moreover, di Pellegrino, Làdavas, and their co-workers (e.g., di Pellegrino, Làdavas, & Farnè, 1997; Làdavas, di Pellegrino, Farnè, & Zeloni, 1998; Làdavas, Zeloni, & Farnè, 1998) have recently shown, in a series of studies, that such extinction of left-hand touch by a right visual stimulus is more pronounced when the right visual stimulus falls close in three-dimensional space to the (unstimulated) right hand. This observation has led to the suggestion that a visual stimulus near one hand may activate a multisensory (visual-tactile) representation of the space near that hand (analogous to the representations of peripersonal space provided by multisensory neurons in the primate brain; e.g., Fogassi et al., 1996; Graziano & Gross, 1995) in addition to a purely visual response. Activating a multisensory representation of the right hand in this way might then in turn compete with activation of the contralesional left hand by touch upon it, hence producing extinction of that contralesional touch. By contrast, when the right visual stimulus is located farther away from the right hand, it may no longer activate a multisensory representation of the space near that hand, hence producing less extinction of touch on the other hand (di Pellegrino et al., 1997; see also Làdavas & Farnè, Chap. 50, this volume).

Given that Iriki and co-workers (1996) have shown, at the level of single cells in the monkey brain, that multisensory representations of space near the hand can extend farther visually when the subject is wielding a long tool, we wondered whether cross-modal extinction in human patients might analogously arise for more distant visual stimuli when the subject wields a tool (see also Farnè & Làdavas, 2000). We studied this question in a single patient, B.V., who showed consistent left extinction after a right hemisphere stroke that affected occipital and temporal cortex, as well as the pulvinar and temporoparietal white matter (Maravita, Husain, Clarke, & Driver, 2001). At the time of testing, a few months after the stroke, B.V. still showed various aspects of left-sided spatial neglect and pronounced left tactile extinction, plus cross-modal extinction of touch on the left hand when a visual stimulus was presented concurrently near the right hand. Indeed, cross-modal extinction occurred on nearly 100% of such trials, but it was much reduced (to only 35%) when the right visual stimulus was presented 50 cm away from the right hand, in the radial plane. A visual stimulus in far space was thus less effective in inducing cross-modal extinction, as was found in the other studies discussed above (di Pellegrino et al., 1997; Làdavas et al., 1998; see also Làdavas and Farnè, Chap. 50, this volume).

We tested in patient B.V. (Maravita et al., 2001) whether reaching to the location of a far visual stimulus on the right with a long stick held in the ipsilesional right hand (Fig. 51.1A, Far Sticks condition) could increase cross-modal extinction of touch on the contralesional hand by that far visual stimulus on the right. If wielding the tool to reach continuously into far space during the experimental blocks was effective in extending the multisensory representation of space around the right hand, then we would expect more extinction from a far visual stimulus at the end of the wielded tool than when that stimulus was not reached by the patient with the tool. A visual stimulus at the end of the tool might then become equivalent, in terms of the cross-modal extinction it can produce, to a stimulus directly presented near the right hand.

B.V. was instructed to wield a stick with each hand and to touch a mark on the table placed by the visual stimulus with the far tip of each stick. B.V. had to maintain this posture throughout the experiment, and he was reminded of this every few trials, or whenever the far tip of the stick drifted away from the target. In a first experiment we tested B.V. by using a variation on the clinical confrontation method (gentle unseen touches generated by the experimenter on the patient's left hand, combined with brief finger movements by the experimenter to produce visual stimulation on the patient's right side), analogous to the procedures used in other recent studies of cross-modal extinction (e.g., di Pellegrino et al., 1997; Làdavas et al., 1998). In a second experiment, we used computerized visual and tactile stimuli (the illumination of LEDs and unseen vibrations, respectively), which allowed more precise control of timing and intensity. Results are shown in Figure 51.1B for Experiment 1 (E1), with manual stimuli generated by the experimenter, and also for Experiment 2 (E2), with computerized stimuli. In both studies, B.V. had to report verbally whether a right visual stimulus, a left touch, or stimulation on both sides (vision plus touch) had been delivered. For both experiments we found (Maravita et al., 2001) that when B.V. reached the location of the far ipsilesional (right) visual stimulus with the stick held in his right hand (Fig. 51.1A, Far Sticks condition), cross-modal extinction of left-hand touch by that far visual stimulus significantly increased, to a level comparable with the extinction from visual stimuli presented directly by the right hand (cf. Fig. 51.1A, Near condition). Critically, this effect required a continuous physical connection between the patient's right hand and the far visual stimulus by means of the wielded stick. Indeed, when the stick instead passively lay on the table, with a small gap between it and B.V.'s right hand (Fig. 51.1A, Far Gap

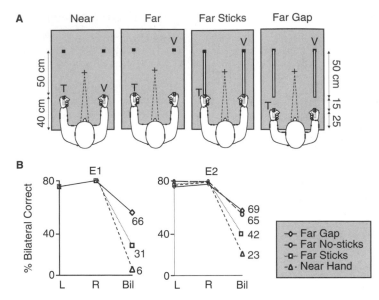

FIGURE 51.1   (A) Schematic drawing of the experimental setup (bird's-eye view). Left tactile (indicated by T) and right visual (V) stimuli were light touch or brief finger movements, respectively, in the first experiment. In the second experiment, touch stimuli were computerized short vibrations (85 ms duration at 70 Hz); visual stimuli were brief flashes (85 ms, with a luminance of 40 cd/m^2, produced by an LED). Vibrators were placed inside a short segment of stick held by the patient throughout the experiment, to which longer sticks were joined when appropriate. The same insertion mechanism was used for the right and left sticks. Conditions varied depending on the position of right visual stimulus: Near (presented directly near the right hand); Far (presented in far space); Far Sticks (at the far end of the stick); Far Gap (same as Far Stick, but with a gap between patient's hand and stick). (B) Results from Experiment 1 (E1, manual stimulation) and 2 (E2, computerized stimuli). Note that the Far condition was present in E2 only. Extinction rate increased going from Far Gap and Far to Far Stick and Near Hand conditions. (Adapted from Maravita et al., 2001, with permission from Elsevier Science.)

condition), the low rate of cross-modal extinction did not differ from a baseline condition that had a far visual stimulus and no stick (Fig. 51.1A, Far condition. This condition was included only in Experiment 2; see Fig. 51.1B [E2] for results).

The critical result of this study was that reaching to the location of a far visual stimulus on the right with a long stick held in the right hand changed the impact of that far stimulus so that it now produced cross-modal effects equivalent to those produced by a near visual stimulus located much closer to the right hand. It seems plausible that when B.V. wielded the stick, the visual stimulus activated multisensory visual-tactile neurons analogous to those described by Iriki and colleagues (e.g., Iriki et al., 1996). Visual RFs of such neurons extend more distantly when a tool is wielded so as to extend reachable space.

No extensive training in use of the stick was necessary to produce the effects we observed in patient B.V. (although, like most people, he would presumably have had a lifetime's experience of wielding various tools in his right hand). This contrasts with the studies in macaque monkeys, where effective tool use had to be trained extensively rather than arising spontaneously (Iriki et al., 1996). Another patient study has also shown

that distant visual stimuli can come to act analogously to near ones for humans when a long tool is wielded, without any need for extensive experimental training. Berti and Frassinetti (2000) described a right-hemisphere-damaged patient, P.P., who showed left visual neglect when bisecting horizontal lines in near space (with bisection errors veering to the right) but not when bisecting lines in more distant extrapersonal space by means of a laser pointer (see also Halligan & Marshall, 1991). However, when far lines were bisected using a long stick, left neglect returned. Thus, once again, when far visual stimuli could be reached with a long tool, they came to act analogously to near visual stimuli (see also Ackroyd, Riddoch, Humphreys, Nightingale, & Townsend, 2002; Pegna et al., 2001).

Farnè and Làdavas (2000) conducted a patient study that is perhaps procedurally closest to the work of Iriki and colleagues in monkeys. As in our study (Maravita et al., 2001), they studied patients with cross-modal extinction. They tested extinction of touch on the left hand by visual stimuli delivered to the far end of a rake held by the subject in the right hand. Critically, patients were tested before and after undergoing 5 minutes of experience in using a long rake with the right hand to retrieve distant visual objects. Shortly after this experience, distant right visual events produced more extinction of left-hand touch than during the pretraining test. This effect dissipated after 5–10 minutes of passive holding of the tool (analogous to the cellular effects found in monkeys; Iriki et al., 1996).

These effects on cross-modal extinction presumably arise because wielding the tool with the right hand links that hand to more distant right visual locations at the end of the tool. In a recent study (Maravita, Spence, Kennett, & Driver, 2002), we tested whether wielding a tool in the left hand to contact distant visual objects in the right hemispace, in crossed fashion (Fig. 51.2A),

might analogously come to generate a link between distant right events and the left hand. If so, distant right visual events might start to activate a multisensory representation of the left hand, rather than competing with it by activating the right hand. As a result, cross-modal extinction might be reduced rather than increased, potentially benefiting the patient. We again studied B.V., in whom parietal cortex, shown to be functionally critical for tool-based spatial remapping in monkeys (Inoue et al., 2001; Iriki et al., 1996; Obayashi et al., 2001), remained structurally intact, even in the damaged right hemisphere. Another virtue of studying

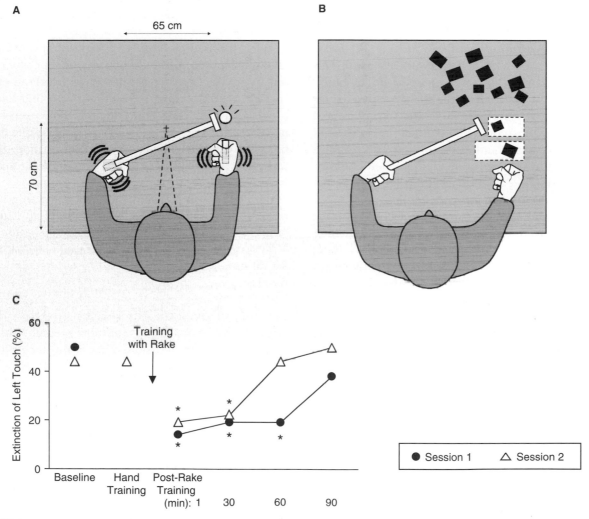

FIGURE 51.2   (A) Schematic of experimental setting in the Baseline-rake situation. Patient fixated a central cross throughout. Single 85-ms touches (represented here by black curved lines) were presented randomly to both hands, with or without visual stimulation on the right (85-ms, 80-cd/m² flashes, represented here as a white circle with black outline in front of the right hand). Bilateral cross-modal stimuli could thus be double (left touch plus right vision) or triple (right and left touches plus right vision). Extinction trials were considered as those double or triple bilateral trials in which left touch was undetected. (B) Schematic of the training phase. Large and small pieces of cardboard (dark patches) on the right side of the table had to be sorted according to their size into two different areas marked on the right of the table, with the patient using the rake in a crossed manner with the left hand held in left hemispace. (C) Extinction results for the two experimental sessions before and after training (Post-rake-training units on x-axis represent minutes elapsed after tool training). *P < 0.05 versus Baseline-rake (as depicted in A). (Adapted from Maravita, Clarke, Husain, & Driver, 2002.)

this patient was that, unlike many patients with right hemisphere damage and left spatial neglect or extinction, B.V. retained relatively intact use of his left limbs when prompted (although he tended not to use his left hand spontaneously, especially for actions that are normally performed bimanually, exhibiting "motor neglect"; see Laplane & Degos, 1983).

In our experiment, B.V. held a long stick with his left hand, reaching to the position of a distant right visual stimulus (Fig. 51.2A). Extinction was tested using the same computerized stimuli as in the experiment described earlier (see Fig. 51.1). B.V. had to report whether a right visual stimulus, a left touch, a left touch plus a right visual stimulus, or bilateral touch plus right visual stimulus was delivered. Within this experimental setting, no difference in extinction rate was found between a baseline condition (with no stick) and the condition in which the stick was held by the left hand. This result contrasted with that observed in the earlier experiment (see Fig. 51.1), in which the stick reaching the far visual stimulus on the right was held with the ipsilesional right hand, and this modulated extinction. However, it should be noted that in addition to showing spatial extinction, B.V. also suffered from complete left homonymous hemianopia (i.e., blindness in the left visual field), some proprioceptive deficit for his left limb, and motor neglect. Thus the patient's input from contralesional space, and his awareness of his left limb, were deficient. It may therefore be less surprising that simply holding the stick with his left hand was insufficient to induce any effective functional link between the left hand and right visual space (where the far end of the stick lay) and thus improve extinction. Such a link evidently did not arise spontaneously simply from holding the stick, unlike the outcome when he held the stick in his right hand. It should also be noted that the previous right-hand result (Fig. 51.1) did not involve a tool held in a crossed arrangement (i.e., with its far end in the hemispace opposite the hand that held it), unlike the situation studied for the left hand.

To determine whether a link to the left hand could be established by more active training, we next implemented a specific motor task to be executed with the tool prior to extinction testing, similar to the rake task used in the monkey studies (Iriki et al., 1996) and in the patient study by Farnè and Làdavas (2000) that was briefly described earlier. In our study, a rake replaced the stick previously used, and B.V. was asked to use this rake with his left hand, resting in left hemispace, to sort small pieces of cardboard scattered on the right side of the table and of his body according to their visible size, dragging them into separate size-appropriate areas marked on the right of the table (Fig. 51.2B). This training lasted for 20 minutes, with B.V.'s cross-modal extinction undergoing computerized testing before and after the training to assess any effect of extended tool use. (Note that all testing for cross-modal extinction was conducted in a fixed static posture, as shown in Fig. 51.2A.) Results now clearly showed an aftereffect of tool use (Fig. 51.2C), with cross-modal extinction of left-hand touch by distant right visual events being significantly reduced following the training, as compared with the tool being absent, or even with the tool being present but prior to training in its crossed use. Further posttraining tests of cross-modal extinction performed 30, 60, and 90 minutes after the end of training showed an enduring effect of training in reducing extinction, with this effect dissipating after 60 minutes (Fig. 51.2C). These results were confirmed in a second experimental session. In this session, only 10 minutes of training was allowed. Moreover, to rule out any nonspecific effects due to prolonged active use of the left hand rather than specific use of the long crossed tool with that hand, in the second session a 20-minute period of control training (*hand training* in Fig. 51.2C) was also implemented first. For this, the sorting task was performed directly with the left hand in right space, without using the rake. Results after training with the rake were similar to those of the first session (Fig. 51.2C). Critically in this session, reduction of extinction was not obtained after the patient used the left hand in right space without the tool. Moreover, the improvement after tool use now lasted for 30 minutes only, as opposed to 60 minutes during the first session, thus suggesting a possible relationship between duration of training and duration of effect. The consistency of the effect in the two experimental sessions and its extended duration in time, although limited, suggest the possible value of this technique for rehabilitation.

To summarize the results of this last study, wielding a long tool in the left hand to contact visual stimuli in distant right space reduced cross-modal extinction between right visual events presented at the end of the stick and touch on the left hand that wielded the tool. Once again, the tool seemed to connect distant visual events to tactile events in peripersonal space, such that the distant visual events came to have a similar effect as events presented close to the hand wielding the tool. Unlike the results obtained when the right hand held the stick, the results for a tool in the left hand depended on extensive recent experience in actively using that tool with the left hand. This constraint could relate either to B.V. having less awareness of his left hand or to the particular situation of using a tool in a crossed arrangement (i.e., holding it with a hand in one hemispace while using it to contact stimuli in the other hemispace). The next section, which reports analogous observations in neurologically intact humans, suggests that the crossing factor may be critical.

EFFECTS OF WIELDING LONG TOOLS ON NORMAL VISUAL-TACTILE SPATIAL INTERFERENCE   Although there have been several studies of the impact of tool use on cross-modal spatial integration in brain-damaged patients, much less work has been done on this issue in normal subjects. We recently conducted two experiments to address this issue (Maravita, Spence, Kennett, et al., 2002). We exploited a visual-tactile interference paradigm previously introduced to study cross-modal attention in normal subjects (Pavani, Spence, & Driver, 2000; Spence, Pavani, & Driver, 1998; Spence, Kingstone, Shore, & Gazzaniga, 2002). In this paradigm, subjects have to make a spatial tactile judgment (typically concerning whether a tactile vibration is delivered to the thumb or index finger of either hand, which is equivalent to an "upper" or "lower" judgment for the posture that is typically used). Visual distracters (LEDs) can be illuminated at any of four positions, one near the index finger (upper position) and one near the thumb (lower position) for each hand, with all these visual possibilities being equally likely regardless of where any concurrent tactile target is presented. The tactile judgments are typically slower and less accurate if the visual distracter is "incongruent" with the location of the concurrent tactile target (e.g., an upper light near the index finger combined with a lower vibration at the thumb). Critically, this cross-modal interference effect is reliably larger if the visual distracter appears closer to the tactile target (e.g., in the same hemifield, or closer within that hemifield to the current location of the tactually stimulated hand). If the hands are crossed over in space, then the cross-modal interference effect remaps accordingly, so that an incongruent visual distracter presented closest to the current location of the stimulated hand will produce the most interference. This remapping is reminiscent of some of the spatial effects found within bimodal visual-tactile neurons in the monkey brain. For instance, multisensory neurons in ventral premotor cortex, IPS, and putamen that have tactile RFs on the hand or arm have visual RFs that tend to follow that body part around in space if it is moved, independent of gaze (e.g., Graziano & Gross, 1995; Graziano et al., 1994; Iriki et al., 1996; Rizzolatti et al., 1997).

The cross-modal visual-tactile interference effects on human performance have been used to study the spatial nature of visual-tactile integration. For instance, not only does the most effective location for a visual distracter shift along with the hands when they are moved,

but the relative contributions of vision and proprioception to this remapping can also be assessed. For instance, by using dummy rubber hands, visual feedback about apparent hand location can be dissociated from proprioceptive information. In this way, Pavani et al. (2000) were able to show some dominance of vision, with visual distracters near dummy rubber hands producing the greatest spatial interference with tactile judgments, provided that the rubber hands were in a plausible posture (see also Farnè, Pavani, Meneghello, & Làdavas, 2000). Moreover, in Pavani and colleagues' (2000) study, the extent of cross-modal interference from visual distracters near the dummy rubber hands correlated with the extent to which subjects "felt" that they actually experienced touch in the location of those dummy hands. Subsequent researchers have dubbed this apparent mislocation of touch toward visible dummy hands the *virtual body effect* (Soto-Faraco, Enns, & Kingstone, 2002).

We adapted the cross-modal interference paradigm to study the effect of wielding tools on the spatial nature of visual-tactile integration in normal adult humans. Specifically, we examined whether wielding two tools in a "crossed" arrangement (Fig. 51.3*B*, left panel) could reverse the impact of left or right visual distracters, so that a right visual distracter might come to have the most impact on judgments concerning left hand touch, and vice versa, when the tools were held crossed, rather than the usual outcome of within-hemifield combinations leading to the greatest cross-modal interference, as is found in the absence of tools.

We remind the reader here that cross-modal interference has repeatedly been found in prior work to be stronger when a tactile target and concurrent visual distracter appear on the same side of external space (i.e., right visual field stimulation paired with vibration on the right hand, or left visual field stimulation with left hand vibration), rather than on opposite sides. In this experiment we tested whether actively wielding a long tool can plastically alter this cross-modal spatial mapping. Our prediction was that when the tools were held straight (Fig. 51.3*A*, left panel), cross-modal interference should, as usual, be greater from a visual distracter on the same side of space as the concurrent tactile target, but that when the tools were held crossed instead (connecting the right hand to the left visual field and vice versa; see Fig. 51.3*B*, left panel), cross-modal interference from visual distracters in the opposite visual field to the tactually stimulated hand might now become larger.

We ran two experiments (Maravita, Spence, Kennett, et al., 2002) that differed in the amount of active use of the tools that was required. If active use is indeed

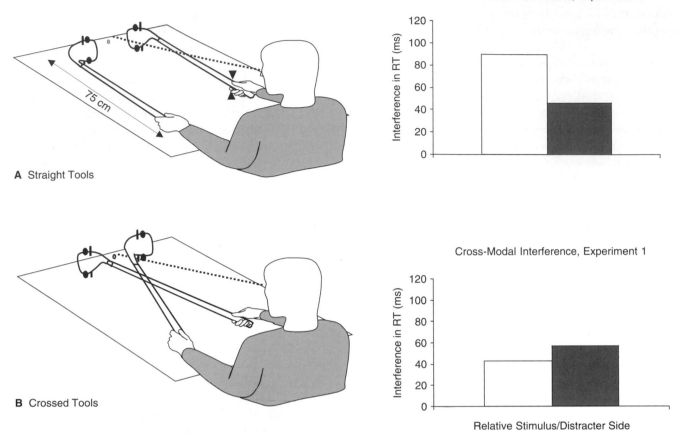

A Straight Tools

B Crossed Tools

Cross-Modal Interference, Experiment 1

Cross-Modal Interference, Experiment 1

Relative Stimulus/Distracter Side

FIGURE 51.3   Line drawing of the experimental setting and mean cross-modal interference effect for response times in Experiment 1. The tools were toy golf clubs. (*A*) Straight-tools condition. (*B*) Crossed-tools condition. In either case, a peg fixed at the far end of the tool (thick black vertical lines) was inserted into a hole to locate it, while hand locations were kept constant with straps. Unseen tactile stimulators were placed below the forefinger and thumb pads on each tool handle (indicated symbolically here with black triangles for the right hand only in the straight-tool situation). Vibrations were 200 Hz sine wave signals presented in three successive 50-ms bursts, each separated by a 50-ms gap. Potential visual distracters (of the same duration and frequency as the vibrations) are shown as black circles. A central LED (small gray circle) had to be fixated (dotted line) during each trial. The noise produced by the vibrators was masked by white noise through headphones. In each experiment, 480 stimuli were delivered, divided into ten blocks, each with crossed or uncrossed tools.

In the panels on the right are shown the mean cross-modal interference effects for response times in the active experiment (tool swapped by participant between uncrossed and crossed positions every four trials). Interference effects were calculated as the difference between incongruent scores (upper vibrations with lower distracters, or vice versa) minus congruent scores (upper vibrations with upper distracters or lower vibrations with lower distracters). White bars indicate results of trials with the visual distracter in the same visual hemifield as the tactually stimulated hand. Black bars indicate results with distracters in the opposite hemifield. Each graph corresponds to the tool situation, straight or crossed, shown at left. Note that the spatial pattern of cross-modal interference (for same versus opposite-side distracters) differs with the different tool situations. (Adapted from Maravita, Spence, Kennett, & Driver, 2002, with permission from Elsevier Science.)

important for modulating visual-tactile links with stimuli in far space (e.g., Farnè & Làdavas, 2000; Iriki et al., 1996; Maravita, Spence, Kennett, et al., 2002), we should expect stronger effects of crossing the sticks in the more active task. Accordingly, in our first experiment, subjects were instructed to change the position of the tools actively from straight (Fig. 51.3*A*) to crossed (Fig. 51.3*B*) every four trials. In our second control experiment, performed with a different group of normal

subjects, the position of the tools was exchanged only every 48 trials, and position changes were done by the experimenter, so that the subjects were passive with respect to tool placement.

The results nicely agreed with our predictions. Data for Experiment 1 are plotted in Figure 51.3 (*A* and *B*, right panel) in terms of cross-modal interference (i.e., the difference in reaction time between incongruent (e.g., lower tactile target on thumb, but upper visual distracter nearby) and congruent conditions (e.g., upper tactile target on finger with upper visual distracter), to provide a measure of the impact of the visual distracter. In the first, *active* experiment, when tools were uncrossed the cross-modal interference was larger from visual distracters in the same anatomical hemifield as the hand receiving the touch. This was found for both reaction times (effects plotted in Fig. 51.3) and for error rates (which showed analogous effects, not plotted). Critically, however, with crossed tools in the *active* experiment, cross-modal interference actually became stronger from visual distracters in the *opposite* hemifield to the stimulated hand, for both response times (Fig. 51.3*B*) and errors. By contrast, in the *passive* control experiment, crossing the tools did not change any of the results. Also, the critical remapping of the results with crossed tools within the *active* experiment took some time to develop, with the crossed-tool results being reversed for the second half (Fig. 51.4*B*) but not the first half of this experiment (Fig. 51.4*A*), across a total of 480 trials.

These results show that after active use of the tools, interference from visual distracters on tactile judgments depended not only on the anatomical locations stimulated but also on links formed between visual locations at the end of each long tool and the hand that wielded that tool. Thus, following extended experience in wielding tools with the right and left hands, visual interference can be stronger either from the same anatomical hemifield as the hand that wields the tool or from the opposite visual hemifield, depending on whether the tools are currently held in a straight or crossed fashion, respectively. With extended use, the tool effectively becomes an extension of the hand that

wields it, so that displacing its far end into the opposite hemispace has similar effects to displacing the hand itself. The fact that these results in normal observers for crossed-tool situations depend on experience in actively wielding the tools accords with the result we described earlier for cross-modal extinction in a brain-damaged patient (see Fig. 51.2).

Our cross-modal results with crossed tools are also reminiscent, in certain respects, of recent tactile findings by Yamamoto and Kitazawa (2001b). In a temporal order judgment (TOJ) task for tactile stimuli delivered at the tips of tools, normal subjects were less accurate when the tools were held in a crossed rather than an uncrossed position, producing a result similar to that observed when tactile stimuli were presented directly to crossed or uncrossed hands (Shore, Spry, & Spence, 2002; Yamamoto & Kitazawa, 2001a). Yamamoto and Kitazawa suggested that tactile stimuli were spatially mapped according to their actual location at the tip of the tool, regardless of the position of the hand sensing them. Crossing the tools (but not the hands) was thus equivalent to actually crossing the hands, for TOJ. Our results go beyond these findings by showing that in a situation with wielded tools, not only can the true external location of tactile sources at the ends of tools be ascertained, but processing of tactile information delivered at the wielding hand can also become cross-modally disrupted by distant visual information at the far end of the tools. Moreover, the spatial nature of this cross-modal interference can be changed by active experience in wielding the tool. In addition, in our task any stimulus-response compatibility effect could be excluded, because only elevation judgments were required and only one effector was used for the response.

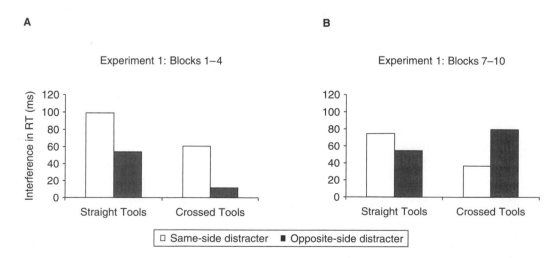

A Experiment 1: Blocks 1–4

B Experiment 1: Blocks 7–10

Same-side distracter ■ Opposite-side distracter

FIGURE 51.4   Reversal of cross-modal interference with crossed tools in Experiment 1 for the first (*A*) and second (*B*) half of the experiment. This critical change in results with crossed tools (to yield more interference from opposite-side distracters) occurred only in the second half (*B*) of the active experiment.

Cross-modal integration modulated by mirrors

CROSS-MODAL INTERFERENCE BETWEEN TOUCH AND DISTANT MIRROR REFLECTIONS IN NORMAL SUBJECTS Because touch is an essentially proximal sense, requiring contact with the body surface, visual information relating to touch often arises from very close to the body surface, in peripersonal space, as during direct sight of an object as it touches you. But wielding long tools provides one relatively common situation in which distant visual stimuli (at the end of the tool) can relate to tactile information on the body surface, picked up by the hand that wields the tool. Another case in which distant visual information can relate to touch on the body crops up when encountering mirrors in daily life. Mirrors are often used to provide visual feedback that would not otherwise be directly in the line of sight. For instance, we often use mirrors to look at ourselves when grooming—shaving, hair dressing, or applying makeup. An intriguing aspect of such situations is that the seen mirror reflections often have the same optical properties as distant visual information, being projected as if they had a source that lay "through the looking glass," and yet such distant visual information can relate to touch felt at the body surface. An example is the distant mirror reflection of a comb running through our hair, for which the actual location is peripersonal but the visual image suggests a distant object. Although this situation might appear to impose a potential conflict between visual and tactile information (suggesting mismatching locations), in practice, the added visual information in the mirror typically increases our efficiency at a grooming task. Localization of the true position of objects seen in mirror reflections is already present, to some extent, even by the age of 2 years in infants (Robinson, Connell, McKenzie, & Day, 1990). Moreover, our daily interactions with reflecting surfaces may lead to highly efficient, possibly even automatic, recoding of the true location of the source for seen reflections.

In a series of experiments, we sought to explore whether automatic cross-modal interference between touch and visual mirror reflections could indeed take the true locations of the sources of the mirror reflections into account. In one study (Maravita, Spence, Sergeant, et al., 2002), we addressed this question in normal adult subjects, using a further variation on the cross-modal interference paradigm introduced earlier, in which the impact of a visual distracter on spatial judgments for a concurrent tactile target (on one or other hand) was assessed. Critically, in our new study, when the visual distracters were placed near the hand, they could be seen only indirectly, as distant reflections in a mirror directly in front of the subject, which also reflected the subject's hands (Figs. 51.5A and B; note that direct view of the hands was prevented by an opaque occluding screen). This Mirror condition was compared with a control Far condition (Fig. 51.5C) in which the visual distracters were presented in far space, beyond the mirror, which was now turned into a window. This was achieved by using a half-silvered mirror along one wall of a box and lighting it from in front (so that it acted like a mirror) or from behind, inside the box (so that it acted like a window). Luminance of the scene and its elements were equal in both situations. Visual distracter lights and other objects could be placed inside the box. The distant distracters placed in the box, and viewed through the window, projected images that were optically equivalent to the mirror reflections of lights that were actually located near the subject's hand. The critical difference was that in the Mirror condition only, each subject knew or could sense that he or she was seeing reflections of the space near the subject's own hand (in part because they were able to make constrained movements with their own hands and so received corresponding visual feedback on their own hand movements only when viewing the mirror, not when looking through the window).

We predicted that if automatic recoding of appropriate distant mirror images as arising from near space occurs, then cross-modal interference from incongruent visual distracters on tactile judgments should be stronger for mirror-reflected stimuli with a near source than for optically equivalent far visual stimuli. In the Mirror condition, visual reflections should be treated as if coming from near space, within which visual tactile integration is typically stronger, as previously shown with both neural and behavioral measures.

We ran three successive experiments with this general method. These experiments differed in the responses made to indicate the tactile judgment and/or in the exact nature of what could be seen inside the box (through the window) in the Far control condition. In the first experiment, subjects made unseen foot pedal responses to indicate whether the tactile target was upper or lower (i.e., on an index finger or thumb). However, between blocks, subjects moved their hands, and thus received occasional feedback that they were viewing reflections of their own hands only in the Mirror condition. No hands were visible in the Far control condition, only distant distracter lights. As predicted, cross-modal interference from visual distracters on tactile judgments was stronger in the Mirror condition (see Fig. 51.6, E1, for reaction times and error rates), in which the visual distracters actually lay close to the hands but were seen only as distant mirror reflections, next to the mirror reflections of the hands themselves.

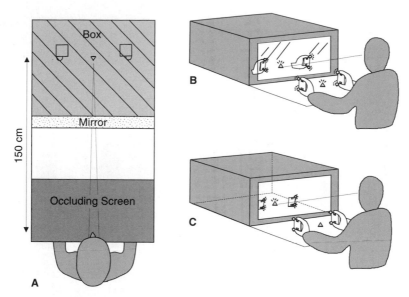

FIGURE 51.5   (A) Bird's-eye view of the experimental setup for the mirror study. An opaque shield prevented direct vision of the hands. Participants looked toward a rectangular box placed 90 cm in front of them. The central part of the facing wall contained a half-silvered mirror. The visual scene presented to the participants varied depending on illumination. (B) In the Mirror condition, the space inside the box was in complete darkness, so that all objects inside it were invisible. Instead, the space around the participants' hands was lit so that participants saw their own hands, the LEDs, and the central fixation light (all oriented toward the mirror) indirectly as reflections in the mirror. In this condition, owing to the physical properties of mirrors, visual stimuli appeared to the observer as if placed at a distance that was double that between the visual stimuli and the mirror (i.e., 120 cm for visual distracter and fixation lights) plus the distance between their actual location and the eyes (30 cm), or a total distance of 150 cm (see A). (C) In the Far condition the box interior was illuminated, thus allowing participants to observe the contents of the box through the half-silvered mirror, as if through a window with no reflection visible on the glass. In the first study, the box contained two sponges, identical to those grasped by the participants, with identical visible vibrators and LEDs mounted on them; an identical fixation light was present as well. The spatial position of the visual distracters and the fixation light were kept identical to their reflection equivalents in the Mirror condition as observed by the participant, thus producing equivalent retinal projections for them across the Mirror and Box conditions. Luminance was matched as well (60 cd/m² for distracters, 28 cd/m² for fixation). The sponges in the box were grasped by rubber hands (in the second study) or by the experimenter's hands (in the third study), with an equivalent posture to that of the participants. (Adapted from Maravita, Spence, Sergeant, & Driver, 2002, with permission from Blackwell Publishers.)

The results of this first experiment might conceivably have been due merely to the sight of some hands in the Mirror condition but not in the Far condition, rather than being genuinely due to recoding of the true peripersonal spatial location for the sources of the mirror reflections. Accordingly, the second experiment included dummy rubber hands in the Far control condition, placed inside the box and thus seen through the window, but at an equivalent distance (and the same posture) as the real hands that were seen as reflections in the Mirror condition. These dummy hands apparently grasped equivalent apparatus to that actually grasped (and seen in the mirror) by the subjects. The stimuli were otherwise as before, but responses were now made manually (with the touched digit), and visual feedback from these manual responses was thus available in reflected form for the Mirror condition only, thus distinguishing sight of the subject's own hands from sight of the dummy hands, which never moved. It should be noted, however, that such visual feedback

from manual responses would be generated only after the response had been initiated, and thus only after the critical latency of responding had been measured on each trial.

The results showed (Fig. 51.6, E2) that, just as in the previous experiment, cross-modal interference from visual distracters on tactile judgments was again larger in the Mirror condition than in the Far (control) condition, even though a pair of hands (either the subject's own or rubber dummies) was now visible for both conditions. However, a critic might suggest that this latest result was due merely to hands that could move attracting more attention than static dummy hands, thereby drawing attention to the visual distracters for the Mirror condition, in a manner that might spill across successive trials.

To assess this possibility, in a final experiment the subjects either viewed their own hands and visual distracters near them reflected in the mirror, or someone else's hands (an experimenter's) at the same distance as

Reaction Times

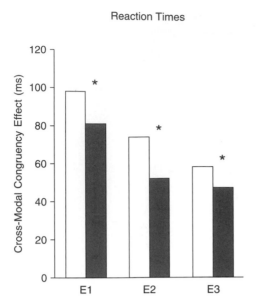

Error Rates

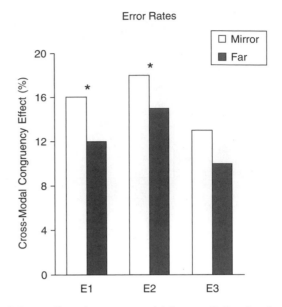

FIGURE 51.6   Cross-modal congruency effects for reaction times (left panel) and error rates (right panel) for the three experiments (E1, E2, E3) on mirror effects in normal subjects. Mirror and Far conditions are represented as white and black bars, respectively. Asterisks indicate significant direct comparisons between these paired conditions. Results are expressed as cross-modal congruency effect, which represents the difference between situations with visual distracters in incongruent (upper light plus lower touch, or vice versa) and congruent (upper or lower touch and light) spatial positions with respect to tactile targets (see text). (Adapted from Maravita, Spence, Sergeant, & Driver, 2002, with permission from Blackwell Publishers.)

the mirror reflections, inside the box through the window. The experimenter sat behind the box, holding equivalent apparatus to the subject and making analogous digit responses that could be seen by the subject through the window, but with an unpredictable delay. Hence, subjects now saw moving hands near the distracter lights in both the Mirror and the Far conditions, but only in the former did the seen hand movements show perfect temporal coupling with their own (because they were mirror reflections of their own). Once again, more cross-modal interference from visual distracters on tactile judgments was found in the Mirror condition than the Far condition (Fig. 51.6, E3), showing that this result depends on seeing one's own hands reflected in a mirror (with temporally coupled visual feedback for any hand movements), not just on seeing any moving hands at a corresponding distance.

These results suggest that visual events near a person's hands, but seen only indirectly as distant mirror reflections together with the reflected hands, can be recoded in terms of their true peripersonal spatial location, and hence come to act like near visual events. It should be noted that in these experiments, the visual modality was task-irrelevant, and the visual distracters could only impair performance when incongruent, as compared to the congruent situation. The evidence that visual mirror reflections were nevertheless recoded in terms of their true peripersonal location thus suggests

that such recoding might be relatively automatic. In the present experimental situation, this led to increased cross-modal interference effects. However, in more naturalistic situations, such as when using combined tactile information and visual mirror reflections to control grooming behavior, the automatic recoding of distant visual images as reflecting peripersonal information that relates to concurrent tactile information would presumably be beneficial rather than disruptive.

It would be interesting to determine in future studies whether our mirror effect specifically depends on close temporal correlations between self-induced hand movements and visual feedback from the mirror reflections, or whether merely being instructed that one is viewing one's own hands indirectly is sufficient to produce the result. The temporal synchrony or asynchrony of visual feedback from hand movements could in principle be manipulated by using video circuits to relay images of the hand. It would be of interest to assess the temporal course of such interactions over successive trials or blocks in the experiment, that is, whether recoding of mirror reflections near the body arises immediately and spontaneously or instead requires practice to build up.

So far we have argued that distant mirror images of the hands and objects near them become recoded as having a source in near peripersonal space. However, in principle one might argue for the reverse recoding (i.e., tactile sensation being referred to distant space, where the mirror images are seen). This could be somewhat analogous to the ventriloquist-like referral of tactile sensation to locations outside the body, as reported by previous authors (e.g., Botvinick & Cohen, 1998; Farnè et al., 2000; Pavani et al., 2000; Ramachandran, Roger-Ramachandran, & Cobb, 1995). However, at present we still favor our hypothesis, for three main reasons. First, in previous studies reporting sensation of tactile stimuli referred to dummy hands, typically the images of the hand had to have a posture compatible with that of the observer (and had to be close to the observer) for the effect to occur (cf. Farnè et al., 2000; Pavani et al., 2000). Mirror reflections of our own body parts, although constituting a familiar sight, are not visually in a location compatible with that of the observer, so they should be unlikely to produce any remapping of tactile perception to their observed position. Second, in our experiment we tested cross-modal interference from vision on touch, which is known to be stronger for visual distracters in near space close to the tactually stimulated hand, and thus a similar mechanism seems likely to apply for our mirror manipulation. Third, our familiarity with mirrors is likely to relate any image of our body to its true source, rather than interpreting distant visual reflections as the spatial location of any tactile stimulation we might receive.

CROSS-MODAL SPATIAL EXTINCTION BETWEEN TOUCH AND DISTANT MIRROR REFLECTIONS The final study we will describe here investigated, once again, cross-modal extinction in a patient (B.V.) with right hemisphere damage. As we described earlier (see also Làdavas & Farnè, Chap. 50, this volume), a number of studies have found that cross-modal extinction of left-hand touch by a right visual event in patients with right hemisphere damage is typically more pronounced when the right visual event falls close to the (unstimulated) right hand. Recall also that we have shown (Maravita et al., 2001) that a distant right visual event can produce more cross-modal extinction of left-hand touch if the visual event is "connected" to the right hand by a wielded tool. In our final study, we sought to determine if an optically distant right visual event that was a mirror reflection of a light source actually positioned close to the right hand (but seen only indirectly, via the mirror) could analogously act as a visual event directly next to the right hand, and hence produce substantial cross-modal extinction.

As described earlier in this chapter patient B.V. showed consistent extinction of touch on the contralesional left hand by ipsilesional right visual stimuli, especially when the latter were located close to the right hand. We carried out two experimental sessions

(Maravita, Spence, Clarke, Husain, & Driver, 2000) using apparatus similar to that described in the preceding section (Fig. 51.5). B.V. sat in a dark, soundproof chamber, with his chin on a rest, facing a box placed 60 cm in front of his hands. In the wall of this box, and facing the patient, a half-silvered rectangular mirror was mounted, with its long axis parallel to the patient's coronal plane (Fig. 51.7A). Again, an opaque screen always prevented direct vision of the hands.

Computerized tactile and visual stimuli were used. Again, the critical experimental manipulation was to vary the source of visual stimulation according to whether the half-silvered mirror was front-lit, so as to act as a mirror (Fig. 51.7C), or back-lit, so as to act as a window (Fig. 51.7B) into the box (the luminance of the scene and its elements was equal for these two situations, as measured by a photometer). For simplicity, we describe only the right side of the visual scene, since the patient had left homonymous hemianopia. With direct illumination of the patient's right hand in front of the half-silvered mirror (Mirror condition), B.V. saw his right hand reflected in the mirror (Fig. 51.7C), projecting a visual image as if lying behind the mirror, 150 cm away from his eyes (Fig. 51.7A). In this condition, the LEDs, which could produce ipsilesional right visual flashes, were close to the patient's own right hand, facing the mirror, where they could be seen on the right when switched on (these LEDs were visible only in the mirror because a horizontal screen occluded any direct view), at the same apparent distance as the mirror reflection of the right hand. A fixation light, again oriented toward the mirror, was placed in alignment with the patient's midsagittal plane, and again was visible only in the mirror, at an apparent distance of 150 cm.

When the inside of the box was illuminated instead (Far condition, Fig. 51.7B), the content of the box behind the half-silvered mirror was now seen as if through a window, and B.V. observed a stuffed rubber hand inside the box, placed at the same spatial location and reproducing the same posture as the mirror reflection of his own right hand in the previous condition. An LED identical to that of the Mirror condition was present near the dummy hand, but now facing the patient directly. An identical central fixation light was also present. The rubber hand served as a control to ensure that any effect from the mirror reflection of the patient's own hand was not due to seeing *any* hand on the right. Particular care was used to match the physical appearance of the visual scene in the two conditions (i.e., Box and Mirror) in order to avoid any trivial explanation of differences in performance. Thus, the distance of the fixation light and LEDs within the box exactly

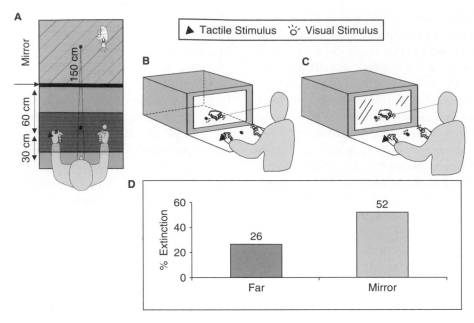

FIGURE 51.7 Experimental setup for the mirror study of cross-modal extinction. (*A*) Bird's-eye view. The patient's hands were concealed from direct view by an opaque cardboard shield (shown as transparent dark gray area). The mirror was in front of the patient (thick black line) and was mounted on one wall of the box that contained the rubber hand (the top section of the box is indicated by diagonal shading). The patient fixated a central point throughout, visible in the distance only (dotted lines). The small triangle close to the left hand represents the tactile stimulus (for simplicity, shown for the left hand only). (*B*) Schematic sketch of the Far condition (with the occluding surface above the patient's hands now removed, for simplicity, but present at all times during the experiment). The patient observed the contents of the box, which consisted of a black interior, a yellow rubber hand holding a small stick with LEDs mounted on it, and a fixation light. (*C*) Mirror condition (real right hand now illuminated, inside of box completely dark). The patient saw the mirror reflection of his own right hand, together with a reflection of the nearby LEDs (held on a small stick in his right hand) and the central fixation point, all of which faced the mirror. (Reflection of the patient's arm and body was prevented by a black cloth; his face was not visible in the mirror either, due to the skewed line of sight.) The positions of the visible mirror reflections exactly matched those of the equivalent items within the box. (*D*) Results. Shown is the extinction rate in the Mirror and Far conditions. It was higher for the Mirror condition. (Adapted from Maravita et al., 2000, with permission from Lippincott Williams & Wilkins.)

matched that of the mirror reflection for the corresponding items in the Mirror condition (i.e., 150 cm from the patient's eyes; Fig. 51.7*A*). The luminance of the fixation light, visual stimuli, and black background were also matched across the two conditions (as in the normal study previously described; Maravita, Spence, Sergeant, & Driver, 2002).

B.V.'s ability to report unilateral stimuli was good on either side (missed stimuli: 6/96 left tactile trials, 3/32 right tactile trials, 2/32 right tactile-visual trials). In agreement with our prediction, extinction of left touches was significantly higher in the Mirror condition than in the Far condition (number of bilateral stimuli with extinction of left touch: 67/128 versus 33/128, respectively; Fig. 51.7*D*). We also found that the extinction rate on preliminary baseline testing with direct vision of the right hand, and any visual events directly next to it, did not differ significantly from that observed in the Mirror condition (66% vs. 52%), but did differ reliably from that in the Far control condition (66% vs. 26%). Thus, a visual stimulus in extrapersonal space

(inside the box) produced much less cross-modal extinction than one viewed directly close to the hand. More important, a stimulus that projected a visual image as if from the same far distance as the light in the box but which was known to be the mirror reflection of an object actually lying close to the true position of the right hand in external space behaved as a visual stimulus viewed directly in peripersonal space, producing substantial cross-modal extinction.

Conclusions

In this chapter we have presented evidence suggesting that, under some circumstances, distant visual stimuli that would fall within conventional extrapersonal space can be recoded as near peripersonal stimuli, to enhance their integration with concurrent tactile stimulation on the body surface. This situation arises both when long tools are wielded and when mirror reflections of one's own body parts (and of visual stimuli near them) are viewed. Both of these situations are illustrations of optically distant visual information being usefully related to tactile information at the body surface (as when the far end of a tool is seen moving across a felt surface, or the mirror reflection of a comb is seen moving across one's own head).

The results obtained when wielding long tools that physically connect the body to visible objects in far space suggest that relatively plastic changes can arise in the multisensory coding of space near the effector that wields the tool. As a result, a visual event at the far end of that tool can come to be integrated with touch as if it were a visual event near the hand wielding the tool. Some of these effects (e.g., those arising with tools held in a crossed fashion) appear to depend on extended recent experience in wielding the tool, whereas others (e.g., with uncrossed tools) may arise spontaneously, in adult subjects at least. These various effects may provide perceptual or behavioral analogues to some of the cellular phenomena uncovered by Iriki and colleagues in regions of monkey parietal cortex, whereby the visual RFs of bimodal tactile-visual cells that are centered on the hand or arm extend into more distant visual space (reachable by the tool) after training in tool use (e.g., Iriki et al., 1996; see Ishibashi et al., Chap. 28, this volume). These same neurons seem to provide a complex multisensory representation of space that is continuously updated, depending on the actual position of the limbs in space, by proprioception or other information about posture (Obayashi, Tanaka, & Iriki, 2000).

The somewhat analogous perceptual/behavioral effects of viewing one's own hands in a mirror that we have uncovered in humans raise the fascinating question of whether analogous cellular results might be observed in monkey cortex, and the further question of whether this (and the human results) might depend on experience in using mirrors (which might be more readily manipulated in laboratory monkeys). In a new series of studies, macaques have been trained to use a rake to retrieve pieces of food out of hand reach while seeing their actions only indirectly on a video monitor (Iriki et al., 2001). After a few weeks of training, these animals succeeded in efficiently controlling their actions by looking at the video image. Moreover, Iriki and colleagues showed that, at this stage only, a visual probe presented in proximity to the video image of the animal's hand, or at the far end of the tool wielded by the animal and observed only indirectly via the monitor, could activate similar multisensory visual-tactile neurons in the anterior bank of the IPS to those activated before training with direct vision of the hand and visual probe. This observation suggests that visual input that is spatially incongruent with the real position of body parts can nevertheless provide similar cues to cross-modal integration as for direct visual observation of such body parts, provided there is some systematic spatial relationship that can be learned.

In the context of video feedback affecting cross-modal influences, it is interesting to note that Tipper and colleagues (Tipper et al., 1998, 2001) have shown that, in normal adult human observers, simple reaction time to tactile stimuli can be enhanced not only by direct vision of the stimulated body part but also by indirect vision of the body part on a video monitor. More recently it has been shown that two-point tactile spatial discrimination thresholds can be enhanced by (noninformative) vision of the relevant part, and even more so if this visual image is magnified (Kennett, Taylor-Clarke, & Haggard, 2001; see also Taylor-Clarke, Kennett, & Haggard, 2002, for related results on somatosensory-evoked potentials).

It will be fascinating to examine the extent to which these recent results and the other phenomena discussed in this chapter depend on experience with particular tactile-visual spatial-temporal correlations, which are extensive in daily life but which could be manipulated experimentally (e.g., via video delay). For now, the existing results already show that it is becoming possible for experiments in this burgeoning cross-modal field to put some psychological and neuroscientific flesh on the skeletal notion of the body schema (Head & Holmes, 1911). We now know that while tactile-visual integration is usually most pronounced within close peripersonal space, such cross-modal effects can be extended into more distant space for both normal and brain-damaged humans, either by wielding long tools or by viewing distant mirror reflections (and possibly video images) of the body.

REFERENCES

Ackroyd, K., Riddoch, M. J., Humphreys, G. W., Nightingale, S., & Townsend, S. (2002). Widening the sphere of influence: Using a tool to extend extrapersonal visual space in a patient with severe neglect. *Neurocase, 8,* 1–12.

Aglioti, S., Smania, N., Manfredi, M., & Berlucchi, G. (1996). Disownership of left hand and objects related to it in a patient with right brain damage. *NeuroReport, 8,* 293–296.

Bender, M. B. (1970). Perceptual interactions. In D. Williams (Ed.), *Modern Trends in Neurology, 5,* 1–28.

Berlucchi, G., & Aglioti, S. (1997). The body in the brain: Neural bases of corporeal awareness. *Trends in Neuroscience, 20,* 560–564.

Berti, A., & Frassinetti, F. (2000). When far becomes near: Re-mapping of space by tool use. *Journal of Cognitive Neuroscience, 12,* 415–420.

Botvinick, M., & Cohen, J. (1998). Rubber hands "feel" touch that eyes see. *Nature, 391,* 756.

Bundesen, C. (1990). A theory of visual attention. *Psychological Review, 97,* 523–547.

Colby, C. L., Duhamel, J. R., & Goldberg, M. E. (1993). Ventral intraparietal area of the macaque: Anatomic location and visual response properties. *Journal of Neurophysiology, 69,* 902–914.

Critchley, M. (1979). *The divine banquet of the brain and other essays.* New York: Raven Press.

Desimone, R., & Duncan, J. (1995). Neural mechanisms of selective visual attention. *Annual Review of Neuroscience, 18,* 193–222.

di Pellegrino, G., Làdavas, E., & Farnè, A. (1997). Seeing where your hands are. *Nature, 388,* 730.

Driver, J., Mattingley, J. B., Rorden, C., & Davis, G. (1997). Extinction as a paradigm measure of attentional bias and restricted capacity following brain injury. In P. Thier & H.-O. Karnath (Eds.), *Parietal lobe contributions to orientation in 3D space* (pp. 401–429). Heidelberg: Springer.

Duhamel, J. R., Colby, C. L., & Goldberg, M. E. (1998). Ventral intraparietal area of the macaque: Congruent visual and somatic response properties. *Journal of Neurophysiology, 79,* 126–136.

Farnè, A., & Làdavas, E. (2000). Dynamic size-change of hand peripersonal space following tool use. *NeuroReport, 11,* 1645–1649.

Farnè, A., Pavani, F., Meneghello, F., & Làdavas, E. (2000). Left tactile extinction following visual stimulation of a rubber hand. *Brain, 123,* 2350–2360.

Fogassi, L., Gallese, V., Fadiga, L., Luppino, G., Matelli, M., & Rizzolatti, G. (1996). Coding of peripersonal space in inferior premotor cortex (area F4). *Journal of Neurophysiology, 76,* 141–157.

Frederiks, J. A. M. (1985). Disorders of the body schema. In J. A. M Frederiks (Ed.), *Clinical neuropsychology* (pp. 207–240). Amsterdam: Elsevier.

Gentilucci, M., Fogassi, L., Luppino, G., Matelli, M., Camarda, R., & Rizzolatti, G. (1988). Functional organization of inferior area 6 in the macaque monkey: I. Somatotopy and the control of proximal movements. *Experimental Brain Research, 71,* 475–490.

Graziano, M. S., & Gross, C. G. (1995). The representation of extrapersonal space: A possible role for bimodal, visual-tactile neurons. In M. S. Gazzaniga (Ed.), *The cognitive neurosciences* (pp. 1021–1034). Cambridge, MA: MIT Press.

Graziano, M. S., Yap, G. S., & Gross, C. G. (1994). Coding of visual space by premotor neurons. *Science, 266,* 1054–1057.

Halligan, P., & Marshall, J. (1991). Left neglect for near but not far space in man. *Nature, 350,* 498–500.

Head, H., & Holmes, G. (1911). Sensory disturbances from cerebral lesion. *Brain, 34,* 102–254.

Inoue, K., Kawashima, R., Sugiura, M., Ogawa, A., Schormann, T., Zilles, K., et al. (2001). Activation in the ipsilateral posterior parietal cortex during tool use: A PET study. *NeuroImage, 14,* 1469–1475.

Iriki, A., Tanaka, M., & Iwamura, Y. (1996). Coding of modified body schema during tool use by macaque postcentral neurones. *NeuroReport, 7,* 2325–2330.

Iriki, A., Tanaka, M., Obayashi, S., & Iwamura, Y. (2001). Self-images in the video monitor coded by monkey intraparietal neurons. *Neuroscience Research, 40,* 163–173.

Ishibashi, H., Hihara, S., & Iriki, A. (2000). Acquisition and development of monkey tool-use: Behavioural and kinematic analyses. *Canadian Journal of Physiological Pharmacology, 78,* 1–9.

Kennett, S., Taylor-Clarke, M., & Haggard, P. (2001). Noninformative vision improves the spatial resolution of touch in humans. *Current Biology, 11,* 1188–1191.

Kohler, W. (1927). *The mentality of apes.* New York: Humanities Press.

Làdavas, E., di Pellegrino, G., Farnè, A., & Zeloni, G. (1998). Neuropsychological evidence of an integrated visuotactile representation of peripersonal space in humans. *Journal of Cognitive Neuroscience, 10,* 581–589.

Làdavas, E., Zeloni, G., & Farnè, A. (1998). Visual peripersonal space centered on the face in humans. *Brain, 121,* 2317–2326.

Laplane, D., & Degos, J. (1983). Motor neglect. *Journal of Neurology, Neurosurgery and Psychiatry, 46,* 152–158.

Leinonen, L., Hyvärinen, J., Nyman, G., & Linnankoski, I. I. (1979). Functional properties of neurons in lateral part of associative area 7 in awake monkeys. *Experimental Brain Research, 34,* 299–320.

Maravita, A., Clarke, K., Husain, M., & Driver, J. (2002). Active tool-use with contralesional hand can reduce cross-modal extinction of touch on that hand. *Neurocase, 8,* 411–416.

Maravita, A., Husain, M., Clarke, K., & Driver, J. (2001). Reaching with a tool extends visual-tactile interactions into far space: Evidence from cross-modal extinction. *Neuropsychologia, 39,* 580–585.

Maravita, A., Spence, C., Clarke, K., Husain, M., & Driver, J. (2000). Vision and touch through the looking glass in a case of crossmodal extinction. *NeuroReport, 11,* 3521–3526.

Maravita, A., Spence, C., Kennett, S., & Driver, J. (2002). Tool-use changes multimodal spatial interactions between vision and touch in normal humans. *Cognition, 83,* B25–B34.

Maravita, A., Spence, C., Sergeant, C., & Driver, J. (2002). Seeing your own touched hands in a mirror modulates crossmodal interactions. *Psychological Science, 13,* 350–355.

Mattingley, J. B., Driver, J., Beschin, N., & Robertson, I. H. (1997). Attentional competition between modalities: Extinction between touch and vision after right hemisphere damage. *Neuropsychologia, 35,* 867–880.

Obayashi, S., Suhara, T., Kawabe, K., Okauchi, T., Maeda, J., Akine, Y., et al. (2001). Functional brain mapping of monkey tool use. *NeuroImage, 14,* 853–861.

Obayashi, S., Tanaka, M., & Iriki, A. (2000). Subjective image of invisible hand coded by monkey intraparietal neurons. *NeuroReport, 11,* 3499–3505.

Paillard, J. (1971). Les determinants moteurs de l'organisation de l'espace. *Cahiers de Psychologie, 14,* 261–316.

Paillard, J. (1993). The hand and the tool: The functional architecture of human technical skills. In A. Berthelet & J. Chavaillon (Eds.), *The use of tools by human and non-human primates* (pp. 36–46). New York: Oxford University Press.

Pavani, F., Spence, C., & Driver, J. (2000). Visual capture of touch: Out-of-the-body experiences with rubber gloves. *Psychological Science, 11,* 353–359.

Pegna, A. J., Petit, L., Caldara-Schnetzer, A. S., Khateb, A., Annoni, J. M., Sztajzel, R., et al. (2001). So near yet so far: Neglect in far or near space depends on tool use. *Annals of Neurology, 50,* 820–822.

Ramachandran, V. S., Rogers-Ramachandran, D., & Cobb, S. (1995). Touching the phantom limb. *Nature, 377,* 489–490.

Rizzolatti, G., Fadiga, L., Fogassi, L., & Gallese, V. (1997). The space around us. *Science, 277,* 190–191.

Rizzolatti, G., Scandolara, C., Matelli, M., & Gentilucci, M. (1981). Afferent properties of periarcuate neurons in macaque monkeys: II. Visual responses. *Behavioral Brain Research, 2,* 147–163.

Robinson, J. A., Connell, S., McKenzie, B. E., & Day, R. H. (1990). Do infants use their own images to locate objects reflected in a mirror? *Child Development, 61,* 1558–1568.

Shore, D. I., Spry, E., & Spence, C. (2002). Confusing the mind by crossing the hands. *Brain Research: Cognitive Brain Research, 14,* 153–163.

Soto-Faraco, S., Enns, J., & Kingstone, A. (2002). *The virtual body effect.* Presented at the International Multisensory Research Forum, Geneva, Switzerland.

Spence, C., Pavani, F., & Driver, J. (1998). What crossing the hands can reveal about visuotactile links in spatial attention. *Abstracts of the Psychonomic Society, 3,* 13.

Spence, C., Kingstone, A., Shore, D. I., & Gazzaniga, M. S. (2002). Representation of visuotactile space in the split brain. *Psychological Science, 12,* 90–93.

Taylor-Clarke, M., Kennett, S., & Haggard, P. (2002). Vision modulates somatosensory cortical processing. *Current Biology, 12,* 233–236.

Tipper, S. P., Lloyd, D., Shorland, B., Dancer, C., Howard, L. A., & McGlone, F. (1998). Vision influences tactile perception without proprioceptive orienting. *NeuroReport, 9,* 1741–1744.

Tipper, S. P., Phillips, N., Dancer, C., Lloyd, D., Howard, L. A., & McGlone, F. (2001). Vision influences tactile perception at body sites that cannot be viewed directly. *Experimental Brain Research, 139,* 160–167.

Vallar, G., Rusconi, M. L., Bignamini, L., Geminiani, G., & Perani, D. (1994). Anatomical correlates of visual and tactile extinction in humans: A clinical CT scan study. *Journal of Neurology, Neurosurgery and Psychiatry, 57,* 464–470.

Yamamoto, S., & Kitazawa, S. (2001a). Reversal of subjective temporal order due to arm crossing. *Nature Neuroscience, 4,* 759–765.

Yamamoto, S., & Kitazawa, S. (2001b). Sensation at the tips of invisible tools. *Nature Neuroscience, 4,* 979–980.

52 Grapheme-Color Synesthesia: When *7* Is Yellow and *D* Is Blue

MIKE J. DIXON, DANIEL SMILEK, BRANDON WAGAR, AND PHILIP M. MERIKLE

Introduction

For persons with synesthesia, ordinary stimuli can elicit extraordinary experiences. For C.S., pain triggers a perception of the color orange, and for M.W., the taste of spiced chicken is pointy (Cytowic, 1993). When H.G. hears a person speak, the voice he hears elicits a multisensory experience of both color and taste. For example, the first author's voice induced the color brown and evoked a taste experience that was "hard to describe, but somewhat like syrup!" All of these extraordinary experiences reflect variants of synesthesia—a union of senses. For synesthetes like C.S., M.W., and H.G., the inducing stimulus leads to experiences that cross modalities (e.g., for H.G., sounds trigger colors and tastes). For others, the inducing stimulus and the synesthetic experience occur in the same modality. For example, in grapheme-color synesthesia, viewing black digits or letters induces a conscious experience of color.

In our laboratory, we have learned much about this extraordinary condition by asking different synesthetes to give detailed subjective descriptions of their experiences (Smilek & Dixon, 2002). When C., a 21-year-old grapheme-color synesthete, is shown black digits or letters (e.g., *1, 3, 7, B, H, Z*) in addition to seeing the black graphemes, she claims that she also perceives colored overlays that appear on top of each digit and each letter. Each grapheme has its own highly specific color (called a photism), and viewing a specific grapheme (e.g., a 7) invariably elicits the perception of that particular photism. As C. relates, "It is difficult to explain . . . I see what you see. I know the numbers are in black . . . but as soon as I recognise the form of a 7 it has to be yellow." Although for a given synesthete the mappings between graphemes and colors remain consistent over time (i.e., for C., a 7 has been yellow ever since she can remember), these mappings tend to be different for every synesthete. For example, when J. is shown a black *7*, rather than seeing yellow, her overlay is "purple with a hint of blue, darkly lit up from behind as though there were a brownish red LED behind."

Two general principles emerge when considering the grapheme-color pairings for different synesthetes (Table 52.1). The first is that the for almost all of the synesthetes we have interviewed (and all those who have been described in the literature), the digit *0* induces a colorless photism appearing to different synesthetes as either white, black, gray, or clear. (Similar correspondences have been noted for the letter *O;* Baron-Cohen, Harrison, Goldstein, & Wyke, 1993.) The second principle is one of diversity: other than *0* and *O,* the grapheme-color pairings appear to be idiosyncratic. These two principles highlight a theme of this chapter, namely, that there are important individual differences among synesthetes, yet in the face of such diversity, there are crucial commonalities. We argue that one key aspect of synesthetic experience, namely, *where* a photism is experienced, allows two important subgroups of grapheme-color synesthetes to be identified.

Based on our interviews of more than 100 synesthetes, we have learned that they can differ markedly in where they experience their photisms. For C., J., and P. D., their photisms appear "out there, on the page," as though a transparency bearing a colored number were superimposed over the black grapheme. We refer to synesthetes like these as *projectors*, an allusion to their photisms being perceived in external space (see also Cytowic, 1989, 1993). For other synesthetes, the synesthetic color is described as appearing "in my mind's eye" or "in my head" (e.g., synesthete G.S., described by Mills, Boteler, & Oliver, 1999). For these synesthetes their experience can be likened to that of a nonsynesthete viewing a black-and-white picture of a stop sign. We "know" the stop sign is red, but do not project this color onto the picture. We refer to synesthetes like G.S. as *associators* because their descriptions of their experiences are more reminiscent of a strong semantic association between a grapheme and a color as opposed to a perceptual experience of color. We believe that this novel distinction between projector and associator synesthetes can be extremely important both in evaluating previous research and in devising new experiments.

TABLE 52.1
A subset of the grapheme-color pairings for three synesthetes

	Inducing Stimulus							
Synesthete	*0*	*1*	*2*	*3*	*A*	*B*	*C*	*D*
C.	White	Gray	Red	Purple	Blue	Yellow	Red	Dark blue
J.	Black	Yellow	Orange	Green	Red	Sky blue	Orange	Light blue
P.D.	Gray	White	Green	Brown	Dark red	Green	Blue	Brown

Here we describe a number of recent experimental investigations from different laboratories designed to further our understanding of synesthesia. Although the research that is reviewed pertains to investigations of grapheme-color synesthesia, many of the principles that emerge are relevant to cases of cross-modal synesthesia where the inducer is in one modality and the synesthetic experience is in another modality. Our main conclusions are the following: (1) photisms are an automatic consequence of viewing alphanumeric characters, (2) projector synesthetes can be empirically distinguished from associator synesthetes by using methods based on the Stroop effect, (3) under certain presentation conditions (e.g., masking, visual search), the photisms experienced by projector synesthetes alter the ease with which black graphemes can be identified, and (4) both the graphemic form and the meaning of alphanumeric characters contribute to determine the color of projected photisms.

Synesthetic photisms are an automatic consequence of viewing graphemes

Synesthetes often claim that their synesthetic experiences occur involuntarily. For example, C. claims that as soon as she sees the digit *2,* she experiences the color red, whether she wishes to or not. In fact, the prevalence of such subjective reports has led some to speculate that the involuntary nature of synesthetic experiences is one of the main diagnostic criteria of synesthesia (e.g., Cytowic, 1993; Dann, 1998). Synesthetes speak also about the "immediacy" of their experiences: they often claim that as soon as they see a digit, they experience the color. Based on claims that their photisms are both immediate and involuntary, researchers have suggested that photisms are an *automatic* consequence of viewing digits. Not surprisingly, researchers have turned to a variant of the Stroop task (Stroop, 1935) to investigate the automaticity of these synesthetic color experiences. Wollen and Ruggiero (1983) were the first to study synesthesia using Stroop methods. They presented A.N., a letter-color synesthete, with cards showing colored disks or letters painted in colors that were either congruent or incongruent with her photisms for the letters. The idea was that if a photism was an automatic consequence of letter identification, then the photism should interfere with naming the ink color of the letters on incongruent cards. Consistent with this hypothesis, A.N.'s color-naming response times were significantly longer for cards containing incongruently colored letters than for cards containing either congruently colored letters or colored disks. Similar methods have been used by different laboratories, with all studies showing photism-induced Stroop interference (e.g., Mills et al., 1999; Odgaard, Flowers, & Bradman, 1999). These findings have been taken to "support the idea that synesthesia is an automatic process" (Mills et al., 1999, p. 186).

Ardent critics of these studies may question the practice of presenting all the stimuli from a given condition on a single card and recording response times for the completion of an entire card using a stopwatch. Because the different conditions appeared on different cards, participants' expectations may have led them to adopt different strategies across conditions. Also, with such a method it is unclear what effect individual errors have on overall response times (i.e., numerous errors may lead to a spuriously fast response time for that card). Finally, Wollen and Ruggiero (1983) failed to report error rates, making it impossible to rule out the possibility that speed-accuracy trade-offs contributed to their results.

Recently, we applied Stroop methods to the study of synesthesia in a way that circumvented the problems associated with previous studies (Dixon, Smilek, Cudahy, & Merikle, 2000). We presented stimuli on a computer monitor rather than on cards. First we presented the digits *0* through *9* beside a color-adjustable square. C. was shown each digit, and we adjusted the red-green-blue values of the colored square until she indicated that the color of the square matched the color of her photism for the presented digit. This procedure allowed us to present stimuli in video colors that were either congruent with C.'s photisms or incongruent with C.'s photisms. (For descriptive purposes we use the term *video colors* for colors that appeared on the video monitor and *synesthetic colors* to refer to the colors of C.'s photisms.) In the Stroop experiment, C. was presented with a colored square (baseline condition) or either a congruently colored digit or an incongruently colored digit (congruent and incongruent conditions, respectively). C.'s task was to name into a microphone the video color of the presented stimulus as fast as possible while maintaining high accuracy. Color-naming response times were recorded to millisecond accuracy, and errors (if any) were recorded. Baseline, congruent and incongruent trials were randomly intermixed, with a total of 144 trials in each condition. C.'s color-naming response times for incongruent trials (797 ms, 2.8% errors) were significantly slower than her response times for either congruent trials (552 ms, 1.4% errors) or baseline trials (545 ms, 0.0% errors). Similar results were found when the experiment was repeated, indicating the reliability of this phenomenon. The markedly slower response times found when C. attempted to name the color of incongruently colored digits suggested that her photisms could not be inhibited. C.'s results were also compared with those obtained in a group of eight nonsynesthetes who showed no differences in their responses to stimuli whose colors were congruent or incongruent with C.'s photisms. These results corroborate previous findings and suggest that synesthetic color experiences do indeed occur automatically.

Whereas each of the Stroop studies discussed thus far used a case study approach, in which only a single synesthete was tested. Mattingley, Rich, Yelland, and Bradshaw (2001a, 2001b) studied the automaticity of synesthetic experiences in a group of 15 synesthetes. The synesthetes who participated in this study reported experiencing colors in response to stimuli consisting of letters, digits, or words. Mattingley et al. (2001a) conducted two separate experiments in which the 15 synesthetes and 15 nonsynesthetes named the video colors of individually presented alphanumeric characters. As in previous studies, the video colors of the stimuli were either congruent or incongruent with the synesthetes' photisms. In one experiment, the congruent and incongruent trials were presented in separate blocks, and in the other experiment, the congruent and incongruent trials were randomly intermixed with baseline trials, consisting of nonalphanumeric symbols that did not induce photisms. The results of both experiments showed that the synesthetes were slower at naming the colors of alphanumeric characters on incongruent trials than on congruent trials. In contrast, the group of nonsynesthetes showed no differences in their responses to stimuli that were congruent or incongruent for the synesthetes. Thus, the results from this study involving a group of synesthetes corroborate the results from the previous single-case investigations of synesthesia. Both

the single case studies and the group study suggest that for those with grapheme-color synesthesia, photisms are an automatic consequence of viewing externally presented alphanumeric digits or letters.

To date, the results of six different studies have shown that synesthetes demonstrate Stroop effects when they name the colors of congruently or incongruently colored letters or digits, whereas nonsynesthetes fail to show any congruent/incongruent response time differences when naming the colors of the same stimuli. Most would agree that these often large Stroop effects shown by synesthetes demonstrate that an alphanumeric stimulus automatically elicits an experience of color.

Empirically distinguishing projector synesthetes from associator synesthetes

Although photisms for grapheme-color synesthetes appear to be an automatic consequence of seeing graphemes, when one listens carefully to the subjective reports of synesthetes, it becomes clear that not all synesthetes experience photisms in a similar fashion. For some synesthetes, like C., the photisms are said to appear as projected color overlays that conform to the shape of the grapheme (projector synesthetes). For other synesthetes the photisms are not projected but appear "in the mind's eye" (associator synesthetes). In our laboratory we have classified projectors and associators based on their subjective reports concerning where they experience their photisms. Using this classification scheme we have found that only 11 out of 100 synesthetes we have interviewed are of the projector subtype.

In addition to asking synesthetes about where they experience their photisms, we have informally interviewed these synesthetes about other aspects of their synesthetic color experiences. These subjective reports of the projector and associator synesthetes studied in our laboratory reveal some intriguing differences. For example, when C. describes viewing an incongruently colored digit, she claims that she perceives two different colors (i.e., the video color and her photism), and that this dual perception is a subjectively jarring experience. Another projector synesthete, J., claims that "having to read something written/typed in a [wrong] color is almost too much for me to handle and upsets/irritates me." When asked to rate the intensity of her synesthetic color experience and the intensity of her experience when viewing a color patch on a computer screen, C. actually reported that the synesthetic experience was more intense than her experience of the video color. By contrast, when associator synesthetes were asked about seeing incongruently colored digits, many claimed that the experience was not disturbing. Further, when asked to rate the intensity of their synesthetic color experience versus the intensity of their experience for video colors when shown a color patch, associator synesthetes claimed that the physically presented video color was by far the more intense experience. Taken together, these first-person descriptions suggest that the photisms experienced by projector synesthetes might differ from the photisms experienced by associator synesthetes on more than just the location of where the photisms are experienced. We postulated that the differences between projector synesthetes and associator synesthetes in terms of how intensely they experienced photisms and how disturbing they found viewing incongruent digits reflected more basic differences in the automaticity with which projectors and associators experienced their photisms and experienced video colors.

It must be noted that although some synesthetes were able to make clear and definitive judgments concerning the relative intensities of their video color and synesthetic color experiences, others found it extremely difficult to do so. Some felt that the two types of color experience were so different that it was extremely difficult to order these experiences in terms of their intensity. Previously, we have argued that certain aspects of experiences may be unavailable for subjective description (Smilek & Dixon, 2002). To appreciate the synesthetes' difficulties in describing these experiences, simply ask yourself whether printed words or patches of color are experienced more intensely. Similar problems would be encountered if the question were framed in terms of automaticity (i.e., based on introspection, which is the more automatic process, word reading or color naming?) To circumvent these difficulties, we sought a more objective means of exploring whether there were differences between projector and associator synesthetes in terms of the automaticity of video color processing and synesthetic color processing.

Our primary hypothesis was that projector synesthetes processed synesthetic colors more automatically than associator synesthetes. In addition, based on the projector C.'s unusual claim that she experienced synesthetic colors more intensely than video colors, we sought to address whether projector synesthetes processed synesthetic colors more automatically than video colors. To address each of these questions, we asked projector and associator synesthetes to perform two different Stroop tasks. In one task, they named the video colors of colored digits. In the other task, they named the photisms that they associated with these same physically colored digits. In both tasks, the digits were presented in video colors that were either congruent or incongruent with the photisms induced by the digits. For each Stroop task, there were 324 incongru-

ent trials and 108 congruent trials. Response times and errors (if any) were recorded on each trial.

Previous research by MacLeod and Dunbar (1988) suggests that the more automatic the process initiated by a stimulus, the harder the subsequent experience is to ignore when it is the interfering dimension in a Stroop situation. Based on this assumption, the critical comparisons in our experiment involved the magnitude of interference from the photism color when projector synesthetes named video colors versus the magnitude of the interference from the photism color when associator synesthetes named video colors (interference being defined as the response time difference between congruent and incongruent trials). We predicted that projector synesthetes would show larger interference effects than associator synesthetes when attempting to ignore their photisms and name the video colors of the digits.

Additionally, we sought to address whether there were differences between projector and associator synesthetes in terms of the magnitudes of interference when ignoring photism colors versus the magnitudes of interference when ignoring video color. Based on C.'s claim that photisms lead to more intense color experiences than viewing video colors, we predicted greater interference from photisms than video colors for projector synesthetes but greater interference from video colors than photism colors for associator synesthetes.

The results from five projector and six associator synesthetes are presented in Figure 52.1. The solid lines in Figure 52.1 shows that when the projector synesthetes named the video colors of digits, the photisms induced by the digits led to significantly greater interference (169 ms) than when associator synesthetes named the video colors of digits (29 ms). This pattern of data indicates that projector synesthetes found their photisms more difficult to ignore than the associator synesthetes did. The left panel of Figure 52.1 also shows that projector synesthetes experienced significantly more interference from photism colors than from video colors. This pattern of results indicates that for projectors, photisms were more difficult to ignore than video colors. This was never the case for any of the six associator synesthetes (means shown in right panel of Fig. 52.1). In fact, three of the six associator synesthetes showed greater interference from video colors than from photisms, a pattern opposite to the pattern of response times shown by the projector synesthetes (the other three associator synesthetes showed equivalent amounts of interference from photisms and video colors).

Previously we distinguished projector and associator synesthetes solely on the basis of their descriptions of their subjective experiences. Now, using Stroop

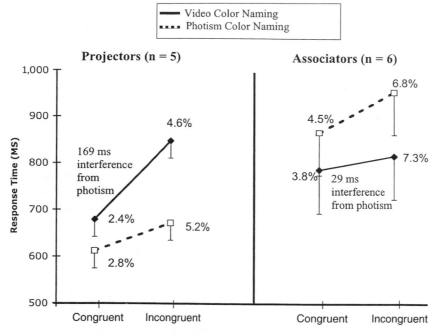

FIGURE 52.1   Mean response times, confidence intervals, and percentage errors for five projector synesthetes and six associator synesthetes.

methods, we have derived a means of empirically distinguishing between these two subtypes of synesthetes. We propose that the relative automaticity of synesthetic photisms reflects a critical difference between these two types of synesthetes, with projector synesthetes processing photisms more automatically than associator synesthetes. The differences in the magnitude of the interference from photisms, and indeed the different patterns of interference that emerge when projector and associator synesthetes engage in photism color naming and video color naming, suggest that care must be taken when interpreting studies that have shown large photism-induced Stroop effects for synesthetes who have named the colors of congruently and incongruently colored digits. It may well be that only projector synesthetes will *invariably* show large Stroop effects when naming such colors. Associator synesthetes may show smaller or possibly no Stroop interference effects from their photisms. Indeed, although the group of synesthetes studied by Mattingley et al. (2001a) was on average faster at naming the color of congruently colored stimuli than incongruently colored stimuli, some synesthetes within this group failed to demonstrate any Stroop effects whatsoever (Mattingley et al., 2001b). The findings that there are different subtypes of alphanumeric synesthetes and that not all associator synesthetes show significant Stroop effects suggest that caution must be exercised when interpreting Stroop effects as a global cognitive marker of grapheme-color synesthesia.

Although we have learned much about the nature of projector and associator synesthetes by using Stroop methods, much remains unanswered. At present, it is unknown whether projector and associator synesthetes show different patterns of Stroop effects because there is a continuum of automaticity, with projector synesthetes processing photisms more automatically than associator synesthetes, or because there is something categorically different about the synesthetic experiences of projector and associator synesthetes that causes these different patterns of Stroop effects. It may well be that a projector synesthete's photism that is perceived in external space may be more difficult to ignore than an associator synesthete's photism that is perceived "in the mind's eye." Consonant with this idea, in the following section we present evidence that projected photisms can, under certain very specific circumstances, actually prevent projector synesthetes from identifying the grapheme that lies beneath the photism.

Assessing perceptual aspects of projected synesthetic photisms

When considering synesthetic experiences, it is important to consider the distinction between the *perception* of color and semantic color associations. When a nonsynesthete sees a color photograph of a stop sign, he or she perceives the color red. When a nonsynesthete sees a black-and-white picture of a stop sign, however, even though he or she knows that the color of the stop sign is red, only an achromatic stop sign is perceived. As noted previously, when projector synesthetes describe their photisms, they claim to *see* colored overlays that adhere to the form of the presented graphemes. What they describe appears more akin to an actual perceptual experience than a semantic association between a number and a color. In a recent study, Ramachandran and Hubbard (2001a) provided evidence for the perceptual nature of this type of synesthetic experience by using a perceptual grouping paradigm.

Ramachandran and Hubbard tested two synesthetes, J.C. and E.R., who reported that they "saw" synesthetic color "spatially in the same location as the form" (p. 979). Based on this description, we would classify J.C. and E.R. as projector synesthetes. In their key experiment, Ramachandran and Hubbard presented J.C., E.R., and 40 nonsynesthetes with matrices comprised of approximately 45 small black graphemes. For example, one matrix was comprised of black *H*s, *P*s, and *F*s. Prior to being shown the matrix, the participants were informed that although the *P*s and *F*s would appear in random locations, the *H*s would be aligned within the matrix to form a shape (a square, a rectangle, a diamond, or a triangle). Participants were then briefly shown the matrix (for 1 s) and asked to indicate what shape was formed by the designated grapheme. The rationale underlying the experiment was that if J.C. and E.R. experienced conscious percepts of color when viewing the displays of black graphemes, then they may perceptually group the graphemes by their synesthetic colors. Thus, J.C., who perceives *H* as green, *P* as red, and *F* as yellow, might, when presented with this matrix, see a green triangle of *H*s stand out against a background of randomly interspersed red and yellow letters. If this were to occur, then J.C. and E.R. should be more accurate at identifying the shape formed by the designated graphemes than the nonsynesthetes who have no synesthetic colors with which to perceptually group the designated graphemes. Ramachandran and Hubbard found that the synesthetes were indeed more accurate at identifying the shapes formed by the designated graphemes than the nonsynesthetes. This finding led them to conclude that synesthetes indeed experience a conscious percept of color when viewing black digits or letters.

In our recent work, we too have focused on assessing the perceptual aspects of synesthetic photisms. As previously noted, when C. is shown a standard black digit, she also sees a projected colored overlay that conforms to the shape of the presented digit. C. describes being able to attend to either the presented black digit or to the photism that overlies the digit. Importantly, however, she reports that the photism is the more dominant of the two perceptions. We used C.'s subjective descriptions of her projected photisms to devise an experiment that would inform us about the perceptual characteristics of these photisms (Smilek, Dixon, Cudahy, & Merikle, 2001). Our premise was a simple one. If C. experiences a black digit in color, then the digit should be more difficult to see when it is presented against a background that is the same color as her photism for the digit than when it is presented against a background that differs in color from her photism for the digit. Concretely, if a black 2 is experienced as red, then this synesthetically perceived "red" 2 should be harder to perceive against a red background than against a green background.

In one experiment, C.'s task was to identify black digits that were presented briefly (32 ms) and followed by a black pattern mask. On each trial, the color of the background of the computer screen was varied so that it was either the same color as or a different color than the photism induced by the black digit. Consonant with our predictions, C. was significantly poorer at identifying black digits when they were presented against backgrounds that were the same color as her photisms for those digits (e.g., a synesthetically perceived "red" 2 against a red background) than when the digits were presented against backgrounds that were different in color from her photisms for those digits (e.g., a synesthetically perceived "red" 2 against a green background). In contrast to C., a group of seven nonsynesthetes showed no difference between their performance on these same-background and different-background conditions. We interpreted these results as showing that C.'s synesthetic experiences influenced her perception of the black digits (Smilek et al., 2001).

In another experiment, C. attempted to localize a black target digit (either a 2 or a 4) embedded among black distracter 8s. As in the previous experiment, the color of the background was varied such that it was either the same as or different from the color of C.'s photism for the target digit. The results showed that C. was significantly slower at localizing target digits in the same-background condition than in the different-background condition. Once again, in contrast to C., a group of seven nonsynesthetes showed no difference between their performance on same-background and different-background trials. These results further corroborated our conclusion that C.'s synesthetic experiences influence her perception of black digits (Smilek et al., 2001).

Wagar, Dixon, Smilek and Cudahy (2002) used the object substitution paradigm developed by Enns and Di Lollo (1997) to provide further evidence that C.'s photisms influence her perception of black digits. Whereas Smilek et al. (2001) showed that black graphemes were more difficult to identify when the photism elicited by a digit caused that digit to blend into a similarly colored background, Wagar et al., sought to show that projected photisms could draw attention to a grapheme and actually aid in the identification of the grapheme. Wagar et al. first tested eight nonsynesthetes. In the key conditions, the nonsynesthetes were briefly (i.e., for 16.67 ms) shown a black target digit (2, 4, 5, or 7) embedded in a display containing 15 black distracter digits (the digit 8). The target digit was surrounded by four black dots, and the nonsynesthetes were told to try and name the digit within these four dots. Critically, on half of the trials the four dots surrounding the target digit disappeared from the screen at the same time as the digits, and on the other half of the trials the digits disappeared but the four dots remained on screen for 320 ms. The nonsynesthetes made significantly more errors (mean of 18 errors on 48 trials) when the four dots remained on the screen for 320 ms than when the four dots disappeared with the digits (mean of 5 errors on 48 trials). The accepted explanation of this finding is that when attention is distributed across multiple items in the display (i.e., a target embedded in 15 distracters), the trailing four dots serve to mask the perception of the target contained within the four dots (Enns & Di Lollo, 1997).

In a second phase of this study (not reported in Wagar et al., 2002), Wagar et al. retested nonsynesthetes but now showed that the trailing four-dot masking effect could be prevented by presenting the target digits in color. When the eight nonsynesthetes were presented with colored targets (e.g., a red 2 surrounded by four black dots, embedded within 15 black distracter 8s), they made on average only four errors—a significant reduction from the average of 18 errors they made with black targets in this same key condition. These findings suggest that nonsynesthetes made fewer errors because color drew attention to the target, thereby preventing four-dot masking from occurring.

In the final phase of this study, Wagar et al. (2002) tested C. using black targets and black distracters. For C., the colors of her photisms for 2, 4, 5, and 7 are red, blue, green, and yellow, respectively, whereas the color of her photism for the digit 8 is black. Thus, if a target digit such as a 2 is embedded among 15 distracter 8s, the colored photism for the target should stand out in this display, since the photisms for the distracters are all black. As such, the prediction was that C.'s endogenously generated synesthetic colors for target digits should act like the externally presented colors for the nonsynesthetes. Thus, even with black targets and distracters, C.'s colored photisms for the digits 2, 4, 5, and 7 should draw attention to these targets and eliminate the masking caused by the four dots even in the most difficult condition. The results showed that in this key condition (15 distracter 8s and a trailing four-dot mask), relative to the nonsynesthetes, who made an average of 18 errors, C. made only five errors. These results are summarized in Table 52.2.

For black target digits and a trailing four-dot mask, C.'s performance (5 errors) was 3 SD below the mean of the nonsynesthetes (18 errors) in this same condition. C.'s error rate was comparable to that of controls attempting to detect *colored* targets in the trailing-mask condition (four errors). From these results we concluded that C.'s *endogenously* generated photisms served to draw attention to the target digits and prevent four-dot masking, just as the exogenously presented colors served to draw attention to the target for nonsynesthetes in the colored-target condition.

The findings reported by Ramachandran and Hubbard (2001a, 2001b), Smilek et al. (2001), and Wagar et al. (2002) are important because they are not easily explained solely in terms of semantic associations between alphanumeric characters and colors. The most straightforward explanation of these findings is that they are a direct result of the perceptual aspects of synesthetic experiences rather than the result of semantic associations between alphanumeric characters and colors. These findings are also interesting in light of our distinction between projector and associator synesthetes. We predict that perceptual effects should only

TABLE 52.2

Errors in identifying black or colored target digits surrounded by four-dot masks that either disappeared at the same time as targets and distracters (No Trailing Mask) or remained on-screen for 320 ms following the disappearance of the targets and distracters (Trailing Mask)

Subjects	No Trailing Mask (48 trials)	Trailing Mask (48 trials)
8 Nonsynesthetes, black targets	Mean = 5 errors (4.31)	Mean = 18 errors (4.07)
8 Nonsynesthetes, colored targets	Mean = 5 errors (4.27)	Mean = 4 errors (4.12)
Synesthete C., black targets	2 errors	5 errors

Note: For nonsynesthetes mean errors (±SD) are presented.

be noted for projector synesthetes—none of these perceptual effects should occur for associator synesthetes. Currently we are conducting experiments designed to provide support for this prediction.

Both form and meaning determine the color of projected photisms

When projector synesthetes are shown black graphemes, in addition to perceiving the black digits or letters they also experience colors that sits atop the graphemes. Two different models have been proposed to account for the projected photisms elicited by graphemes: a cross-linkage model (Ramachandran & Hubbard, 2001a, 2001b) and a reentrant model (Smilek et al., 2001). Although other models have been proposed to account for color experiences triggered by auditory inputs (e.g., Grossenbacher, 1997; Grossenbacher & Lovelace, 2001), we will first discuss the models that have been proposed to account for photisms induced by graphemes, and then integrate our conclusions with the models that account for multisensory experiences.

Ramachandran and Hubbard (2001a, 2001b) recently suggested that photisms stem from abnormal "cross-wiring" between adjacent brain areas. Based on the perceptual grouping experiments conducted with the synesthetes J.C. and E.R., they propose that areas of the fusiform gyrus that deal with the form of a grapheme are directly connected (cross-wired) to adjacent areas implicated in experiencing color (i.e., V4/V8). A concrete example of this cross-wiring is presented in Figure 52.2, depicting a hypothetical account of how a digit may be processed by the visual system. Here the cross-wiring involves an abnormal direct connection between posterior areas of the fusiform gyrus that process form and areas of the fusiform that are associated with color. This abnormal connection is the dashed line in Figure 52.2. According to this proposal, a specific form should automatically activate a specific color and lead to the sensory experience of a projected photism. Importantly, since such cross-wiring would occur *prior* to the activation of later-stage areas that process the meaning of digits or letters, Ramachandran and Hubbard suggest it is the form of the presented grapheme that is crucial, rather than the meaning associated with the grapheme.

A considerably different proposal was recently put forward by Smilek et al. (2001), who described a reentrant model to account for projected synesthetic photisms. Two basic premises of the proposed reentrant model are (1) that information flows through the visual system in cascade form rather than in discrete stages (e.g., Humphreys, Riddoch, & Quinlan, 1988), and (2) that information flows along both feed-forward and

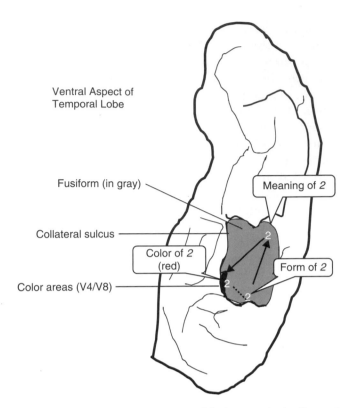

FIGURE 52.2   In the *reentrant model* (black arrows), the form of the digit *2* is processed in posterior fusiform and activates the concept of a *2* in anterior fusiform. Activation of meaning back-activates color areas using reentrant pathways. In the *cross-wiring model* (dashed line), the form of the digit directly activates color areas.

feedback connections (e.g., Di Lollo, Enns, & Rensink, 2000). In terms of the model, when a projector like C. views a black digit, information cascades forward through V1 and V2 to posterior areas of the fusiform gyrus that deal with digit form. Information continues to cascade forward to anterior fusiform and posterior inferior temporal (PIT) cortical areas, where the meaning of the digit is activated (Allison et al., 1994). Information then cascades back from anterior fusiform and PIT areas to V4/V8 using reentrant pathways. Importantly, perception does not occur all at once, but rather accrues over successive cyclical iterations—early-stage areas contact later-stage areas using feed-forward connections, and later-stage areas contact early-stage areas using feedback connections—with these feed-forward and reentrant connections cycling over and over again until a conscious percept emerges.

A concrete example of these feed-forward and feedback connections are presented by means of the black arrows in Figure 52.2. When the various straight and curved line segments that compose a *2* activate the striate cortex and the extrastriate posterior fusiform areas, this information will cascade forward, leading to activation in anterior fusiform/PIT areas associated with the meaning of a *2*. Crucially, on initial iterations the concept of a *2* may be more activated than other concepts (e.g., *3*, *5*, *b*, *d*), but there may be no conscious experience that a *2* was presented. Nevertheless, even though there may be no conscious experience of a *2*, the greater activation of the concept of a *2* relative to other concepts will activate feedback connections that ultimately synapse in areas of V4/V8 corresponding to the color red. Over successive iterations of this reentrant circuit, signals along feed-forward connections will continue to increase the activations for the concept of *2*, and these in turn will lead to signals being propagated along feedback connections that will increase activations for the color red. As the information cascades along feed-forward and feedback pathways, the perception that gradually emerges over successive iterations will be that of a black *2* with a red overlay.

If one assumes that even partial activation of meaning can back-activate color in V4/V8, then one can easily understand why C. would find it easier to identify masked digits when they are presented against background colors that are different from her synesthetic colors. If a *2* is presented against a blue background, the *2* will partially activate the concept of *2*, which will, in turn, activate the experience of a red photism via feedback connections from anterior fusiform/PIT to V4/V8. As a result of the activity in the feed-forward and feedback pathways, C. will ultimately perceive a red *2* against a blue background. If, however, a *2* is presented against a red background, the perception that will emerge over successive iterations is one of a red *2* against a red background. As a result, the digit *2* will be more difficult to segregate from the background and hence it will be harder to identify than when the background color is different from the synesthetic color.

The key difference between the cross-linkage model and the reentrant model is that *concept* activation is necessary to trigger photisms in the reentrant model but not in the early-stage cross-linkage model. To adjudicate between these views, we looked at what would happen when synesthetes were shown "ambiguous" graphemes whose forms could be interpreted as being either digits or letters, depending on the context in which they are presented (the grapheme 5 could be the middle digit in 3 4 5 6 7 or the third letter in M U S I C). In a cross-linked architecture, where form directly activates color and meaning is activated only after photisms are consciously experienced, identically shaped graphemes should elicit the same colors, regardless of whether they are interpreted as letters or digits. In a reentrant feedback architecture, where form activates meaning and meaning back-activates color, the same grapheme could elicit different colors, depending on whether the concept that is activated is a letter or a digit.

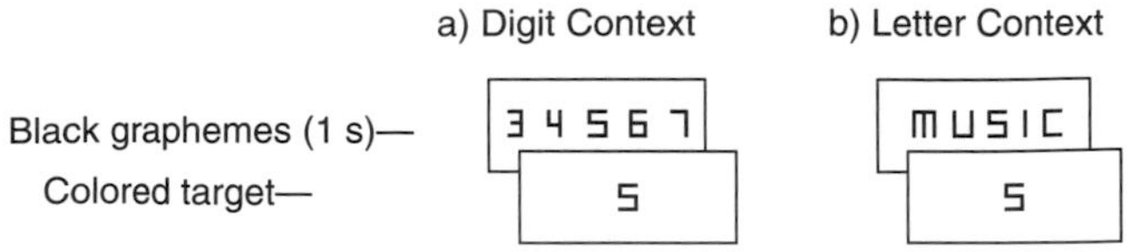

FIGURE 52.3 In the first frame, the entire string was shown for 1 s. In the second frame, all but the ambiguous grapheme disappeared from view. This target appeared in color. For all trials, J. was asked to name the video color of the target as quickly and as accurately as possible. Targets remained on screen until their color was named. Testing was conducted in two sessions. In the digit-context session, J. was presented with 100 digit strings composed of four, five, or six black digits. The letter-context session was identical to the digit-context session except that instead of digit strings, 100 high-frequency words containing four, five, or six letters were presented.

To assess whether the same grapheme can automatically elicit more than one synesthetic color, depending on whether the grapheme is interpreted as a digit or a letter, we devised another method based on Stroop interference. The approach required a synesthete like J., who experiences equally strong photisms for both digits and letters. Figure 52.3 shows the key conditions used in the experiment. Strings of graphemes were presented for 1 s to establish either a digit context or a letter context for subsequently presented colored ambiguous graphemes. For all trials, J. was asked to name the video color of the target as quickly and as accurately as possible. Targets remained on screen until their color was named. The key manipulation involved the congruency between the video colors of the targets and the colors of J.'s photisms. In the digit-context condition, congruent trials entailed presenting the ambiguous graphemes 2 3 H 5 7 in the colors of J.'s photisms for the digits *2*, *3*, *4*, *5*, and *7*, whereas on incongruent trials, the ambiguous graphemes were displayed in the colors of J.'s photisms for the letters *Z*, *B*, *H*, *S*, and *T*. In the letter-context condition, the situation was reversed: congruently colored ambiguous graphemes 2 3 H 5 7 appeared in the colors of J.'s photisms for the letters *Z*, *B*, *H*, *S*, and *T*, but incongruently colored ambiguous graphemes appeared in the colors of J.'s photisms for the digits *2*, *3*, *4*, *5*, and *7*. Crucially, for the ambiguous graphemes, what was a congruent trial in one context was always an incongruent trial in the other context (e.g., a pink 5 would be a congruent trial if this grapheme was interpreted as a digit, but an incongruent trial if this grapheme was interpreted as a letter). If context does determine the color experience elicited by the ambiguous grapheme, then J should respond more slowly on incongruent trials than on congruent trials.

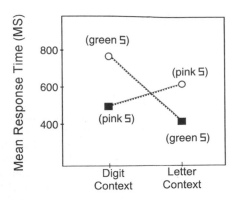

FIGURE 52.4 Mean color naming response times for the synesthete J. Ambiguous graphemes (2 3 H 5 7) were presented in either digit or letter contexts. In the digit context, congruent trials entailed coloring these graphemes using the photism colors for 2, 3, 4, 5, and 7. For incongruent trials, the graphemes were colored using the photism colors of the matching letters Z, B, H, S, and T. In the letter context, graphemes were colored using the photism colors for Z, B, H, S, and T. For incongruent trials, the graphemes were colored using the photism colors of the matching digits 2, 3, 4, 5, and 7. There were 50 trials of each type. The dashed lines join conditions in which J named the colors of *identical* stimuli.

Figure 52.4 shows J.'s color-naming response times in the digit and letter context conditions. Consider her response times in the digit context condition. When the ambiguous graphemes were presented in J.'s colors for the digit interpretation (congruent trial mean = 501 ms), her reaction times were significantly faster than when these same graphemes were presented in her colors for the letter interpretation of these graphemes (incongruent trial mean = 770 ms). This large, 269-ms Stroop effect indicates that J. must have interpreted the ambiguous graphemes 2 3 H 5 7 as the digits *2 3 4 5 7*. Upon viewing these stimuli and interpreting them as digits, we propose that she automatically experienced the photisms that habitually accompany these digits—photisms that facilitated her response times on congruent trials where the color of the photisms were the same as the video colors she had to name, but interfered with her response times on incongruent trials where the color of the photisms were different from the video colors she had to name.

Now consider her response times in the letter context condition. When the ambiguous graphemes were presented in J.'s colors for the letter interpretation of these graphemes (congruent trial mean = 422 ms), her reaction times were significantly faster than when these same graphemes were presented in her colors for the digit interpretation (incongruent trial mean = 633 ms). This large, 211-ms Stroop effect indicates that J. must have interpreted the ambiguous graphemes

2 3 H 5 7 as the letters *Z B H S T* and suggests that J. automatically experienced the photisms that habitually accompany these letters—photisms that would have interfered with her response times on incongruent trials.

The contrasts depicted in Figure 52.4 by the dashed lines show the influence on J.'s response time when she interpreted the same graphemes (e.g., a pink 5) as a digit or as a letter. When the graphemes 2 3 H 5 7 were presented in the digit context and were colored using the color of J.'s photisms for digits, response times were significantly faster (mean = 501 ms) than when exactly the same graphemes were presented in the *letter* context (mean = 621 ms). Similarly, when the graphemes 2 3 H 5 7 were presented in the letter context and were colored using the color of J.'s photisms for letters, response times were significantly faster (414 ms) than when exactly the same graphemes were presented in the *digit* context (770 ms). The rationale is that since identical graphemes (e.g., a pink 5) were presented in each context yet response times differed significantly, what must have changed was the photism that was experienced by J. in the different contexts. That is, these large response time differences between conditions joined by the dashed lines must be attributable to synesthetic color/video color congruency. For example, when a pink 5 was interpreted as a *digit*, J. automatically experienced a pink photism, and response times were facilitated because the synesthetic color matched the video color on the screen that she had to name. When the same pink 5 was interpreted as a *letter*, she experienced a green photism, and response times were increased because now the color of J.'s photism (green) interfered with naming the video color on the screen (pink). Because the stimuli presented to J. in each of the conditions joined by the dashed lines were identical, we conclude that J. must have experienced differently colored photisms for the same ambiguous graphemes in the digit and letter contexts.

Ramachandran and Hubbard (2001a) conducted experiments with two synesthetes whom we would classify as projector synesthetes (i.e., they saw photisms "spatially in the same location as the form"; Ramachandran & Hubbard, 2001a, p. 979). Based on the performance of these projector synesthetes, Ramachandran and Hubbard concluded that the form of a grapheme is more crucial in activating a photism than the concept of a digit or letter. They proposed that areas of the fusiform gyrus dealing with graphemic form are directly linked to fusiform areas dealing with color. Crucially, such linkages occur prior to the activation of meaning. In such an architecture, it is difficult to see how the same form can elicit two different synesthetic colors. Ramachandran and Hubbard (2001b) suggested that, in addition to "lower" synesthetes with early-stage cross-wiring, there are also "higher" synesthetes in whom cross-wiring occurs at later stages in visual processing. For example, brain areas such as the angular gyrus that process abstract numerical concepts may be cross-wired to areas devoted to "more sophisticated color processing" (Ramachandran & Hubbard, 2001a, p. 982). Such late-stage cross-wiring may allow concept activation to activate a specific synesthetic color, a finding in accordance with the present findings. However, it is difficult to see how cross-wiring between late-stage, *abstract* semantic representations could elicit the experience of a perceptual, *projected* photism that occurs in approximately the same spatial coordinates as the presented grapheme. In order for synesthetic percepts to occur in the same spatial location as presented graphemes, it would seem necessary to invoke early-stage areas that support spatiotopic representations. In cross-linkage models, it is always possible that a given synesthete could have linkages at both early and late stages. In order to account for the present findings, however, cross-linkage models would have to include some form of feedback from links involving meaning and links involving form. Importantly, Ramachandran and Hubbard recognized the necessity of accounting for such top-down influences on synesthetic perception, and have even provided some informal demonstrations of how context can ultimately determine the color of photisms (Ramachandran & Hubbard, 2002b). The point here is that cross-wiring models that include reentrant pathways would closely resemble the reentrant feedback models described by Smilek et al. (2001).

When we first postulated an architecture in which form is linked to meaning and meaning is then linked back to color along reentrant pathways, we suggested that the same grapheme could elicit different colors depending on whether that grapheme elicits the concept of a digit or the concept of a letter (Smilek et al., 2001). The present findings provide the first empirical evidence for such top-down context effects. When considering cross-linked versus reentrant models, we suggest that it is easier to account for photisms being perceived as projected overlays in an architecture where later stage areas back-activate early-stage visual areas than architectures involving cross-linkages purely at later stages in visual processing. As such, the finding that the same grapheme can automatically elicit different *projected* photisms depending on whether it is interpreted as a digit or letter, is more consistent with reentrant models than with early- or late-stage cross-linkage models of grapheme-color synesthesia.

Where do associator synesthetes fit into this proposed architecture? We believe the key lies both in the locus of the perceived photism and the degree of spatial correspondence between the presented graphemes and the experienced photisms. For projector synesthetes of the projector subtype, photisms appear to overlie the presented grapheme and to conform exactly to the presented shape of the grapheme that lies beneath. For associator synesthetes, photisms are perceived in "the mind's eye" as opposed to being projected in space. A color representation is consistently activated, but lacks the tight spatial correspondence between the presented grapheme and the photism. This suggests that for associators, areas involved in processing the meaning of graphemes may activate later-stage areas in the anterior fusiform gyrus pertaining to the more conceptual and abstract aspects of color representation, as opposed to the more perceptual aspects of color, which are activated in more posterior fusiform areas such as V4/V8. Such differences suggest that for projector synesthetes, photisms depend on feedbackward pathways from later-stage to earlier-stage visual areas, whereas for associator synesthetes the linkages may be more akin to the later-stage cross-activations proposed by Ramachandran and Hubbard (2001b) when discussing their "higher" synesthetes.

Alphanumeric synesthesia and multisensory processing

In people with grapheme-color synesthesia, unisensory inputs such as black graphemes lead to experiences consisting of the black grapheme plus the experience of a highly specific color. Although the majority of research discussed here has focused on cases where the inducer and the synesthetic experience both lie within the same modality, the general form of the reentrant architecture that we have proposed to account for projected photisms may also account for synesthetic experiences that cross modalities. In fact, such an architecture has been proposed by Grossenbacher (1997) to account for cases in which auditory inducers trigger the experience of colors. According to this architecture, the auditory inducer converges upon a multimodal nexus that also receives input from visual pathways. Importantly, these visual pathways contain both feed-forward pathways that synapse on to the multimodal nexus and reentrant pathways that feed back along the visual pathways to lower-level visual areas. Thus, in a synesthete who experiences photisms for spoken letters, hearing a letter spoken would activate auditory pathways that synapse onto the multimodal nexus and activation within the multimodal nexus would trigger activation visual pathways that feedback to early-stage visual areas associated with color. Such a feedback circuit could explain how the sound of a letter could ultimately induce a visual experience of color. Such an architecture may also be consistent with the findings of brain imagery studies showing that spoken letters induce activation in both auditory association areas as well as early-stage visual areas such as V4/V8 (Nunn et al., 2002). Thus, the architecture we have proposed to account for grapheme-color synesthesia of the projector subtype, and the architecture Grossenbacher has proposed to account for the sound-color synesthesia, bear a striking resemblance in that both rely on reentrant pathways from late-stage to early-stage areas of cortex.

Conclusions

Studies of synesthesia can provide insight into the nature of multisensory processing in humans. Based on the combined evidence from subjective reports and methods based on the Stroop effect, we propose that colored photisms are an automatic consequence of viewing black graphemes, but that not all synesthetes experience photisms in the same way—some synesthetes experience photisms as being projected in space, while others experience photisms as occurring "in the mind's eye." Based on the results of experiments employing a number of different methods from cognitive psychology (masking, visual search, object substitution), we concur with Ramachandran and Hubbard that projected photisms are perceptual in nature rather than a memory association, but would add the cautionary note that such an assertion is correct only when speaking of the experiences of projector synesthetes. Finally, based on the empirical investigation of a projector synesthete who experiences different photisms, depending on whether ambiguous graphemes are interpreted as digits or letters, we conclude that both the graphemic form and the meaning of digits play a role in determining these synesthetic experiences.

REFERENCES

Allison, T., McCarthy, G., Nobre, A., Puce, A., & Berger, A. (1994). Human extrastriate cortex and the perception of faces, words, numbers and colors. *Cerebral Cortex, 5,* 1047–3211.

Baron-Cohen, S., Harrison, J., Goldstein, L. H., & Wyke, M. (1993). Coloured speech perception: Is synaesthesia what happens when modularity breaks down? *Perception, 22,* 419–426.

Cytowic, R. E. (1989). *Synaesthesia: A union of the senses.* New York: Springer-Verlag.

Cytowic, R. E. (1993). *The man who tasted shapes.* New York: Warner Books.

Cytowic, R. E. (1997). Synaesthesia: Phenomenology and neuropsychology. A review of current knowledge. In S. Baron-Cohen & J. E. Harrison (Eds.), *Synaesthesia: Classic and contemporary readings* (pp. 17–39). Cambridge, England: Blackwell.

Dann, K. T. (1998). *Bright colours falsely seen: Synaesthesia and the search for transcendental knowledge.* New Haven, CT: Yale University Press.

Dixon, M. J., Smilek, D., Cudahy, C., & Merikle, P. M. (2000). Five plus two equals yellow. *Nature, 406,* 365.

Enns, J. T., & Di Lollo, V. (1997). Object substitution: A new form of masking in unattended visual locations. *Psychological Science, 8,* 135–139.

Di Lollo, V., Enns, J. T., & Rensink, R. A. (2000). Competition for consciousness among visual events: The psychophysics of reentrant visual pathways. *Journal of Experimental Psychology: General, 129,* 481–507.

Grossenbacher, P. G. (1997). Perception and sensory information in synesthetic experience. In S. Baron-Cohen & J. E. Harrison (Eds.), *Synaesthesia: Classic and contemporary readings* (pp. 148–172). Cambridge, England: Blackwell.

Grossenbacher, P. G., & Lovelace, C. T. (2001). Mechanisms of synesthesia: Cognitive and physiological constraints. *Trends in Cognitive Sciences, 5,* 36–41.

Humphreys, G. W., Riddoch, M. J., & Quinlan, P. T. (1988). Cascade processes in picture identification. *Cognitive Neuropsychology, 5,* 67–104.

MacLeod, C. M., & Dunbar, K. (1988). Training and Stroop-like interference: Evidence for a continuum of automaticity. *Journal of Experimental Psychology: Learning, Memory and Cognition, 14,* 126–135.

Marks, L. E. (1975). On coloured-hearing synesthesia: Cross modal translations of sensory dimensions. *Psychological Bulletin, 82,* 303–331.

Marks, L. E. (2000). Synesthesia. In E. Cardena, S. J. Lynn, & S. Krippner (Eds.), *Varieties of anomalous experiences* (pp. 121–149). Washington, DC: American Psychological Association.

Mattingley, J. B., Rich, A. N., Yelland, G., & Bradshaw, J. L. (2001a). Investigations of automatic binding of colour and form in synaesthesia. *Nature, 410,* 580–582.

Mattingley, J. B., Rich, A. N., Yelland, G., & Bradshaw, J. L. (2001b). *Unconscious priming eliminates automatic binding of colour and alphanumeric form in synaesthesia.* Paper presented at the 12th annual meeting of Theoretical and Experimental Neuropsychology (TENNET-12), Montreal, Quebec.

Mills, C. B., Boteler, E. H., & Oliver, G. K. (1999). Digit synaesthesia: A case study using a Stroop-type test. *Cognitive Neuropsychology, 16,* 181–191.

Nunn, J. A., Gregory, L. J., Brammer, M., Williams, S. C., Parslow, D. M., Morgan, M. J., et al. (2002). Functional magnetic resonance imaging of synesthesia: Activation of V4/V8 by spoken words. *Nature Neuroscience 5,* 371–375.

Odgaard, E. C., Flowers, J. H., & Bradman, H. L. (1999). An investigation of the cognitive and perceptual dynamics of a colour-digit synaesthete. *Perception, 28,* 651–664.

Ramachandran, V. S., & Hubbard, E. M. (2001a). Psychological investigations into the neural basis of synaesthesia. *Proceedings of the Royalty of London, Series B: Biological Sciences, 268,* 979–983.

Ramachandran, V. S., & Hubbard, E. M. (2001b). Synesthesia: A window into perception, thought and language. *Journal of Consciousness Studies, 8,* 3–34.

Smilek, D., & Dixon, M. J. (2002). Towards a synergistic understanding of synaesthesia: Combining current experimental findings with synaesthetes' subjective descriptions. *Psyche, 08* (available: *http://psyche.cs.monash.edu.au/v8/psyche-8-01-smilek.html*).

Smilek, D., Dixon, M. J., Cudahy, C., & Merikle, P. M. (2001). Synaesthetic photisms influence visual perception. *Journal of Cognitive Neuroscience, 13,* 930–936.

Stroop, J. R. (1935). Studies of interference in serial verbal reactions. *Journal of Experimental Psychology, 18,* 643–662.

Wagar, B. M., Dixon, M. J., Smilek, D., & Cudahy, C. (2002). Coloured photisms prevent object-substitution masking in digit colour synaesthesia. *Brain and Cognition, 48,* 606–611.

Wheeler, R. H. (1920). *The synaesthesia of a blind subject.* University of Oregon Publications, No. 5.

Wollen, K. A., & Ruggiero, F. T. (1983). Coloured-letter synaesthesia. *Journal of Mental Imagery, 7,* 83–86.

53 Behavioral and Brain Correlates of Multisensory Experience in Synesthesia

JASON B. MATTINGLEY AND ANINA N. RICH

Introduction

For most people, stimulation within a given sense modality yields a unique and distinctive perceptual experience. For instance, the way a banana looks has a different perceptual quality from the way it smells, tastes, and feels. Even within a single modality, various properties of a stimulus trigger unique sensory experiences. Thus, the visual experience associated with the color of a banana is qualitatively different from the visual experience associated with its shape and surface texture.

Although these distinct perceptual qualities may interact to enhance our knowledge of objects and events in the world, they typically remain clearly distinguishable. For individuals with synesthesia, however, the perceptual experiences elicited by the properties of an object tend to interact in ways that are highly unusual. For such individuals, the taste of a particular food may also elicit a distinct tactile sensation (Cytowic, 1993), or the appearance of a letter or digit may be accompanied by a vivid experience of color (Baron-Cohen, Wyke, & Binnie, 1987; Galton, 1880). Research on synesthesia provides a unique opportunity to examine how the brain represents the sensory and conceptual properties of objects, and how learning and experience shape the neural substrates of these representations.

In this chapter we focus on the most common form of synesthesia, in which letters, words, and digits elicit vivid experiences of color when they are seen or heard. These forms are known as color-graphemic and color-phonemic synesthesia, respectively. Other forms of synesthesia seem to be much more rare (Grossenbacher & Lovelace, 2001) and may even reflect different underlying processes (Rich & Mattingley, 2002). Individuals with color-graphemic or color-phonemic synesthesia typically report experiencing specific colors when they hear or read letters, words, or digits. The colors may be seen as a "mist" or as a colored overlay in space, or as a vivid form of mental imagery "in the mind's eye." Whether these different types of subjective experience reflect different forms of synesthesia is not known, although some authors have drawn such a distinction (see Dixon, Smilek, Wagar, & Merikle, Chap. 52, this volume).

Although the subjective experiences of synesthetes provide important information about the qualitative aspects of the phenomenon, they are difficult to verify experimentally. Our approach has been to use indirect, quantifiable measures of synesthesia to examine its effects on perceptual and cognitive performance. In the first section of this chapter, we review our recent attempts to measure color-graphemic synesthesia objectively and to determine the nature of the representations that give rise to the unusual perceptual experiences. We have found that synesthetic color experiences arise only after substantial early processing of the inducing stimuli (letters and digits), contrary to recent suggestions that synesthetic colors are triggered early in visual processing, prior to the operation of focused attention and explicit recognition of the inducing form (e.g., Palmeri, Blake, Marois, Flanery, & Whetsell, 2002; Ramachandran & Hubbard, 2001a, 2001b). Based on our findings, we have suggested that color-graphemic synesthesia reflects anomalous binding of color and visual form during later, attentive stages of visual processing (Rich & Mattingley, 2002). In support of this hypothesis, we have also shown that synesthetes' color experiences can be substantially modified under conditions of attentional load, or when multiple graphemic forms compete for attention in rivalrous displays.

In the second section of the chapter, we consider the growing evidence from functional brain imaging regarding the neural correlates of synesthesia. Brain imaging studies in color-phonemic synesthetes have revealed significant activity in visual areas of the brain during auditory presentation of words, thus confirming these individuals' subjective reports of vivid color experiences (Nunn et al., 2002; Paulesu et al., 1995). The behavioral tasks used in these studies, however, limit the extent to which they are able to reveal the neural processes that actually give rise to synesthetic experiences. We conclude by suggesting ways in which these limitations might be overcome, and provide some suggestions for future avenues of research.

Measures of the consistency of synesthetic colors

One of the most striking characteristics of synesthesia is the remarkable consistency of the colors experienced in association with specific alphanumeric forms for a particular individual. Thus, although each synesthete possesses an idiosyncratic set of digit-color, letter-color, and word-color pairings, these pairings apparently remain consistent throughout the individual's life. This observation has been reported anecdotally by numerous investigators (e.g., Dresslar, 1903; Ginsberg, 1923) and was confirmed empirically in a landmark study by Baron-Cohen and colleagues (1987). They asked a 76-year-old synesthete, E.P., to provide her synesthetic colors for 103 aurally presented words. Then, 10 weeks later, without warning, she was again presented with the same words and asked to indicate her colors. She provided identical colors for all 103 words on retest, indicating remarkable consistency of synesthetic experiences over time. For comparison, a 27-year-old nonsynesthetic control with an excellent memory was tested on the same set of words but was instructed to try and remember her arbitrary word-color associations for later recall. Just two weeks later, the control subject recalled only 17 of the 103 word-color pairs, a performance that was clearly worse than that of the synesthete E.P.

The apparent consistency of synesthetic color pairings over time has become a litmus test for determining whether an individual actually has synesthesia. We therefore were interested in replicating this result with a group of synesthetes using a standardized list of 150 digits, letters, and words. We had been contacted by more than 150 self-reported synesthetes in response to an article on synesthesia that had appeared in a national newspaper (Dow, 1999). We sent these individuals a questionnaire that included the 150-item list, and asked them to provide their synesthetic color for each. Three months after an individual returned the initial questionnaire, we posted a second copy of the list and asked the participant to again indicate his or her synesthetic color for each item. Figure 53.1 shows the results in a subset of 15 synesthetes and in 15 nonsynesthetic controls, matched for age and sex, who provided arbitrary colors for the same list of 150 items, with a retest interval of just 4 weeks. The individuals with synesthesia were more consistent in their color matches than the nonsynesthetic controls across all categories tested.

These findings confirm that color-graphemic synesthesia is remarkably consistent over time, in keeping with subjective reports and previous literature (Baron-Cohen et al., 1987; Dresslar, 1903; Ginsberg, 1923). They reveal little, however, about how arbitrary symbols such as digits and letters trigger such unusual color experiences, or about the level of processing of the inducing stimulus required for these experiences to arise. In an attempt to address these questions, we have designed a number of tasks to examine

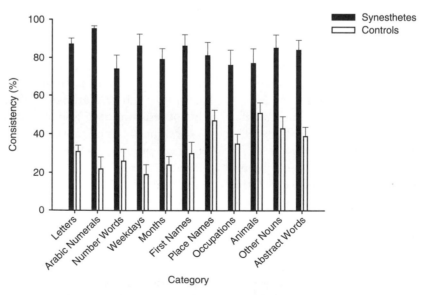

FIGURE 53.1   Consistency of color experiences for a group of 15 color-graphemic synesthetes and 15 nonsynesthetic control subjects, for stimuli in 11 different categories. Synesthetes were retested after 3 months, controls after 4 weeks. (Reproduced with permission from Mattingley et al., 2001a.)

synesthesia indirectly, by measuring its effects on the performance of otherwise unrelated perceptual and cognitive tasks.

Measures of competition: The synesthetic Stroop task

Rather than asking synesthetes about their synesthetic colors directly, several researchers have investigated whether performance on other tasks might be modified by the occurrence of such colors. Anecdotally, most synesthetes claim their colors arise automatically, without the need for conscious thought or effort (Ramachandran & Hubbard, 2001a). If this is true, then it should be possible to contrive artificial situations in which synesthetic colors compete, or are incompatible, with responses on a cognitive task. This should cause a decrement in performance relative to a baseline condition in which there is no competition present. One of the most widely used such tasks is the synesthetic Stroop paradigm (Mills, Boteler, & Oliver, 1999; Odgaard, Flowers, & Bradman, 1999; Wollen & Ruggiero, 1983), in which participants are asked to name the display colors of digits or letters that are colored either congruently or incongruently with the synesthetic colors they normally elicit. For example, one of our synesthetes, T.S., experiences red for the letter *A* and green for the letter *E* (Fig. 53.2*A*). Note that a red *A* is for her "right", as is a green *E*, whereas a green *A* and a red *E* are "wrong", in the sense that their display colors differ from the synesthetic colors elicited by the letters. We might therefore ask, how quickly will T.S. be able to name the color red when it is presented as the letter *A* (congruently colored) versus the letter *E* (incongruently colored)? Clearly, for a nonsynesthete the time required to name a color should not differ depending on the letter (or digit) presented, given that the letters are completely irrelevant to the task. In contrast, if synesthetic colors cannot be fully inhibited, synesthetes should be slower to name colors in the incongruent condition versus the congruent condition.

Following from a series of earlier single case studies (Mills et al., 1999; Odgaard et al., 1999; Wollen & Ruggiero, 1983), we addressed this question in a group study of 15 individuals with color-graphemic synesthesia (the same 15 as those whose consistency data are shown in Fig. 53.1; Mattingley, Rich, Yelland, & Bradshaw, 2001a). In a preliminary phase, each synesthete selected a color that best matched letters of the alphabet and arabic digits from a standard, computer-generated palette. Each letter- and digit-color match was then rated on a 5-point scale for how well it matched the synesthetic color elicited by the character. The six best matching

character-color pairs were used to create ensembles of congruent and incongruent items that were specific to each synesthete and his or her matched, nonsynesthetic control. Participants were then required to name, as quickly as possible, the colors of characters that appeared individually on a computer display, either in separate blocks of congruent and incongruent items or with all stimuli randomly intermingled.

Figure 53.2 shows the group results for this task in the blocked (Fig. 53.2*B*) and randomized (Fig. 53.2*C*) conditions (see also Color Plate 25). Whereas the nonsynesthetic control group showed no difference in color naming times as a function of congruency, the synesthetes were significantly slower in the incongruent trials, both in the blocked and the randomized presentation conditions. These results indicate that synesthetic colors can interfere with the task of color naming, suggesting that the colors induced by alphanumeric characters arise automatically and cannot be fully suppressed under conditions of incompatibility (Mattingley et al., 2001a; Mills et al., 1999; Odgaard et al., 1999; Wollen & Ruggiero, 1983).

The synesthetic Stroop task has proved to be a robust and reliable measure of synesthesia. It has yielded consistent effects despite being implemented in a number of different ways. For instance, Dixon and colleagues found that naming times were significantly slowed when the color of a target patch was incongruent with the color elicited synesthetically by the *concept* of a number, derived arithmetically from two preceding digits (Dixon, Smilek, Cudahy, & Merikle, 2000). Thus, it seems that synesthetic congruency effects occur not only for alphanumeric characters that are physically present, but also for conceptual representations of these inducing stimuli. To further elucidate the level of processing at which inducing stimuli trigger synesthetic colors, we have developed a number of tasks that limit or alter the extent of inducer processing. Each relies on the basic synesthetic Stroop effect described in this section.

The effects of visual masking of inducing stimuli on color-graphemic synesthesia

Considerable low-level processing can occur prior to conscious representation of stimulus information (Snow & Mattingley, 2003). Words and objects that are displayed briefly and masked from awareness may nevertheless undergo substantial unconscious processing, as indicated by participants' responses to subsequently presented target items (Dehaene et al., 1998, 2001). If synesthesia is triggered at early stages of stimulus analysis, prior to the operation of conscious vision, then it

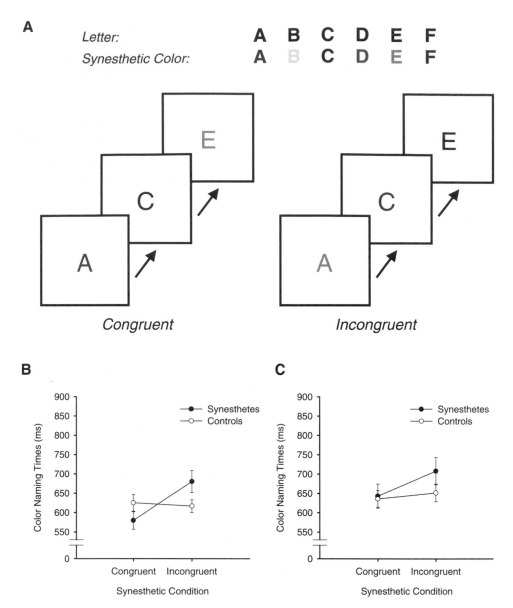

FIGURE 53.2   The synesthetic Stroop task. (*A*) Alphanumeric characters printed in colors that either match ("congruent") or do not match ("incongruent") the synesthetic color experiences of synesthete T.S. (*B*) Mean correct color naming times for 15 synesthetes and 15 nonsynesthetic controls, performing the synesthetic Stroop task—blocked presentation of congruent and incongruent trials. (*C*) Randomized presentation of congruent and incongruent trials. (*A* adapted with permission from Rich and Mattingley, 2002. *B* and *C* reproduced with permission from Mattingley et al., 2001a.) (See Color Plate 25.)

should be possible to elicit synesthesia even when the inducing stimuli are not available for conscious report. If, on the other hand, an inducing stimulus must be perceived consciously before it can trigger a synesthetic color, then masking the inducer from awareness should eliminate the synesthetic experience and reduce any associated congruency effects arising from incongruent character-color pairings.

We tested these competing hypotheses in 15 color-graphemic synesthetes and 15 nonsynesthetic controls, using a masked priming paradigm (Mattingley et al.,

2001a). The basic task required participants to name aloud the color of a target patch, which was composed of several overlapping alphanumeric characters. This target backward masked the single achromatic, alphanumeric character that preceded it (the prime), which under unmasked conditions elicited a vivid synesthetic color. Crucially, the synesthetic color elicited by a prime could be either congruent or incongruent with the color of the target patch to be named, thus allowing an analysis of any cost associated with incongruent prime-target pairs relative to congruent pairs. Since the prime never predicted the color of a subsequent target, participants could simply ignore the prime and focus on their task of target color naming. As in our earlier experiments on the synesthetic Stroop effect, only those characters that induced strong and reliable synesthetic colors and that could be well matched on the computer were used.

The primary aim of the experiment was to determine whether the congruency effect found in the synesthetic Stroop task would persist when the inducing character preceded and was masked by the colored target. We used three different prime durations, 500 ms, 56 ms, and 28 ms. The 500-ms duration was selected because at this duration, the prime remained clearly visible and thus could be processed consciously. The two shorter durations were chosen because they were too brief to

permit reliable, overt reports of prime identity, as confirmed in a separate prime identification task (outlined below). To summarize, then, each trial commenced with a forward mask consisting of a row of hash marks overlaid with @ signs. Following the forward mask, an achromatic prime appeared for one of the three durations, in separate blocks, followed by a colored target, which served as a backward mask (Fig. 53.3A; Color Plate 26).

The results of the priming experiment were clear (Figs. 53.3B and C). At the visible prime duration of 500 ms, synesthetes were significantly slower to name colors on incongruent trials than on congruent trials, whereas controls showed no such congruency effect. This demonstrates that synesthetic interference occurs even when the inducing character is separated

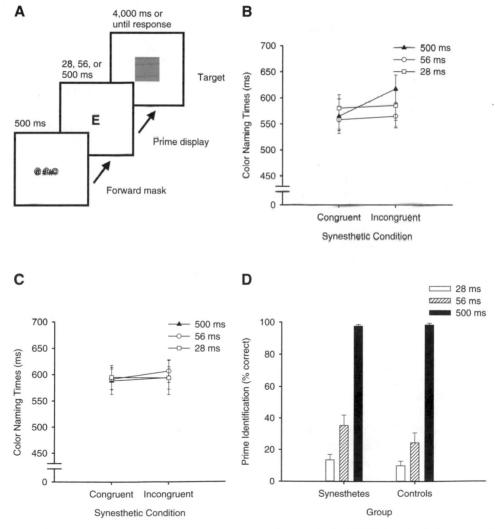

FIGURE 53.3   The synesthetic priming task. (*A*) Sequence of events in a typical trial. The task was to name the target color as quickly as possible. (*B*) Mean correct color naming times for congruent and incongruent trials at prime durations of 28, 56, and 500 ms for synesthetes. (*C*) Nonsynesthetic controls. (*D*) Mean percent correct prime identification for synesthetes and controls. (*B–D* reproduced with permission from Mattingley et al., 2001a.) (See Color Plate 26.)

temporally from the target color to be named. In contrast, at prime durations of 28 ms and 56 ms, the synesthetic congruency effect was absent, suggesting that the synesthetic colors normally triggered by alphanumeric characters are no longer elicited when the characters are unavailable for conscious report.

In a separate experiment, we verified that primes presented for 28 ms and 56 ms could not be identified. Using stimulus displays identical to those shown in Figure 53.3A, we asked participants to focus on the primes rather than the targets, and to try and identify them. As shown in Figure 53.3D, prime identification was poor at 28 and 56 ms but was near ceiling at 500 ms, thus confirming that the masking paradigm was effective in reducing conscious perception of the primes at the shorter durations. Moreover, in a further experiment we showed that although the primes were effectively masked from conscious perception, they were nevertheless processed to the level of letter recognition. In this experiment, the target color patch was replaced by a single uppercase alphanumeric character. This character was preceded by a lowercase alphanumeric prime at one of the original durations (28, 56, or 500 ms). As in the initial priming paradigm, the prime and the target could be either congruent (e.g., $a \rightarrow A$) or incongruent (e.g., $b \rightarrow A$). The participants' task was to name the uppercase target character as quickly as possible. Under the two masked priming durations (28 ms and 56 ms), both synesthetes and controls responded significantly slower on incongruent than on congruent trials. Thus, from the synesthetic priming results, we can conclude that although the identity of alphanumeric characters can be extracted without conscious perception, this level of processing is not sufficient for a synesthetic color to be elicited.

The effects of attentional load and rivalry on color-graphemic synesthesia

The findings from our work with masked priming imply that substantial perceptual processing of inducing stimuli must occur before synesthetic colors are elicited. We have postulated that in order for alphanumeric characters to produce synesthetic color experiences, they must be processed at least to the level of overt recognition, and that this requires focused attention (Mattingley et al., 2001a). According to *feature integration theory* (Treisman, 1998; Treisman & Gelade, 1980), elementary visual properties such as form, color, and motion are extracted rapidly and in parallel across the entire visual field, with no apparent limit in processing capacity. In order for these basic features to be bound into coherent surfaces and objects for overt recognition, however,

focused attention is required, and this is a capacity-limited process. There is considerable evidence to support feature integration theory, or some variant thereof, from studies of normal perception (Treisman, 1999). We believe our findings on synesthesia are also consistent with the key tenets of feature integration theory. Under conditions of focused attention, relevant inducing characters produce vivid synesthetic colors that can interfere with color naming on synesthetic Stroop tasks. When the processing of inducing characters is limited by masking, however, form and color are no longer bound together by focused attention. Under these conditions, synesthetic colors are no longer perceived, and synesthetic Stroop effects do not arise.

If attention plays a crucial role in the manifestation of color-graphemic synesthesia, then it should be possible to modulate the color experiences of these individuals by manipulating the extent to which they can devote their attention to relevant inducing stimuli. We tested this prediction in a recent study of 14 color-graphemic synesthetes using a variation of the synesthetic priming paradigm described above (Mattingley, Rich, & Payne, 2003). The crucial change, however, was that instead of reducing the duration of the inducing characters to modulate prime processing, participants were required to perform a secondary attentional task during presentation of the inducer. We reasoned that if focused attention is required to bind form and color in synesthesia, then diverting attention from the inducer should attenuate any such binding. Letter primes were presented for 400 ms, so that they were clearly visible to all participants (i.e., with overt report near ceiling), followed by a target color patch that again could be congruent or incongruent with the synesthetic color elicited by the letter prime (Fig. 53.4A; Color Plate 27).

The attention task required participants to discriminate the relative sizes of gaps on diagonally opposite sides of a large diamond that surrounded the central inducing prime (Fig. 53.4A). Participants first named the target color as quickly as possible, and then gave their unspeeded gap discrimination response. In a baseline condition ("no load"), participants were instructed to ignore the gaps altogether and to focus exclusively on the color-naming task. This allowed us to verify that the synesthetes experienced the same congruency effects with this altered prime display as in the synesthetic priming paradigm. The sizes of the gaps were titrated in a pilot experiment in order to yield two levels of difficulty. In the *low load* condition, the gaps could be readily discriminated in the time given (400 ms), yielding performances of approximately 98% correct across all participants. In the *high load* condition, the gaps were difficult to discriminate, yielding a mean performance

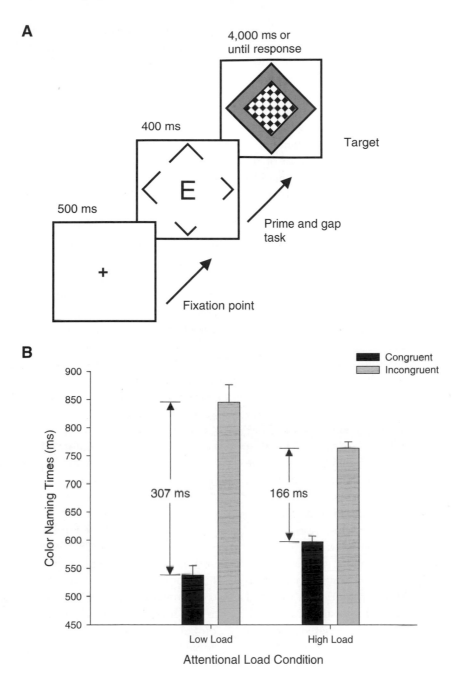

A

500 ms

+

Fixation point

400 ms

E

Prime and gap task

4,000 ms or until response

Target

B

■ Congruent
▨ Incongruent

Color Naming Times (ms)

900
850
800
750
700
650
600
550
500
450

307 ms

166 ms

Low Load   High Load

Attentional Load Condition

FIGURE 53.4   The effects of priming with a concurrent attentional load on color naming in a variant of the synesthetic priming task. (*A*) Sequence of events in a typical trial of the attentional load paradigm. The primary task was to name the target color as quickly as possible; the secondary task in the low- and high-load conditions was to discriminate the larger of two gaps on diagonally opposite sides of the diamond in the prime display. (*B*) Mean correct color naming times in the low- and high-load conditions for a representative synesthete, with separate bars showing data from congruent and incongruent trials. (See Color Plate 27.)

of around 78% correct. Participants were instructed at the beginning of a block to attend either to the upper left/lower right sides of the diamond or to the lower left/upper right sides, corresponding to either the easier (*low load*) or the more difficult (*high load*) gap discrimination. Crucially, on every trial the prime display contained a diamond with gaps on all four sides. Thus, the prime displays were identical for both the *low load*

and *high load* conditions; participants were merely instructed to attend to one pair of gaps or the other. This arrangement of prime displays ensured that any effects on color naming could not be attributed to perceptual differences between the load conditions.

On each trial, a fixation cross was followed by the prime display containing a letter prime in the center of a diamond with gaps in all four sides. A target color patch subsequently appeared (Fig. 53.4A). Participants named the color as quickly as possible, and then, in the two attention conditions, gave an unspeeded two-alternative decision about the position of the larger gap in the prime display. The synesthetic color elicited by the prime could be either congruent or incongruent with the subsequent target color, thus allowing us to use the synesthetic Stroop effect as our dependent measure. Our analyses focused on whether the cost of incongruent relative to congruent trials was attenuated in the high-load condition relative to the low-load condition, as predicted by our attentional explanation for synesthetic binding.

The results from a representative synesthete, M.R., are shown for the two load conditions in Figure 53.4B. For nonsynesthetic controls, there was no effect of congruency in any of the conditions, as expected. In contrast, M.R. was slower to name target colors preceded by incongruent versus congruent primes; that is, she showed a synesthetic Stroop effect. This result is consistent with the group findings from the visible (500 ms) condition of the priming experiment described above (Fig. 53.3B) and confirms that the somewhat different displays in the attention experiment also yielded reliable congruency effects. More important, however, a comparison of her results for the two load conditions demonstrates that attention does indeed have a modulatory role in the synesthetic binding of form and color. As shown in Figure 53.4B, the cost of incongruent versus congruent trials was reduced in the high-load condition relative to the low-load condition. This result, which was also evident in the group as a whole, suggests that synesthetic colors arising from the processing of alphanumeric forms are at least partially dependent on focused attention for their occurrence. When attention is diverted from an inducing form, the usual synesthetic color either is not elicited or is significantly attenuated, and consequently is a weaker competitor when the participant is attempting to name an incongruent color. The fact that the synesthetic congruency effect was not eliminated entirely by the high-load attentional task might be interpreted as implying that synesthetic colors can still arise without focused attention. However, even our high-load condition (which yielded 78% correct performance) probably left residual attentional capacity for processing the alphanumeric prime. This is supported by participants' near-ceiling performance in *identifying* the prime characters under high-load conditions, as revealed in a separate experiment using displays that were identical to those used in the color naming experiment.

The results of our attentional load experiment are reminiscent of findings from studies of the effects of attentional manipulations on the conventional Stroop effect in nonsynesthetes. It has been shown repeatedly that adding one or more irrelevant, "neutral" (i.e., non-color) words to a display containing a color word significantly reduces the magnitude of the conventional Stroop effect (so-called *Stroop dilution;* Brown, 1996; Brown, Gore, & Carr, 2002; Brown, Roos-Gilbert, & Carr, 1995; Kahneman & Chajczyk, 1983). Having participants focus attention explicitly on the color word in such displays eliminates the Stroop dilution effect, whereas having them focus on the neutral word attenuates but does not eliminate the Stroop effect itself (Brown et al., 2002). These findings suggest that word reading is a limited-capacity process and that selective attention mediates the extent to which words activate appropriate semantic representations (Brown et al., 2002). The findings from our experiment on the effects of attentional load on synesthesia are broadly consistent with this view, in the sense that the magnitude of the synesthetic Stroop effect was reduced by a visual attention task presented concurrently with an alphanumeric prime. By limiting selective attention, our manipulation of load may have reduced the efficiency with which the character was able to access relevant semantic representations (including the synesthetic color).

Our hypothesis that selective attention plays a crucial modulatory role in color-graphemic synesthesia is also supported by recent findings from a study involving perceptual rivalry between concurrent inducers, each of which elicits a different synesthetic color (Rich & Mattingley, 2003). We used Navon-type local-global stimuli (Navon, 1977) of the kind illustrated in Figure 53.5A (see also Color Plate 28). When viewing such stimuli, most individuals perceive both the global and local forms but can focus attention voluntarily on either level to enhance its salience. When the task is to discriminate target forms, normal participants typically show a "global precedence" effect, such that information at the global level is processed earlier than information at the local level (Navon, 1977). This effect can be reduced or eliminated, however, by having participants focus their attention preferentially at the local level, demonstrating that attention plays an important part in prioritizing different aspects of a common stimulus array. Anecdotally, when synesthetes view achromatic stimuli composed of different alphanumeric forms at the local and global levels, they typically report seeing the synesthetic color of the letter to which they are currently attending rather than a mixture of the two colors elicited by the different letters (Mattingley, Rich, Yelland, & Bradshaw, 2001b; Palmeri et al., 2002; Ramachandran & Hubbard, 2001b). This again implies that attention plays an important role in binding form and color in synesthesia and that the top-down (endogenous) allocation of

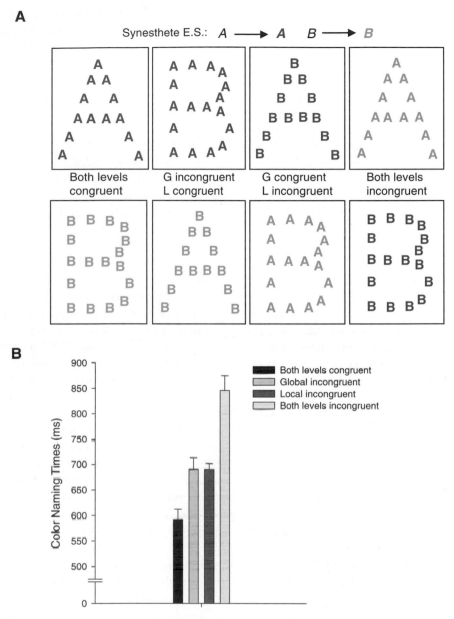

FIGURE 53.5 Synesthetic rivalry induced by global alphanumeric characters composed of local characters. (*A*) Examples of the four stimulus types used to study the effect of rivalry between synesthetic inducers. The task was to name the stimulus color as quickly as possible. Participants never had to name the alphanumeric characters, which were irrelevant and nonpredictive with respect to the display color. (*B*) Mean correct color naming times for each of the four local-global stimulus types, which were randomly intermingled. Data shown are from a single representative synesthete. (G, global; L, local.) (See Color Plate 28.)

attention can alter synesthetic experiences under conditions of rivalry.

In our experiments, stimuli could be composed of the same local and global forms, in either congruent or incongruent colors; or they were composed of two different forms, each of which elicited a unique synesthetic color. In the latter case, the display color could be incongruent with the synesthetic color induced by either the local or the global form, as illustrated in Figure 53.5*A*. We had a group of 14 color-graphemic

synesthetes and 14 nonsynesthetes perform speeded naming of the color (rather than the letter identity) of these local-global stimuli. In the first experiment, the four stimulus types were randomly intermingled and presented individually in the center of a computer display. Participants were told they could ignore the local and global forms, as these were not predictive of the color in which a stimulus would appear.

The color naming times of a representative synesthete are shown in Figure 53.5*B*. The synesthete was slower when both local and global characters elicited a synesthetic color that was incongruent with the display color, compared with each of the other three conditions. In contrast, control subjects showed no significant differences between any of the four conditions, as would be expected for this task of color naming, where letter identity is irrelevant. Interestingly, the synesthete was also slower in the two conditions in which just one level of the hierarchical stimulus elicited an incongruent synesthetic color and the other elicited a congruent color than when both levels elicited a congruent color. Because participants could not predict whether any incongruency would arise at the local or global level, their attention was most likely distributed diffusely over both levels.

In a second experiment, we used the same local-global stimuli to investigate whether synesthetes could use selective attention to filter out a conflicting synesthetic color induced by a local or global form. The task was again to name the display color of the stimulus as quickly as possible, but participants were now instructed to focus their attention covertly on one level of the local-global stimulus throughout a block of trials. In the *attend local* condition, stimuli were either colored congruently with the synesthetic color elicited by the characters at *both* local and global levels (outer left panels in Fig. 53.5A), or they were colored congruently with the synesthetic color elicited by the character at the local level but incongruently with that elicited by the character at the global level (inner left panels of Fig. 53.5A). In the *attend global* condition, the reverse stimulus configuration was used: stimuli were either colored congruently with the synesthetic color elicited by the characters at both local and global levels (outer left panels in Fig. 53.5A) or they were colored congruently with the synesthetic color elicited by the character at the global level but incongruently with that elicited by the character at the local level (inner right panels of Fig. 53.5A). This arrangement of stimuli in each attention condition ensured that synesthetes would benefit from focusing their attention in accordance with the instructions.

Two aspects of our findings are relevant to the present discussion. First, we found that despite the instructions to attend to the local or global level, synesthetes were still significantly slower when the character at one level of the stimulus was colored incongruently with the synesthetic color it elicited, compared to when the characters at both levels were congruently colored. Thus, the synesthetic Stroop effect was not entirely eliminated by the endogenous attentional cue. More important, however, when compared with the congruency effects from the same stimuli in the first experiment, in which there was no attentional cue, having participants focus attention on one level *reduced* the cost associated with an incongruent character at the other level. This finding supports our hypothesis that endogenous attention can be used to modulate synesthetic color experiences elicited by alphanumeric characters.

The implications of our local-global experiments in synesthetes also have parallels with findings from studies of the conventional Stroop effect. Besner and colleagues have examined the effects of cuing participants' spatial attention to individual letters within color-word stimuli. In one such study, Besner, Stolz, and Boutilier (1997) found that the Stroop effect was eliminated when just a single letter was colored instead of the whole word. They suggested that when a single letter is colored, mental processing is biased toward letter-level representations and away from word-level representations, thus reducing the semantic activation associated with the color word. In a further series of experiments, Besner and Stolz (1999a) found that precuing spatial attention to the position of a single letter within a color word significantly reduced the magnitude of the Stroop effect relative to a control condition in which all letters of the word were precued. Based on these findings, the authors suggested that narrowing the focus of spatial attention to a single letter has the effect of reducing the efficiency of word recognition and thus attenuates the detrimental effect of word reading on color naming. Several further experiments by Besner and colleagues (e.g., Besner, 2001; Besner & Stolz, 1999b) have provided results that are broadly consistent with this suggestion. The general message to arise from these cuing studies is that manipulations that divert attention from the word tend to reduce the efficiency of semantic activation, and thus reduce the extent to which conflicting color names are able to interfere with the ongoing task of color naming.

To what extent does this idea relate to the influence of endogenous attention on synesthetic Stroop effects for rivalrous local-global stimuli? It is certainly possible that our manipulations of attention reduced the efficiency with which graphemes were able to activate semantic representations, including any synesthetic color, which in turn might have reduced the synesthetic Stroop effect. This possibility is not incompatible with the established role of selective attention in binding elementary visual features into coherent objects (Treisman, 1998; Treisman & Gelade, 1980) or with our conjecture that attention is crucial for the binding processes that link graphemic forms with synesthetic colors. It is widely accepted that attention operates across multiple levels of perceptual and cognitive processing (Pashler, 1998), and in the absence of evidence to the contrary we assume this also holds true for individuals with synesthesia. Further studies will be required to determine the levels at which mechanisms of selective attention exert their influence over the subjective and behavioral manifestations of synesthesia.

Summary of behavioral findings and relation to other studies

Taken together, the findings from our studies using masked priming, attentional load, and perceptual rivalry paradigms suggest that induction of synesthetic colors arises at a relatively late stage of perceptual processing, following the allocation of selective attention. It would be misleading, however, to imply that all the available evidence supports our conclusion. The reader is directed in particular to the work of the Waterloo group (see Dixon et al., Chap. 52, this volume), which has produced compelling evidence to suggest that color-graphemic synesthesia may arise relatively early in the visual processing hierarchy, at least for some individuals. These authors argue in particular that synesthetes who experience colors projected out in space, such as their synesthete C. (Dixon et al., 2000; Smilek, Dixon, Cudahy, & Merikle, 2001), should be considered as a unique group they call "projectors." These individuals, they suggest, experience color even before they are aware of the alphanumeric form that induces it (Smilek et al., 2001). By contrast, they suggest that in synesthetes who see colors "in the mind's eye," whom they call "associators," the color experience may be triggered at a relatively late stage of processing, after initial recognition of the inducing character is complete. Similar suggestions have been made by Ramachandran and Hubbard (2001a, 2001b), although their conclusions are based on different experiments and are interpreted within a distinct conceptual framework.

We have reviewed the experiments of these and other investigators elsewhere (Rich & Mattingley, 2002), and so will not deal with them at length here. For the purposes of this chapter, however, we would like to add a comment concerning the proposed distinction between "projectors" and "associators." Dixon and colleagues (Chap. 52, this volume) suggest that projectors and associators can be distinguished objectively by comparing their performances on two different versions of the synesthetic Stroop task. In one version, participants are required to name *display* colors of alphanumeric characters that elicit congruent or incongruent synesthetic colors, just as in the typical synesthetic Stroop task. In the other version, participants instead name their *synesthetic* colors for the alphanumeric characters, which are displayed in either congruent or incongruent colors. Their rationale is that the interference produced by

synesthetic colors when naming display colors should be stronger for projectors than for associators, and that the interference from display colors on synesthetic colors should be stronger for associators than for projectors.

The results of their experiment (see Fig. 52.1) reveal clear differences in the magnitude of synesthetic Stroop effects for projector and associator groups (categorized by subjective report). Dixon and colleagues suggest that the large congruency effect shown by projectors on the standard synesthetic Stroop task of display-color naming, combined with the smaller impact of display colors on their synesthetic color naming, indicate that these individuals experience synesthetic colors as more intense and salient than display colors. In contrast, they suggest that the smaller synesthetic Stroop effect for associators, and the impact of display colors on synesthetic color naming, reflects their relatively weak synesthetic experiences and the fact that they find it more difficult to ignore display colors than their synesthetic colors.

These differences alone, however, do not necessarily support an underlying functional distinction between projectors and associators. Instead, they could equally reflect differences in the strength or automaticity of synesthesia that varies along a continuum. Unfortunately, it is not possible to compare the magnitude of Stroop effects directly for our data versus those of Dixon and colleagues, since the proportion of congruent to incongruent trials differed in the two studies, and this difference alone can affect the extent of standard Stroop effects (Cheesman & Merikle, 1986; Logan, 1980). Nevertheless, on considering the individual data from our initial study of synesthetic Stroop effects (Mattingley et al., 2001b), we were impressed by the differences in the magnitude of synesthetic Stroop effects between individuals. According to Dixon and colleagues, projectors will show large synesthetic Stroop effects (a mean cost of 174 ms in their study), whereas associators will show small or absent effects (a mean cost of 19 ms in their study). As shown in Figure 53.6, some individuals in our study showed a very large synesthetic Stroop effect (>200 ms), whereas several showed only a small effect, or even a slight reversal of the overall group pattern. What is remarkable is that *all* these synesthetes described their synesthetic colors as appearing "in the mind's eye" rather than projected, and most spontaneously reported discomfort and tension when they were presented with incongruently colored characters.

We also note that the "reverse" synesthetic Stroop results described by Dixon and colleagues, in which individuals named the synesthetic colors elicited by

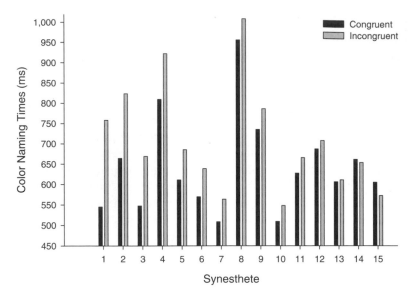

FIGURE 53.6   Size of congruency effects in the synesthetic Stroop task, plotted separately for each of the 15 synesthetes tested by Mattingley et al. (2001a). Participants are arranged from left to right, according to the order of magnitude of the difference between color naming times for congruent and incongruent trials.

alphanumeric characters, do not seem to clearly support the proposed dichotomy. The magnitude of the cost when naming incongruent synesthetic colors was roughly comparable for the projector and associator groups (a difference of just 23 ms; see Fig. 52.1*B*) and would not in itself justify the distinction without a priori evidence based on subjective report.

Although future studies may reveal different subcategories of color-graphemic synesthesia, current data suggest that the strength of synesthetic experience, at least as it is reflected in the relative automaticity of responses in Stroop-type tasks, lies along a continuum from weak to strong. What determines the strength of color-character binding remains unanswered, although we speculate that the intensity of early learning, or ongoing rehearsal (either overt or covert), may play a role. Moreover, our own research suggests that an individual's ability to use focused attention to enhance or suppress particular stimuli plays an important role. The idea that the colors experienced by some synesthetes may be triggered more automatically than those of others is consistent with another aspect of the data of Dixon et al. Their associators are much slower *overall* in naming their synesthetic colors than the projectors, irrespective of congruency. It is not clear why associators should be so much slower to access the color names of their synesthetic experiences simply because they are not projected into space. What seems more likely is that these individuals have weaker associative links between the inducing forms and their synesthetic colors. It remains to be determined in what sense synesthetic colors experienced out in space might be stronger or more salient than

those experienced in the mind's eye. One way forward might be to compare self-reported projectors and associators based on profiles obtained through psychophysical tests of chromatic sensitivity. Changes in the color of synesthetic experiences that are projected out in space should have measurable consequences for an individual's ability to discriminate the hue of isoluminant display colors, whereas such effects would seem less likely to influence the discrimination ability of those with color associations experienced in the mind's eye.

Neural correlates of synesthetic experience

Until recently, the majority of empirical data on synesthesia came from behavioral studies of the kind discussed in the previous section of this chapter. With the wider availability of techniques to visualize the human brain in vivo, however, researchers have turned their attention to the neural correlates of synesthetic experience. Here we will focus only on the most pertinent investigations. In considering the findings from these studies, we shall focus in particular on the stimuli used to elicit synesthesia, and on the tasks required of synesthetes as their brain activity is measured. Although existing studies have provided tantalizing glimpses of the neural correlates of synesthetic experience, much work is still needed to determine which brain areas are critically involved.

To date, virtually all experiments have aimed to show that visual areas of the brain are active during color-phonemic synesthesia, all with seemingly positive outcomes (Aleman, Rutten, Sitskoorn, Dautzenberg, &

Ramsey, 2001; Nunn et al., 2002; Paulesu et al., 1995). In their pioneering study, Paulesu and colleagues (1995) used positron emission tomography (PET) to compare patterns of brain activity in six women with color-phonemic synesthesia and six nonsynesthetic controls. In separate imaging runs, participants listened either to pure tones or to words spoken over headphones, with the latter condition alone inducing synesthetic color experiences. In the spoken-word condition, the synesthetes showed significantly greater activity than nonsynesthetes in several extrastriate visual areas, including the superior occipital and parietal cortices bilaterally, the posterior region of the inferior temporal gyrus bilaterally, and to a lesser extent the left lingual gyrus. Interestingly, there was no evidence for increased activity in area V4 in the synesthetes, which is somewhat surprising, given the documented role of this area in color perception (McKeefry & Zeki, 1997; Zeki & Marini, 1998). On initial reading, these PET results seem to suggest that relevant phonemic stimuli lead to coactivation of higher-order visual areas, but not early areas associated with the perceptual processing of color (such as V4). Unfortunately, the findings remain ambiguous because the study did not include any attempt to measure or quantify the participants' synesthesia, nor were participants engaged in a relevant perceptual or cognitive task during scanning, making it difficult to draw conclusions concerning the relationship between brain activity and behavior. A further potential problem is that the synesthetes were instructed to "let the color perception [for each word] occur automatically" (p. 663), whereas the controls were told simply to listen to the words. Given that the observed extrastriate activity in the synesthetes was very close to that found in studies of color imagery in nonsynesthetes (Howard et al., 1998), the brain activations observed by Paulesu et al. (1995) could reflect the neural correlates of color imagery rather than color-phonemic synesthesia.

More recently, Nunn and colleagues (2002) conducted a functional magnetic resonance imaging (fMRI) study of a group of color-phonemic synesthetes. The major innovation of this study was to train a group of nonsynesthetic controls on a word-color association task, in order to simulate any effects of synesthesia due to associative learning. In one experiment, both groups listened passively to tones or spoken words in alternating blocks (much like the PET study of Paulesu et al., 1995). In a second experiment, the groups viewed colored or achromatic mondrians, again in alternating blocks. Subtraction of activity across the two conditions of this color perception experiment was used to define a region of interest (ROI) within which to examine word-related activity from the first experiment. For the

synesthetes, the only significant activity associated with words versus tones within this ROI involved the left fusiform gyrus, with coordinates corresponding to those previously reported for areas V4 and V8. In contrast, there was no such activity in the nonsynesthetic controls. Moreover, contrary to a previous case study (Aleman et al., 2001), synesthetes showed no significant activity in areas V1 or V2 for words versus tones, suggesting that primary visual cortex does not contribute to induced color experiences in synesthesia. Finally, despite training nonsynesthetes on word-color associations and having them "predict" or "imagine" the color associated with each word during scanning, these individuals showed no significant activity in the V4/V8 region activated in the synesthetes.

The study of Nunn et al. (2002) is unquestionably the most comprehensive investigation of the neural correlates of synesthesia to date, and represents a significant advance on previous research in this area. Nevertheless, it too has a number of methodological features that limit the conclusions that can be drawn from it. First, neither the synesthetes nor the control subjects were required to carry out a relevant behavioral task while listening to words and tones, so it is not possible to determine the perceptual or cognitive factors that gave rise to the differential activity between the two conditions. Second, whereas the synesthetes are likely to have focused attention on their induced colors during the word condition, there was no motivation for controls to evoke color at all during image acquisition (cf. Paulesu et al., 1995). Despite the authors' attempt to address the issue of color imagery by training controls on word-color pairings like those experienced by the synesthetes, the extent to which these participants followed the instructions to "predict" or "imagine" colors was not assessed during scanning; instead, at the end of each run participants simply estimated the percentage of correct associations they felt they had made. It is therefore possible that the absence of significant activity within the color ROI in this experiment was due to control participants' failure to follow the instructions, given the absence of any behavioral motivation to do so. It is perhaps also unlikely that providing controls with a short period of training on arbitrary color-word associations could approximate a lifetime of such experiences in a synesthete.

To conclude, the common outcome of brain imaging studies to date is that extrastriate (and possibly striate) cortical areas are active when synesthetes listen to spoken words (Aleman et al., 2001; Nunn et al., 2002; Paulesu et al., 1995). Given these individuals' subjective reports of vivid color experiences, and the behavioral data that support them, these brain imaging results seem unsurprising. The outstanding questions are *how* and *why* activity in these visual areas correlates with the presentation of inducing forms (seen or heard) and the color experiences they trigger. No study has yet examined brain activity in synesthetes as they perform relevant behavioral tasks, such as the synesthetic Stroop, visual masking, or attention/rivalry paradigms. It would be extremely useful to adopt behavioral tasks such as these, which have already yielded important insights into the cognitive and perceptual mechanisms of synesthesia, in future neuroimaging investigations of the phenomenon.

Conclusions

Despite the many outstanding issues yet to be resolved, synesthesia research is currently enjoying somewhat of a renaissance after languishing as a fringe phenomenon for many decades. In this chapter we have reviewed the results of our own behavioral research and provided a selective appraisal of data from the behavioral and brain imaging studies of others.

We have shown that the synesthetic colors induced by digits, letters, and words, either in their printed or spoken forms, elicit vivid and consistent color experiences (Baron-Cohen et al., 1987; Mattingley et al., 2001a). These experiences can have measurable consequences for cognitive performance, as illustrated by the synesthetic Stroop effect. Under conditions in which the synesthetic color triggered by an alphanumeric character, either seen or imagined, is incompatible with the color of a target to be named, responses are slower and more error-prone than under conditions in which the two are compatible (Dixon et al., 2000; Mattingley et al., 2001b; Mills et al., 1999; Odgaard et al., 1999; Wollen & Ruggiero, 1983). These findings suggest that competition arises between synesthetically induced colors and display colors at some stage of processing between perception of the inducer and production of a response. Precisely where this competition arises, however, remains to be elucidated. We have shown that synesthetic colors, as measured by the synesthetic Stroop task, are eliminated entirely when inducing characters are presented briefly and masked from awareness (Mattingley et al., 2001a). Moreover, such interference is significantly reduced under conditions of attentional load, even though the inducing stimulus itself remains clearly visible and available for overt report (Mattingley et al., 2003). These findings suggest that the competitive interactions in synesthetic Stroop tasks do not occur during early visual processing, prior to grapheme recognition. This is in contrast to the views of some authors, who have suggested that synesthesia can arise very early in visual processing, prior to overt recognition of the inducer (Palmeri et al., 2002; Ramachandran &

Hubbard, 2001a, 2001b; Smilek et al., 2001). These studies have used different tasks from those described in this chapter, however, and may be open to alternative explanations (see Rich & Mattingley, 2002).

In the future, it will be important to determine the extent to which synesthetic color experiences can influence visual perception by using psychophysical tasks with known physiological correlates. We have already suggested one such approach, in which thresholds for discriminating the hue of display stimuli are measured as the individual experiences different synesthetic colors. A further approach could involve the use of perceptual aftereffects, such as orientation-contingent color aftereffects (McCulloch, 1965). If the suggested dichotomy between projector and associator synesthetes is correct (Dixon et al., Chap. 52, this volume), it may be possible to show that the former perceive such color aftereffects following adaptation to appropriately constructed achromatic inducing stimuli, whereas the latter do not. Future studies might also profitably examine the relationship between the graphemic and phonological properties of inducers and the synesthetic experiences they elicit (Ward & Simner, 2003). Is there any relationship between the sound or form of a particular letter and the synesthetic experience it elicits? Finally, many synesthetes report that they use their color experiences to help them remember names and dates, or to perform mental arithmetic. With some notable exceptions (Luria, 1969; Merikle, Dixon, & Smilek, 2002), these aspects of synesthesia have scarcely been addressed to date.

REFERENCES

Aleman, A., Rutten, G. M., Sitskoorn, M. M., Dautzenberg, G., & Ramsey, N. F. (2001). Activation of striate cortex in the absence of visual stimulation: An fMRI study of synaesthesia. *Neuroreport, 12,* 2827–2830.

Baron-Cohen, S., Wyke, M. A., & Binnie, C. (1987). Hearing words and seeing colours: An experimental investigation of a case of synaesthesia. *Perception, 16,* 761–767.

Besner, D. (2001). The myth of ballistic processing: Evidence from Stroop's paradigm. *Psychonomic Bulletin and Review, 8,* 324–330.

Besner, D., & Stolz, J. A. (1999a). What kind of attention modulates the Stroop effect? *Psychonomic Bulletin and Review, 6,* 99–104.

Besner, D., & Stolz, J. A. (1999b). Unconsciously controlled processing: The Stroop effect reconsidered. *Psychonomic Bulletin and Review, 6,* 449–455.

Besner, D., Stolz, J. A., & Boutilier, C. (1997). The Stroop effect and the myth of automaticity. *Psychonomic Bulletin and Review, 4,* 221–225.

Brown, T. L. (1996). Attentional selection and word processing in Stroop and word search tasks: The role of selection for action. *American Journal of Psychology, 109,* 265–286.

Brown, T. L., Gore, C. L., & Carr, T. H. (2002). Visual attention and word recognition in Stroop color naming: Is word recognition "automatic"? *Journal of Experimental Psychology: General, 131,* 220–240.

Brown, T. L., Roos-Gilbert, L., & Carr, T. H. (1995). Automaticity and word perception: Evidence from Stroop and Stroop dilution effects. *Journal of Experimental Psychology: Learning, Memory, and Cognition, 21,* 1395–1411.

Cheesman, J., & Merikle, P. M. (1986). Distinguishing conscious from unconscious perceptual process. *Canadian Journal of Psychology, 40,* 343–367.

Cytowic, R. E. (1993). *The man who tasted shapes.* New York: Putnam.

Dehaene, S., Naccache, L., Cohen, L., Bihan, D. L., Mangin, L. F., Poline, J. B., et al. (2001). Cerebral mechanisms of word masking and unconscious repetition priming. *Nature Neuroscience, 4,* 752–815.

Dehaene, S., Naccache, L., Leclech, G., Koechlin, E., Mueller, M., Dehaenelambertz, G., et al. (1998). Imaging unconscious semantic priming. *Nature, 395,* 597–600.

Dixon, M. J., Smilek, D., Cudahy, C., & Merikle, P. M. (2000). Five plus two equals yellow. *Nature, 406,* 365.

Dow, S. (1999, February 6). Colour-coded. *The Australian Magazine,* 18–21.

Dresslar, F. B. (1903). Are chromaesthesias variable? A study of an individual case. *American Journal of Psychology, 14,* 308–382.

Galton, F. (1880). Visualised numerals. *Nature, 21,* 252–256.

Ginsberg, L. (1923). A case of synaesthesia. *American Journal of Psychology, 34,* 582–589.

Grossenbacher, P. G., & Lovelace, C. T. (2001). Mechanisms of synesthesia: Cognitive and physiological constraints. *Trends in Cognitive Sciences, 5,* 36–41.

Howard, R. J., Ffytche, D. H., Barnes, J., McKeefry, D., Ha, Y., Woodruff, P. W., et al. (1998). The functional anatomy of imagining and perceiving colour. *Neuroreport, 9,* 1019–1023.

Kahneman, D., & Chajczyk, D. (1983). Tests of the automaticity of reading: Dilution of Stroop effects by color-irrelevant stimuli. *Journal of Experimental Psychology: Human Perception and Performance, 9,* 510–522.

Logan, G. D. (1980). Attention and automaticity in Stroop and priming tasks: Theory and data. *Cognitive Psychology, 12,* 523–553.

Luria, A. R. (1969). *The mind of a mnemonist.* London: Jonathan Cape.

Mattingley, J. B., Rich, A. N., & Payne, J. (2003). *Attentional load modulates anomalous colour experiences in colour-graphemic synaesthesia.* Unpublished manuscript.

Mattingley, J. B., Rich, A. N., Yelland, G., & Bradshaw, J. L. (2001a). Unconscious priming eliminates automatic binding of colour and alphanumeric form in synaesthesia. *Nature, 410,* 580–582.

Mattingley, J. B., Rich, A. N., Yelland, G., & Bradshaw, J. L. (2001b). *Investigations of automatic binding of colour and form in synaesthesia,* Paper presented at TENNET, Montreal, Quebec.

McCulloch, C. (1965). Color adaptation of edge detectors in the human visual system. *Science, 149,* 1115–1116.

McKeefry, D. J., & Zeki, S. (1997). The position and topography of the human colour centre as revealed by functional magnetic resonance imaging. *Brain, 120,* 2229–2242.

Merikle, P. M., Dixon, M. J., & Smilek, D. (2002). *The role of synaesthetic photisms in perception, conception, and memory.* Paper presented at the Cognitive Neuroscience Society Ninth Annual Meeting, San Francisco, April 14–16.

Mills, C. B., Boteler, E. H., & Oliver, G. K. (1999). Digit synaesthesia: A case study using a Stroop-type test. *Cognitive Neuropsychology, 16,* 181–191.

Navon, D. (1977). Forest before trees: The precedence of global features in visual perception. *Cognitive Psychology, 9,* 353–383.

Nunn, J. A., Gregory, L. J., Brammer, M., Williams, S. C. R., Parslow, D. M., Morgan, M. J., et al. (2002). Functional magnetic resonance imaging of synaesthesia: Activation of V4/V8 by spoken words. *Nature Neuroscience, 5,* 371–375.

Odgaard, E. C., Flowers, J. H., & Bradman, H. L. (1999). An investigation of the cognitive and perceptual dynamics of a colour-digit synaesthete. *Perception, 28,* 651–664.

Palmeri, T. J., Blake, R., Marois, R., Flanery, M. A., & Whetsell, W. (2002). The perceptual reality of synaesthetic colors. *Proceedings of the National Academy of Sciences, 99,* 4127–4131.

Pashler, H. (1998). *The psychology of attention.* Cambridge, MA: MIT Press.

Paulesu, E., Harrison, J., Baron-Cohen, S., Watson, J. D. G., Goldstein, L., Heather, J., et al. (1995). The physiology of coloured hearing: A PET activation study of colour-word synaesthesia. *Brain, 118,* 661–676.

Ramachandran, V. S., & Hubbard, E. M. (2001a). Psychophysical investigations into the neural basis of synaesthesia. *Proceedings of the Royal Society of London, 268,* 979–983.

Ramachandran, V. S., & Hubbard, E. M. (2001b). Synaesthesia: A window into perception, thought and language. *Journal of Consciousness Studies, 8,* 3–34.

Rich, A. N., & Mattingley, J. B. (2002). Anomalous perception in synaesthesia: A cognitive neuroscience perspective. *Nature Reviews: Neuroscience, 3,* 43–52.

Rich, A. N., & Mattingley, J. B. (2003). The effects of stimulus competition and voluntary attention on colour-graphemic synaesthesia. *Neuroreport, 14,* 1793–1798.

Smilek, D., Dixon, M. J., Cudahy, C., & Merikle, P. M. (2001). Synaesthetic photisms influence visual perception. *Journal of Cognitive Neuroscience, 13,* 930–936.

Snow, J., & Mattingley, J. B. (2003). Perception, unconscious. In L. Nagel (Ed.), *Encyclopedia of cognitive science* (pp. 517–526). London: Macmillan.

Treisman, A. (1998). Feature binding, attention and object perception. *Philosophical Transactions of the Royal Society of London, Series B: Biological Sciences, 353,* 1295–1306.

Treisman, A. (1999). Solutions to the binding problem: Progress through controversy and convergence. *Neuron, 24,* 105–110.

Treisman, A., & Gelade, G. (1980). A feature-integration theory of attention. *Cognitive Psychology, 12,* 97–136.

Ward, J., & Simner, J. (2003). Lexical-gustatory synaesthesia: Linguistic and conceptual factors. *Cognition, 89,* 237–261.

Wollen, K. A., & Ruggiero, F. T. (1983). Colored-letter synesthesia. *Journal of Mental Imagery, 7,* 83–86.

Zeki, S., & Marini, L. (1998). Three cortical stages of colour processing in the human brain. *Brain, 121,* 1669–1685.

54 Synesthesia, Cross-Activation, and the Foundations of Neuroepistemology

V. S. RAMACHANDRAN, E. M. HUBBARD, AND P. A. BUTCHER

Introduction

Certain otherwise normal individuals when presented with a stimulus in one sensory modality may vividly perceive additional sensations in unstimulated sensory modalities, a condition known as synesthesia. For example, a synesthete may experience a specific color whenever he or she encounters a particular tone (e.g., C-sharp may be blue) or may see any given number as always tinged a certain color (e.g., 5 may be green and 6 may be red). One long-standing debate in the study of synesthesia has centered on the issue of whether synesthesia is a perceptual or a conceptual phenomenon. To resolve this issue, we have conducted experiments on 11 grapheme-color synesthetes, with extensive testing on two of them (J.C. and E.R.). These results suggest that grapheme-color synesthesia is a sensory effect rather than a cognitive one (Ramachandran & Hubbard, 2001a).

We have previously reported that synesthetically induced colors are able to influence perceptual grouping, lead to perceptual pop-out, and can be experienced even when the inducing grapheme is not consciously visible (Hubbard & Ramachandran, 2001; Ramachandran & Hubbard, 2000, 2001a). Based on these results, we argued that synesthesia is a sensory phenomenon and that it may be caused by genetically mediated, persistent neural connections, causing cross-wiring between brain maps that process color (V4 or V8) and visual graphemes, which lie adjacent to each other in the fusiform gyrus (see also Hubbard & Ramachandran, 2003).

We identify two different subtypes of number-color synesthesia and propose that they are caused by hyper-connectivity between color and number areas at different stages in processing. "Lower synesthetes" may have cross-wiring (or cross-activation) within the fusiform gyrus, whereas "higher synesthetes" may have cross-activation in the angular gyrus. We then discuss the implications of the study of synesthesia for understand-

ing other aspects of the human mind, such as creativity and metaphor. Finally, we discuss the implications of synesthesia for the philosophical problem of qualia.

Theories of synesthesia causation

Synesthesia was first brought to the attention of the scientific community by Francis Galton (1880, 1883). Artistic, poetic, and philosophical accounts predate Galton's scientific reports; however, Galton was the first to systematically document the phenomenon. Since then, there have been dozens of studies of synesthesia spanning a century (e.g., Gray, Williams, Nunn, & Baron-Cohen, 1997; Paulesu et al., 1995). However, the phenomenon on the whole, has been treated largely as an enigmatic curiosity by mainstream neuroscience and sensory psychology (with a few notable exceptions; e.g., Baron-Cohen & Harrison, 1997; Cytowic, 1989; Grossenbacher & Lovelace, 2001).

One question that has plagued researchers in this field is whether this is a genuine sensory experience or not and how one can establish this operationally (Baron-Cohen & Harrison, 1997; Cytowic, 1989; Harrison, 2001; Ramachandran & Hubbard, 2001a). It is commonplace to hear that these individuals are simply crazy, are trying to draw attention to themselves, are on drugs, or are engaging in vague metaphorical speech, as when normal people say "a shirt is loud" or "cheddar cheese is sharp." One argument is that perhaps when a synesthete says "the chicken tastes pointy" (Cytowic, 1993), he is being no less metaphorical. Another related view, even more common, is the idea that synesthesia is based on childhood memories of colored numerals (and other graphemes) such as might be formed, for example, from playing with colored refrigerator magnets as children.

However, none of these accounts provides a satisfactory explanation of synesthesia. For example, the idea that synesthetes are trying to draw attention to

867

themselves would predict that synesthetes should be telling everyone around them about how different they are. In our experience, it is usually quite the opposite. Synesthetes often think that everyone else experiences the world the same way they do, or else they were ridiculed as children and have not told anyone about their synesthesia for years.

The memory hypothesis also fails as an explanation of synesthesia because it cannot address the questions of why only some individuals have these memories intact, why only specific classes of stimuli are able to induce synesthesia, and why there should be a genetic basis for synesthesia, as discussed later in this chapter.

The problem with the metaphor explanation is that it commits one of the classic blunders in science, trying to explain one mystery (synesthesia) in terms of another mystery (metaphor). Since very little is known about the neural basis of metaphor, saying that "synesthesia is just metaphor" helps to explain neither synesthesia nor metaphor. Indeed, in this chapter we will turn the problem on its head and suggest the very opposite, namely, that synesthesia is a concrete sensory phenomenon whose neural basis we are beginning to understand, and it can therefore provide an experimental lever for understanding more elusive phenomena such as metaphor (Ramachandran & Hubbard, 2001a).

Finally, the idea that synesthesia is a result of drug use is applicable only to a few people and seems to occur only during the "trip." One explanation of this is that certain drugs might pharmacologically mimic the same physiological mechanisms that underlie genetically based synesthesia (see, e.g., Grossenbacher & Lovelace, 2001). However, despite superficial similarities, the phenomenological reports of those who have taken psychedelics differ from the reports of lifelong synesthetes. Psychedelics-induced synesthesia is far less organized than congenital synesthesia. Whereas a congenital synesthete may report that C-sharp is red, someone under the influence of psychedelic drugs will report a sensory confusion in which the individual cannot determine whether a sensation is auditory or visual (Smythies, personal communication, 2002). This suggests that pharmacologically induced synesthesia may not be based on the same neural mechanisms as congenital synesthesia.

Evidence for the reality of synesthesia

GENETIC BASIS OF SYNESTHESIA Estimates of the prevalence of synesthesia vary dramatically. Cytowic (1989, 1997) estimates that it occurs in 1 in 20,000 people, while Galton (1880) placed the prevalence at 1 in 20. More recent, systematic studies have estimated that synesthesia occurs in 1 in 2000 people (Baron-Cohen,

Burt, Smith-Laittan, Harrison, & Bolton, 1996). Our own results indicate that the prevalence may be even greater, perhaps as high as 1 in 200 (Ramachandran, Hubbard, & Altschuler, unpublished observations). Some of this variability is probably due to differences in definitional criteria used by different researchers, but some might also be due to the different subtypes examined by different investigators. For example, Cytowic focused on taste-shape synesthesia, whereas we focus on grapheme-color synesthesia, which is the most common subtype (Day, 2001).

In spite of the variability in estimates of its prevalence, almost every study of synesthesia has agreed that synesthesia seems to run in families. Galton (1880) first noticed this; many of his subjects had relatives who were also synesthetic. More recently, Baron-Cohen et al. (1996) conducted a more formal survey to determine what the genetic component of synesthesia is. They found that synesthesia is more common in females than in males (6:1 ratio) and that approximately one-third of their respondents had family members who were also known synesthetes. Family studies show that the trait seems to be passed along the X-chromosome, and that it may be dominant (Bailey & Johnson, 1997).

However, this model would predict a sex ratio of 3:1, not the observed 6:1, possibly indicating that the effect is polygenetic and that the X-linked component is a necessary trigger factor. Another possibility (Harrison, 2001) is that the synesthesia mutation may be lethal in half of male fetuses that have the gene. This is consistent with Bailey and Johnson's (1997) data showing that synesthetic families have approximately twice as many daughters as sons, although more precise studies are required to determine whether more male infants of synesthetic parents die prenatally. Further investigation into the genetic aspects of synesthesia may clarify some of these questions.

SYNESTHETIC ASSOCIATIONS ARE STABLE OVER TIME Synesthetically induced colors are consistent across months or even years of testing (Baron-Cohen, Harrison, Goldstein, & Wyke, 1993). Baron-Cohen et al. asked nine synesthetic subjects and nine control subjects to give color associations for a list of 130 words. Control subjects were told that they would be tested 1 week later, while synesthetic subjects were retested 1 year later and were not informed prior to testing that they would be retested. Synesthetic subjects were 92.3% consistent, while control subjects were only 37.6% consistent. Although this result shows that the effect is not confabulatory in origin, it does not necessarily show that it is sensory rather than conceptual or based on early memories. After all, if each number triggers a highly specific memory, that memory might have been remembered by the subject with each occurrence of the number over a lifetime, providing plenty of opportunity for rehearsal, even without external reinforcement.

Is synesthesia perceptual or conceptual?

STROOP INTERFERENCE IN SYNESTHESIA Recent studies have demonstrated the reality of synesthesia, but very few studies have adequately addressed the question of whether synesthesia is a perceptual or a conceptual effect. For example, the results of Stroop-like interference tasks are sometimes cited as evidence for the view that synesthesia is sensory (Mills, Boteler, & Oliver, 1999; Wollen & Ruggiero, 1983) and sometimes for the conflicting view that synesthesia is conceptual (Dixon, Smilek, Cudahy, & Merikle, 2000; Mattingley, Rich, Yelland, & Bradshaw, 2001), but neither inference is justified. Stroop interference merely shows that the association between the grapheme and the color is automatic. Because Stroop-like interference can occur at any stage in the system, from perception all the way up to motor output (MacLeod, 1991), it is completely uninformative in determining whether synesthesia is perceptual or conceptual.

PSYCHOPHYSICAL INVESTIGATIONS INTO SYNESTHESIA Contrary to the Stroop results of Dixon et al. and Mattingley et al., our recent studies clearly indicate that, at least for some synesthetes, the effect is indeed perceptual. Our experimental approach is unique in that we have used perceptual tasks in which the experience of synesthetically induced colors should aid the synesthete. Because response bias, demand characteristics, and cognitive influences cannot improve performance on these tasks, they provide unambiguous evidence that these synesthetes' experiences are truly perceptual.

We conducted five experiments with our first two synesthetes (J.C. and E.R.). The results of all of these experiments suggest that grapheme-color synesthesia is a sensory effect rather than cognitive or based on memory associations (Ramachandran & Hubbard, 2001a).

Experiment 1 Synesthetically induced colors can lead to pop-out. We presented subjects with displays composed of graphemes (e.g., a matrix of randomly placed, computer-generated 2s). Within the display we embedded a shape, such as a triangle, composed of other graphemes (e.g., computer-generated 5s; Fig. 54.1; Color Plate 29). Since 5s are mirror images of 2s and are made up of identical features (horizontal and vertical line segments), nonsynesthetic subjects find it hard to detect the embedded shape composed of 5s. Our two synesthetes, on the other hand, see the 2s as one color

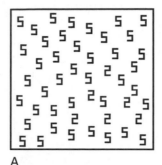 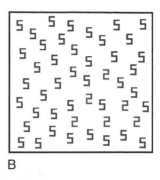

A   B

FIGURE 54.1 Schematic representation of displays used to test whether synesthetically induced colors lead to pop-out. (*A*) When presented with a matrix of 5s with a triangle composed of 2s embedded in it, control subjects find it difficult to find the triangle. (*B*) However, because they see the 5s as (say) green and the 2s as red, our synesthetic subjects were able to easily find the embedded shape. (See Color Plate 29.)

and the 5s as a different color, so they claim to see the display as (for example) a "red triangle" against a background of green 2s. We measured their performance and found that they were significantly better at detecting the embedded shape than control, nonsynesthetic subjects (Ramachandran & Hubbard, 2001a), making it clear that they were not confabulating and could not have been "faking synesthesia." Perceptual grouping and pop-out are often used as diagnostic tests to determine whether a given feature is genuinely perceptual or not (Beck, 1966; Treisman, 1982). For example, tilted lines can be grouped and segregated from a background of vertical lines, but printed words cannot be segregated from nonsense words or even mirror-reversed words. The former is a perceptual difference in orientation signaled early in visual processing by cells in area V1; the latter is a high-level linguistic concept.

Experiment 2 We have found that even "invisible graphemes" can induce synesthetic colors. Individual graphemes presented in the periphery are easily identified. However, when other graphemes flank the target, it is difficult to identify the target grapheme (Fig. 54.2; Color Plate 30). This "crowding" effect is not because of the low visual acuity in the periphery (Bouma, 1970; He, Cavanagh, & Intriligator, 1996). The target grapheme is large enough to be resolved clearly and can be readily identified if the flankers are not present. We have found that the crowded grapheme nevertheless evoked the appropriate color—a curious new form of blindsight (Hubbard & Ramachandran, 2001; Ramachandran & Hubbard, 2001b). The subject said, "I can't see that middle letter but it must be an *O* because it looks blue." This observation implies, again, that the color is evoked at an early sensory—indeed, preconscious—level rather than at a higher cognitive level.

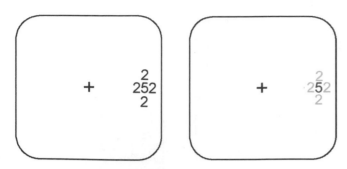

FIGURE 54.2 Demonstration of the crowding effect. A single grapheme presented in the periphery is easily identifiable. However, when it is flanked by other graphemes, the target grapheme becomes much harder to detect. Synesthetic colors are effective (as are real colors) in overcoming this effect. (See Color Plate 30.)

Experiment 3 We have found that when a grapheme was presented near the edge of the screen and scaled for eccentricity (Anstis, 1998), our synesthetes no longer experienced their colors (Ramachandran & Hubbard, 2000, 2001a), even though the grapheme was still clearly visible. If synesthesia were conceptual, as long as the letter was recognized (i.e., the concept was activated), our synesthetes should have experienced their colors. However, despite clearly identifying the grapheme, our synesthetes did not experience their colors, further demonstrating that synesthesia is not based on the activation of the concept.

Experiment 4 We optically superposed two different graphemes and alternated them. Subjects experienced colors alternating up to 4 Hz. At higher speeds, up to 10 Hz, the graphemes could still be seen alternating, but our subjects said they no longer experienced colors (Ramachandran & Hubbard, 2001a). In a third subject the colors started alternating at a much slower rate of once every 2 or 3 s (as in binocular rivalry). Again, because the graphemes could be clearly recognized, the concept must have been activated. However, colors were not experienced. This result further demonstrates that activation of the concept cannot be the critical stimulus for the experience of colors in synesthesia.

Experiment 5 In our first two synesthetes, roman numerals and subitizable clusters of dots were ineffective in eliciting synesthetic colors, suggesting it is the visual grapheme, not the numerical concept, that is critical (but see later discussion for exceptions). Tactile and auditory letters were also ineffective in evoking colors unless the subject visualized the numbers (Ramachandran & Hubbard, 2000, 2001a). Thus, it is the visual grapheme, not the numerical concept, that triggers the perception of color.

Taken collectively, these five experiments prove conclusively that, at least in some synesthetes, the induced colors are genuinely sensory in nature. This leads us to our next question: What causes synesthesia, especially grapheme-color synesthesia?

The cross-activation hypothesis

Since the earliest reports of synesthesia, it has been speculated that synesthesia is a result of crossed wiring of some sort in the brain (Galton, 1883; for reviews see Harrison & Baron-Cohen, 1997; Marks, 1997). Until recently, however, lack of detailed knowledge of human extrastriate cortex severely limited researchers' ability to directly test the neural cross-wiring hypothesis of grapheme-color synesthesia.

Much of what we know about extrastriate visual cortex and visual processing has been obtained through studies on monkeys (e.g., Van Essen & DeYoe, 1995) and through lesion analysis in humans (e.g., Damasio & Damasio, 1989; Feinberg & Farah, 1997). Studies of nonhuman primates suffer from several limitations, including nonhomologous visual areas and differences in anatomical location of homologous areas due to increases in overall brain size and differences in the size of key visual areas (Kaas, 1993). Furthermore, nonhuman primates do not have specific regions of the brain dedicated to the processing of letters or numbers and would not therefore experience grapheme-color synesthesia, even if they were able to tell us about it.

However, the advent of modern imaging techniques has made it possible to study extrastriate visual responses in awake, behaving humans with no pathology. These techniques have led to the identification of the human homologue of macaque V4, the putative color center (Lueck et al., 1989; Wade, Brewer, Rieger, & Wandell, 2002; Zeki & Marini, 1998) in the fusiform gyrus. The precise details of this homology are still debated (e.g., Hadjikhani, Liu, Dale, Cavanagh, & Tootell, 1998; Heywood, Gadotti, & Cowey, 1992; Wade et al., 2002), but these subtle distinctions do not vitiate our main hypothesis concerning cross-wiring in the fusiform.

We were struck by the fact that, remarkably, the grapheme area is also in the fusiform (Allison, McCarthy, Nobre, Puce, & Belger, 1994; Nobre, Allison, & McCarthy, 1994; Pesenti, Thioux, Seron, & De Volder, 2000), especially in the left hemisphere (Tarkiainen et al., 1999) adjacent to V4 (Fig. 54.3; Color Plate 31). When subjects were asked to do a variety of math tasks, the fusiform gyrus, along with other areas (including the inferior parietal lobule and the angular gyrus), was

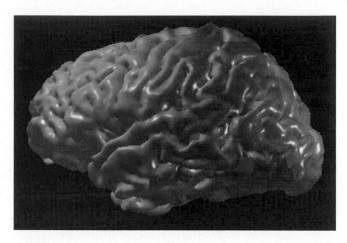

FIGURE 54.3 Schematic showing that cross-wiring in the fusiform might be the neural basis of grapheme-color synesthesia. The left hemisphere of one author's brain (EMH) is shown with area V4 indicated in red and the number-grapheme area indicated in green. (See Color Plate 31.)

activated (Rickard et al., 2000). Using chronically implanted electrodes in epileptic patients, Allison et al. (1994) have shown that the areas of the fusiform involved in number and letter processing are either adjacent to or overlap each other. When number graphemes were explicitly compared against nonsymbolic characters with a similar amount of visual contrast and complexity, the findings of Rickard et al. of activation in fusiform gyrus were replicated (Pesenti et al., 2000).

We were struck by the fact that the most common form of synesthesia involves graphemes and colors, and the brain areas corresponding to these are right next to each other. Based on this anatomical proximity, we propose that synesthesia is caused by cross-wiring between these two areas, in a manner analogous to the cross-activation of the hand area by the face in amputees with phantom arms (Ramachandran & Hirstein, 1998; Ramachandran & Rogers-Ramachandran, 1995; Ramachandran, Rogers-Ramachandran, & Stewart, 1992).

Because synesthesia runs in families, we suggest that a single gene mutation causes an excess of cross-connections or defective pruning of connections between different brain areas. Consequently, every time there is activation of neurons representing number graphemes, there may be a corresponding activation of color neurons.

One potential mechanism for this would be the observed prenatal connections between inferior temporal regions and area V4 (Kennedy, Batardiere, Dehay, & Barone, 1997; Rodman & Moore, 1997). In the immature brain, there are substantially more connections

between and within areas than are present in the adult brain. Some of these connections are removed through a process of pruning, and others remain. There is a much larger feedback input from inferior temporal areas to V4 in prenatal monkeys. In the fetal macaque, approximately 70%–90% of the connections are from higher areas (especially TEO, the macaque homologue of human inferior temporal cortex), while in the adult, approximately 20%–30% of retrograde labeled connections to V4 come from higher areas (Kennedy et al., 1997; H. Kennedy, personal communication, 2001). Hence, if a genetic mutation were to lead to a failure of pruning (or stabilization) of these prenatal pathways, connections between the number grapheme area and V4 would persist into adulthood, leading to the experience of color when a synesthete views numbers or letters.

Even though we postulate a genetic mutation that causes defective pruning or stabilization of connections between brain maps, the final expression must require learning; obviously, people are not born with number and letter graphemes "hard-wired" in the brain (and indeed, different synesthetes have different colors evoked by the same numbers). The excess cross-activation merely permits the opportunity for a number to evoke a color. There may be internal developmental or learning rules that dictate that once a connection has formed between a given "number node" and color, no further connections can form. This would explain why the connections are not haphazard. A given number evokes only a single color.

The cross-activation hypothesis can also explain our finding that in some synesthetes, the colors are susceptible to interference from the edge of the screen. Because memories ordinarily show positional invariance, one cannot argue that synesthesia is just associative memory from childhood. On the other hand, because V4 mainly represents central vision (Gattass, Sousa, & Gross, 1988; Rosa, 1997), if the cross-wiring occurred disproportionately for central vision, one would expect the colors to be evoked selectively in this region.

This idea also explains why, in J.C. and E.R., only the actual arabic numerals evoke colors; roman numerals and subitizable clusters of dots do not. This observation suggests that it is the actual visual appearance of the grapheme, not the numerical concept, that evokes color. This conclusion is consistent with cross-activation in the fusiform, because the latter structure represents the graphemes, not the concept.

Third, our hypothesis can explain why a number rendered invisible through crowding can nevertheless evoke colors. Perhaps perceptual events do not reach consciousness in the fusiform, the place where we postulate the cross-activation to be occurring (i.e., neuronal activity in the fusiform is necessary but not sufficient for conscious awareness; see Dehaene et al., 2001). Perhaps due to crowding, the processing of the graphemes does not extend beyond fusiform, while, since the colors are evoked in parallel by the activity in fusiform neurons (and are not affected by crowding), subsequent color-selective regions could process them.

Fourth, our hypothesis may shed light on the neural basis of other forms of synesthesia. Sacks and Wasserman (1987; Sacks, Wasserman, Zeki, & Siegel, 1988) described a patient who became color-blind (cerebral achromatopsia) after his car was hit by a truck. Prior to the accident, the patient was an artist who also experienced colors when presented with musical tones. However, after the accident, he no longer experienced colors in response to musical tones. Interestingly, the subject also reported transient alexia, in which letters and numbers "looked like Greek or Hebrew to him" (Sacks & Wasserman, 1987, p. 26). This result would indicate that a single brain region might have been damaged in the accident, leading both to the loss of color vision and to the transient alexia, consistent with what is now known from the imaging literature. Perhaps this brain region was also critical for his synesthesia, and when it was damaged, he no longer experienced synesthesia.

Finally, our model may explain why a person with one kind of synesthesia (e.g., number-color) is also more likely to have another kind of synesthesia (e.g., tone-color). The failure of pruning might occur at multiple sites in some people. This possibility leads to our next postulate: Even though a single gene might be involved, it may be expressed in a patchy manner to different extents and in different anatomical loci in different synesthetes. This differential expression of the gene might depend on the expression of certain modulators or transcription factors.

One final piece of evidence for the "hyperconnectivity" hypothesis comes from cases of acquired (as opposed to hereditary) synesthesia. We recently examined a patient who had retinitis pigmentosa and became progressively blind starting from childhood, until he became completely blind at 40. Remarkably, a few years later, he started to experience tactile sensations as visual phosphenes. The tactile thresholds for evoking the phosphenes ("synesthesia threshold") were higher than the tactile thresholds themselves, and the synesthesia thresholds were consistent across intervals separated by weeks, implying that the effect is genuine and not confabulatory in origin (Armel &

Ramachandran, 1999). We suggested that the visual deprivation caused tactile input to activate visual areas; either the back-projections linking these areas became hyperactive or new pathways emerged. If such cross-activation (based on hyperconnectivity) is the basis of acquired synesthesia, one could reasonably conclude that the hereditary disorder might also have a similar neural basis, except that the cause is genetic rather than environmental.

Synesthesia: Cross-wiring or disinhibition?

The cross-activation of brain maps that we postulate can come about by two different mechanisms: (1) cross-wiring between adjacent areas, either through an excess of anatomical connections or defective pruning, or (2) excess activity in back-projections between successive stages in the hierarchy (caused either by defective pruning or by disinhibition).

We use the term cross-wiring somewhat loosely; indeed, the more neutral terms "cross-activation" or "cross-talk" might be preferable. Because of the enormous number of reciprocal connections, even between visual areas that are widely separated (e.g., Felleman & Van Essen, 1991; Van Essen & De Yoe, 1995), the strengthening (or failure of developmental pruning) of any of these connections could lead to cross-activation of brain maps that represent different features of the environment. However, since the length of neural connections tends to be conserved developmentally (Kaas, 1997; Johnson & Vecera, 1996), anatomically close maps are more likely to be cross-wired at birth, thereby providing greater opportunity for the enhanced cross-wiring that might underlie synesthesia (Kennedy et al., 1997). Furthermore, instead of the creation of an actual excess of anatomical connections, there may be merely a failure of inhibition between adjacent regions, causing leakage between areas that are normally insulated from each other (Baron-Cohen et al., 1993).

Our model differs from Grossenbacher's (1997; Grossenbacher & Lovelace, 2001) model of synesthesia as a result of disinhibited cortical feedback in that Grossenbacher's model generally assumes that information is processed up through several levels of the sensory hierarchy to some multimodal sensory nexus before being fed back to lower areas, such as V4. In our model, at least for grapheme-color synesthesia, we propose that the connections are much more local, and that information does not have to go all the way "downtown" before being sent back to color areas, consistent with the bias toward greater cross-wiring in anatomically adjacent maps. Future imaging studies, augmented by ERPs, should help to resolve this issue.

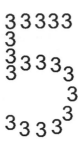

FIGURE 54.4 Hierarchical figure demonstrating top-down influences in synesthesia. When our synesthetic subjects attend to the global 5, they report the color appropriate for viewing a 5. However, when they shift their attention to the 3s that make up the 5, they report the color switching to the one they see for a 3.

Top-down influences in synesthesia

Although to this point we have focused on cross-wiring and early sensory effects, it does not follow that synesthesia cannot be affected by top-down influences. We have conducted several experiments to demonstrate such effects.

First, we have shown that, when presented with a hierarchical figure (say a 5 composed of 3s; Fig. 54.4) our synesthetes can voluntarily switch back and forth between seeing the forest and the trees, alternating between seeing, for example, red and green (Ramachandran, 2000; Ramachandran & Hubbard, 2001b). This shows that although the phenomenon is sensory, it can be modulated by top-down influences such as attention.

Second, when we show our synesthetic subjects a display like THE CAT (Fig. 54.5), they report that they see the correct color for the H and the A immediately, even though the two forms are identical. Hence, although the visual form is necessary for the perception of the colors, the way in which it is classified is important in determining which color is actually evoked.

Third, when we presented another synesthete with a figure that could either be seen as the letters I and V or as the roman numeral IV, he reported that he experienced

THE CAT

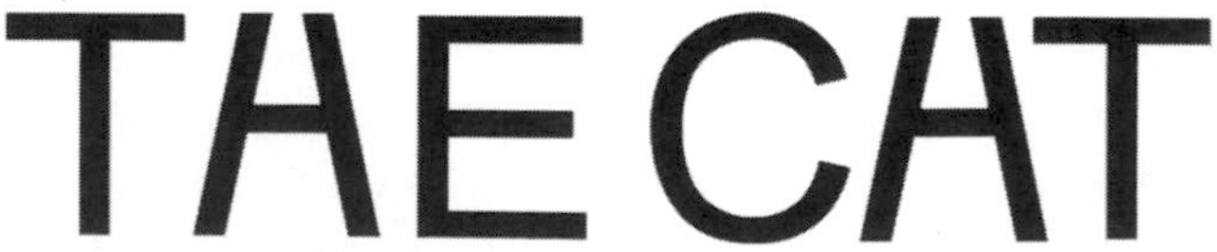

FIGURE 54.5 Ambiguous stimuli demonstrating further top-down influences in synesthesia. When presented with the ambiguous H/A form in "THE CAT," both of our synesthetes reported that they experienced different colors for the H and the A, depending on whether they attended to the T and the E or the C and the T even though the physical stimulus was identical in both cases.

different colors, depending on whether he saw the figure as a letter or as a number.

Taken together, these experiments demonstrate that synesthesia can also be strongly modulated by top-down influences. Some researchers have argued that the fact that synesthesia can be modulated by top-down influences demonstrates that the meaning of the grapheme is in some way critical for the experience of colors (Smilek, Dixon, Cudahy, & Merikle, 2001). However, the presence of top-down influences does not demonstrate that synesthesia critically depends on the concept. Instead, it merely indicates that, like many other perceptual phenomena such as the famous Rubin face-vase or the Dalmatian, cognitive influences can also influence early sensory processing (Churchland, Ramachandran, & Sejnowski, 1994).

Synesthesia and visual imagery

We find that most synesthetes report that when they imagine the numbers, the corresponding colors are evoked more strongly than they are by actual numbers (Ramachandran & Hubbard, 2001b). This result may occur because imagining something partially activates both category-specific regions involved in visual recognition (O'Craven & Kanwisher, 2000) and early visual pathways (Farah, 2000; Farah, Soso, & Dasheiff, 1992; Klein, Paradiso, Poline, Kosslyn, & Le, 2000; Kosslyn et al., 1995, 1999). Depending on the locus of cross-wiring (whether the individual is a higher or lower synesthete), the extent and locus of top-down partial activation, and the extent to which this activation is vetoed by real bottom-up activation from the retina, there may be varying degrees of synesthesia induced by imagery in different subjects.

We are currently investigating these issues using the Perky effect (Craver-Lemley & Reeves, 1992; Perky, 1910), which affords an elegant technique for probing the elusive interface between imagery and perception. In Perky's original experiment, subjects looked at a translucent white screen and were asked to imagine common objects. By means of a slide projector, a real image of the object was back-projected on the screen and gradually made brighter. Remarkably, even though the projected object would have been clearly visible under normal circumstances (that is, it was clearly above threshold), subjects failed to report the presence of the image. More recent work (Craver-Lemley & Reeves, 1992; Segal, 1971) has clearly shown that this is not a simple criterion shift or an attentional effect, but rather a true reduction in perceptual sensitivity.

We have performed an analogous experiment with our two synesthetic subjects, J.C. and E.R. Subjects made a two-alternative forced-choice identification of letters or numbers presented in colors while imagining either consistent or inconsistent graphemes. Their performance on the imagery task was then compared with their performance on the same task with no imagery. We found that synesthetes showed a much greater increase in threshold for detecting the presence of a grapheme when they were imagining another grapheme then did normal subjects, hence a much larger Perky effect. This result further supports the notion that synesthetically induced colors can be experienced due to top-down activation, as in mental imagery.

Cross-wiring and Stroop interference

One advantage of our cross-wiring hypothesis is that it can account not only for our findings but also the findings of Dixon et al. (2000) and Mattingley et al. (2001), which have been taken to show that the experience of colors in synesthesia depends in some way on the activation of the concept of the number. Instead, we would argue that the experience of color depends critically on activation of the neural structures in the fusiform that are involved in processing of the visual form of the grapheme. In the Dixon et al. study, we claim that this activation was achieved through internally generated images, while in the Mattingley et al. study, this activation was present but did not reach conscious awareness because of the masking.

Dixon et al. (2000) presented their subject, C., with addition problems, presenting a digit, an operator, a second digit, and a color patch. C.'s task was to name the color patch and then report the result of the arithmetic problem. When presented with a color patch that differed from her normal concurrent synesthetic color, C. experienced clear interference (a synesthetically induced Stroop effect), whereas control subjects showed no difference between color patches. On the basis of these results, the authors concluded that "an externally presented inducing stimulus is not necessary to trigger a photism and that simply activating the *concept* of a digit is sufficient" (p. 365, emphasis added).

While at first glance, this may appear to demonstrate that synesthesia is conceptual, the inference from Stroop interference to conceptual processing is not licensed. C. may have solved the problem by visualizing the numbers, a strategy that is common in solving arithmetic problems. It is well established that the same neural structures that subserve category-specific visual perception also subserve mental imagery. If C. visualized the number graphemes, we would expect the same areas of fusiform involved with the processing of number-graphemes (Pesenti et al., 2000; Rickard et al.,

2000) to be involved with imagery of the numbers, which would then lead to the experience of synesthetic colors, and therefore Stroop interference. This is consistent with our finding that our two synesthetes report experiencing colors more vividly when asked to visualize the graphemes. Thus, the results of Dixon et al. could be due either to the activation of the numerical magnitude (i.e., the concept) or to the visualized grapheme (i.e., the percept). The experiments described above utilizing the Perky effect will allow us to further explore the relation between mental imagery and synesthesia.

Similarly, our cross-activation hypothesis can explain the Stroop results of Mattingley et al. (2001), which have been taken as evidence that the experience of synesthesia depends critically on the conscious recognition of the digit. Mattingley et al. briefly presented subjects with masked graphemes and then asked them to name a color patch. When the grapheme was presented for 500 ms, robust Stroop interference was found for synesthetes but not for controls. However, when graphemes were presented for 28 ms or 56 ms, no Stroop interference was observed. On the basis of these results, they concluded that "overt recognition of inducing stimuli is crucial" to induce synesthesia.

However, in our model, the visual processing of the grapheme would have been completed in the fusiform, leading to activation of the cross-wired colors areas. The masking may then have interrupted the processing of both form and color information, thereby causing the subjects to fail to consciously experience synesthetically induced colors with masked visual presentation. Consistent with our hypothesis that grapheme-color synesthesia arises from cross-wiring in the fusiform gyrus, recent results have demonstrated that activity in the fusiform gyrus is necessary but not sufficient for conscious awareness of briefly presented graphemes (Dehaene et al., 2001).

Higher and lower synesthetes?

In our experience, as well as from an inspection of older literature, it seems likely that there is considerable heterogeneity in this phenomenon. The findings we have discussed so far were true for the first two synesthetes we tested; they both saw colors only in central vision, and only with arabic numerals. Similarly, a subitized cluster of dots seen instantly as three, four, or five dots did not evoke colors. This implies that it is not the high-level numerical concept or sequence (ordinality, cardinality) that evokes color, but the actual visual arabic numeral grapheme, contrary to Dixon et al. (2000).

However, we have subsequently encountered other synesthetes in whom even days of the week or months of

TABLE 54.1

Synesthetic subjects tested

Subject	Age(yr)	Sex	Description of Synesthesia
J.A.C.	21	M	Grapheme-color synesthete
M.C.	21	F	Grapheme-color synesthete
E.R.	19	F	Number-color (not letter) synesthete
M.T.	19	F	Number-color (not letter) synesthete
R.T.	14	F	Higher synesthete?
L.B.	21	F	Grapheme-color synesthete
S.S.	20	M	Color-anomalous grapheme-color synesthete
B.M.	18	F	Grapheme-color synesthete
A.C.	22	F	Tone-color synesthete
L.S.	22	F	Concept-color/calendar-form synesthete
A.C.2	20	F	Grapheme-color synesthete
C.Z.	54	F	Tone-color synesthete
S.D.	24	F	Grapheme-color/calendar-form synesthete

the year were colored (Table 54.1). Could it be that there is a brain region that encodes the abstract numerical sequence or ordinality, in whatever form, and perhaps in these synesthetes it is this higher or more abstract number area that is cross-wired to the color area?

A suitable candidate is the angular gyrus in the left hemisphere. We have known from several decades of clinical neurology that this region is concerned with abstract numerical calculation; damage to it causes acalculia (Dehaene, 1997; Gerstmann, 1940; Grewel, 1952). Patients cannot do even simple arithmetic such as multiplication or subtraction. Remarkably, the subsequent color areas in the cortical color processing hierarchy lie in the superior temporal gyrus, adjacent to the angular gyrus (Zeki & Marini, 1998). It is tempting to postulate that these two regions—the higher color area and the abstract numerical computation area—are cross-wired in some synesthetes. Indeed, depending on the level at which the gene is expressed (fusiform gyrus or angular gyrus), the level of cross-wiring would be different, so that one could loosely speak of "higher" synesthetes and "lower" synesthetes.

Perhaps the angular gyrus represents the abstract concept of numerical sequence or ordinality, and this would explain why in some higher synesthetes, even days of the week or months of the year elicit colors. Consistent with this hypothesis, Spalding and Zangwill (1950) described a patient with a gunshot wound that entered the brain near the right angular gyrus and lodged near the left temporoparietal junction. Five years after injury he complained of spatial problems and had difficulty on number tasks. In addition, the patient, who experienced synesthesia prior to the injury, complained that his "number-plan" (his forms for months, days of the week, and numbers) was no longer distinct. In view of this result, it might be interesting to see if patients with angular gyrus lesions have difficulty with tasks involving sequence judgment (e.g., days of the week). Furthermore, it would be interesting to see if, in these higher synesthetes, runs of colors corresponding to numerical sequences match up at least partially with runs corresponding to weeks or months.

These results are also consistent with the known role of the parietal lobe in spatial abilities (see, e.g., Burgess, Jeffery, & O'Keefe, 1999; Stiles-Davis, Kritchevsky, & Bellugi, 1998) and in magnitude estimation (Dehaene, 1992; Rickard et al., 2000). Therefore, it would seem that cortical structures involved with spatial abilities and magnitude estimation may also be involved in the experience of number forms (consistent with our hypothesis about "higher" synesthetes).

Since different cortical color areas are involved, the psychophysical properties of the colors evoked in higher synesthetes might be different from those evoked in lower synesthetes. For example, in higher synesthetes the colors might not be produced if crowding masks the grapheme. Another difference is that higher synesthetes might require more focused attention in order to experience their colors. This would be consistent with data supporting the idea that attentional gating is more effective at higher levels of the visual hierarchy (Moran & Desimone, 1985).

Grossenbacher and Lovelace (2001) and Dixon et al. (this volume) have made similar distinctions. Grossenbacher and Lovelace distinguish between "perceptual" and "conceptual" synesthetes on the basis of differences in the stimuli that elicit synesthetic experiences, while Dixon et al. distinguish between "associator" and "projector" synesthetes on the basis of whether they report experiencing colors in the external world or in the mind's eye. Our proposal has the advantage of accounting for both sets of differences under a unified framework and tying these differences to the known anatomical localization of different stages of numerical processing.

Finally, we can consider the so-called number line (Dehaene, Dupoux, & Mehler, 1990). If we ask control subjects which of two numbers is bigger, 2 or 4, or 2 or 15, remarkably, the reaction time is not the same; they take longer in the first case than in the second. It has been suggested that we have an analogue representation of numbers in our brains—a "number line" that one reads off from to determine which number is bigger—and it is more difficult if the numbers are closer on this line (Dehaene, 1997).

Galton (1880) found that some otherwise normal people claimed that when they visualized numbers, each number always occupied a specific location in space. Numbers that were close (e.g., 2 and 4) were close spatially in this synesthetic space, so that if all the number locations were mapped out, they formed a continuous line with no breaks or jumps. However, even though the line was continuous, it was not straight. It was often highly convoluted, even curving back on itself. Two of our subjects have reported exactly this experience.

Unfortunately, other than the subjects' introspective reports, there has not been a single study objectively demonstrating that these subjects really do have a complex convoluted number line. To demonstrate this, we propose the following experiment. One could give them two numbers that are numerically far apart (e.g., 2 and 15) but spatially close together because of the convoluted number line. If so, would the reaction time for responding which number is bigger depend on proximity in abstract number space, or would the subject take a short-cut (e.g., if the convoluted line doubles back on itself, 2 and 15 may be closer to each other in Cartesian space even though more distant along the number line itself)? Such a result would provide objective evidence for their subjective reports in a manner analogous to the texture segregation and crowding experiments for grapheme-color synesthetes described earlier. Indeed, preliminary results with two such synesthetes suggest that this might be the case. Their response times to numbers closer on their synesthetic number line are longer than RTs to nearby numbers that are further in Cartesian space (Hubbard, Escudero, & Ramachandran, 2004).

Finally, it is also possible that the distribution of gene expression and level of cross-activation is not bimodal, hence the heterogeneity of the phenomenon. Indeed, one might expect to encounter mixed types rather than just higher and lower synesthesia.

Synesthesia and metaphor

Related to the question of whether synesthesia is a conceptual or perceptual phenomenon is the relation of synesthesia to metaphor. Traditionally, there have been two extreme views on synesthesia: (1) synesthesia is not a genuine sensory phenomenon; synesthetes are simply being metaphorical; and (2) most people who claim to have synesthesia are merely being metaphorical, but there are also some "genuine" (sensory) synesthetes, who are extremely rare (Cytowic, 1989).

We argue that both these views are wrong. We believe that synesthesia is relatively common and that synesthesia and metaphor may be based on similar neural mechanisms. The notion that synesthetes are just being metaphorical does not help to explain the phenomenon because no one has any idea what the neural basis of metaphor is. It is an example of trying to explain a mystery with an enigma, a strategy that never works in science. Indeed, our preliminary results suggest that we can turn the problem on its head and argue that studying synesthesia—a concrete sensory process whose neural basis can be pinned down—might help explain the seemingly intractable question of how metaphors are represented in the brain.

Artists, poets, and synesthesia

Synesthesia is purported to be more common in artists, poets, and novelists (Dailey, Martindale, & Borkum, 1997; Domino, 1989; Root-Bernstein & Root-Bernstein, 1999). For example, Domino (1989) reports that, in a sample of 358 fine arts students, 84 (23%) reported experiencing synesthesia. This incidence is higher than any reported in the literature, suggesting that synesthesia may be more common among fine arts students than in the population at large. Domino then tested 61 of the self-reported synesthetes and 61 control subjects (equated on sex, major, year in school, and verbal intelligence) on four experimental measures of creativity. He found that, as a group, synesthetes performed better than controls on all four experimental measures of creativity. However, he found only a marginal correlation between vividness and frequency of synesthetic experiences and creativity scores. Although this study has the advantage of using an experimental method to assess creativity, it suffers a severe limitation in that no experimental tests were conducted to assess synesthetic experiences. Further studies making use of our objective experimental measures of synesthesia are clearly required to confirm this result.

How can the cross-wiring hypothesis explain these results? One thing these groups of people have in common is a remarkable facility linking two seemingly unrelated realms in order to highlight a hidden deep similarity (Root-Bernstein & Root-Bernstein, 1999). When we read Shakespeare's "It is the East, and Juliet is the sun," our brains instantly understand the meaning. We do not parse it as "Juliet is the sun. Does that mean she is a glowing ball of fire?" (Schizophrenics might do so, because they often interpret metaphors literally.) Instead, the brain instantly forms the right links: "She is warm like the sun, nurturing like the sun, radiant like the sun," and so on. How is this achieved?

It has often been suggested that concepts are represented in brain maps in the same way that percepts (such as colors or faces) are. One such example is the concept of number, a fairly abstract concept, yet we know that specific brain regions (the fusiform and the angular) are involved. In the case of numbers, the distinction (both logical and anatomical) between the perceptual symbol (the grapheme) and the numerical concept (magnitude) is quite clear. In other cases the distinction between the percept and the concept is not so clear, but there is evidence that certain classes of concepts are represented in regions adjacent to perceptual areas associated with those concepts (Martin, Haxby, Lalonde, Wiggs, & Ungerleider, 1995; Thompson-Schill, Aguirre, D'Esposito, & Farah, 1999; Tranel, Damasio, & Damasio, 1997). If so, we can think of metaphors as involving cross-activation of conceptual maps in a manner analogous to perceptual maps in synesthesia.

This idea could explain the higher incidence of synesthesia in artists and poets. If cross-wiring selectively affects the fusiform or angular gyrus, someone may experience synesthesia, but if it is more diffusely expressed, it may produce a more generally cross-wired brain, creating a greater propensity to and opportunity for creatively mapping from one concept to another (and if the hyperconnectivity also involves sensory to limbic connections, the reward value of such mappings would also be higher among synesthetes).

The angular gyrus and synesthetic metaphors

In addition to its role in abstract numerical cognition, the angular gyrus has long been known to be concerned with cross-modal association (which would be consistent with its strategic location at the crossroads of the temporal, parietal, and occipital lobes). Intriguingly, patients with lesions here tend to be literal-minded (Gardner, 1975), which we would interpret as a difficulty with metaphor. However, no satisfactory explanation has yet been given for this deficit.

Based on what we have said so far, we would argue that the pivotal role of the angular gyrus in forming cross-modal associations is perfectly consistent with our suggestion that it is also involved in metaphors, especially cross-modal metaphors. It is even possible that the angular gyrus was originally involved only in cross-modal metaphor but the same machinery was then co-opted during evolution for other kinds of metaphor as well. Our idea that excess cross-wiring might explain the penchant for metaphors among artists and poets is also consistent with data suggesting that there may be a larger number of cross-connections in specific regions of the right hemisphere (Scheibel et al., 1985) and the observed role of the right hemisphere in processing nonliteral aspects of language (Anaki, Faust, & Kravetz, 1998; Brownell et al., 1990).

We realize that this is an unashamedly phrenological view of metaphor and synesthesia. The reason it may seem slightly implausible at first is the apparent arbitrariness of metaphorical associations (e.g., "a rolling stone gathers no moss"). Yet metaphors are *not* arbitrary. Lakoff and Johnson (1980) have systematically documented the nonarbitrary way in which metaphors are structured and how they in turn structure thought. A large number of metaphors refer to the body, and many more are intersensory (or synesthetic). Furthermore, we have noticed that synesthetic metaphors (e.g., a "loud shirt") also respect the directionality seen in synesthesia (Day, 1996; Ullman, 1945; Williams, 1976)—that is, they are more frequent in one direction than the other, such as from the auditory to the visual modality. We suggest that these rules are a result of strong anatomical constraints that permit certain types of cross-activation but not others.

Finally, one wonders whether the right and left angular gyri are specialized to handle different *types* of metaphors, the right for pervasive spatial and bodily metaphors and the left for more arbitrary ones.

Hyperconnectivity and emotions

Synesthetes often report strong emotions in response to multisensory stimuli (both positive and negative, depending on whether the associations are the "right" or "wrong" ones). Additionally, patients with temporal lobe epilepsy seem to have a propensity toward synesthetic experiences. Why?

One wonders, is their aversion to such stimuli any different from what a nonsynesthete experiences when confronted with, say, a blue carrot or a green rose? Although there is no clear experimental validation of the claim that synesthetes have strong emotional responses to "discordant" sensory inputs, anecdotally we have found this to be true: One of our synesthetes claimed that incorrectly colored numbers were "ugly" and felt like "nails scratching on the blackboard." Conversely, when numbers were the correct color they "felt right, like the 'Aha!' when the solution to a problem finally emerges." Assuming that the claim is true, can we explain it in terms of our cross-wiring or cross-activation hypothesis of synesthesia?

Visual information that is recognized by the cortex of the temporal lobe (e.g., the fusiform) ordinarily gets relayed to the amygdala, nucleus accumbens, and other parts of the limbic system (Amaral, Price, Pitanen, & Carmichael, 1992; LeDoux, 1992). These structures evaluate the significance of the object, so that we may speak of the amygdala and nucleus accumbens as developing an "emotional salience map" of objects and events in the world. If the object is emotionally significant or salient, such as a predator, prey, or mate, the message gets relayed to the hypothalamic nuclei to prepare the body for fighting, fleeing, or mating. Neural signals cascade from the limbic structures down the autonomic nervous system to decrease gastric motility and increase heart rate and sweating (e.g., Lang, Tuovinen, & Valleala, 1964; Mangina & Beurezeron-Mangina, 1996). This autonomic arousal can be measured by monitoring changes in skin conductance caused by sweat, the skin conductance response (SCR), which provides a direct measure of emotional arousal and limbic activation. Typically, when we look at neutral objects such as a table or chair, there is no arousal or change in SCR, but if we look at prey, a mate, or a predator, there is.

We have suggested that a mutation that causes hyperconnectivity (either by defective pruning or reduced inhibition) may cause varying degrees and types of synesthesia, depending on how extensively and where in the brain it is expressed (which in turn is modulated by transcription factors). Now let us imagine what would happen if there were hyperconnectivity between the fusiform gyrus (and other sensory cortices) and the limbic system (especially the amygdala and nucleus accumbens). If we assume that aesthetic and emotional responses to sensory inputs depend on these connections, then presenting a discordant input (such as a grapheme in the wrong color) would produce a disproportionately large emotional aversion ("nails scratching on a blackboard"), and, conversely, harmonious blends of color and grapheme will be especially pleasant to look at (which may involve the nucleus accumbens rather than the amygdala). The net result of this activity is a progressive "bootstrapping" of pleasurable or aversive associations through limbic reinforcement of concordant and discordant inputs (this, by the way, allows us to also invoke a form of learning in the genesis of synesthesia).

In order to test this idea, one could measure the SCR in synesthetes in response to an incorrectly colored number and compare this response to one produced in a nonsynesthetic subject who is looking at blue carrots. A nonsynesthete might be a bit amused or puzzled by the blue carrot but is unlikely to say it feels like nails scratching on a blackboard. We would therefore predict a bigger SCR in the synesthete looking at the incorrectly colored grapheme than in control subjects.

The hyperconnectivity explanation for synesthesia is also consistent with the claim that the phenomenon is more common among patients with temporal lobe epilepsy (TLE). The repeated seizure activity is likely to produce "kindling," causing hyperconnectivity between different brain regions, which would explain reports of synesthesia in TLE (see e.g., Jacome, 1999).

Furthermore, if the seizures (and kindling) were to strengthen the sensory-amygdala connections, then TLE patients might also be expected to have heightened emotional reactions to specific sensory inputs. There are strong hints that this is the case (Ramachandran, Hirstein, Armel, Tecoma, & Iragui, 1997).

Something along these lines may also explain why some famous artists have had TLE, Van Gogh being the most famous example (e.g., Kivalo, 1990; Meissner, 1994). If our scheme is correct, his heightened emotions in response to colors and visual attributes (resulting from kindling) might have indeed fueled his artistic creativity.

Synesthesia and the philosophical riddle of qualia

Finally, the study of the unusual sensory experiences of synesthetes may also shed light on the philosophical problem of qualia. There is a growing consensus that the best way to solve this ancient philosophical riddle is to narrow down the neural circuitry (Crick & Koch, 1995, 1998; Metzinger, 2000) and, especially, the functional logic (Ramachandran & Blakeslee, 1998; Ramachandran & Hirstein, 1997) of those brain processes that are qualia laden as opposed to those that are not (e.g., the reflexive contraction of the pupil in response to light can occur in coma; however, there is no qualia as when the subject is awake and sees a red rose). One strategy used to explore the neural basis of qualia is to hold the physical stimulus constant while tracking brain changes that covary with changes in the conscious percept (e.g., Sheinberg & Logothetis, 1997; Tong & Engel, 2001). In the case of synesthesia, we are making use of the same strategy but using preexisting, stable differences in the conscious experiences of people who experience synesthesia compared with those who do not.

Ramachandran and Hirstein (1997) have suggested three "laws" of qualia, or functional criteria that need to be fulfilled in order for certain neural events to be associated with qualia (a fourth has recently been added; see Ramachandran & Blakeslee, 1998). Of course, this still doesn't explain *why* these particular events are qualia laden and others are not (Chalmer's "hard problem"), but at least it narrows the scope of the problem. The four laws are:

1. Qualia are irrevocable and indubitable. One does not say, "Maybe it is red, but I can visualize it as green if I want to." An explicit neural representation of red is created that invariably and automatically "reports" this to higher brain centers.

2. Once the representation is created, what can be *done* with it is open-ended. There is the luxury of choice. For example, with the percept of an apple, we can use it

to tempt Adam, keep the doctor away, bake a pie, or eat it. Even though the representation at the *input* level is immutable and automatic, the *output* is potentially infinite. The same is not true for, say, a spinal reflex arc, where the output is also inevitable and automatic.

3. Short-term memory. The input invariably creates a representation that persists in short-term memory, long enough to allow time for choice of output. Without this component, there would again be just a reflex arc.

4. Attention. Qualia and attention are closely linked. Attention is needed to fulfill criterion number two, to *choose*. A study of circuits involved in attention, therefore, will shed much light on the riddle of qualia.

Based on these laws, and on the study of brain-damaged patients, we have suggested that the critical brain circuits involved in qualia are the ones that lead from sensory input to amygdala to cingulate gyrus (Ramachandran & Hirstein, 1997).

Synesthesia, or the "blending" of different sensory qualia, obviously has relevance to the qualia problem, as first pointed out by Jeffrey Gray (1998; Gray et al., 1997). In particular we would argue that the lower synesthetes have the qualia of red evoked when they see a 5 or hear C-sharp. But when nonsynesthetes experience red when seeing a black-and-white picture of an apple, the red does not fulfill all four criteria specified above, so there is very little quale (leaving aside the question of whether partial qualia can exist if some criteria alone are fulfilled). And finally, the higher synesthetes may be a borderline case. As such, they can be used to shed light on the nature of qualia (such borderline cases can be valuable in science; we recall here the manner in which viruses have helped researchers understand the chemistry of life).

To understand the importance of synesthesia in illuminating the qualia problem, consider the following thought experiment performed on your own brain. When you are asleep, an evil genius swaps or cross-wires the nerves coming into your brain from your ears and eyes. You then wake up. Consider the following places where the wiring could have been swapped:

1. If the swapping were done sufficiently early in sensory processing, the outcome is obvious; say the pathways from the auditory nucleus of the brainstem are diverted to the visual cortex and the optic radiations to the auditory cortex. Then you would "hear" sights and "see" sounds.

2. If the swapping were done at or close to the output stage (e.g., in Broca's area) where the word "red" or "C-sharp" is generated, again, the answer would be obvious. You might say, "When you play me that tone I know it's a tone and experience it as such, but I feel an irresistible urge to *say* red" (like a patient with Tourette's syndrome).

But now we come to the key question: What if the swapping or cross-wiring were done at some stage in between these two extremes? Is there a critical boundary between these two extremes, so that if the wires are crossed after the boundary, you merely experience an urge, whereas if the wires are crossed before that boundary, you literally see red? Is it a fuzzy boundary or a sharp one? We would argue that this boundary corresponds to the point where the transition is made from the four laws of qualia being fulfilled (before the boundary) to where they are not fulfilled (after the boundary).

Of considerable relevance to this philosophical conundrum is a new observation that we made on a grapheme-color synesthete S.S. (Ramachandran & Hubbard, 2001a). This subject was color anomalous (s-cone deficiency, leading to a difficulty discriminating purples and blues), but intriguingly, he claimed to see numbers in colors that he could never see in the real world ("Martian colors"). This is yet another piece of evidence against the memory hypothesis, for how can he remember something he has never seen? On the other hand, the cross-wiring hypothesis explains it neatly. If we assume that the color processing machinery in V4 in the fusiform is largely innate, then the genetically based cross-activation of cells in this area would evoke color phosphenes even though the colors cannot be seen in the real world because of retinal cone deficiencies.

Indeed, even synesthetes with normal vision sometimes say that the synesthetically induced colors are somehow "weird" or "alien" and don't look quite the same as normal "real-world" colors. Previously, no satisfactory account has been proposed for this. The cross-wiring hypothesis explains this as well. For two reasons, the activation of cells in the visual centers caused by real-world input is, in all likelihood, going to be somewhat different from the spurious or abnormal activation caused indirectly through numbers. First, given that it is abnormal, the cross-wiring is unlikely to be very precise. It might be slightly messy, and this "noise" may be experienced as weird Martian colors. This may be analogous to phantom limb pain (also caused by abnormal cross-wiring; Ramachandran & Hirstein, 1998) and phantom "Martian smells" described by patients with olfactory degeneration (Ramachandran, 2000).

Second, the cross-activation obviously skips the earlier levels of the color processing hierarchy which may ordinarily contribute to the final qualia, and this unnatural stimulation might cause the subject to see Martian colors. The implication of this is that the experience of qualia may depend on the activation of the *whole* visual hierarchy (or a large part of it), not just the pontifical cells at the end of the chain.

Summary and conclusions

Although synesthesia has been studied for more than 100 years, our psychophysical experiments were the first to prove conclusively that synesthesia is a genuine *sensory* phenomenon. Four lines of evidence support this conclusion. (1) Synesthetically induced colors can lead to perceptual grouping, segregation, and pop-out. (2) Synesthetic colors are not seen with eccentric viewing even if the numbers are scaled in size to make them clearly visible. (3) A crowded grapheme that is not consciously perceived can nevertheless evoke the corresponding color. (4) A color-blind synesthete sees colors in numbers that he cannot otherwise see in real-life visual scenes.

Having established the sensory nature of synesthesia in our first two subjects, we propose a specific testable hypothesis: that grapheme-color synesthesia is caused by a mutation causing defective pruning and cross-activation between V4 (or V8) and the number area, which lie right next to each other in the fusiform gyrus. Although the cross-talk idea has been around for some time, no specific brain areas have been suggested, and the idea is usually couched in vague terms that do not take advantage of known patterns of localization.

In addition to the lower synesthetes (J.C. and E.R.), there also appear to be other types of number-color synesthetes in whom the effect may be more concept driven—that is, the effect is conceptual rather than sensory. We suggest that in them, the cross-activation occurs at higher levels, perhaps between the angular gyrus (known to be involved in abstract number representation) and a higher color area in the vicinity that receives input from V4.

We suggest further that synesthesia is caused by a mutation that causes defective pruning between areas that are ordinarily connected only sparsely. Various transcription factors may then influence the exact locus and extent to which the gene is expressed. If it is expressed only in the fusiform, a lower synesthesia results. If it is expressed in the angular gyrus, a higher synesthesia results. The distribution may not be bimodal, however, so there may be mixed types who combine features of several different types of synesthesia.

We suggest also that the study of synesthesia can help us understand the neural basis of metaphor and creativity. Perhaps the same mutation that causes cross-wiring in the fusiform, if expressed very diffusely, can lead to more extensive cross-wiring in the brain. If concepts are represented in brain maps just as percepts are, then cross-activation of brain maps may be the basis for metaphor. This would explain the higher incidence of synesthesia in artists, poets, and novelists (whose brains may be more cross-wired, giving them greater opportunity for metaphors).

The mutation-based hyperconnectivity hypothesis may also explain why many synesthetes exhibit such strong emotional reactions to even trivial sensory discord or harmony. We suggest that this occurs because of hyperactivation of the amygdala, nucleus accumbens, and other limbic structures by sensory inputs. A similar hyperconnectivity (based on kindling rather than mutation) could explain the purported higher incidence of synesthesia as well as heightened emotions in response to sensory stimuli seen in TLE. Such hyperconnectivity (whether caused by genes or by TLE-induced kindling) would also increase the *value* of a reward or aversion, thereby strengthening preexisting associative links (this would allow learning play a role in synesthesia).

Finally, we discuss the relevance of this scheme for more subjective aspects of consciousness such as mental imagery and qualia. While both mental imagery and synesthesia are paradigmatic examples of internal mental states, we have shown how the relation between the two might be fruitfully explored. In addition, we have shown how the cross-wiring hypothesis can explain synesthetes' introspective reports. Because neural activation in the fusiform gyrus bypasses normal stages of processing at the retina, synesthetes can experience qualia that are unavailable to nonsynesthetes. In addition, these results suggest that the *entire* perceptual pathway (or a large portion of it) is essential for the experience of qualia, not merely the final stages.

Thus, far from being a mere curiosity, synesthesia deserves to be brought into mainstream neuroscience and cognitive psychology. Indeed, it may provide a crucial insight into some of the most elusive questions about the mind, such as the neural substrate (and evolution) of metaphor, language, and thought itself, a field of inquiry for which "neuroepistemology" might be a suitable name.

REFERENCES

Allison, T., McCarthy, G., Nobre, A., Puce, A., & Belger, A. (1994). Human extrastriate visual cortex and the perception of faces, words, numbers, and colours. *Cerebral Cortex*, *4*(5), 544–554.

Amaral, D. G., Price, J. L., Pitanen, A., & Carmichael, S. T. (1992). Anatomical organization of the primate amygdaloid complex. In J. P. Aggelton (Ed.), *The amygdala: Neurobiological aspects of emotion, memory and mental dysfunction*. New York: Wiley.

Anaki, D., Faust, M., & Kravetz, S. (1998). Cerebral hemisphere asymmetries in processing lexical metaphors. *Neuropsychologia, 36*(7), 691–700.

Anstis, S. (1998). Picturing peripheral acuity. *Perception, 27,* 817–825.

Armel, K. C., & Ramachandran, V. S. (1999). Acquired synesthesia in retinitis pigmentosa. *Neurocase, 5*(4), 293–296.

Bailey, M. E. S., & Johnson, K. J. (1997). Synaesthesia: Is a genetic analysis feasible? In S. Baron-Cohen & J. E. Harrison (Eds.), *Synaesthesia: Classic and contemporary readings* (pp. 182–207). Oxford, England: Blackwell.

Baron-Cohen, S., Burt, L., Smith-Laittan, F., Harrison, J., & Bolton, P. (1996). Synaesthesia: Prevalence and familiarity. *Perception, 25*(9), 1073–1080.

Baron-Cohen, S., & Harrison, J. (Eds.) (1997). *Synaesthesia: Classic and contemporary readings.* Oxford, England: Blackwell.

Baron-Cohen, S., Harrison, J., Goldstein, L. H., & Wyke, M. (1993). Coloured speech perception: Is synaesthesia what happens when modularity breaks down? *Perception, 22*(4), 419–426.

Beck, J. (1966). Effect of orientation and of shape similarity on perceptual grouping. *Perception & Psychophysics, 1,* 300–302.

Bouma, H. (1970). Interaction effects in parafoveal letter recognition. *Nature, 226,* 177–178.

Brownell, H. H., Simpson, T. L., Bihrle, A. M., Potter, H. H., et al. (1990). Appreciation of metaphoric alternative word meanings by left and right brain-damaged patients. *Neuropsychologia, 28*(4), 375–383.

Burgess, N., Jeffery, K. J., & O'Keefe, J. (Eds.) (1999). *The hippocampal and parietal foundations of spatial cognition.* New York: Oxford University Press.

Churchland, P. S., Ramachandran, V. S., & Sejnowski, T. J. (1994). A critique of pure vision. In C. Koch & J. L. Davis (Eds.), *Large-scale neuronal theories of the brain* (pp. 23–60). Cambridge, MA: MIT Press.

Craver-Lemley, C., & Reeves, A. (1992). How visual imagery interferes with vision. *Psychological Review, 99*(4), 633–649.

Crick, F., & Koch, C. (1995). Are we aware of neural activity in primary visual cortex? *Nature, 375*(6527), 121–123.

Crick, F., & Koch, C. (1998). Consciousness and neuroscience. *Cerebral Cortex, 8*(2), 97–107.

Cytowic, R. E. (1989). *Synaesthesia: A union of the senses.* New York: Springer-Verlag.

Cytowic, R. E. (1993). *The man who tasted shapes.* New York: G. P. Putnam's.

Cytowic, R. E. (1997). Synaesthesia: Phenomenology and neuropsychology. A review of current knowledge. In S. Baron-Cohen & J. E. Harrison (Eds.), *Synaesthesia: Classic and contemporary readings* (pp. 17–39). Oxford, England: Blackwell.

Dailey, A., Martindale, C., & Borkum, J. (1997). Creativity, synaesthesia and physiognomic perception. *Creativity Research Journal, 10*(1), 1–8.

Damasio, H., & Damasio, A. (1989). *Lesion analysis in neuropsychology.* New York: Oxford University Press.

Darwin, C. (1872). *The expression of the emotions in man and animals.* London: J. Murray.

Day, S. (1996). Synaesthesia and synaesthetic metaphors. *Psyche, 2*(32). Retrieved from http://psyche.cs.monash.edu.au/v2/psyche-2–32-day.html

Day, S. (2001). Types of synaesthesia [Web site on synesthesia maintained by Sean Day]. Web site http://home.comcast.net/%7Esean.day/Types.htm.

Dehaene, S. (1992). Varieties of numerical abilities. *Cognition, 44*(1–2), 1–42.

Dehaene, S. (1997). *The number sense: How the mind creates mathematics.* New York: Oxford University Press.

Dehaene, S., Dupoux, E., & Mehler, J. (1990). Is numerical comparison digital? Analogical and symbolic effects in two-digit number comparison. *Journal of Experimental Psychology: Human Perception and Performance, 16*(3), 626–641.

Dehaene, S., Naccache, L., Cohen, L., Le Bihan, D., Mangin, J.-F., Poline, J.-B., et al. (2001). Cerebral mechanisms of word masking and unconscious repetition priming. *Nature Neuroscience, 4*(7), 752–758.

Dixon, M. J., Smilek, D., Cudahy, C., & Merikle, P. M. (2000). Five plus two equals yellow: Mental arithmetic in people with synaesthesia is not coloured by visual experience. *Nature, 406*(6794), 365.

Domino, G. (1989). Synaesthesia and creativity in fine arts students: An empirical look. *Creativity Research Journal, 2*(1–2), 17–29.

Farah, M. J. (2000). The neural bases of mental imagery. In M. S. Gazzaniga (Ed.), *The new cognitive neurosciences* (2nd ed., pp. 965–1061). Cambridge, MA: MIT Press.

Farah, M. J., Soso, M. J., & Dasheiff, R. M. (1992). Visual angle of the mind's eye before and after unilateral occipital lobectomy. *Journal of Experimental Psychology: Human Perception and Performance, 18*(1), 241–246.

Feinberg, T. E., & Farah, M. J. (1997). *Behavioral neurology and neuropsychology.* New York: McGraw-Hill.

Felleman, D. J., & Van Essen, D. C. (1991). Distributed hierarchical processing in the primate cerebral cortex. *Cerebral Cortex, 1*(1), 1–47.

Galton, F. (1880). Visualised numerals. *Nature, 22,* 494–495.

Galton, F. (1883). *Inquiries into human faculty and its development.* London: Dent & Sons.

Gardner, H. (1975). *The shattered mind: The person after brain damage.* New York: Knopf.

Gattass, R., Sousa, A. P., & Gross, C. G. (1988). Visuotopic organization and extent of V3 and V4 of the macaque. *Journal of Neuroscience, 8*(6), 1831–1845.

Gerstmann, J. (1940). Syndrome of finger agnosia, disorientation for right and left, agraphia, acalculia. *Archives of Neurology and Psychiatry, 44,* 398–408.

Gray, J. A. (1998). Creeping up on the hard problem of consciousness. In S. R. Hameroff, A. W. Kaszniak, & A. C. Scott (Eds.), *Toward a science of consciousness II: The Second Tucson Discussions and Debates.* Cambridge, MA: MIT Press.

Gray, J. A., Williams, S. C. R., Nunn, J., & Baron-Cohen, S. (1997). Possible implications of synaesthesia for the hard question of consciousness. In S. Baron-Cohen & J. E. Harrison (Eds.), *Synaesthesia: Classic and contemporary readings* (pp. 173–181). Oxford, England: Blackwell.

Grewel, F. (1952). Acalculia. *Brain, 75,* 397–407.

Grossenbacher, P. G. (1997). Perception and sensory information in synaesthetic experience. In S. Baron-Cohen & J. E. Harrison (Eds.), *Synaesthesia: Classic and contemporary readings* (pp. 148–172). Oxford, England: Blackwell.

Grossenbacher, P. G., & Lovelace, C. T. (2001). Mechanisms of synaesthesia: Cognitive and physiological constraints. *Trends in Cognitive Sciences, 5*(1), 36–41.

Hadjikhani, N., Liu, A. K., Dale, A. M., Cavanagh, P., & Tootell, R. B. H. (1998). Retinotopy and colour sensitivity in human visual cortical area V8. *Nature Neuroscience, 1*(3), 235–241.

Harrison, J. (2001). *Synaesthesia: The strangest thing*. New York: Oxford University Press.

Harrison, J. E., & Baron-Cohen, S. (1997). Synaesthesia: A review of psychological theories. In S. Baron-Cohen & J. E. Harrison (Eds.), *Synaesthesia: Classic and contemporary readings* (pp. 109–122). Oxford, England: Blackwell.

He, S., Cavanagh, P., & Intriligator, J. (1996). Attentional resolution and the locus of visual awareness. *Nature, 383*(6598), 334–337.

Heywood, C. A., Gadotti, A., & Cowey, A. (1992). Cortical area V4 and its role in the perception of color. *Journal of Neuroscience, 12*(10), 4056–4065.

Hubbard, E. M., Escudero, M. R., & Ramachandran, V. S. (2004). The numerical distance effect demonstrates the reality of synesthetic number lines. Eleventh Annual Meeting of the Cognitive Neuroscience Society. San Francisco, CA.

Hubbard, E. M., & Ramachandran, V. S. (2001). Cross wiring and the neural basis of synaesthesia. *Investigative Ophthalmology and Visual Science, 42*(4), S712.

Hubbard, E. M., & Ramachandran, V. S. (2003). Refining the experimental lever: A reply to Shannnon and Pribram. *Journal of Consciousness Studies, 9*(3), 77–84.

Jacome, D. E. (1999). Volitional monocular Lilliputian visual hallucinations and synaesthesia. *European Neurology, 41*(1), 54–56.

Johnson, M. H., & Vecera, S. P. (1996). Cortical differentiation and neurocognitive development: The parcellation conjecture. *Behavioural Processes, 36*(2), 195–212.

Kaas, J. (1993). The organization of visual cortex in primates: Problems, conclusions, and the use of comparative studies in understanding the human brain. In B. Gulyas, D. Ottoson, & P. E. Roland (Eds.), *Functional organization of the human visual cortex* (pp. 1–12). Tarrytown, NY: Pergammon Press.

Kaas, J. H. (1997). Topographic maps are fundamental to sensory processing. *Brain Research Bulletin, 44*(2), 107–112.

Kennedy, H., Batardiere, A., Dehay, C., & Barone, P. (1997). Synaesthesia: Implications for developmental neurobiology. In S. Baron-Cohen & J. E. Harrison (Eds.), *Synaesthesia: Classic and contemporary readings* (pp. 243–256). Oxford, England: Blackwell.

Kivalo, E. (1990). The artist and his illness: Vincent van Gogh 1853–90. *Psychiatria Fennica, 21*, 139–144.

Klein, I., Paradiso, A.-L., Poline, J.-B., Kosslyn, S. M., & Le Bihan, D. (2000). Transient activity in the human calcarine cortex during visual-mental imagery: An event-related fMRI study. *Journal of Cognitive Neuroscience, 12*(Suppl. 2), 15–23.

Kosslyn, S. M., Pascual-Leone, A., Felician, O., Camposano, S., Keenan, J. P., Thompson, W. L., et al. (1999). The role of Area 17 in visual imagery: Convergent evidence from PET and rTMS. *Science, 284*(5411), 167–170.

Kosslyn, S. M., Thompson, W. L., Kim, I. J., & Alpert, N. M. (1995). Topographical representations of mental images in primary visual cortex. *Nature, 378*(6556), 496–498.

Lakoff, G., & Johnson, M. H. (1980). *Metaphors we live by*. Chicago: University of Chicago Press.

Lang, A. H., Tuovinen, T., & Valleala, P. (1964). Amygdaloid after-discharge and galvanic skin response. *Electroencephalography and Clinical Neurophysiology, 16*, 366–374.

LeDoux, J. E. (1992). Brain mechanisms of emotion and emotional learning. *Current Opinion in Neurobiology, 2*(2), 191–197.

Lueck, C. J., Zeki, S., Friston, K. J., Deiber, M. P., Cope, P., Cunningham, V. J., et al. (1989). The colour centre in the cerebral cortex of man. *Nature, 340*(6232), 386–389.

MacLeod, C. M. (1991). Half a century of research on the Stroop effect: An integrative review. *Psychological Bulletin, 109*(2), 163–203.

Mangina, C. A., & Beurezeron-Mangina, J. H. (1996). Direct electrical stimulation of specific brain structures and bilateral electrodermal activity. *International Journal of Psychophysiology, 22*, 1–8.

Marks, L. E. (1997). On coloured-hearing synaesthesia: Cross-modal translations of sensory dimensions. In S. Baron-Cohen & J. E. Harrison (Eds.), *Synaesthesia: Classic and contemporary readings*. Malden, MA: Blackwell.

Martin, A., Haxby, J. V., Lalonde, F. M., Wiggs, C. L., & Ungerleider, L. G. (1995). Discrete cortical regions associated with knowledge of colour and knowledge of action. *Science, 270*(5233), 102–105.

Mattingley, J. B., Rich, A. N., Yelland, G., & Bradshaw, J. L (2001). Unconscious priming eliminates automatic binding of colour and alphanumeric form in synaesthesia. *Nature, 410*(6828), 580–582.

Meissner, W. W. (1994). The artist in the hospital: The van Gogh case. *Bulletin of the Menninger Clinic, 58*(3), 283–306.

Metzinger, T. (Ed). (2000). *Neural correlates of consciousness: Empirical and conceptual questions*. Cambridge, MA: MIT Press.

Mills, C. B., Boteler, E. H., & Oliver, G. K. (1999). Digit synaesthesia: A case study using a Stroop-type test. *Cognitive Neuropsychology, 16*(2), 181–191.

Moran, J., & Desimone, R. (1985). Selective attention gates visual processing in the extrastriate cortex. *Science, 229*(4715), 782–784.

Nobre, A. C., Allison, T., & McCarthy, G. (1994). Word recognition in the human inferior temporal lobe. *Nature, 372*(6503), 260–263.

O'Craven, K. M., & Kanwisher, N. (2000). Mental imagery of faces and places activates corresponding stimulus-specific brain regions. *Journal of Cognitive Neuroscience, 12*(6), 1013–1023.

Paulesu, E., Harrison, J., Baron-Cohen, S., Watson, J. D. G., Goldstein, L., Heather, J., et al. (1995). The physiology of coloured hearing: A PET activation study of colour-word synaesthesia. *Brain, 118*, 661–676.

Perky, C. W. (1910). An experimental study of imagination. *American Journal of Psychology, 21*(3), 422–452.

Pesenti, M., Thioux, M., Seron, X., & De Volder, A. (2000). Neuroanatomical substrates of arabic number processing, numerical comparison, and simple addition: A PET study. *Journal of Cognitive Neuroscience, 12*(3), 461–479.

Pinker, S. (1994). *The language instinct*. New York: Morrow.

Ramachandran, V. S. (2000). Perceptual consequences of cortical cross-wiring: Phantom limb pain and synesthesia. Talk presented at The First International Consensus Meeting on the Management of Phantom Limb Pain, March 24, 2000, Oxford, England.

Ramachandran, V. S., & Blakeslee, S. (1998). *Phantoms in the brain: Probing the mysteries of the human mind*. New York: William Morrow.

Ramachandran, V. S., & Hirstein, W. (1997). Three laws of qualia: What neurology tells us about the biological functions of consciousness. *Journal of Consciousness Studies, 4*(5–6), 429–457.

Ramachandran, V. S., & Hirstein, W. S. (1998). The perception of phantom limbs: The D. O. Hebb lecture. *Brain, 121*(9), 1603–1630.

Ramachandran, V. S., Hirstein, W. S., Armel, K. C., Tecoma, E., & Iragui, V. (1997). The neural basis of religious experience. *Society for Neuroscience Abstracts, 23,* 1316.

Ramachandran, V. S., & Hubbard, E. M. (2000). Number-colour synaesthesia arises from cross wiring in the fusiform gyrus. *Society for Neuroscience Abstracts, 30,* 1222.

Ramachandran, V. S., & Hubbard, E. M. (2001a). Psychophysical investigations into the neural basis of synaesthesia. *Proceedings of the Royal Society of London, B, 268,* 979–983.

Ramachandran, V. S., & Hubbard, E. M. (2001b). Neural cross wiring, synaesthesia and metaphor. Poster presented at the 8th Annual Meeting of the Cognitive Neuroscience Society, New York.

Ramachandran, V. S., & Rogers-Ramachandran, D. (1995). Touching the phantom. *Nature,* 377, 489–490.

Ramachandran, V. S., Rogers-Ramachandran, D., & Stewart, M. (1992). Perceptual correlates of massive cortical reorganization. *Science, 258,* 1159–1160.

Rickard, T. C., Romero, S. G., Basso, G., Wharton, C., Flitman, S., & Grafman, J. (2000). The calculating brain: An fMRI study. *Neuropsychologia, 38*(3), 325–335.

Rodman, H., & Moore, T. (1997). Development and plasticity of extrastriate visual cortex in monkeys. In K. S. Rockland, J. H. Kaas, & A. Peters (Eds.), *Cerebral cortex* (pp. 639–672). New York: Plenum Press.

Root-Bernstein, R., & Root-Bernstein, M. (1999). *Sparks of genius: The thirteen thinking tools of the world's most creative people.* Boston: Houghton Mifflin.

Rosa, M. G. (1997). Visuotopic organization of primate extrastriate cortex. In K. S. Rockland, J. H. Kaas, & A. Peters (Eds.), *Cerebral cortex* (pp. 127–203). New York: Plenum Press.

Sacks, O., & Wasserman, R. L. (1987). The painter who became colour blind. *New York Review of Books, 34*(18), 25–33.

Sacks, O., Wasserman, R. L., Zeki, S., & Siegel, R. M. (1988). Sudden colour blindness of cerebral origin. *Society for Neuroscience Abstracts, 14,* 1251.

Scheibel, A. B., Fried, I., Paul, L., Forsythe, A., Tomiyasu, U., Wechsler, A., et al. (1985). Differentiating characteristics of the human speech cortex: A quantitative Golgi study. In D. F. Beson & E. Zaidel (Eds.), *The dual brain.* New York: Guilford Press.

Segal, S. J. (1971). *Imagery: Current cognitive approaches.* San Diego, CA: Academic Press.

Sheinberg, D. L., & Logothetis, N. K. (1997). The role of temporal cortical areas in perceptual organization. *Proceedings of the National Academy of Sciences, USA, 94,* 3408–3413.

Smilek, D., Dixon, M. J., Cudahy, C., & Merikle, P. M. (2001). Synaesthetic photisms influence visual perception. *Journal of Cognitive Neuroscience, 13*(7), 930–936.

Spalding, J. M. K., & Zangwill, O. (1950). Disturbance of number-form in a case of brain injury. *Journal of Neurology, Neurosurgery, and Psychiatry, 12,* 24–29.

Stiles-Davis, J., Kritchevsky, M., & Bellugi, U. (Eds.) (1998). *Spatial cognition: Brain bases and development.* Hillsdale, NJ: Lawrence Erlbaum Associates.

Tarkiainen, A., Helenius, P., Hansen, P. C., Comelissen, P. L., Salmelin, R. (1999). Dynamics of letter string perception in the human occipitotemporal cortex. *Brain, 122*(11), 2119–2131.

Thompson-Schill, S. L., Aguirre, G. K., D'Esposito, M., & Farah, M. J. (1999). A neural basis for category and modality specificity of semantic knowledge. *Neuropsychologia, 37*(6), 671–676.

Tong, F., & Engel, S. A. (2001). Interocular rivalry revealed in the human cortical blind-spot representation. *Nature, 411,* 195–199.

Tranel, D., Damasio, H., & Damasio, A. R. (1997). A neural basis for the retrieval of conceptual knowledge. *Neuropsychologia, 35*(10), 1319–1327.

Treisman, A. (1982). Perceptual grouping and attention in visual search for features and for objects. *Journal of Experimental Psychology: Human Perception and Performance, 8*(2), 194–214.

Ullmann, S. (1945). Romanticism and synaesthesia: A comparative study of sense transfer in Keats and Byron. *Publications of the Modern Language Association of America, 60,* 811–827.

Van Essen, D. C., & De Yoe, E. A. (1995). Concurrent processing in the primate visual cortex. In M. S. Gazzaniga (Ed.), *The cognitive neurosciences* (pp. 383–400). Cambridge, MA: MIT Press.

Wade, A. R., Brewer, A. A., Rieger, J. W., & Wandell, B. A. (2002). Functional measurements of human ventral occipital cortex: Retinotopy and colour. *Philosophical Transactions of the Royal Society of London B Biological Sciences, 357*(1424), 963–973.

Williams, J. M. (1976). Synaesthetic adjectives: A possible law of semantic change. *Language, 32*(2), 461–478.

Wollen, K. A., & Ruggiero, F. T. (1983). Colored-letter synaesthesia. *Journal of Mental Imagery, 7,* 83–86.

Zeki, S., & Marini, L. (1998). Three cortical stages of colour processing in the human brain. *Brain, 121*(9), 1669–1685.

CONTRIBUTORS

LESLIE ALLISON, M.S., P.T.   Department of Kinesiology, Neuroscience and Cognitive Neuroscience Program, University of Maryland, College Park, Maryland

THOMAS J. ANASTASIO, PH.D.   Department of Molecular and Integrative Physiology, University of Illinois, Urbana, Illinois

RICHARD A. ANDERSEN, PH.D.   Division of Biology, California Institute of Technology, Pasadena, California

EDWARD T. AUER, JR., PH.D.   Department of Communication Neuroscience, House Ear Institute, Los Angeles, California

LORRAINE E. BAHRICK, PH.D.   Department of Psychology, Florida International University, Miami, Florida

DANIEL S. BARTH, PH.D.   Department of Psychology, University of Colorado, Boulder, Colorado

TONYA R. BERGESON, PH.D.   Department of Otolaryngology–Head and Neck Surgery, Indiana University School of Medicine, Indianapolis, Indiana

LYNNE E. BERNSTEIN, PH.D.   Department of Communication Neuroscience, House Ear Institute, Los Angeles, California

ROBERT A. BOAKES, PH.D.   Department of Psychology, University of Sydney, Sydney, NSW, Australia

BARBARA BRETT-GREEN, PH.D.   Department of Psychology, University of Colorado, Boulder, Colorado

PETER A. BUTCHER   Center for Brain and Cognition, University of California, San Diego, La Jolla, California

GEMMA CALVERT, D. PHIL.   University Laboratory of Physiology, University of Oxford, Oxford, United Kingdom

RUTH CAMPBELL, PH.D.   Department of Human Communication Science, University College London, London, United Kingdom

PABLO CELNIK, M.D.   Human Cortical Physiology Section, National Institute of Neurological Disorders and Stroke, Bethesda, Maryland

LEONARDO G. COHEN, M.D.   Human Cortical Physiology Section, National Institute of Neurological Disorders and Stroke, Bethesda, Maryland

YALE E. COHEN, PH.D.   Department of Psychological and Brain Sciences, Center for Cognitive Neuroscience, Dartmouth College, Hanover, New Hampshire

CHRISTINE E. COLLINS, PH.D.   Department of Psychology, Vanderbilt University, Nashville, Tennessee

HANS COLONIUS, PH.D.   University of Oldenburg, Oldenburg, Germany

BEATRICE DE GELDER, PH.D.   Department of Psychology, Tilburg University, Tilburg, The Netherlands

ADELE DIEDERICH, PH.D.   School of Humanities and Social Sciences, International University Bremen, Bremen, Germany

MIKE J. DIXON, PH.D.   Department of Psychology, University of Waterloo, Waterloo, Ontario, Canada

PAUL DIZIO, PH.D.   Ashton Graybiel Spatial Orientation Laboratory, Brandeis University, Waltham, Massachusetts

TIMOTHY P. DOUBELL, PH.D.   University Laboratory of Physiology, University of Oxford, Oxford, United Kingdom

JON DRIVER, D. PHIL.   Institute of Cognitive Neuroscience, University College London, London, United Kingdom

ALEXANDER EASTON, D. PHIL.   School of Psychology, University of Nottingham, University Park, Nottingham, United Kingdom

MARTIN EIMER, PH.D.   School of Psychology, Birkbeck College, University of London, London, United Kingdom

ALLESSANDRO FARNÈ, PH.D.   Department of Psychology, University of Bologna, Bologna, Italy

LEONARDO FOGASSI, PH.D.   Department of Neurosciences, Section of Physiology, University of Parma, Parma, Italy

ALEXANDRA FORT, PH.D.   Mental Processes and Brain Activation, U280-INSERM, Lyon, France

CAROL A. FOWLER, PH.D.   Haskins Laboratories, New Haven, Connecticut

JOHN J. FOXE, PH.D.   Cognitive Neuroscience and Schizophrenia Program, Nathan Kline Institute for Psychiatric Research, Orangeburg, New York

ESTEBAN A. FRIDMAN, M.D.   Department of Neurology, Raul Carrea Institute of Neurological Research, FLENI, Buenos Aires, Argentina

VITTORIO GALLESE, M.D.   Department of Neurosciences, Section of Physiology, University of Parma, Parma, Italy

MARIE-HÉLÈNE GIARD, PH.D.   Mental Processes and Brain Activation, U280—INSERM, Lyons, France

MICHAEL S.A. GRAZIANO, PH.D.   Department of Psychology, Green Hall, Princeton University, Princeton, New Jersey

CHARLES G. GROSS, PH.D.   Department of Psychology, Princeton University, Princeton, New Jersey

YORAM GUTFREUND, PH.D.   Department of Neurobiology, Stanford University School of Medicine, Stanford, California

EDWARD M. HUBBARD, M.A.   Brain and Perception Laboratory, University of California, San Diego, La Jolla, California

ATSUSHI IRIKI, D.D.S., PH.D.   Section of Cognitive Neurobiology, Department of Maxillofacial Biology, Tokyo Medical and Dental University, Tokyo, Japan

HIDETOSHI ISHIBASHI, D.V.M., PH.D.   Section of Cognitive Neurobiology, Department of Maxillofacial Biology, Tokyo Medical and Dental University, Tokyo, Japan

JOHN J. JEKA, PH.D.   Department of Kinesiology, Neuroscience and Cognitive Science Program, University of Maryland, College Park, Maryland

WAN JIANG, PH.D.   Department of Neurobiology and Anatomy, Wake Forest University School of Medicine, Winston-Salem, North Carolina

VEIKKO JOUSMÄKI, PH.D.   Rain Research Unit, Low Temperature Laboratory, Helsinki University of Technology, Espoo, Finland

JON H. KAAS, PH.D.   Department of Psychology, Vanderbilt University, Nashville, Tennessee

YUKIYASU KAMITANI, PH.D.   Department of Neurology, Beth Israel Deaconess Medical Center, Harvard Medical School, Boston, Massachusetts

ANDREW J. KING, PH.D.   University Laboratory of Physiology, Oxford University, Oxford, United Kingdom

ALAN KINGSTONE, PH.D.   Department of Psychology, University of British Columbia, Vancouver, British Columbia, Canada

ROBERTA L. KLATZKY, PH.D.   Department of Psychology, Carnegie Mellon University, Pittsburgh, Pennsylvania

ERIC I. KNUDSEN, PH.D.   Department of Neurobiology, Stanford University School of Medicine, Stanford, California

KIMBERLY S. KRAEBEL, PH.D.   Center for Developmental Psychobiology, Binghamton University, Binghamton, New York

MORTEN KRINGELBACH, PH.D.   Department of Experimental Psychology, University of Oxford, Oxford, United Kingdom

JAMES R. LACKNER, PH.D.   Ashton Graybiel Spatial Orientation Laboratory, Brandeis University, Waltham, Massachusetts

ELISABETTA LÀDAVAS, PH.D.   Department of Psychology, University of Bologna, Bologna, Italy

SUSAN J. LEDERMAN, PH.D.   Department of Psychology, Queen's University, Kingston, Ontario, Canada

JAMES W. LEWIS, PH.D.   Department of Cell Biology, Neurobiology, Medical College of Wisconsin, Milwaukee, Wisconsin

DAVID J. LEWKOWICZ, PH.D.   Department of Psychology, Florida Atlantic University, Davie, Florida

ROBERT LICKLITER, PH.D.   DEPARTMENT OF PSYCHOLOGY, FLORIDA INTERNATIONAL UNIVERSITY, MIAMI, FLORIDA

EMILIANO MACALUSO, PH.D.   Institute of Cognitive Neuroscience, University College London, London, United Kingdom

MAIRÉAD MACSWEENEY, PH.D.   Behavioural and Brain Sciences Unit, Institute of Child Health, University College London, London, United Kingdom

ANGELO MARAVITA, M.D., PH.D.   Department of Psychology, University of Milano-Bicocca, Milan, Italy

LAWRENCE E. MARKS, PH.D.   John B. Pierce Laboratory and Yale University, New Haven, Connecticut

DOMINIC W. MASSARO, PH.D.   Department of Psychology, University of California, Santa Cruz, Santa Cruz, California

JASON B. MATTINGLEY, PH.D.   Department of Psychology, School of Behavioural Science, University of Melbourne, Victoria, Australia

JOHN MCDONALD, PH.D.   Department of Psychology, Simon Fraser University, Burnaby, British Columbia, Canada

M. ALEX MEREDITH, PH.D.   Department of Anatomy and Neurobiology, Virginia Commonwealth University School of Medicine, Richmond, Virginia

PHILIP M. MERIKLE, PH.D.   Department of Psychology, University of Waterloo, Waterloo, Ontario, Canada

JEAN K. MOORE, PH.D.   Department of Communication Neuroscience, House Ear Institute, Los Angeles, California

TIRIN MOORE, PH.D.   Department of Psychology, Princeton University, Princeton, New Jersey

KEVIN G. MUNHALL, PH.D.   Department of Psychology and Department of Otolaryngology, Queen's University, Kingston, Ontario, Canada

DOUGLAS P. MUNOZ, PH.D.   Centre for Neuroscience Studies, Queen's University, Kingston, Ontario, Canada

FIONA N. NEWELL, PH.D.   Department of Psychology, Aras an Phiarsaigh, University of Dublin, Trinity College, Dublin, Ireland

SHIGERU OBAYASHI, M.D., PH.D.   Section of Cognitive Neurobiology, Dept. of Maxillofacial Biology, Tokyo Medical and Dental University, Tokyo, Japan

JOHN O'DOHERTY, D.PHIL.   Wellcome Department of Imaging Neuroscience, Institute of Neurology, London, United Kingdom

AMANDA PARKER, PH.D.   School of Psychology, University of Nottingham, Nottingham, United Kingdom

SARAH R. PARTAN, PH.D.   Department of Psychology, University of South Florida, St. Petersburg, St. Petersburg, Florida

PAUL E. PATTON, PH.D.   Beckman Institute, University of Illinois, Urbana, Illinois

DAVID B. PISONI, PH.D.   Department of Psychology, Indiana University, Bloomington, Indiana

GILLES POURTOIS, PH.D.   Department of Psychology, Tilburg University, Tilburg, The Netherlands

S.C. PRATHER, PH.D.   Department of Neurology, Emory University School of Medicine, Atlanta, Georgia

TOMMI RAIJ, M.D., PH.D.   MGH/MIT/HMS, A.A. Martinos Center for Biomedical Imaging, Charlestown, Massachusetts

VILAYANUR S. RAMACHANDRAN, M.D., PH.D.   Center for Brain and Cognition, University of California, San Diego, La Jolla, California

JOSEF P. RAUSCHECKER, PH.D.   Department of Physiology and Biophysics, Georgetown University Medical Center, Washington, D.C.

GREGG H. RECANZONE, PH.D.   Center for Neuroscience, University of California, Davis, Davis, California

ANINA N. RICH, B.SC. (HONS.)   Department of Psychology, School of Behavioural Science, University of Melbourne, Victoria, Australia

BRIGITTE RÖDER, PH.D.   Biological Psychology and Neuropsychology, University of Hamburg, Hamburg, Germany

EDMUND T. ROLLS, D.SC.   Department of Experimental Psychology, University of Oxford, Oxford, United Kingdom

FRANK RÖSLER, PH.D.   Department of Psychology, Philipps-University Marburg, Marburg, Germany

KRISH SATHIAN, M.D., PH.D.   Department of Neurology, Emory University School of Medicine, Atlanta, Georgia

CHARLES E. SCHROEDER, PH.D.   Cognitive Neuroscience and Schizophrenia Program, Nathan Kline Institute for Psychiatric Research, Orangeburg, New York

LADAN SHAMS, PH.D.   Division of Biology, California Institute of Technology, Pasadena, California

SHINSUKE SHIMOJO, PH.D.   Division of Biology, California Institute of Technology, Pasadena, California

IRINI SKALIORA, PH.D.   University Laboratory of Physiology, Oxford University, Oxford, United Kingdom

DANIEL SMILEK, PH.D.   Department of Psychology, University of Waterloo, Waterloo, Ontario, Canada

SALVADOR SOTO-FARACO, PH.D.   Department of Psychology, University of Barcelona, Barcelona, Spain

CHARLES SPENCE, PH.D.   Department of Experimental Psychology, University of Oxford, Oxford, United Kingdom

TERRENCE R. STANFORD, PH.D.   Department of Neurobiology and Anatomy, Wake Forest University School of Medicine, Winston-Salem, North Carolina

BARRY E. STEIN, PH.D.   Department of Neurobiology and Anatomy, Wake Forest University School of Medicine, Winston-Salem, North Carolina

RICHARD J. STEVENSON, D.PHIL.   Department of Psychology, Macquarie University, Sydney, NSW, Australia

MRIGANKA SUR, PH.D.   Department of Brain and Cognitive Sciences, Massachusetts Institute of Technology, Cambridge, Massachusetts

CHARLOTTE S.R. TAYLOR, PH.D.   Department of Psychology, Princeton University, Princeton, New Jersey

A. JOHN VAN OPSTAL, PH.D.   Department of Biophysics, University of Nijmegen, Nijmegen, The Netherlands

ERIC VATIKIOTIS-BATESON, PH.D.   Department of Linguistics, University of British Columbia, Vancouver, British Columbia; Communication Dynamics Project, ATR Human Information Science Laboratories, Seika-cho, Kyoto, Japan

A. JEAN VROOMEN, PH.D.   Department of Psychology, Tilburg University, Tilburg, The Netherlands

BRANDON WAGAR, M.A.   Department of Psychology, University of Waterloo, Waterloo, Ontario, Canada

MARK T. WALLACE, PH.D.   Department of Neurobiology and Anatomy, Wake Forest University School of Medicine, Winston-Salem, North Carolina

TIMOTHY M. WOODS, PH.D.   The Harker School, San Jose, California

MINMING ZHANG, M.D., PH.D.   Department of Neurology, Emory University School of Medicine, Atlanta, Georgia

INDEX

and neurological deficits related to
peripersonal space, 431–432
role of multisensory integration in,
430–431
F5 area, 426f, 434–435
F5-PF circuit, 434–438, 455
Face, visuotactile interactions near,
807–809
Face features, horizontal size of,
177, 178
Face movements, perception of, 454
Face processing, 213
Face recognition, haptic, 132
Facial affect, perception of, 165
Facial expression(s)
amygdala in processing of, 571–572
of emotions, 582–584
electrophysiological studies of,
585–587
orbitofrontal cortex in processing of,
570–571
Facial gestures, imitation by infants of,
190–191, 192
Facial luminance, in audiovisual speech
perception, 181
Facial motion, in speech perception,
182–183, 184–186
Facial speech gestures
evidence for perception of, 192–194
recognition by infants of, 191–192
Facilitation, 662
multisensory, 674
FAES region, 254
auditory inputs to, 348
excitatory-inhibitory multisensory
neurons in, 351–352
external afferents to, 345, 346
intrinsic cross-modal connectivity of,
349–351
location of, 343
and SIV, 353
in sound localization, 343
Fall-prone elderly population, sensory
reweighting in, 793–795
Far peripersonal space, neuronal bases
for multisensory processing of,
810–811
Fat, mouth feel of, 319–321
Fearful facial expressions, amygdala in
processing of, 571–572
Feature integration information-
processing theories, of
audiovisual speech perception,
215–216
Feature integration theory, 856
and ventriloquism effect, 144
Feedback, in sensory processing,
141, 142
Feedback circuits, for multisensory
convergence, 299–303
Feedback projection, 617
Feed-forward circuits, for multisensory
convergence, 141, 298–303
Feeding behavior, multisensory signals in,
228–229, 230
"Feeling" speech, 777

Ferret(s)
auditory behavior in visually deprived,
695, 697
epigenetic factors that align visual and
auditory maps in midbrain of,
599–610
intersensory integration in, 659
routing visual inputs to auditory
pathway in
behavioral consequence of,
686–690
physiological and anatomical
consequences of, 685–688
technique of, 683–685
Filehne illusion, 50
Filtering task, selective attention as, 86, 91
Fixation neurons, 374–376
Flavor, representation of, 315, 573, 574
Flavor-visual association memory, 336
Flicker-fusion threshold, of visual
stimuli, 38
Flinching, 447–448
FLMP (fuzzy logical model of
perception), convergent and
nonconvergent integration in,
162–163
fMRI. See Functional magnetic resonance
imaging (fMRI)
Focused attention, visual-tactile
interaction in, 405–406
Focused attention paradigm, 396
Focused attention task, integration rule
assumptions for, 404
Food, pleasantness of taste of, 314
Food texture, response of orbitofrontal
taste and olfactory neurons to,
319–321
Fornix, in memory encoding and storage,
337, 338
Foveation-based signal, for auditory space
map, 617
Frame of reference
of somatosensory system, 379
of visual vs. auditory system, 377–378
Free parameters, in bimodal speech
perception, 160
Freezing phenomenon, 146–148
Frontal lobe, multisensory areas
in, 450
Frontoparietal areas, in endogenous
covert spatial attention,
536, 546
Frontoparietal circuit
F2 ventrorostral-V6A/MIP, 432–434
F4-VIP, 426–432
Frontoparietal network, 492, 493
FST (fundus of superior temporal sulcus),
connections to, 288
Functional imaging, of multisensory
spatial representations and cross-
modal attentional interactions,
529–546
Functional magnetic resonance
imaging (fMRI)
of activation of auditory cortex by
visual stimuli, 778

of affective value of stimuli
gustatory, 566–567
olfactory, 568
of amygdala and auditory
reinforcers, 572
of audiovisual associative
learning, 495
of audiovisual interactions relating to
emotion, 495
of audiovisual perception of emotion,
586–588
of auditory areas during visual
processing, 738
of auditory localization with
blindness, 734
of color-phonemic synesthesia, 863
of cross-modal plasticity, 496
deactivation interactions in,
498–499
of detection of changes in sensory
events, 494
of integration at semantic level,
489–490
of integration of phonetic information,
486–488
of language perception with blindness,
728, 729
of linguistic interactions, 485
mapping unimodal and multimodal
brain areas with, 529–530, 531
of multisensory convergence in cortical
processing, 296
of orbitofrontal cortex and amygdala in
emotion, 564
of processing of facial expressions,
570–571
of spatial concordance, 493
of spatial frames of reference for
cross-modal interactions,
543–545
of speech-reading, 774–775
of stimulus-driven cross-modal
interactions, 539–542
of stimulus-reinforcer association
learning, 573–576
of visual cortex
during auditory and tactile
processing, 738
in tactile perception, 705, 706, 707
of visual perception with deafness,
725–726
Functional reallocation, 735, 736–737
Function words, processing by blind
people of, 727, 728–729
Fundamental frequency, in audiovisual
speech perception, 203
Fundus of superior temporal sulcus
(FST), connections to, 288
Fusiform face area, 213
Fusiform gyrus
in audiovisual perception of emotion,
586, 587–588
cross-wiring in synesthesia of, 870–871
in grapheme-color synesthesia,
844–845
in visual speech pathway, 213

F2 ventrorostral-V6A/MIP circuit in, 432–434
F4-VIP circuit in, 426–432
F5-PF circuit in, 434–438
multisensory signals in, 230–231, 232
neocortex of, 285, 286
perception of facial and body movements in, 454
posterior parietal cortex in, 288–289
tool use by, 820
  body image developed through, 455, 456
  brain imaging studies of, 458
  generalization of, 458–459
ventriloquism aftereffect in, 42–45
Macrospatial features, 705
Macular degeneration, auditory localization with, 734
Maevia inclemens, multisensory signals in, 232
Magnetic resonance imaging, functional. *See* Functional magnetic resonance imaging (fMRI)
Magnetoencephalography (MEG), 515–517
advantages of, 515, 517
of audiotactile integration, 518–519
of audiovisual associative learning, 520–522
of audiovisual integration, 518
of auditory processing in musicians, 724
of cross-modal integration and plasticity, 515–524
of cross-modal mental imagery, 522
of cross-modal plasticity, 522–524
of integration of phonetic information, 488
of learning-dependent multisensory processing, 519–522
of multisensory affect perception, 585
of multisensory convergence in cortical processing, 296
principles and instrumentation of, 515–516
of real-time multisensory processing, 518–519
spatial resolution of, 517
temporal resolution of, 517
uses of, 517
of vibrotactile activation of auditory cortex, 777
of visuotactile integration, 519
Magnocellular layer, in visual speech pathway, 213
Magpies, redundant signals in, 228
Manner feature, in speech perception, 204n
Map expansion, 722–723, 736
Mark test, 459
Material properties, multisensory perception of, 108, 109, 120–121
Mating behavior, multisensory signals in, 228, 229, 230, 232, 233, 235–236

Maximum-likelihood integration model, of multisensory texture perception, 119
McGurk effect, 27, 203
in audiovisual speech perception, 177, 205, 207–208, 750
as example of emergence, 234
familiarity with talker and, 207, 208
gaze during, 182
haptic version of, 189
in infants, 662
with low spatial resolution, 180
magnetoencephalography of, 518
and multimodal speech perception, 156, 159
multisensory convergence and, 311, 322, 323–324
positron emission tomography of, 488
sensitivity to asynchrony in, 183
and special nature of speech, 154
in speech perception by infants, 191
McGurk effect tasks, 177–178
Medial auditory belt, connections of, 287–288
Medial geniculate nucleus (MGN)
in audiovisual speech perception, 211, 214
histological tracing of multisensory pathways in, 365, 366, 368
projections to anterior ectosylvian sulcus from, 345
routing visual inputs to, 683–686
Medial intraparietal area (MIP), 426, 433–434
connections to, 288, 289
Medial prefrontal cortex, connections to, 290
Medial pulvinar nucleus
in audiovisual convergence, 483
in auditory speech pathway, 211, 212, 214
Medial superior temporal area (MST)
connections to, 288
multisensory convergence in, 297, 301
Medial temporal lobe, in object discrimination learning, 337
MEG. *See* Magnetoencephalography (MEG)
Memory(ies), episodic, 324–325, 337
Memory encoding and storage, in inferior temporal lobe, 337–339
Mental imagery
magnetoencephalography of, 522
synesthesia and, 873–874
in tactile perception, 707
Mental rotation, of two-dimensional tactile forms, visual cortex in, 704–706
Metaphor, synesthesia and, 876, 877
MGN. *See* Medial geniculate nucleus (MGN)
Microspatial features, 705

Midbrain
epigenetic factors that align visual and auditory maps in, 599–610
multisensory integration in single neurons of, 243–260
visual instruction of auditory space map in, 613–623
Midbrain tectum, with visual deprivation, 696
Middle temporal gyrus (MTG)
in audiovisual perception of emotion, 587–589
in auditory speech pathway, 212
integration at semantic level in, 489–490
in visual speech pathway, 213
Middle temporal visual area (MT), 448
multisensory convergence in, 297, 301, 303, 304
Migration, of birds, 235
Miller's test, 398
MIP (medial intraparietal area), 426, 433–434
connections to, 288, 289
Mirror(s), cross-modal integration modulated by, 828–832
Mirror-image stimuli, discrimination between, 705
Mirror neurons
in audiovisual speech perception, 215
and body schema, 454–455
in circuit for action understanding, 434–435
PF, 436–438
Mirror reflections
cross-modal interference between touch and, 828–831
cross-modal spatial extinction between touch and, 831–832
Mismatch negativity (MMN), 585–586
Misses, 396
Modality appropriateness hypothesis, 27–28, 36
and infants' responsiveness to multisensory compounds, 667
of multisensory texture perception, 116–118
Modality dominance, of cross-modal dynamic capture, 62–64
Modality-specific audiovisual speech perception, 207–210
neural implementation of, 216–218
Modality-specific cues, in perception of amodal invariant, 661–662
Modality-specific stimulus properties
defined, 660
examples of, 644
intersensory redundancy and perceptual learning about, 649
perception by infants of, 644
specification of multisensory object or event by, 660
Model tests, in bimodal speech perception, 161
Modularity, in speech perception, 155
Mole rats, multisensory signals in, 234

Neurogenesis, and compensatory
plasticity, 739
Neuroimaging modalities, 503
Neuroimaging studies
of affective value of stimuli, 564–572
auditory, 572
gustatory, 564–567
olfactory, 567–569
somatosensory, 569–570
visceral and somatic representations
of, 570
visual, 570–572
of cross-modal integration
in amygdala, 572
for emotion, 563–576
in orbitofrontal cortex, 573, 574
of cross-modal plasticity and language
processing in deaf people,
773–780
of representation of flavor, 573, 574
of stimulus-reinforcer association
learning, 573–576
Neuromagnetic inverse problem,
515, 516
Neuromagnetic signals, genesis of, 516
Neuromagnetometers, 516
Neuron(s), multisensory integration in
single, 243–260
Neuronal correlates, of object
recognition, 124–127
Neuronal plasticity, in ventriloquism
illusion, 45–46
Neuroplasticity. *See* Neural plasticity
Neuropsychological evidence, of
integrated multisensory
representation of space,
799–814
Neurotrophin(s), in tool use learning,
457–458
Neurotrophin 3 (NT-3), in tool use
learning, 457
NGF (nerve growth factor), in tool use
learning, 457
Nightingales, learning in, 234
N-methyl-D-aspartate (NMDA)
receptors, 367
in midbrain auditory localization
pathway, 616
in visual and auditory map registration,
606–607
Noisy communication channels, 225
Nonlinguistic interactions, hemodynamic
studies of, 491–494
Non-matching-to-sample (NMS)
task, 334
Nonredundant-cue identification task,
505–509
Nonredundant signals, in animals,
227–228, 230–234
Nose, in smell and taste, 72–74
Novelists, synesthesia in, 876–877
NT-3 (neurotrophin 3), in tool use
learning, 457
Nucleus of solitary tract (NTS), in taste
pathway, 312, 314
Number line, in synesthesia, 875–876

O

Object-based visual search task, attention
in, 326–328
Object constancy, 123, 127–128
Object discrimination learning, medial
temporal lobe in, 337
Object geons, 128
Object recognition, 123–136
behavioral correlates of, 127–130
experimental studies on, 130–135
for multiple objects, 132–135
for single objects, 130–132
haptic, 128–129
lateral occipital cortex in, 31
neuronal correlates of, 124–127
with odor-taste synesthesia, 73–74
spatial constraints on, 135–136
temporal constraints on, 136
verbal mediation in, 134–135
Object segregation, 147
Object similarity, multisensory perception
of, 108
Observation-execution matching (OEM)
system, in audiovisual speech
perception, 215
OC (oral communication), audiovisual
speech perception with, 755,
757–758, 763–765
Occipital cortex, in tactile discrimination
by blind subjects, 711
Occipital visual areas
in blindness, 738
differential activation of, 531
in endogenous spatial attention,
533–534, 536, 538
retinotopic organization of, 530, 543
Occipitotemporal areas, in object
recognition, 126
Ocular dominance columns,
development and plasticity of,
681–682, 683, 699
Oculocentric coordinates
of somatosensory input, 379
of visual input, 377–378, 389
Oculogravic illusion, 411
Odor(s)
defined, 69
sweet, 69–72
liking and, 72
odor-taste learning and, 74
Odor-learning system, 79
Odor-odor learning, 80
Odor perception
odor-taste learning and, 80
role of learning in, 70
Odor-taste learning, 72, 74–78
acquisition and awareness in, 75–76
expectancy test of, 76, 77
extinction procedure for, 76
implicit memory procedures
in, 79–80
and odor perception, 80
preexposure and training in, 77–78
retention and resistance to interference
in, 76–77

successive *vs.* simultaneous associations
in, 75–76
Odor-taste mixtures, configural encoding
of, 78–79
Odor-taste synesthesia, 69–81
language and, 73
and object identification, 73–74
reliability of, 70
validity of, 70–72
OEM (observation-execution matching)
system, in audiovisual speech
perception, 215
Olfaction
orthonasal, 69, 73
retronasal, 69, 72, 73
synesthesia between taste and, 69–81
Olfactory neurons, response to texture of
food by, 319–321
Olfactory pathway, in primate brain, 313
Olfactory representations, in primate
cortex, rules underlying
formation of, 315–316
Olfactory sensory-specific satiety, 318–320
Olfactory stimuli
neuroimaging studies of affective value
of, 567–569
representation of pleasantness of,
318–320
Olfactory-to-taste associations, 311, 315
Omnipause neurons (OPNs), 376
Ontogenetic adaptations, 657
Optic ataxia, 434
Optic tectum (OT), visual instruction of
auditory space map in, 613–623
Oral communication (OC), audiovisual
speech perception with, 755,
757–758, 763–765
Orbital motion, direction of experienced,
419–421
Orbitofrontal cortex
activation of
by auditory stimuli, 572
by gustatory stimuli, 565–567
by olfactory stimuli, 567–569
by somatosensory stimuli, 569–570
by visual stimuli, 570–572
in emotion, neuroimaging studies of,
563–576
imaging methods for, 564
multisensory convergence in, 311,
312, 328
representation of flavor in, 315,
573, 574
representation of tastes in, 565–567
in representing affective value of
stimuli, neuroimaging studies of,
564–572
response to satiety by, 314, 318–320
response to texture of food by, 319–321
rules governing formation of olfactory
representations in, 315–316
secondary taste cortex in, 313
stimulus-reinforcer learning in,
neuroimaging studies of,
563–564, 573–576
visual inputs to, 316–318

Phonetic information, hemodynamic
    studies of integration of,
    486–488
Phonetic module, 195–196
    in speech perception, 154–155
Phonetic processor, in speech
    perception, 196
Photism(s)
    as automatic consequence of viewing
        graphemes, 838–839
    cross-linkage model of, 844, 845
    defined, 837
    form and meaning in determining,
        844–847
    location of, 837
    perceptual aspects of, 841–844
    reentrant model of, 844–845
Physiological plasticity, 721–722
Piriform area, activation by olfactory
    stimulation of, 567, 568
PIT (posterior inferior temporal cortex),
    in grapheme-color synesthesia,
    844–845
Pitch
    and brightness, 90, 91, 98–100
    and lightness, 92, 93, 95–97
    and visual position, 91
Pitch-forward head movements, in
    rotating environments,
    413–414
Pitch-size congruence, 98
Place feature, in speech perception,
    204n, 205
Plasticity
    anatomical, 721–722
    of auditory space map, 616,
        617–620
        model for, 620–622
    of auditory spatial processing in
        superior colliculus,
        604–605, 606
    compensatory
        as consequence of sensory loss,
            719–740
            for language function, 727–731
            mechanisms of, 735–739
            model for investigating, 719–720
            for motor development, 740
            for perceptual functions,
                723–726
            for spatial functions, 731–735
            in developing and adult brain,
                738–739
            maladaptive consequences of,
                739–740
            neural mechanisms of, 698–699
    cross-modal
        and behavioral changes after sensory
            deprivation, 738–739
        with deafness, 773–780
        defined, 711
        hemodynamic studies of, 495–496
        in humans, 690–691
        implications for cortical development
            and function of, 681–691
        intramodal vs., 723

magnetoencephalography of,
    522–524
as mechanism for compensation and
    hypercompensation, 735
period of susceptibility to
    experience, 712, 714, 715
    between visual and somatosensory
        representations, 711–712, 713
intermodal, 723, 735, 738–739
intersystem, 723, 735, 738–739
intramodal, 723, 735, 736
intrasystem, 723, 735, 736
lesion-induced, 736
magnetoencephalography of,
    515–524
neural, 720–723
    classification of, 721–723
    defined, 720, 722
    intramodal vs. intermodal changes
        in, 723
    intrasystem vs. intersystem changes
        in, 723
physiological, 721–722
use-dependent, 736
in ventriloquism illusion, 45–46
Pleasant tastes
    activation of amygdala by, 567
    hunger and, 314
    representation in orbitofrontal cortex
        of, 318–319, 320f, 565–567
PMLS (posterior medial lateral
    suprasylvian cortex), projections
    to anterior ectosylvian sulcus
    from, 344, 345, 346, 347
pMTG (posterior middle temporal
    gyrus), integration at semantic
    level in, 489–490
PMv (ventral premotor) zone
    in control of defensive movements, 443,
        444–448
    multisensory responses of, 289
PO (posterior nucleus), histological
    tracing of multisensory pathways
    in, 365–366, 368
POC (parieto-occipital cortex), in tactile
    discrimination of grating
    orientation, 703, 704
Poets, synesthesia in, 876–877
Polymodal brain areas, reorganization of,
    735, 736–737
Polysensory zone (PZ), in control of
    defensive movements, 443,
    444–448
Pop-outs, in grapheme-color
    synesthesia, 869
Positron emission tomography
    (PET), 564
    of activation of auditory cortex by
        visual stimuli, 778
    of affective value of stimuli
        gustatory, 565–566, 567
        olfactory, 567–568
    of amygdala and auditory
        reinforcers, 572
    of audiovisual associative
        learning, 495

of audiovisual interactions relating to
    emotion, 494–495
of audiovisual perception of emotion,
    587, 589
of audiovisual priming studies, 490
of auditory localization with blindness,
    732–734
of color-phonemic synesthesia, 863
of cross-modal plasticity, 496
of endogenous spatial attention,
    533–536, 538
of integration at semantic level, 489
of integration of phonetic
    information, 488
of linguistic interactions, 485
of orbitofrontal cortex activation by
    auditory stimuli, 572
of orbitofrontal cortex in
    representation of flavor, 573
of spatial concordance, 493
of temporal correspondence, 491
of visual cortex in tactile perception,
    703, 704–705, 706, 707
Postcues, 16n
Posterior cingulate gyrus, in speech-
    reading, 775, 776
Posterior ectosylvian gyral cortex (PEG),
    projections to anterior
    ectosylvian sulcus from, 344,
    345, 346f, 347
Posterior inferior temporal cortex (PIT),
    in grapheme-color synesthesia,
    844–845
Posterior medial lateral suprasylvian
    cortex (PMLS), projections to
    anterior ectosylvian sulcus from,
    344, 345, 346, 347
Posterior middle temporal gyrus
    (pMTG), integration at semantic
    level in, 489–490
Posterior nucleus (PO), histological
    tracing of multisensory pathways
    in, 365–366, 368
Posterior parietal cortex (PPC)
    connections to, 288–289
    eye-centered representations of
        auditory stimuli in,
        473–475
    in movement planning, 464–466
    multisensory representations of space
        in, 463–476
Poststimulus time histograms (PSTHs), of
    auditory/somatosensory evoked
    potentials, 364, 365
Postsynaptic potentials (PSPs),
    364–365, 367
Postural control
    haptic influences on, 421, 422
    multisensory integration in,
        785–796
        ambiguities and, 785–787
        light-touch/vision paradigm and,
            789–793
        sensory reweighting and, 787–789
        in fall-prone elderly population,
            793–795

Postural sway, 787–788, 796
Potential actions, 431
Potentiation, 672–673
PPC. *See* Posterior parietal cortex (PPC)
PPVT (*Peabody Picture Vocabulary Test*),
    after cochlear implantation,
    760, 761
Prairie dog, multisensory signals in, 226
Precentral gyrus, polysensory zone of, in
    control of defensive movements,
    443, 444–448
Preexposure effect, 77
    in odor-taste learning, 77–78
Prefrontal cortex
    in attention, 327
    in audiovisual convergence, 483, 484
    connections to, 290
Prelabeling model, of audiovisual speech
    perception, 209
Premotor cortex
    area F4 of
        anatomical location and functional
            properties of, 426–430, 432–433
        in control of reaching in space,
            432–434
        and deficits related to peripersonal
            space, 431–432
        role of multisensory integration in,
            430–431
    in audiovisual convergence, 483, 484
    connections to, 289–290
    polymodal neurons in, 425
    sensory responses in, 443, 444–448
    spatial representations in, 532
Premotor saccade burst generator, 376
Preparation enhancement model, 400
Presubiculum, and head direction, 326
Primates
    auditory-visual interactions subserving
        gaze orienting in, 373–391
    cross-modal memory in, 333–340
    intersensory integration in, 659
    multisensory signals in, 227
    olfactory pathway in, 313, 315–316
    resurrection of multisensory cortex in,
        285–291
    taste processing in, 312–314, 313f, 315f
Priming, audiovisual, 490
Principal components analysis (PCA), of
    audiovisual speech
    production, 184
Prismatic spectacles, and auditory space
    map, 615–616
Production-based animation, 185–186
Projectors, in synesthesia, 837, 839–841,
    861, 862
Proprioception
    in cross-modal dynamic capture, 62
    visual dominance over, in cross-modal
        modulation, 805
PRR (parietal reach region), 288, 289
    common spatial representation in area
        LIP and, 466–474
    in movement planning, 464, 465
Pseudophone, for ventriloquism
    aftereffect, 40

PSPs (postsynaptic potentials), 364,
    365, 367
PSTHs (poststimulus time histograms), of
    auditory/somatosensory evoked
    potentials, 364, 365
Psychoacoustic accounts, of speech
    perception, 154
Psychometric function, for ventriloquism
    aftereffect, 42, 43
Psychophysical staircase methodology, for
    cross-modal dynamic capture,
    58–60
Psychophysical studies, of cross-modal
    cuing of exogenous spatial
    attention, 16–17
Putamen
    in control of defensive movements, 443,
        444, 450
    in cross-modal integration, 496
    in multisensory processing of near
        peripersonal space, 802
PV region, 287
PZ (polysensory zone), in control of
    defensive movements, 443,
    444–448

Q

Quail(s), sensory development in, 234
Quail chicks
    differential effects of unimodal and
        multimodal stimulation in, 647
    intersensory redundancy and
        perceptual learning in,
        649–650
    responsiveness to multisensory
        compounds in, 672
Quale, 244, 688
Qualia, synesthesia and, 878–879

R

"Rabbit" effect, sound-induced
    visual, 29
Race models
    of response time, 397–400
    of saccade reaction times, 379–380, 388
Random dot kinematogram (RDK),
    apparent motion of, 51
Rat(s)
    learning in, 234
    multisensory signals in, 234
    potentiation in, 673
    trace learning in, 674
Rat cortex, multisensory evoked
    potentials in, 357–368
Rate-based intersensory matching, 670
RBD. *See* Right brain damage (RBD)
RDK (random dot kinematogram),
    apparent motion of, 51
RDLS-III (*Reynell Developmental Language
    Scales, 3rd Edition*), after cochlear
    implantation, 760
Reach, coding of, 464, 465–466
Reaching in space, circuit for control of,
    432–434

Reaching movements, influence of
    Coriolis forces on, 415–417
Reaction times, with event-related
    potentials, 506
Reaction time studies, 16, 16n
Real-time multisensory processing,
    magnetoencephalography of,
    518–519
Receptive fields (RFs)
    maturation of multisensory integration
        and, 631, 633
    multiple overlapping, 246–248
    of multisensory neurons, 633
    in superior colliculus, 246, 247
        consolidation during development
            of, 629–630
Reciprocal stimulus enhancement, 229
Recognition, in speech perception, 155
Redintegration, in odor-taste learning, 79
Red jungle fowl, multisensory signals in,
    225, 226
Redundancy, intersensory
    defined, 664
    in early perceptual development, 647,
        648–651
Redundant-cue identification task,
    505–509
Redundant signal(s), in animals, 227–230
Redundant signal hypothesis, 236
Redundant target effect, 506
Redundant target paradigm, 396
Redundant target task, integration rule
    assumptions for, 404–405
Red-winged blackbirds, multisensory
    processes in, 235
Reed warblers, redundant signals in, 228
Reentrant model, of photisms, 844–845
Reference condition, in hemodynamic
    studies, 497, 498
Reference frame(s), 463
    advantages of common, 475–476
    in area LIP and parietal reach region,
        466–474
    eye-centered, 466–473
        advantages of, 476
        of auditory stimuli, 473–475
        with eye position gain, 468, 473, 474
        transformation of head-centered
            to, 475
    head-centered, 467, 468
        transformation to eye-centered
            of, 475
    intermediate, 467, 468, 475
    limb-centered, 467, 468
    spatial, for cross-modal interactions,
        542–546
Reference-frame transformations,
    463–464
    posterior parietal cortex in, 464–476
Relevant stimuli, 94, 99–100
Reorganization, of polymodal brain areas,
    735, 736–737
Repetitive transcranial magnetic
    stimulation (rTMS), for
    evaluation of visual cortex in
    tactile perception, 712

by infants, 191–192
modularity in, 155
motor theory of, 154–155, 190, 194–197, 206
pattern recognition in, 155–156, 158–159
psychoacoustic accounts of, 154
recognition in, 155
selective adaptation and, 196
as special case of multisensory processing, 153–174
as supramodal, 190–192
theories of, 154–156
visual. *See* Lipreading
Speech production
audiovisual, 184–185
compatibility effects in, 197
as perceptually guided, 189
Speech-reading. *See* Lipreading
Speech signal(s)
in audiovisual speech perception, 209–210
parsing of, 193–194
Speech tutoring
for children with hearing loss, 172–174
in second language, 174
Speeded classification
cross-modal interactions in, 85–103
paradigm of, 85–86, 101
Speeded texture task, 110–111
Spermophilus beecheyi, multisensory signals in, 226
Spiders, multisensory signals in, 227, 228, 233
SPL (superior parietal lobule), in spatial concordance, 494
Split-brain patients, cross-modal dynamic capture in, 55–57
Spoken language, audiovisual properties of, 765–767
Spoken word recognition
after cochlear implantation, in postlingually deaf adults, 752–754
with oral communication *vs.* total communication, 755, 757–758, 763–765
SQUIDs (superconducting quantum interference devices), 516
Squirrels, multisensory signals in, 226
SRTs. *See* Saccade reaction times (SRTs)
Stagewise processing, 141–142
Staircase methodology
for cross-modal dynamic capture, 58–60
for ventriloquism effect, 143, 144–145
Static events
influence on perceived trajectory of motion of, 50
influence on perception of apparent motion of, 49–50
multisensory integration between dynamic and, 49–50, 52
Statistical facilitation, 379–380, 397
STG (superior temporal gyrus)
in auditory speech pathway, 212
in speech-reading, 774–775

Stiffness, multisensory perception of, 113, 120–121
Stimuli, relevant *vs.* irrelevant, 94, 99–100
Stimulus congruence, perceptual *vs.*, 101–103
Stimulus-driven cross-modal interactions, 539–542
Stimulus enhancement, reciprocal, 229
Stimulus information processing, 210–211
Stimulus onset asynchronies (SOAs), 207–208
in multichannel diffusion model, 402, 403
in multisensory integration between moving events, 51, 58–60
in superposition model, 401
in time-window-of-integration model, 404, 406
Stimulus preexposure effect, 77
Stimulus-reinforcer learning, in orbitofrontal cortex and amygdala, neuroimaging studies of, 563–564, 573–576
Stimulus-response compatibility effects, 6
STP (superior temporal polysensory area), 286, 288
multisensory convergence in, 296–297, 301, 303, 304, 305, 306
Streptopelia risoria
multisensory communication in, 226
multisensory signals in, 232
Striate cortex, compensatory plasticity of, 738
Stridulation, in crickets, 227
Stroop dilution effect, 858
Stroop effect, for grapheme-color synesthesia, 861–862
in projectors *vs.* associators, 840–841, 861, 862
reverse, 861–862
selective attention and, 860
Stroop task, for grapheme-color synesthesia, 838–839, 853, 854
Stroop task interference
cross-wiring and, 874
and ventriloquism effect, 142
Structure-based object recognition, 128
STS. *See* Superior temporal sulcus (STS)
Subjective experience, visual cortex in, 125
Subjective impression, 244
Substantia nigra, inhibitory signal to deep superior colliculus from, 279
Subthreshold conditioning, 674
Summation, law of heterogeneous, 229
Superconducting quantum interference devices (SQUIDs), 516
Superior colliculus (SC)
aligning visual and auditory maps in, 600–603
in audiovisual convergence, 483, 810–811
in audiovisual integration, 503, 508, 656
in audiovisual speech perception, 162, 211, 214

auditory consequences of altered visual experience in, 604–606
in coordinated movement, 246
cross-modal interactions in, 508
functions of, 265
location of, 245
modality-specific neurons in cortex send converging inputs to individual neurons in, 254
multiple overlapping receptive fields of multisensory neurons in, 246–248
multisensory development of
absence in early developmental stages of, 630–631, 632
future directions in, 638–640
maturation of corticotectal influences in, 635, 636–638
maturation of integrative properties in multisensory neurons in, 631–634
maturation of receptive fields and, 631, 633
maturation of sensory response properties and, 626–629
mechanisms underlying, 250–252
model of, 245–248
multisensory cortical populations and, 635–638
role of cortical inputs in, 634–635
role of experience in, 637–638, 639, 640
stages of development of, 635, 638
multisensory enhancement in, analysis and modeling of, 265–281
behavioral relevance and decision theory in, 279–280
deriving testable prediction from, 271–274
future directions for, 278–280
information theoretic analysis of, 274–278
for multisensory neuron, 268–271
for unimodal neuron, 266–268
multisensory integration in, 254–257
appearance of, 631
in multisensory processing, 373–376
organization of, 265
in orientation behavior, 245–246
plasticity of auditory spatial processing in, 604–605, 606
receptive field consolidation during development in, 629–630
response enhancement and response depression in, 250, 252–254
in saccadic reaction time, 391
sensory and multisensory development in, 626, 627
sensory map registration in, 599–610
developmental emergence of, 602–604, 605
sensory representations in, 246, 247, 599–601
in temporal correspondence, 491
temporal integration in, 395–396
in visual fixation, 384–386

Superior colliculus (SC) (continued)
  visual instruction of auditory space
    map in, 613–623
  visual signals in shaping of auditory
    responses in, 605–607
  in vitro study of visual-auditory
    convergence in, 607–609
Superior colliculus buildup neurons
    (SCBUNs), 375, 376,
    381–382, 388, 389
Superior colliculus burst neurons
    (SCBNs), 375, 376,
    381–382, 388
Superior colliculus fixation neurons
    (SCFNs), 375, 376
Superior frontal gyri (SFG), in spatial
    concordance, 492
Superior occipital gyrus, endogenous
    spatial attention in, 534–535
Superior olivary complex (SOC)
  binaural neurons in, 250–251
  interaural time delay (ITD) sensitivity
    of, 250–251
Superior parietal lobule (SPL), in spatial
    concordance, 494
Superior temporal gyrus (STG)
  in auditory speech pathway, 212
  in speech-reading, 774–775
Superior temporal polysensory area
    (STP), 286, 288
  multisensory convergence in, 296–297,
    301, 303, 304, 305, 306
Superior temporal sulcus (STS)
  in audiovisual associative learning,
    520, 521
  audiovisual convergence in, 296–297,
    483, 484
  in audiovisual speech perception, 216,
    217, 530
  in auditory speech pathway, 212–213
  in awareness of self and others, 459
  connections of multisensory cortex
    of, 288
  in cross-modal mental imagery, 522
  in endogenous covert spatial attention,
    537, 538, 546
  integration of phonetic information in,
    486–488
  in perception of face and body
    movements, 454
  in spatial concordance, 492
  in speech-reading, 774–775
  in visual speech pathway, 213
Superposition models, 400–402, 403
Supervised learning, of auditory space
    map, 617
Supplementary motor area (SMA), in
    detection of changes in sensory
    events, 494
Suprageniculate nucleus (SG)
  in audiovisual convergence, 483
  histological tracing of multisensory
    pathways in, 365, 366, 368
Supramodal attentional control systems,
    21, 546, 559–561
Supramodal systems, in spatial
    concordance, 492

SV (somatosensory area), projections to
    anterior ectosylvian sulcus from,
    344, 345, 346, 347
SVAR (sinusoidal vertical axis rotation)
    technique, 789
SVD (singular value decomposition), for
    audiovisual speech production,
    184, 185
Sweetness enhancement, 70, 71–72, 74
Sweet odors, 69–72
  liking and, 72
  odor-taste learning and, 74
Syllables, synthetic, 194–195
Synchrony, amodal properties of, 644
Synesthesia
  alphanumeric, and multisensory
    processing, 847–848
  angular gyrus in, 875, 877
  artists, poets, and, 876–877
  auditory-visual, 93
  behavioral and brain correlates of
    multisensory experience in,
    851–864
  color-phonemic, neural correlates of,
    862–863
  color-word, 70
  cross-activation hypothesis of, 870–872
  cross-wiring in, 870–872
    vs. disinhibition, 872
    and Stroop interference, 874
  defined, 93, 837, 867
  evidence for reality of, 868–869
  genetic basis of, 868
  grapheme-color, 837–848, 851
    consistency of, 852–853
    crowding effect and, 869–870,
      871–872
    effects of attentional load and rivalry
      on, 856–861
    effects of visual masking of inducing
      stimuli on, 853–856
    general principles of, 837, 838
    measures of competition in, 853, 854
    photisms in
      as automatic consequence,
        838–839
      cross-linkage model of, 844, 845
      form and meaning in determining,
        844–847
      location of, 837
      perceptual aspects of, 841–844
      reentrant model of, 844–845
    pop-out in, 869
    projectors vs. associators in, 837,
      839–841, 847, 861, 862
    Stroop effect in, 840–841, 860,
      861–862
  higher vs. lower, 874–876
  hyperconnectivity hypothesis of, 872
    and emotions, 877–878
  and metaphor, 876, 877
  neural correlates of, 851–852,
    862–864
  number line in, 875–876
  as perceptual vs. conceptual,
    869–870, 875
  Perky effect in, 873–874

and philosophical riddle of qualia,
    878–879
  psychophysical investigations into,
    869–870
  stability of associations over time in,
    868–869
  Stroop interference in, 869
  between taste and smell, 69–81
  in temporal lobe epilepsy, 878
  theories of causation of, 867–868
  top-down influences in, 872–873
  and visual imagery, 873–874
Synesthesia threshold, 872
Synesthetic colors
  measures of competition for, 853, 854
  measures of consistency of, 852–853
Synesthetic priming task, 853–856
Synesthetic Stroop task, 853, 858
Syntactic priming, with blindness, 729–730
Syntax development, in blind people,
    727, 728–731
Synthetic syllables, 194–195
Synthetic talking face, 172–174

T

Tactile apparent motion, 61–62
Tactile discrimination
  by blind subjects, 712–715
  of grating orientation, visual cortical
    involvement in, 703–704
  visual cortex in, 30–31
Tactile extinction, by visual modulation,
    802–805, 806, 807, 808–809
Tactile forms, visual cortex in
    perception of
  three-dimensional, 706
  two-dimensional, 704–706
Tactile location, vision effect on, 27
Tactile object agnosia, 127, 128
Tactile perception
  with blindness, 724, 725
  contralesional
    enhancing, 804–805
    reducing, 803–804
  cross-modal interactions in, 92–93
  cross-modal modulation of, 805
  with deafness, 726
  visual cortex in, 703–708
    with blindness, 711–716
    for grating orientation, 703–704
    for mental rotation of two-
      dimensional form, 704–706
    for motion, 706
    for three-dimensional
      forms, 706
  visual modulation of, 802–805
    with fake hand, 805–807, 825
    near face, 807–809
Tactile reference frames, 463–464
Tactile-visual-auditory stimulus, test of
    separate activation model with,
    398–399, 400
Tadoma method, of speech-reading,
    vibrotactile activation of
    auditory cortex in, 777
Tadpoles, multisensory signals in, 233

Transverse temporal gyrus
  activation by visual stimuli of, 778
  in auditory speech pathway, 211, 212
Trimodal neurons, 343
  in premotor cortex, 247
  in superior colliculus, 246
Trimodal stimulus, test of separate
      activation model with,
      398–399, 400
Tropical wandering spider, multisensory
      signals in, 232
Turn-and-reach movements, self-
      generated Coriolis forces
      during, 416
TWIN (time-window-of-integration)
      model, of response time,
      403–407
Two-dimensional tactile forms, visual
      cortex in mental rotation of,
      704–705, 706
Two-layer connectionist model, of
      multisensory texture perception,
      119–120
Two-point discrimination tests, 715

U

Umami, 314
Ungulates, multisensory signals in, 227
Unilateral neglect syndrome, 453
Unimodal cortex, multisensory
      neurons in
  contribution of local inputs to,
      348–352
  correspondence with organization of
      external inputs of, 344–348
Unimodal stimulation, differential effects
      of multimodal and, 646–648
Unitization, in odor-taste learning, 79
Unreliable-signal hypothesis, 236
Use-dependent plasticity, 736

V

V6A area, 426, 433–434
VAE. See Ventriloquism aftereffect (VAE)
Vectorview neuromagnetometer, 516
Ventral intraparietal area (VIP)
  anatomical location and functional
      properties of, 426, 430
  in audiovisual convergence, 483, 484
  connections to, 287
  in control of defensive movements, 443,
      444, 448–449
  cortex of, 286
  and deficits related to peripersonal
      space, 432
  multisensory convergence in, 296, 305
  representations of face in, 807
  role of multisensory integration in,
      430–431
  in spatial concordance, 492
Ventral pathway, to temporal lobe, 126
Ventral posterior nucleus (VP),
      histological tracing of
      multisensory pathways in, 365,
      366, 368

Ventral premotor (PMv) zone
  in control of defensive movements, 443,
      444–447
  multisensory responses of, 289
Ventral somatosensory (VS) area,
      multisensory convergence in,
      287, 298, 299–300
Ventriloquism aftereffect (VAE), 40–42
  cognitive strategies in, 143
  experiments in nonhuman primates
      on, 42–45
  functional implications of, 45–47
  persistence of, 45
  spatial disparity and, 45
  in unimodal condition, 46–47
Ventriloquism aftereffect (VAE) ratio,
      43–44
Ventriloquism effect, 35–47, 142–146
  cognitive strategies in, 143
  cross-modal selective attention in, 89
  defined, 36, 142
  dominance of vision in, 27, 28
  examples of, 36
  functional implications of, 45–47
  hemodynamic studies of, 491
  measurement of, 142
  model of neural substrate of
      polysensory integration
      in, 36–38
  with movement, 49, 55–57
  odor-taste synesthesia vs., 73
  parameters necessary for, 36
  perceptual level in, 142–146
  as pre-attentive phenomenon, 146
  response reversals in, 143
  spatial disparity in, 36
  staircase procedure for, 58,
      143, 144–145
  standard explanation of, 142
  strategic or cognitive factors in, 142
  Stroop task interference and, 142
  temporal and spatial dependency of,
      39–40, 41–42
  visual distracter in
      attention to, 144–145
      ignoring of, 142–143
      not conscious seeing of, 145–146
  with visual neglect, 145–146
Ventrobasal complex, in somesthesis, 245
VEPs (visual-evoked potentials), auditory-
      visual interactions in, 30, 31
Verbalism, of language function in blind
      people, 727
Verbal mediation, in object recognition,
      134–135
Vernier acuity, 36–37
Vertical linear oscillation, 417–419, 422
Vestibular system, in postural control,
      785, 786
Vestibulocollic reflexes, 414
Vestibulospinal reflexes, effect of
      gravitoinertial force on, 409–410
Vibrotactile activation, of auditory
      cortex, 777
Video primacy effect, 233
View dependency

in object recognition, 130–131
in scene recognition, 133–134
Viewing distance, in audiovisual speech,
      178, 179–181
VIP. See Ventral intraparietal area (VIP)
Virtual body effect, 825
Visceral representation, of affective value
      of stimuli, neuroimaging
      studies of, 570
Visible speech. See Lipreading
Vision
  alteration by sound of
      in motion perception, 29
      other aspects of, 28
      in temporal aspects, 27–28
  alteration of other modalities by, 27
  cross-modal dynamic capture across
      audition, touch, and, 60–64
  development of cortical networks
      for, 681–683
Vision:place, audition:manner (VPAM)
      hypothesis, 750
Visual agnosia
  and object recognition, 126–127
  recognition of facial expressions in,
      590–591
Visual apparent motion, 50–52, 54–57
Visual association areas, in visual speech
      pathway, 213
Visual-auditory convergence, in vitro
      study of, 607–609
Visual-auditory focused attention task,
      test of separate activation model
      in, 398, 399
Visual bias, in ventriloquism effect,
      144–145
Visual calibration, of auditory space map,
      614–616
Visual capture, 36, 129
Visual cortex
  activation in blind subjects of,
      124, 125
  auditory-visual interactions in, 30–32
  compensatory plasticity of, 738
  connection of auditory cortex with,
      285–287
  cross-modal processing in, 124
  remapping of cross-modal interactions
      in, 544
  simple cells of, 250, 251
  in tactile discrimination, 30–31
  in tactile object recognition, 124–127
  in tactile perception, 703–708
      with blindness, 711–716
      of grating orientation, 703–704
      for mental rotation of two-
          dimensional form, 704–706
      of motion, 706
      of three-dimensional forms, 706
  in visual speech pathway, 213
Visual cues, in auditory spatial
      representations, 731–734
Visual deprivation
  anterior ectosylvian cortex with,
      696–697
  auditory behavior with, 695–696

cross-modal consequences
of, 695–699
Visual discrimination reversal, in
orbitofrontal cortex, 316,
317–318
Visual distracter, in ventriloquism effect
attention to, 144–145
ignoring of, 142–143
not conscious seeing of, 145–146
Visual dominance
cross-modal interactions with,
507–508, 510
in multisensory integration of dynamic
events, 62–64
over proprioception, in cross-modal
modulation, 805
Visual edges, 125
Visual emotion, cross-modal integration
of auditory and, 572
Visual-evoked potentials (VEPs), auditory-
visual interactions in, 30, 31
Visual experience, altered, auditory
consequences of, 604–605, 606
Visual fixation
multisensory integration with, 384–386,
389–390
superior colliculus in, 374
Visual hypothesis, of action
understanding, 454
Visual imagery
magnetoencephalography of, 522
synesthesia and, 873–874
in tactile perception, 707
Visual information processing, in
audiovisual speech perception,
179–184, 180, 181
Visual input(s)
encoding of, 377
to orbitofrontal cortex, 316–318
in postural control, 785, 786
routing to auditory pathway of,
683–685
Visual instruction, of auditory space map
in midbrain, 613–623
Visual localization, errors in, 411–412
Visual masking, of inducing stimuli, in
color-graphemic synesthesia,
853–856
Visual modulation, of tactile perception,
802–805
with fake hand, 805–807, 825
near face, 807–809
Visual neglect
bimodal stimulation for, 811–812
as probe for investigating auditory-
visual interactions, 810
ventriloquism effect with, 145–146
Visual networks, in auditory cortex,
685–686, 687, 688
Visual perception
with deafness, 725–726
enhancement through bimodal
stimulation of contralesional,
811–812
modulations by sound of, 27–32
Visual position, pitch and, 91

Visual processing, cross-modal links with
in endogenous spatial attention,
550–553, 559–561
in exogenous spatial attention, 557–558
Visual projection, to anterior ectosylvian
sulcus, 345
Visual receptive field, in tool use, 455–456
Visual reference frames, 463
Visual reinforcers, amygdala responses to,
571–572
Visual resolution, in audiovisual speech
perception, 181–182
Visual response properties, in superior
colliculus, maturation of,
628–629
Visual responsiveness, in auditory
thalamus and cortex, 659
Visual search task, attention in, 326–328
Visual sensory-specific satiety, 318–320
Visual signals, in shaping of auditory
responses, 605–607
Visual space map(s), 613, 614, 731
aligning auditory and, 599–610, 621
Visual speech pathway, 211, 213–214
Visual speech perception. See Lipreading
Visual stimulation, vertical linear
oscillation and, 417–419
Visual stimuli
activation of auditory cortex by,
778–779
activation of orbitofrontal cortex by,
570–572
flicker-fusion threshold of, 38
representation of pleasantness
of, 318–320
Visual structure, auditory "capture"
of, 28–29
Visual system, spatial acuity in, 36–37
Visual-tactile-auditory neurons, in
polysensory zone of precentral
gyrus, 446, 447
Visual-tactile extinction
cross-modal, 802–805, 826, 827,
828–829
effects of tool use on spatial nature of,
820–825
Visual-tactile integration, 107–111,
113–115
modulated by mirrors, 828–832, 833
modulated by tool use, 819,
820–827, 833
spatial nature of, 825–827
Visual-tactile interaction, in focused
attention, 405–406
Visual-tactile neurons, in polysensory
zone of precentral gyrus,
445–446
Visual-tactile object recognition, 123–136
behavioral correlates of, 127–130
experimental studies on, 130–135
for multiple objects, 132–135
for single objects, 130–132
neuronal correlates of, 124–127
temporal constraints on, 136
Visual-tactile spatial interference, effects
of tool use on, 825–827

Visual target processing, effect of auditory
cues on, 19, 20
Visual-to-taste convergence, 311,
316–318
Visual-vestibular illusions, 244
Visual Wulst area, 647
Visuomotor transformations, 543
Visuotactile integration,
magnetoencephalography
of, 519
Visuotactile interactions, near face,
807–809
Visuotactile processing, reference system
in, 808–809
Vocal expression, of emotion, 165,
582–584
Vocal gestures
evidence for perception of, 192–194
recognition by infants of, 191–192
Vocal imitation, by infants, 191
Vocal tract, acoustic transfer function
of, 206
Vocal tract motion, in audiovisual speech
perception, 184, 185
Voice
dynamic range of, 179
fundamental frequency of, 184
Voicing feature, in speech perception,
204n, 205
Vowels, description of differences among,
196–197
VP (ventral posterior nucleus),
histological tracing of
multisensory pathways
in, 365, 366, 368
VPAM (vision:place, audition:manner)
hypothesis, 750
VS (ventral somatosensory) area,
multisensory convergence in,
287, 298, 299–300

W

Waiting time, 400
Warblers, multisensory processes in,
235, 236
Warning effect, 379
Warning sound, for visual neglect, 812
Weighted average models, of multisensory
texture perception, 119
Wernicke's area
in audiovisual speech perception, 217
in auditory speech, 211, 212
response depression in, 511
in sign language processing,
777–778
"What" pathway, 126
"Where" pathway, 126
Window of integration, 403
Within-compound associations, in odor-
taste learning, 79
Wolf spiders, multisensory signals in,
228, 233
Wood warblers, multisensory processes
in, 236
Wulst area, 647

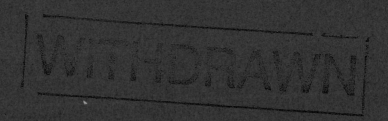